A TEXT-BOOK OF MEDICINE

BY

G. DIEULAFOY

PROFESSOR OF CLINICAL MEDICINE AT THE FACULTÉ DE MÉDECINE DE PARIS; PHYSICIAN
TO THE HÔTEL DIEU; MEMBRE DE L'ACADÉMIE DE MÉDECINE

AUTHORIZED ENGLISH TRANSLATION FROM THE
FIFTEENTH EDITION OF "MANUEL DE
PATHOLOGIE INTERNE"

BY

V. E. COLLINS, M.D. Lond., M.R.C.S., L.R.C.P.

AND

J. A. LIEBMANN, Ph.D., M.A., LL.D.

IN TWO VOLUMES

VOL. II

NEW YORK

D. APPLETON AND COMPANY

1912

PRINTED IN LONDON
BY BAILLIÈRE, TINDALL AND COX.

A TEXT-BOOK OF MEDICINE

VOL. II

CONTENTS OF VOL. II

PART III—*Continued*

DISEASES OF THE URINARY SYSTEM

PART IV

DISEASES OF THE NERVOUS SYSTEM

CONTENTS OF VOL. II

PART V

GENERAL AND INFECTIOUS DISEASES

PART VI

DISEASES OF THE SPLEEN

PART VII

PATHOLOGY OF THE BLOOD

PART XII

THE INTOXICATIONS

APPENDIX ON THERAPEUTICS

PART III

DISEASES OF THE URINARY SYSTEM

CHAPTER I

DISEASES OF THE KIDNEYS

I. ANATOMY AND PHYSIOLOGY OF THE KIDNEYS.

Anatomy.—The kidneys are situated on either side of the spine, on a level with the two upper lumbar vertebræ. They have an average length of 4 inches, a width of $2\frac{1}{2}$ inches, and a thickness of $1\frac{1}{2}$ inches. They weigh about 10 ounces. The kidneys have a thin, transparent, fibro-elastic envelope, which can be detached in the normal condition, but which is often adherent in diseased states. They are surrounded by a fatty layer, in which perinephritic abscesses arise.

A cut section, from the convex edge towards the hilum, presents different parts. In the central or medullary substance ten, twelve, or fifteen striated bundles are seen. These are the pyramids of Malpighi, the summits of which converge towards the hilum. The cortical substance, which is more red and granular, is about $\frac{2}{3}$ inch thick; it is not only peripheral, as its name might seem to indicate, but also central, because it dips in between the pyramids of Malpighi, and forms prolongations which protrude into the hilum, and are known as Bertin's columns.

We find, therefore, at the hilum two kinds of alternating projections : some, red and conoid, are formed by the summit of the pyramids of Malpighi, and are called papillæ; the others, yellowish and rounded, are formed by the prolongation of Bertin's columns. They exist only in the central parts of the hilum, and disappear towards its lateral parts, because Bertin's columns do not there descend so low.

Each papilla is pierced by ten to thirty orifices. Each orifice, visible with a lens, is the opening of an excretory canal, and each of these very short canals is the end of smaller, slightly divergent canals, which are called Bellini's tubes, and unite to form the pyramids of Malpighi. The tubes of Bellini, or collecting canals, ascend, whilst branching out, as far as the cortical substance, where they form straight tubes, called medullary rays, which are the ends of the uriniferous canaliculi.

The canaliculus has a very complicated path. It arises from the glomerulus of Malpighi in the cortical substance. The glomerulus is a small vascular system of a spherical shape, formed by the union of the winding arterioles, and surrounded by a membrane, known as Bowman's capsule.

This system is, as it were, suspended from the interlobular arteries. The afferent arteriole traverses Bowman's capsule, and divides into looped branches. These branches unite to form the efferent arteriole which leaves the capsule in close contact with the afferent vessel, and gives rise to a network of capillaries which envelops the glomeruli, the tubuli contorti, and the medullary rays. Whereas the afferent arteriole is provided with a layer of circular muscle fibres as far as its entrance into the capsule, the efferent arteriole, which is smaller, has only muscular fibres in the neighbourhood of the capsule, and soon loses them, to split up into capillaries. This arrangement forms a kind of sphincter, which probably serves to regulate the blood-pressure in the interior of the glomerulus. The structure of the capillaries in the glomerulus consists of an amorphous wall, lined internally with an endothelium disposed in the form of a protoplasmic membrane with nuclei here and there (Hortolès). The vascular tuft is not free in Bowman's capsule, but has a covering which certain writers look upon as a flattened epithelium. It appears to be rather a membrane of a connective nature, emanating from the connective envelope which accompanies the afferent arteriole at its entry into Bowman's capsule (Cornil, Renaut, Hortolès). This protoplasmic pellicule is interposed between the loops of the vascular tuft.

Bowman's capsule, which surrounds this small vascular apparatus, may be considered as the origin of the uriniferous canaliculi, and is continuous with them by a constricted point, called the neck of the capsule, which is formed by a structureless membrane, provided with flat epithelium.

Immediately after its origin the canaliculus becomes broad and convoluted, whence the name of tubuli contorti. The tubuli contorti are situated in the cortical layer of the kidney, and play a considerable part in the phenomenon of urinary secretion. After a sinuous path, the convoluted part of the canaliculus becomes constricted, plunges into the central substance of the kidney to a variable depth, and is known as Henle's descending branch. The canaliculus then curves (Henle's loop), increases in size, and ascends parallel to its descending branch (Henle's ascending branch); it thus reaches nearly to the surface of the kidney, where, under the name of intercallary tubule and junctional tubule, which is seated in the most superficial layers of the cortical layer of the kidney, it enters into the prolongation of a medullary ray, which is itself, as we have said, but a continuation of a collecting tube of Bellini.

The structure of the canaliculus varies much in each of its parts. The convoluted tubes have a structureless membrane and an epithelium described by Heidenhain. The epithelial cells are so large that they leave only a narrow lumen; their appearance is cloudy and granular, and a portion of their protoplasm is transformed into fine rods, perpendicular to the axis of the tube, which give the section a striated appearance. These rods occupy the part of the cell next to the basement membrane, whilst the protoplasm and the nucleus are on the side of the lumen. The epithelium of Henle's descending branch is pavemented and analogous to that of the bloodvessels. The epithelium of Henle's ascending branch is analogous to that of the convoluted tubes. The epithelium of the intermediary pieces and of the first collecting tubes is somewhat like cylindrical epithelium.

In order to understand the relations of the uriniferous canaliculi with the different elements which enter into the structure of the kidney, it is useful to study them in transverse sections.

1. In a section made in the region of the papillæ we find the large excretory tubes which divide in this region, and some loops of Henle's tubes.

2. In a section made a little higher, in the portion of Malpighi's pyramid called the limiting zone, we meet with three varieties of tubes : Bellini's collecting tubes, Henle's thin or descending branches, and Henle's large or ascending branches. The vasa recta traverse this zone in order to reach the cortical substance.

3. Transverse sections of the cortical substance, starting from the surface of the kidney towards the centre, show the following details : (1) In the most superficial layer we find the capsule of the kidney, hollowed out by cavities which are lymphatic spaces. (2) In a somewhat deeper section we see the sinuous canals, which represent the intercalary and junctional tubules—that is to say, the end of the uriniferous canaliculi in the medullary prolongations ; we also see tubuli contorti. (3) In a still deeper section we see the renal lobule, which is formed of the following elements : In the centre is Ferrein's pyramid, which is composed of the cortical prolongation of Bellini's tube (medullary ray) and Henle's ascending branches. Around Ferrein's pyramid is the labyrinth, and by " labyrinth " must be understood the space between two pyramids with the contents of this space, tubuli contorti, and interlobular arteries with their glomeruli.

It is important to understand the structure of the renal lobule, because it is in this region that most of the pathological phenomena of chronic nephritis take place.

The glomeruli, uriniferous and collecting tubes are embedded in unequally distributed connective tissue. " The communication of this connective tissue with the lymphatic vessels shows that here, as elsewhere, it is made up of lymph spaces, limited by flat cells, and in connection with the lymphatic vessels."

Physiology.—We know to-day that the rôle of the kidney consists in excretion, and not secretion. It does not make the elements of the urine, but finds them ready-made in the blood, and selects them, rejecting some and allowing others to pass. An exception must, however, be made in favour of hippuric acid, which exists in the urine of herbivorous animals, and appears to be made by the kidney (Koch).

In the normal condition, the urine has a pale yellow colour, an acid reaction, and a peculiar odour. Its density is from 1018 to 1020, and the quantity passed by an adult in twenty-four hours varies from 40 to 50 ounces.

Urine is composed of the following elements :

Composition of the Urine.	Passed.	
	Per litre. Gr.	Per 24 hours. Gr.
Organic elements	26–27	35–36
Mineral elements	3·3–10	12–14
Total of dissolved matter	34–37	43–52
Urea { Men	18–24	25–38
Women	10–20	20–32
Uric acid	0·30–0·40	0·50–0·70
Phosphoric acid	1·66	2·50
Sulphuric acid	2·00	3·00
Chloride of sodium	6·6–8·0	10–12
Lime	0·28–0·30	0·33–0·45

Urea, which represents the last stage in the oxidation of the albuminoids, is manufactured in the interior of the tissues, and especially in the liver. I shall not review the numerous theories of the secretion of the urine. It is not certain that the glomerulus has only a mechanical rôle, as was maintained by Ludwig ; the glomerular epithelium seems to play a certain part in the physiological and pathological functions of the glomerulus (Heidenhain). It is through the glomerulus that the aqueous portion, with the salts of the plasma, transudes (Bowman). The glomerulus eliminates the sugar in diabetic patients and the albumin in albuminuric ones. The tubuli contorti and Henle's ascending branch, which are furnished with a special epithelium (Heidenhain), represent the true glandular part of the kidney, and have as their mission the making of urine, by selecting and excreting its principal products.

Chatin and Guinard would give to the kidney, by analogy with other glands, an internal secretion, which appears indeed to exist.

II. CONGESTION OF THE KIDNEYS—CARDIAC KIDNEY.

Congestion of the kidneys may be active or passive. Active congestion is associated with inflammation and new growths of the kidneys, and will, consequently, be described with these various morbid conditions. Passive congestion will be discussed in this section.

Whenever the blood-pressure increases in the area of the efferent veins, or in the vena cava, above the mouth of these veins, the kidneys become congested. Tumours of the abdomen, aneurysms of the abdominal aorta, and pregnancy, may create a mechanical obstacle to the blood-flow in the renal veins. Pleuro-pulmonary affections (pleurisy, emphysema, phthisis) may also form an obstacle to the afflux of the blood from the vena cava to the right side of the heart, and become an indirect cause of renal congestion; but none of these causes can compare with diseases of the heart. As the result of ill-compensated cardiac lesions and in consequence of attacks of asystole, the kidneys participate in the chronic congestion which affects all the viscera, and the **cardiac kidney** (Jaccoud), which is analogous to the cardiac liver, results. Post mortem the kidneys are congested and enlarged; the capsule strips readily; the surface of the organ is red, and streaked with swollen venæ stellatæ; the capillaries and the veins are congested with blood. On section, the surface is of a deep red. Small glomerular and intratubular hæmorrhages are sometimes seen. The tissue of the kidney is indurated, and histological examination shows that the intertubular connective tissue of Malpighi's pyramid is transformed in places into embryonic tissue forming an early stage of cirrhosis. Fatty granules are present in the epithelium of the tubuli contorti, but the cells do not perish. In short, this congested condition causes a slight degree of cirrhosis, but the bloodvessels are hardly ever attacked by endarteritis. The striated epithelium of the convoluted tubes preserves its integrity, and, consequently, the cardiac kidney does not show chronic nephritis, and is not the starting-point of Bright's disease.

This opinion is the most generally accepted, and it must be added that it is correct. Exceptions must, however, be noted, and Fauquez has collected cases which tend to prove that the cardiac kidney may end in the interstitial and parenchymatous lesions of Bright's kidney.

The cardiac kidney reveals itself during life by evident changes in the urine. The urine becomes scanty, thick, and high-coloured. Urates, urea, and uric acid are found in abundance; but albumin, when it exists, is in small quantity. Under the microscope white and red corpuscles, epithelial cells, and sometimes casts of various kinds, are seen.

The insufficiency of urinary depuration, resulting from the lesions just described, is partially responsible for the symptoms of asystole; but it very rarely ends in true uræmia. The treatment described under Mitral Diseases causes the cardiac kidney to resume its functions, and it is, indeed, through the kidney that asystole is in a large part averted.

III. ACUTE NEPHRITIS.

Discussion.—The history of acute nephritis is still somewhat obscure ; the nature of the lesions, the ætiology of the disease, and its modes of termination, have been the subject of such contradictory opinions that it is not possible at the present time to propose a classification of the acute toxi-infections of the kidney. Not long ago acute nephritis was divided into catarrhal and parenchymatous. Catarrhal nephritis had the attributes of being slight and temporary, of limiting its process to the excretory canals, and of leaving the organ unaffected ; whereas parenchymatous nephritis, which was more grave and more persistent, was localized in the epithelium of the secretory canals (tubuli contorti). In order to accentuate this distinction, writers likened catarrhal nephritis of the excretory tubes to common bronchitis, and parenchymatous nephritis of the secretory tubes to lobular pneumonia, or capillary bronchitis (Lécorché). This distinction, however, in no way corresponds to the true lesions of acute nephritis, in which the entire kidney participates more or less in the morbid process. Another division consisted in separating acute nephritis into epithelial and interstitial, the one invading the epithelia of the kidney, and the other the connective tissue ; but this division, so simple in appearance, cannot serve as a basis for a description of the acute infections of the kidney.

The acute process of nephritis was for a long time considered as exclusively vested in the epithelium, whereas the interstitial tissue of the organ seemed to lend itself only to a chronic process (Bartels). It was soon felt that it was wrong to reject interstitial nephritis from the varieties of acute nephritis. The inflammatory nature of the epithelial nephritis was even contested (Klebs) ; it was said that the process in acute epithelial nephritis was not irritative, but only degenerative, and the really active part of the inflammatory process was vested in the interstitial tissue. Nephritis in smallpox (Traube), scarlatina (Klebs), diphtheria, cholera (Kelsch), and typhoid fever was looked on as acute and interstitial, and at this time acute interstitial nephritis may be said to have comprised almost the entire history of acute nephritis.

Fresh researches, however, assisted by experiments and favoured by perfected methods of preparation (Cornil), have enabled us to state the facts more correctly. It is seen that what had been described as an interstitial lesion becomes partially reduced to the diapedesis of the white corpuscles, and, in short, the preponderance of the morbid process remains with the parenchyma. The lesions of acute nephritis are parenchymatous lesions, which attack the various parts of the gland, the excretory tube, the secretory tube, and the glomerulus ; with these lesions there are associated interstitial and vascular changes that are more or less pronounced in different cases.

Do the anatomical forms of acute nephritis vary, according to their cause ? and is the nephritis of scarlet fever, for example, distinct from early syphilitic nephritis, from typhoid nephritis, or from the nephritis which appears after a chill ? The answer is negative. Whether the nephritis be primary (a frigore), which has not been proved ; whether it be of an experimental nature (injections of cantharides) (Cornil) ; or whether it appear during the course of scarlatina, syphilis, smallpox, diphtheria, or pneumonia, it may be said that the acute changes in the kidney do not, in any case, assume a really distinct type. These changes may be more or less extensive, more or less intense, more or less transient, more or less lasting, more or less degenerative, may end more or less quickly in necrosis of the epithelium, and may be more marked in this or that part of the organ ; but they have no particular character, and the topography of the lesions, no more than their ætiology, allows us to divide nephritis into distinct kinds.

I, therefore, unite in one description the varieties of acute nephritis, which were formerly described as catarrhal nephritis, acute albuminous nephritis, acute parenchymatous nephritis, and epithelial nephritis.

In spite of this apparent simplification, the anatomical description of acute nephritis remains surrounded with difficulties, because the lesions show notable differences, according to the cause, the duration, and the intensity of the inflammatory process. As a matter of fact, the changes are sometimes superficial and transitory, and at other times deep and lasting.

In mild cases of acute nephritis the lesion is rather hyperæmic than inflammatory, and we might be tempted to replace the word "nephritis" by the names "congestive œdema," "inflammatory hyperæmia," or "congestive nephritis." In severe cases of acute nephritis the leucocytic infiltration and acute degeneration of the epithelia predominate, while the irritative lesions of the connective tissue and of the glomeruli are but slightly marked. Finally, in some cases the diffuse changes attack the epithelia, the bloodvessels, and the connective tissue.

Furthermore, the division of acute nephritis into congestive, slight, and intense would be purely artificial, for there is no defined limit between these forms, and we pass from one to the other by insensible gradations. There is no absolute relation to be established between nephritis and its cause, for the same cause—scarlatina, for instance —may bring about congestive nephritis, slight and transitory nephritis, or grave and permanent nephritis. It must be added, however, that the intense forms are not common in the course of most infectious diseases, though they are so in scarlatina, syphilis, and perhaps also as the result of a chill. •

In a fatal case of acute nephritis both kidneys will be found equally affected. They are larger than normal. The enlargement is due to the vascular congestion and to the swelling of the cortex. The capsule is easily detached ; the surface of the organ is smooth and mottled. According to circumstances, the kidneys are whitish, greyish, or reddish. In severe inflammation the kidneys may weigh more than twice their normal weight. The tissue forms, as it were, a hernia through the incised capsule. On section, the medullary substance appears normal, while the cortical substance is congested, thickened, and of a yellowish colour, streaked by red striations, and studded with red points.

Let us now study the histology of the lesion in each part of the organ.

1. The collecting tubes which possess cylindrical epithelium and the straight tubes which have cubical epithelium present the lesions of catarrhal inflammation—swelling, multiplication, and desquamation of the cells. The lumen of the collecting tubes is blocked with cells and casts. These catarrhal lesions were long supposed to be the sole lesion in slight nephritis, but we know now that slight nephritis, formerly called catarrhal, also presents changes in the glomeruli and the convoluted tubes.

2. The lesions in the glomeruli are constant. The capillaries become dilated, and an albuminous exudate, which contains white and red corpuscles, passed through by diapedesis, and in some cases hyaline balls, is poured out in the interior of the capsule. The red corpuscles are sometimes

so numerous as to form a glomerular hæmorrhage. The passage of the blood-serum into the capsule explains the presence of the albumin in the urine. When the intracapsular exudate is very profuse, it presses the vascular tuft against the wall, passes under pressure into the convoluted tubes, and may rupture them. These congestive lesions are accompanied by others of an inflammatory nature. In the perivascular protoplasmic layer abundant multiplication of nuclei is noticed (Cornil), and the lining cells of Bowman's capsule swell up and desquamate. According to the duration of the inflammatory process, the vascular coils of the agglutinated capillaries may undergo a connective transformation, the capsule grows thicker, and the glomerulus tends to become fibrous. The neighbouring arterioles of the glomeruli show peri-arteritis and endarteritis.

3. The changes in the striated epithelium of the convoluted tubes and of Henle's ascending tubules have given rise to much discussion. The canaliculi are dilated and opaque ; the epithelium is cloudy, granular, and swollen. The epithelial cells are more or less swollen or broken up. The protoplasm shows cloudy swelling; the nucleus does not stain well with carmine or hæmatoxylin. The condition is necrobiosis of the epithelium. These lesions, according to some writers, are said to be purely degenerative, while others hold that the swelling of the cells, the granular condition, the multiplication of the nuclei, and the secretion of coagulable substances, show an inflammatory process.

In a remarkable article on the condition of the cells of the kidney in albuminuria, Cornil has stated that the epithelial cells of the convoluted tubes showed more or less large vacuoles, containing granules and balls of proteid substance. According to Cornil, the renal cells are said, then, to secrete in the protoplasm " balls of albuminous substance in almost the same manner as the mucous or goblet cells of the intestinal mucosa and of the glands secrete mucus."

These balls of coagulable albuminoid substance are formed of mucin and albumin. They may be granular or hyaline and transparent. These coagulable elements, with the coagulated serum, the red and white corpuscles, the fragments of cells, and the fibrous reticulum, take part in the formation of the **casts.** The formation of the casts commences, then, in the glomeruli, and continues in the tubes. The casts found in the urine will be described under Bright's Disease.

If the inflammatory process is severe, the dilatation of the tubules is very marked. The tubules are filled with granular and colloid exudate, with red corpuscles, which have come from the glomeruli, and with fat corpuscles. The striated epithelium is infiltrated in places with fatty granules.

4. The changes in the connective tissue are but little appreciable at

the commencement of slight nephritis. Œdema of the intertubular tissue and diapedesis of the white corpuscles which infiltrate the intertubular spaces are not indicative of interstitial inflammation, properly speaking. This very marked infiltration (Wagner's lymphomatous nephritis) is accompanied by the glomerular lesions of which I have already spoken, and later by a thickening of the tubular walls. In the end the fibrous element becomes apparent ; the vascular lesions become accentuated, and we have diffuse subacute nephritis. Such are the lesions of acute nephritis. Several writers have held them to be degenerative from the outset (Traube, Klebs, Kelsch). We hold to-day that the lesions are both degenerative and inflammatory. The last word has, I admit, not yet been said on the nature of the lesions in the striated epithelium, but this is no reason for classing the fatty condition of the epithelium amongst the number of purely ischemic and degenerative changes, when it may be the result of an inflammatory process. " The change in the cells of the kidney, which writers have wrongly wished to distinguish from inflammation, behaves like an inflammatory process, for, independently of the fibrino-albuminous exudation which infiltrates the epithelial elements, the latter may return to their primary condition or undergo granulo-fatty degeneration " (Lancereaux). Furthermore, the epithelial degeneration is associated with so many other inflammatory manifestations (glomerulitis, connective irritation, multiplication of the nuclei) that the nature of the process, taken as a whole, is manifestly of inflammatory and necrobiotic origin.

Ætiology.—The causes of acute nephritis are numerous and varied.

1. INFECTIOUS NEPHRITIS.—Toxi-infectious diseases occupy the first place in the pathogenesis of acute nephritis. Scarlatina, syphilis, smallpox, measles, pneumonia, typhoid fever, diphtheria, cholera, influenza, mumps, and erysipelas, predispose to acute nephritis.

The pathogenesis of infectious nephritis has been variously interpreted. It has been asked " whether a profound change in the blood would not be capable of changing the conditions of diffusibility of the albumin," by allowing it to pass through the kidney (Jaccoud), and by irritating the epithelium. The current view of this question is as follows : Microbes have been found in the arterioles of the kidneys and in the coils of the glomeruli. Such are the microbes of anthrax, pneumonia, tuberculosis, typhoid fever, and other organisms, streptococci and staphylococci, which give rise to secondary infections. Researches have since been made as to whether these microbes have of themselves a pathogenic action on the kidneys, or whether the pathogenic action be due to the toxines which they secrete.

When we see certain microbes traversing the kidneys and passing into the urine, staphylococci, pneumococci (in the two first days of pneumonia),

Eberth's bacillus (from the second to the fourth week of typhoid fever), we may well ask whether these microbes are not capable of modifying the anatomical condition of the cells, by ischæmia, congestion, or traumatism.

On the other hand, however, when we know the slight affinity of bacteria for the kidneys and the feeble tendency of the kidneys for the elimination of the microbes *en masse*, we say that the microbes must act chiefly on the renal epithelium through their toxines. Do we not know, too, that certain infectious diseases, such as diphtheria, cholera, or tetanus, cause renal changes, necrosis, or cellular degeneration, though the microbes do not enter the blood ? Have we not seen nephritis supervene in consequence of antitubercular vaccinations with old cultures, and after subcutaneous injections made with Koch's tuberculin ?

Lesions have been produced in the kidney by injecting cultures of Eberth's bacillus (Chantemesse and Widal), and cultures of the pneumococcus (Roger and Gaume), in the same way as experimental nephritis has been produced, by injections of toxines. Charrin observed chronic granular nephritis, with hypertrophy of the left ventricle, in rabbits inoculated with pyocyaneus toxine. In a monkey inoculated with diphtheria toxine Henriquez and Hallion found granular nephritis, with hypertrophy of the left ventricle.

Claude has made a large number of experiments with various toxines (diphtheritic, tetanic, coli - bacillary, streptococcic, staphylococcic, pyocyanic). He has induced acute nephritis (and acute hepatitis) in animals. In the case of intense intoxication we find inflammatory and degenerative changes in the kidneys. In the case of progressive intoxication we find subacute and chronic nephritis, with epithelial, interstitial, and vascular lesions.

These facts prove that the tissues of the kidney are affected by the toxines, just as they are by the mineral poisons. It matters little whether the poison acts directly on the epithelium of the tubules ; whether it acts on the arterioles, causing diapedesis and arterio-sclerosis ; or whether the lesions are associated or independent, degenerative or inflammatory. We know that acute nephritis arises in the infectious diseases, whether the microbes and their toxines are known to us (pneumonia, typhoid fever, diphtheria, tuberculosis, cholera, tetanus, erysipelas, puerperal infection, influenza, appendicitis), or whether the microbes and their toxines are unknown to us (scarlatina, measles, smallpox).

As regards prognosis, it is important to note that these various infections do not attack the kidneys with the same violence nor with the same tenacity. In this respect nephritis in scarlet fever and early syphilitic nephritis are more to be feared than nephritis in diphtheria, typhoid fever, pneumonia, erysipelas, etc. Nevertheless, we must always allow for slight nephritis, because the damaged kidneys may, at a given moment, under the influence of some fresh infection or of cold, become the seat of fresh lesions.

2. NEPHRITIS DUE TO DRUGS.—We must not confound the steatogenous substances (phosphorus, arsenic) which cause fatty degeneration of the organ with the irritating substances (cantharides, blistering fluids) which cause true nephritis.

Serotherapy.—Injections of antidiphtheritic serum are said to cause renal lesions and albuminuria. My view from the clinical standpoint is : If injections of serum, in the case of diphtheria, be administered early, they may prevent albuminuria ; if they be administered when albuminuria is present, they have no retro-active effect, and the statement that they have an ill-effect on the kidneys has not been proved, in my opinion. I am, indeed, disposed, until there be fresh proof, to believe the contrary. It is, in truth, very difficult, when albuminuria is found in a case of diphtheria, to assess the shares of the serum, of the diphtheritic poison, and of the secondary infections.

3. AUTO-INTOXICATION.—The elimination by the kidneys of an excess of tyrosin and of other extractives, which, for divers reasons (diseases of the liver, insufficiency of combustion, slowness of nutrition, cachexia), have a toxic action on the kidneys, may provoke epithelial lesions in the kidneys and albuminuria.

4. PREGNANCY.—We know how frequent albuminuria is in pregnant women. It may be due to congestion from compression of the renal veins, to the presence of special waste products in the blood, or to true nephritis. There is also a variety of nephritis which may be looked upon as one of the numerous complications of pregnancy. A pregnant woman may have simple albuminuria, or albuminuria associated with such symptoms of nephritis as œdema, dyspnœa, headache, and visual troubles. In the presence of the latter symptoms we must beware, because eclampsia may come on during labour. Women who have had no albuminuria during pregnancy have it during labour. This distinction is very important, because albuminuria which appears during labour is transitory, and is not the precursor of eclampsia (Tarnier).

5. NEPHRITIS A FRIGORE.—Cold—and by this word we must understand cold in all its forms—seems to be a cause of acute nephritis. It may even be said that the so-called nephritis *a frigore* is most serious, on account of the intensity and the possible duration of its lesions. Cold, however, *per se* very rarely causes acute nephritis. In many cases it acts as an exciting cause in individuals whose kidneys are predisposed by previous scarlatina, by some infectious disease, by syphilis, etc. In some cases, however, the most minute inquiry fails to establish any other cause but cold. One of my patients was taken ill with acute nephritis, after having

been exposed all day to an ice-cold rain.   Another patient was taken ill with nephritis after going out one very cold night when he was in a state of perspiration.

Symptoms.—Some cases of nephritis are so slight that they escape all description.   Nephritis in diphtheria, mumps, pneumonia, erysipelas, or appendicitis, generally shows no other appreciable symptom except albuminuria, so that many fevers and diseases were said to cause albuminuria without appreciable lesions in the kidneys.

The nephritis of typhoid fever is also insidious and latent, but yet it may be severe and formidable (see Typhoid Fever).   The nephritis of scarlet fever, which will be described under Scarlatina, and which has many symptoms in common with early syphilitic nephritis and with nephritis *a frigore*, is of the utmost importance.

In a general way, the course of acute nephritis is as follows : When the nephritis is severe, the onset is violent.   The patient may have rigors, fever, and lumbar pains ; the urine is scanty and brownish or hæmorrhagic. Œdema appears early.   The anasarca commences, as a rule, in the face, which is pale and swollen, and in a few days invades the lower limbs and the various regions rich in loose cellular tissue, such as the eyelids, the scrotum, the prepuce, and the labia majora.   The œdema is soft, white, and pits readily.

More frequently febrile symptoms are wanting, or, at least, the rigors and the fever are insignificant.   The patient has no pains in the loins. Œdema and dyspnœa, with or without vomiting, are the only signs of nephritis, and even then the onset of the disease is not always clear.   In some cases the œdema is limited to the face and to the malleoli, while one symptom, such as dyspnœa, headache, or vomiting, assumes an especial importance from the start of the disease.

In acute nephritis the amount of urine passed in the twenty-four hours may fall below 30 ounces.   The specific gravity may be normal or increased, and the urinary deposit contains altered epithelial cells, red corpuscles, leucocytes, granular and hyaline casts.   The albumin may exceed 5 or 6 grains per ounce.   The urea diminishes, and may fall to a drachm instead of an ounce, which is the normal quantity.   If the nephritis be very acute, the symptom-complex of acute uræmia may appear within a few days or a few weeks—*i.e.*, dyspeptic troubles (nausea, uncontrollable vomiting), headache, epistaxis, dyspnœa, visual troubles (amblyopia, amaurosis), cutaneous eruptions and itching, nervous symptoms (convulsions, delirium, coma).   Œdema of the lungs or of the glottis and effusions in the pleura and the pericardium may appear.   When the nephritis tends towards a favourable ending, the symptoms improve, the urine increases, the albumin diminishes, and the anasarca gradually disappears.

Prognosis.—Acute nephritis, if slight, may be completely cured with proper care in a few weeks. In other cases it passes into a subacute state, and the symptoms only disappear after several months. Too often, however, it terminates in a chronic condition—Bright's disease. Under some circumstances the disease seems to be cured, and the patient may show hardly a trace of albumin in the urine; but yet one or two years later, under the influence of an infectious disease or of a chill, the symptoms of nephritis all return, as if there were a recurrence of an imperfectly extinct process.

The **prognosis** of acute nephritis is always serious, first, because certain cases (nephritis in scarlatina, syphilitic nephritis, nephritis *a frigore*) may be accompanied by fatal uræmia; and, second, because many cases of acute nephritis, even of fairly benign appearance, end in Bright's disease. Moreover, the prognosis of acute nephritis does not depend on its severity alone, but also on the cause which has given rise to it. The slight nephritis which supervenes during the course of the infectious diseases recovers after a few days or a few weeks, and is not nearly as serious as scarlatinal or syphilitic nephritis. Ætiology alone does not permit us to say that the lesions in the kidneys are slight or grave. Nephritis in typhoid fever and in influenza is usually benign, but yet it may sometimes be of extreme gravity (Renaut). Scarlatinal nephritis, which is often benign, may be very severe, or may become the origin of Bright's disease. The nephritis of pregnancy is serious, because it may lead to eclampsia, or may become chronic.

Diagnosis.—The diagnosis of acute nephritis demands some attention. In many infectious diseases nephritis develops insidiously, and the urine must be carefully examined for signs of renal changes. When the œdema is transient and slight, the other symptoms may be so marked as to cause errors in diagnosis. We must not set down as bronchitis a case of acute nephritis in which the chief symptoms are violent dyspnœa and scattered râles. We must not set down as pleurisy nephritis in which the chief sign is pleuritic effusion. It is sufficient to remember the possibility of these errors to avoid falling into them. Furthermore, albuminuria and œdema, which may be absent in some cases of chronic nephritis, are never wanting in acute nephritis.

Treatment.—The treatment of acute nephritis, consisting of milk diet, cupping of the loins, and general blood-letting in the case of uræmic symptoms, differs little from the treatment of Bright's disease, which is given in the following chapter.

Blood-letting is indicated when we find symptoms of uræmia, epileptiform convulsions, delirium, or coma. In this case 10 to 20 ounces of blood must be withdrawn, and the operation repeated, if necessary. This measure is most valuable, and must never be put off. Many cases of acute nephritis and grave uræmia owe their recovery to free bleeding. I am so convinced of its efficacy in acute nephritis, that I would even advise it in cases of moderate severity. Blood-letting has not only an immediate action on the acute symptoms at the moment, but I believe that it diminishes the risk of subsequent chronic mischief.

Injections of serum and **all foods containing salt** must be proscribed.

Milk diet is of the utmost importance. It must be continued for several weeks **even after the supposed cure** of acute nephritis, and it is one of the most certain means of avoiding chronic nephritis.

IV. APPENDICULAR KIDNEY—TOXIC NEPHRITIS— APPENDICULAR ALBUMINURIA.

I have repeatedly mentioned in this work the dire results of the appendicular toxines on the system. Under Diseases of the Liver I devoted a special section to toxic appendicular hepatitis. I shall now, under Diseases of the Kidneys, discuss toxic appendicular nephritis.

Reduced to its simplest terms, toxic appendicular nephritis reveals itself by a single sign—albuminuria. In nearly all severe cases of appendicitis the effect on the kidneys is at once shown by albuminuria. Since my attention was drawn to this important point, I have found albuminuria in many cases of appendicitis. The albumin may appear on the first, second, or third day, and is sometimes associated with slight jaundice, which also indicates toxic poisoning. We may find only a small quantity of albumin, but at other times we may find 10 to 15 grains, or even more. I have several times followed the gradual disappearance of the albumin after removal of the appendix. To quote examples :

I was asked, at the Hôtel-Dieu, to examine a patient suffering from appendicitis which had been allowed to " grow cold." The disease was of three weeks' duration, and had, unfortunately, been left to the *vis medicatrix naturæ*. After an apparent remission, the fever and vomiting had reappeared, and the situation was critical. I examined the patient, and concluded that the appendicitis had set up peritoneal infection which had spread to the subphrenic region (this opinion was verified at the operation). Examination of the urine revealed over 15 grains of albumin ; no casts in the centrifugal tube. Mauclaire operated, and the condition was relieved. At the same time, the albuminuria gradually diminished, and disappeared in a month, the patient being in good health. Under Appendicular Hepatitis I referred to a patient in my wards with gangrenous appendicitis, albuminuria, and jaundice (toxic appendicitis). He was operated upon on the morning of his arrival. The improvement was slow to show itself, but in a few days the albumin, the pigments, and the jaundice disappeared.

Simple albuminuria, which yields after resection of the appendix, is, I repeat, the only symptom of slight appendicular nephritis. In such cases the renal lesion is neither severe nor lasting, and yet we must not trust this apparent benignity, because this simple albuminuria, whether it be associated or not with jaundice, is at times the first warning of grave troubles, which may end in death.   To quote examples :

I was asked by Marion to see a boy who had been admitted the previous evening into the Hôtel-Dieu.   The disease had commenced suddenly three days before.   He went to bed in his usual health, but woke about two o'clock in the morning with slight umbilical pains, which became more severe.   Next day, in spite of the pains, he went to work again, but was compelled to go to bed.   In the night the pains in the belly became acute, but there was neither nausea nor vomiting.   Next morning (the second day of the disease) the pains were very severe, and his doctor sent him to hospital for appendicitis.

On the third day of the disease he was brought to the Hôtel-Dieu.   The belly was slightly distended, and not quite as painful as on the previous days.   No vomiting ; micturition easy.   Pulse 96 ; morning temperature 101° F. ; evening temperature 103° F. An ice-bag was applied to the belly.

I saw him next morning at ten o'clock (fourth day of the disease).   Pulse was 88, and the temperature, which the previous evening was 104° F., had fallen to 99° F.   In spite of this apparent improvement, I felt that we were face to face with a treacherous calm. The face was earthy ; the features were drawn, and the alæ nasi were working.   He passed gas and urine ; some hiccough ; no vomiting.   The belly was neither tympanitic nor hollow.   Palpation showed that the pain was most acute over the appendix. Hyperæsthesia and muscular resistance were present ; no dullness.

We had to deal with acute appendicitis, but yet, in spite of the bad impression caused by his facies, peritonitis was not the prominent feature in this case.   These forms are suspicious of gangrene of the appendix and of poisoning, which may be severe.   I had the urine analyzed, and the analysis confirmed my suspicions as to the toxic nature of the case.   The kidneys and the liver were affected by the toxines, for the urine contained a fairly large proportion of albumin, granular casts, leucocytes, and bile pigment.

The prognosis appeared to me to be very grave, as it was certain that his system was poisoned, and that removal of the appendicular focus would perhaps be too late.

The operation was performed at once by Fredet.   Opening the peritoneal cavity gave exit to a small quantity of odourless turbid liquid.   No adhesions between the intestinal coils, and but little exudate ; a small collection of fœtid pus behind the cæcum. The appendix was situated in this abscess, and was slightly adherent to the posterior wall of the cæcum ; it was detached without difficulty.   The proximal portion of the appendix adjoining the cæcum appeared healthy, but the remainder was gangrenous ; no apparent perforation.   The wound was left open.   Drainage was effected by means of three large tubes surrounded with gauze.   Next night (Tuesday) he was restless ; on Wednesday repeated vomiting led me to fear hæmatemesis, which is so common in the toxic forms of appendicitis.   On Thursday his face still kept its earthy look ; the pulse was rapid ; albuminuria and bile pigments still present.

On Friday he was worse, being quite prostrate.   Extremities bathed with cold sweat ; urine scanty ; pulse small and quick ; respiration accelerated ; vomiting painful and frequent ; the stomach was quite intolerant of food.   Analysis of the urine showed albumin and a red-brown pigment, which had replaced the bile pigment.   Next night hæmatemesis supervened, and the patient succumbed, after a series of black vomits which persisted until the moment of death.   The temperature did not rise beyond 101° F.

Post-mortem examination : Some fibrinous exudate on the intestinal coils ; no purulent collection, except a tablespoonful of homogeneous pus in the pelvis.   The lungs were of a violet colour and congested with blood, especially at their bases ; no trace of broncho-pneumonia.   Stomach empty ; the entire mucous membrane of the great curvature was covered with hæmorrhagic patches, which in places looked like purpura. The small bloodvessels formed a distended network. No ulceration.

Heart and spleen healthy. The liver and the kidneys were of normal appearance, and not enlarged; had we been satisfied with a superficial examination, these organs might have been considered healthy, but the histological examination revealed marked changes. Letulle undertook the examination, and, in view of the importance of the subject, I give his report *in extenso*.

Portions of the kidneys taken twenty-five hours after death were placed for twenty-four hours in formol (1 per cent.), hardened in alcohol, and cut, after embedding in collodion. The specimens were stained with hæmateine-eosin, thionin, and Kern-schwarz's polychrome blue.

1. Under a low power, the specimens showed necrosis, affecting many of the con-voluted tubes and some of the large branches of Henle's loops, whilst the glomeruli and the straight tubes, as well as the pyramids, had evidently escaped.

2. On careful study of the topography of the necrobiotic zones, the integrity of many of the convoluted tubes in the cortical tissue was evident. The contrast between the dead tubes in the parenchyma and the living ones in the cortical substance was most remarkable, and eliminated the hypothesis of a post-mortem lesion. Furthermore, the examination of the lesions with the high power confirmed this view.

(1) It was easy to see that all the epithelial cells in the section of a convoluted tube were not necrotic, for in some cells the nuclei were more or less deeply stained a lilac colour by the hæmateine.

(2) The epithelial cells in the diseased tubes often bulged into the lumen. They were granular, and even in the necrobiotic regions the elements were on the way to desquamation, whether their nuclei were stained or not.

(3) The cells of the interstitial tissue and the capillaries did not appear to be much affected, and their nuclei were still present.

The glomeruli were engorged with blood; the cavity was filled with rosy serum in some cases; the endothelium of the capsule had proliferated at many spots; the inter-stitial cells of the glomerular loops had not proliferated; the bloodvessels of the cortical substance, and those of the glomerular portion in particular, were dilated, but there was no perivascular diapedesis; there was no trace of serous or fibrinous interstitial exuda-tion. As for the tissue of the pyramids, some of Henle's loops were partially necrotic. There was no inflammation in the collecting tubes, and the nuclei of the epithelial cells were still present.

Fragments stained with osmic acid showed granulo-fatty degeneration, limited to the epithelial cells of the convoluted tubes. This recent lesion was characterized by the desquamation of the renal cells, and the accumulation of fine blackish granules in the protoplasm. These granules were scattered throughout the entire cell, and were not merely accumulated at its base. Appropriate technique showed that in some of the degenerated epithelial cells the nuclei still took the stain.

After staining with thionin, the necrotic cells showed two different types, which did not appear to be two stages of the same lesion, and which never coexisted in the same portion of the tubule.

1. The first type was a fairly good example of coagulation necrosis. The protoplasm of the cell was stained a greyish-blue colour, and was almost homogeneous and trans-lucid. The protoplasm was cut up by large striations with ill-defined edges, and the nucleus no longer took the stain.

2. The second type was more discrete, and characterized by granular fragmentation of all the epithelial protoplasm in the section of any given convoluted tube. The degeneration had led to the disappearance of the outlines of the cells. The granules in the dead protoplasm varied in size; in general, they were fairly large, measuring from 2 to 5 μ. They stained a pale violet with thionin, and were rounded, translucent, and

always distinct one from another. No casts were present in the tubes. It was difficult to say whether all the fatty drops stained by the osmic acid coincided or not with these hyaline masses. It was to be noted that at many points the portion of the tube attacked by the degeneration corresponded with the origin of the uriniferous tube. Some of the

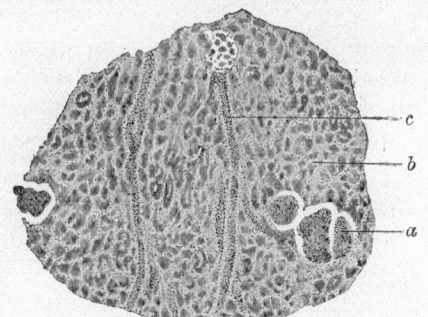

FIG. 62.—SECTION OF KIDNEY.

a, Glomerulus ; *b*, necrosed tubules ; *c*, healthy tubules.

affected convoluted tubules reached even as far as Bowman's capsule. In the degenerated cells the nuclei were, for the most part, refractory to the stain ; some were stained in a diffuse manner, or showed chromatolysis.

In short, the lesions, as a whole, proved that the case was one of **recent superacute degenerative nephritis, the cause of which, through escaping microscopic examination, appeared to be some toxic substance eliminated by the secretory apparatus of the kidneys.**

The liver showed granulo-fatty degeneration of the centro-lobular cells.

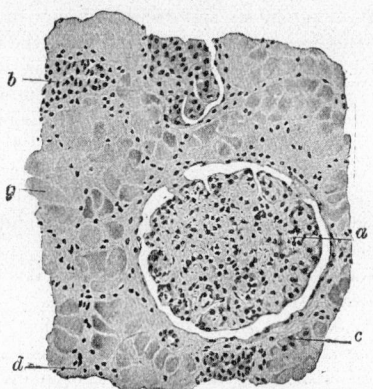

FIG. 63.—SECTION OF KIDNEY.

a, Glomerulus ; *g*, necrosed cells of convoluted tube ; *b*, cells undergoing necrosis, nuclei stiil present ; *c*, normal convoluted tube ; *d*, healthy connective stroma.

In the above case, then, appendicitis caused infection and intoxication of the patient. The lesions due to infection caused slight peritonitis and retrocæcal abscess, but the lesions due to the appendicular toxines caused during life symptoms of intoxication and acute changes found on post-mortem examination.

The patient, therefore, did not succumb to the circumscribed peritonitis, but to the appendicular poisoning, which proceeded more rapidly than the infection, and was in full activity on the fourth day of the disease. Peritonitis is not the all-important complication in appendicitis. We must take count of the toxic complications which sometimes precede the infectious troubles, and are the more to be feared as " temporizing " surgery is power-less against them. When we see these cases (and they are numerous), what are we to think of the short-sighted teaching which only takes account of the peritonitis, and advises an interval operation ? Such teaching fails to recognize that the toxines, by their rapid diffusion, carry off the patient whilst the interval is being awaited.

After I had mentioned this question at the Académie de Médecine,* Routier told of the following case :

A youth was admitted at the Necker Hospital on the evening of July 6. He felt sick two days before, and took a purge to relieve his " indigestion." The pains per-sisted. Next morning Dr. Le Guillant, who was called in, at once diagnosed appendi-citis, and insisted on his immediate removal to the Necker Hospital. Five years before Le Guillant had attended him for appendicitis. He advised operation, and warned the family of the gravity of the disease and of its probable recurrence ; this good advice was not followed.

On admission his temperature was 103° F. Routier saw him next morning. Although the temperature had fallen to 100° F., the case was obviously grave, and toxic symp-toms accompanied those of infection. Pronounced **jaundice,** profuse diarrhœa, and very quick pulse were present. The belly was everywhere painful, with muscular resistance, especially at McBurney's point.

Routier gave a very grave prognosis, and decided on immediate operation ; but as the parents did not consent, the operation was postponed till the next day. The jaundice was still more pronounced. The appendicitis was now four days and a half old. The operation disclosed an enormous abscess below the cæcum, and a large collection of pus in the pelvis. No improvement was manifest after the operation, as the patient was already poisoned. His temperature was 103° F., the pulse 120 ; diarrhœa and **jaundice** persisted. On the 9th extreme restlessness ; on the 10th delirium and death.

In this case, as in the preceding one, it was very important to know exactly the lesions present. Histological examination of the kidneys and of the liver by Nattan-Larrier showed similar lesions to those found by Letulle in the preceding case. In both cases the acute action of the appendicular toxines was evident. I give the histo-logical examination *in extenso.*

The **kidneys** appeared normal to the naked eye, save that the cortical substance was somewhat pale. Histological examination made of fragments taken a few hours after death showed marked lesions. The condition was one of superacute degenerative nephritis ; the lesions were localized to the convoluted tubes and to the ascending limb of Henle's loop. It was a systematized lesion of the whole secretory apparatus. All the convoluted tubules were attacked to the same degree, and presented the same appearance. The cells were large and granular ; the nuclei did not stain. The cell was defined at its base, but was breaking up towards the lumen of the tubule. Cyto-logical stains showed marked reticulation, in the meshes of which large rounded granules were present. At various points, and especially at the base of the cell, there were masses

* *Académie de Médecine,* séance du 8 Juillet, 1902.

of fine fatty granules ; the cells were undergoing granulo-fatty degeneration. The cells of the ascending limb of Henle's loop showed coagulation necrosis. The nucleus did not stain, and the protoplasm, studded with fat globules, was refractile, stained well with eosin, and took a pale blue with polychrome blue. The shape of the cell was changed. It was slightly wrinkled at its base ; its apex was irregular. Desquamation, however, was absent here, as in the convoluted tubes. These cells had necrosed *in situ ;* one section showed the outline of a few cylindrical cells. The cells of the convoluted tubules and of Henle's loop were dead as far as their functional power was concerned. Whilst we could see basal striations and granules which were stained black by iron alum in the normally secreting cell, none of the figures which indicate cellular activity could be detected. The most highly differentiated cells of the kidneys had ceased to be active.

The filtration system of the kidneys was, on the contrary, practically intact, and the glomeruli were normal. At a few isolated points, slight proliferation of the endothelium of Bowmann's capsule was noticed, and osmic acid revealed a few fatty granules in the cells of the straight tubes. These lesions, however, were of minor importance compared with the necrosis and acute degeneration in the convoluted tubules and in Henle's ascending limb—*i.e.,* in the secretory apparatus of the kidneys. The lesion was the more clear

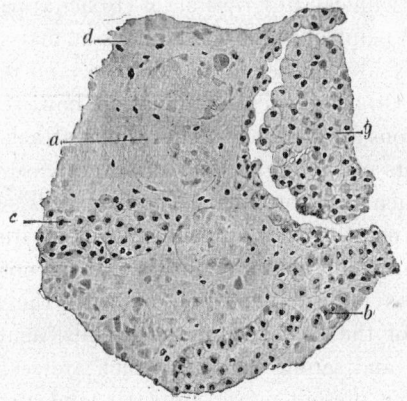

FIG. 64.—SECTION OF KIDNEY.

g, Glomerulus ; *a,* convoluted tubes, with necrosed cells ; *b,* cells in process of necrosis, nuclei still present ; *c,* normal convoluted tube ; *d,* connective tissue.

as it only attacked the glandular cell, while the connective tissue and the bloodvessels were normal. No diapedesis of leucocytes ; no micro-organisms. The lesion was purely toxic, and its localization to the secretory system showed that it was due to the elimination of toxic material by the cells of the convoluted tubes and of Henle's ascending limb.

The liver was very much congested ; the condition of the cells was remarkable, and osmic acid showed that they were crammed with very fine fatty granules. The nuclei, however, took the stain well, but the cells showed evident granulo-fatty degeneration.

Lorrain has published a similar case :

A man who had had two previous attacks was admitted for appendicitis. On his admission, induration was found in the right iliac fossa ; palpation caused acute pain, and the skin was hyperæsthetic ; no vomiting and no fever. Ice and opium were pre-scribed. A few days later, although fever was absent, the belly commenced to swell, the face was drawn, and the pulse was bad. Operation : fœtid abscess between the small intestine and the cæcum, which was gangrenous. A fruitless attempt was made to find the appendix, which was buried in the adhesions. He succumbed, and at the post-mortem examination the gangrenous appendix was discovered. No peritonitis; no collections of pus, except the one opened at the operation. Macroscopic examination of the kidneys showed nothing special, but histological examination revealed the following lesions : The epithelium of the straight tubes was normal, and the nuclei were well stained. The convoluted tubes were much altered ; here and there a few epithelial cells, with a well-stained nucleus, were seen, but in general the nuclei had completely disappeared. The epithelial cells were pale, non-granular, swollen, and had a tendency to fill up the lumen of the tubules. " The condition was one of coagulation necrosis. The lesions affected all the tubes more or less, but some few tubes seemed to have escaped necrosis." The cells of the liver were likewise attacked, and contained ochre pigment in abundance. " In short," says Lorrain, " the clinical course and the lesions in the secretory cells of the kidneys and of the liver showed that the appendicitis of insidious course and necrosing nature caused death, not by infection, but by **profound intoxication of the system.**"

Description.—The cases above quoted give the necessary details for the anatomical and clinical description of toxic appendicular nephritis. From the anatomical point of view, the kidneys at first sight do not appear to be affected. They are neither large nor pale, and do not resemble the large white kidney. On histological examination, however, the situation and the nature of the lesions are striking. The lesions attack almost exclusively the secretory elements of the organ, and in severe cases the cell is rapidly killed by the appendicular cytotoxine. The liver cells suffer the same fate.

From the clinical point of view, appendicular nephritis does not resemble the other known forms of acute nephritis. It is not comparable with scarlatinal or early syphilitic nephritis, or with the so-called nephritis a frigore. Swelling of the face and of the eyelids, acute œdema, dropsy, œdema of the lungs, and serous effusions which are seen in other kinds of acute nephritis, are not present in appendicular nephritis.

As œdema of the eyelids and of the face is absent, and as appendicular nephritis does not show itself, as a rule, by any visible sign, the diagnosis is by no means evident, and, therefore, this variety of nephritis has passed unnoticed. We must make a practice of examining the urine in every case of appendicitis.

Albumin, which is often abundant in other forms of acute nephritis, is generally scanty in the appendicular form. On the other hand, granular casts may be found in the urine as early as the second or third day, and are a bad sign. Albumin alone does not make the prognosis of appendicitis absolutely bad, but it is a sign of poisoning, and a danger-signal. This danger does not come from the nephritis alone (which may end in urinary insufficiency and perhaps oliguria) ; it arises also from the general intoxication of the system—that is, from the **appendicæmia.**

Jaundice, which indicates the involvement of the liver, is fairly often associated with albuminuria. These two signs generally appear early and together. Their signification may not be fatal, and yet no one can say whether the intoxication will confine itself to slight nephritis or hepatitis, or whether it will end in more extensive lesions, such as toxic gastritis, vomito negro, renal and hepatic insufficiency, nervous complications, general poisoning, and death.

What is there to guide us in the **prognosis**? The fever is not a certain guide. The disease may end fatally, and yet the temperature may remain normal. In my first case the temperature oscillated between 99° and 100° F., although the fatal complications were setting in. In Lorrain's patient the temperature was about 99° F. for some days before death. The pulse itself may give no precise information as regards the prognosis.

The history of appendicitis is always deceptive, and the poison often accomplishes its work without giving any sign. We see, then, the errors in the old descriptions of appendicitis as a purely local disease in which the worst complication was peritonitis. Certain pathological classifications on which an exact prognosis was based are now forgotten.

The cases in this section convey a great lesson. They show the gravity of toxic appendicular nephritis, trace the series of toxic complications (hepatitis, gastritis), and prove how rapidly the appendicular toxines may act ; they furnish fresh arguments in favour of **early** surgical intervention, show the danger of delay, and condemn the teaching which advocates an interval operation.

Some day the advocates of delay will have to reply to these arguments otherwise than by words. We have given the precise facts and irrefutable proofs. Let them do the same in support of their teaching. We know how many patients have died because it was not thought advisable to operate before the appendicitis had become quiescent, and we can show the toxic lesions which were the cause of death. Why, then, should we not operate on patients before they are intoxicated and infected ? We ask for an answer based on facts as precise as our own.

I do not wish to close this section without drawing a parallel between the appendicular liver and the appendicular kidney. I described separately early toxic hepatitis, which is non-suppurative, and infective hepatitis, which occurs later, and occupies a prominent place in the history of the appendicular liver. This purulent hepatitis is readily explained, because the infective agents are carried direct from the appendix to the liver by the tributaries of the portal vein. It is not so in the case of the appendicular kidney, which can only become infected by a circuitous path ; consequently, infective nephritis with abscess of the kidney is relatively very rare, whilst toxic nephritis, especially the slight form, is common.

I think the poisoning of the kidneys by the appendicular toxines may in some degree account for the origin of Bright's disease.

V. BRIGHT'S DISEASE—CHRONIC NEPHRITIS— PARENCHYMATOUS NEPHRITIS—INTERSTITIAL NEPHRITIS— MIXED NEPHRITIS.

Discussion.—In 1827 Richard Bright published the results of his observations, and taught that changes are found in the kidneys of patients who die after passing albuminous urine and suffering from persistent dropsy. Bright certainly made use of the researches of Wells and Blackall, but no one had previously described the relation between the symptom and the lesion of the disease which now bears his name. Bright's great merit consists, then, in having grasped the fact that albuminuria and persistent dropsy are dependent upon a lesion of the kidneys; but he took care, with wise reserve, not to state the nature of this lesion, because many years of anatomical research by the English, German, and French schools have not cleared up the nature of these lesions which still give rise to contrary opinions.

All observers agree that post-mortem examination in case of subacute and chronic nephritis reveals the most varied changes in the kidneys, which may be normal or enlarged, whitish or yellowish, or, again, small and atrophied (small red kidney). The question, then, arises whether such dissimilar lesions are not merely successive stages of the same morbid process, which begins in hypertrophy and ends in atrophy; or whether, on the contrary, they represent distinct anatomical forms.

Bright, not wishing to specify the extent and nature of the lesion, abstained from drawing conclusions. In 1840 Rayer, in a work which Rosenstein justly calls the "Archives of Renal Diseases," proclaimed that the various lesions of the kidneys are in reality only successive stages of one inflammatory process. The kidneys are enlarged and congested in the first or acute stage. In the subacute and chronic stages they become anæmic and atrophied. These various stages were divided by Rayer into six successive degrees.

In 1851 Frerichs, who followed in Rayer's footsteps, admitted only three degrees in chronic nephritis; but he, like Rayer, maintained the unity of the inflammatory process, which commenced with congestion of the organ and cloudy swelling of its cells (enlarged kidney), passed on to fatty degeneration of the epithelium, and ended in atrophy of the organ (small kidney). Whether we admit six periods with Rayer, or three with Frerichs, seven with Christison, or five with Martin Solon, it is none the less true that this doctrine, called the doctrine of the unicists, defended by Virchow and by Reinhardt, recognizes one morbid process, which causes successive hypertrophy and atrophy of the kidney. The contrary doctrine maintains the plurality of the forms of this disease: the various conditions found in the kidneys post mortem are not successive stages of one morbid process, but represent absolutely distinct forms. The enlarged white kidney does not give rise to the small contracted kidney, just as the small contracted kidney never commences as a large white kidney. In the small contracted kidney the lesion is an interstitial nephritis, and has nothing in common with the enlarged kidney, just as the enlarged kidney which represents parenchymatous nephritis has nothing to do with the small kidney. These distinct anatomical processes give rise, it is true—to some similar troubles, so the adherents of this theory maintain—but yet their symptomatology is sufficiently distinct for us to say, from the clinical as well as from the pathological point of view, that one patient is suffering from interstitial nephritis, whereas another patient has parenchymatous nephritis.

According to some writers, these two forms, the small and the enlarged kidney, could not be more distinct. The anatomical lesions are dissimilar—in the one, vascular and interstitial; in the other, glandular. The symptoms, course, duration, and complications are said to form a very different *ensemble* in the two cases. The ætiology is held to be distinct; the small kidney is said to be the especial appanage of gout, plumbism, and old age, whereas the enlarged kidney is said to be met with "almost exclusively in tubercular patients, etc."

Some protests were raised against this forced division (Jaccoud). I* fought against it in the name of pathological anatomy and of clinical medicine. For the sake of conciseness, I shall briefly sum up in a few lines our present knowledge of the question as I understand it :

We know that in chronic nephritis the lesions are diffuse, and more or less general in the glandular, vascular, and connective tissues. We need not, therefore, absolutely retain the old division into parenchymatous and interstitial nephritis. It is, nevertheless, true that the lesions may be unequally distributed. We find some cases of nephritis in which the interstitial lesions predominate, and others in which the parenchymatous changes are most marked ; but they are often only varieties, and the nephritis, taken as a whole, is still diffuse.

If we find post mortem large white or small red kidneys, and granular or cystic kidneys, these varieties are due to the rapidity or to the slowness of the process ; to the predominance of epithelial, vascular, or connective changes ; to the nature of the toxines or of the poison ; to the virulence or the attenuation of the infective agents ; but no matter what is the nature of the lesion, as soon as the process runs a progressive course, the final result is the same—viz., a tendency to the destruction of the organ, to the abolition of its functional powers, with gradual or rapid insufficiency of urinary depuration and uræmia.

Numberless discussions have been held as to whether the enlarged kidney may finally become small and sclerotic, and whether the contracted kidneys may have begun with hypertrophy. Divers forms may here present themselves. Certain processes cause hypertrophy of the organ, as well as simultaneous necrosis of its essential parts. In this case the hypertrophic lesion may be considered as the final stage in the nephritis, since it has caused death. On the other hand, when we find the kidneys atrophied to one-half of their normal size, it is evident that the kidney, which was normal at the onset of the disease, has atrophied by this amount. Many discussions have also been held to determine the varieties of nephritis for which the name of Bright's disease should be reserved. The reply seems very simple to me. Every case of chronic nephritis comes under Bright's disease ; "Bright's disease" and "chronic nephritis" are synonymous terms. In making use of the term "Bright's disease," we do homage to an illustrious man who was the first to establish clearly the course of the disease which is at present occupying our attention ; and, furthermore, this term does not prejudge the nature of the lesions : it is, therefore, well adapted to new discoveries.

During the course of this article the word "Brightism" will frequently be used as synonymous with Bright's disease. When I coined the word "Brightism" I applied it more especially to the mild forms of this disease. When I say that a patient is suffering from Brightism, I wish it to be understood that his urinary depuration is insufficient, but that so far mild symptoms only are present ; he does not yet show the grave symptoms of uræmia.

In order to facilitate the anatomical description, I shall describe separately chronic nephritis with enlarged kidneys and chronic nephritis with small kidneys ; we shall see later the intermediary varieties which represent the most common form of Bright's disease.

Parenchymatous Nephritis.

Chronic nephritis with **enlarged kidneys** is generally rapid in its course ; indeed, the name of "subacute nephritis" might be more suitable. "The

* Dieulafoy, *Gaz. Hebdom.*, 1877, Nos. 12 and 14.

size of the kidneys is explained by the severe inflammation, the intra-tubular and interstitial exudates, and the intense glomerulitis. The differ-ence in colour depends on the degree of congestion, on the amount of exudate in the tubes and on the more or less profound change in the epithelial cells of the tubuli contorti " (Brault). These enlarged kidneys, which are generally smooth, may be whitish or hæmorrhagic. On section, they cut readily, are rich in juice, yellowish at certain points, and sometimes studded with small hæmorrhages. The " large white kidney " (Wilks), therefore, represents only one form of the large kidney in Bright's disease. Scarlatina, syphilis and malaria, may give rise to the **enlarged kidney,** by reason of the severe and rapid course of the lesions.

Pathological Anatomy.—The large kidney may weigh three times the normal amount. The capsule strips readily, and we find neither nodules nor cysts, as in the granular kidney. The cortical substance is two or three times its ordinary size.

Under the microscope the glomeruli and the tubuli contorti are two or three times as large as normal. The epithelial cells show cloudy swelling, and the lumen is narrowed. The cells rapidly undergo granulo-fatty de-generation and we find every variety and degree of swollen and " granular cells " (Cornil). In the convoluted tubules, and especially in the straight tubules, we find granular detritus, granular or hyaline casts, white and red corpuscles. It is especially in the interior of the straight tubules that the products of the exudate from the Malpighian glomeruli (corpuscles and plasma), and from the epithelial cells of the convoluted tubes, become coagulated and transformed into **hyaline casts** (Cornil).

The stroma is enlarged, through the diapedesis of the white corpuscles and through the intertubular œdema. Many glomeruli are anæmic and shrunken. We may find abundant multiplication of the nuclei in Bow-man's capsule and in the glomerulus. The cells desquamate and compress the vascular tuft inside the capsule.

Referring to the large white kidney, we might recall the discussion which was held and the doubts which arose as to the inflammatory process in so-called parenchymatous nephritis. According to many writers, parenchy-matous nephritis is really the result of an inflammatory process, the epi-thelium being the chief seat of the inflammation (Rosenstein, Lancereaux, Cornil and Ranvier, Lécorché). Other writers, on the contrary (Johnson, Klebs, Kelsch), hold that the epithelium is not the seat of an inflammatory process, because no trace of new proliferation is found, either in the epi-thelium or in the connective tissue of the diseased kidney. The swelling of the cells and the granulo-fatty degeneration are said to be a primary degenerative process rather than an inflammatory lesion. This explains the name, **enlarged fatty kidney,** given to the large white kidney in England.

Brault, who sums up the question in an important work on nephritis, will not admit the hypothesis of a purely degenerative process. In the first place, says he, the presence of fat in the cells does not prove that the process is degenerative, because fat is always found in inflammations of long duration. The process is really inflammatory, judging from the fibrinous exudate in the tubules, and also from the glomerulitis which is always present. Bowman's capsule is often thickened. The cells lining the capsule encroach upon the cavity of the glomerulus. The loops of the glomerulus are obliterated ; the afferent and efferent arteries near the glomerulus sometimes show endarteritis obliterans.

The preceding description is especially applicable to the large white kidney. In other cases, however, subacute nephritis has a congestive or irritative tendency, and the enlarged kidney presents a different aspect. Its cortical substance is reddish or yellowish ; the glomeruli and the capillaries of the cortical substance are distended with blood ; hæmorrhage occurs in the interior of the glomerulus ; and the convoluted tubule is filled with red corpuscles.

Such is the anatomical description of the enlarged kidney. The name " subacute " nephritis would be more suitable than chronic nephritis. Clinically they present some peculiarities, which I shall now mention.

Chief Symptoms.—The symptoms comprise œdema of the face and legs, anasarca, serous effusions, especially into the pleura, and œdema of the lungs. Headache, dyspnœa, vomiting, epistaxis, and visual troubles are frequently present. The urine, which is scanty, high-coloured, and at times bloody, contains abundant albumin and casts.

The symptoms of Brightism—viz., pollakiuria, dead fingers, cramps in the calves, cryæsthesia, etc.—are less frequent than in other forms of chronic nephritis.

The heart shows little or no hypertrophy. The gallop rhythm is rare. The arteries are not sclerotic, and the pulse is soft, contrasting with the hard pulse found in cases of nephritis with high arterial tension.

Symptoms of uræmia—viz., delirium, convulsions, and coma—are more rare than in the other varieties of chronic nephritis. Pneumonia, pericarditis, erysipelas, and gangrene, occur as secondary infections.

Subacute nephritis with enlarged kidneys terminates in various ways. The lesions are sometimes so severe, the epithelial necrosis is so rapid, that the enlarged kidney represents the final stage, and the patient succumbs in a few months. In some cases the lesions are not so profound, and the nephritis may be cured. The kidney, however, is transformed into an organ of *minoris resistentiæ*. Finally, in other cases nephritis which has commenced with symptoms of an enlarged kidney makes slow progress, and causes a diminution in the size of the organ with the symptoms of an eminently chronic nephritis. In this case the transformation of an enlarged kidney into a smaller one may be admitted.

Interstitial Nephritis.

After having described nephritis **with enlarged kidneys,** I shall now give the description of the opposite type—viz., chronic nephritis with **contracted kidneys.**

Pathological Anatomy.—When toxic or infectious agents (lead, gout, alcohol, secondary infections) act in small and repeated doses, or when the morbid process (arterio-sclerosis, senility) is very slow, it is only after many years that the lesion ends in atrophy of the kidneys. In some cases the kidneys are reduced to one-third of their normal weight. The colour may be greyish, yellowish, or reddish, according to the number of vessels which persist and the condition of the cells. Some have an intense red colour (the old " small red kidney "), which depends on subcapsular ecchymoses and a hæmorrhagic mottling visible to the naked eye.

The kidney is sometimes nodular. The perirenal fat is generally much increased. The capsule is thickened and adherent, so that it is impossible to detach it without removing some portions of the kidney substance. The surface of the organ varies in colour, and is studded with prominent granulations of the size of a millet-seed. These granulations, which are also found deep in the cortex, are formed by the healthy tubules, which are embedded in the fibrous tissue. They must not be confounded with the flat patches in the large fatty kidney which are incorrectly called granulations.

On section, the kidney tissue is resistant. The atrophy principally affects the cortex, which may be only 1 millimetre in thickness. In some cases, indeed, the capsule touches the base of the pyramids. " The region of the glomeruli and of the convoluted tubules disappears, as if there had been absorption of these parts " (Brault). Bertin's columns, which are a prolongation of the cortical substance, do not show such marked atrophy as the cortex.

With the naked eye little **cysts** are seen. They are generally formed at the expense of the convoluted tubules, which are strangled by the fibrous tissue, and dilate above the strangulation, or are at times fused with enlarged tubules. These cysts may become independent. They are often filled with refracting colloid masses. Some are as large as a pea, and project from the surface of the kidney. Other cysts may result from enlargement of Bowman's capsule ; others, again, of an ovoid form, or disposed like a chaplet, arise from the strangulation and enlargement of the straight tubules in the medullary substance. The atrophy is much less pronounced in the pyramids than in the cortex. The calyces and the pelvis are sometimes very dilated. Subcortical nodules of adenoma are found (Tabourin). Small concretions of uric acid and urate of soda are common, especially in the medullary substance and in the interior of the tubules. They will be referred to under Gout.

A section of the cortex, made parallel to the surface of the organ, and stained with picrocarmine, shows considerable invasion by fibrous tissue. In some places the renal lobule has disappeared, and the glomeruli are represented by little spheres of a pale rose colour. Islands and bands of fibrous tissue are found round the tubes, the glomeruli, and the vessels.

The **glomeruli** show enormous thickening of their capsule, which is itself surrounded by a thick fibrous zone. Between the capsule and the vascular tuft flattened cells and fibrous bundles are found. The glomerular tuft is atrophied and fibrous, the arterioles are in part obliterated, and the afferent and efferent arteries are affected with endoperiarteritis. Of certain glomeruli there is only a trace left. Every element has disappeared from their interior, and they blend with the surrounding connective tissue. Hyaline degeneration, which has a lardaceous appearance, is frequently seen.

The membrana propria of the tubuli contorti is sclerotic, and some of the canaliculi are much reduced in calibre. The changes seen in nephritis with enlarged kidney may be met with here (Cornil). When the epithelium of the convoluted tubules has disappeared, it is replaced by cubical cells, which at times fill the lumen of the tubule (Kelsch). Many tubules are filled with granular or waxy casts, while others have almost disappeared, and are only indicated by an islet of round cells.

Theories.—There are many theories to explain the anatomical process in the small granular kidney, according as the lesion is held to begin in the connective tissue, the arteries, the glandular tissue, or these different parts together.

According to the first theory, the process is said to commence in the interstitial connective tissue. In 1850 Traube, following Beer, ascribed the principal rôle in nephritis to the connective tissue of the kidneys, and stated that Bright's disease was the result of an interstitial inflammatory process ; that the changes in the glandular epithelium of the kidneys were consequent on the slow alteration in the connective tissue ; and that the sclerotic process, following its natural course, ended in atrophy of the kidney.

According to the second theory, the lesions of the small contracted kidney were said to be a local form of general **arterio-sclerosis.** Arteriosclerosis had been described by Sutton and Gull under the name of **arterio-capillary fibrosis,** but their description (1872) had been preceded by Lancereaux's work. The walls of the small vessels undergo a transformation, which is not due to hyaline degeneration, as Sutton supposed, but rather resembles the lesions of arteritis. These changes in the small vessels are sometimes associated with atheroma of the larger arteries.

General arterio-sclerosis is said to be the primary trouble, and to cause arterio-sclerosis of the kidneys, fibrous hypertrophy of the heart, cirrhosis of the liver, and the multiple hæmorrhages (cerebral or retinal), which are so common in this form of Bright's disease.

This theory of general arterio-sclerosis, which has been confirmed by many post-mortem examinations, does not explain all the cases of nephritis in which the arteries are chiefly affected—e.g., Brault speaks of a young man who succumbed to sclerotic nephritis. The lesion was entirely confined to the kidneys and to the heart, arterio-sclerosis and atheroma being elsewhere absent.

The third theory holds that the small contracted kidney is the result of epithelial cirrhosis. Charcot, relying on experiments (ligature of the ureter) and on the renal changes produced by the elimination of lead, held that interstitial nephritis belonged to the class of visceral cirrhoses. " The epithelial change, which is due to irritation, and is a primary and necessary fact, reveals itself anatomically by the return of the cells to the embryonic state ; the interstitial lesion, the consequent fact, also reveals itself—in the initial phases, at least—by the production of embryonic tissue. . . ." This theory of epithelial cirrhosis and the return of the cells to the embryonic condition is no longer held (Letulle).

These theories seek to explain the production of the small kidney. It would be wrong to admit or to reject them systematically. It is probable that several of these processes are predominant or concomitant, according to circumstances. As Brault has said, the expressions " glandular," " arterial," and " interstitial " nephritis are inexact ; and I am of the same opinion. One process is not necessarily subordinate to the other. They go on together as the result of the same cause. " This cause creates the reaction of the fibrous tissue, which increases by proliferation, whilst the epithelium of the tubules is destroyed. A slow irritation determines the wear and tear of the epithelium, which gradually disappears, while the connective tissue develops and becomes indurated. " The well-known anatomical picture of general arterio-sclerosis is not affected by the preceding considerations, but the interpretation of them varies. Instead of subordinating the lesions of the kidneys to general arterio-sclerosis, it is more rational to subordinate the lesions both of the kidneys and of other organs to one prime cause (gout, lead, old age, heredity, etc.). " Besides," says Brault, " the importance of the arterial lesions in their relation to the contracted kidney has been much exaggerated."

Symptoms.—Nephritis with atrophied kidneys has a very slow course, and lasts several years. Œdema is rare, and dropsy of the serous membranes is exceptional. On the other hand, the minor symptoms of Brightism, such as dyspnœa, headache, epistaxis, and ocular troubles (hæmorrhage of the retina), are frequent.

Cardiac troubles are almost constant, and examination of the heart generally reveals hypertrophy and a gallop rhythm (Potain).

Dyspnœa is frequent. It may occur in the form of severe attacks like those of asthma ; at other times it shows the Cheyne-Stokes rhythm.

The pulse is hard, and the arterial tension is high. The secretion of urine is increased. The urine is pale. Albumin may be present in small amount, or may be absent. The urea remains at its normal amount, and the other substances are very slightly diminished. The urine contains some casts.

Death frequently follows, with symptoms of uræmia, such as delirium, convulsions, and coma. Cerebral hæmorrhage, hæmiplegia, and apoplexy are frequent complications, due to the rupture of the cerebral arterioles, on which miliary aneurysms are present.

Mixed Nephritis.

We find between the two extreme types already described a host of **intermediate types,** which constitute the **most frequent form** of Bright's disease.

Pathological Anatomy.—In these intermediate types, which are subject to relapse, the kidneys may be normal or enlarged, but are generally on the road to atrophy. The kidney may be nodular, granular, fibrous, or cystic, and of a whitish-yellow, or reddish colour in these intermediate types of chronic nephritis. Compensatory hypertrophy is sometimes met with (Chauffard, Grasset). The capsule is adherent. The cortical substance is atrophied, and the glandular tissue is more or less degenerated.

The histological changes described in the previous section affect to a variable extent the vascular, glandular, or connective tissues. I would, therefore, merely remark that the association or the alternation of these lesions leads to the most varied intermediate types. The mischief may commence as a subacute nephritis, with enlarged kidneys and parenchymatous changes, while the fibrous and vascular lesions later gain the upper hand. In some cases we find at first vascular and connective tissue changes, and it is only later that the parenchymatous lesions modify the nature of the case. These cases are generally of the intermediate type from the start, but in some circumstances they are only the sequel of the forms described in the preceding sections.* These differences depend on the nature and the severity of the causes of the nephritis. We shall return to this question under Ætiology.

* Raynaud has quoted a case which proves the identity and the succession of these lesions. At the post-mortem examination of a woman who had died of Bright's disease at the age of forty-eight years, he found one of the kidneys enlarged and white and the other kidney granular and atrophied. The histological examination showed that the sclerosis was commencing to invade the enlarged kidney (Bartel's "Annotations of Lépine," p. 673).

Lesions of the Heart—Hypertrophy.—While the heart may be hypertrophied in any form of chronic nephritis, enlargement is absent or not so marked in subacute nephritis with enlarged kidneys. The hypertrophy is most pronounced in nephritis with small kidneys. These lesions had not escaped Bright's notice. He thought them secondary to the lesion in the kidneys, and he sought for the mechanism. Later, Traube described these lesions, but he was wrong in believing that they were only present in interstitial nephritis, and he simply took note of the hypertrophy. We know to-day that cardiac lesions may exist in all forms of chronic nephritis, and we also know that the lesions do not always show themselves by hypertrophy of the heart. I would lay great stress on this point, as it is too often said that the heart is always enlarged. The heart may be smaller than normal, and may at first sight appear to be healthy, but yet histological examination shows advanced arterio-sclerotic lesions. I have recently seen a case of this kind.

The renal heart, as it is still called, is generally large. It may be enormous, but in some cases its size is not increased, although its intimate lesions are very pronounced. The hypertrophy chiefly affects the left ventricle, and appears apart from any valvular change, thus differing greatly from the hypertrophy present in lesions of the mitral and aortic orifices. Nevertheless, the heart in Bright's disease may present both its own proper lesions and also chronic endocarditis of the aortic and mitral orifices. The right ventricle, the other parts of the heart, or even the entire organ, may participate in the hypertrophy, and **dilatation** is common.

Histological examination reveals two forms of lesions—the one affecting the vessels and the interstitial tissue, the other affecting the muscle fibre. In a section of the musculi papillares much fibrous tissue is sometimes visible with the naked eye. Under the microscope we see patches of fibrous tissue, forming a kind of network with other bands from the arterioles which are attacked by peri-arteritis. The arterial lesions are probably the starting-point of this fibrous invasion, wherein the muscular tissue has in part disappeared. In other parts of the heart we find hypertrophy of the muscular tissue, which chiefly leads to the enlargement of the heart. The hypertrophy of the muscle, on the one hand, and the arterio-sclerosis on the other, may be combined in various ways. As a result the heart may be enlarged or normal, while the size of the organ gives no information as to the real nature of the intimate lesions. Very marked hypertrophy may coexist with very moderate arterio-sclerosis, and, reciprocally, the arterio-sclerosis may be advanced, while the heart is not hypertrophied.

The pathogenesis of the renal heart has given rise to numerous discussions. Two theories exist: the one supposes that the hypertrophy of the heart is secondary to the renal mischief; the other holds that the cardiac and renal lesions are independent of one another, and arise from a common cause. In the first hypothesis we have to show how the renal lesion produces the cardiac hypertrophy. We may see in this chain of morbid events the result of high arterial tension (Potain). Is this high arterial tension due, as Bright believed, to the incomplete elimination of the waste products of the urine? The answer is negative, because insufficient elimination does not raise the intravascular pressure (Potain); and, furthermore, this explanation would not agree with the fact that hypertrophy is more common and more marked in interstitial nephritis, where the excretion of the solid matter in the urine is but slightly modified (Senator). Are the high arterial tension and the hypertrophy of the heart due to the contraction or the obliteration of the renal arterioles in the atrophied kidneys (Traube)? This is not probable, because experiment has shown that the renal arteries may be ligatured without appreciable increase in the arterial pressure; and, on the other hand, clinical cases testify to advanced cardiac hypertrophy, while the kidneys are not atrophied.

According to the second hypothesis, the kidneys and the heart suffer simultaneously from the action of one cause. According to Gull and Sutton, this cause is the sclerotic thickening (arterio-capillary fibrosis) of the arterioles and capillaries. This change is said to have a twofold action, being the origin of sclerosis in the kidneys, the heart, and other organs, and, on the other hand, placing in the general circulation an obstacle which, by raising the arterial tension, is said to cause the cardiac hypertrophy. Buhl tries to prove that the hypertrophy is the result of myocarditis, which is both interstitial and parenchymatous, and of degenerative lesions of the heart. He adds that the inflammations of the heart and of the kidneys are contemporaneous and independent. Debove and Letulle also think that the cardiac hypertrophy depends upon interstitial myocarditis with sclerotic lesions, but in their opinion the nephritis and the myocarditis are secondary to general arterial fibrosis.

The hypothesis which subordinates the hypertrophy of the heart to the lesion of the kidneys and of the vessels is discussed and in part admitted by Potain. "In a fair number of cases it is clear that the nephritis is primary, and the hypertrophy of the heart is secondary." The hypertrophy, adds Potain, might be the result of exaggerated tonicity of the small vessels— a tonicity of which the kidneys would be, by reflex action, the point of departure. Charcot also holds that the hypertrophy of the heart is consequent upon the lesion of the kidneys. It might, indeed, precede the renal sclerosis if it be admitted that this sclerosis is itself preceded by some functional trouble, the effect of which is to limit the secretory energy of the kidneys.

In some ingenious experiments Strauss ligatured one ureter in a guinea-pig.   He killed the animal some months later, and found the following lesions :

Fibrous atrophy of the kidney on the side of operation ; kidney hypertrophied on the opposite side ; hypertrophy of heart, chiefly of the left ventricle ; myocardium and arterioles healthy.   These experiments prove that the hypertrophy of the heart may follow on the renal lesion, and that we need not expect a special change in the myocardium or general arterio-sclerosis.

In my opinion we must divide the question.   The lesions of the heart in Bright's disease are of two kinds—muscular and arterio-sclerotic.   The muscular fibres in the vicinity of the sclerotic tissue disappear, but at other points they develop, causing the hypertrophy just mentioned.   This hypertrophy is not due to the sclerotic lesions, but to the increased arterial tension, which depends upon the more or less general arterio-sclerosis and the contraction of the small vessels which is so common in Bright's disease.   The fibrosis of the heart results from the cardiac arterio-sclerosis, which is merely a local feature of a generalized process.   It is certain that the muscular lesions and the arterio-sclerosis of the heart may be anterior, parallel, or posterior to the development of the lesions in the kidneys.

Ætiology.—In a general way the infectious diseases (scarlatina, syphilis, pneumonia, influenza, typhoid fever, mumps, erysipelas, diphtheria, malaria, etc.) and puerperal conditions which give rise to acute nephritis may contribute to the ætiology of chronic nephritis.   If the reader will refer to the section on Acute Nephritis, he will find the action of the microbes and of the toxines discussed.   In these various cases, which form the first category, chronic nephritis may be only the end of acute or subacute nephritis.   As a matter of fact, acute nephritis (when it is not fatal) may end in various ways : some cases recover, others apparently do so, but the fire smoulders under the ashes.   Some slight symptoms prove that the process is not yet extinct, until the nephritis ends in the chronic stage.   Others, again, pass insensibly from the acute to the subacute stage, and end in chronic nephritis.

In the second category I place cases which are chronic from the outset. Gout and plumbism hold the first place in this category.   I also include arterio-sclerosis; but here we must remember that partial or general arteriosclerosis depends on a primary cause—viz., gout, syphilis, alcoholism, infectious diseases, advancing age, or heredity.   Heredity plays a considerable part in the pathogenesis of nephritis, as in all chronic diseases ; and by heredity I mean all the hereditary factors which make the organ more vulnerable or which favour auto-intoxication.

We may include in the third category cases of nephritis of **dyscrasic** origin.   The idea of Bright's disease as a primary dyscrasia with secondary renal changes is very old, seeing that Bright himself stated it.   We may place nephritis by auto-intoxication in the group of dyscrasic causes, the renal lesion being due to the elimination of excess of tyrosin and of other poisonous extractives, due to insufficient oxidation (diseases of the liver), too rapid combustion (fevers), impaired nutrition, or chlorosis.

In short, a person may become a sufferer from Bright's disease in many ways. In the first place, an attack of acute nephritis does not recover, but passes into the subacute or chronic stage. In such a case the course of events is clear. In the second place, the invasion of the renal mischief is slow and insidious, the minor or major symptoms of urinary insufficiency being present. This condition obtains in gouty persons and in people suffering from gravel, lead-poisoning, or arterio-sclerosis. In them Bright's disease makes slow progress, and acute attacks are wanting. The renal atrophy is of slow development.

In the third place, the course of events is as follows : An individual has previously suffered from some infectious disease. This disease (scarlatina, diphtheria, mumps) has affected the kidneys, and may have caused but slight and transient nephritis. Although the trouble may have been slight, the kidneys are none the less affected, and the results may long remain. Another person has also been attacked by some infectious disease (pneumonia, typhoid fever, influenza, syphilis, malaria), which has caused only slight nephritis. Although the lesion appears trifling, the kidneys are none the less damaged, and here, as in the preceding case, the effect may remain. These persons whose kidneys have been infected by scarlatina, typhoid fever, influenza, pneumonia or syphilis are liable to acute relapses of nephritis, or to more gradual mischief, which ends in Bright's disease. In one subject the renal lesions may progress slowly ; the symptoms may remain confined to what I have called " the minor troubles of Brightism," and do not end in uræmia. Let them, however, take cold or become pregnant, or let any other cause supervene which severely affects the kidneys, and acute mischief, with all its consequences, will appear.

These persons are most liable to Bright's disease if they are also intemperate, or if their liver, through auto-intoxication, transmits to the urine unchanged waste products. They may also suffer from gout, and their kidneys may be damaged by elimination of uric acid ; or, again, they may show early arterio-sclerosis, or may be suffering from heredity. It is then evident that they are in the best possible condition to fall victims to Bright's disease.

If a young girl suffering from the condition which I have called " chloro-Brightism" marry too early, and become pregnant on one or more occasions, she is more likely to show nephritis gravidarum and eclampsia.

These examples prove that **very different routes may lead to chronic nephritis.** Recovery depends on the nature and the severity of the cause.

The disease may remain stationary or may be split up into latent and acute periods. It may not go beyond " Brightism," but too often it ends in renal insufficiency and fatal uræmia. The onset of uræmia may occur with large granular or cystic kidneys, but it chiefly depends on the severity, quality, and combination of the toxi-infectious agents, and also on the condition of the other organs.

Description of Bright's Disease.—Some years ago, at a period when the different forms of Bright's disease had been artificially separated, it was customary to describe parenchymatous and interstitial nephritis as two distinct diseases, and some writers went so far as to ask for which form the name of Bright's disease ought to be reserved. I do not hold this view of Bright's disease. Typical cases of atrophic interstitial nephritis and of parenchymatous nephritis with enlarged kidneys merit, both anatomically and clinically, the description given above. The chief interest of the question, however, must not be centred in them. I shall, therefore, describe the most common clinical form of Bright's disease which corresponds to the intermediate types of chronic nephritis. We may find glandular lesions complicated by interstitial and vascular changes, or interstitial and vascular changes complicated by glandular lesions. In our description we shall follow the onset, the nature, and the variations of the symptoms and complications which constitute Bright's disease.

Onset.—In some cases Bright's disease follows an attack of acute nephritis. It is, however, more often chronic from the outset. I have often verified the fact that a case of Bright's disease regarded as one of rapid course was really a case of slow evolution, in which an acute stage had supervened. An individual who has always considered his health to be good asks for advice concerning trouble which has affected him for the past few weeks. He has had headache and vomiting or dyspnœa. Œdema of the face and of the legs has appeared. The urine contains albumin and casts. At first sight the case looks like acute nephritis of recent date. On minute inquiry, however, if we look for the symptoms preceding this acute episode, we shall find that some six months or more ago the patient has had headaches, which he calls migraine. He has often suffered from frequent micturition, dead fingers, palpitation of the heart, cramp in the calves, and puffiness of the eyelids. When he blows his nose in the morning, blood is found on the handkerchief. On various occasions he has had buzzing in the ears, defective hearing, itching, cryæsthesia, electric shocks, etc. By grouping these symptoms, which have been practically unnoticed, we can reconstruct the disease which has been slowly maturing, until the marked symptoms make their appearance.

In its most common form, then, Bright's disease has an insidious onset. During a period, which may be of long duration, the symptoms are apparently trifling, and as their origin is not discovered, numerous errors in diagnosis result. Headache, frequent micturition, slight epistaxis, palpitation, cramps in the calves of the legs, breathlessness, pains in the loins, tingling in the ears, defective hearing, vertigo, visual troubles, itching, dead fingers, cryæsthesia, and digestive troubles, may be temporary or permanent, and isolated or associated. They may appear and then disappear for a long time before œdema and other urgent symptoms of Bright's disease make their appearance. During this chronic state, which is intermediate, as it were, between health and disease, acute attacks supervene, and are characterized by asthma-like dyspnœa; by headaches, which resemble those of syphilis; by acute palpitation, such as occurs in diseases of the heart and of the aorta; by digestive troubles, such as we find in ulcer of the stomach; and by œdema of the face and the limbs, which gives a useful clue to the diagnosis. These acute attacks are wrongly taken for the onset of the disease.

Minor Symptoms of Brightism.—Under this name I would include the apparently slight symptoms which may mark the onset or may be present at any stage of Bright's disease.

1. POLLAKIURIA, POLYURIA.—Amongst the urinary troubles peculiar to Bright's disease we find excessive frequency of micturition. In chronic nephritis the patient may urinate six times in the night, or ten times in the twenty-four hours. The desire may be imperative, and the quantity at each evacuation is small. The extreme frequency of micturition is not always due to excess of urine (polyuria), because the quantity is often below the average.

There are two distinct and independent urinary troubles in Bright's disease : the one, polyuria, is a trouble of secretion, and concerns the kidneys ; the other, pollakiuria, is a trouble of excretion, and concerns the bladder. It is indeed remarkable that in many cases the pollakiuria **precedes** the polyuria.

Although these troubles are dissociated by most contemporary writers, they were formerly united under the term " polyuria." This is incorrect, since polyuria deals only with the secretory trouble. The confusion arose from the fact that we had only one word for two symptoms. The frequency of micturition constitutes an independent symptom of importance. It was, therefore, necessary to give it a distinctive name, and I have proposed the term " pollakiuria." Polyuria will, then, be used to indicate abundance of the secretion, and pollakiuria will be reserved for frequency of micturition.

Pollakiuria may appear early or late. In the former case it is an early symptom of Bright's disease. It appears alone as a precursory symptom, but more often it is associated with the other symptoms of Brightism. Pollakiuria appears late in certain cases. At times, especially in women, it is painful. Two patients in my wards showed this peculiarity. They suffered from excessive pollakiuria. The quantity of urine at each micturition only amounted to a spoonful at most, and the pain supervened, not at the moment of emission, but as soon as micturition ended. The pain was acute, and had all the characteristics of spasm of the neck of the bladder. It usually lasted for some minutes, and reappeared after each micturition.

Pollakiuria is no doubt due to exaggerated excitability of the vesical mucosa or muscle, which has been found hypertrophied. When the muscles of the body of the bladder are alone at fault, the pollakiuria shows itself by more or less frequent and imperative desire to micturate. When the sphincter is affected, the emission of urine is often followed by painful spasm. I cannot explain what cause acts thus on the excretory apparatus in a disease where the secretory apparatus only seems to be affected. Is it due to some change in the composition of the urine ? I do not think so, because pollakiuria is often present, while examination of the urine reveals nothing abnormal. Are we to invoke a reflex action which starts in the kidneys and ends in the bladder ? It is possible, but proof is lacking.

Polyuria, or excessive secretion of urine, is chiefly seen in interstitial nephritis, and from the first the patient may pass several pints of urine daily. In parenchymatous nephritis the quantity of urine is notably diminished, and may not be more than 30 to 40 ounces. Variations, however, are frequent, and the quantity may be normal or increased.

2. DEAD FINGERS.—This symptom of Bright's disease has never been noted by other writers. The sensation is similar to that experienced when the hands are exposed to great cold. The patients complain of tingling, pains, and cramps in the fingers. In some cases the tips of the fingers grow bloodless, pale, and numb. This condition lasts for some time, and returns in fits. This symptom affects the fingers and rarely the toes. It is present sometimes in one finger, sometimes in another, or in several fingers. It may be symmetrical. It is not common for all the fingers to be affected. This symptom is seen in all stages of Bright's disease. I have seen it as an initial symptom when the other symptoms were absent or slight. The trouble which I have just described sometimes invades the whole hand or the forearm. This is the symptom of the dead arm. Asphyxia of the limbs, which has been seen (very rarely, it is true) in the course of Bright's disease, might be reconciled with these facts.

3. AUDITORY TROUBLES.—Until I first called attention to the auditory troubles of Bright's disease, this symptom had, I believe, remained unnoticed.* From subsequent observation I now consider the auditory much

* Dieulafoy, *France Méd.*, 1877, No. 16. *Gaz. Hebd.*, 1873, No. 4. Domergue, "Troubles Nutritifs dans la Maladie de Bright," *Thèse de Paris*, 1881, No. 13.

more frequent than the ocular troubles. They are of various kinds. They often take the form of tinkling or buzzing in one or both ears, accompanied or followed by **defective hearing.** As a rule, the half-deafness is transient, and subject to recurrences. It is limited to one ear. The deafness is rarely complete. These auditory troubles may be painless or be accompanied by pains in the ears and the face. They are due to various causes. We sometimes find on examination of the ear sclerosis of the membrane, catarrh of the drum, abnormal vascularity of the malleus, and hæmorrhage into the mucosa of the tympanum. In other cases the lesions are not appreciable, and the auditory troubles are said to result from œdema of the auditory nerve.

Bonnier, struck with the frequency of auditory troubles in Bright's disease, has shown that the ill-defined syndrome called Ménière's vertigo is often only a symptom of Bright's disease. **Vertigo,** therefore, deserves to rank amongst the minor symptoms of Brightism. In some cases the vertigo, after resisting the treatment employed in Ménière's disease, has yielded to milk diet, like most of the other minor symptoms of Brightism.

4. ITCHING —This symptom, which has been ignored by some writers, is frequent, especially in women. The itching* may not differ from ordinary pruritus. It may affect different parts of the body, and last for several days or weeks. In some cases it is so severe as to deprive the patient of all sleep. The patients say that " they scratch themselves till they bleed or rub off the skin." The cause of the itching is not clear, for I do not refer to cases where a cutaneous eruption is present. Rosenstein, who has noticed this symptom, sets it down to uræmia. This explanation does not suffice to solve the problem. It has been suggested that excretion of urea by the skin was the cause of the itching. It is possible, but I have seen sweating of urea without itching. In another variety the itching is compared by patients to the tickling provoked by hairs falling on to the neck, the chest, or the back. In a third variety the patients compare the itching to the tickling caused by an ant. The itchings appear at all stages of the disease. In some cases it appears at the onset, and is then of importance in diagnosis.

5. CRAMPS IN THE CALVES OF THE LEGS are common in Bright's disease. The spasms may occur in the muscles of the shoulder and the neck, and in some cases opisthotonos, with or without articular pains, has been seen (Jaccoud). These latter forms are exceptional, but cramps in the calves are an early and almost constant complication of Brightism. Patients say the cramps are so painful as to wake them up. They may return several times during the same night, or several nights following, and may lead to insomnia.

* Dieulafoy, *Gaz. Hebd.*, 1882, No. 20. Mathieu, *Thèse de Paris*, 1882.

For some years my attention has been drawn to local cramp in the sterno-mastoid muscle. I have called it **torticollis in Bright's disease.** I described two remarkable instances in my lectures. It takes the form of a very painful, permanent contraction in certain muscles of the neck. The pain is not as a rule spontaneous, but is provoked by the least movement. It differs, therefore, from the cramps, which are spontaneous, and last but a few moments. I have repeatedly succeeded in curing the torticollis by milk diet. The intercostal muscles may also be the seat of painful cramps. Writer's cramp, in one of its forms, may have its origin in Bright's disease (Bonnier).

6. EPISTAXIS assumes various forms in Bright's disease. We see profuse epistaxis, which I shall describe later, and also hæmorrhage, which appears with the onset of uræmia. I refer here to the slight epistaxis which appears very early in the disease, especially in the morning. I have called it the " matutinal epistaxis of Brightism."

7. CRYÆSTHESIA.—Another symptom to which I attach some importance is the great sensitiveness to cold of patients suffering from Bright's disease. They suffer, according to their own expression, from " cold skin and cold under the skin." They wear a superabundance of warm clothing, and are wont to rub their thighs and knees to drive away the cold. They are continually warming their feet, which " are like icicles," but yet all these precautions often fail to keep them warm. They do not " shiver with cold." The hyperæsthesia to cold is not only caused by contact with cold objects, but is spontaneous, like the sensation of dead fingers, and independent of the surrounding temperature. In order to emphasize this symptom in patients with Bright's disease, I have proposed the term of " cryæsthesia."

The trouble usually affects the lower limbs—the knees, thighs, feet, and the region of the kidneys. I have published some typical cases.*

8. Amongst the minor symptoms of Brightism I would mention electric shocks, which chiefly occur during sleep. Since my attention was called to this symptom, which has not been previously described, I have found it frequently. The patient who is about to go to sleep, or has just gone to sleep, is suddenly awakened, as it were, by an electric shock. The shock, which is single and violent, is really a convulsion. It represents, in a rudimentary way, the convulsive attacks of uræmia. The electric shock, like most of the other symptoms just described, may appear alone, and may therefore pass unnoticed, unless care is taken to look for it.

9. SIGN OF THE TEMPORAL ARTERY.—I have noticed that in many people with Bright's disease the temporal artery is hard, tortuous, and

* " Contribution à l'Étude Clinique et Expérimentale de la Maladie de Bright sans Albuminurie " (*Soc. Méd. des Hôpit.*, 1886).

dilated. This is the sign of the temporal artery. The distended artery is readily felt as it pursues its tortuous course under the skin. The condition is not due to atheroma, but to **excess of arterial tension,** which affects the whole arterial system. The sign is more evident in the temporal artery, because of its superficial situation. The tension in the vessel varies from one day to another. Post-mortem examination of several cases from my wards has shown that the condition is not atheromatous.

10. I have often noted loss of the senses of smell and taste in patients with Bright's disease.

The above symptoms form the **minor signs of Brightism.** They may exist at all stages of the disease, and are of importance because they often give a clue when œdema, albumin, and symptoms of uræmia are wanting.

Œdema and Serous Effusion.—The œdema generally commences in the face, but it is not possible to assign a reason for this fact. The patient, on awakening, finds that his eyelids are swollen. As the face is slightly puffed, it might appear as if the patient had grown fat. The œdema may be limited to the malleoli, or may involve the legs, the thighs, the scrotum, and the labia majora, and, according to circumstances, it may take months to become general. It is, however, rare in chronic nephritis to find as much anasarca as in acute nephritis. In certain cases the œdema is limited to a single organ (pulmonary or laryngeal œdema). It has been limited to the prepuce (Rosenstein), the spermatic cord (Finger), or to one side of the face or the body (Potain).

In cases of interstitial nephritis œdema appears late, and is transient. It may be limited to the eyelids, the face, or the malleoli, whilst it appears earlier and is more extensive and lasting in parenchymatous nephritis, when it causes not only anasarca, but also effusions into the serous cavities. This distinction is true, **but it is not absolute.** Thus, a patient may have interstitial nephritis without dropsy, when superacute œdema of the lung supervenes.

When the œdema is recent, the tissues are white, soft, and pit on pressure. In the long-run, however, the tissues become thickened, especially in the legs. Because the œdema is sometimes very slight, we must not assume that it is absent. I am convinced that œdema is rarely absent during the course of nephritis. It must, however, be looked for. The marks left by the stethoscope on the thorax, the folds formed by the bedclothes on the skin of the face, the depression caused by spectacles at the root of the nose, will at times indicate œdema, which would otherwise be unnoticed.

Œdema of the viscera and serous effusions may be divided as follows : Out of 406 fatal cases (Frerichs and Rosenstein) we find : Hydrothorax and pleurisy, 82 ; hydropericardium, 21 ; hydrocephalus, 75 ; pulmonary œdema, 115 ; œdema of the glottis, 4. The fluid differs sensibly from the serum of the blood. It is more rich in water, but contains less albumin and mineral salts, and more chloride of sodium. Fibrin is absent, which proves that in such cases of œdema we are not dealing with a simple transudation of serum, as Jaccoud has clearly shown.

Pathogenesis of Œdema—Pre-œdema—Retention of Chlorides.—What are the **causes** of œdema in Bright's disease ? It was long said to depend upon the loss of albumin from the blood (hypo-albuminosis), but we are now less certain of this fact. It is sufficient to quote cases of acute nephritis in which anasarca and albuminuria appear together. Furthermore, how are we to reconcile this hypothesis with cases in which the anasarca is limited to one side of the body (Potain) ? Hydræmia, or an increase in the watery portion of the blood, has been suggested ; but the experiments of Bernard have failed to prove this theory. Lécorché supposes that the œdema is due to atony of the heart muscle, but we see every day renal œdema (scarlatinal and syphilitic nephritis) in which the heart takes no share, and, besides, renal œdema does not behave like cardiac œdema. Can the œdema be due to paralysis of the capillaries (Frerichs) ? Is a reflex action transmitted from the kidneys to the smaller vessels by their vasomotor nerves (Potain) ?

The pathogenesis of œdema in Bright's disease seemed for a long time to defy explanation. Physiology could not show us how simple renal lesions could produce a condition of œdema. The knowledge of the laws of isotonic solutions, the view that chloride of sodium plays the chief part in maintaining the osmotic equilibrium in these solutions, had naturally led to the hypothesis that retention of this salt in certain tissues might attract water from the organism, and cause œdema in them.

Cohnstein, by injecting chloride of sodium into an animal, found that the total amount of this salt reached its maximum at first in the blood and then in the lymph.

Théaulon expressed the opinion that the water in certain cases of œdema is attracted to the tissues by reason of the increased molecular concentration of the lymph plasma.

Hallion and Carrion have produced œdema in the lungs by injection of concentrated salt solutions into the blood of animals.

Reichel has shown that if we inject salt solution in a person suffering from Bright's disease, the absorption of the liquid takes place slowly.

Chauffard, in a case of infective icterus, where the urine was scanty and poor in chlorides, found that after repeated saline injections, the weight of the patient increased by the amount of the liquid injected. Experimental œdema, due, without a doubt, to the retention of the chlorides in the organism, appeared after these injections.

Achard and Loeper, therefore, have suggested that retention of the chlorides may play a part in the production of the œdema. Widal and Lemierre deserve the credit of eliminating theories and of establishing facts. They proved that the ingested chloride of sodium may alone lead to the appearance of œdema, and that the retention in the kidney regulates the appearance of this œdema.

In 1902 these writers proved that the daily ingestion of 10 grammes of chloride of sodium in persons with epithelial nephritis will cause an " experimental œdema."

The appearance of œdema depends on the permeability of the kidney for the chlorides at the moment when the test solution of chlorides is given. If the quantity of chloride eliminated is equal to the quantity ingested, œdema does not supervene, because the salt is not retained. The appearance of the œdema depends, furthermore, upon the degree of chloride saturation of the system, or upon previous lengthy retention, when the supplementary dose of salt is administered.

It is especially in the case of epithelial lesions that the ingestion of chloride of sodium causes œdema, as Widal and Lesné proved in 1900 by cryoscopic examination of the blood. It is in this form of nephritis that the retention is the most marked. Strauss has confirmed the facts advanced by Widal and Lemierre, and has seen œdema diminish when polyuria, and especially polychloruria, were produced.

The appearance of the œdema is preceded by a stage of hydration of the system, inappreciable to the naked eye. Widal and Javal have called it the stage of **preœdema;** and the physician should bear in mind, that by taking the weight of the patient daily, it is possible to estimate the amount of hydration.

The history of a case (Widal and Javal) of epithelial nephritis, in which salt was alternately allowed and excluded from the diet, is interesting. " The weight of the patient varied between 126 and 148 pounds. When on a diet containing salt, his weight exceeded 138 pounds, and œdema appeared ; inversely, when on a salt-free diet the weight fell to 136 pounds, and the œdema disappeared. He had, therefore, a hydration tolerance of 13 pounds, without the appearance of œdema. The scales enabled us to foretell almost to a day the appearance of œdema, by indicating the daily increase of weight during the entire period of pre-œdema."

Finally, Widal and Javal have shown that salt not only affects the œdema, but also the albuminuria, which increases, in certain cases, in a direct ratio to the hydration of the system. We shall see later to what therapeutic deductions these new discoveries may lead.

Albuminuria.—In cases of interstitial nephritis the urine is generally abundant, and the proportion of albumin is very small ; it may, indeed, be absent for a time. In cases of epithelial nephritis the urine is diminished, varies in shade, and may contain from 75 to 450 grains of albumin in twenty-

four hours. The urea, uric acid, salts of potassium, and extractives are
generally decreased. The specific gravity is lowered.

In the deposit we find epithelial débris, red and white corpuscles, and
various casts. The leucocytes are more numerous during an acute attack
(Arnozan). They are of the mononuclear and polynuclear types, and
" their respective proportions are the same in the urine and in the blood "
(Achard). Epithelial and blood casts are rare in chronic nephritis. They
are chiefly found in acute nephritis. The **hyaline** casts, which are homogeneous and transparent like glass, are unimportant. The **colloid** casts
are rigid, brittle, and of a yellow straw colour. The **fibrinous** casts are
especially frequent in hæmaturia. They are opaque, and formed of fibrinous
clots. The **granular** casts differ from the fatty ones in that the granulations
are formed of proteid, and not of fat. As regards prognosis, " the discovery
of granular casts is of value, because it enables us to follow the various
stages of the process." The **composite** casts are formed of colloid material,
and contain the débris of epithelial cells and of red and white corpuscles.
The diagnostic and prognostic value of casts in the urine has been somewhat exaggerated. Granular casts, however, indicate a lesion of the
kidneys, as they do not exist in simple albuminuria.

The urine shows well-defined differences. When the renal lesions are
definitely glandular or interstitial, in most cases the lesions blend, so
that the examination of the urine gives every possible variety. One urine,
for example, though scanty, contains but little albumin ; another urine
contains much albumin, though the secretion is increased. During the past
few years great attention has been paid to the **varieties of albumin** (serine,
globulin, peptone) and their significance in diagnosis. This interesting
research appears so far to have given no positive clinical result, and we shall
see later that albuminuria has no longer the prime importance which it
formerly possessed.

The causation of albuminuria has been variously explained. The
epithelial changes in the canaliculi have been blamed (Lécorché). Recent
researches seem to prove that the transudation of albumin takes place in
the glomerulus. It has not been proved that it is the increase of pressure
in the glomerular circulation which favours the passage of albumin (Stokvis).
The important point, according to recent research, is the slowing of the blood-
stream in the capillaries and the deficient oxygenation which results therefrom.

According to the so-called hæmatogenous or dyscrasic theory, the
origin of the albuminuria is the primary change in the albuminoid matter
of the blood. Jaccoud put forward this idea : The albuminuria recognizes
as its cause a deviation of metabolism from the normal type. This deviation
consists in a transient or lasting disturbance in the metabolism of the

albuminoid matter." In short, the pathogenesis of albuminuria is not yet clear.

Hæmaturia.—The urine in Bright's disease may be of a reddish or brownish colour. Slight or severe hæmaturia may appear in the form of attacks, and disappear later. More rarely the hæmaturia is persistent. I think that hæmaturia, thought to depend upon interstitial nephritis, is frequently due to nephritis, complicated by tuberculosis. Nevertheless, certain cases of nephritis, with hæmaturia, are as yet unexplained. In unilateral nephritis the lesions may affect the glomerulus, and may be accompanied by sharp pain (simulating renal calculus) and persistent hæmaturia (simulating tuberculosis), while the ordinary symptoms of Bright's disease are absent, because one of the kidneys is performing its functions properly. These cases are benefited by nephrotomy, which relieves the pain and the hæmorrhage (see Section VI.).

The symptoms which we shall now discuss, in part blend with those of uræmia. Most of them are dependent upon the insufficiency of the urinary secretion.

Headaches.—Headaches may occur at any stage of Bright's disease. They often appear among the earliest symptoms, and last for weeks or months. In some cases they are acute, and simulate the syphilitic headache. In others they are called " migraine " by the patient. The pain is often much increased when cerebral symptoms of uræmia appear. Leeches to the temples and behind the ears relieve the pain in some cases.

Respiratory Troubles.—The respiratory distress in Bright's disease may be continuous or intermittent, as the following examples show : Some patients suffer from permanent breathlessness, which is increased by exercise. At first sight we think of heart mischief, but careful examination shows that the sufferers have chronic nephritis, which does not, of course, absolutely exclude cardiac lesions. The distress may occur in the form of attacks, which are mistaken by the patient for asthma. The attack may occur by night or by day. It soon becomes acute, and returns on the least movement. It may recur several times during the day, or only reappear at more or less lengthy intervals. In other cases the respiration takes on the Cheyne-Stokes rhythm. This rhythm, which is not confined to the dyspnœa of Bright's disease, is as follows : The respiratory movements are at first quickened in series. They then become slower, and stop completely for a time. After the pause a second series occurs.

Dyspnœa may come on at any stage of Bright's disease, but it is important to remember that the distress may be the initial symptom. The attack may be sudden, like a fit of asthma, or the mischief may come on gradually, like chronic bronchitis. A knowledge of these facts will preclude the despatch of a patient to Mont-Doré or Cauterets for bronchial catarrh and emphysema when he is really suffering from Bright's disease. Amongst the rare, though dangerous, respiratory troubles we must mention **superacute œdema of the lung** and **œdema of the larynx,** which have been already described.

Cardiac Troubles.—The question of hypertrophy of the heart in Bright's disease is most complicated. The hypertrophy, which may be considerable, chiefly attacks the left ventricle, and develops apart from valvular changes. The entire heart may be affected, and dilatation may be also present. When the hypertrophy is marked, as in interstitial nephritis, we find precordial bulging, increased cardiac dullness, and, in the late stages of the disease, **attacks of asystole.** The cardiac troubles are, however, not peculiar to sclerosis of the kidneys. They exist in nearly all forms and stages of Bright's disease. They may precede the other symptoms, and appear as functional troubles, without dilatation or hypertrophy of the heart. The patient suffers from palpitation, precordial distress, and dyspnœa. He feels his heart, and complains of it.

Auscultation may reveal nothing. Sometimes the closure of the sigmoid valves is marked (Traube), indicating the high arterial tension. A *bruit de galop* is often heard. This valuable sign, discovered by Potain, may help us in some cases to recognize Bright's disease, even when albumin is absent. The *bruit de galop*, though more frequent in interstitial nephritis, may exist in all forms of chronic nephritis. It often coincides with hypertrophy of the heart, but yet cardiac hypertrophy is not absolutely necessary for its production. It is made up of three periods—viz., the two normal sounds of the heart and an additional sound which precedes the first sound by a short interval. Potain thinks that the third sound, which forms the gallop rhythm, "results from the suddenness with which the dilatation of the ventricle takes place in the presystolic period." It is, therefore, said to be indirectly "the consequence of the excess of arterial tension," so common in nephritis. The *bruit de galop* is not continuous. It may appear and disappear. It has its maximum of intensity in the ventricular region.

Valvular lesions are common in the course of Bright's disease. **Mitral endocarditis** is a frequent complication. It is convenient here to mention **angina pectoris,** in which lesions of the aorta may or may not be present. In two of my cases the attacks of angina pectoris were for some time the chief trouble, without aortic lesions. Rondot has noted several cases.

Digestive Troubles.—Digestive troubles are seen in all stages of Bright's disease. Some patients have gastric catarrh, with loss of appetite and vomiting of mucous liquid ; others, though not experiencing distaste for food, have pains which simulate ulcer and absolute intolerance of the stomach, so that all food is rejected. In some cases both vomiting and diarrhœa are present. These gastro-intestinal symptoms, which we shall discuss later under Uræmia, are found in all phases of the disease. They may appear as the first sign of Bright's disease, and are said to be due to the elimination of ammoniacal products by the gastro-intestinal mucosa and to ulcerations of this mucosa (Treitz).

Visual troubles (diminished acuteness of vision, amblyopia, blindness) are due to changes in the fundus oculi or to uræmia. The ophthalmoscope reveals retinal hæmorrhages, in the form of red patches around the papilla, whence they radiate in the direction of the bloodvessels, and whitish patches of inflammatory origin. These visual troubles are most frequent in interstitial nephritis. They occur at all stages, and may, indeed, be present when albumin is absent.

Hæmorrhage.—Hæmorrhage is common in interstitial nephritis.

Epistaxis is the most common form of hæmorrhage in Bright's disease. I have already mentioned the slight matutinal epistaxis and the more abundant bleeding which may precede or accompany uræmia. The present variety of epistaxis, as far as I am aware, has not been previously described. For emphasis, I have called it " the great epistaxis of Bright's disease," or " epistaxis *à tamponnement*." I have used this term because plugging of the nasal fossæ is often required to arrest the bleeding. It must not be thought that this epistaxis comes on late in the disease, when the cachexia would theoretically favour the flow of blood. The important feature is that this epistaxis appears quite early in Bright's disease, being at times a prodromal symptom. I am, therefore, accustomed to say " Brightism begins with epistaxis *à tamponnement*."

Some years ago I was called to see a lady of about fifty years of age. She had just been taken ill with profuse epistaxis that nothing would stop. I found her pale and alarmed ; the blood was flowing from both nostrils, and I estimated that she must have lost about a pint. I sent for Berger to plug the nares. All my previous attempts had failed completely, but the epistaxis stopped after plugging. She has since shown most of the symptoms of Bright's disease ; that she has been able to ward off uræmia is due to her strict milk diet.

Ten years ago, with Marquézy, I saw a man of fifty years of age with advanced Bright's disease. On questioning the patient, it was an easy matter to make out the course of events. The disease seemed to date back about eighteen months, but a little while before, the man who was suffering from Bright's disease, had been seized with violent epistaxis.

In 1894 a patient suffering from Bright's disease was sent to me by Grandhomme. Pollakiuria, dead fingers, vertigo, distension of the temporal artery, *bruit de galop*, vomiting, dyspnœa were the symptoms present. It was a case of chronic interstitial nephritis of four years' duration. He said, however, that these symptoms had been preceded by terrible bleeding from the nose, which had lasted for five hours, endangering his life. The bleeding recurred four years later with such violence that it necessitated plugging.

Since my attention has been called to this strange variety of epistaxis in Bright's disease, I have collected several cases from my hospital records.

I cannot give the cause of the bleeding, but we must remember the fact. If a healthy person is, without apparent cause, taken ill with severe epistaxis, and the nasal fossæ do not present any lesion capable of explaining the hæmorrhage, we must think of Bright's disease, and examine for distension of the temporal artery, pollakiuria, dead fingers, cramps in the calves of the legs, and a *bruit de galop*, even if we do not find albumin. We must put the patient on a milk diet, for he is either suffering from Bright's disease or he will fall a victim to it.

Cerebral hæmorrhage is fairly common in patients suffering from interstitial nephritis. Grainger Stewart says that in 100 cases of cerebral hæmorrhage we shall find interstitial nephritis fifteen times. In several cases observed by Bence Jones cerebral hæmorrhage was the only sign of interstitial nephritis, which had reached the atrophic stage without its existence having been previously suspected. This statement would not obtain to-day. In any case, cerebral hæmorrhage and its habitual symptoms—hemiplegia, aphasia, and apoplexy—are seen during the course of Bright's disease.

We have still to mention meningeal and retinal hæmorrhages, and hæmorrhages from the stomach, bowels, and gums. **Broncho-pulmonary hæmorrhage** is not uncommon in interstitial nephritis. I have succeeded in collecting eleven cases. In the great majority of cases post-mortem examinations show the absence of tuberculosis; and pulmonary hæmorrhage directly associated with Bright's disease must not be confounded with hæmoptysis in phthisical patients who are suffering from renal lesions. I have often seen marked hæmaturia in Bright's disease, and on two occasions the hæmaturia was preceded by profuse epistaxis. Some years ago, with Peter, I saw a youth suffering from Bright's disease. The hæmorrhage was at first nasal and then broncho-pulmonary. The bleeding became general, and carried off the patient.

How does chronic nephritis cause hæmorrhage? Are vicious composition of the blood and reduction in the albuminous principles at fault? This is not probable, because hæmorrhage is more frequent in interstitial nephritis when the patient is losing little albumin. Is there some change in the bloodvessels? As far as cerebral hæmorrhage is concerned, the question appears to be settled, because in this case the most common lesion is a miliary aneurysm. As regards the other organs, it is a case of hæmorrhagic necrosis, due to uræmic poisoning. The attacks of hæmorrhage may sometimes mark the onset of Bright's disease.

Condition of the Liver—Ascites.—In speaking of serous effusions in Bright's disease, I omitted to speak of **ascites,** because it is often associated with hepatic lesions. They vary in nature. In 114 cases of Bright's disease Rosenstein found the following lesions: fatty liver, 19; cirrhotic liver, 15 ; nutmeg liver, 11 ; simple hypertrophy, 15 ; amyloid liver, 5. It may be asked whether the hepatic lesion is consequent on the renal lesion, or whether both depend on the same cause. In one of my cases the liver was much enlarged, indurated, and painful. Ascites supervened. I withdrew 14 pints of effusion, which did not reappear.

Cutaneous Symptoms.—In patients suffering from Bright's disease the skin is dry and anæmic, and the perspiration is deficient. In some patients, however, it is limited to a special region—viz., the face, the legs, or the loins ; in others it is general. In some cases the parts subject to cryæsthesia are chiefly affected.

We find at times (I have observed the fact in about a dozen cases of uræmia) **urea in the sweat.** The urea is deposited in crystals on the face, on the forehead, at the roots of the hairs, on the neck, on the chest in the form of a whitish dust analogous to hoar-frost. I consider sweating of urea as of the worst possible prognosis. In the cases I have seen the patient succumbed in a short time.

Some patients with Bright's disease suffer from ptyalism, with or without stomatitis. It is called " uræmic sialorrhœa."

Toxic Inflammations.—We have seen that œdema and effusions take a large share in Bright's disease, and involve the periphery, the viscera (lungs, larynx, brain), the serous membranes (hydrothorax, ascites, hydropericarditis). The phenomena are due to serous transudation. The cases which I shall now discuss are due to inflammation of toxi-infectious origin. We find in the skin erythema, erysipelas, lymphangitis, and cellulitis ; in the lungs, pneumonia ; in the serous membranes, pericarditis, endocarditis, pleurisy, and peritonitis. Out of 406 cases collected by Frerichs and Rosenstein, we find 57 of pleurisy, 46 of peritonitis, 40 of pericarditis, and 52 of pneumonia.

The origin of these inflammations has been variously interpreted. Bright explained the endocarditis, the pericarditis, and other lesions of the serous membranes by the blood changes consequent on the nephritis. His ideas have again become current, and many writers hold that the lesions just enumerated are due to some dyscrasia. They are the result of auto-intoxication secondary to nephritis. Other writers place more importance on the infectious agents, and consider these cases of inflammation to be secondary infections. In reality we have to deal especially with toxic inflammation.

Pleurisy in Bright's disease may or may not be painful. Percussion and auscultation show no difference from ordinary pleurisy as regards friction rub, tubular breathing, ægophony, etc. The important difference is that severe dyspnœa appears early. The dyspnœa is not due only to the effusion, but also to the broncho-pulmonary œdema, which is often present in cases of Bright's disease. Pleurisy in Bright's disease may be observed at any stage of the malady. Cyto-diagnosis shows that it is a form of mechanical and aseptic pleurisy. It is characterized by the presence of large endothelial plaques (Widal and Ravaut).

Pericarditis in Bright's disease is especially common in the uræmic stage, and makes the prognosis hopeless. It is generally painless and apyretic. As it comes on insidiously, it escapes observation, unless careful auscultation is regularly made. The rub is well marked, and a *bruit de galop* may be present. The effusion is scanty. The dullness is in part due to the fluid and in part to the hypertrophy of the heart. The dyspnœa varies according to the presence or the absence of pulmonary œdema and pleural effusion. The fluid may be yellow or bloody (Letulle).

Uræmia.

Pathogenesis.—The theory of uræmia is based on the fact that in consequence of lesions in the kidneys and of insufficient urinary depuration, products of metabolism which should be excreted in the urine accumulate in the blood, and give rise to symptoms of poisoning. As Jaccoud has pointed out, the word "uræmia" does not signify urea, but urine in the blood ($o\tilde{v}\rho o\nu$, urine; and $a\tilde{\imath}\mu a$, blood). This theory is true, but the difficulty arises when we attempt to specify which are the products of metabolism and which are the toxic agents.

Urea has been blamed. In some cases (Bouchard, Brouardel) the onset of uræmia has coincided with a diminution of the urea in the urine and with the presence of an enormous quantity of urea in the blood. On the other hand, however, we have the negative series of blood examinations in which no excess of urea was present (Wurtz and Berthelot, Potain). In the cases of uræmia quoted by Parker, Mosler, and many others, the urine contained either a normal quantity or an excess of urea. I would also remark that injections of urea into the blood of animals do not cause symptoms of uræmia. Feltz and Ritter, Gréhant and Quinquaud, have shown that, in order to kill animals by injections of chemically pure urea, large quantities are necessary. The same fact is evident from the researches of Bouchard, that urea is not capable of reducing the temperature or of producing coma, and that it only accounts for a ninth part of the toxicity of the urine.

Frerichs supposes that the urea is converted in the blood into carbonate of ammonia (Jaccoud calls this condition **ammoniæmia**). Ammonia is present in the vomit and the fæces, and the breath is sometimes ammoniacal, as shown by placing in front of the mouth a piece of wood soaked in acetic acid, on which crystals of acetate of ammonia are deposited.

The **salts of potassium** have been looked upon by Feltz and Ritter as the essential poison in the urine. They proposed the name of " potassi-æmia " for the intoxication produced by retention of the toxic principles of the urine. Bouchard has proved experimentally the toxicity of the salts of potassium, but he does not consider them to be the only factor, and other important substances are likewise at fault.

Some interesting experiments have been made by Lépine and Aubert on the respective toxicity of the organic and saline constituents of the urine. The colouring matters and the ptomaines play a very important part in this question (Bouchard).

I cannot give the details of Bouchard's experiments, but the conclusion is that the intoxication, whether caused by injections of urine into the veins of an animal or by the retention of toxic products in a man whose kidneys are diseased, is not due to one substance contained in the urine, but to all the substances of which some are well known, while others are still under investigation.

From this point of view uræmia depends on insufficiency of the urinary depuration (Jaccoud). It must not, therefore, be considered as a compli-cation of nephritis; it is a symptom. Every patient with acute or chronic nephritis is *ipso facto* threatened with uræmia. He escapes the more serious symptoms if the dose of the toxic agent is small and the lesion of the kidneys is slight; but, as a matter of fact, uræmia, whether slight or severe, only awaits sufficient accumulation of the toxic agent in the blood in order to appear.

The **minor symptoms of Bright's disease**—cryæsthesia, electric shocks, cramps in the calves of the legs, and itching — are, I think, due to mild uræmia. The more marked symptoms—headache, dyspnœa, gastric troubles, and temporary prostration—are due to a more severe uræmic intoxication. Finally, the major symptoms—terrible dyspnœa, violent headache, uncontrollable vomiting, profuse diarrhœa, epileptiform con-vulsions, delirium, and coma—are the consequence of uræmic poisoning in its worst form.

Uræmia has been divided into acute and chronic. It is better to say that the symptoms are sometimes sudden and sometimes slow in their appearance. Some are transient and others are lasting. The symptoms may appear together or in succession. Uræmia does not always begin with the minor symptoms, and pass on to the most severe troubles. In acute or subacute nephritis (cold, scarlatina, syphilis, puerperal fever), when the poison causes rapid changes in the essential elements of the kidneys, the major symptoms may appear early, without any prodromata. On the other hand, in chronic nephritis the major symptoms may only appear late, after a more or less complete series of slight troubles.

Uræmia at times supervenes in the last stage of chronic nephritis, when the kidneys are irremediably disorganized. At other times it breaks out as an acute condition, which may be transient and curable, exactly like an attack of **renal asystole.** In the latter case its causation is not so easy of explanation. A patient is suffering from slowly progressive Bright's disease. Why does the lesion allow sufficient urinary depuration one day, and a week later so change the quantity or the quality of the urine that grave uræmia results ? And, even if the lesion of the kidneys be so advanced as to cause these grave complications, how can we explain the fact that they may be removed, the individual may regain his health, and the urinary depuration prove adequate—at least, for a time ?

It is evident that the lesion *per se* cannot always explain the sudden variations in the urine, and the more or less rapid appearance or disappearance of the uræmic symptoms. I think that other factors are also present. We shall see in the description of Renal Calculus that the presence of a stone in one ureter may cause, by reflex action, **paralysis of both kidneys and anuria,** which is soon followed by uræmia.

In Bright's disease, when the lesion of the kidneys slowly and progressively narrows the field of urinary depuration, a paralysis of the urinary function may diminish or prevent for a time the secretion of urine or its depuration. This factor is, I believe, important in these attacks of renal asystole. I should be quite ready to admit either an affection of the secretory cells of the kidney by the uræmic poison—*i.e.*, renal uræmia—or a spasm of the vessels of the kidneys. As a matter of fact, do we not know the important part played by vascular spasm in Bright's disease ? The dead fingers which are so frequent a symptom, evidently result from vascular spasm. Certain forms of uræmic dyspnœa (*sine materia*) might well be associated with spasm of the small bronchi or of the small bloodvessels (Potain). The high arterial tension which leads to cardiac hypertrophy in Bright's disease, is in part due to the spasm of the peripheral arterioles. Whether, then, the hypothesis of glandular auto-intoxication or of passing renal congestion be admitted or rejected, or the hypothesis of vascular spasm in the kidneys, I maintain that the lesion of the kidneys and the obliteration of the canaliculi by casts will not explain the causation of certain acute and transitory episodes in uræmia.

In the above discussion I have only considered the toxic side of uræmia, but we may find other important factors. Thus, broncho-pulmonary œdema is associated with uræmic dyspnœa. General and local œdema of the brain (Raymond) and hydrocephalus (Coindet) often take their share in the convulsions, the paralysis, and the coma of uræmia.

Description.—I have already said that uræmia in all its forms dominates the history of Bright's disease. Further, in describing the symptoms of Bright's disease we were constantly brought face to face with uræmic troubles. Nevertheless, in order to conform to custom, we have been used, when describing Bright's disease, to comprise under the heading of **uræmia** only the most marked troubles. These I shall now discuss.

Cerebral Uræmia.—In this form we find convulsions, delirium, or coma. The convulsions may occur suddenly, but prodromata are generally present. The urine diminishes in quantity; the patient has severe headache, epistaxis, vertigo, giddiness, auditory and visual troubles, sudden blindness (uræmic amaurosis), and spasmodic movements of the limbs. At a given moment an attack of convulsions, like those of epilepsy, comes on. The sudden loss of consciousness, the tonic and clonic convulsions, the biting of the tongue, and the stage of collapse follow one another, as in epilepsy. There is, however, this difference : that in the uræmic attack the initial cry is often wanting, the seizure is less unilateral, and the temperature falls below normal. This rule, however, is not absolute, and in several cases of uræmia the convulsions have caused a rise in the temperature. This rise of temperature may, however, be due to secondary infections. The number of attacks varies from one or two in twenty-four hours up to fifteen or twenty a day, which end in coma and death.

The **delirium** assumes various forms. As a rule, it appears as an epiphenomenon in the last stages of the disease. In some cases, however, it is of special importance. It may resemble mania. To this form I have given the name of " **folie Brightique.**"* Uræmic delirium sometimes resembles acute mania, with excitement, restlessness, insomnia, constant talking and shouting. The patient cannot sit still, and becomes violent when attempts at restraint are made. The excitement may alternate with phases of torpor and somnolence.

In some cases we find rather hallucinations of hearing and sight. The patient sees squadrons of cavalry manœuvring on the roofs, and hears children, who are carrying brilliant lights or are singing. He may see persons clad in rich robes or hear pistol-shots. In other cases the disease takes the form of melancholia. The patient will not move ; his eye is dull and his face expressionless. He does not speak, and appears quite resigned. He may fear or welcome death, or may show suicidal tendencies.

Ideas of persecution may be marked. He refuses food, for fear of poison. He believes that attempts are being made on his life ; hears persons who wish to kill him, or believes himself guilty of the most horrible crimes, and dreads punishment. More rarely uræmic delirium assumes the erotic and the religious form. These varieties of delirium may exist alone. More frequently they follow one another or occur together.

The **duration** of the delirium varied in the cases which I have published from nineteen days to eight months. Uræmic delirium may break out

* Dieulafoy, Société de Médecine des Hôpitaux, 10 Juillet, 1885.

suddenly, and be most acute from the first, or be ushered in by incoherent words and gestures, and only gradually reach its maximum. In some cases the delirium is practically continuous, and shows but slight remissions. In other cases we find transient improvement. Certain sufferers from Bright's disease are predisposed to delirium by alcoholic antecedents, by previous neuropathic troubles, and by heredity. The delirium sometimes forms one of the general symptoms of Bright's disease, and the diagnosis is easy. At other times it is the **chief** symptom, being so marked that the diagnosis is difficult. This fact is important to remember, lest we should treat as a lunatic a patient who is really suffering from Bright's disease. The delirium does not supervene only in confirmed Bright's disease ; it may appear while the other signs are but slight. De Fleury has reported four cases of mental troubles in the early stage of Bright's disease. "The patients were not improved by the ordinary treatment of these affections, but the symptoms were markedly relieved by milk diet, with or without injections of pilo-carpine. The symptoms reappeared when the milk was discontinued."

Coma.—The patient is in an apoplectiform condition. He suffers from drowsiness, from which it is difficult to rouse him, and which often ends in coma, the usual termination of the various forms of cerebral uræmia. The coma is rarely primary ; it generally follows the preceding forms.

Uræmic Paralyses.—In some cases we find definite paralyses in patients suffering from uræmia. The paralyses are of various kinds—hemiplegia, simulating that due to cerebral hæmorrhage ; right hemiplegia, with aphasia, simulating embolism of the left Sylvian artery ; hemiplegia, with epilepti-form convulsions ; monoplegia, with or without Jacksonian epilepsy, simulating a lesion in the motor convolutions ; aphasia, without hemiplegia ; facial hemiplegia ; partial paralyses of the third and seventh pairs of nerves ; crossed hemiplegia ; laryngoplegia. Some of these paralyses are due to focal lesions (hæmorrhage or softening), changes in the cerebral vessels being frequent in the course of chronic nephritis. I am not here alluding to these cases, but to the curable or fatal cases of paralysis which are due to none of the above-mentioned lesions. We must admit that in such a case the paralysis is due either to œdema or to intoxication of a definite cerebral region. Cerebral œdema, with or without serous effusion into the ventricles, is found in a fair number of post-mortem examinations, renal lesions being always present. In spite of the opposition of Charcot, cerebral œdema and the anæmia resulting therefrom, admitted by Frerichs, Jaccoud, and Rosenstein, is now a definite entity, which post-mortem examinations have verified (Carpentier, Raymond, Chantemesse and Tenneson).

Nevertheless, sufferers from Bright's disease have succumbed to paralysis, and post-mortem focal lesions, disease of the cerebral arteries, and œdema of the brain have been absent (Chauffard, Level). It is probable that the paralysis is of toxic origin, like the paralysis due to sulphide of carbon, lead-poisoning, etc. But how can we explain the fact that general uræmic poisoning may cause partial paralysis and hemiplegia ? We are reduced to theories.

Dyspnœa.—I have already mentioned respiratory troubles due to toxines or to œdema. The nature of the dyspnœa has not been clearly understood, because it was wrongly thought that the dyspnœa must naturally assume the Cheyne-Stokes rhythm. Now, this rhythm represents only one form of uræmic dyspnœa. We may find every grade, from slight distress to the most marked continuous dyspnœa, from breathlessness on exertion to severe attacks which come on suddenly, like those of asthma (uræmic asthma). Uræmic dyspnœa may be most severe, and yet no signs are found on auscultation. It is toxic dyspnœa *sine materia*. In other cases we find signs of bronchitis, broncho-pulmonary œdema or pleural effusion, which accompany the dyspnœa and modify its characters. Superacute œdema of the lungs has been previously discussed.

Gastro-Intestinal Uræmia.—In some cases of Bright's disease we find vomiting of mucus or food, as in chronic gastritis ; uncontrollable vomiting, as in pregnancy ; and even hæmatemesis, as in ulcer of the stomach (gastric uræmia). We also find dysenteric diarrhœa. These troubles comprise the chief features of gastro-intestinal uræmia, which has been explained by the passage of urea through the mucosæ of the stomach and of the intestine. The digestive passages assist in the elimination of urea. Bernard proved this by ligaturing the ureters in animals. In man we find urea or its compounds in the excreta. At the post-mortem examination of patients who died of uræmia, Rosenstein has found numerous ulcers in the bowel. In a case of Bartel's the ulcers had given rise to a perforation 6 inches above the ileocæcal valve. Fatal peritonitis followed. In one of Méry's cases the ulcers of the small intestines were numerous. One had perforated, and caused death by peritonitis. Letulle has found several ulcers scattered through the ileum. They were irregular, clean-cut, and varied in size from a sixpence to a shilling. They were all seated on the free edge of the intestine, and did not specially affect Peyer's patches. Two ulcers had perforated, causing peritonitis.

There is such a thing as **renal** uræmia, although the term seems redundant. By this term I do not refer to the lesions of the kidney or to the obstruction of the tubules, but to the uræmic poisoning of the organ, which diminishes or destroys its functions, causing oliguria or anuria. This toxic anuria may, I believe, be cured by subcutaneous injections of **nephrin,** as I first suggested some years ago.

Cardio-aortic uræmia exists. It is characterized by tendency to collapse and by pain, recalling angina pectoris.

The different forms of uræmia, which are separated for purposes of description, may occur together, or follow one another in the same subject. A patient at first suffers from fits of suffocation, visual troubles, violent headache, and uncontrollable vomiting. In time coma or convulsions appear. In some cases, however, the mischief spends its force **on one organ,** although it is not possible to explain the reason of this selection. Thus, the dyspnœa may be so severe as to kill the patient, quite apart from other uræmic troubles. The same remark applies to gastric uræmia, as in the following case, which I saw with Potain :

A patient who had Bright's disease was taken ill with general œdema. The urine became scanty, about 3 ounces daily. Uncontrollable vomiting set in, and all food was vomited. Vomiting of greenish watery fluid occurred, even when no drink was given. The uræmic poisoning was accompanied by intolerable itching. In spite of all treatment, the patient succumbed in three weeks ; headache, dyspnœa, delirium, convulsions, and coma were all absent. It was a pure case of gastric uræmia.

We can often distinguish clinically moist and dry forms of uræmia. The former is due to retention of the chlorides ; the latter results from retention of the urea.

If in the course of Bright's disease the kidneys do not eliminate the chlorides, the excess retained in the body does not remain long in the blood, which always tends to maintain its molecular equilibrium, but passes into the tissues (Achard and Loeper). As salt is a hygroscopic substance, it takes up water from the tissues, and preserves by dilution the isotonic condition of the protoplasm. Chloruræmia, then (Widal), tends to the moist form which is characterized by multiple œdema. Deformity results when the œdema is superficial. If the œdema is deep-seated, it leads to visceral disorders, which affect the lungs and the brain, and reveal themselves by nervous and respiratory troubles.

When the free discharge of urea is impeded by the affected kidney, it does not pass back suddenly, as the chlorides do, into the tissues, but accumulates in the blood, and all the molecules tend unceasingly toward the epithelium of the tubules. In order to overcome the resistance opposed by the kidneys to the passage of the urea, the blood becomes mechanically surcharged with a certain quantity of this substance. An urea-pressure is established, which varies in amount according to the extent of the renal lesion and to the quantity of albumin ingested. Owing to this regulating mechanism, the kidney performs its functions better, and practically regains the permeability necessary to assure the free passage of the urea that it has to eliminate.

We see, therefore, that the molecules of urea follow in order to accumulate in the blood, an inverse course to that which the molecules of the chlorides pursue in order to accumulate in the tissues. The retention of the molecules of urea does not give rise to œdema, but only to dry uræmia.

A patient with Bright's disease, therefore, may be of the azotæmic or chloruræmic type. The signs of azotæmia are loss of appetite, which may amount to invincible distaste for food, fatigue, and torpor, which may end in complete coma. The presence of an excess of urea in the blood is the best evidence of the retention of this substance (Widal and Javal).

Just as retention of chlorides may exist alone for a lengthy period, so may retention of urea appear at any stage of the disease, quite apart from any retention of chlorides. Patients may die of uræmia, although they have never shown any trace of œdema. These cases are exceptional, for in most instances we find that the retention of both substances has an influence on the renal insufficiency.

We see, therefore, that there are several varieties of uræmia. The disease may be sudden in its onset, or may come on insidiously, simulating some other malady, and causing difficulties in diagnosis, which we shall now discuss.

Diagnosis.—The following remarks on diagnosis are applicable both to the symptoms of Bright's disease and to the most marked forms of uræmia. As I have already remarked, Bright's disease in its slow and insidious forms, which are the most common, shows itself by headaches, which are wrongly spoken of as migraine ; by gastric troubles and by fits of vomiting, which are wrongly put down to dyspepsia or alcoholic gastritis ; by fits of suffocation, which are confounded with attacks of asthma ; by difficulty in breathing, which is called emphysema ; by cardiac troubles, which are mistaken for heart disease ; by pleural effusion, which simulates ordinary pleurisy ; by bronchial catarrh of undetermined nature ; by mental troubles, which are mistaken for mania, and for which the patient is sent to an asylum ; by auditory troubles and vertigo, which are confounded with Ménière's disease ; by nervous phenomena, which are charged to neurasthenia ; by frequent micturition, which is attributed to some lesion of the bladder or of the prostate.

A thorough knowledge of the symptoms of Bright's disease reveals its nature, and allows us to group around some symptom which has attracted the attention of the patient other symptoms which have passed almost unnoticed. In this way we arrive at the diagnosis. I am well aware that, as far as the diagnosis is concerned, there are two signs of the utmost importance—**œdema** and **albuminuria.** As regards albuminuria, however, I must mention certain restrictions. Albuminuria has been looked upon as so important in the diagnosis of nephritis that we cannot rid our minds of this idea. It commenced with Bright himself. Under the influence of Bright and of Rayer, whose great authority I delight in acknowledging, albuminuria was for a long time considered as the decisive factor in the diagnosis of nephritis. I am of opinion that this view is incorrect, although I am neither the first nor the only one to think so.

In **acute** nephritis albuminuria is of the utmost importance. In chronic interstitial nephritis, on the other hand, albuminuria is an inconstant sign. Not only may albuminuria be absent in the initial phase of Brightism, but it may be wanting when Bright's disease is confirmed, and even in the grave forms of uræmia.

In my communication to the Société Médicale des Hôpitaux on the clinical and experimental study of Bright's disease without albuminuria,* and in my communication to the Académie de Médecine† regarding Brightism and the dissociation of the morbid processes in the kidneys, I quoted cases, some verified by post-mortem examinations, in which the albumin had completely disappeared for some considerable time.

It is, therefore, proven that albuminuria has a somewhat secondary value in Bright's disease. It is only an unreliable sign, because it may either be absent, or because it may exist apart from any condition of Bright's disease.

We should, then, be very liable to errors in diagnosis if we looked upon albuminuria as being the decisive sign.

The remarks which I have just made on albuminuria also apply to **œdema.** Sufferers from Bright's disease, especially if they have arteriosclerosis, may show no trace of œdema for a long time, whilst œdema of rheumatic origin (Potain) simulates that due to Bright's disease, though it has nothing to do with Bright's disease, and is of good prognosis.

In order to distinguish the defaced forms of Bright's disease (œdema and albuminuria being absent), and to recognize its initial stage or its presence when the more marked symptoms are absent, I have tried for many years to bring into relief certain signs which I have named the " minor symptoms of Brightism." I have described them in the course of this article. They have little value when they are isolated. Because a patient presents isolated pollakiuria, cryæsthesia, dead finger, cramps in the calves of the legs, electric shocks, or auditory troubles, we must not at once put him down as suffering from Bright's disease. If, however, a patient complains of violent headache of which we cannot find the cause, of attacks of dyspnœa which are not due to asthma, of gastric troubles or vomiting due to some unknown cause, etc.; and if he also suffers from pollakiuria, dead fingers, cramps in the calves of the legs, morning epistaxis, cryæsthesia, auditory troubles, itchings, electric shocks, etc.—in short, if, after a minute inquiry, we succeed in **grouping** some of these signs, whether they have shown themselves successively or simultaneously, if the arterial tension is raised, if we find the *bruit*

---

* Société de Médecine des Hôpitaux, Séances du 11 Juin et du 22 Octobre, 1886.
† *Bulletin de l'Académie de Médecine*, 6 Juin et 20 Juin, 1893.

de galop, we have then good reason to say that he has **Brightism,** even when œdema is absent and the urine does not contain albumin. The minor symptoms of Brightism appear in the first period of Bright's disease in subjects who have not yet suffered from the more severe symptoms, and who will perhaps never have them. They are often present throughout the whole of the disease. They are not recognized because they are not looked for. I am convinced that many people, though healthy in appearance, are really affected with Brightism.

I think these facts should be included in our descriptions of Bright's disease. Many gouty persons, who perchance suffer from renal colic or albuminuria, are for a long time afflicted with the minor symptoms of Brightism before the appearance of the grave symptoms of uræmia. Many syphilitic patients show symptoms which are put down to syphilis, while they are really due to Brightism, and form the prelude to more severe mischief, unless appropriate measures are employed. In many people, after an infectious disease (typhoid fever, pneumonia, and especially scarlatina), the symptoms of Brightism run an insidious course, until, for want of treatment, the more severe troubles of Bright's disease appear. Many women who appear to suffer from anæmia, with pallor, headaches, breathlessness, palpitation of the heart, etc., and are considered chlorotic, are really suffering from chloro-Brightism, a special form, which I shall discuss later. In many cases, therefore, a knowledge of the slight symptoms of Brightism and of the existence of high tension and of a *bruit de galop* helps us to make the diagnosis of incipient Bright's disease, even in the absence of œdema and albuminuria. In my own wards I constantly see patients in whom the minor symptoms are present without œdema or albuminuria. Some months later the diagnosis is verified, when the patient returns with obvious symptoms of Bright's disease, including œdema and albuminuria.

Renal Insufficiency and Laboratory Researches.—The three methods which we are about to consider are employed in the diagnosis of renal insufficiency, and in the estimation of its amount (Achard). They comprise the study of the urinary toxicity, the study of the permeability of the kidneys, and cryoscopy.

URINARY TOXICITY.—Bouchard, as the result of many experiments, has shown that if the urine of a healthy adult be collected for twenty-four hours and injected, after filtration and neutralization, into the veins of a rabbit weighing $3\frac{1}{2}$ pounds, death follows after the injection of about 3 ounces. These figures are, of course, relative, as normal urine may vary in its toxic power. A rabbit weighing $3\frac{1}{2}$ pounds may die after the injection of from 1 to 2 ounces. On the other hand, it may not die till after the injection of 4 ounces, for many conditions, even in the normal state, modify the toxicity of the urine. Under correct experimental conditions, with proper precautions, it may be said that a rabbit weighing 1 pound will be killed by 1 ounce of normal urine.

I have repeated these experiments with similar results—namely, that as the quantity of the injection is increased, the animal suffers from myosis, acceleration of the respiratory movements, weakness or abolition of the eye reflexes, lowering of the temperature, tetanic rigidity, salivation, convulsive movements, and exophthalmos. The less toxic the urine the greater must be the quantity injected in order to kill the animal. It might *a priori* be supposed that as the urine in Bright's disease is less toxic, because the urinary depuration is imperfect, we should have to inject a large quantity to kill an animal. This is, as a matter of fact, just what Bouchard found. The urine of patients suffering from Bright's disease (in various degrees and under certain conditions) has but little toxic power. These experiments, repeated with the urine of patients who had Bright's disease but no albuminuria, have helped me to a correct diagnosis* in many difficult cases.

A complete investigation of the toxicity must, however, take both the urine and the blood into account, says Achard. The conclusion is, says this writer, that, "besides practical difficulties, the investigation is also liable to theoretical objections. As the results obtained with the same liquid are liable to variation, no exact value can be attributed to a single trial. In practice it is impossible to make more than one experiment in each case. The uncertainties and the technical difficulties must, therefore, limit this method to the laboratory, and prevent it from becoming an ordinary clinical method."

Renal Permeability through Provoked Elimination.—It has long been known that certain drugs, and also the normal constituents of the urine, are not so readily eliminated by the kidney in cases of nephritis. Various authors had investigated the elimination of certain substances, when Achard and Castaigne proposed a practical method, based on the use of methylene blue. This method has led to systematic researches on renal permeability. A hypodermic injection of 1 grain of methylene blue is given, and the urine is then examined repeatedly for traces of the pigment.

The passage of the blue into the urine shows the following features : (1) Under normal conditions it begins to appear within half an hour ; in pathological conditions it may be delayed for several hours. (2) The elimination in normal subjects varies from thirty-five to sixty hours ; in pathological conditions it is either shortened or prolonged. (3) The quantity of the substance eliminated is, according to Achard and Clerc, the most important element of the test. This is difficult to estimate. The whole of the urine must be carefully collected, and the amount of the blue eliminated

* Dieulafoy, "Étude Clinique et Expérimentale de la Maladie de Bright" (Société de Médecine des Hôpitaux, Séances du 11 Juin et du 22 Octobre).

must be estimated by chromometric tests. Under normal conditions the rate of elimination in the first twenty-four hours (methylene blue and chromogen united) amounts at least to half of the quantity injected. The quantity eliminated in the first twenty-four hours is the most interesting. The amounts are, nevertheless, estimated every twenty-four hours, if need be, until the end of the elimination. (4) The rhythm of the elimination, which, under normal conditions, at first increases regularly and then decreases, after having attained a maximum. Chauffard has shown that intermittent elimination is characteristic of hepatic insufficiency.

The pathological results furnished by the methylene blue test are as follows : In interstitial nephritis the permeability is diminished, though some cases have been recorded in which it was practically normal. The explanation given is that a small portion of the parenchyma capable of eliminating the dye still remains. In parenchymatous nephritis, on the contrary, Bard, and, later, Léon Bernard, Widal, Achard and Clerc, have shown that the permeability remains normal, or may be increased.

The test, therefore, often gives a general idea of the permeability of the kidneys ; but, as Bernard and Widal have pointed out, the variations in the elimination in nephritis are far from being always proportional to the degree of the renal lesion and to the intensity of the uræmic symptoms. Widal has reported a case of syphilitic nephritis in which the permeability was normal, in spite of severe uræmia. To interpret these facts we must remember that the permeability of the renal epithelium varies for different substances. On the other hand, we must remember that methylene blue is a substance which may undergo considerable reduction in the body. Bard and Bonnet have shown that, in certain cases, there may be disassociation between the elimination of the blue and that of the iodide of potassium. Widal and Ravaut have shown a similar dissociation for the elimination of salicylate of soda. On the other hand, they have shown that salicylate of soda injected in doses under the skin has the advantage of being eliminated more rapidly than methylene blue or iodide of potassium—viz., in fifteen to twenty hours under normal conditions. The quantity eliminated may be tested with great accuracy in the urine discharged at each micturition. Taken as a whole, the elimination of these substances by the kidneys does not furnish in the diagnosis of renal insufficiency results precise enough to enable us to estimate the degree of this insufficiency.

It is not the same with the elimination by the kidneys of a natural substance like chloride of sodium. In epithelial nephritis the elimination of methylene blue may be normal, while the elimination of the chlorides is much disturbed.

Widal has shown that differences of permeability might be noticed even between substances naturally eliminated—between urea and chloride of

the blood-serum, it is easy to establish their relation. The variations in the latter will indicate the differences of concentration which result from the pathological condition of the kidneys." These researches and all the calculations which they necessitate (Claude and Balthazard) have little practical value, and are too complicated for everyday use.

Duration.—The duration of Bright's disease is very variable : one or two years, and still less, in parenchymatous nephritis ; five, six, or seven years, and even more, in interstitial nephritis and in cases of mixed nephritis. Remissions are fairly frequent. We meet with patients who appear cured, and in whom the disease returns after a few years. It may be asked whether the return of the disease is not the result of some fresh cause.

Cases of cure which are frequent in instances of acute nephritis are less common in Bright's disease, especially if the arterio-sclerosis is more or less general. Death may result from hæmorrhage, apoplexy, cardiac and pulmonary lesions. In some cases cutaneous and visceral inflammation and gangrene (secondary infections) hasten the end, and if the patient escape these complications, he may be carried off by uræmia, dyspnœa, apoplexy, epilepsy, or coma.

Prognosis.—We must remember, in dealing with the prognosis, that albuminuria may last for years without being due to Bright's disease, or may be the only evidence ; and, on the other hand, Bright's disease may run its course without albuminuria. The following examples illustrate this :

I had under my care a youth who has suffered for many years from scarlatinal albuminuria, without Bright's disease. I placed him on a milk diet ; and I may remark, in passing, that milk diet, which is so efficacious in uræmia, is of less benefit in albuminuria. I am at present attending a child ten years of age who, after scarlatina, has had albuminuria for several years. The face is pale, and the eyelids are sometimes puffy, but no symptom of Bright's disease has appeared. I saw a lady in consultation with a colleague ; she has had scarlatinal nephritis for seven years. The albumin disappeared at intervals, and then reappeared, but no symptoms of uræmia had ever appeared. As opposed to these cases, I can quote two others : one refers to a woman of twenty-five years, and the other to a youth of seventeen years of age. Both have scarlatinal nephritis with albuminuria ; the symptoms of Bright's disease persist, although the albuminuria has disappeared for some time.

This dissociation of the morbid acts of the kidneys is fairly common in chronic nephritis. Caussade told me of a naval surgeon who had been suffering from pneumococcal nephritis for the past five years. During these five years albuminuria had been the only symptom. The minor troubles of Brightism then began to appear.

Syphilis also presents analogous forms. It is common to find during the first year after infection albuminuria without other symptoms of Bright's disease. On the other hand, we see syphilitic patients suffering from symptoms of uræmia, while albuminuria is for the time being absent.

We shall study this dissociation of the morbid acts of the kidneys under Chloro-Brightism, Syphilo-Brightism, and Gouty Brightism. A subject with articular gout may have albuminuria for years without any other symptoms of Bright's disease. I am acquainted with gouty persons who have passed albumin for several years, and yet have none of the minor troubles of Brightism. I have often spoken to a foreign doctor who attended my clinic at Necker Hospital. He was very gouty, and for seven years passed large quantities of albumin, without having experienced the least symptom of Bright's disease. I recently saw a young man who was subject to attacks of acute articular gout, and who, to his own knowledge, had for three years passed albuminous urine. His urine actually contained 30 grains of albumin to the quart, but its toxicity was absolutely normal. I have questioned him most minutely, and find that he has had no signs of Bright's disease. There is, therefore, a gouty albuminuria, which may last for years without leading to Bright's disease. These facts are important from the point of view of the prognosis.

A patient suffering from albuminuria due to gout, syphilis, scarlatina, etc., has, consequently, nothing to fear as long as the urinary depuration is sufficient—that is to say, as long as the albuminuria is not accompanied by the minor troubles of Brightism, or by a lowering of urinary toxicity. I say there is nothing to be feared, provided that he diets himself and avoids as far as possible infectious conditions, influenza, colds, etc., which may light up a latent nephritis in which albuminuria has been the only sign.

On the other hand, a patient, although he has no albumin in the urine, but only the minor symptoms of Brightism, must be continually on the alert, because his urinary depuration is insufficient.

The presence of these minor symptoms does not absolutely imply a grave prognosis. Fortunately, many syphilitic, gouty, or anæmic persons have only Brightism, and fatal uræmia does not set in. When, however, a patient is suffering from these minor symptoms of Brightism, it is a warning that he must be careful whether albuminuria be present or not.

Summary.—My view of the question is as follows : Every case of sub-acute or chronic nephritis implies a greater or less change in the urinary depuration. It matters little whether the nephritis is interstitial, epithelial, or mixed, and whether the lesion is limited to the kidneys or whether other organs are more or less affected : the condition is Bright's disease.

Bright's disease may follow on acute nephritis, but in most cases it is chronic from the outset. Exacerbations and remissions may or may not occur. Finally, it may be cured. Whatever the order and the course of the lesions and of the symptoms, the patient is suffering from Bright's disease ; the renal lesion and the insufficient urinary depuration then expose him to the minor and the major troubles which I have enumerated above.

We must not, however, look upon the urinary insufficiency and the consequent poisoning as the only symptoms. Other complications are dependent on the nephritis, or march side by side with it : œdema of the lungs and of the brain; effusions into the pleura, the peritoneum, and the pericardium; hypertrophy and fibrosis of the heart; miliary aneurysms, cerebral and retinal hæmorrhage; lesions of the liver, secondary infections, pneumonia, suppuration, and gangrene, are complications which may be present and which may modify the complex symptomatology of Bright's disease.

When these symptoms are present, the albuminuria is of minor importance, and, therefore, the names " albuminuric dyspnœa," " convulsions," and " retinitis " are bad. Instead of remarking that a man is suffering from Bright's disease, we often say he is albuminuric. This is incorrect, because many people suffering from albuminuria have not Bright's disease, and in certain cases of Bright's disease albuminuria may not be present at times.

The terms " albuminuria " and " Bright's disease " are not only not synonymous, but albuminuria itself, during the course of Bright's disease, gives only uncertain information as to the course and the prognosis of the disease. As a matter of fact, it is not in the cases with the most marked albuminuria that we find the major troubles. The albumin sometimes disappears at the gravest moment, and, on the other hand, it may persist in spite of the apparent cure of Bright's disease.

In a word, the key to the whole situation **is not what passes through the kidneys, but what does not pass.** It is not because the kidneys allow some albumin to pass every day that there is danger. The danger lies in the fact that the diseased kidneys do not allow the elements of depuration to pass in proper quantity. The poison retained in the system may accumulate rapidly and in large amount if the urinary depuration be much affected, and the major symptoms of uræmia then appear. If the effect on the urinary depuration is slight, the poison takes longer to accumulate in the system, and the patient is threatened with the condition which I have just described under the name of " Brightism," or " minor uræmia."

The appearance or the disappearance of albumin in all stages of Bright's disease condemns the theory of Mahomed, who had described a pre-albuminuric period, as if Bright's disease must perforce commence with a stage in which albumin was absent.

Treatment.—Milk diet is of prime importance in Bright's disease in most cases. The patient should take 5 or 6 pints of milk at equal intervals and in equal quantities—for instance, $\frac{1}{2}$ pint every two hours. If the patient does not like the milk, it may be sweetened or be flavoured with a spoonful of coffee. If the milk does not agree well, small quantities should be given at first, care being taken to make it alkaline with lime-water or Vichy. According to the taste of the patient, cow's milk, goat's milk, ass's milk, koumiss, kephyr, or milk aerated with carbonic acid by means of a sparklet, may be given. In some cases the milk diet must be absolute. A few eggs may, however, be allowed, as well as a little cream-cheese, milk foods, cream flavoured with vanilla or chocolate, and some fruit. As milk diet readily produces constipation, simple enemata or laxatives such as manna or cascara should be prescribed.

The result is that the urine becomes more abundant, the œdema diminishes, and the dyspnœa disappears. It is a remarkable fact that milk diet, which has such a marked action on the toxic symptoms and the œdema, has less effect on the albuminuria. I have often seen patients suffering from Bright's disease in whom an absolute milk diet for months worked marvels, but yet moderate albuminuria persisted.

Some patients are literally poisoned as soon as they substitute a meat diet for a milk one. One of my colleagues, whose health is excellent as long as he strictly follows his milk diet, suffers from headache, breathlessness, and vomiting if he swallows even a few cups of broth.

Experiments have been made to account for the good effects of milk. Gilbert and Dominici have shown that the number of bacteria in the intestinal tract is much diminished with a milk diet. There is, therefore, a quasi-asepsis of the digestive tube, and the auto-intoxication is diminished in proportion. We shall see later that one advantage of the milk cure is to reduce the chlorides in the food.

The milk diet should be continued for months; if it does not agree well, it should be replaced by a mixed diet of fresh vegetables, farinaceous foods, cakes, fruits, with little or no meat. Tonics and injections of cacodylate of soda, may prove useful at this period.

The skin should be stimulated by massage, but I do not advise vapour baths. The cutaneous stimulation must be methodical and constant (Semmola). Blisters over the kidneys and dry-cuppings are also indicated.

Iodide of sodium or of potassium which is recommended when the arterio-sclerosis is present does not appear to me to be necessary. Both have the disadvantage of upsetting the patient. They cause a " bad mouth and stomach," and their curative value, except in syphilis, is questionable, in my opinion.

Other drugs, such as tannin, gallic acid, or fuchsin, which have been so highly lauded, are of no value.

If the œdema is persistent, the heart is failing, in spite of the milk diet, and the urine too scanty, diuretics should be employed. We may give Trousseau's wine, digitalis, digitalin, diuretin, or theobromin. The last-named drug, in doses of 30 grains daily, is best. It produces diuresis and dechlorination. In many cases the urine becomes abundant, the chlorides diminish, and the œdema disappears. " Furthermore, the diuretics most powerful in Bright's disease have proved themselves to be the best agents in causing dechlorination. Theobromin is a renal diuretic, which re-establishes the passage of chlorides through the kidneys, produces polyuria, and rids the body of the excess of chlorides." These conclusions are deduced from the convincing researches of Widal and Javal. Digitalis should be given if the heart is at fault. If the serous effusions are abundant, they must be drawn off.

We may here consider the **dechlorination cure** proposed by Widal and Javal. It refers especially to Bright's disease with œdema. In some patients it also seems to have an influence on the albuminuria. We have already seen that Widal and his pupils have proved the rôle of chloride of sodium in the production of œdema in Bright's disease. The practical deductions followed quite naturally. As they have proved that the salt is the dangerous element in many cases, it is natural to restrict it in the diet of persons with Bright's disease.

Milk, which has long been known for its good effect in nephritis, no doubt owes a part of its qualities to its small chlorination. Widal and Javal have shown that the addition of chloride of sodium rendered the milk injurious as a food, and that in the same subject a mixed diet, though rich in proteids, sugar, and fats, did not hinder (if salt were not added) the disappearance of œdema and albuminuria, and might, therefore, help in the dechlorination cure. Rice, pastry, and food pastes give similar results, provided no salt be added in their preparation. As these foods contain only traces of chlorides, we can employ them to vary the diet in certain cases of Bright's disease. We know that chloride of sodium is absolutely prejudicial to patients suffering from Bright's disease, especially to those who have œdema, and the salt must, therefore, be excluded from their diet. As to the diet : milk alone, or lacto-vegetarian diet, to which meat may be added. It is varied to suit the patient, and is, indeed, almost a question of experiment.

In uræmia with acute delirium, epileptiform convulsions or coma, and acute œdema of the lungs, bleeding should be employed up to about 10 ounces, and repeated as may be necessary. Bleeding, if properly employed, gives excellent results, and often arrests the convulsions, which are prone to be fatal. The improvement obtained is due to two causes : first, bleeding facilitates the absorption of the visceral œdema ; and, secondly, it withdraws a considerable quantity of the uræmic poison. In the absence of blood-letting, leeches may be applied behind the ears or in the lumbar region.

I formerly asked myself whether transfusion might not be of service in uræmia, and whether the pure blood so introduced might not modify the vicious composition of the blood in the body. I have performed transfusion on ten occasions. My cases are too few for any definite conclusions, but they seem to show that the transfusion of 3 or 4 ounces of blood has a beneficial influence on uræmia, and may hold it in check for a period which varies with the nature and the severity of the lesions. This result was very clear in my first case.* It is evident that the transfusion of 4 ounces of blood could not modify the renal lesions, but the headache, vomiting, convulsions, and coma were kept in check. For the time being we cannot draw any other conclusions, but we may well ask what might happen if, instead of performing a single transfusion, a series of them were performed.

In Stohr's case transfusion was performed for acute uræmia. The patient succumbed thirteen days later from pleuro-pulmonary trouble, but the operation, says Bartels, was a brilliant success as far as the uræmic symptoms were concerned. Belina Swiouthowsky performed transfusion in a woman with puerperal eclampsia, and the success was complete and lasting.

In **uræmic dyspnœa,** which may be most severe, we may use various means, especially bleeding. Small injections of morphia should be given, each injection containing $\frac{1}{6}$ to $\frac{1}{4}$ grain. I do not share the prejudice of certain physicians as to the use of morphia in Bright's disease. It gives good results when it is properly used.

Some years ago I decided to try ipecacuanha in uræmic dyspnœa. The drug succeeded the better because the dyspnœa is rather toxic, and not so much dependent on œdema of the lung. I gave pills of ipecacuanha and opium every two hours. The drug is stopped as soon as vomiting threatens, and is given again on the following days, if necessary. I have seen several cases which were much relieved. Inhalations of oxygen have also been extolled in uræmic dyspnœa.

Uræmic headache is relieved by the application of leeches behind the ears and by antipyrin in doses of 15 to 30 grains daily.

Uræmic vomiting is sometimes very difficult to relieve. The patient must be placed on starvation diet—no water, no milk. He may be allowed a few pieces of ice; enemata, containing 5 ounces water, $\frac{1}{2}$ ounce lactose, the yolk of an egg, and 3 drachms peptone, are prescribed. As soon as the stomach has become more tolerant, a wineglassful of iced water, preceded by a teaspoonful of the following solution, is given :

Lime-water	3 ounces.
Hydrochlorate of cocaine	1 grain.
Hydrochlorate of morphia	$\frac{1}{6}$ grain.

* Dieulafoy, "Étude sur la Transfusion du Sang dans la Maladie de Bright" (*Gaz. Hebd.*, 18 Janvier, 1884).

Oliguria and **anuria** are fairly frequently met with in Bright's disease. They are the direct cause of the uræmic symptoms. As I remarked above, it is not the extent of the lesion which of itself is the cause of oliguria or anuria in Bright's disease. If the oliguria ran a parallel course with the renal lesions, we should not have, as is sometimes seen, periods of oliguria alternating with periods in which the secretion is normal or in excess. It is, therefore, evident that in Bright's disease the urinary secretion is not only dependent on the lesions of the kidneys and the obstruction of the tubules, but also on an intoxication which at times affects or destroys the functions of the kidneys. Anuria in Bright's disease is, therefore, difficult to relieve by blood-letting or by means of diuretics, and it is because I had failed in anuria or oliguria due to Bright's disease with the known diuretics that I was anxious to try as a diuretic an extract of the cortical substance of the kidney.

With this object in view, my assistant prepared the following solution, to which I have given the name of nephrin : A fresh bullock's kidney is placed in a sterile vessel ; the cortical substance is removed with every antiseptic precaution. It weighs about 200 grammes. The cortical substance is pounded in a mortar, and to it are added 300 grammes of neutral glycerin and 200 grammes of sterile water containing 0·5 per cent. of sea-salt. The whole is then macerated for five hours in a vessel surrounded by ice. The filtration is carried out in two parts : (1) filtration of the whole mass through a filter of Chardin paper ; (2) filtration of the liquid thus obtained through a Chamberland candle (sterilized in the autoclave at 115° C.). This filtration is made with compressed air at a variable pressure by means of D'Arsonval's ingenious apparatus. We thus obtain 50 to 55 grammes of a yellowish, transparent, viscid, and absolutely sterile liquid, and eight, ten, or twelve subcutaneous injections are given daily, each injection containing 50 centigrammes of nephrin and 50 grammes of sterilized water.

We are so helpless in cases of oliguria and of anuria that I felt compelled to try this new means, in the hope that it might be not altogether useless. It is not possible to pass judgment after a single case. If, however, the reader will peruse the account of this case, he will see that the urinary secretion, which had stopped completely for five days, reappeared after the injections of nephrin. At the same time as the urinary secretion reappeared, there was a notable improvement in the patient's condition. The stupor passed off, and he took his milk ; the sweating of urea diminished. I noticed that after each injection of nephrin, especially after the first ones, the symptoms were improved. It is, therefore, permissible to believe that subcutaneous injections of nephrin may be of some service in cases of anuria, especially in Bright's disease.* Nephrin

* Dieulafoy, Société de Médecine des Hôpitaux, Séance du 14 Octobre, 1892.

has since been employed in many cases. Gonin reports the following case :

In a woman forty-nine years of age, with Bright's disease, symptoms of uræmia appeared : dyspnœa, uncontrollable vomiting, oliguria, and abundant albuminuria. As the condition did not yield to bleeding and other measures, an injection of nephrin was given every day. The urine gradually rose to 80 ounces, and vomiting ceased. When the remedy was discontinued, the former symptoms reappeared, and again gave way to the remedy.

Schiperovitsch, of St. Petersburg, has given fresh kidney extract to thirty-five patients suffering from nephritis, with or without uræmia. The patients were not given any other drug, and took a meat diet. The conclusions arrived at by the author are : In 40 per cent. of the cases the albumin disappeared from the urine. The remedy caused marked improvement in the general condition, and cessation of the uræmic symptoms. When the remedy was suspended, the symptoms returned after a period which varied in each case. The kidneys of the animals, therefore, possess diuretic properties.

Injections of serum are very harmful, on account of the chloride of sodium contained in the serum. I advise injections of sterilized water.

These different remedies may, therefore, be of service in uræmia. Drastic purgatives must not be given to uræmic patients, because the purgative robs the system of fluid necessary for the secretion of urine. Blisters should be avoided. Opiates must be given in strict moderation, and injections of morphia should be reserved for dyspnœa. We must not forget that remedies given in excessive doses and imperfectly eliminated by the diseased kidney may cause symptoms of poisoning (Bouchard, Chauvet). This fear, however, must not be exaggerated, and in syphilitic nephritis there must be no hesitation in prescribing mercury and iodide of potassium, whilst carefully watching the action of the remedies. The surgical treatment of Bright's disease will be discussed in the next section.

Sufferers from Bright's disease, on account of their insufficient urinary depuration, must avoid food rich in ptomaines—game, certain kinds of fish, mussels, shell-fish, etc. I witnessed, in company with Potain and Boncour, the onset of fatal trouble in a patient with Bright's disease who was poisoned by bad shell-fish.*

VI. DISCUSSION ON UNILATERAL NEPHRITIS—SURGICAL TREATMENT OF NEPHRITIS.

Can one of the kidneys remain healthy whilst its fellow is attacked by nephritis, or, in other words, can unilateral nephritis occur ?

These questions are the more important in that surgery now claims a large share in the treatment of nephritis. At first its intervention was

* Dieulafoy, "Brightism et Toxhémie Alimentaire" (*La Presse Médicale*, 1896, p. 205).

limited to certain cases of **unilateral** nephritis—tuberculosis, suppurating infarcts, and abscess of the kidneys, stone in the kidney, and floating kidney. Since then it has intervened in acute and chronic nephritis. Numerous papers on this subject have been published in France and abroad. It will suffice to quote the names of Pousson (France), Israel and Rose (Germany), Rovsing (Denmark), Fergusson and Edebohls (United States), Newman and Harrison (England), to show the importance of the work which has been undertaken in this direction. These works should fix our attention, and we physicians must ask ourselves what is the exact value of surgical intervention, and how far is it beneficial in acute and chronic nephritis ?

In unilateral nephritis the conditions are particularly favourable for surgical intervention, and in such cases an operation is often indicated. We must, therefore, review the pathological conditions which favour unilateral lesions in the kidney, and see which cases lend themselves best to operation.

1. Ascending infection frequently affects one kidney alone. The infectious agents which start from the genito-urinary passages, especially from the bladder, sometimes affect both kidneys ; at other times one kidney only. Statistics show that the lesion is unilateral 19 times in 150 cases (Godhardt), 19 times in 71 cases (Weir). Unilateral nephritis has been experimentally reproduced (Albarran). It is favourable for surgical intervention, as in the following examples :

Pousson had a patient who suffered for a long time from purulent cystitis ; acute inflammation of the right kidney supervened ; pain intense, fever very high, lumbar region indurated and very painful on pressure. Pousson operated. The perirenal cellular tissue was healthy, but at the upper end of the kidney a small abscess was found, and incision along the convex edge disclosed a large number of small miliary abscesses, due to the coli bacillus. The operation was followed by recovery.

Pousson quotes several other cases of unilateral ascending nephritis cured by surgical intervention. A case of Jordan refers to a man who, after gonorrhœa, was taken ill with pains in the right kidney, high fever, albumin and pus in the urine. Weir opened the kidney, and found it riddled with small abscesses. He performed nephrectomy. The coli bacillus was present. A few weeks later the patient was cured.

Potherat performed a successful nephrotomy in nephritis of the right kidney, following on gonorrhœal cystitis.

Wilms operated on, and cured, a young girl suffering from acute ascending pyelo-nephritis which was secondary to cystitis. The incision of the kidney disclosed purulent tracts. The coli bacillus was the infective agent.

Le Nouëne has collected eleven cases of abscess secondary to infection of the bladder, and treated by surgical intervention. The coli bacillus was the most common agent. These eleven cases are as follows : Eight cases of nephrotomy, seven recoveries, and one death ; two cases of nephrectomy, one cure and one death ; one case of decapsulation, cured. In one of the fatal cases the nephritis was double ; in the other it was probably double and tubercular. It is certain that the chance of a cure is much greater when the nephritis is unilateral. The clinical symptoms (localization of the pain, swelling of the region) do not show that the nephritis is unilateral. It is necessary, when possible, to separate the urine by Luys's segregator, which indicates the condition of each kidney.

2. Infection by the blood-stream is also likely to cause a unilateral lesion. Castaigne and Rathery quote the following examples :

In a patient who died on the nineteenth day of typhoid fever the post-mortem examination revealed two abscesses as big as a large nut in the right kidney, but no pus in the left kidney. In the case of a young man who died of staphylococcic infection, due to osteomyelitis, the left kidney was riddled with miliary abscesses. Finally, in the case of a patient who died of pneumococcal infection with suppurating pneumonia, they found three small abscesses in the left kidney, whilst the right kidney was healthy.

Surgical intervention has sometimes given good results in cases due to blood infection. Israel operated successfully for nephritis of the left kidney, secondary to a carbuncle. He removed the kidney, which contained miliary abscesses.

Monod has reported the case of a young girl who was taken ill " with quick pulse, temperature 104° F., and incessant vomiting, and painful mobile tumour in the region of the right kidney." The urine contained neither albumin nor pus. Monod performed nephrectomy, and recovery followed. The kidney was enormous, and contained miliary abscesses.

Pousson performed nephrotomy on a woman with acute nephritis of the right kidney, probably due to influenza. The urine contained pus, and the pain was acute in the right lumbar region. Pousson found an enlarged kidney, of a dead-leaf colour, with an abscess at its upper end. Incision of the kidney showed no pus anywhere else. The case was followed for four years, and recovery was maintained.

Routier has communicated the following case to the Société de Chirurgie :

A young woman was sent to him with the diagnosis of pyelo-nephritis. Her temperature was very high. The urine was not purulent, and did not show any trace of albumin. Much pain in the right renal region. A lumbar incision disclosed a somewhat enlarged kidney ; on opening it, scattered points of pus were found.

In nephritis due to blood infection and to ascending infection it is necessary to segregate the urine in order to ascertain the condition of the kidneys. We may not find any pus in the urine from the affected kidney, but it is rare not to find albumin.

In some cases of infective nephritis pus does not appear. We find simply congestion of the kidney, which is perhaps an early stage.

3. **Tuberculosis** of the kidney is often unilateral. This question will be discussed in Section IX. Vigneron, collecting the statistics of Roberts, Dickinson, Gaultier, Morris and Gergon, found that the lesions were unilateral in 99 out of 205 cases of tuberculosis of the kidney. Albarran found that the lesions were bilateral in 15 to 20 per cent. of the cases. According to Tamayo, the lesions were unilateral in 32, and bilateral in 59 cases. Unilateral tubercular nephritis, if operated upon early, is amenable to surgical inter-

vention. It is essential to examine the urine from each kidney separately, in order to know the condition of the kidney which is healthy, or is supposed to be so. The healthy kidney may show compensatory hypertrophy, and as pain is present, we might make a mistake in the absence of segregation of the urine.

4. I shall refer in greater detail to unilateral nephritis, which is sometimes associated with a movable kidney. This question is still under discussion, and I must, therefore, give details. For a long time a movable kidney was considered to be exempt from lesions. Tuffier has, however, said that, if in operating for movable kidney, we find the capsule of the organ to be fibro-lipomatous or indurated, we must think of an infective lesion. This point must never be lost sight of in these cases. In certain cases we find albuminuria. The organ is often enlarged, and may show nephritis. A few years ago, in company with Guyon and Robin, I saw a lady whose right kidney was movable. The kidney was enlarged, painful, and the albumin was abundant. Œdema and other complications led me to suppose that both kidneys were affected by nephritis. This question of nephritis in movable kidney has entered a new phase since the works of Edebohls, Box and Newmann. These writers performed nephropexy in subjects suffering from floating kidney and albuminuria, and found that the albuminuria disappeared after the operation. Box quotes a case of floating kidney with chronic nephritis and albuminuria. After the operation every sign of nephritis disappeared.

The most complete work in this field is due to Edebohls.* He had occasion to perform nephropexy in five cases of floating kidney with coexisting chronic nephritis. The nephritis was undeniable, being proved *de visu*. The urine contained albumin and casts. In three out of the five cases operated on, the kidney was fixed, and the nephritis was also cured, the albumin and the casts disappearing from the urine. Edebohls performed bilateral nephropexy on a woman in whom one kidney was affected by chronic nephritis. The urine became normal, and she was cured simultaneously of all her trouble.

Although the cases reported by Edebohls do not give all the medical details of the question, it is none the less true that people with movable kidney have albuminuria. The albumin is present in 14 per cent., according to Schilling. There are also people who have albuminuria, casts and coexisting nephritis, as proved by surgeons. It must, therefore, be admitted that a direct relation exists between movable kidney and the development of nephritis. "It is incontestable," says Lépine, "that a displaced kidney is predisposed to the development of nephritis. Kinking of the ureter may cause not only changes in the excretion of urine, but also stasis of the urine in the canaliculi,

* *Medical News*, April 22, 1899.

which is very favourable to infection of the kidneys." In conclusion, the association of nephritis and of floating kidney is one of the most interesting facts in the pathogenesis of chronic unilateral nephritis on the one hand and the surgical treatment of chronic nephritis in general on the other. When Edebohls found that he could cure chronic nephritis by fixing the kidney, he hoped to employ this mode of treatment successfully in all forms of chronic nephritis. We find, however, chronic unilateral nephritis and chronic bilateral nephritis (Bright's disease), which is very different.

5. Chronic unilateral nephritis (leaving aside calculi, tuberculosis, and syphilis of the kidney) is found not only in floating kidney, but also under other conditions.

A kidney may be infected without the infection leading to the formation of pus. The toxines may cause an infecting sclerosis which leads to the death of the renal cells and to the proliferation of the connective tissue. This process may be confined to one kidney only and we have a unilateral nephritis.

In many cases surgeons have been able to examine these cases. Thus, Edebohls, on exposing both kidneys, has often found that only one kidney was attacked by nephritis. On referring to the statistics of nineteen cases of chronic nephritis operated on by him, we see that in several cases where both kidneys were exposed, the chronic nephritis was unilateral. The existence of chronic nephritis was here beyond doubt, because, in addition to the albumin and the casts found in the urine, the condition of the decapsulated kidney was verified, and histological examination made of the portions removed during the operation. Several of the patients operated on recovered, while others were much improved.

In some of the published cases of chronic unilateral nephritis the chief symptoms were pain and hæmaturia. The pains are at times very acute, and the hæmaturia is often persistent or abundant. In these cases of mixed nephritis the lesions chiefly affect the glomerular system and the connective tissue. I am of opinion that some of these cases are due to tuberculosis. In some of the published cases, nevertheless, it does seem that tuberculosis was not present, and that they were really cases of chronic unilateral nephritis, with pain and hæmaturia. They were cured by the operation.

6. We now come to a side of the question which has not yet been elucidated. Our discussion so far has referred principally to unilateral nephritis and its surgical treatment. On reading the reports of the surgical treatment, we find that the operation has been frequently performed in Bright's disease. The term " Bright's disease " implies the idea of bilateral nephritis. The presence of albumin and casts in the urine is not sufficient to prompt the diagnosis of Bright's disease. Albumin and casts may be found when

only one kidney is affected. If the other kidney is healthy, the urinary depuration is sufficient, and there is no need to fear uræmia. This condition is not Bright's disease. We must, therefore, not speak of having operated on a case of Bright's disease when only one kidney is involved. This confusion is sometimes made by surgeons. It may falsify our ideas. A case is called Bright's disease (which presupposes bilateral nephritis), and, on reading the report, we find that it is a case of unilateral nephritis.

Surgical intervention has, however, been frequent in Bright's disease (chronic bilateral nephritis). This question is well put by Bassan. I quote verbatim :

"In an article which appeared in the *British Medical Journal* of November 23, 1902, Edebohls compared decapsulation of the kidney with nephrotomy and nephrectomy. He carried out decapsulation in 40 cases of Bright's disease—23 cases in women, 1 case in a child, and 16 cases in men, of whom 6 were doctors. In 16 cases Edebohls removed the capsule and fixed the kidney. In 4 cases the right kidney was operated on, and in the other 12 cases both kidneys were decapsulated. In the 24 other cases double and total decapsulation was performed, which brings the number of bilateral interventions carried out by Edebohls to 36. In other words, 36 persons were operated on by him for Bright's disease (bilateral chronic nephritis), and from that time Edebohls announced new facts."

What is the nature of these operations ? It is not usual in a text-book of medicine to describe operative technique, and I shall therefore rest satisfied with pointing out that these operations were nephrotomy, decapsulation, nephropexy, etc. By nephrotomy we remedy the increased tension in the kidney. The loosening of the inextensible capsule frees the kidney and favours proper circulation and functional activity. According to Edebohls, the operation assists the insufficient circulation of the blood in the kidney. With this object in view, he performs decapsulation or decortication of the kidney (partial or extensive ablation of the capsule). He calls this operation " nephrocapsectomy."

According to Edebohls, " decortication renders the circulation of the kidney more active, and brings more arterial blood to the diseased organ through the bloodvessels of the perirenal fat, the vessels being increased in size and in number. Decapsulation, which places the entire cortical surface in direct contact with this area, rich in vessels, is said to result in the formation on a large scale of a vascular network between the kidney and the fatty tissue. In this way there arises an active **arterialization** of the diseased kidney, which, by the creation of a new circulation, would tend, if not to an absolute cure, at least to an improvement of the lesions in Bright's disease."

It is certain that the results of surgical intervention are often excellent in a case of acute or chronic unilateral nephritis, and they appear to be worthy of consideration in Bright's disease. It is, however, indispensable to state clearly the indications and the contra-indications of surgical intervention, and to select cases that are amenable to operation. For the time being we are unable to answer this question, because many of the published cases are incomplete from a medical point of view. I am convinced, however, that this gap will soon be filled. In Bright's disease, which makes progress in spite of treatment, we are so often at a loss that we must try to ascertain as clearly as possible the proper time for surgical intervention.

VII. CASES OF ALBUMINURIA NOT DUE TO BRIGHT'S DISEASE.

We have seen that albuminuria may be absent for a time in Bright's disease. The opposite is also true, and just as in Bright's disease albuminuria may be absent, so also may albuminuria occur, quite apart from Bright's disease. Cases of albuminuria not due to Bright's disease have become more and more numerous since they have been sought for. This question has been discussed by Senator, Lépine, Noorden, and other writers.

Physiological albuminuria may occur aside from any lesion of the kidneys and any general affection. It is probable that absolutely physiological albuminuria does not exist, and that in a final analysis these cases of so-called physiological albuminuria are associated with a vicious process in the proteids or in the uropoietic system. If, however, they are not physiological in the true sense of the word, they are at least compatible with good health, which, clinically speaking, leaves nothing to be desired. To quote examples :

I attended a young man who for some years had noticed a fair amount of albumin in his urine. He examined his urine himself, and drew up a comparative table of the albuminuria, according to the time of day, the hours of rest or work, and the nature of the food taken at meals. The quantity of albumin varied, but his health was good, and **symptoms of Bright's disease never appeared.**

A doctor who was expert in laboratory work tested his own urine, and was surprised to find albumin. His health is excellent; his urine shows a normal toxic coefficient, as I have satisfied myself **by experiment ;** and he has never experienced any symptom of Bright's disease.

A friend of mine was anxious about his little daughter, because she had had albuminuria since she was four years old. This condition lasted for sixteen or seventeen years. She has now been married for some years, and has never had any sign of Bright's disease.

Amongst these cases, I know of none more interesting than those reported to the Clinical Society of London by Hawkins. A robust man, forty-nine years of age, had albuminuria for twenty-five years. A doctor passed albumin for forty-three years, but remained free from Bright's disease, though Bright, whom he had consulted thirty years previously, had predicted early death.

Our difficulty commences when we try to interpret the facts. Noorden has classified these cases into several groups, according as albumin alone is found in the urine or associated with globulin or mucin ; according, also, as the albumin is met with in the morning or at any hour of the day ; or as it appears independently of any external cause ; or as it varies with meals, exercise, malaise, fatigue, etc. (intermittent albuminuria, cyclic albuminuria).

Tessier classifies these cases as follows : (1) intermittent albuminuria in apparently healthy subjects ; (2) albuminuria in youths, which is generally intermittent and cyclical ; (3) albuminuria of a digestive or hepatic kind ; (4) neuropathic albuminuria, and especially albuminuria of the erect position or orthostatic albuminuria.

These cases of albuminuria may be slight, intermittent, or continuous. and may have different origins, but they are perfectly compatible with good health. It is important to find out whether albuminuria is or is not due to Bright's disease, because the prognosis is different. Absence of granular casts and of the minor symptoms of Brightism, together with normal toxicity of the urine and physiological permeability of the kidney, shows that the albuminuria is not due to Bright's disease.

Linossier and Lemoine give the following differential characteristics :

1. In absolutely normal kidneys orthostatism only reveals its noxious action by moderate diminution of the watery secretion. The excretion of the solids undergoes no regular modification. The urea only is eliminated in greater abundance, but this is due rather to increased production than to excessive elimination.

2. If the kidneys are incompetent, the diminution in the watery secretion by the erect position is much more marked than when the kidneys are normal, so that an exaggeration of the **orthostatic oliguria** may be looked upon as a sign of functional insufficiency of the kidney. In this case it is combined with diminished secretion of the solids, and especially of the urea. There is, therefore, **oliguria** and also **orthostatic hypo-azoturia.**

3. If the kidneys are even more incompetent, the influence of orthostatism is still further revealed by the appearance of albumin or by the exaggeration of an already existing albuminuria.

Nevertheless, it is at times very difficult to diagnose between simple albuminuria and that due to a renal lesion. Nephritis limited to a part of the kidney (tubercular lesion) may have albuminuria as its sole sign. We only discover later that this simple albuminuria was in reality the precursor of renal tuberculosis.

Some cases of nephritis, especially of unilateral nephritis, may for a long time give no sign save albuminuria. We have no proof that some forms of Bright's disease are not primarily limited to one kidney, the lesion passing later to the other one.

In a difficult case of albuminuria it is well to segregate the urine by Luys's apparatus, in order to study the conditions of each kidney.

The treatment of simple albuminuria varies. The milk cure is not so essential as it is in Bright's disease. The diet must be carefully regulated, and the food selected on the basis of practical experience. Rest, or even the supine position, must be prescribed, and tonics, alkalis, or the cure at Évian be recommended.

VIII. AMYLOID KIDNEY.

Pathological Anatomy.—We mean by amyloid degeneration the deposit in certain organs (kidney, spleen, liver, intestinal mucosa) of a transparent homogeneous substance, which, by its chemical reaction, is allied to the carbohydrates, but which, by the presence of nitrogen, is also allied to the proteids. This substance is readily detected in the kidney and other organs by certain reactions. A section of the kidney is made, and the surface washed with water. An aqueous solution of iodine and iodide of potassium is poured over it. The healthy parts assume a pale yellow tint; the affected parts become a mahogany colour, distinct striæ (arterioles) and points (glomeruli) being visible. Several writers include the **amyloid kidney** under Bright's disease, and, as a matter of fact, amyloid disease of the kidney is in many cases associated with parenchymatous or interstitial nephritis. Cornil and Ranvier even state that in diffuse subacute nephritis with enlarged kidney amyloid lesions are always present in the vessels and the walls of the tubules, the parenchymatous nephritis preceding the amyloid degeneration. These mixed forms are included in Bright's disease. In other cases (Cohnheim, Weigert, Straus) the amyloid change occurs alone, and therefore deserves special mention. The amyloid kidney may be enlarged or of normal size. Its surface is smooth and whitish or yellowish. On section, it is waxy, and its capsule is easily detached. Atrophy is rare. The atrophy, if present, is anterior to the amyloid degeneration.

The microscopic examination is made easy by the use of gentian violet, which stains the amyloid substance violet and the normal tissue pale blue. Amyloid degeneration attacks, in order of frequency, the glomeruli, the vasa recta, and the interlobular capillaries. The membrana propria of the canaliculi is not invaded except in advanced cases. The disease may exist for a long while before the function of the kidney is affected. When parenchymatous nephritis is also present, we find the lesions previously described under Nephritis. When the kidneys are affected, we generally find that the spleen, the liver, and the muscular coat of the intestine are also involved.

Description.—The symptoms may be the same as in Bright's disease. At other times they are practically absent. This diversity in the appearance and the succession of the symptoms is due to the anatomical condition of the kidney, and varies according as the amyloid degeneration is pure or associated with more or less marked parenchymatous lesions. When it is pure, the symptoms may be limited to urinary troubles (polyuria, diminution of urea, uric acid, phosphoric acid, and of most of the salts) (Lécorché). When it is mixed, other symptoms appear. The permeability for methylene blue, according to Achard and Loeper, is normal or increased in amyloid disease. This fact may help in the diagnosis between it and chronic nephritis.

The question of **albuminuria** in amyloid degeneration of the kidney deserves special mention. According to certain writers, it is always present. Others maintain that it only supervenes when inflammatory lesions are also present.

Straus, in his interesting monograph, has collected cases of amyloid degeneration in which albuminuria was both present and absent. Straus explains this apparent contradiction by the occurrence of the degeneration in the vasa recta in the former case, and in the glomeruli in the latter case. In some cases as much as 10 to 20 grammes of albumin have been found per litre. Urinary casts only appear at an advanced phase of the disease. They are colloid, but they never give the true amyloid reaction.

Uræmia is rare in amyloid kidney. The patient is carried off by other complications—uncontrollable diarrhœa, pulmonary tuberculosis, pneumonia, cachexia, or coma. The prognosis is fatal.

As regards **diagnosis,** in amyloid kidney we must look for its cause. Persons with tubercular or syphilitic cachexia, children with caries, abscess of bone, or tubercular glands, are liable to suffer from amyloid disease. Examination of the other organs helps us in the diagnosis : enlargement of the liver and the spleen ; diarrhœa, due to amyloid disease of the intestine.

Amyloid degeneration of the kidneys is usually due to caries, prolonged suppuration, tuberculosis, or syphilis. Gout, chronic rheumatism, malaria, and alcoholism have also been incriminated.

Charrin, in his experiments on the *Bacillus pyocyaneus*, found that after inoculation, rabbits and guinea-pigs were attacked by paralysis, nephritis, and, in the long-run, by amyloid degeneration, though there was no suppuration.

IX. TUBERCULOSIS OF THE KIDNEY.

Acute miliary tuberculosis, which accompanies general infection, merely deserves mention. In general tuberculosis, especially in children, both kidneys are often riddled with miliary tubercles. Tubercles are found in the cortical and medullary substance. They are small, transparent, and white or greyish. They occur in " the perivascular connective tissue, along the bloodvessels, and in the glomeruli, or the space corresponding to several adjacent tubules" (Brault). This form of miliary tuberculosis often spares the ureters, the bladder, and the genito-urinary organs.

I shall now describe chronic tuberculosis of the kidney. The infection may reach the kidney by the blood-stream (primary form), or may begin in the bladder, prostate, testicle, or epididymis (ascending or secondary form). It may invade both kidneys, or, as usually happens, it may be limited to one kidney. In any case the lesions finally end in caseation.

Pathological Anatomy.—The removal of the kidney is not always easy, because numerous adhesions fix the organ to the lymphatic glands of the hilum and of the lumbar chain, to the renal vein, the vena cava, and the aorta, in the case of the right kidney; to the intestine and the peritoneum, in the case of both kidneys. The tumour, after removal, is bulky, because it comprises the kidney and the perirenal fat. The kidneys have not the shapeless look seen in certain cases of cancer. The surface is smooth or at times nodular from the projection of cavities, and is perforated by sinuses which connect the cavities with the perirenal tissue. The capsule is thickened, fibrous, and adherent to the perirenal fat, which is of great importance in certain diseases of the kidney. By reason of the overgrowth of fibrous and adipose tissue the perirenal fat may be some inches in thickness, especially in the pelvis, where it forms lipomata. The fibro-fatty tissue around the kidney prevents the renal lesions from spreading to the rest of the body, but this barrier is not insurmountable, and, either by direct propagation or by the lymphatics, infection from the kidney may reach the perirenal tissue. In this way a perinephritic abscess is formed.

The abscess is sometimes limited, and of small size. At other times it extends into neighbouring regions, reaches up to the diaphragm, opens into the thoracic cavity, and causes a vomica, or else the pus descends towards the iliac fossa, and points at the crural ring or small trochanter. It may open into the intestine or into the bladder. The fluid in these collections is sero-purulent or sanguinolent, evil-smelling, and mixed with caseous débris. A guinea-pig inoculated with this pus contracts tuberculosis. On section of the kidney, we find the following lesions : tubercular granulations ; caseous foci, which are beginning to soften ; cavities containing caseating matter ; cavities which look like abscesses ; and transformation of the kidney into a putty-like mass, the ureter being obliterated.

Tubercular lesions in the kidney run a different course, according as the infection takes place by the blood-stream—the bacillus first affecting the cortex, and being transported thence by the renal or capsular arteries—or as it takes place by the ascending path of the bladder, ureter, pelvis, and calices, thus affecting first the medullary substance.

The tubercles may be few or many, and may exist in every part of the organ. They usually invade the cortical substance in the case of blood infection, whilst they first become localized in the medullary substance, in the case of ascending infection. In cortical tuberculosis Durand-Fardel found tubercle bacilli in the parenchyma, prior to the formation of tubercles. The bacilli are usually found in the glomeruli and the terminal arterioles of the cortex, and may reach the uriniferous tubules, which they may invade from without and from within.

The fused tubercles or the infiltrated tubercular tissue form caseous masses of the size of a hazel-nut or of a walnut. These masses soften and give rise to cavities. The cavities are anfractuous and well defined. They contain débris, pus, and at times phosphatic calculi. The topography of these cavities presents some variation, according to the process which has caused them. When the tuberculosis is cortical, the cavities are formed in the cortex, and open by narrow or broad orifices into the pelvis, which is not dilated. When the tubercular infection follows the ascending path, the pelvis, which is first invaded, is much dilated, and we find, instead of several more or less gaping cavities, one large festooned excavation, formed at the expense of the dilated pelvis and the pyramidal substance of the kidney. The calices and the pelvis are bathed in purulent caseous liquid, and in some places the organ is reduced to a fibrous shell, infiltrated with lime salts.

In some cases the kidney, including the calices and the pelvis, is transformed into a putty-like mass, compared by Tuffier to the contents of a large dermoid cyst. This degeneration *en masse* is due to the obliteration of the ureter, which is blocked up by the tubercular débris. I found this condition in a patient who died in my wards. The kidney was transformed into a caseous, putty-like mass, and surrounded by a fibrous shell.

This obliterating ureteritis may cause true hydronephrosis. In a case published by Tuffier the obliteration of the ureter was absolute, the pelvis, the calices, and the kidney being converted into a pseudo-cystic cavity, containing transparent sterile fluid. Similar cases have been published.

Renal tuberculosis may then present the following forms : (1) The tubercular infiltration is confined to the cortex (blood infection), and causes foci, cavities, or abscesses, which empty into the pelvis. (2) The tubercular lesions are ascending, and cause pyelonephritis. We may find obstruction of the ureter, distension of the gland, retention of pus and urine, and tubercular lesions in the medullary substance and in the cortex. (3) Tubercular ureteritis leads to obliteration, and is associated with tubercular degeneration of the kidney *en masse*. (4) Ureteritis obliterans is associated with

72—2

sodium, for instance—and that there was, as far as the kidneys were concerned, a very special mechanism for elimination of the chlorides, which
might be disturbed, while the other mechanisms were still intact.

The permeability of the kidneys for chlorides is most interesting, because the retention of this salt may, as we have already seen, lead to œdema.
If we know the approximate quantity of chloride of sodium in the diet taken
for some days by the patient, and compare it with the quantity of the
chlorides eliminated in the urine, we can deduce the degree of renal permeability.

Toxicity of the Serum.—Researches into the toxicity of normal or pathological serum injected into the veins or the subcutaneous cellular tissue have
so far given contradictory results. Widal, Sicard, and Lesné have experimented with the serum of normal or uræmic subjects by the method of intracerebral injections. They have shown that in healthy people or in persons
suffering from symptoms of uræmia there exists a convulsive poison, which
causes certain symptoms when injected into the brain of a guinea-pig but
none in the case of the rabbit. The nerve cells of allied species of animals,
such as the guinea-pig and the rabbit, may thus react quite differently to
the same systemic poison. If the serum of uræmic patients injected into
the brain of rabbits is not more toxic than the serum of normal subjects,
we may ask whether this anomaly is not due to the fact that poisons which
affect the nerve cell of man do not affect the cell of a different species, such
as the rabbit.

The following experiment of Widal and Lesné is in favour of this hypothesis. They produced parenchymatous nephritis in a rabbit by the injection of chromic acid. The serum of the animals thus treated was toxic
when used as an intracerebral injection—for the guinea-pig in a dose of
$\frac{1}{10}$ c.c., and for the rabbit in a dose of $\frac{1}{2}$ c.c. Before the appearance of the
renal lesion the serum was harmless to the guinea-pig after intracerebral
injection of $\frac{1}{4}$ c.c., and for the rabbit after injection of $\frac{1}{2}$ c.c.

Cryoscopy.—" The object of cryoscopy," says Achard, " is to overcome
the insurmountable difficulty which the chemical comparison of the blood
and of the urine presents, by substituting the estimation of a physical
quality for a chemical value. Instead of estimating the relative proportion
of the substances in the blood and the urine, this method estimates the total
quantity of the molecules contained in these two liquids, and does not distinguish their nature. The relatively simple procedure which yields the
molecular concentration of a liquid consists in determining its freezing-
point. As a matter of fact, according to Raoult's law the lowering of the
freezing-point of a solution is proportional to the number of molecules dissolved in unit volume of the solvent, irrespective of the size and nature of
these molecules. Given the molecular concentration of the urine and of

tubercular hydronephrosis. (5) The cellulo-fatty layer which surrounds the kidney is attacked by sclero-lipomatous or by suppurative perinephritis. All these lesions are seen in the tubercular kidney, and if their topography differs at first, according as the infection is cortical or ascending (secondary), we may say that at a given moment the lesions become fused.

The **ureter** is usually affected. In ascending tuberculosis it is always so. It is enlarged, indurated, constricted, or obliterated, and sometimes adherent to the peritoneum, to the utero-ovarian vessels, or to the ileum on the right and to the sigmoid on the left side. It forms a large hard cord, which can be felt through the abdominal wall.

In the **bladder** we find tubercles at any part of the mucosa. In descending tuberculosis we may see tubercles at the level of and below the ureter of the diseased kidney (Albarran, Israel). Ulcers eventually appear, but their evolution is very slow.

In the male, the vesiculæ seminales, prostate, vas deferens, and epididymis are frequently attacked. Genital tuberculosis is one of the most common origins of secondary disease in the kidney. On the other hand, tuberculosis of the genital system in woman is exceedingly rare.

I have already stated that tuberculosis of the kidney is often **unilateral.** From post-mortem examinations—i.e., when the infection has had time to become general—we find that the lesion is unilateral in half of the cases. From the statistics of surgical intervention we see that the second kidney is immune in three-quarters of the cases—a point in favour of operative interference. Albarran estimates that in 15 to 20 per cent. of the cases both kidneys are tubercular. And though the second kidney is not tubercular, at a fairly advanced period it frequently shows other lesions —e.g., pyelonephritis, calculous pyelitis, and amyloid degeneration. Koch's bacillus is found in the early stages of the renal lesion. Later we usually find the coli bacillus, streptococcus, and staphylococcus.

The **lungs** are often infected, either before or after the invasion of the kidney.

Description.—Tuberculosis of the kidneys is insidious and latent in its commencement. It may remain almost latent until an advanced period, especially if the ureter be obliterated. When I say that it remains almost latent, it would be more correct to say that it may fail to be recognized, as it is sometimes masked by tuberculosis of the bladder. In some cases, after remaining latent for a time, the mischief reveals itself by certain symptoms. The patient passes pus or blood; he has acute pains; a perinephritic abscess appears. In any case, bladder symptoms—hæmaturia, pyuria, albuminuria, pain, and renal tumour—are the most common symptoms.

BLADDER SYMPTOMS.—Albarran has shown that tuberculosis may at first simulate cystitis. Frequency of micturition, pain, and diminution of the capacity of the bladder are the symptoms. They may be due to concomitant cystitis, but in most cases they are only reflex. It is not rare to see patients who have urinary troubles, and who complain of frequent and painful micturition when the bladder is absolutely healthy, as a cystoscopic examination will prove. I recently saw a case with Albarran. The bladder symptoms were marked, while the kidney alone was affected.

HÆMATURIA.—Hæmaturia is a frequent symptom. Here, as in pulmonary tuberculosis, hæmorrhage may be the first sign. We find cases of early hæmaturia, which precedes the appearance of renal tuberculosis by months and years, just as "defensive hæmoptysis" precedes the appearance of phthisis. The hæmaturia is, as a rule, neither abundant nor obstinate. We do not find, as in cancer, long fibrinous clots in the ureter, which cause pain or retention of urine. Tubercular hæmaturia supervenes without appreciable cause. It is not brought on, like calculous hæmaturia, by violent exercise, riding, or driving. When it is over, it may not appear again, or it may reappear only at intervals of several weeks or months.

Such is the usual course of events, and tubercular hæmaturia has not the same importance as the hæmorrhage seen in cancer. We must not, however, trust too much to this feature. In some cases the hæmaturia is abundant; it may last from two or three months up to four years.

ROUTIER'S CASE.—A young woman was taken ill, without cause and without pain, with hæmaturia. The urine was blackish, and the quantity of blood lost considerable. After five weeks she was pale and cachectic, and could not stand. She repeatedly had renal colic, followed, not by the expulsion of calculi, but of clots. The right kidney was painful and enlarged. Cystoscopy showed that the blood came from the right ureter. She was threatened with death. Nephrectomy was performed by Routier six weeks after the appearance of the hæmaturia. The bleeding stopped, and the patient regained her health. Her husband wrote a few months later : " The urine is always clear ; she looks splendid, and has grown fat." The kidney examined by Pilliet showed only one tubercular focus, in a calyx, on a level with the arterial arch of the kidney, but this focus had caused profuse hæmaturia, due to the erosion of the vessels and to the arterial tension. It was, in short, a case of primary tuberculosis, which was circumscribed and favourable for operation.

POUSSON'S CASE.—In a young man the first symptom was hæmaturia, which lasted for seven months and a half without interruption, and increased in severity. He had sharp attacks of hæmaturia, with blackish urine and renal colic, caused by the expulsion of the clots and retention of urine due to obliteration of the ureter. Rest or exercise had no influence on the hæmaturia. Other symptoms, such as pyuria or enlargement of the kidney, were absent. Koch's bacillus was found in the urine. Exploration of the ureters, the bladder, the vesiculæ, the prostate, etc., was absolutely negative. It was, therefore, a case of primary or cortical tuberculosis of the right kidney, which was painful during the attacks of bleeding. The hæmaturia was gradually replaced by pyuria ; the infection took a descending course. The patient declined operation, and the tuberculosis spread to the vesiculæ seminales and the neck of the bladder.

TUFFIER'S CASE.—A woman, without premonitory symptoms, was taken ill with abundant hæmaturia. It was quite temporary, because the urine soon regained its normal colour, but for **four years and a half** the attacks recurred every few months.

lasting on each occasion for ten or twelve days. In the intervals the urine was absolutely normal. She had no pain. The final attack was so severe that the patient had
to stop for two weeks in a railway-station. She was pale and cachectic. Cystoscopy
showed that the blood came from the left ureter. Tuffier decided to remove the left
kidney. The operation was most successful. The kidney was of normal size ; on the
convex edge and at the two extremities tubercular abscesses were present ; the fluid,
when inoculated, caused tuberculosis. On section, three other abscesses were seen at
the junction of the cortex and the medulla ; they did not communicate with the pelvis.
The pelvis and the ureter were absolutely healthy. It was, therefore, a case of primary
or cortical tuberculosis, which had revealed itself by hæmaturia. These recurrent
attacks had caused no symptoms ; pain, pyuria, albuminuria, fever, and tumour being
absent.

These cases prove that we may find the classical form of the disease, in
which the hæmaturia is painless, transient, and of little importance, and
also other forms. The latter show numerous intermediary stages, in which
hæmaturia is the sole or the chief symptom. It may be profuse and painful,
the clots in the ureter simulating renal colic or causing retention of urine.
The patient loses flesh, and becomes cachectic, and the symptoms thus
recall those seen in hæmaturia due to cancer. These cases constitute the
hæmaturic form. In some cases the bleeding is continuous, and the patient
passes blood without interruption for several months. In other cases the
bleeding is intermittent, and the patient passes blood during periods of
three days or more for years (Tuffier). And as these attacks of profuse
hæmaturia are almost always associated with primary tuberculosis due to
blood infection, and as the lesion is limited to the cortex—for some time,
at least—and does not invade the calices and the pelvis, it follows that this
form can produce only one symptom—viz., hæmaturia. The other symptoms of pyuria, pyelonephritis, and fever are here absent, though they are
rarely so in tubercular pyelonephritis of the ascending type.

The nature and the amount of the hæmorrhage *per se* are not, then, of
much help in showing the nature of the renal lesion (cancer, calculus, cyst,
essential hæmaturia), but they furnish valuable information when we have
to decide upon an operation. Surgical intervention is very successful in
limited cortical tuberculosis.

PYURIA.—Pus in the urine is especially associated with ascending tuberculosis when the lesion assumes the aspect of suppurative tubercular pyelonephritis. Pyuria likewise occurs in cortical tuberculosis when the cavities
or abscesses have opened into the pelvis, or when the calices and pelvis
take part (descending infection) in the process. In a general way, pyuria,
which is an early, or, indeed, the chief symptom in ascending tuberculosis
of the kidney, is, on the contrary, an inconstant or late symptom in the
cortical form. It may, indeed, be absent, as in some of the cases already
cited.

The urine is turbid or clearly purulent, and sometimes rich in caseous matter. When we allow the urine collected during twenty-four hours to stand in a test-tube, the deposit of pus and phosphates is sometimes considerable. It is much larger in pyelonephritis than in cystitis. The pus may vary in amount at different times, but once it is installed, it never disappears, unless the ureter is obliterated. In half the cases Koch's bacillus is found in the urine.

PAIN.—Many people with renal tuberculosis do not feel the least pain. Others experience a sensation of heaviness or of tearing, and the pain may radiate to the other kidney, to the bladder, to the groin, or to the testicles, which are retracted, as in renal colic (Guyon).

These pains are sometimes spontaneous, and appear to be the result of nephralgia. Under other circumstances here, as in pericholecystitis with adhesions, perihepatitis, perigastritis, or peri-appendicitis, the pains may have their origin in the adhesions. In some cases, too, they are due to the passage of caseous fragments, phosphatic concretions, or fibrinous clots consequent on nephrorrhagia. In some patients the pains are so severe and persistent as to form the chief symptom. They constitute a **painful type** of renal tuberculosis (Tuffier), and supply a motive for surgical intervention. These cases are quite exceptional. To quote examples :

Tuffier reports a case treated for some years for renal colic. The pains began in the lumbar region, spread into the flanks and the groin, with repeated fits of vomiting, and ceased after a few hours. These crises returned several times every month. Urine contained pus, but not gravel. Slight hæmaturia appeared. As the pains recurred at shorter intervals and became more severe, the patient asked for an operation. Tuffier removed the kidney, and the operation confirmed the diagnosis. The kidney showed diffuse tuberculosis and some caseous centres. The pelvis was quite healthy. It was a case of primary tuberculosis of the kidney ; caseous foci in the cortex had opened into the pelvis. The patient was cured of all pain, and resumed his work.

In Cormak's case (reported by Tuffier), renal colic had appeared four years previously, and the pain had remained the chief symptom. Some months prior to the operation the urine had contained pus and blood, but no bacilli. A calculus in the right kidney was suspected. The patient was operated on, and the kidney was found to be studded with tubercles. A small cavity existed in the cortex. The pelvis and the ureter were healthy. This was also a case of primary tuberculosis of the kidney. The patient recovered quickly.

There is, therefore, a painful as well as a hæmaturic form of renal tuberculosis. Continuous or paroxysmal pain is the chief element. It may be the only symptom, pyuria, hæmaturia, and renal tumour being absent. When pain is present and the bacilli are absent, we may think of renal calculus ; but the crises are not followed by the expulsion of gravel, unless the patient pass phosphatic concretions formed in the tubercular centres. The urine must be repeatedly centrifugalized and examined for bacilli.

RENAL TUMOUR.—The tumour is not, as a rule, of large proportions. It is partly due to the distension of the organ and partly to the sclero-lipomatous perinephritis. The tumour projects below the costal margin by some inches; it may even extend below the umbilicus. It may be more or less movable or it may be fixed by adhesions. Bimanual palpation will reveal the size, situation, and mobility of the renal tumour (Guyon).

General Symptoms.—I have just reviewed the various symptoms which may accompany the evolution of renal tuberculosis. When the renal trouble is secondary, the extent or the age of the lesions (bladder, prostate, vesiculæ seminales, ureter) accelerates the course and the gravity of the symptoms. When the condition is primary, the patient's general health remains good for a long time. Fever is usually absent—or, at least, it does not appear until later. Slight symptoms of fever, with a rise in temperature to 100° F., indicate mild infection; but severe rigors, sweating, pyrexia of 103° F. and pyuria, point to complications, and indicate here, as in all cases of pyelo-nephritis, either the onset of perinephritic abscess or, more frequently, the formation of a closed cavity in the kidney.

As long as the pus can make its exit through the ureter, retention of the organisms and toxines does not take place, and the fever is slight. If the ureter becomes blocked, or an abscess is shut off in the kidney, the **retention of the infectious agents in a closed cavity**—just as occurs in appendicitis—betrays itself by renal pain, rigors, and attacks of intermittent fever, followed by sweating and by rapid loss of strength. An apparent improvement in the urine often coincides with this aggravation of the symptoms. The urine, which was turbid, ammoniacal, and purulent, becomes clear, because it is derived from the healthy kidney alone. If the ureter again becomes patent, or if a quantity of pus is passed, the complications will cease for a time. Similar complications occur in calculous pyelonephritis. As the disease progresses, the patient grows weak and loses his appetite. The cachectic stage commences with œdema, diarrhœa, and sweating, and becomes the more marked as the tuberculosis invades the other parts of the genito-urinary system and the lungs.

Complications.—Perinephritic inflammation may appear early or late in tubercular kidney. It is sometimes the first indication of insidious or latent renal tuberculosis. Suppuration in the fatty tissue around the kidney is not always accompanied by acute fever. It may be apyretic and insidious, like a cold abscess, or may begin with pain, rigors, fever, and induration or swelling in the loin. Under Pathological Anatomy I have already mentioned the various terminations of perinephritic abscess.

Tuberculosis of the bladder is a collateral phenomenon rather than a complication. Still, in almost every case of primary renal tuberculosis which is localized to the cortex and is not accompanied by descending lesions the bladder is free. This condition also obtains in cases where early obliteration of the ureter prevents the renal infection from passing down to the bladder. On the other hand, in ascending or surgical tuberculosis the disease of the bladder first attracts attention. It may, indeed, be so marked that the secondary mischief in the kidney is not discovered. The chief symptom is painful and frequent micturition. I saw with Guyon a young girl who had tuberculosis of the bladder. She passed water more than 100 times a day. She passed at each micturition a few drops of turbid, bloody urine, while the spasms of the neck of the bladder were most acute, and the pain radiated to the bladder, the anus, and the urethra. The unfortunate patient attempted in vain, by various changes in position, to lessen the agonizing pain of these spasms. This painful form is, fortunately, the exception. It will be understood that it masks the onset of ascending renal tuberculosis.

Tuberculosis of the bladder is not always easy to recognize at its outset. Micturition is frequent and painful. The passage of a catheter causes pain, and rectal examination reveals the induration at the lower part of the bladder. "In a patient from twenty to thirty-five years of age, suffering from the bladder without appreciable cause, examine the condition of the chest, palpate the epididymis, and explore the prostate and the vesiculæ seminales. Inquire into his past history for scrofulous manifestations in childhood, and ask about the health of his parents and his relatives" (Guyon). These points must not be forgotten in a difficult case.

Tubercular and Paratubercular Nephritis.—The **complications of Bright's disease** now demand our attention, and I make use of the opportunity to present this question, as I did during my course of lectures at the Faculté :* Are persons with renal tuberculosis liable to complications and to uræmia, like those who are suffering from chronic nephritis ? In other words : Is there such a thing as tubercular Bright's disease ? The kidney may be affected with cavities, tubercular pyelonephritis, or degeneration *en masse;* it may be destroyed, with total loss of function, and yet the patient does not show either the symptoms of Bright's disease or of uræmia, because the other kidney is usually able to do the work. The urinary insufficiency seen in nephritis and the symptoms of Brightism and of uræmia depend on the fact that in nephritis, whether it be due to infection, diathetic causes, or poisoning, the lesion always affects both kidneys. As the glandular substance of both kidneys is affected, we have not a healthy kidney to supplement its diseased fellow, and the insufficiency or the suppression of the function brings minor or major uræmia.

In renal tuberculosis, when one of the kidneys is compromised, the other one is healthy or sufficiently sound to carry out the urinary depuration. The patients do not show symptoms of Bright's disease, and do not succumb

* Dieulafoy, " Cours de Pathologie Interne," Février, 1896.

to uræmia. If uræmia does occur (this is very rare), it is because the other kidney is injured by amyloid degeneration or other lesions. Hence, in spite of the destruction of the tubercular kidney, the patient hardly ever dies from uræmia, because the other kidney can carry out the work of urinary depuration. I hold the same opinion as regards cancer and other unilateral lesions, which, in spite of the destruction of one kidney, do not cause Brightism or uræmia, provided the other kidney is sufficiently healthy.

But, it will be asked, can there not be **tubercular nephritis** in the true sense of the word, both kidneys being attacked simultaneously with diffuse nephritis, as they are in infectious, syphilitic, or scarlatinal nephritis? In phthisis, it will be asked, do we not see patients suffering from symptoms of Bright's disease—viz., œdema and albuminuria—the albuminuria having here nothing to do with hæmaturia or pyuria? Are these cases of Bright's disease or of tubercular nephritis? In the first place, it is a well-established fact that phthisical patients—and they are numerous—**very rarely** die of uræmia. The infection does not easily spread to the kidneys and cause nephritis. We see a difference from other infectious diseases—scarlatina and syphilis, for example—which may cause acute or chronic nephritis. We do not see this result in phthisis. We do not find phthisical patients contracting chronic tubercular nephritis with symptoms of Brightism and of uræmia. I have seen but few tubercular patients who suffered from acute nephritis with much œdema and symptoms of uræmia. It is, therefore, certain that tubercular infection does not, as a rule, lead to nephritis, and yet patients suffering from tuberculosis often have albuminuria. A pretubercular form of albuminuria has been described. They also suffer from œdema, which is not the result of venous thrombosis or cachexia. Their kidneys may show diffuse epithelial and amyloid lesions, and, therefore, tubercular nephritis exists in the true sense of the word. It would, however, be more correct to call it **nephritis in tubercular patients** —in fact, I should prefer the epithet " **paratubercular**," which is similar to Fournier's " **parasyphilitic** " troubles. This paratubercular nephritis is due to the action of the tuberculin on the kidneys, as experiments have proved. The kidneys are tuberculinized rather than tuberculized, and Koch's bacillus is absent (Du Pasquier). This form of nephritis causes albuminuria and œdema, but it is usually an indefinite condition, and rarely ends in uræmia. The conclusion, therefore, is that **renal tuberculosis is common, whereas tubercular nephritis is very rare.**

Diagnosis.—The previous description of renal tuberculosis clearly shows the difficulties in diagnosis. In ascending tuberculosis, when we have found the bacillus in the urine or the pus, the diagnosis is much simplified. The presence of the bacilli, although eliminating all doubts as to the nature of the disease, does not always indicate its exact seat This examination is much more delicate than the examination of the phthisical sputum, and the absence of bacilli, even in centrifugalized urine, does not eliminate all idea of urinary tuberculosis. Albarran has shown that **the search for the bacillus must be made in acid urine**—that is to say, in a fresh specimen, and not in a specimen taken from the total urine discharged during the day.

Experiments may help us in difficult cases. We should make cultures of the tubercle bacillus on glycerinated blood, as already described. The urine must be absolutely free from the organisms of secondary infection. These microbes develop, as a matter of fact, more rapidly than Koch's bacillus, and would invade the entire surface of the culture medium before the colonies of tubercle bacilli have time to appear. It is a good plan to centrifugalize the urine, and to sow only the deposit.

Nattan-Larrier's method is often of service. He injects 1 c.c. of the suspected urine into the mammary gland of a suckling guinea-pig. A few days later tubercular mammitis appears, and Koch's bacilli can be found in the milk, collected by squeezing the gland.

The diagnosis is still more difficult when the trouble is limited to the cortex, and reveals its presence by pains like those due to calculus or by hæmaturia, as is seen in cancer of the kidneys. It has been suggested that **tuberculin** might help in diagnosis, but Guyon and Albarran condemn this method as being both harmful and inconstant. It is better to employ **radioscopy.** In several cases the presence of calculi has been thus revealed (Albarran and Contremoulin). According to these writers, calculi may be thus classified in order of decreasing opacity : oxalic, phosphatic, and uric acid. **Cystoscopy** is of value when the bladder itself is invaded by tuberculosis ; in such a case examination with the cystoscope may reveal a patch or a tubercular swelling at the mouth of the ureter.

Catheterization of the ureter may also assist us in the differential diagnosis between tuberculosis and calculosis. The catheter passes readily in calculus, whereas tubercular lesions of the ureter, which are common in renal tuberculosis, make the ureter practically impermeable (Guyon and Albarran).

In order to complete the diagnosis, it is necessary to ascertain which kidney is affected and the condition of the other kidney. The diagnosis of the diseased kidney is difficult when neither kidney is painful nor hypertrophied. It is even more difficult when the healthy kidney is painful and affected by compensatory hypertrophy (Albarran). In such a case cystoscopic examination may show blood or pus issuing from the ureter on the diseased side. The ureter may be catheterized in order to collect the urine from the affected kidney, but it is better to use the ingenious apparatus of Luys, which segregates the urine of each kidney. Amongst other services rendered by the segregator in tubercular nephritis Luys quotes the following case :

A young woman whose urine contained pus and tubercle bacilli complained of her right kidney, which was enlarged. As the left kidney was painless and not perceptible on palpation, the right kidney might have been removed for tuberculosis, if the segregator had not shown that, contrary to the clinical evidence, the urine came almost entirely from the right ureter. It was therefore clear that, in spite of the clinical signs, the left kidney was much affected ; nephrectomy revealed atrophy of the organ. We can imagine what might have happened if the operator, relying on the clinical evidence alone, had removed the right kidney. As a general rule, segregation of the urine should always be performed, and no operation be performed until the diagnosis has been thus confirmed.

This method shows that in early renal tuberculosis the diseased kidney sometimes secretes more urine than the healthy kidney. Furthermore, the urine secreted by the diseased kidney is not so rich in urea, phosphates, and chlorides. It generally contains pus and some bacilli.

The condition of the other kidney (which is supposed to be healthy) must be ascertained prior to any operation. It is not permissible to remove a tubercular kidney unless we are sure that the other kidney is carrying out its functions normally (Albarran). Absolute precision in diagnosis can only be obtained by ureteral catheterization. I have recently proved this fact in a patient whom I saw with Albarran.

A young man who had no hereditary antecedents, and was free from pulmonary or genital tuberculosis, had for four months complained of painful pollakiuria. The urine was turbid and contained pus ; bacteriological examination revealed the presence of Koch's bacillus. The kidneys were neither enlarged nor painful on pressure. The bladder was of normal size, and cystoscopic examination showed that it was healthy. By catheterization of the left ureter, Albarran in an hour and a half collected 2 ounces of turbid urine, whilst the right kidney only secreted 1½ ounces of clear urine. Pus and Koch's bacilli were found in the urine from the left kidney ; neither pus nor bacilli in the urine from the right kidney. Urea, phosphates, and chlorides were 30 per cent. higher in the urine from the left or diseased kidney than in the urine from the right kidney. It was evident that the left kidney only was tubercular, and that the lesions were not advanced. Albarran removed the left kidney. At first sight it appeared to be healthy, but on section he found the following lesions : a hard tubercle at the base of a pyramid, a small cavity of the size of a pea in the cortical region, tubercular granulations in the pelvis. The patient recovered.

The **prognosis** is much graver in the secondary than in the primary form. Recovery is possible, because the cicatrices of cavities have been met with. The disease generally lasts for one or more years if early intervention has not been made, and the patient succumbs to hectic fever, tubercular invasion of the genito-urinary organs, septic fever, or tubercular complications in the respiratory system.

Treatment.—The medical treatment of renal tuberculosis is reduced to hygienic considerations. As surgical treatment, which is the only rational one, has no detailed place in a text-book of medicine, I refer the reader to works on surgery. This article, however, gives some idea of the principal indications for operation. We have seen that the cases of primary tuberculosis of the kidney are more favourable for intervention than the secondary cases, in which the bladder, the ureter, and other organs are already infected.

Two different operations are performed in tubercular kidney : (1) **Nephrotomy,** or simple incision of the kidney, the object being to evacuate the pus which has accumulated in the pelvis in case of retention. It is an operation of necessity which has the great drawback of leaving a permanent fistula. (2) **Nephrectomy,** or extirpation of the kidney. The results of this operation have much improved, owing to the more accurate diagnosis rendered possible by ureteral catheterization. Vigneron in 1892 found the mortality to be 34 per cent. Albarran lost only one patient, who died of meningitis, out of thirty-one cases of nephrectomy. These results are the more remarkable in that several patients had fever or advanced cachexia. Several of the cures have been maintained for five or six years.

X. RENAL SYPHILIS—SECONDARY SYPHILITIC NEPHRITIS— TERTIARY SYPHILIS OF THE KIDNEY.

According to a certain theory (Güntz), mercurial treatment is largely responsible for the nephritis which occurs in syphilitic patients. In a monograph on syphilosis of the kidney Mauriac rightly protests against this statement. To refute it, we have only to study mercurial poisoning in workmen who employ this metal. Except in acute poisoning, due to the ingestion of large quantities of the drug, mercurial intoxication does not affect the kidney. Gilders, looking-glass manufacturers, miners, and many other workmen who use mercury, may suffer from stomatitis, disease of the jaws, tremors, and other symptoms, but their kidneys remain healthy. Mercury differs from lead, which does cause nephritis. In this section I shall cite cases of acute nephritis in syphilitic persons, appearing three or four months after the chancre, when they had not taken mercury. I shall also speak of cases in whom syphilis of the kidney appeared fifteen years after the chancre. The patients had not taken any mercury for many years. The question is therefore settled. The cause of this nephritis is not mercury, but syphilis.

The syphilitic toxine is very poisonous to the renal filter. It exercises a harmful or even deadly action on the kidneys, but it acts differently, according as the kidney is attacked in the secondary or in the tertiary stage of the disease. This fact is easily seen from an analysis of the cases, and I shall, therefore, follow the division indicated by writers, and also employed in my pathological and clinical lectures.

Early infection causes **nephritis** in the true sense of the word. Both kidneys are attacked, as they are in acute infective nephritis—*e.g.*, scarlatinal nephritis. This early form may show itself by slight or moderate symptoms. In some cases the symptoms are acute, and the mischief proves fatal.

Late infection, which supervenes in the tertiary stage, does not reveal itself only by the lesions of nephritis, in the true sense of the word. It engenders gummatous or amyloid lesions, which are sometimes predominant, or are at other times associated with the lesions of ordinary nephritis.

In these various cases, therefore, the clinical picture differs. **Syphilitic nephritis** is most suitable for the early cases, and **tertiary syphilis of the kidneys** for the late cases. Between these two extremes there are, of course, intermediate types.

1. Early Syphilitic Nephritis.

In a first category of cases the nephritis is so slight as to pass unnoticed. It appears a few months after infection, and albuminuria is almost the only symptom (Jaccoud). From 3 to 5 grains of albumin are found daily. The urine is of normal toxicity ; the amounts of urea and extractives are normal ; and histological examination reveals the presence of hyaline casts. The albumin is present for a longer or shorter period, which may be lessened by specific treatment, and then disappears without further complications. In this form of nephritis the functions of the kidneys are not deranged. The urinary depuration is sufficient, and the patient does not suffer from " symptoms of Brightism." Another symptom, however, often accompanies the albuminuria—viz., slight puffiness of the eyelids or of the face. There may also be slight œdema over the malleoli.

This attenuated form of nephritis, revealing itself only by albuminuria and perhaps slight œdema, is not strange, for we find in influenza, typhoid fever, scarlatina, or pneumonia, that the renal changes may for a time be indicated only by albuminuria, with or without œdema. I am of opinion that this mild form is due to the weakness of the toxi-infectious agent, and perhaps to the previous integrity of the kidneys. These cases must be carefully treated by antisyphilitic remedies, and must be closely watched, because they do not always recover at once. They sometimes recur in a more severe form.

Syphilitic nephritis, however, does not always run such a favourable course. It is sometimes very much more severe. I shall cite cases which prove that early syphilitic nephritis may be as severe as the other forms of infective nephritis. It may run an acute and fatal course, and at the post-mortem examination we find diffuse nephritis, the kidney being enlarged and pale or showing hæmorrhages. The histological examination shows swelling and necrosis of the glandular tissue, and sometimes enlargement of the glomeruli, irritative lesions of the capsules and the bloodvessels, and glomerular hæmorrhage. It would be wrong to suppose that acute syphilitic nephritis, which is often fatal, and the lesions of which are especially limited to the secretory and excretory elements of the kidneys, is only seen in malignant syphilis. It usually appears during the first months of an ordinary attack of syphilis, while the other manifestations are only roseola and mucous patches.

Case I.—The best example which I can give is a case mentioned in my clinical lectures.* A young man was sent to me by Mauriac. Puffiness of the face and œdema of the legs had appeared suddenly two days previously. On admission, the eyelids were swollen and the œdema of the lower limbs was considerable. The œdema, which was white and soft, extended as far as the loins. Abundant albuminuria. The urine, which was fairly coloured, was normal in amount ; no hæmaturia. It contained 6 drachms of albumin in the twenty-four hours. No other symptoms. It was a case of acute nephritis, which had come on suddenly, without pain in the loins, rigors, or fever. I agreed with Mauriac that it was a case of early syphilitic nephritis. As a matter of fact, he had had a chancre on the penis two months previously. The slight induration of the tissues, their colour, and the hard, painless glands in the groin were corroborative evidence. Mucous patches were present in the throat and round the anus.

As this acute nephritis appeared nine weeks after the chancre in a man who previously had not had a chill, scarlatina, influenza, typhoid fever, or any infection capable of affecting the kidneys, it was quite natural to set it down to syphilis. It was no doubt a case of acute nephritis, and not an outburst of nephritis during the course of chronic Brightism, because no symptoms of Brightism were discovered in the previous history. There could, therefore, be no possible doubt as to the diagnosis.

Although alarming symptoms were absent, I gave a guarded prognosis, because experience has led me to beware of early syphilitic nephritis. I prescribed milk diet and a dessertspoonful of the following preparation night and morning :

Iodide of potassium	..	..	..	..	1 ounce.
Biniodide of mercury	..	..	..	..	3 grains.
Distilled water	..	..	..	..	12 ounces.

The effects were rapid and successful : in a fortnight the œdema had completely disappeared. As the œdema diminished, the patient lost weight in proportion. The amount of fluid taken and the quantity of urine passed, were measured daily. The latter exceeded the former, and the excess passed by the kidney agreed with the loss of weight due to the diminution in the œdema. In a fortnight he got rid of 21 pounds of liquid from the tissues. The albumin had all disappeared by the seventeenth day.

I have seen him several times since he left the Hôtel-Dieu ; his recovery is maintained. I kept him on milk diet for two months, and then I allowed him to take soup, vegetables, and bread. The mixture was given for a fortnight, and then suspended for a fortnight. Six months later he was perfectly well, and could eat ordinary diet. The albumin never reappeared.

Case II.—On March 16, 1898, a man, thirty-four years of age, was admitted for anasarca. About a month before, whilst in perfect health, he noticed that his eyelids were puffy. Next day his whole face was œdematous, and in twenty-four hours the œdema had reached the lower limbs. The anasarca showed a tendency to become

---

* "Néphrite Syphilitique : Syphilis Tertiaire du Rein" (*Clinique Médicale de Hôtel-Dieu*, 1898, 13me et 14me leçons).

general. His doctor examined his urine, and prescribed milk diet. In spite of the milk diet, the anasarca spread, and reached the scrotum. It was solely for dropsy that he came to the Hôtel-Dieu, as he had no other symptoms. At first sight he looked like a healthy man with a clear and rosy complexion. His arms were muscular, but the abdomen, the scrotum, and the lower limbs were œdematous. The urine was rather high-coloured; 4 pints were collected in twenty-four hours, and contained 120 grains of albumin per pint. We diagnosed acute nephritis.

The only discoverable cause for this nephritis was recent syphilis (eight months old). In June, 1897, he had been treated at the Hôpital du Midi by Mauriac for a chancre on the penis with pills of proto-iodide; a few months later he returned to the hospital with mucous patches in his throat. In the absence of any other cause, it was quite natural to diagnose specific nephritis, which had set in seven months after the chancre.

I put him on milk diet, and prescribed injections of biniodide of mercury. During the next few days the situation did not improve; the œdema persisted, the urine increased in quantity, and the albumin varied from 250 to 300 grains in the twenty-four hours. After the seventh injection, the biniodide of mercury was stopped. The patient, who was of a very optimistic nature, felt neither discomfort nor pain, and readily took his 8 pints of milk. The œdema unfortunately increased, and reached the loin. The scrotum and penis was as large as a fœtal head. I gave iodide of potassium in small doses, but stopped it, because no benefit resulted. The injections of biniodide were given again, and then suspended. On April 4—that is to say, twenty days after his admission—he passed 135 instead of 250 grains of albumin. The anasarca, however, still increased; this seemed a bad sign to me. On April 13 he complained of distress, and on auscultation I heard râles, due to pulmonary œdema. He had gained 11 pounds in weight since his admission, this increase being due to the œdema, which was gaining ground. On April 20 he was not so well, disliking his milk, and feeling nausea. The urine increased in quantity, but the pulmonary œdema made progress. On April 24 he felt pain in the right side of the abdomen; it was due to diffuse lymphangitis and a patch of erysipelas. This complication was most dangerous, in my opinion, because in several cases of early syphilitic nephritis death has been due to erysipelas. During the evening cyanosis and severe dyspnœa came on. In spite of all the means taken, he became rapidly worse: the pain in the erysipelatous areas was severe; the pulse grew threadlike and irregular, and the heart-beats were tumultuous. The face was pale and mottled, and he died next day, after retaining consciousness almost to the last. Results of the post-mortem examination: In the lungs œdema and congestion were fairly extensive. The cavities of the right side of the heart were filled with a large clot; it was white, solid, and formed of pure fibrin. It was not a post-mortem clot, but had certainly formed during the death-agony. It filled the entire right auricle, passed into the ventricle through the tricuspid valve, and from the ventricle into the pulmonary artery, where it ended in a point a short distance from the bifurcation.

The kidneys were enlarged. The right kidney weighed 7 ounces, the left one 6 ounces. The cortex was pale, and showed a well-marked network of vessels. The capsule stripped readily. The pyramidal substance was congested and of a bluish tint.

The histological examination showed that the lesions were most marked in the cortex. The epithelial cells which lined the convoluted tubules, instead of forming a row of equal cells, with well-stained nuclei, were irregular in form and size. The protoplasm was uniformly cloudy; the nuclei had either disappeared or were ill-defined and unstained. In some of the tubules there were several rows of these altered cells. Elsewhere desquamated cells or cellular débris blocked the tubules; in other places the cells had disappeared, leaving the basal membrane in direct contact with the lumen of the tube at certain points. The basal membrane of the tubules was not affected, and the tissue between the tubules showed no lesion. The glomeruli, with their arterioles, were healthy. The arterial and venous anastomoses at the junctions of the cortical and pyramidal substances showed no change. The pyramidal substance showed both tubules with changes similar to those in the convoluted tubules and narrow tubules which were healthy. The interstitial tissue of the pyramids was healthy. The capsule of the kidney showed no change.

In conclusion, in this case of syphilitic nephritis the lesion was purely epithelial. The glomeruli were intact, the narrow tubules were healthy, and the lesion affected only certain portions of the secretory and excretory systems. These lesions were marked in the convoluted and straight tubules, the epithelial cells being changed or destroyed.

CASE III.—A young man contracted syphilis, which appeared at first to be mild ; the rash was slight, and from the outset Siredey gave mercury. Nephritis appeared six months after infection, with symptoms of headache, nausea, and weakness. The urine contained nearly an ounce of albumin in 35 ounces. In spite of milk diet and specific treatment, he grew rapidly worse, suffering from drowsiness and fœtid diarrhœa. The tongue was dry, and the pulse rose to 120. The dropsy made rapid progress, involving the lungs and the abdominal cavity. In spite of treatment, the vomiting and diarrhœa were still severe. The milk was continued, and mercury was rubbed in over the kidneys. The situation was now so satisfactory that the patient took 6 pints of milk a day, and he passed, on an average, 6 to 7 pints of urine. The albumin diminished from 1 ounce to 45 grains, the pulmonary œdema improved, the headache disappeared, the anasarca grew less, constipation replaced the diarrhœa, and his nights were much quieter. This phase of relative calm lasted a fortnight, when the anasarca returned ; the skin was much affected, the legs and thighs being three times their normal size, and the scrotum as large as a man's head. Pain soon appeared in the left side, and pleural effusion showed itself. The ascites, which was very slight at first, now became marked. We estimated that the peritoneum contained about 15 pints of fluid. The vomiting was acute ; the vomited matter was mucous, blackish, and there was slight hæmatemesis. Dyspnœa now became the chief symptom. The pleural effusion on the left side increased, and fluid also formed on the right side. We decided to aspirate the fluid at several sittings, in order to prevent acute œdema of the lungs. At the first sitting I drew off 8 ounces. The patient, who was much relieved, asked for a second, and later for a third, puncture. Each time we withdrew some 10 ounces of fluid, and this gave temporary relief. The fluid, however, reformed, the heart grew weaker, and the torpor almost merged into coma. The dyspnœa grew worse, and in a few weeks this early syphilitic nephritis proved fatal.

Analysis of the Symptoms.—We may now consider the history of **early** syphilitic nephritis of the grave type. The first point of importance is that the nephritis is early. In syphilis it is customary to look upon the secondary troubles as being much less serious than the tertiary lesions. This is true in the majority of cases. The grave troubles (cerebral, aortic, laryngeal, or pulmonary syphilis) do not appear, as a rule, till some years after the infection. Many exceptions to this rule, however, occur. Amongst the early visceral lesions nephritis stands out, even when the kidneys were healthy before the attack of syphilis. The syphilitic poison kills the epithelium of the organ or destroys its functions, and renal insufficiency, with its grave symptoms, appears. In order to emphasize this fact, I give the dates when the nephritis appeared in seventeen cases : In two cases eight months after infection ; in two, six months ; in two, four months ; in five, three months ; in five, two months. According to these statistics, syphilitic nephritis usually appears **in the second and third months after the chancre.** It is often contemporary with the roseola and the first mucous patches. It is less common from the eighth to the twelfth month after infection, and after the first year the patient is practically safe from this terrible eventuality. I do not assert that acute nephritis cannot appear later, but this is an exception.

The next point is the **sudden onset** of the nephritis and its tendency to cause **general infiltration**—anasarca, œdema of the lung, pleural effusions, and ascites. In my first case puffiness of the face and considerable œdema of the leg appeared suddenly. I estimated the infiltration to be about 20 pints. In my second case the œdema appeared suddenly, and in a few days, judging from the weight of the patient, the infiltration was about 30 pints. The young man, whom I saw with Siredey, had such marked anasarca that he resembled a toy manikin of goldbeaters' skin. Furthermore, he had pulmonary œdema, double pleural effusion, which promptly reformed after thoracentesis, and ascites. In a case published by Gastou the anasarca became general in a day, and was soon followed by effusion into both pleuræ and by ascites. The sudden onset of anasarca and of pulmonary œdema is noted by Jaccoud. The above examples prove that rapid œdema, with serous effusion, is one of the principal characteristics of early syphilitic nephritis. I agree with Jaccoud that scarlatinal nephritis can alone be compared with it.

The **abundance of the albumin** is another peculiarity of early syphilitic nephritis—345 grains in my first case, in the second case 240 grains, and in the third case 500 grains in twenty-four hours.

This excessive albuminuria in early syphilitic nephritis agrees with the extent of the epithelial lesions, which may exist to the exclusion of any interstitial or vascular lesion in the kidney. The lesions in Case 2 were strictly limited to the epithelia of the convoluted and straight tubules. In another case (Darier and Hudelo) glomerulitis was associated with parenchymatous changes. In a case reported by Horteloup and Wickham the histological examination showed similar epithelial lesions with interstitial changes. In two cases published by Brault the glomerular and arterial lesions occupied an important place. They differed notably from the lesions found in my patient. Indeed, here the epithelial changes were practically exclusive, whilst elsewhere the changes were especially vasculoconnective. It is possible that the lesions may present some differences, according to the duration of the nephritis. In two cases reported by Brault the nephritis had in the one instance lasted five or six weeks and in the other four months.

Description.—The following are, in general terms, the most salient features of early syphilitic nephritis : An individual has contracted a chancre a few weeks or a few months previously. The roseola has hardly faded, and mucous patches have just made their appearance, when puffiness of the face, œdema of the lower limbs, and general anasarca suddenly appear. The urine contains a quantity of albumin and perhaps blood. The infiltration tends to reach the organs, and we find œdema of the lungs, pleural effusion, and ascites. During this phase œdema and albuminuria are often the only appreciable symptoms. After a few weeks of treatment improvement and cure may supervene, without any other incident, as in the first case quoted. In other cases the œdema and the albuminuria are accompanied by headache, dyspnœa, vomiting, and profuse diarrhœa. The urine becomes scanty, and if the disease progress, the patient succumbs in a few weeks or months. Death may result from general dropsy, dyspnœa, and coma, from some intercurrent infection (lymphangitis, erysipelas), or from uræmia. Uræmic symptoms (convulsions, coma, etc.) are, however, not as common here as in cases of chronic nephritis.

Syphilitic nephritis often appears to be cured. The œdema and albuminuria disappear ; the patient, tired of treatment, and believing himself to be henceforth invulnerable, wrongly resumes his ordinary life, without troubling about his former illness. The nephritis, although apparently cured, sometimes leaves sequelæ, which will, at the first opportunity, result in an outbreak of acute nephritis. I have seen a young man with severe Bright's disease, following upon acute syphilitic nephritis, which was considered cured, and which was too soon left to itself. It is not sufficient to limit the nephritis. It must be closely watched, even after the disappearance of symptoms, because the condition may end in chronic nephritis. In this respect it does not differ from the other forms of acute nephritis, which may become chronic.

The **diagnosis** is not difficult. Two symptoms are generally present— rapid œdema and abundant albuminuria. We must not mistake syphilitic nephritis for nephritis *a frigore*. I do not absolutely deny nephritis *a frigore*, which is allowed by the most eminent writers. I believe that I have seen undoubted cases of it, but, on closer scrutiny, we are forced to admit that the so-called nephritis *a frigore* has sometimes an origin other than cold, and that syphilis plays an important part. If we look for the cicatrix and the induration which point to a recent chancre, and search for the enlarged glands which persist after the chancre, we shall, then, find that in a supposed case of nephritis due to cold the condition is really syphilitic nephritis, which has appeared a few months after infection.

Our prognosis must be guarded in this event, because experience shows that we may find cases of early syphilitic nephritis in which the œdema and albuminuria are slight and treatment is successful, and also cases in which the œdema, effusion, albuminuria, and uræmic symptoms are severe, and fraught with danger because treatment fails. This does not mean that grave syphilitic nephritis cannot be cured. It is curable, even though the anasarca is great and the albuminuria severe, as we have seen in the first case quoted. The amelioration is announced by diminution of the œdema and albuminuria. On the other hand, persistence of the albumin and increase in the œdema, in spite of the treatment, demand reservation as to the ultimate issue of the disease.

The gravity does not arise solely from the uræmic troubles, which are less frequent here than in the case of chronic nephritis. The patients die from the general anasarca, which involves the pleuræ, the peritoneum, the lungs, and the larynx. Secondary infection often shows itself, and hastens death. My second case died of erysipelas, with œdema of the lung and a clot in the heart. The young man whom I attended with Siredey, died from pulmonary œdema, pleural effusions, which thoracentesis failed to relieve, and coma, probably due to cerebral œdema.

Treatment.—In early syphilitic nephritis we must first prescribe absolute milk diet, which, though far from being sufficient, is, nevertheless, indispensable. I question as to whether, from the prophylactic point of view, milk diet ought not to be prescribed for some months in every case of chancre, just as it is in every case of scarlatina. When we see the rapidity and intensity with which the renal epithelium is affected by the syhilitic toxine, it may be asked whether the kidneys would not benefit by a preventive regimen which renders them more able to resist the poison. Milk diet is even more necessary when syphilis attacks an individual whose kidneys are already affected. Many people have had their kidneys damaged by scarlatina, influenza, puerperal condition, malaria, plumbism, gout, calculus, etc. And though every trace of the former nephritis has apparently disappeared, we must not forget that the kidneys under these conditions present a *locus minoris resistentiæ* to syphilis for a long time. It is, therefore, a good rule to recommend milk in every case of syphilitic chancre. This regimen must be followed for three or four months, because syphilitic nephritis usually appears some two or three months after infection. Mercurial preparations are indicated, but we must prescribe them in moderation. As to the mode of administration, we have a most varied selection to choose from : proto-iodide of mercury in the form of pills, in daily doses of $\frac{1}{2}$ to 1 grain ; or biniodide of mercury, in solution or as an injection. I use an aqueous solution of biniodide of mercury. Fifteen minims of this solution contain $\frac{1}{16}$ grain of the active principle ; 10 to 15 drops of the solution are injected daily for a week to a fortnight. The injections are then stopped, and again given if need be. Other mercurial preparations may be recommended, with or without iodide of potassium—Gibert's syrup, for instance, in doses of 1 to 2 drachms daily; iodide of potassium, in doses of 15 to 30 grains per day. Mercury and iodides, which give such marvellous results in many syphilitic lesions, are less certain in acute syphilitic nephritis. We see both cases of undoubted and rapid success, and others in which these drugs do little good. In any case, we must use care in prescribing mercury, because the kidneys are weak, and the filter is bad. If rapid improvement occur (as in my first case), we may rest content; but if, in spite of mercury and milk diet, the disease remain stationary or become worse (as in my second case), we may well feel alarmed lest we have exceeded the proper dose or have not reached it. The drug is stopped, and, then, given again, but the disease progresses. It would appear that the epithelial lesions of the kidneys caused by the syphilitic toxine are irreparable.

The œdema and the effusions demand relief. This point requires some words of explanation. The patient who has pleural effusion on one or both sides has certainly also œdema of the lung, which helps to cause the symptoms of dyspnœa. The effusion is rightly tapped, but we must not withdraw 2 or 3 pints at a time, because a circumscribed œdema of the lung may, immediately after thoracentesis, become a superacute œdema of the gravest kind. In such a case let us be satisfied with withdrawing 8 to 10 ounces of the liquid. The operation may be repeated several times a week, as was done in my third case. Thoracentesis with a No. 2 needle is of no more consequence than a puncture made with a Pravaz syringe. Repeated withdrawals of small amounts of fluid protect against every complication, and relieve the patient. Unfortunately, the pleural liquid is often quick to reform.

When the anasarca is abundant, we should favour the exit of the liquid by acupuncture of the legs, thighs, and scrotum. We can, by this means, draw off several pints of fluid in the day, and give the sufferer great relief. The puncture may, however, in spite of every aseptic precaution, become the starting-point of erythema or lymphangitis; and, indeed, erysipelas, and lymphangitis (apart from any puncture) often cause death in patients with dropsy due to early syphilitic nephritis. If, then, lymphangitis or fatal erysipelas supervene in consequence, we may be held responsible for a fatal result.

2. Tertiary Syphilis of the Kidneys.

Late renal syphilis is a variety of chronic nephritis sometimes associated with gummatous, fibrous, or amyloid lesions, which appear many years after the chancre. It may be called " syphilitic Bright's disease." I know that under such circumstances it is often difficult to decide the share of syphilis as an ætiological factor. If a syphilitic patient has Bright's disease, and at the same time we find from his history one or more causes of nephritis (scarlatina, influenza, typhoid fever, plumbism, renal calculus, or gout), it is difficult to decide how far syphilis is concerned. If, however, he has chronic nephritis, and we find in his history no other cause than syphilis, and if, *a fortiori*, the nephritis is contemporaneous with other tertiary lesions (gummata of the skin or tongue, nasal syphilis, osteoperiostitis, etc.). it is logical to set down the kidney trouble to syphilis.

Pathological Anatomy.—Pathological anatomy has specified the various forms which tertiary syphilis of the kidneys may assume. We find chronic nephritis, with or without gummatous, fibrous or amyloid changes. They may exist alone or in combination. Let us first consider the gummata. "Syphilitic gummata," says Cornil, "are not common in the kidney. In 1864 I saw a kidney with about twenty in the cortex. The patient was an old woman who had died from albuminuria and anasarca. The liver was riddled with typical gummata. The kidneys showed amyloid degeneration, and the gummata presented the characteristic three zones."

Cüffer showed a case of syphilis of the liver at the Société Anatomique characterized by a large grey and homogeneous gumma. Wagner has published a case of gumma in the right kidney, which was small, dark, and smooth, whilst the left kidney was enlarged and pale. Püngel, Lancereaux, Lailler, and Key have found gummata of the kidney associated with other syphilitic lesions. Chronic syphilitic nephritis with interstitial fibrosis may end in atrophy of the organ. In sixty-three cases of syphilitic nephritis Wagner in eight cases found that the kidney was small, granular, and atrophied. Sometimes, on the other hand, the kidneys are enlarged, and show parenchymatous lesions. In some cases one kidney shows atrophic nephritis, whilst the other is enlarged and amyloid. Lancereaux has seen renal syphilis, characterized by gummata, interstitial nephritis, amyloid degeneration, and deep cicatrices. In two cases of syphilosis of the kidney Key noted that the atrophic fibrosis was limited to the lower part of the kidney. Weigert has published six cases of unilateral atrophy of the kidney in syphilitic patients. These various quotations, borrowed from Mauriac's monograph, prove that, while early syphilitic nephritis is general and uniform, tertiary syphilis may not affect both organs to the same extent. It may limit itself to one kidney or to a portion of the kidney. Amyloid degeneration is a very common lesion in renal syphilis, and often coincides with similar degeneration of the liver and spleen.

These gummatous, fibrous, and amyloid changes are associated to an unequal degree with chronic nephritis. We often find chronic nephritis alone, without any trace of gummatous or amyloid change. In other words, the kidney in tertiary syphilis may differ much in shape and appearance. It may be enlarged, or atrophied, nodular and furrowed.

Description.—The following cases will give an idea of the clinical features :

CASE I.—A man was admitted into my wards for chronic nephritis. The disease had appeared a year previously with the minor symptoms of Brightism. Œdema supervened later. At this period the patient was examined by Charrier, who found Bright's disease and prescribed a milk diet. The symptoms persisted, in spite of treatment ; the attacks of headache became more acute, the œdema of the legs increased, and Charrier asked me to admit him. I found, as a matter of fact, chronic nephritis, which in no wise differed as regards its course from common Bright's disease.

Headache and dyspnœa were the chief symptoms. The urine, which was normal in quantity, contained albumin. The patient finally admitted that sixteen years previously he had had syphilis, for which he had been treated at the Hôpital du Midi. As he had had no other infectious disease capable of explaining this nephritis, I considered that the trouble was syphilitic, and prescribed accordingly : daily inunction of mercury and iodide of potassium in 45-grain doses, which were soon increased to 90 grains daily. Although the milk diet which had already been given had by itself produced no improvement, it was continued. In a fortnight the situation was very different, and in a month the patient was discharged at his own request, all symptoms having disappeared. The albumin gradually diminished, and after eighteen days there was not a trace in the urine.

CASE II.—A man, forty-six years of age, was sent to me by Sauvineau, who had found retinitis. On his admission to the St. Christopher Ward, the strain of walking upstairs caused such marked dyspnœa that he could hardly speak. He told us that his breathing had been difficult for a long time, and slight effort caused fits of suffocation. Auscultation immediately revealed the cause : in both lungs râles due to œdema were audible. His face was puffy, especially about the eyelids ; and the legs were also œdematous. This information, together with abundance of albumin in the urine, confirmed the diagnosis of Bright's disease.

Examination of the heart revealed a *bruit de galop*, and analysis of the urine showed 1 drachm of albumin per pint. He had chronic nephritis, because the duration of the minor symptoms of Brightism showed that the disaese had commenced about a year and a half before. The visual troubles disturbed the patient more than the dyspnœa. He was able to walk about, but could not distinguish the features of persons nor the hands of the ward clock. Sauvineau found, with the ophthalmoscope, that the visual troubles were due to albuminuric retinitis.

As he had a history of syphilis, I ordered mercury, iodide of potassium, and milk diet. Anyone not familiar with the extraordinary results which at times follow this treatment would certainly have had reason to be surprised at the rapid improvement. After three days, his condition began to improve. He breathed more easily, and could walk without feeling breathless (he had not done this for a year). In six days he was able to distinguish the features of those around him. He was a different man at the end of twenty-five days, during which time he had had twenty-five injections of mercury and had taken 5 ounces of iodide of potassium. He was able to read a newspaper, and felt no distress. During this same period the albumin fell to 6 grains per pint, the pulmonary œdema disappeared, and he felt so well that he left the hospital.

In the two preceding cases the history made a diagnosis possible, but there are cases in which the patient who has well-marked uræmia is incapable of giving any information.

A man was admitted for coma. We noted no distortion of the face and no sign of hemiplegia. As Charrier, on examining him, found marked œdema of the face and legs, he thought of uræmic coma due to Bright's disease. He cupped the loins, and drew off about 8 ounces of blood. A letter from the doctor who had attended the patient informed me that he had found as much as 12 grains of albumin per ounce, and that for the past ten days the man had been suffering from violent frontal headache. This information was sufficient to confirm the diagnosis of uræmic coma. I prescribed milk. I managed to collect some urine, which contained 7 grains of albumin per ounce. During the next few days his somnolent condition did not change, and he replied imperfectly to questions. I learnt that he had had syphilis fifteen years previously, and was, therefore, hopeful that his condition was dependent on syphilis. In consequence, I prescribed mercury and iodide of potassium—the mercury in the form of the oily solution of biniodide of mercury by injection, and the iodide in doses of 60 grains daily.

In four days improvement was manifest : he passed twice as much urine, and the amount of albumin, which had been 12 grains per ounce, now fell to 5 grains. In the next few days, progressive improvement. The drowsiness and headache disappeared ; the patient spoke without difficulty ; the amount of urine reached 6 pints in twenty-four hours, and contained only a trace of albumin. Eighteen days before he was comatose, and his condition was most grave, but he could now get out of bed and talk like a normal person. This result was due to eighteen injections and to 3½ ounces of iodide of potassium. The specific treatment was stopped for the time being, and resumed a fortnight later, but the patient objected to the strict diet. He now considered himself cured (this idea was premature, as he had still a trace of albumin), and asked to leave the hospital. Six months later he was in good health, the albumin being the only evidence of his nephritis. He was again put under the mercurial and iodide treatment, but left without having the patience to wait for a definite cure.

These cases prove that tertiary syphilis of the kidney shows all the symptoms of ordinary Bright's disease. It is a type of Bright's disease which often commences in a more or less insidious manner. In this type, as in the other types of chronic nephritis, the minor symptoms of Brightism open the scene without otherwise disturbing the patient. During the course of this " syphilo-Brightism," which is intermediate between a state of health and of disease, we find severe epistaxis, attacks of dyspnœa simulating asthma, digestive troubles with vomiting, like those seen in chronic gastritis and œdema of the face and limbs, which help us to clear up a doubtful diagnosis. The tertiary form of renal syphilis may not be chronic from the outset, but may follow acute syphilitic nephritis ; and yet, whatever its mode of onset, it usually ends, in the absence of careful treatment, in grave complications—dyspnœa, coma, delirium, or convulsions.

In some cases, which are fairly common (especially in the case of untreated syphilis), the lesions in the kidney are complicated with syphilis of the liver (painful and deformed liver, jaundice, ascites, etc.). The association of hepatic and renal syphilis, in which amyloid degeneration plays a large part, has been pointed out by Mauriac. Rayer had already noted this fact. Naegel and Wagner have reported cases of it. Brault has reported the following case :

A woman of forty-eight years had albuminuria with œdema of the limbs, which gradually reached the hypochondriac region, and at the same time the liver became painful. The abundant ascites called for repeated paracentesis. She was jaundiced throughout the disease. Post mortem the liver, which only weighed 30 ounces, showed numerous fissures, dividing it into several lobes. The intrahepatic fibrous tissue contained gummata—some almost healed, others large, confluent, and in full growth. The chief change in the liver was diffuse hepatitis of long standing, with amyloid degeneration of the large bloodvessels. The kidneys, which were of normal size, showed amyloid degeneration in almost all the glomeruli.

In some instances the syphilitic lesions are not limited to the kidneys and liver, but invade several organs. The following case, taken from Naegel, will give an idea :

A man, thirty-six years of age, had a chancre at the age of eighteen, and was treated with mercury and iodide of potassium. Ten years later ulcerous syphilides appeared, and seventeen years after the first infection nephritis showed itself. The appearance of œdema and albuminuria was followed by uncontrollable vomiting and most intense dyspnœa; the disease advanced so rapidly that at the end of a year the patient succumbed from cachexia. At the post-mortem examination the kidneys showed interstitial nephritis and amyloid degeneration of the arterioles and of the glomeruli. The arterioles in the liver and spleen were infiltrated with amyloid matter. The heart was enlarged, and the left ventricle, which was hypertrophied, showed no fibrosis, but simply amyloid degeneration. The lungs were œdematous and congested.

It will be well to sum up the question of tertiary renal syphilis briefly.

In the first variety, the disease is attenuated. It does not cause the grave symptoms of Bright's disease, but only the minor symptoms of Brightism and albuminuria, with or without œdema. This form is " **syphilo-Brightism.**"

In the second variety, which is the most common, the course is that of ordinary Bright's disease. It commences more or less insidiously in the form of Brightism, with albuminuria and moderate œdema. Epistaxis, headache, vomiting, dyspnœa, visual troubles, cardiac hypertrophy, etc., may supervene at some later date, and the major symptoms of uræmia only appear if the disease is not suitably treated. Sometimes the onset and the progress of the disease are more sudden and rapid. The œdema is more general (œdema of the lung included); the albumin is more abundant, and the dyspnœa appears earlier. It is probable that severe epithelial lesions are present, in addition to the other changes in the kidneys.

In the third variety, the kidneys are not alone affected. The syphilis also attacks the liver, a coexistence which must always cause grave alarm. Hypertrophy or atrophy of the organ, pain, urobilinuria, icterus, and ascites point to hepatic lesions. Finally, in the fourth variety, the infection is even more general, and several organs are invaded. The liver, spleen, intestines, and heart are invaded by amyloid degeneration, and the patient succumbs from cachexia.

Tertiary syphilis of the kidney may appear some few years after infection or much later—ten, twenty, or thirty years after the chancre. It sometimes shows itself by repeated outbreaks, with intervals of arrest. The symptoms are at first those of syphilo-Brightism, and soon improve, as though the disease were cured ; yet we must not be led astray by this fact, because severe nephritis may reappear later.

A few words more concerning **hereditary** syphilis of the kidneys. We have not at present full data on this subject. It may appear during the course of the first year of life or only fifteen to twenty years later (Fournier). It reveals itself by symptoms similar to those of the acquired disease.

The **diagnosis** is a matter of supposition, because the onset, course, and complications of syphilitic nephritis do not differ from ordinary Bright's disease. If the patient has had syphilis, we may assume that the nephritis is syphilitic. The simultaneous or previous appearance of specific lesions in other regions (gummata of the skin and the mouth, tertiary ulcerations, osteoperiostitis, etc.) has a bearing on the diagnosis—at any rate, in case of Bright's disease. We should always look for syphilis, and if we find evidence in favour of a specific origin for the nephritis, we should at once give specific treatment.

I have now to discuss those obscure cases in which syphilitic albuminuria exists alone, without other symptoms of chronic nephritis. These cases realize what I have called " **the dissociation of the morbid acts of the kidneys.**"

In chronic nephritis albuminuria and insufficient depuration usually appear together, and are connected with renal changes. In other instances, which are more numerous than we might at first think, these two morbid conditions—albuminuria and symptoms of Bright's disease—may remain dissociated for a long time. This dissociation presents itself in various forms : A person may have Bright's disease for a long time without passing albumin ; on the other hand, he may pass albumin for years without getting Bright's disease. I have discussed this question in Section VII., but I mention it again with regard to chronic syphilitic nephritis.

Syphilo-Brightism may exist without albuminuria, and, on the other hand, syphilitic albuminuria may persist without any other symptoms of nephritis. To quote examples :

In 1897 a man came into my consulting-room supporting himself on a stick and dragging his legs. He had paraplegia. He told me that some months before he had. experienced formication, pain, and heaviness, which made walking difficult. These symptoms had been preceded by pains in the loins. His doctor found much albumin present in the urine. Absolute milk diet was prescribed for two months. A second examination of the urine showed that the albuminuria had increased, in spite of the milk diet. When I examined the patient, I found symptoms of slowly progressive paraplegia. As an infantry officer, he was accustomed to long marches, but was now unable to walk fifty steps without stopping. The patellar reflexes were much diminished, especially on the right side. The bladder was sluggish, and although true retention was not present, micturition was slow and difficult. As he had had syphilis eight years before, it was evident that the paraplegia was due to syphilitic mischief in the cord. And as the albuminuria and the paraplegia had come on together, it might be presumed that the kidneys had been attacked simultaneously by syphilis. I found plenty of albumin, but no other symptom of nephritis. Œdema, pollakiuria, cryæsthesia, cramp in the calves of the legs, increased arterial tension, *bruit de galop*, dyspnœa, and any indication of insufficient urinary depuration, were all absent. The kidneys, there-fore, were normal as regards the function of depuration, though they allowed the passage of albumin. There was, therefore, dissociation of the morbid acts of the kidneys.

I ordered mercury and iodides. Six weeks later the improvement was so marked that he could climb several flights of stairs or walk a mile without any fatigue. Although I stopped the milk diet from the first, the albuminuria diminished. The mercurial treatment was resumed, and six months later he rejoined the service, marching several miles without fatigue, and having regained his health. The albuminuria still persists, without any other symptom of Bright's disease. These are probably the cases which Jaccoud had in view when he wrote : " This form of nephritis in which the symptoms of the renal localization are limited to the change of the urine—at least, for a very long time."

Treatment.—Mercury and iodide of potassium are the two best drugs in tertiary syphilis of the kidney. The mercurial preparations are, however, to be preferred. I give injections of an aqueous solution of biniodide of mercury. Iodide of potassium may be given in daily doses of 30 grains. The action of these remedies must be closely watched, because the renal filter is compromised. If only the kidneys are attacked by syphilis, the liver and other organs being free, the treatment gives the best results. We can restore health to patients who have advanced Bright's disease when the disease is due to syphilis.

To bring about complete cure, however, the treatment must be stopped and resumed several times. Tertiary lesions of the kidneys or elsewhere rarely recover at the first attempt. The improvement is often rapid, some-times surprising, but definite cure is difficult to obtain. Sometimes the improvement stops while treatment is being taken ; sometimes the disease reappears at a shorter or longer date after supposed cure. The disease leaves some traces. The nephritis must, therefore, be watched, even when it appears to be cured, and treatment must be resumed when necessary. The cures at Luchon, Uriage, and Aix-la-Chapelle, where thermal baths and mercurial inunction are combined, are of much service. Hospital patients are rarely completely cured, because they leave as soon as they feel some-what better, being unwilling or unable to wait longer. Relapses are also frequent.

The milk cure is not as important in syphilitic as in other forms of nephritis. One of my patients was cured by specific treatment after an absolute milk diet had given no result. Milk is, nevertheless, a useful adjunct. Dechlorination (of which I spoke under Bright's Disease) must be employed in syphilitic nephritis, especially when œdema is present.

XI. CYSTS OF THE KIDNEY—ENLARGED POLYCYSTIC KIDNEY.

Cysts of the kidney may be congenital or acquired. To the latter variety belong (1) the small cysts of interstitial nephritis ; (2) blood cysts ; (3) cystic degeneration in the adult ; (4) hydatid cysts.

1. Congenital Cysts.

Cystic degeneration of the kidney in the fœtus may assume such dimensions as to cause dystocia. The enlarged kidneys press upon and push back the neighbouring organs. The surface is nodular, and a section of the kidney shows a number of pockets of variable dimensions. These pockets contain a clear or dark liquid. Many theories have been propounded to explain the formation of these cysts : atrophy of the medullary substance, constriction and obliteration of the straight tubules, distension of the glomeruli (Virchow), or faulty development of the urinary system (Koster). In certain cases this cystic degeneration coincides with other malformations of the fœtus.

2. Cysts of Interstitial Nephritis.

They are of the size of a pin's head or a small pea, and are found on the surface and in the interior of the kidney. They contain a colloid substance, and are due either to enlargement of the tubules, which are constricted by the fibrous tissue, or to dilatation of the glomeruli.

3. Blood Cysts.

Blood cysts probably have their origin in obliteration of a tubule. They become fairly large. Hæmorrhage takes place from the vascular lining membrane, and the liquid, which is more or less clear, contains granules of hæmatosin and crystals of hæmatoidin (Lancereaux).

4. The Enlarged Polycystic Kidney—Cystic Degeneration.

Pathological Anatomy.—Cystic degeneration of the kidneys in the adult somewhat resembles that seen in the fœtus. Both kidneys are always affected, but to a different extent and at a different time. Each kidney may weigh 30 or 40 ounces. The polycystic kidney often looks like a bunch of grapes. The single grapes are not of the same shape and size, and are said to be formed by the cystic pockets. These anfractuous pockets, which may be isolated or fused, are filled with opaque or transparent fluid of various colours and kinds. The fluid may be serous, albuminous, gelatiniform, or purulent, and often contains urea, chlorides, and phosphates. In a cyst of average size fibrous bands divide it into compartments. The walls are thin, and the renal parenchyma between the cysts may be healthy or may undergo fibrous change. The renal tissue is finally replaced by fibrous or cystic tissue. The cysts arise in the cortex, and extend into the medullary substance.

The polycystic kidney often contracts adhesions with the liver, diaphragm, spleen, lumbar fascia, or duodenum. They are sometimes surrounded by a shell of fibro-adipose tissue, such as is seen in all chronic affections of the kidneys, and arises in the perirenal fat. A perinephritic abscess may be found. When the organ is not kept in place by adhesions, it becomes movable. The ureter and the pelvis are of normal size and patency—a condition opposite to that found in hydronephrosis. The left side of the heart may be hypertrophied, just as in chronic nephritis.

The liver often shows cystic degeneration. This simultaneous degeneration of the liver and of the kidneys is fairly common. Lejars has collected seventeen cases. The changes in the liver are similar to those seen in the kidney. The organ becomes enormous and may weigh 8 or 10 pounds (Sabourin). Its surface is studded with reddish or brownish transparent cysts, from the size of a pea to that of an apple. The cysts commence on the surface under the capsule, and spread into the deep tissue of the organ. On section, the liver has the appearance of a hive, the cystic pockets being more or less shut off.

The lesions in the kidneys and the liver may be successive or simultaneous, but have no tendency to become general. The lesion of the kidneys remains confined to that organ. It invades neither the glands nor the neighbouring tissues.

The formation of the polycystic kidney is a matter of supposition. " In spite of its character as an epithelial tumour which establishes its relation to the new growths, cystic degeneration of the kidneys does not tend to become general. It never, therefore, resembles a cystic epithelioma of invading tendency. It is a transformation of the organ in situ, analogous to that which may be found in the liver, breast, or testicle " (Brault).

Description.—The symptoms show extraordinary variation. I shall describe some of the various forms. They will also give an idea of the extreme difficulty in diagnosis.

In the first variety the disease is latent. A post-mortem examination is performed on a patient who has died of some other malady, such as tuberculosis or pneumonia, and the surprise is great on finding two polycystic kidneys. This latency is not difficult to explain. As long as one of the kidneys performs its functions sufficiently well, or as long as there remains in the kidneys sufficient renal substance to assure urinary depuration, the cystic disease, which is harmless in nature, may pass unnoticed. It may not cause pain, hæmaturia, or uræmic symptoms, and the patient may die from another disease before the renal lesion has given rise to symptoms. I am of the opinion that, while the renal substance is completely atrophied or fibrous in some cases, it is hypertrophied in others. Chantreuil has published a case of this kind. This compensatory hyperplasia, if verified, would be analogous with the compensatory hypertrophy of the liver, described under Hypertrophic Alcoholic Cirrhosis and Hydatid Cysts of the Liver.

In the second variety hæmaturia is the first and most important symptom of polycystic kidney. Slight or severe hæmaturia, which comes on in attacks, and is often accompanied by pain, is a frequent symptom in poly-cystic kidney ; but there are other cases in which hæmaturia is the chief symptom, and, indeed, causes errors in diagnosis. For example :

A woman, forty-two years of age, had sharp pains in the loins and attacks of hæma-turia, which lasted for about a month. After an interval, the pains returned, together with the hæmaturia. A year later pains in the lumbar region and the right hypochon-drium, accompanied by hæmaturia, lasting a fortnight. Pneumonia came on a year later ; it commenced and ended with attacks of hæmaturia, which lasted from two to three days. An indefinite swelling was now found in the right hypochondrium, and as profuse hæmaturia occurred, cancer of the right kidney was suspected. Later, the patient was taken ill with fever, vomiting, and coma, which proved fatal. At the post-mortem examination polycystic degeneration of the right kidney and of the liver was found. The left kidney was also polycystic.

In the third variety pain is the initial or chief symptom. It is common in polycystic kidney, and may be attributed to various causes—to the size of the tumour, to its mobility, to its displacement, to its adhesions, to cystic or perirenal suppuration ; but in other cases the pain appears from the first without evident cause. For example :

A man, thirty-seven years of age, was admitted, under Hanot, for acute pains in the left side and vomiting. As the pains radiated into the groin and testicle, they seemed to indicate renal colic. Three days before, the pain in the loin had been so severe that the patient applied a blister. On admission, the pain was most marked in the left flank, was increased by pressure, and radiated into the right hypochondrium. For some eighteen years he had felt, without apparent cause, acute pains in the hypo-chondria or the flanks. The pains lasted for several days, and the patient was com-pelled to keep his bed. During the attack the pains were continuous. The urine contained albumin. Vomiting and diarrhœa appeared. In spite of milk diet, dyspnœa, and prostration, vomiting and diarrhœa, and almost complete anuria were present, and the patient succumbed in coma. At the post-mortem examination polycystic de-generation of both kidneys was discovered ; the left kidney was most affected, and weighed 40 ounces, while the right one weighed 25 ounces.

In the fourth variety symptoms of uræmia or of Bright's disease are from the outset predominant. As a rule, they supervene at an advanced stage of the disease, when the glandular substance of the kidneys is no longer equal to effecting urinary depuration ; but in other cases the degeneration of the kidneys is latent until the ordinary symptoms of chronic nephritis appear. Legrand quotes the following case :

A man, forty-nine years of age, admitted for violent headache, causing insomnia. He seemed stupefied, and answered with great difficulty. He had never been ill until two years before, when he showed signs of Brightism : buzzing in the ears and defective hearing, violent cramps in the calves of the legs, the sensation of dead fingers, acute itchings, cryæsthesia in the legs, and matutinal epistaxis. The more serious symptoms of uræmia then appeared : continuous headache, paroxysms of dyspnœa, vomiting, and diarrhœa. Œdema of the face and legs had appeared at intervals during the past two years. The urine was clear and abundant, but did not at the time contain any albumin ; it, however, contained about 3 grains to the pint ten days later ; dissociation of the morbid acts of the kidney. These symptoms pointed strongly to interstitial nephritis. He was put on milk diet, but the mischief made rapid progress, and ended in fatal coma. Post-mortem : no chronic nephritis, but only polycystic degeneration of both kidneys, which resembled large bunches of grapes, and were composed of cysts of various sizes and colours.

Polycystic degeneration of the kidneys not only gives rise to symptoms of urinary insufficiency, but also to all the symptoms which are at times seen in chronic nephritis—viz., high arterial tension, hypertrophy of the left side of the heart, with *bruit de galop*, profuse epistaxis, and cerebral hæmorrhage, followed by apoplexy or hemiplegia.

The polycystic kidney is not always evident on palpation. A tumour was noticed but eighteen times in sixty-two cases collected by Lejars. It is almost always in a **forward direction** that the polycystic tumour must be sought, because all renal tumours usually have a tendency to project forwards. The tumour, whether mobile or not, may be felt on bimanual palpation (Guyon). While both kidneys are enlarged, one is, as a rule, so much larger than the other that it is hardly ever possible to feel both organs. The discovery of a tumour on each side simplifies the diagnosis.

Course of the Disease.—The cases above mentioned show that polycystic degeneration of the kidneys does not run a regular course. Hæmaturia and pain are generally early symptoms. A tumour which can be felt gradually appears after some time. At a given moment the signs of Brightism, albuminuria, and œdema appear, and patients are carried off by uræmia, in the absence of some other intercurrent affection. While this is the usual course of events, the polycystic degeneration is insidious in other cases. The predominance of symptoms of Bright's disease causes it to simulate chronic nephritis. The predominance of pains, with or without attacks of hæmaturia, causes it to simulate renal calculus. The abundance and obstinacy of the hæmaturia (with or without a renal tumour) cause it to simulate cancer of the kidney. Diagnosis, therefore, is often extremely difficult, especially as cystic degeneration of the liver may also complicate the situation. Rigors and high fever in the course of polycystic degeneration indicate purulent infection. Pus may form in the cystic cavities, and give rise to abscesses, which open into the pelvis (pyuria). Sometimes the suppuration leads to a perinephritic abscess.

The course of polycystic degeneration is very slow, and its duration indeterminate, but its termination is fatal, because surgery is powerless in a disease which gradually destroys both kidneys.

XII. HYDATID CYSTS OF THE KIDNEYS.

Pathological Anatomy.—In order of frequency hydatid cysts of the kidney come next to those of the liver and the lungs. The proportion is as follows: Liver, 166; lungs, 42; kidneys, 30 (Davaine). The disease is usually limited to one kidney—the left more frequently than the right. The lesion commences, as a rule, in the cortex. The cyst may be multilocular or unilocular, and in the latter case it varies in size from an egg to a child's head. The structure and the life-history of the cyst have been fully described under Hydatid Cysts of the Liver. The only peculiarities to be noted are that the cysts of the kidney sometimes contain crystals of uric acid or phosphate and oxalate of lime, which have penetrated into the cyst by dialysis.

The hydatid cyst of the kidney sometimes contracts adhesions with the liver, the spleen, the stomach, the mesentery, and the intestine; these adhesions become vascular, and interfere with surgical intervention. The affected kidney is sometimes reduced to a fibrous shell; at other times some glandular substance is preserved. The remnants of the renal tissue may show interstitial or parenchymatous nephritis. In some cases a few pieces of the glandular tissue escape destruction, and undergo compensatory hypertrophy. The question of compensatory hyperplasia in the glandular organs is very interesting, and is becoming well known as far as certain organs are concerned. It will be found described in detail under Alcoholic Hypertrophic Cirrhosis and Hydatid Cysts of the Liver. I have seen it in hydatid cysts of the spleen, and it is also met with in cysts of the kidney. We might say that the organ regenerates, to supplement the destroyed portions. Regeneration of the glandular substance sometimes takes place in a cystic kidney. Sometimes the healthy kidney is hypertrophied. In this respect Braillon quotes a case of Blackburn. The kidney and ureter were absent on the right side. The left kidney became affected with a hydatid cyst, and post mortem it was found that the glandular substance not invaded by the cyst had increased threefold in size.

The **pathogenesis** of hydatid cysts of the kidney is still somewhat obscure. Neisser and Boeckel have, nevertheless, attempted to explain it as follows:

The eggs of the tænia are introduced into the digestive passages by the food. When they reach the intestine, they may follow various routes. They may be transported to the liver by the portal vein, which explains the presence of cysts in the liver. They may be transported to the mesentery by the lymphatics (cysts of the mesentery). They continue their wanderings through the lymphatic networks, and give rise to cysts of the peritoneum and of the pleura. They follow the track of the lymphatic vessels as far as the thoracic canal, which empties them into the venous system and the right side of the heart. Thence they penetrate into the lungs (hydatid cysts of the lungs). They may continue their path through the lungs, reach the left side of the heart, and be launched into the general circulation (hydatid cysts of the brain, muscles, spleen, and kidneys).

Symptoms.—The hydatid cyst of the kidney develops slowly, until it has acquired a fair size, and the patient only feels slight pain and heaviness in the lumbar region. Sometimes, however, hæmaturia appears early in the history of the case, resembling the hæmoptysis that is so frequent at any early stage in hydatid cyst of the lung. After a variable time a tumour becomes manifest. If the tumour is formed at the upper pole of the kidney, it may be in such close relation with the liver or the spleen that the diagnosis becomes very difficult. If it develops at the lower pole, it projects into the iliac fossa. The cyst may suppurate, as described under Hydatids of the Liver, and the pus then escapes by various routes.

Rupture is almost always preceded by suppuration in the cyst. Perforation is commonly preceded by pain, rigors, fever, anorexia, and prostration, which indicate infection of the hydatid cyst.

Perforation usually takes place into the pelvis and ureter. It may be spontaneous or brought on by trauma. At the moment of perforation the patient experiences a sharp pain, a sensation of tearing in the lumbar region. Liquid débris of membranes and small hydatid vesicles soon become engaged in the ureter, and give rise to violent pains along the ureter, in the perineum, in the penis, and in the buttock, with retraction of the testicle, nausea, and vomiting. Nothing is wanting. If the foreign body passes into the bladder, the colic ceases. Arrest of the membranes or the vesicles in the ureter may cause hydronephrosis or pyonephrosis. Their retention in the bladder may cause pain and frequent micturition. Their arrest in the urethra may cause retention of urine, and necessitate catheterization. If after rupture the contents pass freely through the urinary tract, the patient passes, according to circumstances, colourless or turbid purulent liquid (which may be offensive), blood-stained fluid, bits of hydatids, vesicles, or phosphatic concretions. Examination of the liquid shows hooklets and characteristic stratified membranes. The evacuation of the cyst by the urinary passages, however, may not take place at one time. The same troubles will be repeated each time a fresh discharge occurs. The fluid will pass readily. Such is not the case with the hydatids, the shreds of the cyst wall, and the débris, rich in cholesterin and phosphates, found in old cysts. We must also remember the possible infection of the urinary passages.

In other cases the hydatid opens into the small intestine or the colon. The patient has acute abdominal pains, and passes foul-smelling liquid, membranes, and at times many hydatid vesicles. As the intestine offers a free passage to the hydatids, recovery generally occurs.

Rupture of the cyst into the bronchi is much less favourable. The symptoms are in every respect similar to those seen when a hydatid of the liver ruptures into the bronchi. The cyst has been known to open through the skin of the lumbar region. The perforation is, then, preceded by the formation of an abscess, and is followed by a fistula.

The **diagnosis** is a matter of supposition. A feeling of heaviness or pain and hæmaturia appear, and later a tumour is felt. This tumour varies in size, and may be mobile or fixed. It tends to project either backwards, towards the lumbar region, or forwards, into the abdominal cavity. We must decide whether it is a floating kidney, a hydronephrosis, a cyst of the spleen, mesentery, or liver, an ovarian cyst, or a lipoma of the mesentery. The records of cases show the difficulties in diagnosis, and mistakes have often been corrected by puncture, operation, or post-mortem examination.

Hydatid cyst of the kidney, though grave, is infinitely less serious than polycystic degeneration, because the latter lesion is always double and the former is almost always single. Symptoms of Bright's disease and death from uræmia, which are the rule in polycystic degeneration, are, therefore, not met with in hydatid cyst. Such a condition might, however, arise if by chance the hydatid cyst is bilateral, and if the lesion so affects both kidneys as to cause insufficient depuration, as in a case I saw with Berger.

A woman was suffering from an enormous hydatid cyst of the left kidney. Profuse hæmaturia was the first sign. The bleeding recurred on several occasions, and was accompanied by a feeling of weight, sharp pain radiating in various directions, and the appearance of a tumour. The tumour was at first thought to be malignant. After a slow course, it quickly increased to an enormous size, and became fluctuating. Berger drew off by puncture a large quantity of clear, non-albuminous hydatid liquid. As the liquid reformed, two more punctures were made, and injections of sublimate were given, without any better result. As the tumour occupied the left flank and a part of the umbilical region, and was therefore difficult to attack by the lumbar route, the abdomen was opened. The descending colon was in front of the tumour, which was clearly retroperitoneal, and on incision contained a large number of hydatid vesicles, but no pus. The lining membrane was removed piecemeal, and recovery was complete at the end of two months. A little later I noticed symptoms of Brightism, with albuminuria, cardiac hypertrophy, and a *bruit de galop*. I should say that albuminuria had been present from the first. In any case, it was evident that the opposite kidney, which had apparently been healthy, was now invaded either by the hydatid or by concomitant nephritis. Uræmia set in, and the patient died in convulsions.

The only treatment in hydatid cyst of the kidney is surgical intervention. Simple aspiratory puncture without injection may be enough, but in the case of failure an operation must be performed.

XIII. CANCER OF THE KIDNEY.

Pathological Anatomy.—Cancer of the kidney may be primary or secondary. The secondary form is consequent on cancer of the testicle, uterus, or stomach, and is made up of nodules, which are usually situated in the cortex, and are of the same nature as the primary growth.

The primary form is almost always unilateral, and it does not spare youth, with the exception, well understood, of cases of sarcoma, which are peculiar to childhood. The growth may be encephaloid, scirrhous, colloid, or melanotic, but the encephaloid form is the most common. " Whether the cancer of the kidney is soft (encephaloid cancer), of an elastic consistency (adenoma), or fairly firm (scirrhous variety), it is always formed of epithelial tissue ; and we have never met with a cancer of the kidney which was not a well-marked epithelioma " (Brault).

The kidney generally preserves its shape. Its weight varies from 2 to 20 pounds. Nodules covered with vessels are often seen. On section, the consistency of the organ varies. The newly-formed portions often have an adenomatous appearance. The furrows which separate them from the healthy portions are almost always festooned (Brault). Compensatory hypertrophy has been noted by Albarran. The cancer sometimes forms a mass, encysted, as it were, in the distended capsule, and no trace of the pelvis or the orifice of the obliterated ureter can be found. Cancerous vegetations which have perforated the mucosa, frequently project into the pelvis.

The growth often commences in the upper pole of the kidney, first attacking the cortex and then spreading into the medulla. The tumour is diffuse, or is composed of nodules, and the tissue between them undergoes fibrous thickening. The capsule of the kidney may resist the onset of the growth for some time. Secondary infection occurs late, as a rule, and, therefore, the patient in some cases may survive five or six years. In the statistics compiled by Roberts secondary growths occurred in thirty-one of his fifty-one cases. In Ebstein's statistics they were found in almost half the number of cases.

The ureter is often obliterated, and converted into a rigid mass by the growth. The hilum of the kidney is often invaded by the cancer. The glands are large and adherent, and the arteries resist for a long time, but the veins of the hilum are sometimes perforated by cancerous nodules. A nodule has been found to start in the renal vein, and, then, to assume such dimensions that it penetrated the inferior vena cava, and reached up into the right auricle, which it partly filled (Brault). The vessels of the hilum, if not invaded, may be compressed by the cancerous mass. This compression may give rise to thrombi, which form in the renal vein, and reach into the inferior vena cava and right auricle, thus causing œdema of the lower limbs and of the lower half of the trunk.

The growth may spread by contiguity or by infection through the veins and lymphatics. The fibrous capsule offers such resistance that propagation by contiguity is relatively rare. When the infection takes place through the bloodvessels and lymphatics, it affects the lungs, the liver, the lumbar and mesenteric glands, and the suprarenal capsule. The vertebræ are also invaded by the cancer. If cancer of the kidney rarely invades the genito-urinary organs, it is on account of the direction of the lymph flow. For a similar reason cancer of the genito-urinary organs very often invades the kidney (Guillet). The heart is often dilated and hypertrophied—a fact which, by the way, is seen in the various tumours of the abdomen.

Description.—Pain, hæmaturia, the development of an abdominal tumour, and symptomatic varicocele are the general symptoms of renal carcinoma. The first point to remember, however, is that cancer of the kidney may be absolutely latent.

Renal Cancer of the Latent Type.—The kidney at times shows such great toleration that Rayer gave a special description of "latent cancer." Secondary cancer is no doubt more often latent than primary cancer, but still latency may occur in both cases. Tuffier gives a clear account of latent primary cancer :

A patient, over fifty years of age, gradually lost his strength, and became of a pale yellow colour, although no viscus appeared to be diseased. The urine showed a very slight trace of albumin at times. The weakness became extreme, and the anorexia was complete. Signs of compression appeared, affecting the pleuræ, the lungs, and the mediastinal organs, and the patient succumbed. The post-mortem examination showed a primary cancer of the kidney, which had destroyed the entire organ, and had given rise to cancerous nodules in other organs.

Secondary cancer of the kidney is frequently quite latent. Tuffier reports the following case :

A labourer, twenty-six years of age, was admitted to hospital for a tumour in the right iliac fossa. The patient had been growing weak for the past three months, when a painless tumour was discovered by accident in the right flank. He continued his work, when he was taken ill with pain and symptoms of phlebitis in the right leg. On examining the patient, a tumour was found filling the right hypochondrium, reaching up as far as the umbilicus, and descending into the iliac fossa as far as Poupart's ligament. The tumour was hard, nodular, adherent to the deep parts, dull on percussion, and absolutely painless. The only symptom was increasing weakness. He died without having shown any renal symptoms. Post-mortem : primary cancer of the right suprarenal capsule, and in the enlarged right kidney seven to eight hard or soft cancerous tumours, which had destroyed almost all the glandular substance of the kidney.

Renal Cancer of the Painful Type.—Cancer of the kidney causes pain, which may be due to adhesions, displacement of the enlarged organ, or compression of the neighbouring nerves. These pains are more or less severe, and generally paroxysmal. They may be felt in the lumbar region or the hypochondria, and may radiate towards the intercostal spaces, like intercostal neuralgia. The pains sometimes precede or accompany the hæmaturia, and the clots in their migration through the ureter often provoke renal colic.

These varieties of pain in renal cancer are classical. There are, however, cases in which pain becomes the chief symptom of renal cancer, the other symptoms being of minor importance. To quote an example :

A man, aged forty, was admitted under Brault for severe pains in the hypochondrium, the flank, and the right side. These pains were continuous, and radiated into the epigastrium, the buttock, and the testicle, resembling the lightning-like pains of tabes. Walking, palpation, and pressure, brought on pain, which was so acute that the patient was doubled up in agony. Careful examination of the organs revealed neither albumin nor an abdominal tumour. Fever, however, appeared. The situation grew worse ; the patient became thin, the pain was most intense, and the patient finally succumbed. The post-mortem examination revealed cancer of the right kidney. The kidney was normal in size. It was adherent to the vertebral column, against which it was flattened by the growth in the peritoneal tissue ; a prolongation of the growth sheathed the aorta and vena cava, and penetrated the psoas. The pressure on the lumbar and sacral nerves by the perirenal tumour explained the persistence, violence, and radiation of the pains.

This case supports the idea put forth by Roberts that, as far as renal lesions are concerned, sharp and continuous pain in the area supplied by a given nerve indicates that the tumour extends beyond the normal limits of the kidney. These obstinate cases of neuralgia may depend upon attacks of congestion, which for a time increase the size of the kidney, and thus assist in the compression of the nerve trunks. In one of Tuffier's patients the pains became terrible within the sphere of the crural nerve just before an attack of hæmaturia, and grew better as soon as there was free flow of blood—that is to say, as soon as the congestion ceased.

Renal Cancer of the Hæmaturic Type.—Cancer stands first among the lesions of the kidney, accompanied by bleeding. Hæmaturia is frequently met with. It sometimes appears suddenly at the onset of the affection in subjects who are in good health ; at other times it appears only at an advanced stage. It lasts for a few days or weeks, and, then, disappears completely for one or two months. It may or may not reappear. The colour of the urine varies from pale red to black, according to the amount of the hæmorrhage. Clots which are moulded in the ureter may be present. They are very thin, and measure 5 or 6 inches in length. Such clots are never seen in vesical hæmorrhage The passage of the clots through the ureter sometimes causes pain like that of renal colic, and, on the other hand, in obstruction of the ureter by a clot the urine may be quite clear, because the bladder only receives urine from the healthy kidney. Obstruction of the urethra by a clot may cause retention of urine, calling for the use of the catheter.

The hæmaturia sometimes is so profuse that it becomes the chief symptom. As an example :

A man of about fifty years of age, who had always been in excellent health, had been taken ill three years previously (without cause, warning, or pain), with such profuse hæmaturia that the liquid voided filled half a chamber with blood. Next day there was retention of urine, which yielded on the passage of a catheter ; long clots were passed for several days following. For six months the patient was quite well, and then, without the least warning, he passed blood and clots for several days. Nothing happened for eight months, and then the same trouble occurred : passage of blood and clots, pain, and retention of urine. Since that time the hæmaturia appeared for several days every month. Hæmaturia had been so far the only sign. Two years after the first attack of hæmaturia the physicians in St. Petersburg discovered a tumour of the right kidney, which was confirmed in Vienna and in Paris. Guyon diagnosed cancer of the right kidney ; fresh attacks of hæmaturia appeared. The tumour was now as large as a fœtal head, and occupied the right flank. Above, it reached up to the false ribs ; below, it descended to within an inch or two of the iliac crest. The tumour was movable in all directions, and absolutely painless on palpation. Hæmaturia remained the chief symptom of this renal cancer. The fragments of cancer and the cells which are so frequently met with in the urine when cancer of the bladder is present are not found in cancer of the kidney. The appearance of a varicocele is a fairly frequent symptom (Guyon). It is especially apparent during walking or standing. Its development is rapid and is sometimes unknown to patients.

Tumour.—The development of a tumour, though a fairly late symptom, is rarely wanting. The tumour is at first deeply seated in the flank, and is not easily made out. It may, however, be discovered on bimanual palpation. One hand is placed behind, in the costo-vertebral angle, and the other hand is placed in front, on a level with the rectus muscle. The examiner gives repeated pushes to the lumbar wall with the posterior hand, and the kidney transmits a feeling of ballottement to the other hand. When the tumour is somewhat larger, it has a tendency to leave the lumbar region, and project in a forward direction. In this case the posterior hand pushes the tumour against the anterior hand. The tumour is, then, felt to move with difficulty. When the tumour grows very large, it fills the iliac fossa, crosses the median line, and invades the other side of the belly.

The cancerous tumour has a " renal " shape. It is hard and resistant. It pushes the intestine forwards, and a resonant note is, therefore, obtained over its anterior surface. Sometimes the resonance is replaced by dullness when the cæcum and the colon remain internal to the kidney, and the tumour comes in direct contact with the abdominal wall, after having pushed aside the resonant intestine (Tuffier).

Diagnosis.—The signs just enumerated will help us to diagnose a renal cancer. Nevertheless, in many cases we meet with great difficulties. On what symptom can we rely ? Take hæmaturia, for instance. If it appears before a tumour is present, it tells us nothing, because the hæmorrhage caused by calculi, tuberculosis, etc., may simulate the early hæmorrhage of renal cancer. If it appears when a tumour has formed, it also tells us nothing, for the kidney may be enlarged by tuberculosis, calculi, or cysts, and hæmaturia may occur in these conditions, just as in cancer. These remarks hold good in the case of the pain and tumour. It is sometimes difficult to know whether the tumour is or is not renal. The diagnosis from sarcomatous and fatty subperitoneal tumours is so difficult that in several cases the error has only been discovered at the operation. Although tumours of the ovary and uterus are readily distinguished from tumours of the kidney, mistakes have been made, and Billroth wrongly took myxosarcoma of the kidney for fibroma of the uterus. It is also hard to distinguish cancer of the kidney from tumours of the spleen. In the latter case we do not find the resonance of the colon. Examination of the urine is important in diagnosis, and in the absence of marked hæmaturia, we can generally find **histological hæmaturia.** The microscope reveals red corpuscles in the centrifugalized urea, and the ingenious segregator of Luys allows us to collect the urine from each kidney. By comparison of the urines we can ascertain the side of the lesion.

Amongst the complications of renal cancer I may mention compression of the portal vein (ascites), of the inferior vena cava (œdema of the legs), and of the common bile-duct (icterus), lesions of the spine and compression of the spinal cord (paraplegia), pulmonary embolism, intestinal occlusion, peritonitis, and pulmonary tuberculosis. Cancer and calculi often occur together, just as in cancer of the gall-bladder, we frequently find gall-stones. A new growth in the pelvis may lead to infection of the kidney, by causing retention of urine.

Cancer of the kidney develops very slowly, and has the least tendency to become general of the visceral cancers. Its average duration is from two to three years, and may even extend to five or six years. Death is caused by cachexia or by one of the complications already enumerated. The treatment consists in removal of the kidney.

XIV. RENAL CALCULI.

Precipitation of the salts in the urine leads to concretions in the kidneys, which are termed, according to size, "infarcts," "gravel," or "calculi." The infarct is an intracanalicular deposit, more frequent in the medulla than in the cortex. It is calcareous or uratic, and is chiefly seen in new-born children and in gouty subjects.

Gravel and calculi very rarely exist in the actual substance of the kidney. It is in the calices and the pelvis that they are found. They may be of all sizes, from sand to stones as big as a hen's egg. They are situated in the depressions around the papillæ, the calices, the pelvis, in which they mould themselves, and even in the ureters. The small gravel is rounded, polyhedral, irregular, raspberry-shaped, or faceted. The large stone is mammillated, of an hour-glass shape, angular, or branched like coral, taking the shape of the calices and of the pelvis. The large stone may be single, but more frequently it is accompanied by one or more pieces of gravel. In about half the number of cases only one kidney is affected.

Pathogenesis.—It is usual to describe secondary and primary lithiasis. The former variety supervenes during the course of a suppurative lesion of the kidney. Pyelonephritis may occur in renal tuberculosis, polycystic degeneration of the kidney, or in ascending infection, and the suppuration and fermentation in the urine, then, furnish most favourable soil for the development of secondary calculi. The phosphates impregnate the necrosed matter, the organic waste products become calcified, and a phosphatic concretion forms. Litten has produced these calculi experimentally by interrupting the circulation in the kidney of a dog. The epithelium began to calcify, and the canaliculi were filled with calcareous salts. Secondary calculi are almost always formed of ammonio-magnesium carbonates and phosphates. They are greyish, chalky, and friable. Their presence explains the renal colic sometimes seen in people suffering from suppurative lesions of the kidney.

The primary calculi are of a different composition and origin, being composed of urates and oxalates. They may be small or large, and are hard and resistant. The small stones are rounded, smooth, and brownish. They are mulberry-shaped and reddish if oxalic acid predominates. The large stones are branched like coral or moulded in the shape of the renal pelvis. Uric and oxalic gravels may occur together, the oxalic acid being derived from the uric acid by more complete oxidation. The uric acid gravel is favoured by generous living, want of exercise, and inactivity of the skin—in a word, by circumstances capable of increasing the quantity of uric acid. It is likewise favoured by all causes which lead to imperfect metabolism and diminished solubility of the uric acid (Bouchard). While this theory is true, in practice we meet people living under the best hygienic conditions who suffer from gravel and renal colic.

In most cases the dominant factor in primary lithiasis is the gouty diathesis. This side of the question has been clearly put by Trousseau. Renal gravel may be transmitted directly, and a father suffering from gravel may beget children who suffer from gravel ; but the factor which is especially transmitted is the special predisposition that reveals itself in the descendants by various manifestations—gout, asthma, migraine, obesity, eczema, gallstones, and intestinal lithiasis, and I would add appendicular lithiasis.

An individual who during his youth has suffered from migraine, hæmorrhoids, or eczema, may later be troubled with gout, asthma, and renal colic. Renal lithiasis is often related to the gouty diathesis. " I have nephritis and you have the gout," Erasmus wrote to one of his friends. " We have married two sisters." Gout and gravel commonly occur in the same subject. Renal lithiasis is common in children.

The puerperal state favours the formation of calculi, and I have quoted several cases in a clinical lecture on the relation of pregnancy and lithiasis.* Renal colic may supervene during pregnancy or after accouchement. At first sight it simulates the onset of labour or peritonitis. A careful study of the case will clear up the diagnosis. However violent the pains of renal colic may be, the prognosis is good, and the woman goes to full term without accident.

The greater frequency of gravel in certain countries (England, Holland) and in certain localities has given rise to the view that local conditions (drinking-water, nature of the soil) play some part in the pathogenesis.

We cannot absolutely separate secondary or phosphatic lithiasis from primary or uric-acid lithiasis. Many calculi are both phosphatic and oxalic. Arthritic patients suffering from so-called primary lithiasis and renal colic pass phosphatic and uratic calculi, and examples are not wanting of secondary lithiasis characterized by oxalic and phosphatic stones. Speaking generally, in this, as in every other kind of lithiasis, the genesis of the calculi does not consist only in a deposit and an agglomeration of mineral substances. Two elements in variable proportions—the one organic and the other inorganic—are always required. In renal calculi the organic substance is formed of albuminoid matter—peptone, mucus, epithelial cells, and perhaps micro-organisms. Traces of all of these are found in the nucleus or in the reticulum of the calculus. The inorganic element has been described under the different varieties of Uratic, Oxalic, and Phosphatic Calculi.

I have just given an idea of lithiasis of the kidneys and of the mode of formation of the calculi. The kidneys may tolerate for a long time the presence of one or more calculi, but for multiple reasons, which I shall enumerate, certain troubles may appear. They are as follows:

1. **Mobile calculi—renal colic.**
2. **Fixed calculi—pain and hæmaturia.**
3. **Calculous anuria—uræmia.**
4. **Calculous pyelonephritis.**
5. **Calculous perinephritis.**
6. **Calculous fistulæ.**
7. **Fibrosis and renal atrophy.**

1. Renal Colic—Mobile Calculi.

Description.—Gravel which is too large or too anfractuous to pass freely through the ureter may cause the syndrome of renal colic. The attack may come on suddenly, without prodromata, or it may be preceded by a

* *Clinique Médicale de l'Hôtel-Dieu*, 1898, 15me leçon.

prodromal period of a few hours or a few days, well known to persons who have already had renal colic. This period is characterized by the following symptoms : Dull or acute pains, simulating lumbago ; a feeling of weight in the kidneys or the anus ; painful swelling of the testicle ; burning at the tip of the penis ; frequent desire to make water ; discharge of sand and blood-stained urine ; and abdominal tympanites. In some cases renal colic comes on during violent exercise, or after the use of diuretic water in the course of a cure.

The attack commences with sharp pain on one side in the lumbar region. After some time the pain becomes more severe, and spreads to the flank. Marked retraction of the testicle is seen from the first. The pain is of a stabbing character, and radiates along the ureter to the penis, the urethra, the glands, the perineum, the rectum, and the buttocks. The patient suffers the greatest agony, and tries by every possible means to lessen the pain. The pulse is small ; the face is pale and covered with sweat ; the extremities are cold. Nausea and vomiting are frequent, and the patient, after much straining, passes a few drops of urine. Fever is generally absent.

The attack may last for six or eight hours, or longer, without intermission. The end of the attack is often announced by a violent paroxysm, with or without vomiting, and when the gravel, after its difficult passage through the ureter, enters the bladder, all the symptoms at once cease, and the patient experiences an unspeakable feeling of relief, often falling asleep. After the attack, the patient passes either abundant clear urine or dull, brownish urine. The lumbar region remains painful. Slight hæmaturia may persist for several days. The patient often passes not only gravel, but also coarse sand, blood, and thin fibrinous clots, which may be coloured or colourless, and which float in the urine like worms.

Gravel is not, as a rule, present in the first urine discharged after the attack of colic. It may not appear for a day or two. The urine must be carefully examined in a specimen glass, and when we see the fine yellowish or blackish gravel, no larger than a grain of rice, we may well ask how so small a body can cause such terrible pain. The gravel is sometimes large enough to obstruct the urethra and to cause retention of urine. It must, then, be removed. In a patient who had previously suffered from nephritic colic I noted retention of urine from a large piece of gravel which was arrested in the urethra, preventing the flow of the urine.

In some cases the termination of the attack is not followed by the complete relief already mentioned, and the pain does not entirely cease. The kidneys remain sensitive. The desire to pass water is frequent, and during the same day or the next one fresh attacks occur, so that the colic may last for several days. One of my patients, who was gouty and subject to nephritis had an attack which lasted for twenty days, and ended with the expulsion of a large calculus.

These prolonged attacks of renal colic, comprising a series of ten, fifteen, or twenty successive fits, are, fortunately, very rare. In one of my gouty patients renal colic lasted three weeks, and the calculus was not passed until six weeks after the disappearance of the acute pain. When the expulsion of the calculus occurs as late as this, we may well ask whether the patient is suffering from renal colic due to a calculus or from an attack of renal gout, without a migratory stone. We may also ask whether the calculus in the bladder has not been there for some time, forming the nucleus of a vesical calculus. In the case just mentioned, the pain lasted for three weeks, with an interval of relative calm, and then a second period of three weeks supervened, with gouty pains in the limbs, frequent passage of uric acid, abundant night-sweats, but no fever. It may be said that an attack of gout and an attack of renal colic were combined.

During the attack of colic the patient sometimes experiences throbbing pain in the kidney, in the flank, or along the ureter, analogous to the pain of an abscess which is about to open. Happily, there is no question of an abscess, and the throbbing ceases with the termination of the attack. I have noticed this important symptom in several patients. Renal colic has not always the severe form just described. It may be defaced or reduced to an isolated symptom, such as vomiting. Some patients pass fairly large-sized gravel without any pain. About twenty years ago I attended a patient who was suffering from calculous pyelitis, from which he recovered. He had been previously operated on by Sanson for stone in the bladder, and since that time he passed calculi almost as large as peas without the slightest colic. He had collected a bushel.

Some individuals have but one attack of renal colic during their life, and they are fortunate. In others the attacks occur every year, several times a year, or at intervals of several years. A consoling feature is that the first attacks of colic are the most painful. I do not know whether this is due to tolerance or to a greater extensibility of the ureter, but it is certain that a patient who has suffered terribly can later expel gravel of the same size with much less distress. Renal colic is never bilateral at first, but after attacks of colic caused by calculi in the right kidney attacks of colic may be caused by calculi in the left kidney.

Between the attacks some patients experience a feeling of discomfort and heaviness in the lumbar region, and complain of lumbago. The urine contains coarse reddish sand. In other patients, without warning, the testicle corresponding to the affected kidney becomes painful and swollen. Palpation shows that the testicle is painful, hard, and swollen. These symptoms last some hours, and show that something is happening in the

kidney. It does not always mean the onset of renal colic, but it is often
the signal of congestion of the kidney; and if we examine the urine, we find
that it is of a brownish colour, and contains a blackish deposit of blood and
uric acid. A discharge has just taken place, and, then, everything becomes
normal for the time being. In certain gouty persons the kidney
is nearly always in trouble, and perhaps the above-mentioned discharges of
uric acid and blood act as a safety-valve. In any case, the testicle fairly
often gives us warning, as I have long since noticed.

Renal and biliary gravel often alternate in the same subject.

Diagnosis.—Even moderate care will prevent us from mistaking renal
colic for hepatic colic, appendicitis, or lumbago. It is sometimes very
difficult to distinguish renal pseudo-colic from true colic due to a calculus.
Let me explain.

Maurice Raynaud has shown that certain sufferers from tabes have renal
crises. These renal crises absolutely resemble in symptoms renal colic, and
careful examination for the other signs or stigmata of tabes is necessary for
a diagnosis. Many people having no renal calculus may nevertheless have
the most classical symptoms of renal colic—viz., radiating pains in the loin,
pain, swelling and retraction of the testicle, vomiting, oliguria or anuria
sudden onset and sudden cessation of symptoms. I am not speaking of
attacks of colic due to the passage of blood-clots through the ureter (cancer of
the kidney), but I have in view certain diseases of the kidneys in which the
syndrome of renal colic arises. Such are tuberculosis or new growths of the
kidney, polycystic degeneration, movable kidney, with or without intermittent hydronephrosis and pyelitis. Tuffier has carefully described these
cases of pseudo-colic, showing that it is possible to suffer from severe attacks
of renal colic without renal lithiasis, and even without appreciable lesions
in the kidney or ureter. He groups these cases into two categories, according
as there is or is not an obstacle to the passage of urine through the ureter.

The first category includes all lesions capable of causing sudden and
total obstruction of the ureter, with distension of the pelvis. Such are
pyelonephritis, including renal tuberculosis and intermittent hydronephrosis due to displaced kidney, kinking of the ureter, etc. In such cases
it is probable that the sudden obliteration of the ureter and the stretching
of the pelvis of the kidney produce the syndrome of colic.

In the second category Tuffier places cases of pseudo-colic in which there
is no sign of ureteral obstruction. He quotes an absolutely convincing case:

A young woman had for two years had attacks of renal colic, without hæmaturia
or discharge of gravel. The attacks became more frequent, and the pain was unbearable.
She was looked upon as a neurasthenic patient suffering from neuralgia. Under chloroform, the kidney was felt to be slightly displaced, and Tuffier diagnosed pseudo-colic,
probably symptomatic of a slightly movable right kidney. The medical means employed
(suggestion included) produced no effect. Later, as the pain became worse, an operation

was decided on. The kidney was found to be absolutely healthy, without any adhesions. Acupuncture in all directions failed to reveal any calculus. The kidney was fixed, and complete recovery followed.

The pathogenesis of these forms may, perhaps, be due to congestion of the kidney, consequent on bending of the renal vein. Experiments seem to prove the correctness of this hypothesis.

In any case, the foregoing series of facts proves that nothing resembles renal colic due to calculus more than the attacks of pseudo-colic that have no connection with any calculus. When an individual suffering from renal colic is neither arthritic nor of gouty stock, so that we fail to discover any other stigmata of the gouty diathesis; when the renal colic is never accompanied by the hæmaturia, and is never followed by the discharge of gravel; when the urine, in spite of diuretic treatment, never contains uric acid, it is almost certain that this individual has only pseudo-colic.

Prognosis.—The serious feature is not the colic, but the renal lithiasis, because we are never sure of our ground in these cases. We can readily grasp the truth of this statement by reading of the mishaps and complications. There is, however, a certain inherent gravity, due to the anuria, in renal colic itself.

Treatment.—The first object is to lessen the pain. Injections of morphia, syrup of chloral, or inhalations of chloroform, are used. Tepid baths are of service, and alkaline diuretic drinks (milk with Vichy water) should be given. Aspirin gives excellent results. At the time of the attack two to four cachets, each containing 7 grains, may be given daily, and it is well to use also injections of morphia. Between the attacks the treatment is that of urinary lithiasis. Diet and hygiene fill an important place. Vegetables rich in oxalic acid must be avoided (sorrel or asparagus). Alcoholic beverages, truffles, and game must be forbidden. Carbonate of lithia, in doses of 10 to 20 grains daily, and bicarbonate of soda, in doses of 15 to 30 grains, should be prescribed. A cure at Vittel (Boulomie), at Contrexéville, Châtelguyon, Évian, Vichy, or Carlsbad is of benefit.

2. Large Fixed Calculi—Pains—Hæmaturia.

Renal lithiasis only causes colic when the stones are sufficiently small to engage in the ureter. The larger stones which are fixed in the pelvis may for a long time give rise to no symptoms. Legueu has collected several cases proving that fixation of the calculi under aseptic conditions is favourable to renal tolerance. Do we not find patients in whom anuria, hydronephrosis, pyelitis, and perinephritic abscess are the first indication of renal calculi which have been latent for years? Clark in his statistics has noted thirteen cases of latent calculi in twenty-four cases of stone in the kidneys. Legueu's second case refers to a patient in whom several renal calculi were present, without having given rise to hæmaturia or pain. A fixed stone generally gives rise to two chief symptoms—pain and hæmaturia.

Pain.—A patient with a large calculus experiences a sensation of heaviness in the lumbar region. The pain is increased by pressure, palpation, or percussion, and reappears as the result of exercise. The pain is not, as a rule, continuous, and there is sometimes a truce lasting for weeks or months. In some cases the pain lasts without cessation for years. I had a patient in hospital who had had practically continuous pain for eleven years. Lentz speaks of a young man, eighteen years of age, who had suffered for ten years from pain in the left renal region without other symptoms. The kidney was resected and a large calculus was removed.

The pain caused by a fixed calculus is generally much less severe than the pain of renal colic. It may, however, be very acute, and as it radiates it may simulate the pain of renal colic. Pain is not limited to cases of large calculi. In Le Dentu's case small fixed gravel in the kidneys gave rise to acute pains that rendered an operation necessary. In Moty's case, quoted by Legueu, the pain was almost unbearable for ten years, and yet only one small coral-like calculus was found in the ulcerated kidney. The intensity of the pain is not, therefore, always in proportion to the number or the size of the calculi. It is also due to the hyperæsthesia of the kidney, the renal infection appearing to make the kidney less tolerant.

In many cases the pain due to large calculi is not limited to the lumbar region, but radiates to the testicle, and simulates renal colic. It may radiate towards the abdominal wall, in the form of lumbo-abdominal neuralgia, to the opposite kidney (reno-renal reflex), or to the bladder (vesico-renal reflex). The pain in the bladder may, indeed, be so severe that the diagnosis of vesical, and not of renal, calculus may be made. The pain, radiating into the right iliac fossa, may lead to a diagnosis of appendicitis.

Hæmaturia.—Hæmaturia is the important symptom of calculus. I have already spoken of the slight bleeding which supervenes at the onset of renal colic, and after or between the crises. In such a case hæmaturia forms, so to say, a part of the renal colic, announcing or surviving it. In other cases hæmaturia appears as an isolated symptom of calculi of the kidney, but here again it supervenes in an individual who has previously had renal colic. In such circumstances the pathogenic diagnosis is clear, because hæmaturia is evidently due to the calculi fixed in the kidney. In other cases calculous hæmaturia supervenes in persons who have never had nephritic colic, and the pathogenic diagnosis is, then, more difficult. Pousson's case proves this point :

A farmer, thirty-four years of age, without personal or hereditary disease, having never had renal colic or gravel, complained for several years of pain in the region of the right kidney. These pains did not radiate along the ureter or to the testicle ; they disappeared when the patient rested, and came on when he worked. The urine, which was limpid when the patient did not exert himself, became bloody in consequence of work. These attacks of hæmaturia weakened the patient, and had none of the characteristics of vesical hæmaturia. Palpation of both kidneys revealed no enlargement, but the right kidney was painful on pressure. An operation was performed. Exploratory incision of the kidney revealed a rounded calculus of the size of a hazelnut. The patient recovered completely. "Since that time," says Pousson, "I have repeatedly heard that he has had no more hæmaturia."

Sydenham, who was gouty, writes thus of his own case :

A Dissertation on the Discharge of Blood caused by a Stone in the Kidney.— In the year 1660 I had an attack of gout in the feet, the most severe and longest attack I have ever had. The attack terminated in a dull pain, which I commenced to feel in the left kidney. The gout disappeared, but the pain in the kidney remained. It increased at intervals, but was by no means unbearable, because I never had a single attack of renal colic—a disease always accompanied by vomiting and by acute pain along the ureter towards the bladder. I was, however, quite convinced that I had in the pelvis of one of my kidneys a stone of considerable size, which did not cause symptoms of renal colic, because it was too large to pass through the ureter. What happened at the end of several years proved to me that I was not mistaken, because during the winter of 1666 after a long walk during a great thaw, I passed urine mixed with blood. The same thing happened every time I took long walks or drove in a carriage over a paved road, but it did not happen when the road was not paved. The urine passed was alarming, because it seemed to be nothing but pure blood, and in the deposit the blood was collected in clots at the bottom of the chamber.

This case is typical of hæmaturia, due to a large calculus, and it is marvellous to see with what accuracy Sydenham states the important features of the case—the remarks on the association of gout and renal lithiasis ; the distinction between large and small calculi ; the calculus being unable to pass through the ureter, and not producing colic ; hæmaturia brought on by the jolting of the carriage. Nothing is wanting in this description that is nearly two centuries and a half old. In my lectures at the Faculté I have given the name of "Sydenham's hæmaturia" to hæmorrhage caused by large calculi in the kidney.

In conclusion, large calculi of the kidney may give rise to no symptoms. In most instances, however, they provoke pain and hæmaturia. Pain may exist without hæmaturia, but hæmaturia is always preceded or accompanied by pain. The pain is felt chiefly in the lumbar region ; it is brought on by pressure, and is made worse by violent exercise. The bleeding rarely occurs during rest, but is readily brought on by running, strains, or riding.

Radioscopy is of service, especially in the diagnosis of large calculi. Ringel has made the following experiments on the cadaver : Three varieties of calculi were placed in the pelvis of the kidney, and photographed under identical conditions. The result showed the degree of permeability. The oxalate stone gave as clear an image as a bullet ; the image of the uric-acid stone was not so clear ; the phosphatic stone gave no image. Wagner has employed radiography in the following case : A girl was suffering from a fistula in the left lumbar region. The X rays showed four calculi—one large, and three as big as split-peas. Wagner does not share Ringel's opinion as to the permeability of calculi to the X rays; he considers that uric-acid calculi are very permeable. Léonhard considers that the phosphatic calculi are most permeable; next come the uric-acid stones, and last the oxalate calculi. Hermann and Alsberg report cases of calculi diagnosed by the X rays, the diagnosis being verified at the operation. Lauenstein diagnosed a calculus by means of radioscopy; the stone was composed of carbonate of lime. This case is of much interest because this variety of calculus is not considered favourable for X-ray diagnosis.

The treatment of large renal calculi is purely surgical; many persons, after suffering for several years, have been cured by operation. There is no more justification for leaving a stone in the kidney than there is for leaving one in the bladder.

3. Calculous Anuria.

Description.—Let us first consider calculous anuria, which supervenes during an attack of renal colic.

A lady, forty-three years of age, had for some years suffered from attacks of renal colic; in every attack she had passed gravel and bloody urine. In the last attack she had been suffering for two days from acute pain in the left loin. The pain radiated to the thighs and to the bladder, and was increased by the least movement. The attack was similar to the preceding ones, except that she had passed no urine for two days. On the third day she passed half a wineglassful of urine; on the fourth day the pain was as bad as ever: the patient was anxious, her face was pale and bathed in sweat, the extremities were cold, and she vomited bilious fluid. On the fifth day the lumbar pain was very acute, but no tumour was present; the headache was severe, the vomiting continued. The patient passed some urine which was not blood-stained. On the ninth day the situation became worse, dyspnœa setting in, and the patient died coma-tose on the tenth day.

A man who had in five days passed only a few drops of bloody urine was admitted to the Necker Hospital. As the bladder was empty, it was a case of anuria. The patient had suffered three years before from renal colic, the secretion of urine being totally suppressed for four days. He had had two subsequent attacks of colic, due to the passage of a stone. In the present instance he had suffered for some days from hæmaturia, but he had had no pain. Acute pain in the left flank suddenly came on, and the flow of urine was arrested. The ureter was evidently blocked by a calculus. Uræmic vomiting soon appeared, mental dullness and loss of strength being also present. The kidneys did not appear to be enlarged, but the left flank was painful, and the muscles were contracted on this side. As the uræmic symptoms were threatening, Legueu operated. The kidney was exposed and incised along the convex edge; several friable stones were extracted from the pelvis. A calculus was felt in the ureter, about an inch from the pelvis. It was pushed back into the pelvis and extracted. The excretion of the urine was re-established, and rapid recovery followed.

Calculous anuria may also occur in persons who have never had an attack of renal colic.

A healthy man, fifty-six years of age, was surprised to find that he could not pass water. As the bladder yielded no urine on the passage of a catheter, it was a case of anuria. The anuria went on for some days without pain or other incidents, and the patient was then admitted under Tennessen. The anuria had then existed for ten days, and the bladder was empty. Calculous anuria was at first suspected, but the patient's answers were negative as to previous colic or hæmaturia. On palpation of the abdomen, no tumour, and no tenderness on pressure. Symptoms of uræmia, then, appeared, and the patient died on the fourth day. At the autopsy the bladder was empty ; the right ureter was blocked by a calculus as large as a pea. Hydronephrosis was absent, except that one of the calices was dilated. The left ureter was quite patent. A stone was found in one of the calices. The anuria had, therefore, supervened during latent renal lithiasis.

From these cases we see that calculous uræmia does not always supervene in renal colic, as we are too ready to suppose ; in most cases it forms a part of renal colic, but in other cases it occurs in persons who have never had any sign of renal colic.

Two periods are seen in the evolution of calculous anuria : the one of tolerance, the other of uræmia. During the period of tolerance, the suppression of the urinary secretion is not revealed by any symptoms ; the patient feels well, and has no pain ; he either passes no urine, or only a little urine of low specific gravity, poor in urea, and sometimes blood-stained. This period lasts from three days to a week ; the passage of a few ounces of urine and the absence of uræmic symptoms induce hope of recovery. After a variable period the first symptoms of uræmia appear—vomiting, torpor, and cramps in the calves ; at the same time, or shortly afterwards, we find epistaxis, headache, visual troubles, dyspnœa, diarrhœa, and, in rare cases, œdema, and the patient dies in convulsions or in coma from two to six days after the onset of uræmia.

Pathogenesis.—Legueu has collected some thirty cases, which show the courses of events both in the affected and in the healthy kidney. In thirty cases of calculous anuria, the obliteration was situated twenty-three times in the ureter and seven times in the pelvis ; in the latter case the obliteration was due to large calculi, fitting into the orifice of the ureter. The kidney showed various changes—pyelitis, hydronephrosis, fibrosis, etc.

As regards the opposite kidney the findings were :

Congenital absence ..	..	..	.. 3	cases.
Calculous changes ..	..	..	.. 14	,,
Atrophy and fibrosis	..	..	.. 6	,,
Obliteration of the ureter	..	..	.. 6	,,
Kidney quite healthy	..	..	.. 1	,,

These cases show that calculous obliteration does not always occur in the ureter ; small calculi cause blocking of the ureter, because their small size allows them to enter it, while large calculi obstruct the orifice of the ureter in the pelvis. Accordingly anuria, accompanied or preceded by renal colic, is usually due to blocking of the ureter, while anuria, which is only associated with signs of a large calculus, or which is not accompanied by signs of renal colic, is usually due to intrarenal obliteration; exceptions, however, occur, as Tennessen's case, already quoted, shows.

How does obliteration of one ureter bring about total suppression of urine ? The anuria has been explained by lesions of the other kidney, and it has been argued : It is not surprising to find anuria ; one kidney is obstructed, and the other is diseased. This is true, but yet the kidney was secreting before the obliteration of its fellow-organ ; for a kidney may be calculous, and still the secretion of urine is not quite suppressed; and how can we explain complete anuria when the opposite kidney has no lesions, or when the lesions are slight ? We are driven to admit a functional paralysis of both kidneys, which causes total abolition of the secretory function. This secretory paralysis may affect the opposite kidney, although it is practically healthy. The proof of this functional paralysis is that the kidney on the side of the obliteration practically never shows hydronephrosis ; the urine, therefore, is not secreted by the kidney, because its function is suspended, and the suppression of function spreads reflexly to the other kidney. That the suppression is functional and due to reflex action is proved by Broca's case, in which anuria was present : although the obliteration was due to a small cancer of the bladder affecting only the left ureter, the flow of urine reappeared half an hour after nephrotomy.

Diagnosis.—The diagnosis of anuria is obvious, but it is sometimes difficult to say whether the anuria is calculous. There is no room for doubt when anuria accompanies or follows an attack of colic or of hæmaturia. We have, however, to remember cases in which anuria supervenes in persons with calculi that have given no warning ; in this event we must attempt to provoke lumbar pain, and we must inquire carefully into the pathological history of the case. Hysterical anuria is revealed by the discovery of the symptoms and stigmata of hysteria. Anuria due to compression of the ureter by an abdominal or pelvic tumour is characterized by gradual diminution of the urine passed, and by the presence of hydronephrosis.

It is not always easy to say on which side the obstruction exists, and it is even more difficult to recognize its exact seat. " As regards the exact seat of the obstruction, aside from cases in which the foreign body can be felt by rectal or vaginal examination, the most skilled observer has to rely on the fact that most stones are arrested in the upper part of the ureter " (Demons and Pousson). Catheterization of the ureter may be of great help in making a diagnosis (Albarran).

The prognosis of calculous anuria is most grave, since recovery (in the absence of operation) occurs in only 28 per cent. of the cases. It is difficult, however, to say exactly when the prognosis becomes grave.

Many sufferers from renal colic have transient suppression of urine, lasting for some hours. Are we to count them as recovering from calculous anuria? The answer is negative. Anuria lasting for twenty-four hours after an attack of renal colic should cause alarm; if it lasts forty-eight hours, the situation is dangerous; after three or four days intervention is indicated.

Treatment.—Medical measures are of service; bleeding over the kidneys is to be commended, because many observations in cases of nephrotomy for calculous anuria show that the kidney is very congested and vascular. Valuable time should not be lost, and it is better to operate too soon than too late. We must not wait for uræmia to set in before we decide on surgical intervention.

4. Calculous Pyelonephritis.

Pathogenesis.—Pyelitis is usually due to calculus. Suppuration does not occur as long as the medium in which the calculi develop remains aseptic. Renal calculi may exist for years without causing pyelitis, just as gall-stones may be present in the gall-bladder without causing cholecystitis. Persons have ten or twenty attacks of renal colic without suppuration occurring in the urinary tract; a large stone may remain for years in the kidney without causing infection of that organ. Calculi, then, may remain for a long while in the pelvis or in the calices, and give rise to fibrous changes; but as they are aseptic, they do not *per se* provoke suppuration. Furthermore, this tolerance of the kidneys for aseptic calculi has been experimentally demonstrated. Legueu, repeating the experiments of Tuffier, has introduced aseptic gravel into the pelvis of a dog's kidney; after two months the pelvis showed no trace of suppuration, and the bacteriological examination was negative. If pyelitis is to occur, the infection must be carried from outside. In 1886 Clado found that the pathogenic organism of urinary infection was a bacterium which he called the *Bacillus septicus*. At the present day this organism is called the *Bacillus coli*, which is often associated with other species—streptococci, staphylococci, etc. These organisms enter the urinary tract through lesions of the urethra (stricture, gonorrhœa, diseases of the prostate, use of septic catheters), lesions of the bladder, and lesions of the ureter. The infection is an ascending one, and the micro-organisms reach the kidney, which is in a condition of morbid receptivity on account of the traumatism produced by the calculi; pyelitis then results.

Pathological Anatomy.—In mild cases of calculous pyelitis we find congestion of the calices and of the pelvis, with hypersecretion and desquamation of the epithelium. In more severe cases and in the chronic form, the mucous membrane is thickened, ulcerated, and covered with muco-pus. The diphtheritic form is characterized by a pseudo-membranous or fibrinous deposit spread over the mucosa. The calices and the pelvis at times form an anfractuous, multilocular pocket, containing branching calculi, purulent fluid and caseous débris. This pocket may be of large size, especially if the ureter is blocked ; the kidney substance is, then, reduced to an atrophied fibrous shell. The ureter often shares in the inflammation and dilatation of the pelvis ; it becomes tortuous. If the lesion is unilateral, the healthy kidney hypertrophies, and is thus able to carry on the secretion of urine ; if the lesion is double, anuria and uræmia soon appear. The contents of the pocket may undergo calcareous change, the walls becoming thickened and forming a fibrous shell, while the ureter is converted into a fibrous cord.

The kidney may be enlarged and cystic, or atrophied, wrinkled, and fibrous. If suppuration has invaded the kidney, we find in the medulla abscesses of the straight tubules, which under the lens are characterized by greyish striæ, and in the cortex resemble miliary abscesses. The kidney, which at first sight appears to be large, sometimes owes its enlargement to hypertrophy of the perirenal tissue. In some cases we find at the autopsy perforation of the pelvis, perinephritic abscess, urinary infiltration and fistulæ, communicating with the adjacent organs or with the skin.

Description.—Pyelitis generally occurs late in renal lithiasis supervening in persons who have suffered for a long time from renal colic, hæmaturia, or symptoms of large calculi. In some instances, however, intrarenal or perirenal suppuration may occur in persons with calculi which have been latent.

Pyelitis usually sets in insidiously, without fever or pain ; after a while the patient finds that the urine is slightly turbid, and feels pain in the loin, while the region corresponding to the kidney is tender on pressure. He suffers from dyspepsia, loss of appetite and dryness of the mouth, but fever is absent or moderate. This condition may be interrupted by attacks of hæmaturia or of colic. The disease may not grow worse. The patient takes a cure at Vittel, Evian, or Capvern, and for many years the pyelitis does not become worse ; recovery may even follow. This is the mild form.

In other cases the symptoms are severe. The urine contains abundance of muco-pus ; the quantity of urine passed in the twenty-four hours varies, being in most cases above the normal. The passage of much turbid urine is the cardinal symptom of polyuria. The mucus and pus give to the urine a milky look. The urine clears slowly, but never completely, the purulent matter gradually falling to the bottom of the glass, though never completely so, as in the case of the mineral sediments. The pyuria is not fortuitous ; the admixture of pus and urine is constant and occurs daily. The urine in pyelitis is nearly always alkaline ; it sometimes contains imbricated plaques of epithelium from the pelvis.

Severe pyelitis is usually accompanied by fever ; in some cases rigors occur, and the temperature rises to 104° F., these symptoms indicating retention and infection. These complications may supervene in every variety of pyelitis. I have already mentioned them under Tubercular Pyelitis, and they are even more common in calculous pyelitis. As long as the pus can pass through the ureter, retention of the septic products does not occur, and the fever, if present, is moderate. If, however, the ureter or a suppurating pocket becomes blocked, we have the formation of a closed cavity, with retention of the infective products, and we find as the result renal pain, rigors, and attacks of intermittent fever, followed by sweating and rapid wasting. An apparent improvement in the urine often coincides with this aggravation of the symptoms. Urine, which was purulent and ammoniacal on the previous day, is now clear, the reason being that the clear urine comes from the healthy kidney, while the purulent urine from the diseased kidney cannot pass through the obliterated ureter. If the ureter regains its permeability, so that the pus can pass freely, the complications may disappear. I saw a typical case some years ago :

A lady, fifty years of age, had suffered for nine years from renal calculi, colic, and hæmaturia ; for the last year pyelitis had also been present. The urine contained some pus, but fever was absent, and the patient's health was fair. One day the urine diminished in quantity, and became clear instead of turbid ; severe attacks of fever set in, with rigors, rise of temperature to 104° F., and profuse sweating. I found the left kidney enlarged and painful. I expressed the opinion that the kidney was the seat of obstructive infection, and advised prompt surgical intervention. Pozzi operated, and the fever at once disappeared after the nephrotomy.

When the pyelitis is secondary to ureteritis we may be able, by rectal or vaginal examination, to feel the dilated or indurated ureter. If the obliteration of the ureter is progressive and final, fresh symptoms appear : the secreted products accumulate and form a renal tumour, which may contain several pints of fluid, and project into the abdominal cavity or into the loin. In order to ascertain the nature of this tumour, we must inquire into the patient's history, and find out whether he has passed pus and blood in the urine, or whether he has been subject to renal colic.

The prognosis of calculous pyelitis is benign in mild cases, but in other instances the pyuria grows worse, the suppuration invades the parenchyma of the kidney, the fever becomes hectic, and the patient dies from cachexia.

Medical treatment consists in milk diet, cures at Vittel, Contrexéville, Evian, or Capvern, and balsamic remedies ; surgical intervention is often necessary, and must not be too long delayed. The ureteral catheter or Luys' segregator will indicate the condition of the kidneys. Nephrotomy or nephrectomy is necessary, according to the condition found.

5. Calculous Perinephritis.

The kidneys are surrounded by cellular tissue, which may be called the renal fascia, and which is an offshoot of the fascia propria. This sac, which surrounds the entire organ, is composed of connective tissue in the fœtus. Later, an invasion of fatty tissue occurs, and in the adult the cellulo-fatty layer acquires a considerable thickness. The fatty capsule of the kidney is especially abundant over the posterior surface of the organ. Below it is continuous with the cellular tissue of the iliac fossa and of the pelvis.

The perirenal tissue rarely remains perfectly normal in long-standing pyelonephritis. In some cases its lesions are of more import than those of the kidney. Rayer coined the term " perinephritis " to designate inflammation of the perirenal tissue ; but perinephritis does not always show itself by suppuration, and we also see chronic lesions which are fibrous or fatty.

Fibro-Fatty Perinephritis.—This form runs a chronic course ; the process ends in induration of the connective tissue and in overgrowth of the fatty tissue. These two lesions vary in degree according to the particular case. At first the cellular tissue is thickened, indurated, and adherent to the capsule of the kidney and to the ureter. At a later stage the lesions are more marked and more extensive.

When the fibrous tissue predominates, the envelope of the kidney is thickened and creaks under the knife. In a case quoted by Tuffier the fibrous induration invaded the muscles and the abdominal wall as far as the skin. When the fatty tissue predominates, we find masses of fat, forming tumours, separated by thick fibrinous septa. Hartmann has described fatty tumours situated around the pelvis ; they may compress the vessels in the hilum, producing thrombosis in the veins, while the arteries are atrophied. The fatty tissue may invade the kidney, which is converted into a sclero-lipomatous mass, the kidney substance being represented by some remnants of glandular tissue around the pelvis, which contains one large or several small stones.

The sclero-lipomatous form of perinephritis is important ; it is met with in several diseases of the kidney (tuberculosis, pyelitis), but it is most common and most marked in renal lithiasis. This form sometimes causes a calculous kidney to have the appearance of a very large tumour ; examination of the patient reveals a large tumour, and when we examine the specimen we find that sclero-lipomatous degeneration makes up the major part of it. I had a remarkable case in hospital :

A young woman had suffered from abdominal pain for eleven years. The left kidney was enlarged and painful, and pain was also felt in the lumbar region. The urine had contained pus for eight months, but the patient had not had either renal colic or hæmaturia. A diagnosis was necessary. Cancer was eliminated, because the patient had suffered for eleven years, and had not had hæmaturia. It was not a polycystic kidney, because polycystic degeneration would certainly have affected the other kidney in eleven years. As the centrifugalized urine did not contain Koch's bacillus, and as the disease was of many years' standing, tuberculosis could be eliminated. I, therefore, made the following diagnosis: calculous kidney, with pyelitis and sclero-lipomatous perinephritis. As the patient had never had renal colic, I concluded that the calculus was a large one, giving rise to but moderate pain for several years, the pain being increased for some months by the pyelitis. The operation proved the correctness of my diagnosis.

Suppurative Perinephritis.—Calculous pyelonephritis may at any time cause perirenal suppuration. The abscess may, indeed, be the first sign of a latent pyelitis due to stone.

Pathogenesis.—Perirenal suppuration is due to the invasion of the perirenal tissue by pyogenic organisms. Albarran, in his bacteriological researches, has given the following results : In seven cases of perinephritic abscess the *Bacillus coli* was in pure culture in four, and in the other three cases it was associated with other organisms.

We can show experimentally the invasion of the perirenal tissue by injecting micro-organisms into the ureter. They pass through the lymphatics. Albarran has caused suppurative nephritis and perinephritis by injecting pyogenic organisms into the blood of the rabbit, after bruising the kidney and the perirenal tissue.

Pathological Anatomy.—Perinephritis is nearly always unilateral, and more common on the right side. The abscess wall is thickened, anfractuous, and covered by organized false membranes. In some cases the abscess sends prolongations into the psoas, latissimus dorsi, and external oblique muscles. The pus contained in the cavity may be laudable, or mixed with gravel and sloughy shreds. The abscess gives off a fæcal odour, even when it does not communicate with the bowel. The invaded muscles are reduced to a greyish pulp. The kidney shows calculous pyelonephritis. If the abscess is confined beneath the capsule of the kidney, the purulent collections may be small and multiple, or may completely surround the kidney, which is bathed in pus (subcapsular abscess) ; in this case the pelvis is external to the abscess, because the capsule ceases at the hilum.

Symptoms.—Pain and fever are usually the first symptoms. The pain, situated in the lumbar region, is spontaneous, and is always increased by pressure, especially if the painful region is compressed between the two hands. It is important, because it may be for days or weeks the only local sign. The fever is continuous, with periodical paroxysms ; at night the patient has a rigor, followed by a hot stage and sweating ; vomiting sometimes occurs. Wasting and loss of appetite follow ; the constipation is absolute.

Other signs appear after a week to a fortnight when the course of the disease is acute, and after several weeks if the course is chronic. " More or less brawny induration appears in the lumbar region, which becomes more and more tender on pressure ; the ilio-costal hollow fills up, and when the patient lies on his back, the examiner, by pushing his hand into the loin, can feel a more or less marked prominence. The induration in the loin is often accompanied by œdema, which may extend to the dorsal and gluteal regions ; slight redness of the skin is also present " (Trousseau).

Diagnosis.—The diagnosis presents no difficulty when the abscess has been preceded by renal colic, pyelitis, hæmaturia, or the passage of muco-purulent urine. When we have this history, and when the patient suffers from sharp pain in the loin, with daily attacks of fever, and when we find induration and œdema in the lumbar region, we can say that a perinephritic abscess is forming.

The diagnosis is not, however, always so easy; in some cases the prime cause of the abscess passes unnoticed, and for several days the only symptom is more or less acute lumbar pain, accompanied by remittent or intermittent fever. Calculous pyelitis may present the same symptoms, and even end in the formation of a tumour (pyonephrosis); the diagnosis is, then, most difficult. In pyonephrosis, however, the tumour is mainly abdominal; in perinephritis the tumour is mainly lumbar. In pyonephrosis the tumour is more rounded and more clearly limited, while the perirenal abscess is more diffuse, and blends with the œdematous abdominal wall. The prognosis is more serious in the acute and septic forms than in the phlegmonous forms.

The treatment is purely surgical.

6. Renal and Perirenal Fistulæ.

We have seen that a perinephritic abscess may open in the loin, at the navel, into the intestine, or into the bronchi; when the opening does not close, a fistula results.

When the fistula originates in the kidney, it is called renal; when it originates in the perirenal tissue, it is called perirenal. The fistula is called purulent or urinary, according as the discharge is pus or urine. If the fistula opens on the skin, it is called reno-cutaneous; if it discharges into an organ, it is called reno-intestinal, reno-bronchial, etc.

Reno-Cutaneous Fistulæ.—These fistulæ usually open in the loin, the discharge being purulent or urinary; the external opening is funnel-shaped, with fungating edges, and the canal, which has thick fibrous walls, ends in a deep renal or perirenal focus. The ureter is nearly always constricted or obliterated, and the discharge, then, contains urine and pus; the flow is continuous, and has a characteristic odour; the edges of the wound are raw, erythematous, and painful, so that frequent dressing is required.

Intestinal Fistulæ.—These fistulæ are fairly common, especially those which open into the colon. They are preceded by symptoms of enteritis; the dejecta are purulent and fœtid; the patient wastes and finally succumbs.

7. Fibrosis and Atrophy.

Fibrous atrophy may or may not be accompanied by hydronephrosis. While pyonephrosis due to calculus is common, hydronephrosis is rare. Brault and Cornil have studied the changes in the kidney consecutive to compression, ligature and obstruction of the ureters; the changes end in atrophy of the kidney. When the ureters and the pelvis are dilated and contain fluid, the kidney appears to be enlarged ; it is œdematous, and the limit of the cortex and of the medulla is no longer clear ; the calices, pushed back by the pressure of the fluid, in their turn push back the cortex. On making a section of the kidney we find calculi which often betray their presence by bosses on the surface. The cortex is hollowed out. Some of the cavities communicate with the dilated calices and pelvis, while others are isolated in the form of independent cysts.

On histological examination the kidney presents lesions, divided by Jardet into three stages. At first the renal lesion is characterized by stasis of the urine, with dilatation of the tubules from the glomerulus to the papilla. The arteries are thickened from arteritis. At a more advanced stage the fibrosis invades the medulla and the cortex in an irregular fashion ; the lumen of the tubules is sometimes enlarged, sometimes constricted, and the glomeruli are fibrous and atrophied. In the final stage the fibrosis ends in atrophy ; the kidney tissue may be atrophied, although the organ as a whole is enlarged by reason of the distension of the calices and of the pelvis. In the opposite case the atrophic fibrosis causes diminution in the size of the organ. Jardet has pointed out that these atrophic lesions are not always consecutive to mechanical obliteration of the ureter ; it is probable, on the contrary, that the fibrous lesions precede the obliteration.

" When the kidney has been destroyed by atrophic nephritis, the other kidney is usually hypertrophied, but the hypertrophy is less marked and less regular than it is after nephrectomy. The kidney as a whole appears to be larger, but we can nearly always see with the naked eye traces of partial fibrosis. The microscope shows fibrosis at some spots, and at others enlargement of the canaliculi and of the glomeruli ; in short, compensatory hypertrophy exists, but only at certain parts of the kidney. This peculiarity appears to be due to the fact that the nephritis is frequently bilateral in the case of a calculous kidney ; the fibrous lesions so common in these cases are due not only to the presence of calculi in the pelvis, but also to the irritant action of the urine, the composition of which is altered by the special mode of nutrition of the patient " (Albarran).

As long as the fibrosis is limited to the diseased kidney, the secretion of urine is assured by the opposite kidney; but when both are the seat of lithiasis or of fibrosis, the minor symptoms of Brightism appear, and, later, the major symptoms of uræmia. Raymond has published a case in point. An elderly man who had never suffered from renal colic or from symptoms of calculus died from uræmia. The autopsy revealed large calculi in both kidneys and atrophy of the cortex, with interstitial nephritis.

XV. PYELITIS—PYELONEPHRITIS.

Pyelitis is inflammation of the mucous membrane of the calices and pelvis ; it may be acute or chronic, and nephritis may or may not be present. The word " pyelitis " has been preserved, although its etymology (πύελος, pelvis) bears no relation to the morbid localization. Pyelitis may supervene as a secondary infection in such diseases as typhus, scarlatina, measles, smallpox, or cholera. In some cases it follows poisoning by turpentine, cubebs, and especially cantharides.

Affections of the genital organs in women, cancer of the uterus, infections of the urethra, bladder, and ureter (gonorrhœa), often cause pyelitis ; the micro-organisms take the urine for a culture medium, and the infection nearly always spreads by the ascending path.

Tubercular pyelitis has been described (p. 1126 *et seq.*). The most frequent cause of pyelonephritis is renal calculus. The question has already been fully discussed.

XVI. SUPPURATIVE NEPHRITIS.

Pathological Anatomy.—I shall here describe suppurative nephritis properly so called and metastatic abscesses of the kidney. The history of suppurative nephritis is often associated with that of pyelitis, the two lesions being successive stages of the same infection.

The nephritis may be unilateral or bilateral. It is due to many causes. Some are exceptional, such as contusions, wounds, and adjacent abscesses ; others are more common, and include infection by the ascending path and by the blood-stream. Cystitis, enlarged prostate, strictures of the urethra, and operations on the urethra or on the bladder, may cause nephritis by ascending infection.

In nephritis due to blood infection the course of events is as follows : The primary affection of the urinary tract induces general infection, and the organisms carried by the blood form emboli in the renal vessels. Albarran, by injecting the colon bacillus into the ureter of the rabbit, has produced ascending nephritis. Furthermore, any blood infection (staphylococcus, pneumococcus, streptococcus, etc.) may cause abscesses in the kidney. The suppuration may be diffuse or collected in the form of an abscess ; these two forms at times occur together. Diffuse nephritis commences with congestion of the organ ; the kidney is swollen, red on section, and studded with ecchymoses, caused by parenchymatous and interstitial hæmorrhages. Pus then forms, and infiltrates the cortex and pyramids of the kidney. The organ is yellowish and opaque on section, and homogeneous pus can be squeezed out on pressure.

The nephritis may be infiltrating or radiating. In the diffuse infiltrating form the parenchyma is a mottled red and grey; abscesses of different sizes are found in the cortex or at the base of the pyramids. In the radiating form the pyramids are marked with perpendicular striæ of a greyish colour, standing out against the dark red background. Some of the striæ are larger, forming a cone with a peripheral base, and containing a drop of pus. The centre of the foci is usually a tubule dilated by the microbes which are found in the glomerulus between the tuft and the capsule.

The recent abscesses contain homogeneous pus, and their walls are formed by the kidney tissue. The old abscesses contain pus mixed with lime salts, and their walls are formed by a membrane of connective tissue. When the lesion is old, the kidney is more or less deformed and nodular. These abscesses are rarely larger than a hazel-nut; the large abscesses are chiefly seen in suppuration of the pelvis. The abscesses may open into the pelvis; into the duodenum; in the lumbar region; into the peritoneum, where they cause acute peritonitis; or into the bronchi, after perforating the diaphragm. In case of cure cicatrization and atrophy of the kidney follow. The metastatic abscesses occur in the form of isolated or agglomerated miliary abscesses. The latter are found both in the cortex and in the medulla; their shape is conical, the base being peripheral; the topography depends on the distribution of the renal arteries.

Description.—Acute suppurative nephritis is ushered in by rigors and fever, which is sometimes of an intermittent type; nausea and vomiting are frequent. The patient complains of sharp pain, situated in the loin and radiating along the ureter to the bladder and to the testicle. The desire to micturate is urgent, and the patient usually passes but a small quantity of high-coloured acid urine, containing albumin and blood. In some cases the onset is insidious, and the disease is of a typhoid type, with adynamia, dry tongue, and sweating. In old people suppurative nephritis, like suppurative pneumonia, may be apyretic. The gravity of the disease depends on the age of the patient, on the cause and extent of the suppuration, on the duration of the disease, and on the condition of the other kidney. If both kidneys are affected, death may result from uræmia.

Diagnosis.—Suppurative nephritis rarely has a sudden onset. The seat and the radiation of the pain, as well as the urinary troubles, are in favour of nephritis. We can ascertain by means of Luys' segregator whether the nephritis is unilateral or bilateral. The pain of nephritis may simulate that of renal colic, but as the latter is apyretic, this fact decides the point. In pyelitis the urine is purulent from the first, and remains so. In nephritis the pus appears late, and is not constantly present.

Acute nephritis demands antiphlogistic measures. Leeches over the kidneys are indicated; soothing and diuretic drinks are to be given; the pain is to be relieved with morphia, and the vomiting with iced beverages. We must be ready to employ surgical intervention (see Section VI.).

XVII. PRIMARY AND SECONDARY PERINEPHRITIC ABSCESS.

A perinephritic abscess is an abscess in the fatty tissue around the kidney. This tissue is most abundant behind and at the extremities of the kidney. It is continuous with the subperitoneal tissues, and with the cellular tissue in the iliac fossa and in the pelvis. On the other hand, it is continuous with the cellular tissue in the lumbar region, external to the quadratus lumborum, between the borders of the latissimus dorsi and external oblique muscles. The pus may remain limited to the perirenal focus, but in some cases it extends to the cellular tissue of the lumbar, dorsal, or gluteal regions, to the tissue in the iliac fossa, and even into the vesical and rectal cellular tissue.

Secondary Abscess.—This form occurs in lesions of the neighbouring organs, and especially in certain affections of the kidney. In the first place stands renal lithiasis, with or without pyelo-nephritis; the infection extends by propagation or by perforation. Tuberculosis of the kidney also favours the occurrence of perirenal suppuration. Other causes are: pyelonephritis of various origins, including ascending infection by the gonococcus; hydatid cysts and cancer of the kidney; suppuration in the liver, the gall-bladder, the psoas, and the cellular tissue of the pelvis; perforation of the colon, appendicitis, and pancreatitis. Perinephritis may be associated with other diseases, such as typhoid fever, typhus, and puerperal conditions.

When the kidneys are at fault and pyelonephritis is already present, we can readily understand the occurrence of suppuration, on account of the proximity of the lesions. In other cases, however, the original focus of infection is far more remote; this fact leads me to mention the relations between perirenal infection and pleuro-pulmonary infection. This side of the question was recognized by Rayer and Trousseau. The following case is taken from Rayer's work:

A woman, sixty-five years of age, who had suffered from renal colic, had been ill for some months, with pain in the right kidney, fever, and malaise. The right loin was very tender on pressure, and palpation revealed an ilio-lumbar tumour. The diagnosis of extrarenal abscess was made. An incision gave exit to a pint of foul-smelling pus. Digital examination showed that the focus was behind the kidney, and the abscess was therefore perinephritic. Much relief followed. On the thirteenth day, however, the patient was taken ill with pneumonia of the right lung. The attack subsided in a few days; the lumbar wound still discharged some pus. The patient finally recovered.

Trousseau has repeatedly insisted on the relations between perirenal suppuration and pleuro-pneumonia. " Perinephritic abscesses may cause pleurisy and pneumonia. I would have you remember that in cases where a perinephritic abscess is complicated by pleuro-pneumonia, the latter is always on the same side as the abscess. Desruelles found a perinephritic abscess in an old woman convalescent from gangrenous pneumonia."

Recent researches have explained the pathogenesis of these reciprocal infections. Tuffier and Lejars have described a costo-lumbar hiatus, through which the subpleural fat communicates with the perirenal fatty tissue. The hiatus is traversed by veins and lymphatics, which establish communication between the perirenal tissue and the thoracic cavity; in this way pleuro-pulmonary infections may become perirenal, and *vice versa*. Tuffier has published a case of pneumococcal perinephritic abscess secondary to pneumonia.

Injury plays an important part in the causation of diseases. The occurrence of pneumonia and the appearance of tuberculosis after injury are well known, although it is not always easy to explain the pathogenesis. A similar ætiology obtains in the history of perinephritic abscess. The following example is from De Mussy's lectures :

A woman, forty years of age, who had been kicked in the loin by a horse, was taken ill six months later with acute pain, fever, and rigors. The pain spread from the loin to the iliac region. The symptoms improved under sedative measures, but reappeared a week later. In the space between the last rib and the iliac crest a swelling, with induration of the cellular tissue, could be made out. Pressure in the lumbar region caused unbearable pain. The fever was continuous, with an evening rise and rigors. The diagnosis was perinephritic abscess. Nélaton made a puncture, giving exit to a quantity of pus. After a transient improvement, the rigors and the fever reappeared, because the pus did not find a free exit. The patient finally succumbed.

Bergounhioux speaks of a peasant who fell from a tree, sustaining a severe bruise in the right lumbar region. The urine contained blood for several days. The patient felt deep-seated pain in the loin, and fever set in. The passing of blood then ceased, but the bruised region swelled up, and fluctuation became evident. An incision was made, giving exit to pus. Recovery followed.

Appendicitis is fairly often a cause of perinephritic abscess, either by continuity or by remote infection; the *Bacillus coli* is the organism usually present. I have named this variety " appendicular perinephritic abscess."

Suppurative pancreatitis has been noted as a cause of perinephritic abscess.

Primary Perinephritic Abscess.—I shall now quote two cases from one of my clinical lectures :*

I saw a young girl who at first sight appeared to be suffering from typhoid fever, the temperature being 104° F. The chief symptom was pain in the left lumbar region. The illness had commenced a month before with lumbar pain, so that lumbago was at first suspected. The suffering soon became so great that the patient could only

* *Clinique Médicale de l'Hôtel-Dieu*, 1899, 8me leçon.

walk with her body bent. About the eighteenth day the patient felt shooting pains in the left lumbar region, the fever became severe, and vomiting set in ; this condition persisted until her admission to hospital.

Inspection revealed some induration in the lumbar region, which was evidently the seat of the mischief. The evolution of the symptoms led to the diagnosis of perinephritic suppuration. The abscess was primary, since no cause for a secondary abscess was present. There was no history of calculus, tuberculosis, pyelonephritis, appendicitis, injury, pleuro-pulmonary infection, or furunculosis. Accordingly the most likely lesion was a primary perinephritic abscess. The diagnosis was confirmed next day. The urine suddenly became turbid, with a marked deposit. The urinalysis showed the presence of pus, and the exclusive existence of the *Staphylococcus aureus*. The abscess had opened into the urinary passages.

Marion operated. In front of the quadratus he opened an abscess cavity, passing down into the iliac fossa, and upwards into a long track. The kidney appeared to be of normal size. The pus contained the *Staphylococcus aureus*.

After transient improvement, pneumonia appeared on the left side, the infection being secondary to the perirenal mischief. Shooting pains were felt in the hypogastrium, and a swelling was found above the pubes. This abscess was opened, the pus containing the *Staphylococcus aureus*. The fever persisted for some days ; the two incisions discharged some pus, and showed a tendency to close ; but the pyuria persisted. Recovery finally followed.

A man, thirty-five years of age, was admitted for pain in the left lumbar region. It had come on suddenly ten days before, without appreciable cause, and was so acute that the patient was confined to bed. On admission the temperature was 102° F., the tongue dry, and the urine scanty. There was marked tenderness on pressure in the loin and in the iliac fossa. The muscular resistance rendered abdominal palpation difficult. Within the next few days the loin became indurated, and some swelling appeared. I diagnosed primary perinephritic abscess, because there was no history of any cause for a secondary abscess.

An operation was decided upon, when a new incident supervened. The urine suddenly became purulent. At the same time the temperature fell to 98° F., the pain diminished, and the patient felt much relief. The abscess had evidently opened into the urinary tract. It was impossible to say whether this incident meant a favourable ending to the disease, or whether the suppuration might not continue.

The patient was given fluids in abundance. The pus diminished progressively, the swelling in the loin disappeared, and the pain yielded. The patient left the hospital cured.

Description.—The same description holds good for primary and secondary abscesses. The initial symptom is pain in the loin ; its situation simulates lumbago. This mistake has often been made. The patient complains of lumbar pain. Fever rarely appears at the same time as the pain ; at an advanced period it is acute, and accompanied by rigors. Pain and fever, and at times vomiting, are the only symptoms at the onset of perinephritic abscess. Rigors, swelling, and œdema of the lumbar region appear later.

The course of the abscess has been well described by Trousseau. The patient suddenly feels deep-seated and diffuse lumbar pain, which may be acute or dull. The pain, though spontaneous, is always made worse by pressure, especially bimanual pressure. The pain may disappear for some weeks or months, until a fresh cause brings on another attack. As a rule, however, the suffering is persistent, and increases until the pus is let out. This pain is of the highest importance, because for a considerable period it is the only local sign; certain general troubles show that the suffering depends on an organic cause; the fever is continuous, and an evening rigor often occurs. The patient loses appetite and wastes rapidly; vomiting sometimes occurs at the onset of the febrile paroxysm, and obstinate constipation is nearly always present.

" For a week or a fortnight the only symptoms are local pain, general weakness, and fever, with a daily paroxysm. Other local signs of deep inflammation then appear : the region becomes more and more tender on pressure, and more or less extensive induration develops ; at the same time the ilio-costal hollow is effaced, and bimanual palpation—the patient being in the dorsal decubitus—reveals a deep swelling continuous with the subcutaneous cellular tissue. The tumour does not move with respiration, thus proving that it is independent of the liver, which moves up and down on respiration. The induration of the lumbar region is often accompanied by œdema, which may extend to the dorsal and gluteal regions ; the skin may be slightly reddened. The redness is erysipelatous when the inflammation extends to the cellular tissue " (Trousseau).

The above description portrays in a striking way the onset and the evolution of the perinephritic abscess. In the absence of surgical intervention the following varieties may be seen : (a) The suppuration reaches the subdiaphragmatic cellular tissue, and pleurisy or pneumonia follows, or the pus opens into the bronchi. Rupture into the pericardium has been noted. (b) More often the suppuration extends into the iliac fossa, which becomes painful, and a swelling appears either above or below Poupart's ligament ; in the latter case, the pus follows the sheath of the vessels and points in Scarpa's triangle. In some cases the pus follows the sheath of the psoas down to the lesser trochanter, and may invade the hip-joint. (c) The suppuration spreads into the pelvis, and the abscess opens into the bladder or the vagina. (b) Rupture into the colon is followed by the expulsion of muco-purulent or bloody, foul-smelling stools, while the gas from the intestine, entering the abscess cavity, may produce emphysema of the dorsal region. (e) Rupture into peritoneum is exceptional, a fact explained by the distance between the peritoneum and the abscess, which is usually behind the kidney. (f) Rupture at the umbilicus is fairly common.

Perinephritic abscess, then, may terminate in the foregoing ways. The course of events may, however, be different. The invasion may be marked by repeated attacks of pain and fever, occurring weeks or months apart, as though the first attacks were followed by resolution. In other cases the symptoms are sudden and severe, resembling acute septicæmia : the rigors are violent, the temperature is much raised, the sweating is profuse, the diarrhœa is fœtid, the abdomen is tympanitic, the pulse is bad, delirium is present; the general condition becomes alarming in a few days, and death may result unless intervention is most prompt.

Diagnosis.—The diagnosis is at first very difficult, especially in the primary form. The secondary form is not so difficult, because the provoking cause gives valuable information. Let us suppose an injury to the renal region. Some days or weeks later we are told of pain at the injured spot, with rigors and fever ; the lumbar region becomes very tender on pressure, and is indurated and swollen, while the fever increases. Our attention being aroused by the injury, we diagnose an abscess in process of formation. Let us suppose that a patient has suffered from calculus, with renal colic, hæmaturia and pyuria, pointing to pyelitis. We can readily diagnose perine-phritic abscess, if lumbar pain, rigors, and fever appear, and are followed by tenderness on pressure and by induration in the loin. The same remark applies to cases of perinephritic abscess secondary to appendicitis, or to other well-known causes.

If, however, the abscess is primary, and appears when the patient is in good health, the diagnosis remains obscure. Our only guide is pain : as the movements of the trunk are painful, the muscles are hard and contracted ; we suspect lumbago, and order rest, massage, cupping, morphia, and anti-pyrin. The condition remains unchanged for several days. The lumbar pain is the chief symptom, and examination is rendered difficult by the muscular contraction. The patient complains of malaise, insomnia, and loss of appetite, and feels that there is something more than lumbago ; he suffers from rigors and sweats, vomiting comes on, the temperature rises to 102° F., and the diagnosis commences to be obvious.

The situation is at times rendered obscure by the fact that the patient is prostrated with diarrhœa and epistaxis, as in enteric fever. In this event the lumbar pain and the fever are our best guide. Bimanual palpation of the loin causes intense suffering. The fever points to suppuration. Blood examination shows marked polynucleosis : 20,000 to 30,000 polynuclear cells in place of 6,000. Sooner or later the painful region becomes brawny and œdematous, and the diagnosis of perirenal abscess is clear. Immediate intervention is necessary, and, though in some cases recovery may follow spontaneous evacuation of the pus by the urinary tract, we must not trust to this event, because many complications may occur.

XVIII. HYDRONEPHROSIS.

The term " hydronephrosis " is applied to dilatation of the calices and of the pelvis caused by accumulation of urine. If the urine becomes purulent, the term " pyonephrosis " is employed. When the obstruction to the flow of urine is low down in the urinary passages, the ureter becomes dilated. Hydronephrosis in the fœtus is usually double, and obstructs delivery; it is dependent on a congenital malformation. In the adult hydronephrosis is due to compression of the ureter by a tumour of the bladder, of the uterus, or of the ovary.

Cancer of the uterus, by spreading to the trigone or to the ureters, produces more or less complete obstruction of these ducts ; the obstruction and the resulting anuria are sometimes intermittent ; hydronephrosis may result. Obliteration of the ureter due to the migration of gravel is rarely followed by hydronephrosis.

Pregnancy is a cause of hydronephrosis. The enlarged uterus may press upon the ureter, especially on the right side, bringing on dilatation of the ureter and of the pelvis. Cruveilhier found marked dilatation of the ureters in women who had died at the end of pregnancy or after delivery. If infection occurs during delivery, the micro-organisms carried by the circulation infect the kidney, which is in a state of receptivity by reason of the retention.

Hydronephrosis is generally unilateral. Although the dilatation may be limited to one of the calices, it is usually general, the kidney being flattened and converted into a pouch containing several pints of fluid, while the remnants of the kidney tissue have undergone fibrous atrophy. When the ureter takes part in the dilatation, it may be as large as a coil of gut. The fluid in hydronephrosis contains scarcely any of the elements of the urine, but it is often albuminous, and in some cases purulent, the infection taking place either by the ascending path or by the blood-stream.

Hydronephrosis is not appreciable until the tumour reaches a certain size ; we then find an abdominal tumour that can also be felt in the loin. The tumour may be fluctuating, and may invade the neighbouring regions in every direction. The diagnosis is difficult, but the patient's history may be of value; thus previous renal colic would point to obstruction by a calculus. Radioscopy may help in making a diagnosis. The prognosis is very grave in double hydronephrosis, on account of the risk of uræmia ; it is not so serious in unilateral hydronephrosis as long as the other kidney is healthy. The treatment is surgical.

XIX. HÆMATURIA—CHYLURIA.

Hæmaturia denotes the passage of blood in the urine ; we speak of vesical or renal hæmaturia, according as the lesion is situated in the bladder or in the kidney. The colour of the fluid passed is rosy, reddish, brownish, or blackish, according to the amount of the blood passed and of the urine with which the blood is mixed. More or less elongated clots float in the liquid. These clots may form a mould of the ureter, being 8 or 10 inches in length ; in their passage through the ureter they may cause renal colic and temporary retention of urine. I shall describe secondary hæmaturia and essential hæmaturia.

1. Secondary Hæmaturia.

Secondary hæmaturia may be associated with some general disease or with a local lesion of the kidney.

Hæmaturia in General Diseases.—Many general infections may cause the kidney to bleed, the most common being scarlet fever. In some cases variola, measles, purpura, erysipelas, and erythema, assume the hæmorrhagic form, and the hæmaturia is simply an episode in the general hæmorrhagic process. Acute rheumatism may cause hæmaturia.

This form of hæmaturia is due to micro-organisms, or to their toxines. They may lead to hæmorrhages in the skin and the mucous membranes, or from the kidneys. The renal hæmorrhage is nearly always associated with nephritis.

Hæmaturia associated with Renal Lesions.—In the preceding sections on tuberculosis, cysts, cancer, and lithiasis we have seen that any one of these affections may give rise to hæmaturia.

Tuberculosis of the kidneys often causes hæmaturia, the blood appearing at the onset or at a more advanced stage of the lesion. The bleeding is usually slight, of short duration, and independent of external causes (riding, driving, or exercise). In other instances it is so severe and so obstinate as to constitute a hæmorrhagic form of renal tuberculosis.

Cysts of the kidney, especially polycystic degeneration, are often accompanied by hæmaturia. The bleeding, though usually slight, may be serious in amount. Of all the renal affections cancer causes the most copious bleeding ; the hæmorrhage may appear early or late. It is generally profuse and obstinate, whether the kidney is or is not enlarged.

Renal lithiasis very frequently causes hæmaturia. The stones may be so small as to produce renal colic, or so large that they remain fixed in the kidney. The bleeding, though moderate as a rule, is readily brought on by shocks or exercise, and is at times so profuse and continuous as to constitute a hæmorrhagic form of renal lithiasis.

This enumeration, and the details already given in the preceding sections on the diseases of the kidneys, show that hæmaturia is a symptom of but little value in distinguishing between the lesions of the kidneys. Profuse and obstinate hæmaturia is not solely the appanage of cancer, because it is also met with in tuberculosis and in lithiasis of the kidney. Hæmaturia, with enlargement of the kidney, is not always the result of cancer, since we also find it in enlargements of the kidney due to perinephritis or to cysts.

Hæmaturia, in spite of its abundance and its obstinacy, in spite of the long clots which accompany it, and in spite of the size of the kidney, whether enlarged or normal, may give no hint as to the nature of the renal lesion producing the bleeding. It may also happen that the hæmaturia is not associated with any of the lesions above mentioned. A patient may have profuse and repeated hæmaturia, so that we suspect tuberculosis, cancer, cyst, or calculus of the kidney, and yet the patient has not any one of these diseases.

Acute and chronic nephritis may be accompanied by hæmaturia, but it is not a case of pure hæmaturia ; the urine (apart from the hæmaturia) contains albumin, and the usual signs of nephritis are present.

I believe that the hæmaturia of interstitial nephritis has not always been correctly interpreted. According to my observations, hæmaturia considered as dependent on interstitial nephritis is frequently dependent on tubercular mischief. The nephritis is often unilateral and amenable to surgical intervention.

Pregnancy is sometimes accompanied by hæmaturia, due to congestion ; in some cases nephritis gravidarum may be the cause.

Parasitic hæmaturia is endemic in Brazil, Cape Colony, India, and the islands of Maurice and Réunion. It occurs chiefly in young persons under the following conditions : Sometimes the urine becomes bloody without prodromata being present, and this symptom recurs for months and years without affecting the health ; at other times the hæmaturia is accompanied by lumbar pain, fatigue, and anæmia. In many instances the patient, after passing bloody urine for some days or weeks, begins to pass milky, rose-coloured urine ; this is called chylous hæmaturia. The urine forms three layers in the test-glass : a bottom layer, composed of blood ; a middle layer of urine ; and a top layer of the chylous matter. The urine becomes clear on shaking with ether. The fat is present in the form of an emulsion, and examination of the blood shows that it does not contain any excess of fat. The prognosis is fairly good, and the hæmaturia may disappear if the patient emigrates to a temperate clime.

The pathogenesis of chylous hæmaturia is obscure. Bilharz, Griesinger, and other writers, have shown that the endemic hæmaturia of hot countries depends on the presence of various parasites in the blood. The parasite in Northern and Southern Africa is a distoma; in Guadeloupe and in Brazil it is usually a strongylus. The parasites are said to cause the hæmaturia by producing changes in the mucous membrane of the urinary passages. In some cases the parasite has been found in the blood passed *per urethram*.

How can we explain the chyluria so often associated with the hæmaturia ? Some authorities say that the presence of the chyle is due to changes in the red corpuscles, which break up, and allow the fat to escape in the form of granules. Gubler holds that the chyluria is due to lymphatic varices which open into the urinary tract.

The distinction between vesical and renal hæmaturia is not always easy. In case of doubt cystoscopy will indicate the exact origin of the hæmorrhage.

2. Essential Hæmaturia.

Essential hæmaturia resembles congestive epistaxis, which supervenes without appreciable lesions of the nasal mucosa. Essential hæmaturia, though very rare, certainly occurs, as the following example shows :

A patient, twenty-eight years of age, who had no previous history of hæmophilia or of tuberculosis, was taken ill with pain in the right lumbar and hypochondriac regions during an attack of hæmaturia, which had lasted for six months. The urine had always been more or less blood-stained ; the blood was intimately mixed with the urine, and from the first the hæmaturia, instead of diminishing, became more profuse. The renal pain was bilateral, slight, and transitory on the left, but continuous on the right side. It never had the character of renal colic, being rather a feeling of heaviness and painfulness in this region.   No oliguria, no gravel, no deposit of uric acid in the chamber. These symptoms were quite consistent with an organic lesion, such as tuberculosis or cancer.   Broca found that the right kidney was neither hypertrophied nor pushed down ; it was painful on pressure in the costo-vertebral angle. Micturition was painless, frequent, and the urine always contained blood. The hæmaturia was not affected by walking or by jolting in a carriage. The patient looked well, and had not lost flesh. Rest in bed, instead of improving the situation, caused a reappearance of the pain and hæmaturia. The urine did not contain Koch's bacilli. Broca decided to operate. The kidney was found to be quite normal ; the pelvis and ureter were normal. Terrier and Hartmann examined this kidney with the same result ; they could not discover any lesion.   It was considered unnecessary to carry the operation further ; the result was most satisfactory, though most unexpected. The hæmaturia ceased, and the patient when seen three years later was in perfect health.

Broca, in his work, has collected seven cases which in various ways resemble his own case, and whether we speak of hæmophilia, or of congestive vasomotor troubles, matters very little. The interesting and undeniable fact remains that persistent and copious hæmaturia, with or without pains, may appear independently of any known lesion, and may be cured by surgical intervention. The following case may be included under this variety of hæmaturia :

Some years ago a boy of fifteen years of age came into the Necker Hospital for hæmaturia of two years' duration. The hæmaturia, of renal origin, was not continuous ;

it sometimes came on without apparent cause, at other times as the result of the least exertion. He told me that he could not stand for two hours without his urine becoming blood-stained. If he took a short walk, the bleeding appeared; it often lasted for several days in spite of rest. The persistent hæmorrhage had made the patient so weak and anæmic that he was quite prepared to undergo any operation. The kidneys were not especially tender, and I found it impossible to formulate any pathogenic diagnosis; lithiasis, tuberculosis, and cancer were all possible. There were no renal colic and no tubercle bacilli; the general condition was not such as a cancer of long standing would have caused.

I put the patient on turpentine in increasing doses; the hæmaturia disappeared completely. In five years it has only recurred once. After two years and a half of illness the cure was definite. The patient can now take long walks, and work standing throughout the day, sometimes doing overtime at night. His health is excellent in every way, and there has not been the slightest reappearance of hæmaturia. He continues to take turpentine. These examples and this discussion with regard to hæmaturia prove that the pathogenic diagnosis of renal hæmaturia is often difficult, and at times impossible.

XX. HÆMOGLOBINURIA.

Description.—Hæmoglobinuria is a false hæmaturia. The urine in hæmoglobinuria owes its colour to hæmoglobin, and never contains red corpuscles, or only in quite an insignificant quantity—a condition very different from hæmaturia, where the blood is passed in its natural state.

Hæmoglobinuria is only a symptom, but it shows itself in such various conditions that three varieties may be considered: (1) Paroxysmal or essential hæmoglobinuria; (2) hæmoglobinuria symptomatic of infectious diseases; (3) hæmoglobinuria symptomatic of poisoning.

Essential hæmoglobinuria (also called "primary" or *a frigore*) was first described by Harley in 1864, and seems to constitute a definite morbid entity. In consequence of a chill, an individual, otherwise in good health, is taken ill with rigors, malaise, and pain in the loins and the epigastrium. These more or less pronounced phenomena are accompanied by a rise in temperature, which may reach to 102° F. During these attacks, which last from six to eight hours, the urine gradually becomes darker. The urine first passed is of a pale red; the subsequent discharges are the colour of Bordeaux or of Malaga wine. After the attack the urine gradually loses its colour, and some hours later it is quite normal.

The urine is albuminous. The microscope reveals no red corpuscles and no débris of corpuscles; the spectroscope reveals the two lines of oxy-hæmoglobin. The transformation of these two bands into the single band of reduced hæmoglobin may be observed. In some cases a third line—the line of methæmoglobin—is seen. This methæmoglobinuria is not constant (Hénocque). The urinary deposit is formed by a reddish sediment, composed of granules of hæmoglobin, of casts, and of epithelial cells. The examination of the blood made during the attack shows a delay in the

formation of the fibrinous coagulum, and a feeble tendency of the corpuscles
to form rouleaux (Hayem).

At the moment of the crisis there is a slight increase in the number of
white corpuscles and a notable diminution in the red corpuscles. Two
days later hæmatoblasts and dwarf corpuscles appear. The study of the
serum will be discussed under Pathogenesis.

Paroxysmal hæmoglobinuria is especially frequent in male adults. The
attacks may occur at intervals of several days, or even of several months.
Cold favours its appearance, whence the name " winter hæmoglobinuria,"
and I have often seen Mesnet bring on an attack in his patient by making
him go into the hospital garden when the thermometer stood at 0° C. In
addition to these symptoms, which are constant during the attacks, there
are others which, though not constant, are of much value from the pathogenic point of view. These are : (1) urticaria and purpura ; (2) acute,
painful, and temporary swelling of the spleen and of the liver ; (3) a subicteric tint, that lasts for several days after the disappearance of the other
symptoms.

The attack is not always so severe. It is sometimes characterized by
a few rigors, lassitude, and slight albuminuria. Side by side with these
abortive attacks we find, on the contrary, others which are very severe,
and it is especially in these cases that we see the foregoing inconstant symptoms. After the attack the urine is normal ; the patient is more or less
anæmic, but he soon regains his health, and never becomes cachectic. Widal
and myself have seen a case in which death supervened during an attack
of hæmoglobinuria.

The most typical form of hæmoglobinuria due to infection is seen in
malaria, when it is known as " hæmoglobinuric fever." It appears only
in those who have lived for a long while in fever-stricken countries. The
attack is most frequently preceded by a slight attack of simple or of bilious
fever. The duration is generally twelve to thirty-six hours. Hæmoglobinuria generally appears with the rigor and diminishes with the defervescence. At the same time as hæmoglobinuria appears we find
bilious symptoms of much severity, characterized by vomiting, bilious stools,
lumbar pain, jaundice, and bile in the urine. The attack may be slight or
severe, and it may end in collapse, anuria, or uræmia. In the opinion of
Kelsch and Kiener, hæmoglobinuria in this case always indicates rapid destruction of the red corpuscles. Jaundice is a contingent phenomenon, resulting
from the direct action of the malarial organism on the biliary secretion.

Hæmoglobinuria may occur in the ox as an infectious disease, due to
a bacterium, described by Babès. It can also be reproduced by experimental infections in the laboratory. It has been noted in typhus, scarlatina,
and perhaps it would be found more frequently if it were looked for in

the infectious diseases of man. The introduction into the system of certain vegetable or mineral substances, such as mushrooms, carbolic acid, arseniu- retted hydrogen, chlorate of potash, pyrogallic acid, iodine, and glycerine, may cause so-called toxic hæmoglobinuria. The simple injection of water, the injection of dissolved hæmoglobin or of bile acids, into the blood of animals also causes experimental hæmoglobinuria. Under the influence of the toxic agent the hæmoglobin leaves the red corpuscles and dissolves in the serum. The researches of Ponfick, and also those of Marchand, Lebe- deff, and Litten, have revealed three varieties in the preliminary hæmoglo- binæmia. In the first one, the hæmoglobin dissolved in the blood is in such small quantity that it is destroyed, and does not appear in the urine. In the second, the spleen and the marrow of the bones contribute to change the corpuscular detritus into pigments. In the third, the destroying organs are insufficient, and we see hæmoglobinuria, with jaundice, and oliguria, or anuria from obliteration of the tubules of the kidney.

Pathogenesis.—The pathogenesis of malarial and toxic hæmoglobinuria has been cleared up within recent years by means of anatomical and experi- mental research. We shall see how, in a certain degree, it may help us to understand the disputed mechanism of paroxysmal hæmoglobinuria *a frigore.* In malarial, as in experimental, hæmoglobinuria we find a phase of hæmo- globinuria followed by a phase of renal change.

In order that hæmoglobinuria may occur, the destruction of corpuscles must correspond to about a sixth of the total mass of the red blood-corpuscles. It must be rapid, and take place in less than twenty-four hours at the most. The renal changes are due to the excretion of the pigment by the tubuli contorti. The pigment is not seen in Henle's descending loop, in the straight tubules, in the collecting tubules, or in the glomeruli. It is only found in the epithelium of the convoluted tubules and in Henle's ascending loop. The localization simulates that of colouring substances injected into the circulation, as in Heidenhain's well-known experiment with indigo. The cells, infiltrated by the indigo, become opaque ; the nuclei and the divisions of the cells are no longer visible. The pigmentary inundation may be such that in the interior of the tubes we find a fine granular dust of the same aspect as the pigment, sometimes forming large masses that may block the canaliculi and cause anuria.

Two theories have been propounded as to the pathogenesis of paroxysmal hæmoglobinuria : renal congestion and primary hæmoglobinæmia. The renal theory, supported in France by Hayem and Robin, rests on pure theory. According to Robin, it is due to local congestion in the kidney, assisted by disordered nutrition, consequent on rheumatism, syphilis, or malaria.

The partisans of the second theory say that the process is that of experimental toxic hæmoglobinuria. Hæmoglobinæmia is said to be the initial phenomenon, while the renal change is secondary. The question to be solved is, then, whether in an attack of paroxysmal hæmoglobinuria there is previous hæmoglobinæmia, and consequent renal lesion, characterized by pigmentary infiltration of the cells of the convoluted tubules. If, as certain writers have maintained, there are cases in which the serum of the blood presents no changes, there are other authors, such as Lépine, Rodet and Salle, Ehrlich, de Cazal, Boas, and Lichteim, who have proved hæmoglobinæmia beyond a doubt by collecting blood during the attack.

The often quoted experiment of Ehrlich is most significant. He was able to reproduce, apart from a crisis, alteration of the blood in a limited zone. He plunged a finger into iced water, after having applied an elastic ligature, and produced a circumscribed hæmoglobinæmia in the superficial capillaries.

Hayem, though a partisan of the renal theory, admits that the congestion of the kidney must be assisted by a change in the blood. In his opinion, the cherry-red colour of the serum, stated to be characteristic of hæmoglobinæmia, is only produced after the blood has remained some time *in vitro*. It is said to indicate that the blood is certainly changed, because this coloration of the serum does not take place in normal blood. If, on the other hand, we shake a tube four hours after having poured some blood into it, the central clot is completely dissolved, and gives a red colour to the mixture —a phenomenon, says Hayem, not observed in any other disease.

The previous change in the blood (hæmoglobinæmia) is not a matter of doubt, but in order to know whether, during an attack of paroxysmal hæmoglobinuria, the renal lesions are similar to those seen in other varieties of hæmoglobinuria, we needed a post-mortem examination, where, death having occurred during the attack, we could observe the renal lesion at the moment when the hæmoglobinuria began. The lacuna has been filled by a unique case which Widal and myself were fortunate enough to observe :

A woman died during an attack in the Necker Hospital. At the autopsy we found the entire renal cortex of a marked sepia colour. Under the microscope the glomeruli were healthy ; the cells of the convoluted tubules and of Henle's ascending loop alone showed hæmoglobinic infiltration ; large granules of hæmoglobin were met with even in the lumen of the tubules. The localization corresponded to that of the pigments, previously dissolved in the general circulation, and eliminated by the kidney, in the well-known experiment of Heidenhain. This post-mortem examination, then, furnishes one of the proofs which the hæmoglobinæmic theory lacked.

What is the cause of this instability of the blood ? Cold or fatigue seems to be the most common determining cause, but, furthermore, patients with hæmoglobinuria have nearly all had malaria or syphilis. One of my patients had suffered from both these diseases. He improved on the mercurial treatment which I ordered.

Donath and Landsteiner have shown that " Ehrlich's experiment of the cold finger " may be reproduced *in vitro* with the plasma from a case of hæmoglobinuria. These authors mix human red corpuscles with the serum or oxalate plasma collected from a case of hæmoglobinuria in the interval of the attacks. They subject the mixture for half an hour to a temperature of 0° C., and then place it in the oven at 37° C. for two hours. They find after this treatment marked hæmatolysis, but when the mixture is submitted to a temperature of 37° C. without previous cooling, the hæmatolysis does not occur.

This experiment of cooling *in vitro* closely reproduces an attack of hæmoglobinuria resulting from cold. Widal and Rostaine have shown that this phenomenon is due to a lack of the anti-immune body which the blood normally contains in order to protect its corpuscles by neutralizing the action of the immune body which it constantly carries. If the red cells remain whole in their own proper serum, or in serum from an animal of the same species, it is because of this anti-immune body, which is powerless to protect them against a strange serum.

Bordet has proved the existence of an anti-immune body specific for the corpuscle of a given species in serum from animals of a different species, treated with injections of red cells or serum from the first species. Widal and Rostaine have injected horses with massive doses of human serum, obtained by bleeding for therapeutic purposes. In the serum of animals thus treated there developed an anti-immune body specific for the amboceptor of human red corpuscles. These authorities have shown that a very minute quantity of this serum heated to 55° C., in order to remove its cytose, and added to the plasma of a patient with hæmoglobinuria, sufficed to remove its power of affecting human red corpuscles after exposure to cold. The anti-immune body, by uniting with the immune body, which was attached to the corpuscles by the action of cold, has thus neutralized this action.

As it is sufficient to add to the plasma of a patient with hæmoglobinuria a relatively small amount of the anti-immune body in order to prevent the solvent action on the red corpuscles that cold produces, it was natural to see whether injection of the anti-immune body would not prevent an attack *a frigore* in man. Widal and Rostaine have been able, by means of large injections of their horse serum, to prevent the attack *a frigore* in hæmoglobinuric patients.

The protection of the organism varied directly with the dose injected, and for a given dose the resistance to hæmoglobinæmia was the greater, the less severe the cold and the less prolonged its action. So far in human pathology, serotherapy has only furnished results in diseases due to micro-organisms and toxines. It is therefore interesting to note the action of serum upon a humoral trouble such as hæmoglobinæmia. We can in this way confer but a transient immunity, lasting some three weeks. After this period it is necessary to inject large doses of serum when the patient is very sensitive to cold.

Another variety of hæmoglobinuria occurs. It is due to the elimination of the muscular hæmoglobin. There exists in muscle a special hæmoglobin, which gives it its red colour. In these cases there is no hæmoglobin-æmia, as may be proved by examination of the blood-serum. This is because the muscular hæmoglobin passes through the kidneys far more readily than the corpuscular hæmoglobin does. Furthermore, it is eliminated as soon as it is set at liberty, and does not accumulate in the blood. As with the hæmoglobin of the red blood-corpuscles, the freeing of the hæmoglobin in muscle is caused by cold. The attack is accompanied by pain in the muscles, which may cause paresis (Camus and Pagniez).

Finally, false hæmoglobinuria may follow on nephrorrhagia or cystorrhagia. The red corpuscles are dissolved in the contents of the bladder, and the proper character of the hæmaturia then disappears. This occurs in certain kinds of urine, which dissolve the red corpuscles with great facility. We then speak of "cythæmolytic urine." This property is especially marked in watery urine. It is remedied by administering chloride of sodium to the patient, the elimination of which increases the density of the urine, and transforms false hæmoglobinuria into hæmaturia (Camus).

Patients with hæmoglobinuria must avoid cold or sudden changes of temperature, and live as far as possible in temperate climates. These measures will at least prevent the attacks.

If the patient has had malaria, we should give quinine and arsenic. The mercurial preparations should be reserved for syphilitic patients.

XXI. MOVABLE KIDNEY—COEXISTENT UNILATERAL NEPHRITIS.

Pathogenesis.—In order to gain a clear idea of displacements of the kidneys we must first consider how the organ is fixed. The kidney is held in its normal position by a cellulo-fibrous envelope, rich in adipose tissue. The kidney is buried in this envelope, to which it adheres by fine threads. According to certain writers, the fibrous element is said to form a sort of transverse shelf, ensheathing the kidney in front and behind, and uniting below the organ, but absent inside and below. It is, in fact, in these directions that the kidney escapes. In its migration it covers itself with the peritoneum, which it pushes in front of it. It may even descend very low between the intestinal coils.

According to Trocart, it is not the cellulo-fatty envelope, but the peritoneum, which is the principal obstacle to displacement of the kidney. This writer has found that, in order to draw a kidney covered by its peritoneum downwards or forwards, a force of 20 to 25 pounds is required, whilst the resistance of the cellulo-fatty capsule does not exceed 5 pounds.

Renal ectopia (floating kidney, nephroptosis) is much more frequent in women than in men. It affects the right kidney more often than the left, and rarely both kidneys. Repeated pregnancies, tight corsets, relaxation of the abdominal walls, contusions, strains, and absorption of the cellulo-fatty layer around the kidney, have been assigned as causes. The influence of sex is undoubted, because we find that in 100 cases of renal ectopia about 86 cases occur in women. The right kidney is displaced four times as often as the left one. As to **pregnancy,** its influence has been singularly exaggerated, since in 94 cases (Küttner) the kidneys were displaced in 40 women who had never borne a child. Glénard, who included nephroptosis under the more general theory of enteroptosis, supposes that the movable kidney is a digestive syndrome. Potain thinks that the mobility of the kidney is due to inflammatory phenomena. He says that displacements of the kidney by sliding are the most common; they are often associated with muco-membranous colitis. The displacements by anteversion are often associated with biliary lithiasis.

Pathological Anatomy.—As people do not die of renal ectopia, the pathological anatomy is based upon the operation findings. In a thousand post-mortem examinations, made in different diseases, we may not find one case of movable kidney (Schultze). When the kidney is much displaced, it may be found in the iliac fossa, epigastrium, or hypochondria, but the suprarenal capsule never accompanies the kidney in its displacement. The kidney is sometimes fixed in its new position by adhesions. The kidney may be cystic or cancerous. It is sometimes affected by chronic nephritis.

Description.—Many patients have a displaced kidney without being aware of the fact; this is the latent form. An individual complains of dyspeptic troubles, belching, or abdominal tympanites. On examination we find dilatation of the stomach and of the colon, and also a movable kidney. Another individual is neurasthenic, and complains of vertigo, hot flushes, headaches, loss of appetite, weakness, and loss of flesh. Examination reveals a displaced kidney. A third subject has discovered a tumour in the belly, but experiences no symptoms. Examination reveals a floating kidney. In these various cases the displaced kidney is associated with diverse morbid conditions, without causing its own symptoms.

The floating kidney has two chief symptoms—**pain** and **abdominal tumour,** with more or less pronounced general troubles. Renal ectopia is sometimes sudden in its onset. In consequence of fatigue or strain, or even without appreciable cause, the patient is taken ill with acute pain in the abdomen. The usual story is : " I fancy that something has got loose in my inside." The kidney may be replaced, and the patient is cured. This sudden displacement of the kidney, sometimes accompanied by a tendency to syncope, may be of traumatic origin.

In other cases the symptoms come on gradually. The pain, limited to the hypochondrium or to the lumbar region of the affected side, is often accompanied by a feeling of weight or dragging. The pain is dull, or pulsating like an abscess, and is brought on by walking, riding, or exercise, and relieved by the horizontal position. Very painful attacks may supervene as the result of strain or of menstruation. They are accompanied by rigors, vomiting, and syncope (Lancereaux). Rest in bed generally puts an end to these attacks. In some people the pains simulate hepatic or renal colic ; in the latter event they radiate to the ureter, bladder, loins, or thighs. Anorexia, gastralgia, gastro-intestinal distension, pyrosis, eructations, nausea, and vomiting, are frequent in patients with movable kidney. The same remark applies to the neurasthenic, hysterical, and hypochondriacal symptoms.

The displaced kidney forms a tumour, which can be felt deep under the costal margin and toward the lateral part of the abdomen. This tumour is reniform, painful on pressure, and generally so mobile that it can be displaced in all directions. In some cases, however, the kidney is fixed by adhesions.

Strangulation of the Kidney.—I must now refer to an acute complication which appears in the following manner : An individual with a displaced kidney is taken suddenly ill, without appreciable cause, with symptoms resembling acute peritonitis. Sharp pains in the belly, nausea, vomiting, feeble pulse, cold sweats, abdominal tympanism, pinched face, and syncope occur, closely simulating the picture of acute peritonitis caused by perforation. The first thought is perforation of the stomach or duodenum by an ulcer, or appendicular peritonitis ; but a more careful examination reveals in the abdomen a mobile, reducible, and painful tumour, which is the displaced kidney. The organ is for the time being enlarged by hydronephrosis, which is a complication of renal strangulation. The attack may last for several hours or days, with intervals of calm, and then everything again becomes normal if the patient has been ordered to rest in the horizontal position. The attack ceases suddenly with the passage of abundant urine and the disappearance of the fluid tumour in the belly. Although the name " renal strangulation," invented by Dietl, is not absolutely true, it sums up fairly well the pathogenesis of the troubles due to torsion of the ureter, with intermittent hydronephrosis and venous stasis, caused by temporary arrest of the circulation in the renal vein. These attacks, which are extremely painful, may occur frequently. They were well known to Trousseau, who, at the commencement of his lecture on "Movable Kidney," gives a description to which nothing remains to be added.

The **diagnosis** of renal ectopia, though easy in some cases, may present much difficulty. Many abdominal, renal, mesenteric, hepatic, and ovarian tumours may simulate a displaced kidney. The diagnosis of renal strangulation is simplified by the recognition of the displaced kidney ; we must always think of it in these cases of pseudo-peritonitis, which simulate appendicitis, internal strangulation, and gastro-intestinal perforations.

The **prognosis** is not grave, and yet its indefinite duration, its serious effect on the system, and the complications that it may cause (nephritis), deserve careful consideration.

Rehal Lesions — Albuminuria — Nephritis.—It was for a long time believed that the composition of the urine was not affected in movable kidney. A floating kidney was said to be exempt from lesions. These ideas must be modified, as Tuffier has already shown. In a patient with movable kidney albuminuria is fairly common (according to Schilling, in 14 per cent. of the cases). The presence of casts is sometimes noticed, in addition to albuminuria.

I had a woman in my wards with symptoms of movable kidney at the fourth month of pregnancy. After her confinement she was attacked by puerperal infection, with phlebitis, cystitis, and ascending nephritis, which grafted itself on to the movable kidney (*locus minoris resistentiæ*). Three months later the patient resumed duty as infirmary nurse, but she had still pains in the right loin and slight pyæmia. It was interesting to ascertain the composition of the urine from each kidney ; this was readily done with the segregator. The analysis of the quantity of urine passed in twenty minutes was made by Gouraud :

	Right Movable Kidney.	*Left Kidney.*
Quantity	180 minims	360 minims
Urea	1·5 grains	4 grains
Chlorides	1·5 grains	5 grains
Albumin	abundant	notable
Cells from the kidney	absent	absent
Casts	absent	absent
Cells from the bladder	numerous	numerous
Red corpuscles	numerous	numerous
White corpuscles	numerous	numerous
Streptococci	abundant	absent

This table shows that the activity of the movable kidney is diminished by one-half, and that it is from this kidney, infected by the streptococcus, that nearly all the albumin comes.

The researches of recent years have shown that movable kidneys fairly often show slight or severe lesions, amounting even to chronic nephritis. I have discussed this unilateral nephritis in Section VI. It has often been noticed by surgeons, particularly by Edebohls.

The **medical treatment** of movable kidney has as its object the maintenance of the organ in position by appropriate bandages. Massage may give good results. Nephropexy is often necessary. This operation consists in provoking adhesions between the kidney and the abdominal wall.

Tuffier's figures read :

	Perfect cure			86
	Lasting improvement			25
In 163 cases	Satisfactory results			24
	Temporary improvement			8
	Failures			20

If the reader will refer to Section VI., he will see the results obtained by Edebohls in cases of movable kidney, complicated with nephritis. In several cases the ectopia and the coexistent nephritis have been cured simultaneously.

CHAPTER II

DISEASES OF THE SUPRARENAL CAPSULES

ADDISON'S DISEASE—DEFACED TYPE OF ADDISON'S DISEASE

Description.—Addison's disease is characterized, in a typical case, by marked asthenia, bronzed colouring of the skin, pain, and gastro-intestinal troubles.

Asthenia is generally the first symptom, and has a special character. It is characterized by muscular weakness, which makes every effort impossible, and which at its commencement presents the peculiar feature "that, when the disease is primary and isolated, it is not accompanied by albuminuria, hæmorrhage, leucocytosis, or even by the customary diarrhœa" (Jaccoud). This kind of asthenia, then, is very different to cachectic asthenia.

One of my patients repeated incessantly : " I am done for ; my strength is gone ; I am incapable of any effort." It is certain that the patient realizes the weakening of his muscular strength. As far as he is concerned, there can be no question of walking or riding. At a more advanced period of the disease any movement causes absolute horror. Speaking and eating cause fatigue. The patient lies down, so that he may not be obliged to move, and has hardly sufficient strength to remain standing. There is no paralysis, but the muscular system is incapable of any sustained effort. If the patient's first attempt registers 40 pounds on the dynamometer, the second and third attempts will give not more than 20 or 10 pounds. A fourth or fifth attempt will not show any registration at all ; his muscular strength is exhausted. One of my patients registered a force of 80 pounds at his first attempt, but his fifth and sixth efforts only registered 20 and 10 pounds. This rapid muscular exhaustion has been accurately registered by means of Mosso's ergograph. Several of these charts are to be found in Dupaigne's thesis. They show not only the work " which has produced the fatigue, but also the rapidity and the form of this fatigue."

This muscular weakness is due to the suppression of the function of the suprarenal capsules. Animals after the removal of the suprarenal capsules

1199

become intoxicated by their mechanical work. Their muscles become less and less capable of effort; but if suprarenal extract is injected, it destroys in part the muscular toxines, and for a time prevents the muscular exhaustion (Langlois).

Pain.—The pains are felt in the epigastrium, the loins, the region of the kidneys, the hypochondrium, the limbs, the muscles, and the joints. They are sometimes very severe, being lancinating and radiating as far as the groins along the small branches of the ovarian or spermatic plexus. They may simulate the gastric crises of tabes, with or without vomiting. They remain fixed in the region of the kidneys, and simulate lumbago; and as they cause hyperæsthesia of the entire belly, they give the idea of peritonitis (Wurtz). They invade the muscles and the joints, just as rheumatism does. These pains generally appear after the onset of the asthenia, In some cases, however, they may be the first symptom of Addison's disease.

Gastro-Intestinal Troubles.—Anorexia, vomiting, and diarrhœa supervene, either from the commencement or during the course of the disease. The vomit may be mucous, as in alcoholism, or it may consist of foodstuffs; it may be uncontrollable and accompanied by gastralgia. Diarrhœa is a frequent symptom. It may be paroxysmal or continuous, sometimes lasting for several weeks. It disappears and reappears without interruption, especially at an advanced period of the disease. Loss of flesh usually supervenes from the first in Addison's disease; sometimes it is rapid and considerable.

Melanodermia.—Pigmentation of the skin is very rarely the initial symptom of Addison's disease (six times in 144 cases—Jaccoud). Melanodermia is, as a rule, preceded by asthenia, pain, and gastro-intestinal troubles. The appearance of melanodermia decides the diagnosis, which has been previously impossible or doubtful. The pigmentation appears at first on the exposed parts of the body—the face, neck, forearms, dorsal surface of the hands, and wrists—and next on the parts normally pigmented—the breasts, the genital organs (glans, labia minora), the groins, and the axillæ. At first the skin is not bronzed, but of a light slate colour, and looks dirty; it is only later that it acquires the mulatto tint. Trousseau's patient observed that for some three months his hands had been bistre-coloured and dirty, in spite of repeated washing. His face had a smoky look. This brownish tint showed itself on different parts of the body, and prolonged baths caused no change. At first the discoloration is limited to brownish patches, but later it becomes general, and resembles the complexion of the mulatto. Darker patches sometimes stand out on the uniform background. There are sometimes patches where the pigment is entirely absent (vitiligo). The colouring also affects some of the mucous membranes; the lips, gums, tongue, palate, and internal surface of the cheeks are mottled with black patches, such as are seen inside the mouth of certain dogs.

Course of the Disease.—As Trousseau says, the onset is slow, and the disease at first passes unnoticed. The patient cannot fix exactly the commencement of the symptoms. There is general malaise, with weakening of the physical and moral forces. The appetite grows less, the digestion is disturbed by uncontrollable vomiting. At the same time gastric and lumbo-abdominal pain supervenes. Pigmentation of the skin soon shows itself. As the disease progresses, the bronzed tint becomes more and more pronounced. Cachexia appears, prostration becomes extreme, and the patient is confined to bed, unwilling to move and refusing all food. He suffers from irrepressible vomiting, with continual diarrhœa. He has a sensation of vertigo, fainting, or syncope, and complains of a feeling of cold in the limbs, which persists in spite of everything, and he dies, emaciated to the utmost degree, in marasmus or coma.

In some cases Addison's disease has a rapid course, and death may supervene in a few weeks or months (Starr). Generally, however, its course is slower. According to Ball's statistics, the duration was less than a year in thirty-nine cases, and in thirty-nine other cases it was more than a year. In any event, the disease ends in death.

If the patient is attacked by secondary or primary pulmonary tuberculosis, the symptoms of tubercular cachexia are added to those of Addison's cachexia, the loss of flesh and the course of events being more rapid. Addison's disease does not always go through all its phases without periods of arrest. Remissions of longer or shorter duration may occur. These remissions follow as the result of absolute rest, and cease at once as soon as the patient resumes his ordinary work.

Sudden Death.—Patients with Addison's disease do not, as a rule, die suddenly; they gradually become cachectic and die of marasmus or coma, the pulmonary and suprarenal lesions helping to this end.

In such circumstances death is not unexpected, and the physician can foretell the fatal termination. In some cases, however, the march of events is different, and an individual with Addison's disease is suddenly seized with convulsions, coma, or syncope, and death rapidly follows. To quote examples :

Hiller : A man suffering from pulmonary tuberculosis had also an anal fistula, which was operated on. Next morning the patient's condition was good. The patient was suddenly seized with epileptiform convulsions and loss of consciousness. The convulsive attack recurred during the day, and the patient died. At the post-mortem examination a few tubercles were found at the apices of the lungs. All the other organs were normal, with the exception of the suprarenal capsules, which showed tubercular degeneration. The patient **had no bronzed tint.** (The case is an example of the defaced type.)

II.   77

Chauffard : A lady, thirty-five years of age, had all the symptoms of Addison's disease : the asthenia was so great that she could not drive in a carriage without fatigue ; the patient passed her days stretched out on a long chair, incapable of the least muscular movement ; the pigmentation was typical. Without warning the patient was seized with angina, pain, and acceleration of the pulse to 160, and she succumbed, intoxicated by the toxine, acting here " like curare, and causing paralytic tachycardia."

Letulle : A man, twenty-eight years of age, who for some weeks had felt great lassitude and depression, was admitted to St. Antoine Hospital. His skin was of an earthy colour ; this was ascribed to an old attack of malaria. The examination revealed a suspicious tubercular lesion at the left apex. Nine days later, without apparent cause, death supervened suddenly, just as the patient was about to sit up. The post-mortem examination showed that each suprarenal capsule was transformed into a fibro-caseous block of the size of a small tangerine orange. The man had died suddenly of Addison's disease.

Sudden death has been noted in children, who may also suffer from Addison's disease. With regard to this point, Variot relates the following case :

A thin little girl, fourteen years of age, was admitted into the Trousseau Hospital for weakness and a tired feeling in the legs. Her uncle was said to have noticed that the skin had been getting brown. The hyperpigmentation of the skin was, in fact, general. Addison's disease was diagnosed. One morning the child got up to use the chamber ; she got back to bed, became pale, and died. At the post-mortem examination miliary tubercles were found in both lungs. Both suprarenal capsules were enlarged, and converted into tubercular tissue.

These cases show that Addison's disease may terminate in sudden death. This sudden ending may happen in the cachectic stage, or at a period of the disease when nothing could have caused it to be foreseen.

I consider it important to mention that sudden death has been noted several times in Addison's disease of the defaced type, where the patient had no bronzed tint. The importance of these cases will be apparent from the medico-legal point of view. An individual dies suddenly, and as the bronzed tint is wanting, attention is not called to the nature of the disease. The post-mortem examination reveals the fatal lesion in the suprarenal capsules.

Defaced Type.—In one of my clinical lectures* I proposed the name **defaced** for cases of Addison's disease in which pigmentation of the skin and of the mucosæ was absent. I quote the case upon which the lecture was based :

In January, 1898, a youth of seventeen years of age came into my wards very much exhausted. He understood the questions put to him, but his answers were slow and difficult. He awoke from his somnolence, as it were, with regret, and fell back into it again as soon as I ceased questioning him. I was, nevertheless, able to obtain some information. He had come to the hospital for extreme lassitude. He was not paralyzed, but the slightest movement was an effort. He was pale, remarkably thin, motionless, and lay in his bed like a dying man.

The patient gave the following history : Six months previously he began to

* " Forme Fruste de la Maladie d'Addison " (*Clinique Médicale de l'Hôtel-Dieu*, 1898, 9me leçon).

cough; no fever, no hæmoptysis; rapid loss of flesh and extreme weakness. At the Tenon Hospital tubercular bronchitis was diagnosed. After a fortnight's treatment the patient returned home. The cough was almost gone, but his strength was gradually failing; he was so tired that he never wished to leave his bed. This condition of weakness and of loss of flesh became still more pronounced during the fortnight preceding his admission into my wards. There was no other symptom to be noticed excepting slight vomiting of food.

It was necessary to make a diagnosis. The signs of pulmonary tuberculosis were undeniable, but the tubercular lesion was not sufficient to account for the asthenia and lassitude. The clinical picture was not that of early phthisis. Diabetes sometimes causes similar symptoms, but the patient was not diabetic. All the organs, with the exception of the lungs, were healthy; the skin showed no patches and no eruption; and we were perhaps face to face with complications such as meningeal or miliary tuberculosis. The prostration, vomiting, constipation, and retraction of the abdomen, were in favour of meningitis; but meningitis, even supposing it were present, would not have accounted for the progressive asthenia, which in six months had ended in marasmus. The following morning, the situation remained the same. At eleven o'clock in the morning he took a glass of milk, and fell back again into his apathy. At half-past two o'clock the nurse on duty found him dead.

The results of the post-mortem examination were quite a surprise. At the apices of the lungs the ordinary tubercular lesions were met with. The brain, liver, kidneys, and spleen were absolutely healthy, but both suprarenal capsules were enlarged and converted into tuberculo-caseous tissue. They were superimposed on the kidneys like large mushrooms. The left suprarenal capsule was hypertrophied, indurated, and calcareous, with soft points; the lower portion was much harder, of a golden yellow colour, and had undergone cretaceous change. The right suprarenal capsule was likewise transformed into tuberculo-caseous tissue; it was indurated and calcified in places.

As the post-mortem examination showed that the patient had died of Addison's disease, we searched with the greatest care, both on the skin and on the mucosæ, for some traces of pigmentation. **There were none at all.** The disease had been **defaced.** Other examples are :

Lancereaux : A woman who had been ill for a month with vomiting and loss of flesh came to the hospital in a condition of complete prostration. Vomiting and weakness were the chief symptoms. The patient was so weak that she would not even move in her bed, and was afraid of changing her position. **The skin was normal.** The urine contained neither sugar nor albumin. The patient succumbed. At the post-mortem examination three little tubercular masses were found at the apex of the left lung. The suprarenal capsules were hard, indurated, yellowish, and tuberculo-caseous. Death was due to Addison's disease, which had caused melanodermia.

Carpentier : A man within six months had grown so thin and weak that he lay motionless on his bed, except when he took a little food. The urine contained neither sugar nor albumin. The temperature was normal. The successive examination of the various organs gave only negative results. There was no pigmentation. For a fortnight no change was noticed. One morning he experienced a feeling of distress and cold. Half an hour later the pulse became thready, the extremities grew cold, and the patient died, remaining conscious until the very end. The post-mortem examination revealed old tubercular foci at the apex of the lungs. The suprarenal capsules were attacked by tuberculosis. The skin and mucous membranes were examined most carefully, but no trace of pigmentation could be found. It was a case of Addison's disease without melanodermia.

Diagnosis.—It is quite impossible to diagnose Addison's disease before the appearance of melanodermia. The character of the muscular asthenia furnishes a strong presumption in favour of Addison's disease, especially if gastric troubles and pains are also present. The appearance of melano- dermia decides the diagnosis, for the syndrome is then complete ; and yet, when melanodermia occurs in an anæmic or neurasthenic patient, we must not diagnose Addison's disease before making a careful examination. Some syphilitic patients (women especially) show in the secondary period a pig- mentation of the skin of the neck (pigmentary syphilides), and suffer from muscular weakness. In malarial cachexia the pigmentation of the skin is less pronounced, the patches on the mucosæ are wanting, the spleen is hypertrophied, and the causes of the disease are known. Patients who have been treated for a long time with nitrate of silver, either through the diges- tive passages or by injections, have sometimes an indelible bluish tinge, which is especially marked on the face and hands, since they are exposed to the light. In **bronzed diabetes** there is a lesion of the liver, and more or less abundant glycosuria. In the **defaced** forms of Addison's disease the diagnosis presents the greatest difficulty.

Addison's disease must not be confounded with vagabond's itch, in which the pigmentation is due to *Pediculi corporis*, and affects the parts in contact with the clothes. The presence of the parasites and the scratch- marks give the diagnosis. The diagnosis may, however, be difficult on account of the pigmentation of the buccal mucous membrane that sometimes occurs in vagabond's itch. In such a case, however, asthenia, gastro- intestinal troubles, pain, and low arterial tension are absent.

In Addison's disease the pseudo-peritoneal symptoms sometimes simu- late appendicitis.

Pathological Anatomy.—The essential lesions of Addison's disease are seated in the·suprarenal capsules and in the neighbouring nerve plexus. The nature of the lesion matters little ; the important point is the seat of the lesion. In fact, the changes of the capsules are very diverse. Tuber- culo-scrofulous lesions are the most common ; then come cancer, suppurative inflammation, cystic degeneration, and the echinococcus. The lesion is almost always bilateral. The capsules are often hypertrophied and adherent to the neighbouring organs. In tubercular degeneration they are mammil- lated, and their substance is converted into a lardaceous mass, showing opaque yellowish portions, tubercular granulations, caseous and cretaceous masses, and islets or bands of connective substance. In a certain number of post-mortem examinations, lesions of the semilunar ganglia and of the solar plexus (sclerosis and fatty degeneration) have been noted. The melanodermia is due to accumulation of pigment in the corpus mucosum.

Ætiology—Pathogenesis.—Addison's disease is most frequent between the ages of twenty and forty years. It is sometimes primary, and super- venes in the midst of good health. Sometimes it is secondary, and supervenes in a patient who is already tubercular. In any case, the syndrome of Addison's disease does not answer to any one lesion of the suprarenal capsules. The essential factor is that the suprarenal region must be affected. The lesion is, it is true, most frequently tuberculo-caseous, but it may be malignant or fibrous.

The pathogenesis of the disease may be stated thus : Brown-Séquard, Abelous, and Langlois have proved that complete extirpation of both supra-renal capsules in the frog, guinea-pig, or dog, causes death in a few days. If only a sixth part of the suprarenal capsules is left, this part is sufficient to carry on the function, and the animal may not die. The animal, after complete extirpation of the capsules, succumbs after suffering rapid loss of strength, similar to the muscular asthenia of Addison's disease.

It is a question of toxic symptoms. The deficiency or the suppression of the suprarenal function allows the accumulation of a poison in the blood. This toxine is identical with the toxine obtained from the muscles of an overworked animal, and seems to have the effect of curare. It attacks the motor nerve endings (fatigue and muscular paresis, rapid exhaustion of the motor excitability). It may even involve the cardiac nerves, and cause paralytic tachycardia (Chauffard). The suprarenal capsules have, then, an antitoxic action upon the waste products of muscular combustion, neutralizing or destroying the poisons of the curare type that are elaborated during muscular work.   They belong to the group of glands having an internal secretion.

Most of the symptoms of Addison's disease, including the grave and fatal symptoms, are due to suprarenal insufficiency, to the resulting auto-intoxica-tion, and to the nature of the toxines, which are no longer neutralized or destroyed when the suprarenal function is suppressed (experiments on animals), or when the function is destroyed by lesions (tuberculosis, cancer, fibroid and calcareous changes, or abscess).

The melanodermia has still to be explained. It is said to be due, not to the suprarenal insufficiency, but to the nervous lesions of the plexus around the capsules (Jaccoud, Alezais, and Arnaud). Melanodermia is said to be absent when the lesion is confined to the interior of the gland. It is said to appear when the lesion involves the ganglia and the nerve plexus in the fibrous covering of the suprarenal capsule. It will, therefore, be understood that a lesion may attack either the gland or the nerve plexus. Lesions of the nerve plexus without direct lesions of the gland might reproduce the syndrome of Addison's disease, as the glands only function definitely through their nerves (Caussade).

Treatment.—Hygiene occupies a prominent place in the treatment of Addison's disease. A few days of complete rest are sometimes sufficient to make a patient recover who appears to have reached an advanced state of asthenia. The most approved line of treatment consists in supplementing the insufficiency by giving suprarenal extract. Brown-Séquard deserves the highest credit as the pioneer in this branch of therapeutics. Suprarenal insufficiency causes symptoms of auto-intoxication in much the same way as thyroid insufficiency causes an auto-intoxication. The introduction of thyroid extract into the system has an extraordinary effect on myxœdema. It was, therefore, reasonable to hope that the introduction of suprarenal extract into the system would give good results.

The first attempts in this direction were not encouraging (Abalous, Langlois, Charrin, and Chauffard). Several cases have since been published (Béclère, Dupaigne, Gilbert, and Marie). I made use of this remedy in the following case :

A man, twenty-nine years of age, was admitted into my wards on June 14, 1895, for muscular exhaustion, preventing any effort. The muscular asthenia began four months after the military manœuvres. Three months before admission vomiting and pain appeared, and soon after diarrhœa. The vomit contained bile and food-stuff ; the vomiting recurred several times daily for several weeks. The pains were very sharp in the epigastric region, in the hypochondria, and in the calves of the legs. The diarrhœa had been continuous for several days—up to twelve and fourteen stools a day. The patient was very thin. On looking at him we were immediately struck with the bistre colour of his face, neck, forearm, and the dorsal surface of his hands. There were pigmentary patches on the lower limbs. We also found bronzed patches on the buccal mucosa, on the velum palati, and behind the labial commissure. The patient told us himself that during the past few months his skin had " become the colour of gingerbread."

It was a case of Addison's disease. We had still to discover the nature of the lesion in the suprarenal capsules. As the left subspinal fossa showed some signs of early tuberculosis, it was evident that the suprarenal capsules were invaded by tuberculosis. An injection of 1 c.c. of glycerinated suprarenal extract was administered every other day. The symptoms rapidly improved ; the vomiting, pain, and diarrhœa disappeared. The appetite was excellent, and the muscular asthenia diminished so much that the patient, who during his first days in hospital could not leave his bed, now helped to clean the floors. He asked to be discharged. He returned three months afterwards in a state of muscular asthenia more pronounced than on his first visit. He was carried on a stretcher. The vomiting, diarrhœa, and pains had reappeared, the bronzed tint had increased, and the loss of flesh was so great that the patient only weighed 110 pounds. The signs of pulmonary tuberculosis were unchanged, and bacilli were found in the sputum. I again prescribed suprarenal extract, but in view of threatening lymphangitis I replaced the injections by capsules, each capsule containing 1½ grains of dried suprarenal gland. Four capsules were administered daily. The improvement was even more rapid than on the first occasion, all the symptoms yielding in a few days. The patient put on flesh visibly, gaining 20 pounds in a month. He again left the hospital and resumed his work, but he was obliged to come back on December 5, for the same symptoms ; he only weighed 106 pounds. For a third time the treatment, to which large doses of cod-liver oil were added, caused the symptoms (except the pigmentation) to disappear, and two months and a half later the patient, who had regained his strength, weighed 125 pounds. The pulmonary lesions had improved, the expectoration was almost absent, and contained no more bacilli.

Surgeon-Lieutenant Pech, of Sidi-bel-Abbès, sent me the following notes of a patient suffering from advanced Addison's disease, and treated with grilled suprarenal capsules from bullocks.   After taking this food for a few days the improvement in the patient was surprising.   He felt strong and well.   The vomiting did not reappear, and the striking thing was that he was losing his bronzed complexion.   He walked up the stairs and about the garden, although he had been incapable of the slightest movement. He ate voraciously and without vomiting, although he had been a prey to uncontrollable vomiting.

The amelioration obtained by suprarenal opotherapy is, unfortunately, not of long duration—at least, we are not absolutely certain as to the value of the remedy.   In a case published by Béclère, however, the pigmentation disappeared, the dynamometric force increased to quite an unexpected degree, and the cure was maintained three years afterwards.   Whatever the future may have in store for opotherapy in Addison's disease, it remains none the less true that the remedy has given undeniable results.   I propose, therefore, in cases of Addison's disease of the masked type to clear up the diagnosis by the remedy in question.   Grilled suprarenal capsules, or else subcutaneous injections of glycerinated extract of the capsules, will be given, and if the asthenia is improved in a few days, there is a valid reason for making a diagnosis of Addison's disease.

We must not, however, be too ready to regard this treatment as a specific.   Account must be taken of the hygienic conditions and of absolute rest, which are such a valuable auxiliary ; and yet it appears to me undeniable that the ingestion of suprarenal extract is in certain forms of Addison's disease a means to which we must have recourse.   I do not advise the use of subcutaneous injections, because glycerinated extracts, even if aseptic, cause necrosis of the tissues.   I recommend the fresh pulp of the suprarenal glands, or capsules of the dried extract.   The suprarenal capsules of young calves are the best (Pettit).   For many reasons they are preferable to the suprarenal capsules of other animals.

II. INSUFFICIENCY OF THE SUPRARENAL CAPSULES— HÆMORRHAGE—SUPRARENALITIS.

The rôle of the suprarenal glands in the human economy is so important that any change in their function may bring on certain toxic troubles.   We thus have a syndrome of suprarenal insufficiency, comprising the following elements : asthenia, arterial hypotension, vomiting, diarrhœa, cerebral phenomena, and abdominal pains.

They are met with in almost all more or less pronounced capsular lesions, but they do not always appear with the same severity.   Sometimes suprarenal insufficiency manifests itself suddenly in a few days or in a few hours. This is acute insufficiency, very analogous to that seen after the ablation or the sudden destruction of both glands in an animal.

It sometimes appears in an insidious manner.   This is chronic insufficiency, resulting from the slow destruction of the glands by diverse poisons and in particular those of the tubercle bacillus. Caseous tuberculosis and epithelioma of the suprarenal capsules were for a long time considered as the only lesions capable of causing insufficiency. The syndrome was complete, being acute or chronic, sudden or progressive, and causing sudden death or gradual weakening, according as some superadded infection did or did not hasten the course of events.

Recent researches, however, have shown that this syndrome is also found in other affections of the suprarenal capsules.

There are, first of all, cases of primary hæmorrhage or hæmatomata, caused by rupture of an atheromatous vessel, and destroying the glandular parenchyma partially or entirely.

The symptoms in these cases are those of internal hæmorrhage, rather than those of profound intoxication.

Next infections and profound intoxications follow: in the animal, diphtheritic and phosphorus poisoning and pneumo-bacillary infection (Roger, Oppenheim and Loeper); in man, erysipelas, small-pox, measles, scarlatina, diphtheria, icterus gravis, and appendicitis, may be the origin of acute suprarenalitis (Oppenheim and Loeper).

The suprarenal syndrome is not always easily recognized in the symptom-complex of the infection, or of the intoxication that has given rise to it. Sometimes there is a very marked fall in the arterial tension, sometimes there is a sudden and rapidly fatal weakening, sometimes there are cerebral troubles. At other times, as in some of Oppenheim and Loeper's cases, death is sudden.

The post-mortem examination then reveals intense congestion, which may go so far as to cause hæmorrhage, abscesses, and very extensive cellular necrosis.

The frequency of these lesions in individuals who have died of infection or of grave intoxication testifies even more than the suprarenal symptoms to the part which the suprarenal insufficiency must play side by side with the renal and hepatic insufficiency.

The only rational treatment of suprarenal insufficiency appears to be opotherapy. The very rare trials which have been made do not allow us to draw any precise conclusion.

PART IV

DISEASES OF THE NERVOUS SYSTEM

CHAPTER I

DISEASES OF THE SPINAL CORD

I. PROGRESSIVE LOCOMOTOR ATAXY—TABES DORSALIS—DUCHENNE'S DISEASE.

UNDER the names of **tabes dorsalis,** and **spinal paralysis,** the German school had studied the disease which Duchenne had called **progressive locomotor ataxy,** and though the researches undertaken at Vienna and at Berlin concerning this question (Romberg, Wunderlich, Rokitansky) are of undoubted value, we must nevertheless recognize that our present knowledge of this malady is largely due to Duchenne. " Progressive abolition of the co-ordination of the movements and apparent paralysis, contrasting with the integrity of muscular force, are the fundamental characteristics of the disease which I propose to describe. Its symptoms and its course make of it a distinct morbid entity. I propose to call it 'progressive locomotor ataxy.' " This sentence from Duchenne's monograph proves how this accurate observer had at the outset brought into relief the striking features of the disease which bears his name.

Description—Classical Form.—Locomotor ataxy presents two types: the classical and the defaced.

It is customary to describe three periods, although the clinical picture of the disease does not lend itself well to this arbitrary division, created to meet the needs of pathology.

First Period.—In the **classic type** the scene opens with pains. They are rapid and ephemeral, and are known as " lightning pains." They shoot through the lower limb, and follow one after the other in the shape of fits, that sometimes leave as a mark of their passage various eruptions and ecchymotic patches on the skin. The attacks are repeated day and night for several days in succession. They then disappear, and leave the patient in peace for weeks and months. At other times the pains are lancinating, as though caused by a pointed instrument which is plunged into the flesh and bones and twisted. Sometimes they are seated around a joint, and have a grinding character.

In the **body** they take the form of girdle pains, the patient feeling as

1209

though he were being held in a vice. The extension of the disease to the upper limbs is announced by pains in the ring and little fingers (area of the ulnar nerve). In the **face** the pains may be continuous or intermittent (area of the trigeminal nerve). They are often lancinating, and affect in some cases the temporal or the occipital region (exit point of the suboccipital nerve). These troubles in the area of the trigeminal nerve are said by Collet to exist in two-fifths of the cases.

The **viscera** are not exempt from these crises. In the **stomach** they sometimes take the form of very severe gastralgia, accompanied by great distress and vomiting of mucus, food, bile, or blood. These gastric crises appear and disappear suddenly ; they last a few hours or a few days without remission, and recur on taking any food. The intensity of the pains and of the vomiting sometimes induces collapse. The gastric crises are purely nervous in most cases, although they may be associated with lesions of the stomach. I had under my care a patient who suffered from agonizing gastric crises. The autopsy revealed the characteristic lesions of tabes, and also marked atrophy of the stomach, which was reduced to the size of a coil of gut. Histological examination showed the lesions of subacute gastritis (Crouzon).

In the case of the **kidneys** the crises cause lumbar pains, with retraction of the testicle and vomiting, as in renal colic. In certain patients the crises are vesical and urethral, simulating stone in the bladder. The patient suffers from pollakiuria, sometimes accompanied by dysuria and temporary retention of urine. In other cases the crises invade the rectum, causing the sensation of a foreign body, or of burning and tearing. Attacks of angina pectoris have even been noticed. They are due to changes in the cardiac plexus found post mortem. I have given full details, under Angina Pectoris and in one of my clinical lectures, of the relations between angina pectoris and **tabes.** Amongst these different painful manifestations of **tabes,** the lightning pains in the lower limbs are the most common and the earliest to appear.

At this period, and sometimes even from the very first, we notice the absence of the patellar reflex (Westphal). If, in the normal condition, we cross one leg over the other, the upper leg being allowed to hang with the muscles relaxed, a smart blow with the ulnar border of the hand on the tendon of the patella causes contraction of the quadriceps extensor, the leg rising and falling with an oscillatory movement. The absence of the patellar reflex is one of the earliest signs of tabes dorsalis. In consequence of the degeneration of the posterior columns of the spinal cord, the nerve ending in the tendon no longer transmits stimuli to the cells of the anterior cornua. Side by side with the patellar reflex we must mention the reflex of the tendo Achillis. This reflex is obtained in the following manner :

The patient kneels on a chair, and the muscles of the calf are felt to make sure that they are relaxed. The tendo Achillis is percussed with a plessor, and we see that the foot is extended on the leg. The absence of the reflex of the tendo Achillis is an early sign of tabes (Babinski).

To this first period of the disease also belong the cerebral symptoms and the ocular symptoms which constitute the tabetic eye. The **tabetic eye** may show itself by paralytic troubles, disorders of accommodation, or visual troubles. The ocular paralyses may occur early or late ; they affect the motor muscles of the eyeball and the levator palpebræ superioris (fourth, fifth, and sixth pairs of nerves). The early paralyses (preataxic period) are generally slighter and more transient than the late paralyses. They last only a few weeks or even only a few hours ; they appear and disappear rapidly. Their characteristic feature is that they are monocular and partial, affecting only a single terminal branch, or a few terminal branches, of the motor nerves of the eye. According to the nervous branch involved, the patient is affected with very troublesome diplopia or with ptosis. These passing troubles are subject to recurrences. The late ocular paralyses, which occur during the course of confirmed tabes, behave very differently to the early paralyses. They run a slower course, and they do not generally retrocede. They often affect both eyes, involving especially the muscles supplied by the common ocular motor nerve, the levator palpebræ (ptosis), the recti, and the oblique muscles. The muscles supplied by the fourth and sixth pair are less often affected. The late paralyses of the four recti and of the two oblique muscles cause diplopia and permanent strabismus, the characters of which vary according to the muscles attacked. If all the muscles are affected, the eyeballs are absolutely immovable. This condition is external ophthalmoplegia.

The late ocular paralyses differ, then, in their course from the early paralyses. They differ likewise in the lesion which causes them, the early and transitory paralyses being due only to peripheral neuritis* (Kahler,

* The transient oculo-motor troubles have been looked upon by P. Bonnier as reflex phenomena, which most frequently depend on systematic lesions of the labyrinthine nerve, of its nuclei in the brain, and of the fibres which pass from it to form a system homologous with the system in the posterior columns of the cord. The system of the labyrinth, in fact, peripheral as well as central, is very frequently diseased in tabes. It may be asked whether certain symptoms may not be caused by the tabetic lesion of this system when we remember the frequency with which these same symptoms appear during the course of ear affections that are absolutely independent of tabes. To deafness, buzzing, vertigo, agoraphobia, nystagmus, ptosis, diplopia, myosis, and amblyopia, which have been noticed in non-tabetic diseases of the ear, Bonnier has added Romberg's sign, uncertainty of walking in the dark, incoherent movements of the balls under the closed eyelids, slowness of accommodation to light, paralysis of accommodation, and, finally, mydriasis, observed for the first time during the course of otitis in a nurse in my wards. All these troubles exist in tabes, and it is by relying on the well-established anatomical relations between the labyrinthine nuclei and the

Dejerine), whilst the late and permanent paralyses are due to the lesions of the nuclei in the bulb. Certain patients with tabes are attacked by hyper-secretion from the conjunctiva (Trousseau), which generally coincides with the lightning pains (Féré, Berger).

Disorders of the pupils and of accommodation are likewise very important. The pupils are frequently contracted, often unequal, and it is a curious fact that in cases of myosis consequent on tabes dorsalis the contracted pupils still react to accommodation. They dilate if the patient looks at a near object, whilst they remain insensible to the action of light (Argyll-Robertson).

Robertson's sign is of the utmost importance in the diagnosis of tabes. It is not, however, pathognomonic of the affection, being also found in general paralysis. According to Babinski and Charpentier, this sign does not exist only in these two affections, which they look upon as syphilitic diseases of the nervous system, but it may also be associated with other syphilitic manifestations in the nervous system (hemiplegia, paraplegia, etc.). It may even exist alone in syphilitic patients. In a word, it is said to be a function of syphilis.

The power of accommodation, properly so called, may also be paralyzed, making it impossible for patients whose eyes were normal or hypermetropic to see clearly near objects. It is only distant vision that is still intact. Paralysis of accommodation generally accompanies paralysis of the two reflexes of the iris (light and accommodation), and the union of these symptoms in the same eye constitutes internal ophthalmoplegia.

I must now refer to atrophy of the optic nerves. Visual troubles due to optic atrophy are found in the proportion of 15 to 20 per cent. The atrophy sometimes develops rapidly, and blindness may supervene in less than a year. At other times the lesion progresses slowly. The lesion is not bilateral from the first. It invades one eye after the other. The keenness of the sight grows weak (amblyopia), and the field of vision becomes contracted from the circumference in the form of notches. The sense of colour is affected in the following order: disappearance of green, red, yellow, blue, and white. The blindness is then complete. If the fundus is examined with the ophthalmoscope, we see at first paleness of the optic papilla, the normal rosy tint tending to become of a bluish-white. This change is especially marked in the external half (temporal) of the disc. The papilla shows no change, either in shape or size. The outlines are always very clear. At a more advanced period, " in consequence of a change

oculo-motor centres, and by relying also on the physiological necessities of this association, and on the systematic character of the tabetic affection, that he has been able to propose a labyrinthine phase of tabes side by side with tabes dorsalis, cerebral tabes, and bulbar tabes itself.

in the texture of the optic nerve, and especially in consequence of the dis-appearance of the myeline cylinder, the papilla ceases to be transparent. It reflects the light strongly, and does not allow the vessels to be clearly seen in its depths. Accordingly it does not present the normal rosy tint, but is of a chalky-white colour " (Charcot). The central vessels become more slender. The arteries are attacked before the veins.

Optic atrophy is often an early symptom of tabes. There is, indeed, a type of tabes (tabes superior) in which the symptoms are limited to atrophy of the optic nerves and some other cephalic signs (pupillary signs, ocular paresis, etc.). The late appearance of optic atrophy is far less common. It has been said that optic atrophy may arrest the lesions in the cord.

The aural troubles are sometimes characterized by weakening of the sense of hearing, with or without buzzings in the ears, and in such a case there is a lesion of the auditory nerve. In other cases the buzzings and ringings in the ears are accompanied by vertigo, by impulsion, and even by falling, and by agoraphobia, although the sense of hearing is not affected. It is then probable that the lesion does not involve the fibres of the auditory nerve which govern the hearing of sounds, but the fibres which come from the semicircular canals, and govern the sense of space (De Cyon), or, more exactly, the sense of the position of the head and of the rest of the body (P. Bonnier).

Laryngo-bronchial troubles may supervene from the first in tabes. They are characterized by attacks of cough, with spasms of the glottis and a sensation of choking. These attacks are sometimes violent, accompanied by vertigo, vomiting, and even in some cases by epileptiform convulsions, loss of consciousness, and falling down of the patient. The attack is sudden or preceded by prodromata. It lasts a few seconds or minutes, and it may recur several times in the twenty-four hours. These laryngeal crises are due to hyperæsthesia and to spasms of the glottis. In one case they dis-appeared after tracheotomy. In some patients the disease affects the larynx, causing paralysis of the muscles, especially of the posterior crico-arytenoids.

Genital troubles—spermatorrhœa, impotence, venereal excitement, etc. —occur in all phases of the disease. They may, indeed, precede the other symptoms. Clitoridean crises have also been noticed, the patients being attacked, **without cause,** with voluptuous sensations, frequently repeated, and often preceding the other symptoms of the disease by several years. We shall see later, when describing the defaced types of locomotor ataxy, that many other symptoms may precede the painful phase of the first period. It would be more true to say that there is not a single symptom, rare or common, that may not appear before the stage of ataxy.

Second Period.—Although inco-ordination may exist from the com-mencement, it usually marks the second phase of the disease. It is the chief, but not the exclusive, symptom, because the pains and other symptoms previously described also belong to this period. The ataxy is characterized by gradual abolition of the co-ordination of movements. It shows itself at indeterminate periods, sometimes many years after the appearance of the lightning pains and the cerebral troubles.

The ataxy commences in the lower limbs, the patient having less control of his movements and experiencing difficulty in standing erect. If he is asked to stand erect, with the feet close together and the eyes shut, he becomes unsteady, and may even fall over (Romberg's sign). The patient with tabes finds it difficult to stand on one leg, turns round with difficulty, and readily loses his equilibrium. If he is lying in bed, and is asked to cross his legs, he will suddenly throw his leg forward, because he can no longer control the force, the direction, or the extent of the movement. In the patient suffering from ataxy the movement exceeds the object, or does not reach it. Thus in walking the patient has his eyes continually fixed on his feet, in order to guide them, and this explains why the lack of co-ordination is more pronounced in the dark, or when the patient is made to walk with his eyes closed. Later, walking becomes difficult and disordered, the patient being unable to take a step without the aid of a stick or other support. He thrusts his legs wildly forward, and strikes the ground with his heel, until the disease makes such progress that walking and standing erect become impossible. Brissaud has drawn attention to the impossibility of patients assuming the position of semi-genuflexion. The sudden giving way of the legs which the patient fears, and which takes him unawares, obliges him to keep his legs stiff when walking and standing erect. Prior to Duchenne's researches, those patients were looked upon as suffering from paraplegia, but there is no question of paralysis—or, at least, the paralytic symptoms are secondary and late. An attempt to flex or to extend the leg of a patient suffering from ataxy at once shows the power of resistance. The integrity of the muscular force is retained until a late stage. The want of co-ordination of the muscular force is the striking feature.

When the ataxy involves the upper limbs, it causes disorder in the use of the hands. If it is a question of shaving, tying a knot, or taking a small object in the fingers, the patient is awkward, and his mode of prehension is fairly characteristic.

At this period, and even earlier, the sense of touch is changed. The sensations of touch, pain, and tickling are diminished, abolished, or perverted; it is only the sense of cold which is exaggerated. Furthermore, we notice retardation of the sensibility. Thus a patient whose foot or whose leg has been pricked only feels the prick three, four, or five seconds later.

The stereognostic sense—that is to say, the faculty of recognizing the shape of objects by palpation—may be diminished or abolished. Anæsthesia is not limited to the skin; it also attacks the mucosæ, notably that of the larynx and the entire locomotor system—muscles, tendons, and articulations.* In the normal condition sensibility renders us an account of the effort of our muscles less by the sensation of contraction (muscular sense of Bell, sense of muscular activity of Gerdy), than by the measure of the resistance opposed to this effort by the tendons, the ligaments, the articular surfaces, and the integument. As a matter of fact, Trousseau was the first to establish an important distinction "between the consciousness of the accomplished movement and the consciousness of the muscular contraction that accomplishes the movement." Trousseau in no way denies the sensibility which the muscle possesses, like all living tissues, but he denies the sentiment of muscular activity. The thing appreciated, and consequently ruling the muscular expense itself at every moment, is movement properly so called, and this movement is perceived in that it causes a change in the attitudes.†

Side by side with these various forms of anæsthesia certain varieties of visceral analgesia may be observed—testicular, epigastric, or mammary analgesia, described by Pitres, and also tracheal and lingual analgesia, pointed out by Sicard.

* This appreciation of muscular force may be easily noticed with a dynamometer. Jaccoud makes use of another method. To the feet of a patient lying in bed he suspends bags of known weight, and whilst a healthy man lifting these weights with his foot can recognize perfectly a difference of 100 to 150 grammes, a patient suffering from ataxy, on the contrary, fails to recognize differences of 1,000 to 3,000 grammes.

† P. Bonnier in various publications (*Le Vertige*, Paris, 1893) proposes to replace the too exclusive expression **muscular sense** by the more exact idea of the **sense of the attitudes.** Whether there is muscular contraction or not, whether the attitude is realized actively or passively, it is always the attitude which is perceived, and in no wise one of the numerous sensorial operations, the composition of which defines the attitude for us. The writer distinguishes **segmentary attitudes**—that is to say, the respective positions of the various segments of the trunk and of the limbs, of the attitudes of the head, and the attitudes of the whole body. The pictures of the segmentary attitudes are transported by the nerve roots, and the posterior columns to the cerebrum and the cerebellum. The pictures of the attitudes of the head and of the whole body, of a labyrinthic origin follow the vestibular nerve, and likewise end in the brain and in the cerebellum.

There exists, then, a **medullo-cerebral** system serving for the **conscious** adaptation of partial movements and for voluntary equilibration, and a **medullo-cerebellar** system, devoted to the **reflex** working of these movements and of equilibration. In tabes, which is a medullo-labyrintho-cerebral affection (Bonnier), the movements are said to remain co-ordinated, but they are badly adapted. Tell a patient to close his eyes, and immediately the absence of sight betrays itself by the loss of voluntary equilibrium, by the disturbance of equilibrium (Romberg's sign), by the exaggeration of the ataxic movements, and by the sensation of vertigo. In Friedreich's disease, and in cerebellar heredo-ataxia, which are medullo-cerebellar affections, the sense of the attitudes is affected as far as the reflex acts are concerned, but it is preserved as far as the conscious act that supplements the reflex act. Thus, the closing of the eyelids scarcely affects the equilibration, and only slightly influences the adaptation of the movements.

Cerebral symptoms may appear at various periods of tabes, preceding in a third of the cases, says Fournier, the pains and the ataxia—a further proof that the lesions of this disease are not only limited to the medullary axis, as the original meaning of **tabes dorsalis** wrongly indicates; they are spread over the entire nervous system. These cerebral symptoms may be divided into two principal varieties, motor and psychical. To the motor troubles belong vertigo, impulsion, gyration, epileptiform convulsions, and apoplectiform attacks, and certain kinds of paralyses, to which I shall refer in a moment.

To the psychical troubles belong aphasia, intellectual torpor, loss of memory, intellectual troubles, constituting a sort of tabetic madness, and most of the symptoms of general pseudo-paralysis. These troubles may be temporary or permanent. They sometimes appear in the last stage of tabes; at other times they are the first symptoms (Fournier).

Alienists have for a long time noticed in patients suffering from general paralysis the following symptoms : Lightning pains, oculo-pupillary and genito-urinary troubles, anæsthesia, localized paralysis, arthropathy, abolition of the reflexes, etc.—manifestations indicating the participation of the cord or of the peripheral nerves in the morbid process. Neuro-pathologists, on their side, had noticed in several cases of ataxy the appearance of apoplectiform and epileptiform attacks, followed or not by hemiplegia, buzzing, delirium of an ambitious or depressed type, all pointing to anatomical changes in the brain centres. We may add to these Ménière's vertigo, due to labyrinthine apoplexy.

The result was that a patient considered to be suffering from general paralysis at the commencement of the disease was later classed as a case of ataxy. Often, too, a patient with ataxy was admitted into an asylum, and condemned to end his days amongst lunatics. The study of these complex cases has recently been resumed. Some regard them as the casual union of two distinct diseases in the same subject ; others, on the contrary, consider them as localizations in the brain and in the cord of a single morbid entity.

The partisans of the dualist doctrine rely on pathological anatomy to support their opinion. According to them, tabes is an affection of central origin, characterized by a progressively systematic lesion of the cerebrospinal sensory system, whilst general paralysis is characterized by an essentially diffuse lesion of the cerebrospinal axis. The same difference is said to exist between these two affections as exists between amyotrophic lateral sclerosis and disseminated sclerosis. Ballet goes even further, and admits that tabes is an affection with a perivascular onset. Finally, one of these diseases ends in induration of the nerve centres, and the other in softening. The dualists recognize, however, that if these two diseases differ as to their essential nature, they both develop in subjects who are identical, as far as the medium is concerned—that is to say, in neuropathic individuals, especially in those with hereditary predisposition, and often also in syphilitic and alcoholic persons.

The partisans of the unicist theory, on the contrary, turn this question of the medium to account, and especially the neuropathic medium on which syphilis has been grafted, in order to prove the identity of tabes and general paralysis. According to them, the frequency of the cerebral and spinal manifestations in the same subject is too great to be simply a coincidence. Finally, they rely on the fact that in tabes the systematization of the lesions is not as rigorous as some maintain. They say that in a large number of cases manifestly diffuse changes are found in the lateral columns, in the anterior cornua, and in the peripheral nerves. The unicists say that, as for stating precisely the histological starting-point of the lesions in general paralysis, and making it an argument by which to differentiate the two diseases, histological research is not sufficiently advanced to permit of such a demarcation.

Let us now pass to the motor troubles. We may notice in all phases of Duchenne's disease paralyses of various kinds ; such are hemiplegia, monoplegia, paraplegia, facial and radial paralysis, and paralysis of the muscles of the eye. These paralyses are often incomplete and transient, subject to recurrences, and deserve rather the name of " paresis." Some, nevertheless, have other characters ; thus we find persistent hemiplegia associated with cerebral lesions, hemiplegia with sensitivo-sensorial hemi-anæsthesia, due to the association of tabes with hysteria. Tabetic paraplegia sometimes has a sudden onset, improves, and may be cured after a few weeks or months. Central lesions, peripheral neuritis, and hysteria play various parts in the causation of these paralyses. Another category includes choreiform movements and athetosis, generally accompanied by contractures, and depending on an accessory lesion of the lateral columns.

Third Period.—After some ten to fifteen years or more the disease may improve, but more frequently it ends in the final period of paralysis and cachexia, often complicated with ulcerative cystitis, bedsores, pulmonary tuberculosis, bulbar phenomena, and general paralysis. This period really merits the name of **tabes,** the patient dying of cachexia if he is not carried off by some intercurrent disease.

Trophic Troubles.—Trophic and vasomotor troubles may appear at any period of the disease. The lightning pains in the limbs and in the face are sometimes accompanied by cutaneous eruptions, ecchymoses, and temporary œdema. Shedding of the nails is noticed, especially of the nail of the big toe. The shedding of the nail may or may not be preceded by subungual ecchymosis, with pain or numbness, and the nail falls off without ulceration, " like a crust of ecthyma," being replaced by a friable nail, which falls off in its turn. Vitiligo, ichthyosis of the skin, and perforating ulcer of the foot are often seen.

One of the first cases of perforating disease of the foot was reported by my uncle, Paul Dieulafoy. Tabes accounts for 75 per cent. of the cases of perforating disease. It usually attacks the head of the first and fifth metatarsal bones ; it may be superficial or deep. In some cases it affects the palm of the hand, the face, the mouth, the aortic valve, the œsophagus, the intestine, or the buttock. In a case at the Hôtel-Dieu, perforating disease of the sacro-coccygeal region produced a large cavity. The area around the cavity was anæsthetic; the incontinence of urine and fæces, the lightning pains, and the abolition of the reflex of the tendo Achillis, proved the diagnosis of tabes. The autopsy showed the characteristic lesions in the lumbo-sacral cord and ascending degeneration in the posterior columns.

From the commencement of the disease well-marked arthropathies may be seen, affecting the knee, the foot, and the hip (Ball, Charcot), and sometimes appearing almost suddenly. They are generally painless, and very rapidly accompanied by hydarthrosis, hard œdema, and swelling, which gives to the affected limb the appearance of elephantiasis. In spite of this invasion, the movements are practically normal for some time. When the arthropathy is benign, there may be resolution ; but when it is grave, the swelling and the œdema persist, the capsule, the ligaments, the cartilage, the ends of the bones, and the articular cavities are destroyed by the trophic disorders, and dislocations and intra-articular fractures occur. These disorders cause considerable deformity, and allow the most weird movements of the diseased joint. The arthropathy is not always of the atrophic type. Thickening of the synovial membrane and osteocartilaginous tumours are also seen.

Let us also notice as trophic troubles fractures due to rarefying osteitis. These fractures particularly attack the bones of the limbs, but they have also been observed in the vertebræ. The characteristic feature is that they occur without pain. They are sometimes multiple, and result from very trifling causes, but they become consolidated, and the callus is exuberant, shapeless, and resisting. Osteoporosis of the maxillæ causes the painless falling out of healthy teeth. I had in my wards a patient suffering from tabes who lost seven teeth in a few days. This shedding of the teeth is sometimes followed by the absorption of the alveolar border, the first degree of perforating disease of the mouth, already described under Syphilitic Perforations of the Vault of the Palate. Let us also note ulcerations of the nose (Giraudeau), velum palati, pillars of the fauces (Bonnier) and face (P. Marie).

In sufferers from tabes we sometimes see deformity of the foot analogous to the congenital flat-foot. The internal edge of the foot is thickened, the dorsal surface is prominent, especially in the tarso-metatarsal region, and the plantar arch is flat and weakened. The foot is shortened. These deformities, easily recognized in footprints, are caused by trophic lesions of the tarsal bones, which become friable, atrophied, and disjointed. "There is rather osteopathy than arthropathy" (Chauffard). This **tabetic foot** may supervene from the commencement of the disease. It must not be confounded with the **tabetic club-foot,** due to atrophy of certain muscles of the leg, the deformity of the foot being constituted by an exaggerated extension, with an inward curve of the internal edge, and a deviation of the toes towards the middle line of the body (Joffroy).

The name **hypotonia** is given to a condition in which the muscles are relaxed, and abnormal mobility of the articulations follows. In certain cases of hypotonic tabes we can produce hyperextension of the leg on the thigh, so as to form an obtuse angle. When the patient is lying down, it is possible to abduct the legs to such an extent that their axes lie in a straight line. In the hands it is possible to cause hyperextension of the phalanges on the metacarpus and of the phalanges on one another.

Muscular atrophy appears chiefly at an advanced period. It is usually symmetrical, and always commences in the muscles of the limbs, more often in the hands than in the feet. In the lower limbs the atrophy causes pes equinus, with plantar flexion of the toes. In the upper limbs it takes the Aran-Duchenne type, but very rarely the scapulo-humeral or antibrachial one. The muscular atrophy is not accompanied by fibrillary contractions. The idio-muscular contraction is diminished or abolished, but the reaction of degeneration is not common.

Atrophy of the muscles of the eye and of the upper eyelid has also been noticed, as well as hemiatrophy of the tongue. Lesions of the aorta (atheroma and aortic insufficiency) are fairly common in tabes. It may be asked whether they are due to trophic trouble or to syphilis and rheumatism, which are often associated with tabes.

The **secretory troubles** are **diarrhœa,** occurring in a continuous form, or in crises, with or without colic—it may last for months and years—**sialorrhœa,** and **vomiting,** which supervene apart from the gastric troubles. The sweat is sometimes suppressed, sometimes abundant. The sweating may be limited to the feet, the hands, one side of the body, or the head.

Defaced Form.—In more instances than we are wont to think the disease is defaced at its commencement, and remains defaced for months and years. It only reveals itself then by an isolated symptom, which at first sight seems to have no relation with locomotor ataxy, of which, however, it is the precursor. Patients may, for example, suffer from progressive amblyopia, while the other manifestations of locomotor ataxy do not show

78—2

themselves till months and years later. The same remark applies to the ocular paralyses and visceral neuralgia. The crises of gastralgia, with vomiting, which so closely simulate ulcer of the stomach; the vesical, urethral, and rectal crises; the lumbar pains, with retraction of the testes, which might readily be taken for renal colic, are all manifestations which may mark the commencement of tabes with an isolated symptom. Auditory troubles; deafness, with or without vertigo (lesion of the auditory nerve); laryngeal troubles; spasms of the glottis, with or without falling of the patient; and angina pectoris, are all early manifestations of tabes dorsalis.

Bladder troubles (dysuria, incontinence, and retention), **genital troubles** (impotence, spermatorrhœa, satyriasis, and clitoridean crises), **secretory troubles** (diarrhœa, sialorrhœa, sweating, and polyuria), **trophic troubles** (shedding of the nails or teeth, "mal perforant," and ichthyosis), may precede the customary and classical troubles of tabes.

Even the painless arthropathy of the first period may be looked upon as a local joint affection, when it really belongs to the trophic troubles of ataxy. It will be important to remember these facts when we have to discuss the diagnosis.

Course—Diagnosis.—Locomotor ataxy has been divided into three periods, but these periods lend themselves but little to a methodical division, for they are extremely variable as to duration and as to their time of appearance. In some exceptional cases the disease runs a rapid course, reaching the stationary stage within the first year, but more frequently it lasts from six to twenty years, or even longer. In some circumstances the ataxic symptoms only appear years after other tabetic troubles. Generally speaking, the cerebral troubles are consecutive to the medullary troubles, but in some cases the contrary is observed, and the patient is attacked at first by cerebral troubles (apoplectiform congestion, paralysis, or madness), and only becomes ataxic later (Fournier).

The **prognosis** of locomotor ataxy, though very grave, is not absolutely fatal, because the posterior sclerosis is sometimes arrested. Under the name of **benign tabes,** Charcot has collected cases of people who had only some few tabetic symptoms, developing with extreme slowness, and possibly ending in recovery.

The **diagnosis** is especially difficult in the defaced cases. An error is most frequently avoided if care is taken to inquire into the nature of the painful crises, if the absence of the reflex of the tendo Achillis is found, if the patient is carefully questioned on some phenomenon which he has failed to notice, and if this phenomenon is joined to another phenomenon which has passed unnoticed. The patient must be asked whether he has ever had lightning pains, or suffered from diplopia, strabismus, achromatopsia, amblyopia, deafness, or some of the numerous genital, vesical, trophic, and secretory troubles which we have reviewed. The condition of the reflexes and the various kinds of muscular sense must be carefully examined. It is rare if, after a minute examination, we do not succeed in discovering the correct diagnosis.

The cerebro-spinal fluid should be examined in most cases. Lymphocytosis is the rule in tabetic patients, and the exception in pseudo-tabes due to peripheral neuritis. We must, further, assure ourselves of the almost constant presence of albumin in the cerebro-spinal fluid in tabetic patients. On boiling the liquid, we see a marked albuminous cloud, while in the normal condition heat only produces very slight opalescence.

Examination by cyto-diagnosis and the albumin test will be considered in conjunction with the clinical signs in doubtful cases and in cases of pseudo-tabes. Pseudo-tabes associated with polyneuritis is seen after infectious diseases, in diabetes, and in chronic poisoning, especially by alcohol. It is well to remember the possibility of error, in order to avoid it. In alcoholic pseudo-tabes the paresis, the ataxic symptoms and the pains are early, rapid, and dominant. They are associated with symptoms of alcoholic intoxication (trembling of the hands, dreams, nightmare, etc.). They are sometimes followed by muscular atrophy, but they are hardly ever accompanied by lightning pains, visceral crises, ocular paralyses, disorders of the sphincters, etc., which in true tabes form the preataxic period.

Locomotor ataxy (Duchenne's disease) should not be confounded with Friedreich's disease. The latter malady has been wrongly called " hereditary ataxy." It is indeed hereditary, and especially common in families, but heredity also plays a considerable part in Duchenne's disease. The muscular ataxy described by Friedreich is an affection which has somewhat indefinite anatomical characters, although its clinical features are well recognized. It is an affection of childhood and puberty. While it is not locomotor ataxy, disseminated sclerosis, or a combination of these two diseases, it borrows from the former the motor inco-ordination of the limbs and the absence of the knee-jerk, from the latter nystagmus and scanning speech. It differs, however, from both in its other symptoms, its ætiology, its mode of evolution, and its prognosis (Charcot). The lightning pains, the vesical crises, the anæsthesias, and the trophic troubles met with in Duchenne's ataxy are absent in Friedreich's ataxy. Vertigo, epileptiform attacks, and optic neuritis, are also absent in Friedreich's disease.

The diagnosis becomes very difficult if other affections of the nervous system are juxtaposed with tabes. These affections associated with tabes include general paralysis, syphilis of the nerve centres, hemiatrophy of the tongue, progressive muscular atrophy, Friedreich's disease, syringomyelia, and hysteria. Under such circumstances the diagnosis may present serious difficulties, for the similar signs are more numerous than the differential ones.

Pathological Anatomy.—We know to-day that the lesion of locomotor ataxy is a sclerosis, affecting to an unequal extent the spinal cord, the mesencephalon, the encephalon, the great sympathetic, and the nerves.

1. With regard to the encephalon, the changes, though frequent, are not constant, and the localization takes place without order and without system, thus differing from the medullary lesion, which is **systematic.** We meet with sclerosis in the inferior peduncles of the cerebellum, and in certain cranial nerves, such as the optic, the auditory, and the common oculo-motor nerve. The most common and the best known encephalic lesion is that of the optic nerves. It commences in one nerve before invading the other. Like peripheral neuritis, it advances progressively from

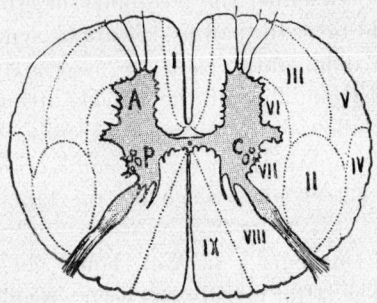

Fig. 65.—Section of the Spinal Cord in the Dorsal Region.

A, anterior cornu ; *P*, posterior cornu ; *C*, Clarke's column ; *I*, direct pyramidal tract ; *II*, crossed pyramidal tract ; *III*, anterior radicular tract ; *IV*, direct cerebellar tracts ; *V*, Gowers' tract ; *VI*, motor and vasomotor portion of the mixed tract ; *VII*, sensory portion of the mixed tract ; *VIII*, Burdach's tract, containing in its external third the fasciculi cuneati of Charcot and Pierret ; *IX*, Goll's column.

the periphery towards the optic tracts and the geniculate bodies, and gives rise to grey induration of the nerves ; and as the lesion of the nerve fibre seems to precede the invasion of the connective tissue, the neuritis might be called parenchymatous.

Locomotor ataxy may precede, follow, or coincide with general paralysis of the insane. In these special forms we then find the lesions of diffuse meningo-encephalitis. These forms are of great interest from the point of view of prognosis.

2. As regards the bulb and the pons, we see in some cases that the sclerosis of the posterior columns continues under the floor of the fourth ventricle. It invades the nuclei of the restiform bodies, the substantia gelatinosa of Rolando, the ascending root of the trigeminal nerve, and

sometimes causes atrophy of the sensory nuclei of the glosso-pharyngeal, spinal accessory, and pneumogastric nerves.

Dejerine has often observed atrophy of the nucleus of the sixth pair and of the corresponding radicular fillets. Several writers have noticed atrophy of the auditory nerves and of the nuclei.

Before describing the lesions of the spinal cord, I give here a diagram of a section of the cord, in order to facilitate the description of these lesions.

3. Of the changes in the spinal cord, some are constant and others inconstant. The latter are situated in the anterior cornua and the lateral columns. We shall return to them later.

The constant and characteristic changes in tabes dorsalis invade the posterior spinal system—that is to say, the posterior columns, the most posterior portion of the grey matter, the posterior nerve roots, and the adjacent meninges. The scierosis of the posterior columns commences in the lumbar region, where in general it is more pronounced than elsewhere. It ascends into the cervical and bulbar regions, and it may even reach the floor of the fourth ventricle.

When the sclerosis is of long standing, the posterior columns are indurated, greyish, and atrophied. They are soldered together " by the formation of new connective tissue, at the expense of the pia mater, which thrusts itself into the furrow separating them in the healthy condition " (Cornil and Ranvier). This chronic posterior meningitis is constant, according to Vulpian, who questions whether it does not play an important rôle " as a productive cause in the pathogenesis of tabes dorsalis." According to Dejerine, the meningitis and cortical meningo-myelitis explain the propagation of the lesions to the lateral columns in cases where lateral sclerosis complicates posterior sclerosis.

P. Marie and Guillain attribute the chief part in the development of tabetic lesions to posterior meningitis, and to the changes in the posterior lymphatic system of the spinal cord.

Is the grey matter of the posterior cornua affected ? At first sight it would seem as though it must be so, on account of its intimate relations with the posterior columns. And yet the cells of the posterior cornu are almost unaffected, but the radiating fibres from the posterior column are involved (Lissauer). In Clarke's columns, tabes attacks the reticulum, but not the cells.

The **posterior roots** of the spinal nerves are shrunken to less than half their normal size. We know that as soon as the fibres of the posterior roots enter the cord they divide into two terminal branches. One descends in Burdach's column, which in its external third contains the external band of Charcot and Pierret, and soon ends in the cord ; the other ascends vertically in the posterior cord, to end at different levels in the posterior cornu. Some fibres reach the bulb. These terminal branches give out collateral branches, which penetrate the grey matter by fine arborizations. The shortest soon terminate around the nearest cells. Those of average length form a rich plexus around the cells of Clarke's column, which send a tract of fibres to the cerebellum. Others pass through the posterior grey commissure, and lose themselves in the posterior cornu of the opposite side. Finally, there are long collaterals forming Köllicker's reflex collateral bundle (sensitivo-motor tract of Ramon y Cajal), and ending in the anterior cornu.

This collateral system, described by Ramon y Cajal, is the seat of constant and early lesions in tabes, as Lissauer and Weigert have shown. Pierret, in 1871, had noticed the degeneration of the nerve fibrils in the grey matter of the posterior cornua. The degeneration of the reflex collaterals and of the collaterals of Clarke's column exists from the commencement of tabes (Marinesco). It always coincides with the change in the posterior cords.

The posterior roots are the seat of very evident lesions in old tabes; their integrity has only been noted at the commencement of tabes. Vulpian, in 1874, and Schultze, Leyden, and Dejerine later, held that the medullary lesion was due to neuritis of the posterior roots. The lesions of the ganglia are much more vague and uncommon. The result of Vulpian's interesting researches is that the posterior roots, which are much affected between the spinal cord and the ganglion, are perfectly healthy beyond the ganglion. This fact would seem to prove that the lesion does not commence in the periphery of the nerves, in order to ascend towards the spinal cord, any more than it commences in the roots, because we find the posterior roots almost healthy, while the posterior columns are diseased. Tabes commences, then, in the posterior columns, and extends to the neighbouring parts, and this systematic sclerosis leads us to suppose that the myelitis is at first parenchymatous (Hallopeau), before becoming interstitial, the initial irritation affecting the nerve fibre before it attacks the connective tissue.

The primary and constant lesion, as we have said, is the systematic sclerosis of the posterior column of the spinal cord. This fact, however, requires explanation. The posterior column of the spinal cord is itself divided into several independent territories, the distinct lesions of which cause various symptoms. Knowledge gained from embryology, anatomy, and pathology shows us that each posterior column of the marrow is divided into two secondary bundles, the one median and the other external, the respective size of the bundles varying according to the regions of the spinal cord.

The **median bundle,** which is thin in the lumbar region, larger in the dorsal region, and threadlike in the cervical region (Goll's column), ends in the posterior pyramids. This median bundle exists, then, throughout the entire length of the spinal cord. It is composed of longitudinal fibres, arising in the grey matter at various levels and in relation with the cells of Clarke's vesicular columns. The longer the tract that these longitudinal fibres have to pass through, the more superficial they are. Some of them are of sufficient length to unite the lumbar swelling with the posterior pyramids.

The external or Burdach's column contains in its outer third the fasciculus cuneatus, which is also found throughout the entire length of the cord. It is formed, on the one hand, of commissural fibres, that establish intimate relations between the various points of the posterior grey matter (Todd, Vulpian), and, on the other hand, of fibres having a transverse and oblique direction, arising in the posterior roots of the nerves, and joining the cells of the posterior cornu.

The posterior columns of the cord are formed by Goll and Burdach's columns, containing the fasciculi cuneati. In tabes dorsalis does the change invade the entire posterior column, or does it remain limited to one of the two secondary bundles? And in this case which one of them is affected? Is it Goll's or Burdach's column? When post-mortem examinations are performed at an advanced period of the disease, we find that the sclerosis affects all of the posterior bundles; but when the anatomical examination is carried out at less advanced stages, the lesion may be observed in various phases of its evolution (Pierret), and we see side by side with the primary, characteristic and constant lesion other lesions that are secondary and inconstant.

The characteristic and constant lesion is in Burdach's column. Amongst the secondary lesions we find degeneration of Goll's column. Isolated sclerosis of Goll's column in the cervical region occurs as a secondary ascending sclerosis when the dorsal portion of the spinal cord is affected (Pott's disease, tumours). It is accompanied neither by lightning pains nor by ataxy. This is a proof that the isolated sclerosis is not dependent on the tabetic symptoms, and if it is frequently found post mortem in tabes dorsalis, it is simply consecutive to the dorso-lumbar lesion of tabes (Pierret), just as it is consecutive to a tumour or to Pott's disease. We must not, therefore, seek for the lesion of tabes in the sclerosis of Goll's column.

The constant and characteristic lesion of tabes is situated in the fasciculi cuneati, and Pierret has collected several cases in which the disease was only in the stage of lightning pains and sclerosis was present in the fasciculi, without any change in Goll's columns. The medullary lesion commences, then, in the fasciculi cuneati of Burdach's column, invades the posterior spinal roots and the posterior grey matter, and causes, secondarily, ascending sclerosis of Goll's columns.

Philippe stained a series of sections of the cord according to the Weigert-Pal process. He was thus able to determine the early and the more advanced lesions of tabes. At the commencement the fasciculi cuneati are the first to be attacked in their middle radicular fibres. If the disease is of long duration, the lesions constantly affect the descending bundle, and in a lesser degree the ascending bundle. The invasion of the endogenous bundles is characteristic of advanced tabes. Goll's cord undergoes a secondary degeneration in the cervical region (Pierret), but it may be primarily attacked in the lumbar region. The histological process is essentially parenchymatous. "The parenchymatous lesions exist from the commencement of tabes in the nerve fibre. The cell of the vertebral ganglion remains intact. The parenchymatous lesions are especially primary " (Philippe).

4. The lesions of the **great sympathetic** are at present imperfectly worked out. Lesions of the ganglia have, however, been met with, which is not to be wondered at, seeing that the spinal origin of the great sympathetic appears to be in the posterior vesicular columns and in Clarke's intermedio-lateral tract (Pierret). Neuritis has been noticed in various plexuses.

5. **Peripheral Neuritis.**—Some of the peripheral nerves are attacked by neuritis. This lesion, though not constant, is very frequent. These changes affect the periphery of the nerves, and are most frequently peripheral from the outset. As a matter of fact, the corresponding spinal ganglia, up to a certain distance, are healthy. The peripheral neuritis may be very pronounced, even in early tabes, and, inversely, the peripheral nerves may be healthy in cases in which the posterior columns of the marrow have for a long time been sclerosed. In some cases peripheral neuritis has been met with on one side only, whereas the lesion in the spinal cord is symmetrical. These facts prove that peripheral neuritis in tabes may evolve on its own account parallel with the lesion in the cord, but without being directly associated with it. Besides, this autonomy of peripheral neuritis does not affect Waller's law, but proves that peripheral lesions of the nerves may arise independently of lesions in the trophic centres.

The peripheral neuritis may attack the sensory, mixed, or visceral nerves. It is very frequent in the cutaneous nerves, and has also been met with in the branches to the muscles. Amongst other nerves attacked by peripheral neuritis I may mention the nerves of the levator palpebræ superioris (Dejerine), the recurrent and the pneumogastric (Oppenheim), the cardiac plexus, the cœliac plexus, and the abdominal sympathetic (Grocéo and Fusari). The neuritis is of a parenchymatous nature—atrophied nerve fibres, or fibres in course of destruction, interstitial lesions, and perineuritis. In some cases the peripheral neuritis is curable (Pierret).

Pathological Physiology.—Is the appearance of the symptoms of loco-motor ataxy in relation with the systematic invasion of the lesion ? This question will now be discussed.

Pain.—In the stage of the lightning pains the lesion is confined to the fasciculi cuneati in the shape of a very thin and limited band of sclerosis. As the posterior roots of the spinal nerves are not attacked at this period, it must be admitted that the pains of tabes dorsalis are due to the change in the posterior roots during their intraspinal course. These lesions fully explain the pains in the limbs and in the trunk, but when it is a question of the crises of the stomach, bladder, rectum, and kidneys, it is probable that we must refer them to peripheral neuritis in the corresponding visceral plexuses. Peripheral neuritis of the laryngeal and pneumogastric nerves explains the laryngeal crises.

Anæsthesia.—The diminution, loss, and perversion of the senses of touch, pain, temperature, and orientation, as well as of the muscular and articular sensibility, are phenomena observed only at a fairly advanced period of the disease. The anæsthesia and analgesia are often patchy. They are sometimes complete (foot, leg, and face), and there is often a delay of several seconds in the perception of the sensations. What are these phenomena due to ?

This question has been carefully discussed by Vulpian. It may be thus summed up : The impressions received at the periphery are carried by the fibres of the posterior nerve roots to the grey matter of the spinal cord. It is probable that the impression passes from the grey matter, in which it is elaborated, into the posterior columns, which transmit it to the brain ; and if these columns are destroyed for a certain extent, it is the grey matter which undertakes to re-establish the path of the sensory impressions. One thing is certain—viz., that the sensory impressions have not an exclusive route in their medullary passage. The path of transmission may vary according to the need, and the paths of communication supplement one another so well that sensory troubles presuppose an already extensive lesion in the cord. The diminution and the loss of sensibility are conse-quently due to the multiple lesions of the posterior cords, of the posterior grey matter, and of the corresponding spinal roots ; and as to the delay in the transmission of sensory impressions, it may be asked " whether it is not due to the atrophy of the posterior columns, and to the necessity of the impressions abandoning the direct path of the white bundles, to follow more slowly the tortuous path of the grey matter " (Vulpian).

Another cause, no doubt, exists to explain the patches of hyperæsthesia and of anæsthesia and the delay of the sensations—viz., the neuritis of the peripheral cutaneous nerves. We must admit the important part played by peripheral neuritis, because the disturbances in the senses of touch, pain, and of temperature are more marked at the extremities, and diminish from below upwards (Dejerine).

Ataxy.—It is exceptional for the loss of co-ordination of movements to appear from the commencement of the disease. It shows itself two or three years, and even longer, after the lightning pains and visceral crises. Raynaud has found that in certain cases where visceral crises were present, to the exclusion of the pains in the extremities, the symptom of ataxy was indefinitely delayed. However this may be, ataxy of the lower or upper limbs always shows itself by the same symptoms. Muscular force persists as to quantity at least for a long time, but it lacks regulating power, the movements either exceeding their object or failing to reach it. The patient with ataxy cannot regulate the quality nor the amplitude, so that we find want of co-ordination of the voluntary movements and "disorder of mechanical co-ordination" (Jaccoud). The pathogenesis of this ataxy has given rise to much discussion.

According to Charcot and Pierret, the ataxy appears when the sclerosis of the fasciculi cuneati extends, both internally and externally, and they interpret this fact by admitting that the commissural fibres and the fasciculi cuneati "serve in the co-ordination of the movements of the limbs." This hypothesis is not yet based on a sure foundation.

Other writers have advanced a theory, based on cutaneous **anæsthesia,** both muscular and articular. The troubles of sensibility destroy, on the one hand, the source of the reflex actions, and, on the other, they deprive the muscles of the ideas of force, resistance, extent, and duration, which govern the synergy of the contractions (muscular sense). This theory, which at first sight is seductive, appears to be overthrown by these two facts. We find hysterical patients who are deprived of sensibility, and who do not suffer from ataxy, and also patients suffering from ataxy who have very advanced motor inco-ordination, when their sensibility is almost normal (Duchenne). Nevertheless, the peripheral lesions of the sensory nerves and the consequent anæsthesia might well be connected with the troubles of inco-ordination.

According to Jaccoud, sclerosis of the posterior columns produces ataxy by causing disturbance of the reflex actions and of the spinal radiations—that is to say, by destroying the nerve fibres which, arising from the posterior roots, extend as far as the anterior cornua of the grey matter (reflex motor fibres), or as far as Gerlach's nervous network. These fibres appear to have a regulating action on the previously established synergic contraction of the groups of muscles.

According to Pierret, "the prime cause of locomotor ataxy is said to be an irritation of the sensory fibres of the nervous centres." The irritation of these fibres has the effect of paralyzing certain muscles, or groups of muscles, by reflex action, and " as soon as an attempt at movement is made in which the paretic muscle is antagonistic to the healthy muscle, the former overrides the latter, and the movement exceeds its object." The ataxy would thus be explained. " There is no need for me to dwell," says Grasset, " on the objections to this theory, which has need of fresh proofs."

Onimus has put forward the view that the want of co-ordination is due to contractures. The word " contracture " must not be taken here in its most common acceptation, which supposes rigidity of the muscular fibre. There are less marked degrees, and it may be said that contracture exists in a muscle as soon as its natural suppleness is lessened, and as soon as it experiences a difficulty in relaxing after voluntary contraction. In patients suffering from ataxy these phenomena of muscular rigidity accompany the disease throughout its course, but they are more marked as the malady progresses. What happens then ? When the patient suffering from ataxy wishes to make a movement, he experiences a certain resistance, due to this state of contraction, and in order to overcome this resistance he employs a force that outstrips the desired object, because the disturbance of the muscular and cutaneous sensibility gives wrong information to the spinal cord.

Leyden has more recently sought for the point of departure of tabes in the periphery itself, in the irritation of all kinds which develops a centripetal process of degeneration, attacking and paralyzing the ganglion cells.

Brissaud attributes the want of co-ordination to the constant ignorance of the patient as to the extent of the resistance experienced. The muscular effort, therefore, is always excessive. He is of opinion that the primary lesion of tabes is an affection of " the centripetal protoneuroma "—that is to say, of that part of the centripetal system which is made up of the afferent nerve fibres, the ganglion cell, and its afferent fibres.

Bonnier opposes the idea of motor inco-ordination in the strict sense of the word. The elementary movements are said to be well co-ordinated, but ill advised. A military officer, ignorant of the ground over which he is manœuvring, of the forces to which he is opposed, and of the condition of his troops, might give ill-advised orders, which will, however, be perfectly executed by his men. The sufferer from ataxy executes movements that prove the co-ordination of muscular efforts, but these movements are unsuitable to the end in view, because the sufferer from ataxy does not know how to begin, is ignorant when he reaches the point of arrival, and cannot grasp the various attitudes required. It is not the muscular sense that is affected, but the sense of the attitudes.

The diversity of these theories proves that the pathogenesis of ataxy is still a matter of speculation. Taking up the question, not from the pathological, but from the physiological, point of view, we see that the explanation of the co-ordination of the movements given by Duchenne is true. Even the simplest movement can only be carried out by the co-operation of several muscles. It requires the contraction of the muscles which are to produce this movement, and the contraction of the antagonistic muscles which are to limit this movement. The flexor muscles have the extensor muscles as antagonists, just as the adductor muscles have the abductor ones. The regularity of a movement supposes, then, the harmony of contraction of the muscles which produce the movement, and the harmony of the antagonistic muscles destined to limit this movement. If one of these factors is wanting, the movement is no longer co-ordinated, and ataxy results.

Why are one or both of these factors compromised in posterior spinal sclerosis? The preceding theories are attempts to solve this problem.

Paralysis and Atrophy.—I have said that in the different periods of muscular ataxy we sometimes see transient or persistent paralyses. These paralyses may be due to focal lesions in the brain, to the extension of the posterior sclerosis to the lateral columns of the cord, to the peripheral changes in the motor nerves, and to the association of hysteria with tabes. The muscular atrophies are in some cases due to change in the cells of the anterior cornua, especially in those of the external group. According to certain observations, however (Dejerine), the muscular atrophy is said to be due to peripheral neuritis, the motor cells and the grey matter of the cord being intact. In hemiatrophy of the tongue degeneration of the bulbar nucleus of the hypoglossal nerve has been found.

Trophic and Secretory Troubles.—It seems certain that most of the trophic and secretory troubles are due to lesions in the roots, the ganglia, and the terminal branches of the great sympathetic. The peripheral neuritis will explain the trophic troubles in the skin—various eruptions, œdema, perforating disease, and shedding of the nails. Peripheral neuritis may also be responsible for the spontaneous fractures and arthropathies, which, according to some writers, are put down to the lesions of the anterior cornua or of the root zones. The trophic influence of the trigeminal nerve and the neuritis of the branches of this nerve explain the troubles affecting the teeth and the maxilla.

Ætiology—Treatment.—The causes of locomotor ataxy are obscure. The disease is more frequent in men than in women, and almost always occurs in middle age—from twenty to forty years. According to certain writers (Fournier, Vulpian, Erb, Marie), syphilis is almost always to be blamed. Fournier has sustained this opinion, which is now accepted, but it remains to be seen whether syphilis can of itself produce locomotor ataxy, or whether it only acts as a provoking agent. A patient whom I attended some years ago at the Necker Hospital for syphilitic hæmoptysis had at a later date come back into the Hôtel-Dieu with confirmed tabes. Heredity is an important factor. Sometimes it is direct, and then it is a case of heredo-syphilis; otherwise it is indirect. How many sufferers from tabes are there not in whose family we find madness, general paralysis, epilepsy, and diabetes associated with the preceding causes ! Traumatism plays an important rôle in the development of tabes, and the first symptoms have often appeared after a fall or a violent contusion. Cases of conjugal syphilitic tabes have been noticed.

Treatment.—Raymond has discussed the treatment of tabes in detail. According to him, true tabes is a disease, the cure of which is most problematical.

Pain.—The pains may be relieved with the following remedies : Injections of morphia, antipyrin, acetanilide, phenacetin, chloral, or salicylate of soda. These remedies are of undoubted value, but their constant administration may have bad results. It will be enough to remember that sufferers from tabes furnish an important contingent of morphomaniacs. Other remedies have also been recommended—faradization, continuous currents, refrigeration, massage, and especially suspension. Intraspinal injections of cocaine can only be given under exceptional conditions.

The means of treating the anæsthesia and paræsthesia are reduced to faradization and carbonic acid baths.

The remedies for the ocular troubles are multiple. In order to limit papillary atrophy and amblyopia, we may use subcutaneous injections of cyanide of gold, silver, or platinum (Galezowski). The paralyses are amenable to faradization, and especially to specific treatment with mercury and iodide of potassium, when the patient has recently had syphilis.

The ataxy should be treated, on the one hand, by suspension, and, on the other, by the so-called Fraenkel method, based on the re-education of the muscles. Raymond speaks of the value of this method. It consists in the systematic execution of movements which at first are simple, and become gradually more and more complicated, thus bringing into play the dexterity, and not the muscular force, of the patient. Its use is especially indicated in cases of tabes with early ataxy, when the lower limbs are from the first so severely affected that standing and walking are impossible without a support. It is contra-indicated when the tabes has a rapid onset, with acute and obstinate lightning pains. It is likewise contra-indicated in patients suffering from spontaneous fracture, rupture of tendons, arthropathy or cardiopathy, and in obese patients poisoned by morphia or alcohol. The remedy always fails in tabetic patients suffering from amaurosis, motor paresis, and muscular atrophy.

Suspension has a great advantage over Fraenkel's treatment, in that it aims at the improvement of the ataxy, the lightning pains, and the genito-urinary troubles. On the other hand, the method is more severe. It requires special education on the part of the physician, and it exposes the patient to fatal risks. Its use is counterindicated in tabetic patients suffering from cardio-vascular troubles (valvular lesions, and especially aortic lesions); in tubercular, emphysematous, or stout persons; and, finally, in those who have had apoplectiform or epileptiform attacks, or who have a tendency to vertigo or syncope.

Does a curative remedy for tabes exist? Raymond thinks there is none, and I share his opinion. I have seen tabes persist indefinitely, without causing death. I have seen some cases of tabes remain stationary, and others improve up to the point of an apparent cure, but I doubt whether true tabes can be cured. Nitrate of silver, bromide of potassium, preparations of phosphorus, hydrotherapy, injections of artificial serum and of testicular fluid, have all enjoyed well-merited favour. They are excellent aids in treatment, but they do not bring about a cure. A place apart must be reserved for the antisyphilitic treatment, as far as the cure of tabes is concerned. Nearly all tabetic patients are syphilitic. This fact cannot be questioned (Fournier). Are we to say that the antisyphilitic treatment has chances of curing tabes, or of markedly improving the syphilitic patient suffering from tabes? If syphilitic tabes is of recent date, intensive anti-syphilitic treatment, continued for a long time, may be of real service. If the tabes is inveterate, heroic antisyphilitic treatment rarely gives good results.

II. FRIEDREICH'S DISEASE AND HEREDITARY CEREBELLAR ATAXY—SPASMODIC FAMILY PARAPLEGIA.

This disease, first described by Friedreich, was considered by its author as a variety of locomotor ataxy. Others regarded it as a variety of disseminated sclerosis, but it was Brousse who affirmed its autonomy, and gave it the name of "Friedreich's disease."

Description.—Friedreich's disease commences in early life. Difficulty in walking opens the scene. The child walks with heavy, irregular steps and legs apart, so that the staggering gait recalls drunkenness, or the walk due to lesions of the cerebellum. Some lack of co-ordination is also present, and the gait was therefore called "tabeto-cerebellar" by Charcot.

There is also difficulty in standing, which Friedreich calls "static ataxy." The child, having some difficulty in standing erect and motionless, on account of the oscillations of its body, is obliged, in order to maintain equilibrium, to change its feet frequently. The line of march, instead of being straight, is directed alternately to the right and to the left. To these troubles are added choreiform movements and intention tremors, resembling those of insular sclerosis. In some cases athetoid movements are present.

Sensory troubles, which play such a prominent part in Duchenne's disease, are absent or insignificant in Friedreich's disease. Lightning pains are exceptional, but have nevertheless been noted (Brissaud). Anæsthesia and analgesia are very rare and but slightly marked.

The **muscular sense**—or, rather, "the sense of attitudes" (Bonnier)—the abolition of which is characteristic of locomotor ataxy, seems to be intact in Friedreich's disease. Choreiform instability is, however, noticed.

The **tendon reflexes** are abolished. The cutaneous reflexes are preserved. Babinski's phenomenon is seen.

The ocular troubles principally affect the muscular system of the eye. Nystagmus is frequent. Paralysis of the muscles, with or without diplopia, is extremely rare. Vision is normal, whilst it is often affected in tabes.

The genito-urinary troubles are practically absent. The cerebral troubles are slight. The intelligence remains intact throughout the disease. Speech is somewhat halting, as in ataxy.

Muscular atrophy is sometimes seen in certain muscles of the trunk or of the limbs.

Deformities may exist in the trunk in the form of scoliosis, and are common in the feet, the type being that of equino-varus, with exaggerated extension of the big toe. This deformity is known as "the foot of Friedreich's disease."

Such are the symptoms of Friedreich's disease. After some years the troubles involve the upper limbs, and the patient is absolutely helpless, being condemned to remain indefinitely in bed or in a chair. The disease is rarely fatal.

The diagnosis of Friedreich's disease is given under Insular Sclerosis and Tabes.

Ætiology.—Friedreich's disease is a **family** disease—that is to say, it attacks several children of the same family. It is also hereditary, and Friedreich therefore called it hereditary ataxy. These two conditions are, however, not absolute. The disease commences before the age of fourteen years in two-thirds of the cases (Sottla), and in the same family the "age at which the disease commences is the same for each member attacked."

Pathological Anatomy.—The lesions found have not always been constant in the few post-mortem examinations that have been performed. Sclerosis is found in Goll's and Burdach's columns, in the direct cerebellar tract, and the lateral tracts (combined sclerosis). The grey matter in the reticulum of Clarke's columns is affected. Some writers have noticed changes in the anterior cornua. The posterior roots only show irregular lesions.

II·

According to Dejerine and Letulle, the sclerosis of the posterior columns in Friedreich's disease is said to be a gliosis, whereas that of the cerebellar and of crossed pyramidal tracts is said to be a vascular sclerosis. These views are not generally accepted (Marie).

Treatment seems to have no effect on the disease.

Hereditary Cerebellar Ataxy.

Let us now refer to a morbid condition having many relations with Friedreich's disease, and described by Marie under the name of " hereditary cerebellar ataxy." Marie thus describes this morbid condition : " Hereditary cerebellar ataxy is a family disease, like Friedreich's disease. It attacks several generations more often than Friedreich's ataxy does—that is to say, it is more directly hereditary. Its onset usually occurs at a more advanced age than Friedreich's disease, either after the twentieth or sometimes after the thirtieth year. The initial symptom consists in motor disturbances in the lower limbs, perfectly analogous to those of Friedreich's disease— staggering gait, difficulty in standing erect with or without Romberg's sign, pseudo-tremors of the upper limbs, and nystagmus. So much for its resemblances to Friedreich's disease. The principal differences consist in the exaggeration of the patellar reflexes; in the existence of various spasmodic phenomena ; in visual troubles, consisting in dichromatopsia, restriction of the visual field, diminution of visual acuity, and changes in the papilla ; in the loss or diminution of the light reflex ; and, finally, in the presence of objective troubles in the cutaneous sensibility, as well as in the absence of trophic troubles, such as scoliosis, or the club-foot of Friedreich's disease."

The fundamental lesion is atrophy of the cerebellum. The atrophy is general or partial. The cerebellum may be reduced to half its normal size. It is not a question of sclerosis. Perhaps even, says Londe, it may be possible, according to the nature of the lesion, to establish a difference between sclerotic, accidental, non-family atrophy of the cerebellum and the family atrophy of hereditary cerebellar ataxy. Spinal lesions, which were clearly defined and constituted the sole anatomical substratum in the cases of Vincelet and Switalski, Thomas and Roux, have been noticed. The condition was a combined sclerosis of the posterior columns, of Gowers' tracts, and of the direct cerebellar tracts.

To sum up, as Londe says, hereditary cerebellar ataxy and Friedreich's disease seem to be two forms of hereditary ataxy. The lesion in the one is said to commence in the cerebellum, the lesion in the other in the spinal cord. They may both limit themselves to the organ first attacked, but they may also be complicated, the one with spinal lesions, the other with cerebellar lesions, thus forming types of transition frequent in family diseases (Charcot).

Spasmodic Family Paraplegia.

Strümpell noticed spasmodic paraplegia in two brothers, and at the post-mortem examination of each one he found in the spinal cord lesions in the posterior and lateral columns. The condition was a primary combined systematic sclerosis. Other writers have seen cases of spasmodic family paraplegia, and in some cases other symptoms were superposed on this syndrome, giving to the disease an aspect different from the primary type—either that of spasmodic tabes or of insular sclerosis. We may agree with Lorrain that this disease may be regarded as a group of family affections, united one with another in transition forms.

III. COMBINED SCLEROSIS.

We designate under the name of combined scleroses, not a clinical entity, but an anatomo-pathological grouping which is the substratum of several clinical types. The characteristic feature is the combination of sclerotic changes in the posterior and in the lateral columns of the spinal cord.

Description of the Clinical Types.—The clinical types of combined scleroses may be classified in the following manner:

1. **Combined Congenital or Family Sclerosis.**—These are Friedreich's disease, hereditary cerebellar ataxy of Pierre Marie, and spasmodic family paraplegia of Strümpell.

2. **Combined Acquired Sclerosis.**—These are : (a) Combined tabetic sclerosis (in the form of ordinary tabes and combined tabes) ; (b) the combined scleroses of general paralysis ; (c) the combined scleroses of spasmodic form ; (d) the subacute combined scleroses, and those due to anæmia and intoxication.

Tabetic Form (Combined Tabes).

The clinical aspect of patients attacked by this form is as follows : A patient has all the classical signs of tabes—Robertson's sign, Romberg's sign, loss of tendon reflexes, lightning pains, urinary troubles, etc. There is no reason a priori to suspect an abnormal form of tabes, and patients suffering from this form were for a long time considered as cases of ordinary ataxy, although the post-mortem examination revealed the presence of combined lesions in the posterior and the lateral columns.

Marie and Crouzon have shown that it is possible to make a diagnosis of combined sclerosis by the three following signs :

1. **Gait, with Dragging of the Feet.**—The patient does not push his feet forward, as in ataxy, and does not walk on his heels. He walks on crutches or rides in a carriage. When he moves, he drags his legs behind

him, the body bent forward. Each leg moves forward with difficulty, dragging the point of the toe, as though it were dragging a heavy weight.

2. **Paraplegia.**—A patient suffering from tabes whose muscular power in the lower limbs is either diminishing or is so weak that he remains confined to his bed, like a paraplegic patient, has not only lesions in the posterior columns, but also lesions in the lateral columns. The excessive want of co-ordination, or the muscular weakness that may be associated with the amyotrophy seen in some patients, must not always be taken for paraplegia.

3. **Babinski's Sign.**—Babinski, in 1900, noticed this sign in certain tabetic patients, and put forward the hypothesis that it showed the presence of combined sclerosis. Marie and Crouzon have verified this view by post-mortem examination. The three cardinal signs just enumerated enabled Marie and Crouzon to prove combined sclerosis once in every thirteen cases of tabes. This clinical form is therefore relatively frequent.

Combined Scleroses of General Paralysis.

Combined spinal lesions in the course of general paralysis were noticed by Westphal, and later by Raymond (1892). They were present seventy-three times in 145 post-mortem examinations made by Fürstner.

These lesions, however, are difficult to trace clinically. Crou on, considering them solely from the point of view of the clinical signs of lesions of the posterior columns in patients suffering from general paralysis (Féré and Seglas's wards at Bicêtre), found them only in one out of every four cases, while the spinal lesions existed in two-thirds of the post-mortem examinations.

Combined Spasmodic Scleroses.

The fundamental character of this form is the existence of spasmodic phenomena, combined with symptoms of tabes, due to the lesions in the posterior columns. We may thus have to deal with a tabetic patient who shows some of the classical signs of tabes—Romberg's sign, Robertson's sign, lack of co-ordination, urinary troubles, etc. The tendon reflexes are examined, and we expect to find them abolished; but we find, on the contrary, preservation or exaggeration of the patellar reflexes, ankle-clonus, and Babinski's sign.

Another patient is attacked by spasmodic paraplegia and lack of co-ordination of the movements, but, unlike the preceding patient, he does not show the other phenomena of classical tabes—no lightning pains, no Robertson's sign, no Romberg's sign, etc. This type was described by Gowers in 1886 under the name of **ataxic paraplegia.**

Finally, Strümpell, Dejerine, and Sottas have been able to verify the presence of combined sclerosis at the post-mortem examination of patients who during their lifetime had only shown slow and progressive spasmodic paraplegia, without any sign of associated tabes.

Ataxo-Spasmodic Paraplegia in Old People.—Marie and Crouzon have seen at Bicêtre a certain number of old men suffering from spasmodic paraplegia, with inco-ordination and cerebellar symptoms. This disease developed at an advanced age and ran a slow course. Crouzon has described this clinical type, and has classed it with the cases formerly described by Demange under the name of " progressive tabetic contracture." Recent autopsies have shown that the lesion to which this morbid entity corresponds is a primary parenchymatous atrophy of the cerebellar cortex.

Subacute Combined Scleroses.

In certain cases post-mortem examination has shown the existence of a combined sclerosis of the spinal cord, causing a disease with the following symptoms :

The patient has first of all trouble in walking, with slight inco-ordination and spastic paraplegia. In the second stage the paraplegia becomes marked, and anæsthesia of the lower limbs and of the trunk is noticed. In the third stage the paraplegia becomes complete and flaccid. The tendon reflexes are abolished, and muscular atrophy, with incontinence of the sphincters, appears.

In this disease we notice more or less marked, but not characteristic, anæmia. Death supervenes in one to three years. This form was described in 1900 by Risien Russell, Batten, and Collier, under the name of " subacute combined degeneration of the spinal cord." It has not yet been observed in France, although it is not rare in London. The total number of cases observed in the Queen's Square Hospital since 1898 numbers over twenty.

We also see in pernicious anæmia combined sclerosis of the spinal cord, which may be recognized clinically, or may be revealed only at the post-mortem examination. When the clinical signs exist, they are, according to Dejerine and Thomas, most frequently troubles of subjective and objective sensibility, as well as motor troubles, which are a mixture of ataxy and paraplegia. The reflexes are usually abolished, though they are sometimes exaggerated. The course is rapid, and death occurs in a few months.

Finally, in pellagra, ergotism, lathyrism, and cachexia we find combined sclerosis, the clinical picture being sometimes that of pseudo-tabes, at other times that of spastic paraplegia.

Pathological Anatomy.—The definition of the disease indicates the topography of the lesions. The following combinations may be seen : (a) Combined lesions of the posterior columns and of the crossed pyramidal tracts ; (b) combined lesions of the posterior columns and of the direct cerebellar tracts ; (c) combined lesions of the posterior and lateral columns with lesions of the anterior pyramidal tracts.

Pathogenic Varieties.—Combined scleroses are divided into two large classes, according as they are localized in a system of fibres or are diffuse, having only a systematic appearance.

The systematic scleroses may be created by changes in the nerve cells, producing exogenous (spinal ganglia) or endogenous degeneration. This type of combined sclerosis is seen in general paralysis and in tabes (lesions of the direct cerebellar tracts, consequent on lesions of the cells in Clarke's columns). The sclerosis may, however, be primary, and independent of any cellular atrophy, as well as of any meningeal or vascular lesion (Dejerine and Sottas).

The combined pseudo-systematic scleroses have only a systematic appearance. In reality they are diffuse, and associated with meningeal or vascular lesions. In the pseudo-systematic scleroses of meningeal origin the sclerosis penetrates the cord from the surface towards the deep parts in the form of marginal sclerosis. Some cases of combined tabetic sclerosis are due to a process of this kind (meningitis by propagation). The value of posterior meningitis in the theory of Marie and Guillain relative to tabes helps to confirm this pathogenesis.

The combined scleroses of vascular origin are explained by the distribution of the vessels in the spinal cord. They coincide with toxic changes in the cord (pernicious anæmia, cystoma, lathyrism, etc.).

Ætiology.—Syphilis plays an important part in the combined scleroses. It is almost always the cause of tabes and of general paralysis. According to Gowers, it is rare in ataxic paraplegia. The senile form seems to depend on atheroma, and the subacute scleroses are associated with the anæmias and the intoxications.

Treatment.—In the combined syphilitic scleroses of tabes and of general paralysis we employ, as in tabes and general paralysis, the intensive mercurial treatment.

IV. SYRINGOMYELIA.

The word **syringomyelia** (σύριγξ, canal ; μυελός, marrow) signifies a canal in the marrow. This expression, employed for the first time by Ollivier, of Angers, in 1827, was almost abandoned, when the recent labours of Mlle. Bäumler, and especially of Schultze and Kahler, rescued it from oblivion. These writers did more : whilst rehabilitating the word they also applied it to a morbid entity, having its own symptomatology and pathological anatomy. Their researches, which were at first favourably received (Debove, Bruhl), were later criticized, especially as regards the nature of the lesions (Charcot, Joffroy, and Achard), and the pathological interpretation of the symptoms (Dejerine, Zambacco).

Pathological Anatomy.—The cord, when removed from the spinal canal, becomes flat like a ribbon. The consistency is less firm, and the cut section is diffluent, so that we must be very careful lest we should render any further examination impossible. The changes are sometimes limited to a small segment. In most cases they measure from 3 to 4 inches, but the spinal cord may be affected throughout its entire length. The lesions are chiefly situated at the cervico-brachial enlargement of the cord.

In the centre of the spinal cord we find a cavity, containing a fluid analogous to the cerebro-spinal fluid, and of the size of a knitting-needle, of a probe, or of a pencil. The cavity is sometimes double or triple, and presents several diverticula. This cavity was for a long time thought to be formed at the expense of the central canal (hydromyelia). Schultze and Kahler held that it is due to a glioma commencing in the deep parts of the spinal cord. This glioma generally develops at the expense of the posterior half of the cord, pushing back the grey and white matter, first in the posterior half, and then in the anterior half of the spinal cord.

This tumour is formed of proliferated neuroglial elements. A felting is thus formed of fine cells, with a central swelling and multiple interlacing prolongations, plunged into the midst of a thin fibrillary network. At the central canal we find some trace of a limiting membrane, but in general this is merely neuroglial cells piled up one against the other. Sometimes, however, an incomplete layer of cylindrical cells is found, arising from the central canal of the spinal cord. The arteries are often thickened, and their lumen is constricted. This peculiarity has led several writers (Joffroy and Achard) to ask whether all cases of syringomyelia are really caused by gliomata, or whether certain of them are not due to a central myelitis of vascular origin. The latter would be related to periependymal myelitis (Hallopeau). Finally, Charcot recognizes three varieties of syringomyelia : (1) medullary malformation ; (2) periependymal myelitis ; (3) medullary glioma.

Description.—From what we have just said, it follows that the symptoms of syringomyelia vary according to the seat of the lesions and the direction of their development. As, however, the lesions chiefly affect the posterior half of the spinal cord, especially at the commencement, the principal manifestations are of the sensory type.

These sensory troubles, in the absence of which it is almost impossible to make the diagnosis, consist in a special anæsthesia of the upper limbs, though it often attacks in a less degree the lower limbs. It may be exclusively limited to them. The anæsthesia is frequently more marked on one side than on the other, never following the distribution of the nerves and ceasing suddenly in certain regions, which vary according to the particular case. The anæsthesia sometimes occupies the hand, and ends like a ruffle. It sometimes reaches to the elbow, or even as far as the shoulder, terminating then like a sleeve. It invades the legs, in the shape of a stocking, or it attacks the whole lower limb, like a pair of drawers. It sometimes attacks the whole body, leaving the face intact. This last character, for a long time regarded as pathognomonic, loses its value in view of certain recently published cases.

This special anæsthesia consists in a dissociation of the various forms of sensibility. The sense of heat and cold is abolished, or simply blurred. Patients often have burns for which they cannot account. The sense of pain is likewise abolished, so that patients may be pricked and pinched without feeling any pain. Some of them have even fractured an anæsthetic limb without feeling any pain. The anæsthesia is both superficial and deep-seated. In some cases thermo-anæsthesia exists alone; in one case the sense of heat only was abolished (Dejerine). The sense of touch is, on the contrary, preserved; the patient feels the ground when walking, but a pin-prick is interpreted as a tactile sensation.

These troubles of sensibility are divided in zones, the upper limit being perpendicular to the axis of the body or the axis of the limbs. There is no agreement between these girdles of anæsthesia and the topographical distribution of the nerves. The anæsthesia may be limited to the hand, in the shape of a glove, and the three nerves affected (ulnar, radial, and median) have quite a different peripheral distribution. This circular distribution of the anæsthesia can only be explained by the persistence of the primary metamerism of the nerve centre (Brissaud). I must also mention spinal metamerism and the distribution of herpes.

The **motor troubles** are likewise subordinate to the regions of the spinal cord, compressed from within outwards. They consist in muscular atrophy of the Aran-Duchenne type. It is usually limited to the hands and the forearms. It sometimes affects only the lower limbs, and is accompanied by fibrillary tremors. When the antero-lateral columns are attacked, contractures appear; the reflexes are then exaggerated. Sometimes the ataxic symptoms predominate, being most common in the lower limbs.

The existence of dorso-lumbar scoliosis has often been noted. The skin shows trophic lesions—blisters, puffiness, white or blue œdema of the limbs, glossy skin, eschars, repeated whitlows, shedding of the nails, phlegmons, etc. The trophic troubles in the bones are fractures, with rapid consolidation, and depression of the anterior thoracic wall. In the joints we find arthropathies like those seen in ataxy. Ulceration and perforation of the bladder also occur.

The nervous troubles sometimes reach the superior cervical region, and even the region of the bulb: sensory troubles in the tongue, dyspnœa, and palpitations. We must also remember inequality of the pupils, unilateral paralytic mydriasis, myosis, and Argyll-Robertson's sign. Nystagmus is fairly frequent. Paralysis of the motor muscles, ptosis, and diplopia are more rare. Concentric narrowing of the field of vision is due to the con-comitant hysteria rather than the syringomyelia.   Finally, we must mention defaced cases—unilateral nature of the lesions, complete loss of all kinds of sensation, absence of atrophy, etc.

Guillain has isolated a spasmodic form of syringomyelia, characterized by contractures and exaggeration of the reflexes in all four limbs. The three last fingers are firmly flexed, so that the thumb and the index-finger, which are almost free, can alone be used by the patient (*main en pince*).

Syringomyelia commences generally in the young. Its course is very slow, and, at the end of many years, death is due to exhaustion, syncope, or some intercurrent disease. Syringomyelia is not hereditary, and, accord-ing to those who admit only the existence of the central glioma, it is a disease of evolution.

Diagnosis.—The special troubles of sensation distinguish syringomyelia from progressive muscular atrophy, amyotrophic lateral sclerosis, and the various forms of progressive myopathy. In hysteria the dissociation of the sensory troubles may exist, as may also the limitation of the anæsthesia to the wrist, to the shoulder, etc. Constriction of the field of vision and atrophy are likewise common to both diseases. It is obvious how difficult the diagnosis may be in the absence of any convulsive attack, or of any hysterogenous zone. Their presence even does not settle the question, because syringomyelia and hysteria may exist in the same subject.

Morvan's disease, or painless whitlow, is considered by some authors as a variety of syringomyelia. In this disease recurrent whitlows, with loss of the phalanx, finally causing marked mutilation, and evolving without pain, constitute the capital syndrome. Although the anæsthesia is almost always complete, it may happen that dissociation of the sensory troubles may be found in certain patients with painless whitlows. The unilateral nature of the lesions is only an element in the diagnosis, because it may exist in certain cases of syringomyelia. Besides, Joffroy and Achard have twice found gliomatous changes in the spinal cords of patients with painless whitlow.

The existence of peripheral neuritis, characterized by nodules on the nerves, and particularly on the ulnar nerve at the elbow, the sensory troubles, and the mutilations that accompany them, have led Zambacco to unite syringomyelia and Morvan's disease under one heading. He holds that they are an attenuated form of leprosy. The microscopic examination of a nodule on the ulnar nerve made by Pitres revealed the leprosy bacillus, but this finding does not prove that all cases of nodular neuritis are of leprous origin.

In five patients with hæmatomyelia of traumatic origin Minor has noted most of the symptoms of syringomyelia ; the patient's gait alone permitted the diagnosis to be made.

Compression of the spinal cord (Charcot) may lead to confusion. One of Charcot's patients showed, as a distinctive sign, thermo-anæsthesia in the region of the internal cutaneous nerve of the arm, but it did not terminate in a ruffle.

Thermo-anæsthesia has been noticed in alcoholism and diabetes (Vergely). In these two diseases neuroses are frequent, and cause sensory troubles. The diagnosis will be facilitated by the symptoms peculiar to these diseases. The coexistence in the same subject of exophthalmic goitre and syringomyelia has been observed by Joffroy and Achard. The coexistence of syringomyelia and spasmodic hemiplegia has been noted by Charcot and Brissaud.

Certain lesions causing cavities in the spinal cord have clinical signs identical with those of syringomyelia (Dejerine and Thomas).

V. PROGRESSIVE MUSCULAR ATROPHY.

The muscular atrophies play an important part in the diseases of the spinal cord which we are now about to describe. They are, furthermore, met with in many cases of myelitis. They are due to a lesion in the cells of the anterior cornua of the spinal cord. The muscular atrophy is sometimes inconstant, slight, and appears without order and without any fixed date in the course of myelitis (insular sclerosis). At other times the atrophy is the most important, whilst being at the same time associated with other symptoms which of themselves are of great value (amyotrophic lateral sclerosis, syringomyelia, atrophic paralysis of infants). Finally, in other cases the muscular atrophy shows a systematic and progressive course. It forms a well-defined morbid entity, and is known as Duchenne's progressive muscular atrophy.

And yet, whatever the kind and the variety of these muscular atrophies, they are all of spinal origin, and are myelopathic atrophies, whilst there are other diseases of the muscular system which are also progressive, and run their course with or without atrophy of the muscle, but which are primary and independent (at least, in appearance) of lesions in the spinal cord. These family myopathies are described later. There are two kinds : (1) pseudo-hypertrophic muscular paralysis (Duchenne's type) ; (2) progressive atrophic myopathy (Landouzy-Dejerine type).

These muscular atrophies of myelopathic and myopathic origin must be contrasted with the muscular atrophies of neuritic origin, as exemplified in alcoholic paralysis and lead palsy.

The existence, however, of a progressive muscular atrophy, which occurs in families and is of myelopathic origin (Werding and Hoffmann), seems to establish a bond of union between the Aran-Duchenne type and the various primary myopathies, and to bring us back to the unitary doctrine (Raymond). " There is no insurmountable line of demarcation between the progressive family amyotrophies and the progressive muscular atrophy of the Aran-Duchenne type. The various types of progressive muscular atrophy are but varieties of the same morbid entity. It has as a substratum the same organic system, the spino-muscular neuron, and its prolongation, the muscle. The weak portion of this organic system seems to be the muscle in the early stages of life, and the tropho-motor cell of the neuron in adult age. This does not prevent in exceptional cases the dystrophy, which gives rise to progressive muscular atrophy, from commencing in the tropho-motor cells of the spinal cord and manifesting itself in the first years of life; just as it may commence in the muscles and limit itself there in an adult subject. Progressive muscular atrophy, as Duchenne conceived it, is therefore placed on a new basis, which appears to me to be permanent " (Raymond). I shall now describe progressive muscular atrophy of the Aran-Duchenne type.

Description.—The disease commences insidiously with atrophy of the abductor pollicis; the atrophy spreads to the muscles of the hand, invading both hands symmetrically, and then affects the upper limbs and the trunk, so that in five to ten years the muscles of these various regions have almost entirely disappeared, the patient preserving the absolute integrity of the other functions until the atrophy lays hold of the muscles of respiration, of mastication, and of deglutition.

This disease has received from Aran and Duchenne the name of **progressive muscular atrophy.** The work published in 1850 by Aran has largely contributed to its recognition. It must, however, be added that in 1849 Duchenne had already presented a monograph to the Institute which establishes the question of priority, and leaves him the honour of the discovery.

Progressive muscular atrophy almost always commences in the upper limbs. In 159 cases collected by Duchenne it commenced only twice in the lower limbs, and twelve times in the muscles of the trunk; it never attacks the face. On the other hand, there is an amyotrophy which often commences in the face, especially in children. Duchenne wrongly considered it to be a progressive myelopathic amyotrophy, and included it under progressive muscular atrophy. It should be classed with the primary myopathies, and we shall meet with it in the diseases of the muscular system under the name of progressive atrophic myopathy (Landouzy-Dejerine type).

In progressive muscular atrophy the **atrophy** of the muscle is the prominent feature. The muscle loses its function, not because it is paralyzed,

but because it is destroyed. The atrophy does not attack a limb or a group
of muscles; it attacks certain bundles of the muscle, whilst the neighbouring
bundles are intact, but they will be attacked in turn. As soon as the
muscle is affected, it loses its consistency, becoming soft and contracting
with less vigour ; but the intact bundles of the muscle contract and preserve
the electrical reaction. Although the muscle on the way to atrophy has
preserved its electrical contractility, this electrical excitability is exhausted
quicker than in the healthy condition. According to some writers, the
diseased muscle is said to have a momentarily exaggerated electrical excitability (reaction of degeneration).

As a general rule, when a muscle or a group of muscles becomes atrophied,
the succession of the phenomena is always the same. The atrophy of the
muscle modifies the shape of the affected part, the bones becoming prominent,
while flattening replaces the muscular contour. Furthermore, as the antagonistic muscles are rarely atrophied at the same time, their action becomes
predominant, and hence vicious attitudes result, which are nowhere more
appreciable than in the hand.

Atrophy of the Muscles of the Hand.—The atrophy commences most
frequently in the thenar eminence of the right hand (Aran). The short
abductor muscle of the thumb is the first affected. The action of this
muscle, abductor and extensor of the last phalanx, is to oppose the ball of
the thumb to the ball of the index finger and of the middle finger when
flexed (Duchenne). This muscle is therefore indispensable in holding a pen
or a pencil, and in working with a brush or a graver. Its atrophy is
therefore quickly noticed, and the hand immediately becomes useless.
As the atrophy also invades the other muscles of the thenar eminence, the
normal prominence is replaced by a flattening ; the opposition of the thumb
is impossible, and the antagonistic muscle, the long extensor of the thumb
being unopposed, draws the first metacarpal backwards and outwards.
The hand then assumes the aspect of a monkey's hand (Duchenne).

When the lumbricales and the interossei are atrophied, the metacarpal bones appear to be stripped of the flesh, and adduction and abduction
of the fingers become impossible. The interossei and the lumbricales, however, have another action : they flex the metacarpal phalanx and extend
the two last phalanges. Their antagonists are the flexors and extensors
of the fingers, which flex the two last phalanges and extend the metacarpal
phalanx. As the action of these antagonistic muscles is unopposed, the
interossei being atrophied, we find the *main en griffe* (Duchenne).

At a later period the hand is so emaciated that it resembles the hand of
a skeleton.

Atrophy of the Muscles of the Arm and of the Shoulder.—In the
forearm the muscles of the anterior and external regions are first attacked.

In the arm the triceps is the muscle which resists longest. In the shoulder the three bundles of the deltoid are invaded, so that elevation of the arm becomes impossible (Duchenne).

Atrophy of the Muscles of the Trunk.—The upper part of the trapezius, which receives its nerve supply from multiple sources, is not atrophied, the atrophy being limited to its lower part; the scapula stands out from the spinal column. The pectoral muscles, the serrati, the rhomboid muscles, and the sacro-lumbar muscles, become atrophied without any fixed rule. When the pectoral muscles are atrophied, the normal mass of the muscles is replaced on each side of the sternum by a hollow. The atrophy of the extensor or flexor muscles of the trunk displaces the centre of gravity, and to remedy it curvatures of the spinal column are produced. The head falls in every direction after the atrophy of the extensor and flexor muscles. The contrast is striking when we examine, on the one hand, the wasted trunk and the emaciated upper limbs, and, on the other, the lower limbs, still clothed with masses of muscles. The lower limbs are either spared or do not become atrophied until a very advanced period.

The chief functions of the general economy are so far intact. The general symptoms are trifling; they are fibrillary contractions in the muscles on the road to atrophy, some pain and a sensation of cold in the atrophied limbs, with actual lowering of the temperature. At a more advanced period of the disease, usually after several years, the atrophy lays hold of the depressors of the jaw, and mastication becomes impossible. Sometimes the muscles of deglutition are invaded. More frequently the muscles of respiration become atrophied, the intercostals first, and costal respiration is abolished. Later the diaphragm is attacked, and respiration then becomes so laboured that any lesion of the respiratory apparatus, even the least bronchitis, may carry off the patient. The duration of the disease is variable, being rarely less than two years, and most often more than ten or twelve years.

The above description applies to a typical case, but there are cases in which we find anæsthesia, contractures, bulbar paralysis (glosso-labio-laryngeal paralysis), or external ophthalmoplegia.

In some cases progressive muscular atrophy, instead of commencing in the muscles of the thenar eminence, attacks at first the muscles of the shoulder and of the arm. This is Vulpian's scapulo-humeral type. The atrophy is generally symmetrical, and remains confined for a long time to the root of the limb before attacking the other regions. It never affects the face.

Pathological Anatomy.—The atrophy of the muscles has been said by some writers to be fatty, but recent researches (Hayem) have established that it is most often simple, without fatty degeneration. The muscles preserve their striation till the last moment; they gradually diminish in size and take on a dead-leaf colour, whole bundles finally disappearing. In some cases the nuclei of the sarcolemma proliferate and give rise to fibrosis. The fatty elements sometimes accumulate in the interior of the sheath, giving rise to a steatosis, which may mask the disappearance of the muscle, and at first cause a belief in its preservation.

In fact, as Ranvier has shown, the fundamental lesions of the muscles in muscular atrophy of myelopathic origin are equivalent to those seen in muscles separated from their trophic centres. The non-differentiated protoplasm of the primary fibre becomes hypertrophied; the nuclei of the sarcolemma proliferate; their phagocytic action is then exercised, and causes the differentiated tissue to disappear.

It was at first thought that the lesion of the muscles comprised the entire disease, but Cruveilhier soon showed that the lesions of the nervous system claimed a preponderant part, and in a post-mortem examination that has remained celebrated he discovered the atrophy of the anterior roots of the spinal cord.

Cruveilhier went even farther, and, divining the lesion which he did not see, announced that the grey matter of the spinal cord must be involved. To Luys belongs the honour of having been the first to describe clearly the real lesion of muscular progressive atrophy. In 1860 Luys stated that the anterior cornua of the grey matter were partially destroyed at points corresponding to the anterior roots of the atrophied nerves; and, in fact, subsequent post-mortem examinations (Hayem, Charcot, Vulpian, Joffroy, etc.) have proved that the primary and constant lesion of muscular atrophy is seated in the anterior cornua of the grey matter. The cells of the anterior cornua disappear by pigmentary or by sclerotic atrophy, the capillary vessels are thickened, and connective proliferation is found in the neuroglia of the anterior cornua. There is, then, a lesion which is at first localized in the nerve cell, but it is difficult to say whether this lesion is irritative or degenerative. In any event the disease may be regarded as a systematic affection of the medullary parenchyma.

The morbid process, starting in the nerve cells of the anterior cornua (atrophic degeneration of the cell, with connective proliferation), extends to the anterior roots of the nerves (atrophy of the roots), and ends in the muscles (simple atrophy, with or without sclero-fatty transformation). The change in the anterior roots of the spinal nerves is often visible to the naked eye. The roots are obviously atrophied, and in some cases are greyish. Under the microscope healthy nerve fibres are found side by side with diseased fibres, irregularly distributed. Lesions of the great sympathetic have been noticed, but they are inconstant and secondary. Why does an irritative lesion of the anterior nerve cells of the spinal cord cause muscular atrophy? The spinal cord, by means of its anterior grey matter, exercises a trophic action on the muscles.   The fact is evident, but the question arises as to how this action is exercised.

It is not transmitted from the spinal cord to the muscles by the vaso-motor fibres, because section of the fibres of the sympathetic or tearing out of the ganglia does not produce muscular atrophy (Vulpian).   It appears to be transmitted by the motor nerves, because crushing or section of a motor nerve—the sciatic nerve, for example—causes atrophy in the corre-sponding muscles.   According to some authors, muscular atrophy is said to be due to irritation of the nerve.   There is an excess of action, and this excess of function is said to lead to malnutrition (Brown-Séquard, Charcot). According to another theory (Vulpian, Hayem), the muscular atrophy is due, not to an excess of action, but to a deficiency of action, the affected nerve no longer transmitting, or transmitting imperfectly, to the corre-sponding muscle the trophic power received from the spinal cord.   It appears evident that the nutrition of the muscles is connected with the cells of the anterior cornua, and the situation of the muscular lesion always corresponds to a definite site as regards the medullary lesion.   When the muscular atrophy was limited to the muscles of the hand on one side (Prevost*), atrophy of the anterior cornua of the same side was found in the region of the spinal cord, extending from the seventh cervical to the first dorsal pair (exit of the roots of the median and ulnar nerves).

Muscular atrophy with atrophy of the anterior cornua of the spinal cord has been produced by injection of cultures of streptococci into animals.

Diagnosis—Ætiology—Treatment.—Progressive   muscular   atrophy must not be confounded with secondary atrophy supervening in a more or less irregular manner during the course of other affections of the spinal cord, either in posterior or in lateral sclerosis.

Progressive myopathy often commencing in children in the face was for a long time described as forming part of progressive muscular atrophy. We shall see under Diseases of the Muscular System that this progressive atrophic myopathy (Landouzy-Dejerine type) has nothing in common with progressive muscular atrophy.

The atrophy of the muscles of the hand, due to a lesion of the ulnar nerve at the elbow or at the wrist, presents the following characters : The muscles of the hypothenar eminence, the interossei and lumbricales, are atrophied, but the muscles of the thenar eminence supplied by the median

* Prevost and David, *Arch. de Physiol.*, 1874, p. 595.   This case is as conclusive as it is remarkable.   The muscular atrophy was limited solely to the muscles of the right thenar eminence, and this atrophy dated from infancy.   At the autopsy there was evident atrophy of the right anterior root of the eighth cervical pair, and under the microscope there was seen atrophy of the anterior cornu of the grey matter at this level throughout a length of from 2 to 3 centimetres.

nerve are normal. The claw only extends to the last two fingers, because the interossei and lumbricales of the two first spaces have a double supply from the ulnar and the median nerves.

Progressive muscular atrophy will not be confounded with atrophic rheumatism of the deltoid and with muscular atrophy in the neighbourhood of rheumatic joints. In such a case the painful stage at the onset of the disease sufficiently indicates its nature. The deformity of the hand, consequent on nodular rheumatism or on contraction of the palmar fascia, simu lates but very imperfectly the claw-like hand of muscular atrophy.

The paralyses of the brachial plexus are accompanied by atrophy of the deltoid, the biceps, the brachialis anticus and supinator longus, the infraspinatus, the teres major and minor, and the rhomboid muscles in the superior type, and by the other muscles of the upper limb in the inferior type. In the latter type the sensibility of the hand is abolished, while it is preserved over the inner side of the arm, and to some extent on the posterior surface, these parts being supplied by the branches of the first intercostal nerves. The existence of oculo-pupillary troubles (inferior type), of trophic troubles, and of the reaction of degeneration are signs of lesions in the brachial plexus, and are not met with in Aran-Duchenne's disease.

Charcot and Marie's progressive muscular atrophy commences in the muscles of the feet and legs. The atrophy is for years limited to these regions before invading the upper limbs. In the arms it first attacks the muscles of the thenar and hypothenar eminences and the interossei, producing the claw hand. The muscles of the trunk, shoulders, and face remain free, and those of the arms and of the thighs are relatively normal. The atrophied regions only show slight fibrillary contractions. At an advanced period the reaction of degeneration is seen. Sensory troubles are sometimes seen in the form of a dissociated anæsthesia, which leaves the tactile sense immune. The disease commences in childhood, more rarely in youth ; it is a family disease. These characteristics suffice to distinguish it from atrophy of the Aran-Duchenne type.

Syringomyelia presents numerous points of resemblance to progressive muscular atrophy (Aran-Duchenne type). In both diseases the muscular atrophy commences in the upper limbs, attacking by preference the thenar and hypothenar eminences, the interossei, next the muscles of the forearm, and finally those of the arm. In both cases the deformities and the vicious attitudes of the hand and of the forearm are similar. Finally, in both cases fibrillary contractions are seen in the diseased muscles. In syringomyelia, however, we notice sensory troubles, which are always absent in progressive muscular atrophy. Certain trophic troubles are also present—glossy skin, eschars, fragility of the bones, swelling of the epi physes, articular lesions, panaris with loss of the phalanges, and increased sweating over the anæsthetic regions. From the anatomo-pathological point of view, the recent researches of Kahler, Debove, and Dejerine have shown that in syringomyelia there is not a lesion limited to the cells of the anterior cornua; either a glioma develops in the circumference of the central canal, and compresses the cornua of the spinal cord from within outwards, or there is a central myelitis, which produces a cavity (Joffroy and Achard). If the effects are more marked in the upper limbs, it is because the lesion is especially localized in the cervical region of the cord.

The **ætiology** of progressive muscular atrophy is very obscure. Heredity and excessive muscular fatigue have been invoked. Charrin and Claude, by repeated injections of pyocyanic toxine, were able to produce progressive muscular atrophy in animals. The post-mortem examination revealed a lesion of slow evolution in the grey matter of the spinal cord. The diseases of the anterior cornua, and especially infantile paralysis, are regarded as favouring the ulterior development of progressive muscular atrophy. According to certain authors, however, the appearance of Aran-Duchenne's disease is said to be independent of any anterior cornual affection. Both diseases are said to develop successively, in consequence of a congenital weakness of the spinal cord (*locus minoris resistentiæ*). Rendu has further pointed out that in these cases the muscular atrophy is not essentially progressive, but that it rapidly attacks certain muscles or groups of muscles, while progressive atrophy generally involves small bundles of fibres. The atrophy caused by lead-poisoning differs markedly from the classic disease just described. The prognosis, though grave, is not always fatal. The disease sometimes has long periods of arrest; it may, indeed, stop in its evolution. Faradization is the most efficacious treatment for progressive muscular atrophy.

VI. SECONDARY AND PRIMARY LATERAL SCLEROSIS— SPASMODIC TABES DORSALIS.

Sclerosis of the lateral columns of the spinal cord may be unilateral or symmetrical, primary or secondary, and isolated or associated with other medullary changes.

Sclerosis of the lateral columns is generally only an episode in the course of some cerebral or spinal disease; at other times the whole interest of the question is concentrated in the lateral sclerosis. The following forms are seen:

(*a*) Descending secondary lateral sclerosis.
(*b*) Symmetrical lateral sclerosis; spasmodic tabes dorsalis.

Lateral Columns.—The lateral columns of the spinal cord contain the longitudinal nerve fibres, some long, others short, which cause the anterior grey matter of the spinal cord throughout its entire length to communicate with the brain, and which unite the various segments of this grey matter. The crossed pyramidal tract (described in detail under Cerebral Hæmorrhage) forms the bulk of the lateral columns. It is by means of the fibres of the pyramidal tract, situated in the posterior portion of the lateral columns, that the anterior grey matter of the spinal cord receives from the brain the order for contraction, which it subsequently transmits to the muscles by means of the motor nerves (voluntary movement). It is therefore clear that the destruction of these tracts will be followed by paresis or paralysis of the voluntary muscles. It is also clear that the chronic irritative lesions of these columns (descending or primary sclerosis), by causing abnormal excitability in the anterior grey matter, will give rise to abnormal muscular action, or tonus, which by its intensity or permanence constitutes contracture. In a disease of the cord, transient or permanent contractures, the tendon reflexes and the tremors that so often accompany the contractures are phenomena associated with irritative lesions of the lateral columns. The motor troubles of paralysis and of contracture may exist at the same time, or may follow each other in diverse degrees. If they are often found together, although the paralysis is the result of a destructive lesion and the contracture of an irritative lesion, it is because both kinds of lesion are present in lateral sclerosis.

1. Secondary Descending Lateral Sclerosis.

When the crossed pyramidal tract is diseased at any point in its cerebral or spinal course, the portion of the cord subjacent to the lesion (hæmorrhage, softening, tumour, etc.) may become the seat of a secondary descending sclerosis. The lateral sclerosis thus constituted is situated on the side of the provoking lesion, if the lesion is in the spinal cord, and on the opposite side if the provoking lesion is above the decussation of the pyramids. This secondary sclerosis is generally unilateral. Its form and its extent vary according as its origin is cerebral or spinal, but it reveals itself by constant symptoms, which are : (1) Exaggeration of the tendon reflexes ; (2) contracture. The contracture, which is at first temporary and then permanent, attacks the upper and the lower limb, according to the extension of the spinal lesion. This contracture is frequently accompanied by Babinski's sign and tremors (spontaneous or provoked) of varying intensity.

The lesion in the lateral columns does not, however, always remain limited to the territory first invaded. The irritation sometimes spreads into the anterior cornua of the grey matter, with which these columns are directly related (change in the motor cells), in which case we notice atrophy of certain muscles or groups of muscles. This variety of sclerosis of the lateral columns is secondary and descending ; and if it is sometimes complicated with muscular atrophy, this atrophy is limited, and has no progressive tendency.

2. Symmetrical Lateral Sclerosis—Spasmodic Tabes Dorsalis.

Description. — This sclerosis, which, according to certain writers (Richter), is said to be a double primary sclerosis of the lateral columns, has been described under the name of spasmodic paralysis (Erb) and of spasmodic tabes dorsalis (Charcot). No proof, however, exists that it is a distinct morbid species—a simple primary sclerosis systematically confined to the pyramidal tracts—and it is quite possible that this affection is really a variety of disseminated sclerosis. In some cases, followed by post-mortem examination, the degeneration of the lateral columns was secondary and was caused by foci of myelitis, by cerebral lesions, by lesions of both capsules, or by the meningeal lesions of general paralysis.

According to Little and Marie, the existence of spasmodic tabes may be admitted, but it must be considered as a congenital disease, due to imperfect development of the pyramidal tract throughout its whole length. In four cases of Little's syndrome, Philippe and Cestan found the pyramidal tract absolutely normal, both in the bulb and in the spinal cord. The symptoms commence in infancy. The disease always makes its appearance in the lower limbs, and may be confined to them indefinitely.

Both lower limbs are attacked, either simultaneously or subsequently, by paresis. The loss of power is complicated by exaggeration of the tendon reflexes, muscular spasm, and later by contractures, which are at first transient and then permanent. The legs are placed in the position of extension and adduction. These symptoms are often accompanied by twitchings and spinal epilepsy, which are sometimes spontaneous, sometimes provoked by the patient's movements. It is very rare for these symptoms to invade the upper limbs. Stiffness of the neck, strabismus, and speech troubles may be observed. The disease lasts indefinitely, until some intercurrent affection carries off the patient. This form of sclerosis is not, as a rule, accompanied by muscular atrophy.

Of the affections which may evolve under the outward appearance of spasmodic tabes, some may recover (Raymond).

VII. AMYOTROPHIC LATERAL SCLEROSIS.

Since the date of Charcot's work we designate under the name of **amyotrophic lateral sclerosis** primary and symmetrical sclerosis of the lateral columns, accompanied in the invaded segment of the cord by a change in the cells of the anterior cornua. The symptoms of lateral sclerosis are also associated with the symptoms of invading muscular atrophy.

Pathological Anatomy.—According to Charcot, " the lesion of amyotrophic sclerosis commences at the level of the olivary bodies in the pyramidal tract. The sclerosis spreads along the direct and crossed tracts in such a manner as to cause total atrophy. This anatomical period corresponds to the clinical period of paralysis." The sclerosis does not remain confined to the pyramidal tract. It also attacks the mass of the anterolateral tracts and Goll's columns. Later or simultaneously changes supervene in the grey matter of the spinal cord, and extend through the entire extent of the anterior cornua, causing atrophy of the large ganglion cells.

These spinal lesions are always accompanied at a given moment by bulbar lesions, such as sclerosis of the pyramids, degeneration with pigmentation, or more or less complete disappearance of the cells in the inferior

nucleus of the hypoglossal and of the facial nerves. The nuclei of origin of
the mixed nerves and of the trigeminal nerves are not always exempt from
lesions. The pyramidal tract may show lesions in its course through the
peduncles, the internal capsule, and as far as the motor convolutions, which
in some cases are said to have presented atrophic lesions, with disappearance
of the nerve cells through pigmentary degeneration. The anterior roots of
the nerves are generally atrophied, and the small intramuscular nerves are
often sclerosed, whilst the trunks of the motor nerves are often healthy.
The atrophied muscles show simple atrophy. According to these data,
latent amyotrophic sclerosis might be considered as an affection attacking
primarily the pyramidal tract, and affecting by choice a portion of this tract,
but in some cases attacking the entire tract, and even the motor cells in
various regions of the brain, medulla, and cord. The primary lesion in
the antero-lateral column is not subordinated to the cellular changes.
Cellular atrophy causes simple atrophy of the white bundles, but not
sclerosis. The disease, therefore, is a **primary lesion** of the antero-lateral
tract (Philippe and Guillain).

Symptoms.—In amyotrophic lateral sclerosis paralytic and spasmodic
troubles open the scene, and show themselves in nearly every case in the
upper limbs. The patient experiences paresis in the arms, often preceded by
pains and accompanied by spasmodic phenomena. The muscles preserve
their electrical contractility, but muscular rigidity, exaggeration of the
tendon reflexes, spasms, and contracture are early troubles.

The exaggeration of the tendon reflexes is general; it is observed in the
knee, the heel, the wrist, and the masseter. The muscular contracture
exists more frequently in the condition of stiffness than in the condition of
true contracture.

In the **first period** of the disease—that is to say, a few months after the
commencement of symptoms—the upper limbs show invading muscular
atrophy (lesions of the anterior cornua) and permanent contracture (lesion
of the lateral column). The fingers are bent in the hand. The forearm is
semiflexed on the arm, and the arm is forcibly adducted to the side. These
symptoms are naturally less pronounced in proportion as the muscular
atrophy progresses. The atrophy especially affects the muscles of the
hands and of the forearms.

In the **second period**—that is to say, ten to twelve months after the
commencement of the disease—the lower limbs are involved. Paresis,
exaggeration of the tendon reflexes, contracture, and tremors (lesions of
the lateral columns) are, however, the dominant symptoms, and the muscular
atrophy (lesion of the anterior cornua) is much less pronounced than in the
upper limbs. The lower limbs are extended and rigid, with inward rotation
of the internal edge of the feet.

The paresis, contracture, and atrophy may also attack the muscles of the neck. The positions of the head vary according to the muscles most affected.

Finally, in the **third period**, the bulbar phenomena supervene. The patient looks like a crying child ; the saliva drools from the mouth ; the tongue, which is often atrophied, moves with difficulty ; the velum palati is paralyzed ; the lower jaw loses its movements of diduction ; and we find successively or simultaneously troubles of speech, of mastication, of deglutition, and of respiration (atrophy of the nuclei of the hypoglossal, of the facial, of the motor branch of the trigeminal, and of the pneumogastric nerves). Sometimes the onset is **bulbar,** difficulty in the articulation of words and embarrassment of speech being the first symptoms (Raymond).

The sphincters remain intact. There are no sensory or trophic troubles. When the patient is not carried off by an intercurrent disease, he dies of asphyxia, syncope, or inanition.

The special feature of amyotrophic lateral sclerosis is the rapidity of its evolution. In two or three years, sometimes in one year, it runs its course, ending without exception in bulbar phenomena. What a difference from progressive muscular atrophy and spasmodic tabes, which have a slow invading course, and which may even become stationary without threatening the patient's life for a long time ! Although writers have wished to cast these two affections into a single disease, the distinction must be rigidly maintained (Raymond and Ricklin).

Ætiology—Diagnosis.—Nothing is known as to the causes of this disease. It is almost special to adult age. The absence of all cerebral symptoms, the presence of bulbar symptoms, and the evolution of muscular atrophy distinguish it from insular sclerosis. Spasmodic tabes differs from it in the absence of muscular atrophy and in the initial localization of the disease to the lower limbs. In Duchenne's progressive muscular atrophy the initial stage of paresis and the contractures are absent.

VIII. INSULAR SCLEROSIS.

Pathological Anatomy.—The various forms of myelitis so far described are both systematic (Vulpian) and parenchymatous (Hallopeau) : **systematic** —that is to say, they are limited to a system of fibres or cells (posterior or lateral columns, anterior cornua) ; **parenchymatous**—that is to say, the irritative process seems to commence in the nerve fibre or cell before reaching the neuroglia.

Insular sclerosis, on the contrary, is a diffuse and interstitial chronic myelitis. It is diffuse because it invades, in the shape of islets, the white matter of the nerve centres and the columns of the spinal cord without taking account of the furrows. It is interstitial because the irritative process seems to commence in the vascular element and in the neuroglia. The grey matter is less affected than the white matter. The patches of sclerosis may be superficial or deep, greyish, rosy, of a firm consistency. clearly circumscribed, and rich in vessels. The sclerotic lesion is very pronounced in the centre of the patch, and disappears at the circumference by insensible transitions. The meninges are, as a rule, neither thickened nor adherent.

The nerve tubes are affected in the midst of this proliferating connective tisue. The axis-cylinder remains even in the centre of the patch until a very advanced period (Charcot), which is not customary in scleroses of the tracts. The myelin, however, disintegrates, and the leucocytes, which have passed out of the bloodvessels by diapedesis, become charged with drops of myelin, converted into granular bodies, which infiltrate the lymphatic sheaths. The destruction of the sheaths of myelin, formerly supposed to be due to compression of the nerve fibres by the new connective tissue, appears to result from the nutritive activity of the neuroglial and lymphatic cells.

The neuroglia of the grey matter also undergoes a sclerotic process ; the nerve cells degenerate, become atrophied, and their processes disappear. The bloodvessels show periarteritis and endarteritis, the wall becoming thickened and the lumen constricted. It has, indeed, been asked whether the vascular lesions were not the origin of the patches of sclerosis. The patches are discrete or confluent ; they may be found throughout the whole extent of the nervous centres (spinal cord, bulb, pons, cerebellum, cerebrum and cranial nerves), and their predominance in certain parts explains the spinal, cerebral, and cerebro-spinal forms of this disease. The cerebral variety is the least common, the cerebro-spinal form the most common. The lesions of insular sclerosis are rarely followed by secondary degenerations, doubtless because the axis-cylinders are almost always intact.

Description.—The irregularity and the predominance of the patches in various parts of the nervous system make this form of sclerosis essentially a polymorphous disease. I shall nevertheless base my description on the most common or cerebro-spinal type.

In some cases the disease makes its appearance suddenly by hemiplegia, with or without apoplexy, by vertigo, or by visual troubles. The commencement is generally slow and progressive, the dominant symptom consisting in speech troubles, tremors, particularly of the hands, and increasing difficulty in walking. The last-named trouble is the most common initial symptom. The patient experiences paresis in the lower limbs, which gradually becomes more marked, but which presents, as its characteristic, remissions that may last for several months.

At an earlier or later period the paresis in the lower limbs is complicated by rigidity and contractures, at first temporary and then permanent. The contracture places the legs in the position of extension and of adduction, causing the spasmodic gait. As the rigidity of the leg does not allow flexion of the knee, the patient has to walk forward by alternately raising the pelvis and the trunk on each side, and even then the point of the foot which is not properly raised from the ground causes a dragging to be heard at every step. The tendon reflexes being exaggerated, Babinski's sign may show itself when the patient stands on the soles of his feet. The walk is not only of a spasmodic character, but often assumes a cerebellar type, the patient walking like a drunken man, with legs apart and staggering steps (cere bello-spasmodic gait). The motor troubles, called cerebellar asynergy by Babinski, have been verified by Campbell and Crouzon at Bicêtre in patients with insular sclerosis. In some cases walking is rendered even more difficult by a general tremor, which appears as soon as the patient tries to rise and walk.

The contracture is not so marked in the arms as in the legs, but spas-modic paresis is, however, noticed in them, and makes the movements very awkward. The chief factor, however, in the upper limbs is a tremor which has a special character in insular sclerosis. As long as the patient is at rest, the tremor is not seen ; it is **intentional,** and only produced on the occasion of voluntary movements. If a patient is told to drink a glass of water, he will seize the glass and clutch it tightly. The arm commences to tremble, and makes the glass shake. The amplitude and the rapidity of the oscillations increase as the patient brings the glass to his mouth, the water is spilt in all directions, and the head and body, which have been bent forward to meet the glass, are seized with rhythmic oscillations as the glass reaches the mouth. It knocks against the teeth, the nose, and the chin, and the patient can only take the glass between his teeth by making a fresh attempt with both hands. This intentional tremor may invade every part of the body.

Ocular troubles are frequent and generally well marked ; they are of great importance from the diagnostic point of view. Let me first mention **nystagmus,** which is present in half the number of cases, and which consists in rapid involuntary oscillations of the eyeballs, in the horizontal plane. Besides true nystagmus, due to a bulbar or cerebral lesion, Uhthoff has noticed a false nystagmus, due to paresis of the motor muscles. The paralyses of the oculo-motor muscles are usually incomplete and associated —associated in that they affect in both eyes the muscles entrusted with the function of movement. They are sometimes temporary, and have a preference for the external or internal recti. As in tabes, we notice the inequality of the pupils and myosis. Whilst, however, in tabes, myosis **is** accompanied by Argyll-Robertson's sign, in insular sclerosis the pupil reflexes are preserved. Amblyopia is frequent, but, contrary to that of tabes, it rarely ends in blindness. The ophthalmoscope shows that the external segments of the optic discs are pale; atrophy is rare. Retro-bulbar neuritis may provoke similar functional troubles. The field of vision fairly often shows a central scotoma. The dyschromatopsy may be compared to that of tabes. Red and green are the first colours to disappear.

Embarrassment of speech is almost constant, and closely resembles that of general paralysis, although the words are more scanned, spasmodic, and monotonous than in the latter disease.

Sensory troubles do not form a part of the clinical picture of insular sclerosis (Charcot). Trophic troubles are quite exceptional. Glycosuria has been noticed; it indicates a lesion in the fourth ventricle. For several years these symptoms follow one another, combine, improve, or grow worse, and finally there comes a period characterized by the appearance of loss of flesh, anorexia, frequent diarrhœa, and progressive weakening of the intelligence. The excessive embarrassment reduces the speech to an unintelligible sputtering. Eschars form, the sphincters become paralyzed, and the patient succumbs in cachexia.

Insular sclerosis lasts from two to twenty years. The course of this disease is most irregular. In the first place, it may be cured. In other cases it improves, with long intermissions, or else events are rapidly precipitated. The patient is sometimes carried off by phthisis or pneumonia; sometimes he succumbs with symptoms of glosso-labio-laryngeal paralysis or of general paralysis. Temporary or persistent hemiplegia, accompanied or not by apoplexy and aphasia, may be observed in all stages of insular sclerosis (Blanche, Edwards). Apoplectiform attacks sometimes supervene at the onset or during the course of the disease, and may be followed by death. The important point is that they cause a rise in temperature (Charcot), unlike apoplexy from cerebral hæmorrhage, at the commencement of which the temperature is lowered.

Diagnosis.—In addition to the various forms already described, insular sclerosis sometimes presents a defaced form, in which the ordinary symptoms are absent. In several cases it has simulated the clinical picture of **spasmodic tabes** so closely that certain writers have considered spasmodic tabes to be a variety of insular sclerosis rather than a distinct morbid entity, due to the primary and symmetrical sclerosis of the lateral columns. Insular sclerosis is sometimes complicated by muscular atrophy, and these cases of atrophy, with contractures, so closely resemble **amyotrophic lateral sclerosis** that it has been asked whether the latter disease deserves to be placed as a morbid entity in diseases of the spinal cord. The anatomical lesions, however, justify this distinction.

Insular sclerosis was for a long time confounded with **paralysis agitans,** but in the latter disease, amongst other distinctive signs, the tremor particularly affects the wrists and the fingers, and is continuous, whilst in sclerosis it is intentional. Although the speech is more scanning and less tremulous in insular sclerosis than in **general paralysis,** it must nevertheless be noted that the speech troubles are sometimes identical. But in general paralysis we do not find the same tremors or contractures, and the psychical troubles often appear early.

The mercurial tremor has many analogies with that of insular sclerosis. It has a certain amplitude, and it may be exaggerated by voluntary movements, but in insular sclerosis the tremor is absent as long as the patient is at rest.

In some cases gastric crises, thoracic pains, and troubles of equilibrium recall **locomotor ataxy.** In several instances predominance of the **paralytic** troubles has been noted—partial hemiplegia, with a sudden or slow onset, monoplegia, and paraplegia—so that the diagnosis from cerebral hæmorrhage and softening of cerebral tumours sometimes causes much difficulty. This difficulty is all the greater as the attacks of paralysis (hemiplegia or paraplegia) sometimes supervene from the commencement of the disease. **Hysteria** may simulate insular sclerosis ; it may, indeed, be associated with it.

Ætiology.—The ætiology of insular sclerosis is very obscure. It is chiefly seen in adults, but it is not rare in children. The infectious diseases (variola, scarlatina, typhoid fever, diphtheria, dysentery, and pneumonia) appear to act as a determining cause. As Jaccoud has shown, these diseases are, as a matter of fact, capable of causing the symptoms of insular sclerosis, but we must wait for further cases, followed by post-mortem examination, before we can say that they may produce the disease.

IX. ACUTE MYELITIS IN GENERAL.

Before describing the different varieties of acute myelitis, it will be well to discuss these affections in general terms. As regards localization, we find cases of diffuse myelitis, in which the lesions are scattered, attacking both the grey and the white matter. In some forms of myelitis the lesions confine themselves more to the grey matter, especially to the anterior cornua. They are called " poliomyelitis " ($\pi o \lambda \iota \acute{o}s$, grey). Other forms of myelitis confine themselves to the white matter, and are called " leucomyelitis " ($\lambda \epsilon \upsilon \kappa \acute{o}s$, white).

As regards pathogenesis, myelitis is divided into two great classes—myelitis due to infectious or toxi-infectious agents (and we must mention here all the infections—typhoid fever, influenza, diphtheria, cholera, coli bacillus, streptococcia, staphylococcia, gonorrhœa, syphilis, and tuberculosis), and myelitis due to toxic substances (alcohol, lead, ergot, pellagra, arsenic, etc.). We shall see how these questions in human pathology have been cleared up by experiments.

Myelitis due to Infection.

Experiments.—Myelitis has been produced by Charrin with the *Bacillus pyocyaneus ;* by Roux and Yersin with the diphtheria toxine ; by Grancher, Martin, and Leroux-Rebard with avian tubercle bacilli ; by Gilbert and Lion with human tubercle bacilli ; by Thoinot and Masselin with the *Staphylococcus aureus ;* by Gilbert and Lyon with the *B. coli ;* by Vincent with the *B. typhosus ;* by Roger, Bourges, Widal, and Besançon with the streptococcus ; by Marinesco with the tetanus toxine.

These cases of experimental myelitis may be produced either by injecting into the bloodvessels the microbes themselves or their toxines. When the experiment is made with living cultures, the pathogenic microbes may be found in the spinal lesions. Thoinot and Masselin found the *Bacillus coli* and the staphylococcus. On the other hand, they did not find the streptococcus. The presence or the colonization *in situ* of a microbe is not therefore an essential condition for the determination of the lesions. It has, indeed, been proved that most of the pathogenic microbes act by means of their toxines, as, for example, in the special lesions provoked by the pyocyanic toxine (Charrin), by the diphtheritic toxine (Enriquez and Haillon), and by the streptococcic toxine (Manfredi and Traversa). The pathogenic microbe may have disappeared, and its toxine may still persist. The microbe may have been cultivated in a spot remote from the spinal cord, and its toxine may nevertheless poison the bulbo-spinal axis (diphtheria).

Paralytic troubles occur in experimental animals at indefinite periods ; they may be early or late. The paralysis is sometimes the first manifestation of the infection, the animal appearing to be in no wise affected by the infectious agents with which it has been inoculated. Events usually take this course in the human being. The paralytic troubles may be contemporary with the infectious disease, or may not appear till later, so that the infection having passed unnoticed, the myelitis appears to be an essential or spontaneous disease.

The **medullary troubles** vary greatly in the experimental animals. One animal has flaccid paraplegia ; another one has spasmodic paraplegia, with permanent or paroxysmal contracture. In one animal the paralytic lesions remain confined to the hind-quarters ; in another one they invade all the limbs, becoming general, like Landry's ascending paralysis ; or else they may assume a hemiplegic type. Sometimes the muscles remain normal ; at other times they are atrophied (amyotrophia). These various types do not depend solely on the nature of the infective agent, since in the animals under experiment the streptococcus, for example, may produce the flaccid or spasmodic, paraplegic or general, amyotrophic or non-amyotrophic, varieties of paralysis. The same fact is observed in human pathology. The same provoking agent (typhoid fever, influenza, streptococcia, infection by the

Bacillus coli) may cause various medullary lesions, and consequently diverse symptoms.

In the animals experimented on, the duration and the severity of the troubles are very variable—transient and curable paralysis, rapid and fatal complications, or slow and chronic evolution of the disease. Here again clinical medicine is in agreement with experimental research.

The **medullary lesions** in animals present many forms. Sometimes we find no lesion in the nerve centres, the nerves, or the muscles. This apparent absence of lesions, in spite of severe symptoms, has been noticed by Charrin and Babinski in paralyses caused by infection with the *Bacillus pyocyaneus*, and by Gilbert and Lion in paralyses caused by infection with a bacillus obtained from a case of endocarditis. Similar conditions may exist in the human being, but as a rule the medullary lesions found in animals " are concentrated in an almost exclusive manner in the ganglion cells of the grey matter, and particularly in the large cells of the anterior cornua " (Vaillard). Granular degeneration, changes in the protoplasm and in the nucleus, vacuolar condition of the cell, atrophy of the cell and of its prolongations are seen. The disaggregation of the chromatophile elements is said to be the first change in the nerve cell, the chromatolysis being either peripheral, perinuclear, or diffuse (Marinesco). It is said to be accompanied by lesions of the achromatic substance, which shows molecular disintegration, has a vitreous aspect, and stains readily. The white matter of the spinal cord presents less constant and less characteristic changes. Nevertheless in rabbits infected with the streptococcus the white columns are attacked, the cylinder-axis is changed, and the nerve fibres are atrophied (Widal and Besançon). In rabbits infected with the *Bacillus coli* the white matter is also affected (Thoinot and Masselin).

The neuroglia is almost always free. The bloodvessels show no lesion in their walls, although they are dilated and cause hæmorrhage. These different changes are generally disseminated throughout the entire length of the spinal cord, being more pronounced at the medullary swellings.

These cases of experimental myelitis have the greatest analogy with acute infective myelitis in the human being. The infection and the toxi-infection are the proved or disguised cause of myelitis, whether the myelitis is produced by a specific pathogenic agent or by pathogenic agents acting as a secondary infection. Sometimes the microbe is still present in the medullary lesions, as in the cases of Curschmann and Vaillard, due to the *Bacillus typhosus*, and the cases of Auché and Hobbs, due to streptococcal infection from the spinal cord of smallpox patients. Most frequently, it is true, the pathogenic microbes have not reached the cord, or they may have disappeared, and it is their toxines that have provoked the lesions. In clinical medicine, as in experimental research, the infection may cause acute diffuse

myelitis, with disseminated lesions (white and grey matter), or with localized
lesions (poliomyelitis).   In clinical medicine, as in the animals experimented
on, the infection of the cord may show several forms, with or without amyotrophy, contractures, and sensory troubles.   The symptomatic picture
may be very varied, although the disease is due to the same pathogenic
agent, as in three cases quoted by Mossé of influenzal myelitis and polyneuritis, the disease running a different course, according to the soil in
which the infection developed.

We now have some idea of the ætiology and pathogenesis of certain
obscure forms of myelitis, which were formerly called essential, spontaneous,
or a frigore—not that cold is not an important agent, of which count must
be taken, but it is an agent incapable per se of provoking an infection. Such
must be certain cases of myelitis attributable to the Bacillus coli, and supervening in infections due to this germ (enteritis, diarrhœa, cystitis, pyelitis),
and to streptococcal infections.

Although the known infectious agents have but little tendency to produce
chronic myelitis from the outset, it is none the less true that the acute
infective process may be transformed into a slow process, which finally
becomes chronic.

Myelitis from Intoxication.—The history of myelitis due to toxic
substances is less extensive and less interesting than that of infective
myelitis, but nevertheless it comprises certain developments which are
referred to under the Intoxications (ergotism, pellagra, etc.).

X. INFANTILE POLIOMYELITIS—ATROPHIC SPINAL PARALYSIS OF CHILDHOOD.

Description.—Infantile poliomyelitis (infantile paralysis) occurs chiefly
in children from one to three years of age.   It begins with fever and paralysis, and terminates in a chronic stage with atrophy.   The onset is quite
insidious.   One child is taken ill with severe or slight fever, lasting a few
hours or a few days; another child has convulsions; and yet another has
gastro-intestinal troubles, and the case is thought to be one of simple indisposition, because other symptoms capable of giving a clue to the diagnosis
are absent.   In some cases we find, as initial symptoms, pains in the spine,
the trunk, or the limbs; hyperæsthesia or anæsthesia.   The child complains,
but as it is unable to state precisely the seat and the nature of the pain,
the physician perhaps suspects rheumatism.   Sometimes from the commencement we notice contractures, especially in the muscles which are
paralyzed later.

A few days after this obscure onset—sometimes, indeed, the next day—
paralysis appears.   It does not assume the progressive form, but rapidly

strikes all the parts which are to be attacked. The paralysis rarely affects all four limbs. Sometimes it is limited to a leg or an arm. It most often assumes the form of paraplegia.

The physician who on the previous evening considered the child to be suffering from simple indisposition, rheumatic pains, or a chill, is told next day : " The child is paralyzed, and cannot move his legs. He can scarcely rise up in bed on account of the paralysis in the arms." As a matter of fact, the paralysis is obvious in the legs ; and will soon reach some of the muscles of the arm. The muscles of the trunk and of the neck may be involved, and the child's head wobbles in all directions. In a case that I attended with Joffroy these symptoms were accompanied for several days with fits of suffocation and continuous and paroxysmal dyspnœa, that caused us the greatest anxiety. The bulbar nuclei were doubtless involved. The affection sometimes extends to the nuclei in the medulla and pons, causing double paralysis of the external oculo-motor muscles.

The tendon reflexes are diminished, but the sphincters are intact. Electrical examination from the first gives the following results : Increased reaction to the galvanic current, and reaction of degeneration in the muscles which are to remain paralyzed ; rapid disappearance of galvanic excitability in these same muscles. The persistence of Faradic contractility after a fortnight is a good sign.

The paralytic period is followed by a kind of slow remission. From two to six months after the commencement of the disease the paralysis leaves certain muscles and becomes limited usually to the extensor longus digitorum, the peronei, and the tibialis anticus. It is likewise observed in the triceps femoralis, the serratus magnus, the infraspinatus, the rhomboids, etc. When the paralysis persists in the upper limbs, the deltoid is usually attacked.

The period of atrophy then commences. The atrophy, which may appear from the first month, involves the paralyzed muscles. Trophic troubles also affect the osseous system. Certain bones—the femur or tibia— are arrested in their development, and remain thinner and shorter than those on the healthy side, thus giving rise to a limp. There is no relation between the change in the bones and that in the muscles. The bone may be affected in the segment of a limb without any lesion in the muscular system, and vice versa, just as if the bones and the muscles had different trophic centres. In the paralyzed and atrophied limb, marked coldness (Charcot) and a diminution in the calibre of the bloodvessel have been noticed. These partial atrophies are followed by deformity of the limbs. The overaction of the antagonistic muscles that have remained healthy causes vicious positions, such as club-foot, especially equino-varus, forcing the patient to walk on the outer edge of the foot. When the atrophic lesion is more extensive, the legs become slender and deformed, the unfortunate patients being obliged to drag themselves on their ischia. In the upper limbs we meet with club-hand; and in the trunk, with scoliosis. The arrested development of the bones on one side causes limping. The **prognosis** of this disease is not dangerous as regards the life of the patient, but incurable infirmities are the consequence.

Diagnosis.—The tender age of the patients explains the difficulty of the diagnosis at the commencement of the affection. Several diseases may simulate infantile paralysis. We find **infantile cerebral hemiplegia,** with paralysis and atrophy of both limbs on the same side; but infantile paralysis is flaccid, while contracture is present in the case of cerebral paralysis. Infantile pseudo-paralysis of **syphilitic** origin, like spinal paralysis, may affect one limb or several limbs, but this syphilitic pseudo-paralysis is due to the separation of the diaphysis from the epiphysis (Parrot, Troisier). It is recognized by sharp pains on movement, and by the swelling of the joints, accompanied or not by crepitus.

Obstetrical paralyses, due to the application of the forceps, have a special localization to the deltoid, infraspinatus, biceps, brachialis anticus, supinator longus, and coraco-brachialis. **Hysteria with atrophy** is very rare in very young children. The diagnosis can be made by remembering that the tendon reflexes are normal and the electrical reactions are preserved in hysteria.

Ætiology.—The ætiology of infantile paralysis is most obscure, and the various causes invoked—cold, dentition, etc.—are anything but proved. The disease generally appears in children between the first and the third year. In some cases it has followed infectious conditions (measles, scarlatina, etc.). Everything leads us to believe that infantile poliomyelitis is the result of an infection. It has a febrile onset, accompanied by general symptoms, and it sometimes appears in epidemics (Marie). As a matter of fact, the accounts of several epidemics have been published. In 1885 Cordier saw within a few months thirteen cases of infantile paralysis at Sainte-Foy-l'Argentière, in a population of 1,500 inhabitants. In 1888 Medin noted in six months forty-four cases of infantile paralysis in the same district. In 1890 Leegard reported eight cases of infantile paralysis in a small Norwegian town where the disease had hitherto been unknown. Finally, Pasteur saw infantile paralysis attack seven children of the same family in three weeks.

Pathological Anatomy.—The lesions of infantile paralysis closely resemble those of progressive muscular atrophy, except that the former are acute and the latter chronic. The atrophy of the muscles is most often a simple atrophy, with or without fatty infiltration.

The foci of myelitis are often multiple; they may be 3 or 4 inches in length. The appearance of the focus varies according as the post-mortem examination is made in the acute or in the chronic period. In the acute stage we find inflammatory softening. It is a **systematic anterior myelitis,** which appears limited, or nearly so, to the anterior cornua of the grey matter, although it is not easy to explain why an apparently identical lesion should at one time produce isolated muscular atrophy (progressive muscular atrophy) and at another muscular atrophy preceded by paralysis and accompanied by atrophy of bone (spinal paralysis of childhood).

The lesion of the anterior cornua consists in atrophy of the large motor cells, with proliferation of the connective tissue. The cells are invaded *en bloc,* and are not picked one by one, as in progressive muscular atrophy. The nerve fibres running in the grey matter of the anterior cornua are attacked. The bloodvessels are thickened and dilated. Marie thinks that the arterioles are responsible for the foci of poliomyelitis : " It seems that the central artery of the anterior cornua is most frequently, if not exclusively, affected by the process." In some cases the foci are also found in the bulb or the brain, but then, according to the localization of the lesions, and according to the symptomatic aspect, the affection ends in infantile cerebral hemiplegia, in idiocy, or in epilepsy.

The anterior roots of the nerves are even more affected than in progressive muscular atrophy. When the examination of the spinal cord is made, not at the time of the acute lesions, but many years later, the focus of softening is replaced by corresponding atrophy, which does not stop at the anterior cornua, but also attacks the antero-lateral columns, the posterior columns, and even the posterior cornua. The inflammatory focus of the acute condition is replaced by a fibrillary tissue of a neuroglial nature.

This atrophic paralysis of childhood has the greatest affinity with progressive muscular atrophy, with acute spinal paralysis of adults, and with anterior spinal general paralysis. The proof of the affinity of these various affections of medullary origin is found in that patients who in their infancy have had an attack of atrophic paralysis have later suffered from spinal paralysis, from progressive muscular atrophy, from all three diseases, or from anterior spinal general paralysis. Other analogous cases have been published.

Treatment.—As soon as the period of retrogression begins, if not before, slowly-interrupted currents should be employed ; they form the most rational method of treatment. The treatment must be carried out with care and perseverance. Massage, salt baths, and a cure at Salies should also be employed.

XI. POLIOMYELITIS IN THE ADULT—ACUTE SPINAL PARALYSIS IN THE ADULT.

Acute poliomyelitis in the adult—that is to say, myelitis with a tendency to limit itself in the region of the anterior cornua (πολιός, grey)—does not form as well-marked a morbid entity as infantile poliomyelitis. Some writers question whether many cases of spinal paralysis in adults are nothing but polyneuritis. I am of the opinion that polyneuritis must claim some cases formerly considered to be spinal paralysis. I also think that it is sometimes difficult to classify the spinal paralyses of adults, the disease being often curable, and the post-mortem examination being then lacking; but it is none the less true that the spinal paralyses of adults rest on a group of pathological and clinical facts which assures their autonomy. This autonomy is rightly claimed by Grasset, who quotes in its favour, not only former researches, but the much more recent writings of men like Franz Müller in 1880, of Blocq and of Marinesco, and the publications of Blocq, referring to two incontestable post-mortem examinations made by Schultze and Rissler. Blocq is, furthermore, quite positive in his conclusions. "It is permissible," says he, "after the recent example of Raymond and Marie, according to the teaching of Charcot, and, relying, moreover, on demonstrative cases, to admit the existence of an acute spinal paralysis in adults clinically and anatomically similar to infantile paralysis."

1. Acute Spinal Paralysis of Adults.

A form of paralysis very similar to infantile poliomyelitis may develop in adults. It is called acute spinal paralysis.

Duchenne was the first to describe it. "I have long thought," says he, "that the symptomatology of the atrophic paralysis of childhood would not be met with in the adult, but having sometimes seen this same symptomatology in the adult, I have naturally concluded that the paralysis must be produced by a similar anatomical lesion. This consideration induced me, therefore, to call it acute anterior spinal paralysis of adults, due to atrophy of the anterior cells."

The disease commences with diffuse pains in the limbs, rigidity, muscular contractures, and gastro-intestinal troubles. Rapid and more or less extensive paralysis then appears. After a few days atrophy appears in some of the muscles, and becomes localized in them, whilst the paralysis disappears. The sphincters of the bladder and of the rectum are intact. The tendon reflexes are diminished or abolished. The sensory troubles are more marked than in infantile paralysis; they are due to lesions of the posterior cornua and of the commissures, in addition to the essential lesion in the anterior cornua.

The electrical reactions (loss of faradic reaction) are seen here, as in the child. One single factor distinguishes the disease in the adult from that in the child—viz., in the adult the **deformities** are less frequent and less marked than in the child, because growth has finished when the disease occurs.

The **diagnosis** from Landry's disease (acute ascending paralysis) is the more difficult in that this affection specially involves the anterior cornua ; but acute spinal paralysis has a much slower course, and the atrophy follows closely on the paralysis, confining itself to a few muscles.

2. Anterior Spinal General Paralysis.

Under this name Duchenne has described a distinct morbid entity with the following characteristics : An individual, without appreciable cause, is seized with paralysis, commencing in the lower limbs, and becoming general in all the muscles of the body, except those of the face.   The paralysis is flaccid, without contractures ; the sphincters are normal ; sensation is intact ; the tendon reflexes are abolished, and the application of the faradic current has practically no effect.   The muscular atrophy appears during the course of the paralysis.   It is very marked, and affects all the muscles without distinction, so that the patient is confined to his bed, and incapable of making the slightest movement.   After a few weeks the movements gradually reappear, and the atrophy in turn diminishes.   This disease is usually slow in its course, and Duchenne therefore called it subacute.   The characteristic of this affection is that it terminates by a restoration to health.   The paralysis and the atrophy disappear completely without leaving any trace.

The anatomical lesion is seated in the motor cells throughout the entire length of the spinal cord.   It remains confined to these cells, but this myelopathy is of a special nature, and does not end in irremediable lesions, like the myelopathies of atrophic paralysis of childhood.   Landouzy and Dejerine, in a remarkable monograph, have reported several cases.   I give a summary of two of them :

CASE 1.—A man, fifty-five years of age, was taken ill with paralysis and atrophy affecting all the muscles of the body, except those of the face.   The principal features of this case were : Rapid evolution of the paralysis and of the muscular atrophy ; old deformity of the left leg, due to infantile paralysis ; abolition of the tendon reflexes in all the diseased muscles ; reaction of degeneration ; marked exaggeration of the idiomuscular contractility ; integrity of the general and special sensibility ; integrity of the sphincters ; complete cure of the paralysis and of the muscular atrophy after a duration of ten months.   The patient died of miliary tuberculosis.   At the post-mortem examination the spinal cord showed the following lesions : An old focus of infantile paralysis in the lumbar swelling on the left side ; slight changes, and probably of recent date, in the **anterior grey matter** of the rest of the spinal cord ; integrity of the anterior and posterior roots; integrity of the intramuscular peripheral nerves.

CASE 2.—A woman, thirty years of age, was taken ill with paralysis and atrophy of all the muscles of the body, the disease having commenced with temporary paralysis of the left facial nerve, abolition of the patellar reflex, alteration of the faradic contractility, integrity of sensibility, integrity of the sphincters and of the nutrition of the skin, paralysis and atrophy of rapid evolution, ending in recovery after seven months. No return of the disease four years later.

Discussion—Diagnosis.—We may notice, therefore, in adults spinal paralysis of acute or subacute course, producing muscular paralysis with more or less general atrophy, not causing the death of the patient, recovering completely in some cases, and sometimes leaving indelible stigmata of muscular atrophy. These cases have a tendency to confine themselves to the anterior grey matter of the spinal cord. They are cases of poliomyelitis. Although their infective origin is not clearly proved, we may readily admit it, and the systematization of the spinal lesions is certainly due to the selective action of the toxi-infection for the anterior grey matter (Marie).

The diagnosis between acute spinal paralysis and polyneuritis presents great difficulties. Confusion has often arisen between polyneuritis and acute poliomyelitis. I would even say that in many cases it is almost unavoidable, because the two diseases, polyneuritis and acute poliomyelitis, may differ very slightly. As a general rule, such is not the case. A neurologist will find sufficient to distinguish with a degree of certainty between polyneuritis and anterior poliomyelitis, and I cannot do better than take as my guide the admirable lectures given by my colleague Raymond at La Salpêtrière.

The manner of the onset and of the evolution of the disease presents certain distinct features. In acute anterior poliomyelitis the motor paralysis commences in the root of the limbs. It is far from being symmetrical, and it may confine itself to one limb (monoplegia) or to a single segment. Furthermore, it reaches its maximum in a few days. It then ceases to extend. In the first phase the muscles are simply paralyzed, and not atrophied. In this paralytic phase, however, electrical tests will show which of the paralyzed muscles will later be atrophied. Atrophy will invade those muscles which have lost from the first their faradic excitability. Furthermore, the diminution of the faradic excitability is proportionate to the degree of paralysis.

In polyneuritis the onset is much less sudden ; even the course of events is slower. The paralysis spreads from the periphery towards the centre— that is to say, from the extremities of the limbs to their roots. It shows its maximum of intensity at the extremities (feet, hands). The hands and feet therefore drop. Polyneuritis is ushered in with numbness and tingling in the toes and fingers. It is also announced by painful twitchings of the limbs. In this phase the polyneuritis may extend to the areas supplied by the cranial nerves, giving rise to alarming symptoms—paralysis of the phrenic nerve (fits of suffocation and death from paralysis of the diaphragm), paralysis of the vagus nerve (tachycardia, death from cardiac paralysis). During the second phase of these two diseases the dominant symptom is **muscular atrophy,** which behaves differently according as it depends on anterior poliomyelitis or on polyneuritis.

In acute anterior poliomyelitis the atrophy strikes *en masse* the muscles which have lost their faradic excitability, and respects the neighbouring muscles, whether paralyzed or not. In places where it is severe, it is proportionate to the degree of the paralysis. It is irremediable, and causes a kind of mummification in the atrophied parts. At an advanced period the atrophied segments of the limbs show a livid tint and a lowering of the local temperature.

In polyneuritis the atrophy almost always accompanies the motor paralysis, but it is generally later. It never strikes *en masse* a group of muscles to the exclusion of the neighbouring ones. It always affects a character of diffusion, contrasting with the distribution of the atrophy in poliomyelitis. It invades the muscles which have preserved their faradic excitability at the onset of the first phase. Finally, it is curable, in spite of the paralysis.

Other differential characters require notice. Thus, in poliomyelitis the abolition of the tendon reflexes is constant in the paralyzed and atrophied limbs. Exaggeration of the cutaneous reflexes is never seen. In poly-neuritis the tendon reflexes may be preserved and the cutaneous reflexes may be exaggerated.

In poliomyelitis the sensory troubles play a very minor part. In poly-neuritis, independently of the early paræsthesias, we notice diffuse pains, often of myosalgia. The compression of the nerve trunk and of the muscles is always painful. This last sign is of great diagnostic value. The same may be said of the cutaneous hyperæsthesia, of the anæsthesia, and of the delayed sensation, which are far from being constant. Lowering of the temperature in the paralyzed parts may also be noticed, as well as herpetic, bullous, and eczematous eruptions, alopecia or hypertrophy of the hair, deformity or shedding of the nails, but especially subcutaneous peri-articular œdema, which, being associated with the pains, may lead to a suspicion of articular rheumatism.

In anterior poliomyelitis paralyses of the cranial nerves are quite excep-tional; the absence of psychical troubles is the rule. In polyneuritis paralyses of the cranial nerves are relatively frequent. The same may be said of the intellectual troubles, which in some circumstances assume the triple character of amnesia, intellectual weakness, and delirium (Korsakoff's polyneuritic psychosis).

Finally, acute poliomyelitis is not subject to relapses, but it always leaves irreparable traces. Polyneuritis, essentially a curable affection, is subject to recurrences.

Such are the distinctive characters of acute poliomyelitis and poly-neuritis. I have verified their value and their correctness in a patient with polyneuritis whom I saw with Raymond.

M. X., a cavalry officer, was a powerful man. In his history, as far as morbid conditions were concerned, we only found traumatic arthritis of the right knee, with muscular atrophy of the quadriceps extensor. The arthritis and the atrophy were both cured. During the May manœuvres M. X. was seized with violent rigors, fever, and lassitude. The doctor found an influenzal condition, with high fever (104° F.). Four days afterwards the patient noticed a weakness in his lower limbs; twenty-four hours later the weakness invaded the upper limbs. At the same time the pains in the lumbar region had disappeared. Nothing abnormal in regard to the sphincters.

The febrile condition gradually passed away, the appetite came back, and the patient, though almost completely paralyzed, was brought back to Paris. At our first visit the general condition was good. We found total paralysis of the four limbs, but the patient could abduct the right arm by a snake-like movement. The paralysis was limited to the limbs. At this period the muscular atrophy was scarcely apparent. On the other hand, pressure at the points of exit of the nerves caused pain. No hyper-æsthesia and no anæsthesia of the skin. By extending and raising the legs vigorously, sharp pains were felt along the sciatic nerves. The reaction of degeneration was present in most of the muscles. The reflexes were completely abolished. The functions of the sphincters were normal.

In spite of appropriate treatment, the patient was unable for several months to perform the slightest movement. The muscular atrophy was extremely pronounced. Improvement gradually supervened; less pain, less marked reaction of degeneration. Tonic treatment with strychnine, phosphate of lime, arsenic, etc., was associated with carefully applied electrification and massage. Six months after the commencement of the disease the patient was well on the road to recovery.

The foregoing discussion proves that in many instances we can distinguish between acute poliomyelitis and polyneuritis. Too absolute a division must not, however, be attempted between these different nervous localizations of infectious diseases. While in certain cases the toxi-infection affects the nerves or the spinal cord exclusively, in other cases the process involves the spinal cord and the peripheral nervous system successively or simultaneously. Poliomyelitis is, then, associated with polyneuritis, and their symptoms blend. This association of polyneuritis and poliomyelitis has been noticed by Grasset, Lépine, Mossé and Dastarac, and by Mossé in an interesting study of influenzal paralyses.

XII. ACUTE DIFFUSE MYELITIS.

The forms of myelitis already described, insular sclerosis excepted, tend to limit themselves to a system of fibres or cells (posterior column, anterior cornua), and their respective symptoms (locomotor ataxy, progressive muscular atrophy, atrophic paralysis of infancy, acute spinal paralysis of adults) lend themselves to clinical types that are almost constant. This is not the case in diffuse myelitis, which strikes indifferently the various parts of a medullary segment, grey matter or white columns, while the meninges are always involved. It invades the spinal cord in its various regions, and consequently offers a very variable symptomatology.

Pathological Anatomy.—Diffuse and interstitial acute myelitis forms **foci** of variable dimensions (focal myelitis). It sometimes extends to an entire region of the spinal cord. When it is superficial, the meninges are always invaded. In some cases it is limited to the grey matter of the spinal cord (central myelitis). Post mortem we find changes varying according to the age and the acuteness of the morbid process. The spinal cord is generally softened. In some cases it is fluctuating and converted into a pulp of varying consistency and colour. It often happens that the lesion is much less advanced, and even so little apparent that it can only be recognized by histological examination.

In the first period the myelitis is characterized by congestion, swelling of the invaded portion, and sero-fibrinous exudate into the connective tissue. The vessels are dilated and filled with blood; the lymphatics are blocked with red corpuscles and with leucocytes that have emerged by diapedesis. The axis-cylinder is very much swollen; the nerve cell is enlarged, and the connective tissue is undergoing proliferation.

In the second period we meet with abundant embryonic cells formed by the neuroglia, and on the second or third day the inflamed part becomes softened. This softening is at first red, becoming yellow or white from alteration of the colouring matter of the blood, and from the addition of new elements. Granulo-fatty bodies are formed in this focus of softening. These granulo-fatty bodies, with which the leucocytes become charged, are in part derived from the myeline of the nerve fibres. Hæmorrhages are not uncommon in these foci of softening; they are secondary hæmorrhages, primary hæmorrhages of the spinal cord being quite exceptional.

In the third period we find yellow or white softening, and the various terminations of the anatomical process—the passage of the myelitis into the chronic state, cicatrization of the focus, or progressive extension of the lesion.

Symptoms.—Acute myelitis is characterized by motor, sensory, and trophic troubles of varying degree. Let us take as our type myelitis of the dorso-lumbar region. Rigors and fever open the scene. The patient complains of pain, formication, and cramps in the legs. Girdle pains are marked, and exploration of the spine with the hand or with a sponge soaked in hot water often causes pain in the dorso-lumbar region. Weakness of the lower limbs, accompanied or not by contractures, immediately appears, and increases to such a degree that walking soon becomes impossible (paraplegia). In some cases the loss of movement in the lower limbs is absolute. The reflex movements are increased in the initial period, and disappear later; the electrical reactions undergo the same changes as the reflex movements. Sensation is affected or lost in the parts below the lesion.

Incontinence of urine (paralysis of the vesical sphincter) is generally preceded by retention (paralysis of the detrusor). The urine rapidly becomes ammoniacal, blood-stained, and purulent. Retention and incontinence of the fæces are also observed.

The trophic and vasomotor troubles are numerous, and early eschars appear on the scrotum, over the malleoli, and the sacral region. The sacral eschar (decubitus acutus) quickly increases in depth and extent. To the same period belong œdema, transient rise in temperature, and later considerable fall of the temperature in the legs. Copious sweatings of the upper limbs have also been noted (Mannkoff).

Dorso-lumbar myelitis may kill in a few days (apoplectiform myelitis). Death often supervenes in the second to the fourth week. When the issue is to be fatal, respiratory troubles make their appearance, and, the patient, plunged in marasmus and coma, is generally carried off by asphyxia. Acute myelitis is rarely cured. I have, however, seen one case of a complete cure in a patient with acute non-syphilitic myelitis. It sometimes passes into the chronic condition.

Varieties.—Acute myelitis of the dorso-lumbar region is the most common variety, but myelitis may affect other parts of the spinal cord. When it involves the brachio-spinal region, from the fifth cervical to the sixth dorsal vertebra, the upper limbs show motor and sensory troubles analogous to those of the lower limbs, and the patient often experiences gastric pain and vomiting, which resemble the gastric crises of ataxy. The pupils are sometimes dilated and the eyeballs are prominent, but these symptoms of excitation are transient, and constriction of the pupil follows the dilatation.

Myelitis of the cervical region shows itself by special symptoms—pains in the nuchal region, contractures of the muscles of the neck, trismus, paralysis of the four limbs or of the arms alone,* pain and œdema in the upper limbs, dysphagia, slowing or quickening of the pulse, syncope and apoplectiform troubles, hiccough, dyspnœa, and attacks of suffocation.

Optic neuritis is seen in acute myelitis. It is usually bilateral, and it precedes or accompanies the onset of the myelitis. It may affect the retro-bulbar type—that is to say, it gives rise to a central scotoma, with slight or no ophthalmoscopic signs. Recovery is possible.

Acute myelitis does not always remain confined to the region primarily invaded. It may commence in the dorso-lumbar region, and spread up to the cervical region. Acute ascending paralysis (Landry) is probably an ascending myelitis. I say probably, for side by side with cases in which the lesions are indisputable there are others in which the histological examination has not shown anything (Vulpian). Some cases are simply polyneuritis. Widal and Le Sourd have described a case of acute ascending

* In order to explain the paralysis of the upper limbs before that of the lower ones Brown-Séquard points out that the motor tracts of the upper limbs are more superficial than the motor tracts of the lower ones. But why not admit, says Hallopeau, that the lesion first destroys the grey nuclei of the upper limbs, prior to attacking the lateral columns, which contain the motor tracts of the lower limbs ?

paralysis, characterized from the histological point of view by an inflammation exclusively limited to the anterior roots, without meningeal changes and without lymphocytosis of the cerebro-spinal fluid. Landry's disease may be very rapid or slow. It is apyretic, and presents, as it were, superposed from the lumbar to the cervical region, the symptoms just described under the various forms of myelitis.

Ætiology—Duration.—Acute myelitis is primary or secondary. Cold is a very rare cause of myelitis. Secondary myelitis is at times due to the spread of a neighbouring lesion, such as Pott's disease. It may also super·vene in chronic myelitis. Sometimes it is consecutive to an irritation of the peripheral nerves (ascending neuritis). This morbid process has been produced experimentally (Hayem), but clinically we do not always meet with the lesion intermediate between myelitis and the supposed provoking organ. In the majority of cases acute myelitis is due to toxi-infectious agents, and belongs, therefore, to the class of infectious diseases. This ætiological and pathogenic question was fully discussed in Section IX.

The **course** and **duration** of acute myelitis are not subject to any fixed rule. Apoplectiform myelitis is fatal in four or five days, and the suddenness of the events is due to various causes. Thus at the post-mortem examination we find a hæmorrhagic focus or an inflammatory lesion which from the outset involves a large part of the spinal cord. Sometimes, on the contrary, we find lesions that have followed an ascending course, and are not well marked, as if they had not had time to evolve. In some cases the myelitis is of the recurrent type ; in others it runs a subacute or chronic course ; and in a few exceptional cases recovery may occur.

Epidemic Paraplegia.—About twenty years ago a form of epidemic paraplegia was described in Spain. It was, up to a certain point, comparable with epidemic cerebro-spinal meningitis. This acute or chronic disease was characterized by incomplete paraplegia, with much pain, incontinence of urine, and conservation of the electro-muscular contractility. Similar cases have been met with in France.

XIII. CHRONIC DIFFUSE MYELITIS.

Pathological Anatomy.—The history of chronic diffuse myelitis in part blends with that of acute diffuse myelitis. The pathological anatomy of the lesion is summed up in two words—sclerosis or softening. The softening is most often the last stage of an acute myelitis, and the sclerosis realizes the most common change in chronic myelitis. Proliferation of the neuroglia leads to progressive sclerosis. The connective network and the wall of the vessels become thickened, the nerve fibres diminish in size, the myeline becomes segmented and separates out, the nerve cells lose their

processes and become atrophied. The spinal cord becomes indurated,
assumes a greyish tint, and stains readily with carmine.

This sclerosis (induration of the connective tissue, and consequent
atrophy of the nerve elements) is not always irregularly diffused. It sometimes occupies a well-defined segment of the spinal cord, affecting either
the whole (transverse myelitis) or only one-half of the spinal cord (hemilateral myelitis—Brown-Séquard). It takes the form of a ring, the meninges
being affected while the grey matter is free (annular sclerosis—Vulpian).
It surrounds the ependymal canal, which becomes constricted or dilated
(periependymal sclerosis—Hallopeau), and invades various regions in
succession (ascending or descending myelitis—Hallopeau); but all these
varieties are exceptions, and in the most common form the inflammation
predominates in the antero-lateral parts of the cord on a level with the
dorso-lumbar enlargement, and gives rise to chronic paraplegia. Chronic
myelitis often provokes secondary ascending or descending scleroses, which
at length complicate the initial picture of the disease. The causes are
those of acute myelitis, to which heredity may be added.

Description.—Aside from cases in which the symptoms of excitation
(acute phase) open the scene, the disease commences with disturbance of
locomotion.

The patient soon becomes fatigued, the legs feel heavy, walking is
painful, and especially difficult when plantar anæsthesia is also present
(walking on down). Later the patient can only walk with a stick or other
support. His feet hardly leave the ground; he glides rather than walks,
and in the end locomotion becomes impossible and the paraplegia complete.
The reflex movements, which were at first increased, persist as long as the
grey matter of the spinal cord is not destroyed.

The reproductive functions are generally abolished. Troubles of the
bladder and of the rectum (retention and incontinence) are not early, unless
the genito-crural enlargement is invaded. Retention of urine precedes
incontinence, because paralysis of the detrusor precedes paralysis of the
sphincter; but " the function of the sphincters sometimes remains intact,
in spite of the existence of cervico-dorsal lesions, provided they are superficial, whence it may be inferred that the cerebro-vesical cord occupies in
the anterior system of the spinal cord a deeper position than the cords of
the lower limbs " (Rollet).

In conclusion, paraplegia, accompanied by paralysis of the sphincters,
forms the common picture of chronic dorso-lumbar myelitis; but it is not
uncommon for this picture to be modified by the appearance or by the
predominance of some new symptom, such as pain (lesion of the posterior
cords), anæsthesia (lesions of the grey and posterior white matter), contractures (primary or descending lesions of the lateral cords), muscular

atrophy (lesions of the anterior cornua). The average duration of chronic myelitis is six years. Death is due either to the extension of the paralysis or to complications, such as cystitis, phthisis, or pneumonia.

Varieties.—I have already indicated, under Acute Myelitis, the diversity of the symptoms, according as the lesion is in the lumbar, dorsal, or cervical regions. I shall now describe certain rare varieties in which the myelitis is hemilateral, central, or cortical.

1. **Hemilateral Myelitis.**—When one-half of the cord is affected by traumatism, compression, tumour, or sclerosis, we see certain special symptoms, well described by Brown-Séquard. The salient features are as follows : (1) paralysis on the side of the body corresponding to the lesion in the spinal cord (hemiparaplegia) ; (2) anæsthesia of the side of the body opposite to the lesion (crossed hemianæsthesia). The dissociation of these two symptoms, one of which is direct and the other crossed, is due to the fact (Brown-Séquard) that the motor fibres have already crossed in the bulb. The higher the lesion is in the spinal cord, the more extensive are these symptoms.

2. **Central Myelitis.**—In this variety of periependymal myelitis the grey matter is especially attacked in front of the central canal of the spinal cord. The symptoms consist in paralysis, followed by muscular atrophy and diminution of the electrical contractility. This variety of myelitis closely resembles syringomyelia.

Blisters, cauterization, and the use of electricity sum up the treatment of chronic myelitis. Iodide of potassium, in large doses, and mercurial preparations must always be tried when syphilis is proved or suspected.

XIV. SYPHILITIC MYELITIS.

Ætiology.—Syphilis of the spinal cord independent of any other lesion in the nerve centres is not very frequent. In 1,085 cases of syphilitic lesions of the nerve centres, we find 416 cases of cerebro-spinal syphilis, and only 77 cases of pure medullary syphilis (Fournier, Boulloche). The time of the syphilitic infection is of great importance. The spinal cord may be attacked from the commencement of the disease. In fifty-eight cases of early medullary syphilis (Moinet), myelitis was rare before the third month, fairly common from the third to the tenth month, and frequent in the sixth month. In two-thirds of the cases (Fournier) myelitis is seen from the third to the tenth year of the syphilitic infection. It is very rare in women, but frequent in men between twenty and forty years of age. As contributory causes, alcoholism, venereal excesses, traumatism, and overwork may be mentioned.

Does syphilis, if not treated, predispose to myelitis ? Fournier's answer is affirmative ; Mauriac's answer is negative. Severe syphilis is often accompanied by acute and early myelitis.

Pathological Anatomy.—The lesions differ in acute and in chronic syphilitic myelitis. Acute syphilitic myelitis presents the same lesions as ordinary acute myelitis. In the spinal cord we find one or more foci of softening, usually in the middle regions of the spinal cord. The lesions are diffuse, attacking the white and the grey matter. The meninges frequently participate in the process which realizes the diffuse embryonic meningo-myelitis of Gilbert and Lyon. In these cases of acute myelitis with a sudden onset the vascular lesions predominate, phlebitis and arteritis representing the initial element of the inflammatory process. There is a true syphilitic arteritis, analogous to cerebral arteritis, followed by vascular obliteration, with softening of a more or less extensive area of the spinal cord.

When medullary syphilis is subacute or chronic, we also find lesions of meningitis, embryonic infiltration of the meninges and of their prolongations, gummata, hyperæmia, and dilatation of the bloodvessels. The degenerated parenchyma sometimes becomes sclerotic, and the disease incurable. Myelitis is sometimes accompanied by cerebral changes, especially meningitis of the base of the interpeduncular region and of the chiasma. Medullary syphilis in some cases affects the entire length of the spinal cord. Most often, however, it is limited to the dorso-lumbar region.

Symptoms.—Syphilitic myelitis shows so many clinical types that its description must be separated into the acute and chronic forms and a rare form.

Acute Myelitis.—The acute form of medullary syphilis is almost always an early trouble. This form usually commences very suddenly.

In one patient, twenty-seven years of age, the myelitis announced itself nine months after the chancre by formication in both legs, with unusual weakness. Next day the patient could not even stand. He also had complete retention of urine, abolition of the patellar reflexes, total anæsthesia of the lower limbs, and slight pain in the lumbar region. These symptoms had appeared within thirty-six hours with the suddenness which seems to be the principal characteristic of this acute and early form. Ten days later incontinence of urine followed the retention, and at the end of a fortnight incontinence of fæces appeared. The patient was submitted to a very active treatment (inunction of 90 grains of mercurial ointment and 240 grains of iodide a day). Three weeks later movement reappeared in the legs. In ten weeks the patient left the hospital cured, never having had either trophic troubles or contractures.

The termination of acute syphilitic myelitis is far from being always as favourable as in the preceding case. With Hammonic, I attended a man of fifty-five who was taken ill, a year after the chancre, with such rapid syphilitic myelitis that death supervened in six weeks.

In its acute and early form syphilitic myelitis presents the clinical picture of transverse meningo-myelitis: onset with sensory troubles, formication, numbness of the lower limbs, and girdle pains, followed by motor troubles, weakness of the legs, paresis, paraplegia with or without contractures, retention and incontinence of urine and of fæces, trophic troubles, bed-sores, and general symptoms.

Chronic Myelitis.—This form may be chronic from the outset or may follow on acute or subacute myelitis. In the form which is chronic from the first the onset is very different from that of subacute myelitis. It is much slower, and the functional impotence comes on gradually.

In one of my patients, twenty-two years of age, the myelitis declared itself three years after the chancre with incontinence of urine, formication in one leg, and muscular spasms when the foot touched the ground. In a short while the legs grew stiff and painful, and in three months' time walking was impossible. Contracture was accompanied by exaggeration of the patellar reflexes and by the phenomenon of spinal tremor. Sensibility was intact. After active treatment (inunction of 90 grains of mercurial ointment and 240 grains of iodide a day) the improvement was progressive. A sacral bed-sore which had appeared a few days after the patient's admission, and which had led me to fear a fatal termination, healed rapidly. The pains disappeared. Walking was possible after three weeks, but the leg remained somewhat stiff, as the contracture had not completely ceased.

I have just described the common symptoms of syphilitic myelitis, but in some forms, which are very **much rarer,** medullary syphilis resembles sclerosis of the antero-lateral cords, progressive muscular atrophy, insular sclerosis, or Brown-Séquard's paralysis (paralysis of one limb and anæsthesia of the other).

Under the name of **syphilitic spinal paralysis** Erb has described a variety of chronic medullary syphilis, characterized by incomplete spastic paraplegia of progressive course. The disease commences with pains in the legs, weakness, and muscular rigidity. It takes months and years to end in spastic paresis of the lower limbs, and hardly ever goes on to complete paraplegia. The patients continue to walk, but they have a spastic gait, with exaggeration of the tendon reflexes and ankle-clonus. The sensory troubles consist in numbness, formication, and anæsthesia. The bladder troubles consist in retention or incontinence of urine, with urgent desire to urinate. The genital functions are weakened.

Trophic troubles are absent; no amyotrophy and no bed-sores. This form may remain stationary for an indefinite period. Specific treatment, if early applied, may lead to good results. In spite of its relatively benign appearance, this variety of chronic myelitis may be complicated by multiple lesions of the spinal cord or of the brain, which render the prognosis more serious. This form of syphilitic spinal paralysis is frequent. It does not, as a rule, appear at as early a period as acute syphilitic myelitis; it supervenes nevertheless in the first few years of the syphilitic infection. The absence of post-mortem examinations has prevented our tracing its pathological anatomy. It is certainly a transverse myelitis of the dorso-lumbar region.

Early or late syphilitic myelitis is often accompanied by syphilitic manifestations in other regions (cerebro-spinal syphilis and bulbo-spinal syphilis).

I saw with Fournier* a remarkable case of syphilitic myelitis simulating acute tabes. A man who had been syphilitic for about ten years was taken ill with heaviness in the legs, difficulty in walking, and the following symptoms : ptosis of the left eye, patches of anæsthesia on the buttock, diminution of the patellar reflexes, paresis of the bladder, impotence, and Romberg's sign. All these symptoms disappeared in two months and a half, through active specific treatment.

Diagnosis.—The diagnosis must be promptly made in order that treatment can be commenced at once. If a man is suddenly seized with paraplegia, contracture of the lower limbs, and incontinence or retention of urine, we must think of syphilis. Careful examination will at times enable us to recognize characteristic cicatrices, specific eruption, cutaneous gummata, enlarged glands, violent headache, etc. We can then have no doubt as to the syphilitic nature of the affection. This is the true manner of making a diagnosis, because to differentiate in any other manner between syphilitic myelitis and the diseases most resembling it (insular sclerosis, tabes, and transverse myelitis) is often a very difficult matter.

Cyto-diagnosis of the cerebro-spinal fluid gives interesting results in syphilitic meningo-myelitis. It is clearly positive with pronounced lymphocytosis (Sicard and Monod), whereas it is often negative in Pott's disease with chronic pachymeningitis (Widal and Le Sourd).

The **prognosis** of untreated syphilitic myelitis is grave. In the acute form death has been noticed eighteen times in fifty-eight cases in consequence of the myelitis. In seven cases there was slight improvement, in seventeen cases marked improvement, and only sixteen cases of cure. In the chronic forms death is not so common, but recoveries are rare, because the treatment is often delayed. Too often the syphilis passes unnoticed, and the most energetic medication cannot then remove the lesions of sclerosis.

Hereditary Spinal Syphilis.—Hereditary syphilis of the spinal cord had until recently been little studied. This lacuna has been filled by Gilles de la Tourette, whose conclusions I quote verbatim.

Hereditary syphilis may attack the spinal cord during the first years of life (heredo-syphilis), during intra-uterine life (early congenital heredo-syphilis), during adolescence and adult age (late heredo-syphilis).

When syphilis attacks the infant before birth, the accouchement is often premature. The child may be stillborn or alive. If the child is stillborn,

* Dieulafoy and Fournier, " Accidents Syphilitiques Cérébro-spinaux de Forme Tabétique " (Société de Dermatologie, 1890).

or if it rapidly succumbs, we cannot with certainty attribute death to the spinal lesion, because we find in almost every case fatal lesions in the viscera. The clinical signs are then completely absent. In such a case the lesions of the spinal cord consist in a diffuse embryonic meningo-myelitis, analogous to the interstitial hepatitis of congenital syphilis. Congestion with leuco-cytic stasis is never absent, and may attain an extreme degree, leading even to rupture of the vessels (Gasne).

If the child survives the congenital lesions, symptoms appear, but they blend in part with the symptoms of cerebral sclerosis. Anatomically, the lesions end in sclerosis. The symptoms reveal themselves, as far as the spinal cord is concerned, by spasmodic paralysis. When hereditary syphilis attacks the spinal cord in childhood or in youth, the brain may also partici-pate in the process (cerebro-spinal syphilis), but the spinal lesion is especially associated with lesions of the mesencephalon. In these cases of early or late hereditary syphilis the clinical types are more varied than in congenital spinal syphilis. In fact, as the patient advances in years, the tissues be-come more and more differentiated, and take on a more marked functional individuality. The spinal cord, the meninges, and the vessels seem to be more individually affected. The embryonic infiltration collects more readily, in order to end in perivascular or meningeal gumma. The clinical field becomes enlarged, and, leaving the general tendency to become cerebro-spinal on one side, early or late hereditary syphilis does not sensibly differ from the numerous expressions of acquired spinal or cerebro-spinal syphilis. At times it causes brachial monoplegias, with flaccid paralysis and consequent muscular atrophy of an amyotrophic form (Raymond).

Treatment.—Medullary syphilis demands very active treatment. For a fortnight or three weeks I give daily mercurial injection of 90 grains of Neapolitan ointment, or, better still, injections of biniodide of mercury. Large doses of iodide of potassium are also given. By these active measures I have cured three patients, and owing to the precautions taken (incessant cleansing of the mouth and of the teeth with chlorate of potash, and the same drug taken internally), I have never seen any complication arise. The utility of this energetic treatment is, in my opinion, proved, for two of my three patients had been taking mercury and iodide of potassium for months, but in too small doses.

XV. AFFECTIONS OF THE CAUDA EQUINA AND OF THE FILUM TERMINALE.

The spinal cord terminates below the lumbar enlargement in a conical extremity, the filum terminale, which is threadlike, and descends as far as the coccyx. From the lumbar enlargement the lumbar and sacral nerves arise, and follow a long course in the spinal canal before traversing the conjugate foramina. These nerves, disposed like a fan (the lumbar nerves being external to the sacral nerves), form the cauda equina, surrounding the filum terminale. The lesions of these regions, studied in France by Raymond and by Dufour, give rise to very curious symptoms.

Pathological Physiology.—If the exit of the third pair of sacral nerves is considered as the upper limit of the cauda equina (Raymond), the lesions of this region provoke the following symptoms: Paralysis of the bladder, with integrity of the involuntary sphincter; syndrome of paradoxical ischuria, comprising retention of urine, followed by incontinence through overflowing; paralysis of the anal sphincter; anæsthesia of the urethra, of the perineum, of the anus, of the inner surfaces of the buttocks, and of the postero-superior region of the thigh; hypoæsthesia of the penis and of the scrotum, or of the labia majora; incomplete paralysis of the gluteus maximus, of the plantar muscles, and of the posterior surface of the leg; power of erection, but diminution of voluptuous sensation from anæsthesia of the urethra; slowness of ejaculation.

If the lesion is higher in the lumbar swelling or in the roots of the cauda equina, we find total suppression of erection, complete paralysis of the sphincter of the bladder, with incontinence, and paralysis of the gluteus medius and minimus (Dufour). If the lesion is seated in the lowest portion, or filum terminale, there is paralysis of the bladder and of the rectum, or of only one of these viscera (Lachmann).

Ætiology.—Trauma is the most frequent cause of these affections. Direct injury (crushing or gunshot wounds of the lumbar region) and indirect trauma (falls on the feet, buttocks, chest or hips, fracture and luxation of the lumbo-sacral column) are often present. I must likewise mention hydatid cysts either extra- or intraspinal, tumours (epithelioma, sarcoma, neuroma, or gummata), and syphilitic or tubercular spinal meningitis. Injuries are especially met with in men, and hydatid cysts in women.

Pathological Anatomy.—The lesions are due to the medullary hæmorrhage and to the compression. The cauda equina is flattened. The white columns and the grey axis may disappear completely. Histologically, we find atrophy of the cells of the grey cornua, presence of granular bodies, disappearance of the myeline of the nerve fibres, perivascularitis, with thickening of the sheaths and of the bloodvessels. The roots present identical lesions. Above and below the point attacked Wallerian degeneration takes place, with all its consequences.

Symptoms.—Sensation is always affected. Pains are never absent. They usually involve the lumbar or sacro-coccygeal region, and radiate into the lower limbs, the groins, the buttocks, the knees, and the ankles, often corresponding with the distribution of the sciatic nerve. The pains may be spontaneous or provoked by percussion of the sacro-lumbar region, walking, and flexion of the leg. The sacrum, the coccyx, the legs, and the feet, often present zones of hyperæsthesia. Anæsthesia is the rule; it varies from the slightest hypoæsthesia to complete loss of sensation. Its distribution admits of four categories, which are important in diagnosis (Dufour):

(1) Anæsthesia of the ano-rectal and vesico-urethral mucosæ; anæsthesia of the perineum, of the scrotum, of the penis, of the inferior and internal half of the buttocks, and of the posterior part of the thighs (the anæsthesia affects a triangular form, with the apex pointing downwards). (2) Anæsthesia of the skin supplied by the sciatic nerve, with or without participation of the perineo-scrotal and visceral branches. The persistence of sensation on the internal edge of the foot and at the root of the big toe is of much diagnostic value. (3) Anæsthesia of the anterior and internal regions of the thigh and of the leg. (4) Anæsthesia of the entire lower limb, of the bladder, and of the rectum. The testicles are always sensitive to pressure.

Paralysis with muscular atrophy attacks the region of the buttocks, the posterior muscles of the thigh, the muscles of the legs, and the muscles of the perineum; in rare cases the quadriceps and the adductors of the thigh. I have already referred to the importance of the muscles attacked as regards the localization of the lesions. The paralysis is always flaccid; it explains the disturbance of equilibrium, of walking, and of movements. The reflexes are diminished or abolished.

Of all the trophic troubles, the most frequent are bed-sores on the buttocks, sacrum, and trochanters. The syndrome of paradoxical ischuria (retention of urine with incontinence) and obstinate constipation, with or without involuntary passage of fæces, make up the vesical and rectal troubles. The **genital functions** are abolished; most frequently desire and sensation are weakened. The erections continue, but ejaculation does not occur, the ejection of the semen being hindered by the paralysis of the muscles of the perineum.

The onset and the course of the disease depend essentially on the cause. In the case of traumatism, pains and paralysis are sudden; improvement and cure are possible. The only complications arise from the infection of the bladder and from the bed-sores. In the case of tumour the course is progressive, and whether the tumour is malignant or benign, it causes death in the absence of surgical intervention.

Diagnosis.—Toxic neuritis (lead, alcohol, oxide of carbon, etc.) is distinguished from affections of the cauda equina and of the filum terminale by the predominance of the paralysis in the antero-external muscles of the leg, and by its symptoms. Double sciatica may lead to confusion, but

careful examination of the patient, analysis for glycosuria, the presence of
a neoplasm in the pelvis, or of a prostato-pelvic carcinoma (Guyon), will
clear up the diagnosis. The same remark applies to dorso-lumbar rheumatic arthritis, muscular lumbago, amyotrophia (Charcot-Marie's type),
and all the spinal affections that have some analogy with those of the cauda
equina. The position of the lesion as regards height has been discussed
under the Pathological Physiology.

Treatment.—The pains must be relieved by analgesics, such as antipyrin and pyramidon. If syphilis is suspected, immediate recourse must be
had to injections of biniodide of mercury. In the case of tumours and of
traumatism, surgical intervention is indicated. Several cases of success
fully justify it (Thorburn, Renn, Schaw, and Busch).

XVI. HÆMATOMYELIA.

Ollivier of Angers in 1827 applied the term **hæmatomyelia** to hæmorrhage into the spinal cord.

Ætiology.—According as the hæmorrhagic rupture occurs in healthy
or diseased tissue, the hæmatomyelia is primary or secondary. Secondary
hæmatomyelia is met with in acute myelitis, in meningo-myelitis consequent
on Pott's disease (Raymond), in abscesses of the spinal cord, and in softening
by thrombosis or embolism. We may also note the share of syphilis
(Siemerling), of syringomyelia, of gliomata, of myxomata, and of sarcomata.

Primary hæmatomyelia may follow on fracture, dislocation, or violent
movements of the vertebral column, exaggerated flexion of the head backwards (Thorburn), and elongation of the spinal cord by the application of
the forceps. Concussion is an undoubted cause of slight hæmatomyelia.
In the genesis of so-called spontaneous hæmatomyelia we always meet with
strain, fits of whooping-cough, poisoning by tetanus or strychnine, stoppage
of the menstrual flow, cold (Hochhaus), and the vascular changes of syphilis
and alcoholism.

I must mention as a more singular and interesting cause sudden decompression in divers. The caissons used for sinking piles are certainly the most
dangerous of these apparatus. The accidents always happen at the moment
of decompression, when the divers are about to leave the water. " They
only pay on leaving " (Pol and Watelle). In sudden decompression the
spinal lesions are due to the liberation of the nitrogen which under pressure
has accumulated in excess in the blood, and which is then set free (Bert).
Decompression is harmless if care is taken to make it last several minutes
for each atmosphere. Several causes generally unite to produce hæmatomyelia, and it seems that the vascular system of the spinal cord must have
a " relative fragility " (J. Lépine).

Pathogenesis.—J. Lépine has caused experimental hæmatomyelia by various means. Injection of blood into the posterior columns in the neighbourhood of the centre of the spinal cord spreads the hæmorrhage upwards in the grey matter and the central canal. The nerve tissue becomes partially softened. Punctures of the spinal cord are accompanied by myelitis, with vascular dilatations and capillary extravasations in the grey matter. Spinal concussion is followed by intense congestion of the injured region, leading to hæmorrhage. Later it may provoke myelitis. It is a curious fact that animals can be accustomed to spinal concussion (J. Lépine). By placing rabbits and guinea-pigs in a large autoclave, under a pressure of ten atmospheres, and decompressing them in a few seconds, J. Lépine found in the spinal cords gaseous emboli, hæmorrhagic infarcts, and primary hæmorrhages due to rupture of the vessels. The vascular distension is due to the liberation of the gases of the blood *in situ*, and to the great afflux of the blood in the abdomen, driven out by the gaseous distension of the intestines.

Pathological Anatomy.—The grey matter is the seat of election for medullary hæmorrhages, because it is much more vascular than the white matter. The capillaries of the branches of the anterior spinal artery supply the anterior cornu, Clarke's column, and the most anterior portion of the posterior cornu. The remainder of this cornu is supplied by capillaries coming from the posterior radicular arteries, which send prolongations forward as far as Clarke's column. This column also receives the branches of the artery in the posterior sulcus. I have considered it right to dwell on this intensive vascularization, as it is in part responsible for the localization of the hæmorrhage. I must also mention the existence of septa which limit the effusions of blood to exact regions of the grey matter (Goldscheider and Flatan).

The medullary hæmorrhages are capillary or focal. The former are punctiform, of the size of a pin's head, and close to the vessels of the grey matter. The latter are composed of a clot broken up into several secondary clots, separated by more or less torn nerve-tissue. The grey matter is destroyed in Clarke's column, in the posterior grey commissure, and in part of the posterior cornu ; the anterior cornua may be immune. The central hæmorrhages are elongated, and known as tubular hæmatomyelitis (Levier). When the lesions have time to evolve, softening follows the hæmorrhage, which is eliminated, causing a lacunar condition, and sometimes ascending degenerations. At a more advanced stage hæmatomyelia may give rise to syringomyelia, according to Minor, Raymond, and Brissaud. Certain forms of hæmatomyelia produce symptoms of syringomyelia.

Symptoms.—The onset of traumatic hæmatomyelia is instantaneous. The paraplegia is complete, sudden, and associated with corresponding anæsthesia. In spontaneous hæmatomyelia the onset is more or less sudden

II.   82

and the disease is established in a few hours, without pain or fever. Sensation in the lower limbs and in the trunk is completely lost. The paraplegia is total, and often accompanied by paralysis of the abdominal muscles. Incontinence of urine and of fæces is often preceded by retention. The reflexes are abolished. A slight tendency to collapse, with a lowering of the central temperature, is sometimes noticed. After a few hours or a few days the symptoms improve ; sensation reappears, the abdominal muscles regain the power of movement, and the reflexes reappear. We hope for recovery, but it is only relative, the improvement ceasing after a few weeks. " The affection becomes fixed " (Jean Lépine), and leaves behind a pareto-spasmodic condition of the lower limbs, with atrophy and sensory troubles. Slight incontinence is almost the rule as regards the sphincters. Recovery is, however, possible. Acute decubitus, consecutive myelitis, and urinary infection may cause death. Early death depends on the abundance of the hæmorrhage and on its localization in the cervical cord, near the bulb.

Central hæmatomyelia (Minor) reveals itself by slight motor troubles and by important sensory signs. The syringomyelic dissociation of the sensibility is constant, and persists after the more or less complete return of the motor functions.

Hæmatomyelia with Brown-Séquard's syndrome is not often accompanied by zones of hyperæsthesia ; the syndrome is almost always incomplete. Cervical hæmatomyelia, according to its localization, provokes either diplegia of the upper limbs, with muscular atrophy, pseudo-hypertrophy, vasomotor troubles, and arrest of development (Raymond), paralysis of the diaphragm, or complete paralysis of the brachial plexus. Recovery is exceptional. Death supervenes in a few hours or in a few days.

Hæmatomyelia of the filum terminale is characterized by integrity of the mobility in the lower limbs, anæsthesia of the inferior region of the buttocks and of the middle portion of the posterior surface of the thigh, anæsthesia and vesico-rectal paralysis, disturbance of the genital functions.

The **diagnosis** must be made from the apoplectiform affections—hæmatorrhachis, consequent on gunshot wounds ; Pott's disease with sudden bending; rapid syringomyelia, acute apoplectiform myelitis, and traumatic hysteria. The difficulties are often very great, and the ætiological data must always be borne in mind.

The **treatment** depends on the cause. In cases of fracture, dislocation, or Pott's disease, surgical intervention may be successful. Care must be taken to avoid the use of counter-irritants, because they may produce a deep, incurable, and even fatal bed-sore (Brissaud).

XVII. COMPRESSION OF THE SPINAL CORD.

Does compression exist ?   And if so, what is the nature of this compression ?   Is the spinal cord deeply or superficially affected, or is it simply inhibited ?   Where is the seat of the compression ?   Must we intervene surgically ?

The positive diagnosis of medullary compression rests on the following symptoms : Girdle pains, pains in the lower limbs ; paraplegia, which is generally spastic ; vesical and rectal troubles ; sensory disturbances ; trophic phenomena ; deformity of the vertebræ ; and radiography of the suspected region.

Meningo-myelitis, whether toxic, infective, influenzal, syphilitic, etc., from the fact that it especially affects the meninges, may exercise some compression on the parenchyma of the spinal cord ; but this is not, properly speaking, compression of the cord, especially from the surgical point of view.   The most frequent causes of compression are fractures or dislocations of the spine, having their seat of election at the twelfth dorsal and the first lumbar vertebræ.   Next come meningeal and extrameningeal tumours (sarcomata, fibromata, myxomata, hydatid cysts, tubercles, etc.), vertebral tumours, and Pott's disease.

The diagnosis of compression being made, we must next ascertain how far the cord is affected.   Are the pyramidal tracts degenerated ?   This problem is of interest, and it is sometimes a difficult problem to solve. The question must be divided ; the case is sometimes one of sudden compression, at other times one of slow compression.

Sudden Compression.—This variety is due to falls, injuries, or bullet-wounds, and the paraplegia appears suddenly.   If a few days after the onset of paraplegia we find trophic phenomena (vasomotor troubles), important sensory troubles, retention of urine, and fever, it may be said that the spinal cord is seriously affected.   When under these conditions the paraplegia remains indefinitely flaccid, with complete loss of the reflexes and absolute superficial and deep anæsthesia, complete division of the spinal cord must be diagnosed.   The spinal cord cannot become regenerated, and the lesion is irremediable.   The patient soon dies from extensive bedsores and urinary infection.   Intervention is useless in this case, as will be readily understood.   It would only put a quicker end to the patient's life by fresh traumatic shock.

If, on the contrary, after the accident, more or less pronounced paresis alone persists, with exaggeration of the tendon reflexes and slight sensory and trophic troubles, the spinal cord is compressed rather than destroyed. Intervention is indicated, and the patient may recover.

Slow Compression.—In the case of slow compression the severity of the paresis, and especially of the objective sensory symptoms, the trophic phenomena, the reflex movements of defence, rather than the spastic features and the exaggerations of the reflexes, will indicate the gravity of the spinal lesion.

In the long run slow compression, provided it is progressive, may lead to complete section of the spinal cord. In this case, do the clinical symptoms vary ? Authorities do not agree on this point, and the entire discussion (Limoges Congress, 1901) turns on the condition of the tendon reflexes. The classical theory of Charcot states that even in complete section there is always an exaggeration of the reflexes below the lesion. Bastian's theory denies this opinion. According to Bastian, Bruns, and Borolby, there is certainly contracture and exaggeration of the reflexes when the lesion of the spinal cord is not complete; but as soon as this section is complete, the paralysis becomes flaccid and the reflexes are abolished. The importance of this discussion from the surgical point of view will be understood.

When surgical intervention has been deemed necessary, we look for the signs that will localize the situation and extent of the compression. Notice must be taken of pain on percussion over a vertebra, of the prominence or the deformity of certain spinous processes, and, in some cases, of radiography. Nothing, however, can replace the study of the upper limit of the anæsthesia. To it our final appeal must be made. We know, for example, that a band of anæsthesia through the umbilicus corresponds with the eighth dorsal root, and if we remember that this root arises at the level of the eighth dorsal vertebra, we can immediately map out the exact seat of the lesion.

Regarding the relations between the spines, the bodies of the vertebræ, and the spinal nerve roots, Chipault says : " In the cervical region it is always necessary to add one to the number of the spine determined by palpation to find the number of the roots which arise at its level ; in the dorsal region we must add two ; in the inferior dorsal region, three. The lower part of the eleventh dorsal vertebra and the subjacent interspinous space correspond to the last three lumbar pairs. The twelfth dorsal spine and the subjacent interspinous space correspond to the sacral roots." The lesion having been thus mapped out, laminectomy may be performed.

XVIII. SPINAL MENINGITIS.

Spinal meningitis is acute or chronic. Amongst its causes I would mention lesions in the neighbourhood, vertebral caries, tumour, abscesses, and bed-sores of the sacrum. Tubercular spinal meningitis is allied to cerebral meningitis of the same nature. I may say the same of pneumonic spinal meningitis. To complete this section, the one on Cerebro-spinal Meningitis must be studied. It will then be seen how the infection of the meninges takes place, and what are the causes of this infection.   This general survey of spinal meningitis leaves much to be desired.   I shall deal with a few generalities, but as regards the description of the various forms of meningitis, I refer the reader to the respective sections in which they are described.

Pathological Anatomy.—The inflammation affects all the meninges, and principally the pia mater, which is thickened and infiltrated with fibrino-purulent deposits, while the subarachnoid space is invaded by a flaky or purulent sero-fibrinous liquid.   When the meningitis is chronic, there are, furthermore, adhesions between the meninges and the spinal cord, amounting in some cases to meningo-medullary sclerosis.   The spinal cord is sclerosed at its periphery, principally in its posterior columns (Vulpian).

Description.—(1) **Acute Meningitis.**—The phenomena of pain and of contracture may be attributed to the excitation of the nerve roots emerging from the spinal cord (Jaccoud) and to the excitation of the nerves of the meninges, the pia mater being richly supplied (Vulpian).   Moderate fever first appears, and is accompanied later by spinal and girdle pains, pains in the limbs, cutaneous hyperæsthesia, and cramps, which vary in situation with the localization of the meningitis.

Meningitis of the cervical region is at times accompanied by opisthotonos, and meningitis of the dorso-lumbar region may in its first period cause retention of urine and of fæces from the contraction of the sphincters of the bladder and rectum.   The reflex movements and the muscular contractility are normal.

For some years past the study of meningitis has been aided by new signs—Kernig's sign, lumbar puncture, and cyto-diagnosis.   These signs will be discussed under Cerebro-Spinal Meningitis.   Kernig's sign is as follows : As long as the patient is in the dorsal decubitus, the legs may be extended, and will remain extended, without the least muscular resistance. If the patient is made to sit down (this is sometimes painful on account of the stiffness in the nuchal and dorsal muscles), the legs are flexed on the thighs and the thighs on the trunk ; in other words, whilst he is being placed in a sitting position the patient draws his legs and his thighs towards him. Lumbar puncture consists in making a puncture in the subarachnoid space, between the laminæ of the third and fourth lumbar vertebra.   Cyto-diagnosis gives the cellular formula of the cerebro-spinal fluid.

The early phenomena of excitation, which last thirty-six to forty-eight hours, are succeeded by diminution of the pains and by paretic symptoms. The **prognosis** is very grave.   The meningitis may be cured or pass into the chronic state.   If it attacks the cervical region, the patient dies of asphyxia.

Acute Spinal Perimeningitis.—Cases have been reported in which trauma produced spinal perimeningitis, not meningitis.   The inflammation is primarily limited to the perimeningeal cellular tissue, without the dura mater being involved, and a phlegmon develops. The symptoms are not those of meningitis, but rather those of myelitis due to compression and softening of the spinal cord.

(2) **Chronic Meningitis** is usually primary ; it also presents a phase of excitation and a phase of paralysis. The phenomena of excitation are hyperæsthesia, cramps, and pains throughout the limbs and the spine. These pains are not as severe as those of acute meningitis, and simulate rather rheumatic pains. The phenomena of paralysis are symmetrical and appear slowly. Most frequently chronic cortical myelitis develops and the troubles of myelitis appear.

Chronic meningitis has a predilection for the cervical region (cervical pachymeningitis). The primary change affects the dura mater, which becomes dense and fibrous. It subsequently invades the cervical cord, and chronic meningo-myelitis is the result, the entire thickness of the cord undergoing the changes of diffuse transverse myelitis. The disease commences with pain and terminates with paralysis. To the painful period belong the pains in the neck, head, and upper limbs, with rigidity and contracture simulating Pott's disease. To the paralytic period belong the increasing paralysis of the upper limbs and their muscular atrophy (lesions of the anterior cornua). The contracture of the lower limbs (descending sclerosis of the lateral columns) is a late symptom. The disease, though very grave, may end in recovery.

Myelitis and spinal meningitis have many signs in common, and the former is often complicated by the latter. Nevertheless to myelitis belong the early paralytic troubles, anæsthesia, and trophic troubles, which we do not find in meningitis.

The **treatment** of meningitis consists in local blood-letting, counter-irritants to the affected region, the administration of calomel, subcutaneous injections of morphia, etc.

CHAPTER II

POLIOENCEPHALITIS

DISEASES OF THE PONS, CRURA, AND BULB

Anatomy.—Before describing polioencephalitis (πολιός, grey), I shall mention briefly the distribution of the grey nuclei in the bulb, pons, and crura.

When the spinal cord passes into the bulb, it opens out posteriorly, and its central canal, having become superficial, spreads out and continues to form the floor of the fourth ventricle. The result of this expansion of the spinal cord is that the parts which were posterior in the cord become external in the bulb. Accordingly, the nuclei of the motor nerves in the bulb (which are the upward continuation of the spinal motor nerves) are situated along the median line under the floor of the fourth ventricle, while the nuclei of the mixed nerves are situated a little more outside. The bulbar motor nuclei include the nuclei of the hypoglossus below and the nuclei of the facial and of the sixth nerves above.

Higher still in the crura are the nucleus of the fourth pair (pathetic nerve) and the superposed nuclei of the third pair (common oculo-motor). The mixed nuclei are those of spinal accessory, pneumogastric, glosso-pharyngeal, and the motor portion of the trifacial nerves. Let us add the nucleus of the auditory nerve. In short, all these nuclei are grouped, some around the central canal of the spinal cord when it passes into the bulb, others in the ventricular floor near Flourens' vital node. The accumulation of these nuclei in such a restricted space, and the extreme importance of the organs which the nerves supply, explain the invading course of the symptoms and the gravity of the lesions in this region.

The nuclei of the oculo-motor nerves in the crura and the nuclei of the motor nerves in the bulb represent the prolongation of the anterior cornua of the grey matter of the spinal cord. Systematic degeneration of the anterior grey column of the spinal cord (anterior poliomyelitis) causes in its chronic form progressive muscular atrophy (Duchenne-Aran's type). If the lesion, instead of first affecting the anterior cornua of the cord, attacks the grey nuclei in the bulb, we observe the symptoms of labio-glosso-laryngeal paralysis. Similarly, if the lesion, instead of first affecting the spinal or bulbar column, attacks the grey matter in the crura and pons, the symptoms of ophthalmoplegia develop.

Chronic progressive ophthalmoplegia is, therefore, in the crura and pons the equivalent of labio-glosso-laryngeal paralysis in the bulb and of progressive muscular atrophy in the spinal cord—that is to say, the expression of a systematic change limited to the cells of the grey motor substance in one of these three regions. As the grey motor column may be affected throughout its entire length in the spinal cord, in the bulb, in the pons, and in the crura (polioencephalo-myelitis), causing at the same time progressive muscular atrophy, labio-glosso-pharyngeal paralysis, and progressive external ophthalmoplegia, so, too, may one of these three segments be affected separately. Thus, by analogy with poliomyelitis, where a lesion involves the anterior cornua of the spinal

1287

cord, Wernicke proposes to call the corresponding affection of the bulbar, pontine, and crural nuclei **polioencephalitis** (πολιός, grey). He distinguishes two varieties— superior polioencephalitis, the lesion being in the nuclei of the oculo-motor nerves, and causing ophthalmoplegia ; and inferior polioencephalitis, the lesion being in the bulbar nuclei, and giving rise to labio-glosso-laryngeal paralysis. Polioencephalitis, like polio-myelitis, may have an acute, subacute, or chronic course.

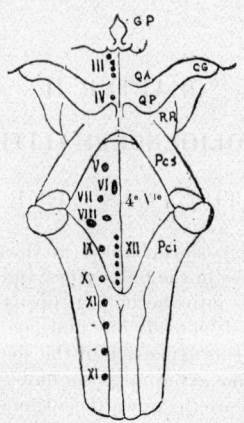

FIG. 66.—FOURTH VENTRICLE AND NUCLEI OF THE CRANIAL NERVES.

GP, Pineal gland ; QA, anterior quadrigeminal body ; QP, posterior quadrigeminal body ; CG, external geniculate body ; Pcs, superior peduncle of cerebellum ; Pci, inferior peduncle of cerebellum ; RR, Reil's band ; III-XII, nuclei of cranial nerves ; 4^e V^{le}, fourth ventricle.

I. GLOSSO-LABIO-LARYNGEAL PARALYSIS—INFERIOR CHRONIC POLIOENCEPHALITIS.

Glosso-labio-laryngeal paralysis, described in 1864 by Duchenne with the exactness found in all the descriptions of this keen observer, com-mences insidiously without fever and without pain, and progressively invades the tongue, the lips, the velum palati, and the larynx. After having destroyed the functions of deglutition and of phonation, it often ends in asphyxia or syncope.

The following typical case occurred under my care :

A man, aged seventy-three years, had preserved his understanding, although he was unable to speak a word. His speech was reduced to a mumbling of inarticulate sounds. Deglutition was practically impossible, the lips were wide open, and the saliva drooled away. The velum palati was flaccid, and the tongue, flattened against the floor of the mouth, was motionless. The extrinsic muscles of the larynx were paralyzed. The condition was bulbar, and not pseudo-bulbar. Against the hypothesis of pseudo-bulbar paralysis we had the progressive course of the disease without any stroke, and the absence of paralysis in the limbs. The absence of any nervous trouble eliminated the hypothesis of any previous affection of the nervous system, such as tabes, syringo-myelia, or amyotrophic lateral sclerosis. The condition in this case was rather that due to a primary lesion in the bulb.

The trouble had commenced eighteen months before with some difficulty in mastication and deglutition. As treatment was futile, and the man was doomed to die of hunger, I advised gastrostomy, which gave a fair measure of relief.

1. **Paralysis of the Tongue.**—Glosso-labio-laryngeal paralysis generally commences in the tongue, the superior lingualis being the first muscle attacked, just as in progressive muscular atrophy the abductor of the thumb is first affected. The muscles of the tongue being paralyzed (nerve supply from the hypoglossus and the facial), difficulties in pronunciation and in deglutition result. The patient pronounces *t* and *d* like *ch*, on account of the paralysis of the superior lingual muscle, which normally raises and presses the tip of the tongue against the upper teeth. As the tongue has lost its lateral movement and cannot be applied to the palate, the first phase of deglutition is much impeded, and the saliva is swallowed with difficulty. It accumulates in the mouth, and drools away. At a more advanced period the movements of the tongue are completely abolished, and it appears fixed to the floor of the mouth. When the atrophy is fairly considerable, the tongue is wrinkled.

2. **Paralysis of the Velum Palati** increases still more the difficulties in pronunciation and deglutition. *B* and *p* are articulated like *m* for the following reasons : In the normal condition the letters *b* and *p* are formed by the column of expired air, which suddenly separates the lips and causes them to vibrate. When the velum is paralyzed, the column of expired air loses its force by being separated into two parts : one gently separates the lips, and only succeeds in producing *m*, while the other passes into the nasal fossæ, where it gives rise to a nasal intonation. The patient can remedy this inconvenience by pinching his nose. Deglutition, already impeded by the paralysis of the tongue, becomes still more difficult. In fact, the stage of deglutition when the bolus is passing from before backwards between the tongue and the palate can only be carried out properly when the velum, being made tense by the tensor palati (fifth pair), is drawn downwards by the palato-glossi (facial nerve), and, finally, when the floor of the mouth is stretched by the mylohyoid muscles (mylohyoid branch of the inferior dental nerve), which, acting like a girth, press the base of the tongue firmly against the velum. As most of these conditions are abolished in glosso-labio-pharyngeal paralysis, the dysphagia is excessive, and, in spite of every effort on the part of the patient, the lightest meal becomes a painful and laborious operation, and deglutition is often accompanied by the passage of food into the nasal fossæ or into the larynx, which causes fits of suffocation and of asphyxia. Paralysis of the velum also betrays itself by other symptoms, such as impossibility of sucking, of gargling, etc.

3. **Paralysis of the Lips.**—When the lips are paralyzed, the patient can neither whistle nor pronounce the vowels *o* and *u*. [This, of course, is the

French *u.*—Translator.] The paralysis of the orbicularis allows the over-action of the motor muscles of the commissures. The mouth becomes widened ; the physiognomy is that of a crying child ; the food is held in the mouth with difficulty, and the saliva flows incessantly.

4. **Paralysis of the Pterygoid Muscles.**—These muscles (supplied by the trigeminal nerve) preside over the grinding movements of the jaw (movements for grinding the food). The paralysis of these muscles is generally the precursor of grave trouble (Duchenne).

Paralyses of the tongue, of the velum, of the lips, and of the pterygoid muscles combine to abolish (1) phonation, (2) deglutition. At length deglutition becomes extremely difficult, and speech is merely an unintelligible growl with a nasal tone. As these paralyses are **symmetrical,** they do not cause deviation of the mouth, of the tongue, or of the uvula. The other muscles of the face are not affected (superior facial branch), and the intelligence remains intact, but other troubles are soon added to those already described.

5. **Laryngeal Troubles.**—Anæsthesia and loss of the reflex excitability of the mucosæ of the pharynx, larynx, and trachea may exist from the commencement of the disease (Krishaber). The muscles of the larynx are sometimes attacked by incomplete paralysis. The voice is weakened, but not extinguished.

6. **Respiratory Troubles.**—At an advanced period of the disease the respiration is compromised, and the least effort causes breathlessness. Expiration is incomplete and coughing is difficult. The mucus accumulated in the bronchi is brought up with difficulty. Furthermore, the mildest bronchitis may cause grave complications. This respiratory insufficiency, which Duchenne attributes to paralysis of the bronchial muscles, is complicated by attacks of dyspnœa, which become more frequent as the disease progresses.

7. **Cardiac Troubles.**—Cardiac troubles also supervene at an advanced stage of the disease. The patient complains of a feeling of faintness, with angina and palpitations, and fatal syncope often ends the scene.

Course—Prognosis.—Glosso-labio-laryngeal paralysis commences insidiously and without fever. It attacks successively the tongue, the soft palate, the orbicularis oris, the pterygoid muscles, the larynx, the respiratory muscles, and the heart, and after a duration varying from a few months to three years the patient is carried off rapidly or slowly by various complications. Sudden death supervenes from syncope or asphyxia. It is also caused by the passage of food into the trachea, or by some intercurrent disease, such as bronchitis or pneumonia. Slow death is due to the wasting from which the patient would suffer unless fed with the œsophageal tube. Respiratory and cardiac complications mark the second phase of the disease. They are generally preceded by paralysis of the pterygoid muscles, which seems to indicate that the bulbar lesion spreads from the motor nucleus of the fifth nerve to the nucleus of the vagus.

Diagnosis and Varieties.—Cases in which the tongue, the lips, and the soft palate, are separately paralyzed must not be confounded with glosso-labio-laryngeal paralysis. Simultaneous paralysis of the facial nerves has some symptoms in common with glosso-labio-laryngeal paralysis ; the difference lies in the paralysis of the muscles of the upper part of the face. Diphtheritic paralysis of the soft palate is distinguished by the previous existence of croup or angina, by the sudden onset of the trouble, and by the integrity of the movements of the tongue and of the lips. General paralysis presents amongst its symptoms hesitation in speech and peculiar tremor of the lips, which have nothing in common with the initial troubles of phonation seen in glosso-labio-laryngeal paralysis.

I have so far described the primary form of glosso-labio-laryngeal paralysis, but the disease is often secondary to progressive muscular atrophy, insular sclerosis, and amyotrophic sclerosis. It may even be said that in many cases it forms such an integral part of these diseases that the idiopathic form of glosso-labio-laryngeal paralysis is doubted by some writers. When it is associated with the different affections just enumerated, it becomes joined to the symptoms peculiar to each of these morbid conditions, and we have the bulbo-spinal form (Hallopeau).

In certain cases the syndrome of glosso-labio-laryngeal paralysis has supervened suddenly, consequent on hæmorrhage or softening of the bulb. In this case the appearance of the glosso-labio-laryngeal paralysis coincided with sudden death (embolism of the vertebral artery—Hayem), or with hemiplegia and recovery.

The syndrome of glosso-labio-laryngeal paralysis may also find its cause, not in a bulbar, but in a cerebral lesion. This has been described under the name of pseudo-bulbar paralysis of cerebral origin. The cases of Lépine and those published later prove that there really exists a glosso-labio-laryngeal paralysis of cerebral origin. Oppenheim, having found slight bulbar lesions associated with cerebral lesions in several post-mortem examinations, has described a mixed form, to which he has given the name of paralysis of cerebro-bulbar origin. No matter how we may regard Oppenheim's cases, the pseudo-bulbar form with a cerebral localization really exists. In which region are we to localize the cerebral lesion ? A priori, it seems that the lesion ought to be bilateral, and that it ought to affect the centre for the movements of the lips (inferior facial nerve), which is situated in the lower part of the ascending frontal convolution, the centre for movement of the tongue (hypoglossal nerve), and the centre for the muscles of mastication (motor branch of the fifth nerve), which are all close together. It seems that the lesion ought likewise to affect the centre for the movements of deglutition, which is near the foot of the ascending frontal convolution, and the cortical centre, which probably lies at the junction of the foot of the ascending frontal and the foot of the third frontal convolutions. And, as a matter of fact, in several cases of pseudo-bulbar paralysis the cortical or subcortical lesions were seated in the above-mentioned cerebral region. A bilateral lesion of the optic thalamus and corpus striatum, and a cortical lesion of the right hemisphere, with a lesion in the left thalamus and corpus striatum, or *vice versa*, also give a similar syndrome (Halipré).

The interpretation of these pseudo-bulbar paralyses, however, is more difficult when the cerebral lesion is situated in the external segment of the lenticular nucleus. Sometimes, even, there is no symmetry of the lesions. In such a case, for instance, there is a focus of softening in the head of the nucleus on the right side, and another focus in the white matter of the middle lobe of the left hemisphere. These facts, though difficult to interpret, have been ingeniously explained by Halipré and Brissaud. In any event, glosso-labio-laryngeal paralysis of cerebral origin is distinguished from the bulbar form by the absence of atrophy in the paralyzed muscles, and by the preservation of the reflex movements, which spares the patient the troubles in respiration and circulation that are always a source of danger in true bulbar paralysis.

Asthenic bulbar paralysis (Erb's syndrome) closely resembles Duchenne's glosso-labio-laryngeal paralysis, but distinctive features are not wanting. The constancy of ptosis, of paresis of the muscles of mastication and of the nape of the neck, the alternation of periods of remission and aggravation, the myasthenic electrical reaction (Jolly), form the principal characteristics of Erb's syndrome, and furnish the points for diagnosis.

Pathological Anatomy.—It was first believed that glosso-labio-laryngeal paralysis is not accompanied by muscular atrophy. It is true that paralysis is the chief feature, but there is also atrophy of the muscles, which is sometimes visible with the naked eye, and always under the microscope. This atrophy, often well marked in the tongue, is similar to that described under Progressive Muscular Atrophy.

The atrophy of some of the bulbar nerves has been noticed, but the initial lesion of the disease is seated in the bulbar nuclei of these nerves (Charcot), just as the initial lesion of progressive muscular atrophy is seated in the anterior cornua of the spinal cord. The organs of phonation, of deglutition, of respiration, and of circulation, which are progressively invaded by the disease, are supplied by the hypoglossal, facial, trigeminal, spinal accessory, and pneumogastric nerves. The initial lesion of the disease must, therefore, be sought in the nuclei of these nerves.

The lesion in the nuclei consists in atrophy of the nerve cells, with or without pigmentary degeneration. It is analogous with the lesion in the anterior cornua of the spinal cord in progressive muscular atrophy. The bulbar nuclei are unequally affected by the atrophy; the nucleus of the hypoglossal nerve is the most affected (Joffroy), and in a section of the bulb we find the large cells of this nucleus replaced by some deformed cells.

II. CHRONIC SUPERIOR POLIOENCEPHALITIS.

Ophthalmoplegia is called external or internal, according as the paralysis affects the motor muscles of the eyeball or the internal musculature of the eye (iris and ciliary muscle). All the ocular paralyses must not, however, be classed under this rubric, even though they are of nuclear origin. It is useful to distinguish from ophthalmoplegia, and to classify separately— (1) the classical paralyses of each of the nerves of the eye (paralysis of the third, fourth, and sixth pair); (2) associated paralyses which affect in both eyes the muscles producing similar movements.

External ophthalmoplegia is a special clinical type, due to paralysis of all the motor muscles of the eye, and characterized in typical cases by absolute immobility of the eyes. "When however, the paralysis of the third pair is coexistent with that of the sixth pair, and when the superior oblique only is intact (fourth pair), the slight movement in a downward and outward direction scarcely changes the clinical picture. On the other hand, when the third and fourth pairs are paralyzed, it is very rare for the sixth pair to be absolutely free. For these reasons, the term ' external ophthalmoplegia ' may also be applied to cases in which the muscles supplied by two different nerves in the same eye are paralyzed, one of them being constantly the common oculo-motor nerve " (Sauvineau).

Internal ophthalmoplegia is paralysis of the entire internal musculature of the eye.

These two forms, when present in the same eye, constitute mixed or total ophthalmoplegia. Each one of these three forms may be unilateral or bilateral.

Ophthalmoplegia may be divided according to the situation of the lesion in the course of the fibres from the cerebral cortex to the orbital branches of the motor nerves of the eye. These varieties will be described under the Paralyses of the Motor Muscles of the Eye. We are only concerned at present with ophthalmoplegia of nuclear origin—that is to say, arising from a progressive change in the nuclei of the motor nerves of the eye. A short account of these nuclei will lead to a better understanding of the subject.

Anatomy.—The common oculo-motor nerve arises in the grey column under the floor of the aqueduct of Sylvius. This column forms, not a single nucleus, but a series of distinct nuclei (Hensen and Valkers, Kahler and Pick, Westphal). Each one of these little nuclei constitutes a motor centre corresponding to one of the terminal branches of the oculo-motor nerve, and corresponding, therefore, to one of the muscles of the eye supplied by the third pair. This grey column under the aqueduct of Sylvius forms the principal part of the oculo-motor nucleus. It comprises five separate nuclei, which control the four extrinsic muscles supplied by the third pair and the levator muscle of the eyelid.

In front of the principal portion of this nucleus there exists another smaller portion, formed of smaller nerve cells. It is not under the aqueduct of Sylvius, but under the floor of the third ventricle, and a little separated from the median line. It comprises two nuclei for the sphincter of the iris and the ciliary muscle.

As regards the disposition of the nuclei, the scheme proposed by Kahler and Pick is generally followed:

Median side.
1. Ciliary muscle.
2. Sphincter of the iris.
3. Internal rectus.
4. Inferior rectus.
5. Levator palpebræ.
6. Superior rectus.
7. Inferior oblique.
Lateral, or external side.

The nucleus of the fourth nerve is just below.
Lower still the nucleus of the sixth nerve is found.

Symptoms.—The onset of ophthalmoplegia is insidious, and the muscles are affected one after the other without regular order.

When the ophthalmoplegia is complete, the physiognomy of the patient has a special character, known as Hutchinson's facies. The eyelids are half closed, so that the patient appears to be asleep; they partially cover the cornea. As the patient tries to remedy this blepharoptosis by contraction of the frontalis muscle, the brow is wrinkled and the eyebrows are arched. If the upper eyelids are raised, the eyeballs are immovable, "as though formed of wax" (Benedickt). When the paralysis affects all the external muscles, the eyes are directed straight forwards. The look is, however, somewhat vague, because the optical axes are not absolutely parallel.

If the patient's head is held so that he cannot make up for the absence of movement in the eyes by moving the neck, and if he tries to fix an object and to follow it upwards, downwards, outwards, and inwards, we find that the eye remains absolutely immovable. The ophthalmoplegia, however, is not always so complete, and more or less limited movements may be performed in the direction of the action of one or of several of the muscles of the eye. In order to be more certain, we may have recourse to the examination of the field of fixation.

Diplopia only shows itself when there is a considerable difference in the paralysis of the various motor muscles.

The nuclear affection most frequently remains limited to the extrinsic muscles, the internal musculature being unaffected. The sphincter of the iris and the ciliary muscle respectively continue to react to light and to accommodation.

Finally, let us notice the absence of vertigo, of headache, and of every cerebral reaction.

Such is, in broad outline, the aspect of a patient suffering from external ophthalmoplegia.

The features of internal ophthalmoplegia are as follows : the pupil is moderately dilated ; it does not react to light or to accommodation. The ciliary muscle is also paralyzed. The patient can no longer accommodate, the punctum proximum being brought forward and confounded with the punctum remotum. Internal ophthalmoplegia may be primary and exist alone, being later accompanied by external ophthalmoplegia. It may be secondary to the latter. Finally, it may appear at the same time as external ophthalmoplegia.

Course—Prognosis.—The course of nuclear ophthalmoplegia, in its chronic form, varies. It sometimes remains stationary for years ; sometimes, on the contrary, it follows a progressive course. The course varies according to the nuclear region in which the lesion starts, and whether the lesion remains confined to these nuclei or extends farther.

In the first case the ophthalmoplegia, which is purely external, becomes complicated with internal ophthalmoplegia. The ophthalmoplegia becomes total. The inverse course (which commences in the intrinsic muscles of the eye) is far less common. The affection may not remain limited to the nuclei of the oculo-motor nerves, but may also attack the other nuclei (motor and sensory nuclei of the fifth nerve), the vasomotor centres (glycosuria, albuminuria, polyuria), the bulbar nuclei (labio-glosso-laryngeal paralysis), and even the anterior spinal cornua (progressive muscular atrophy).

In other cases we see that ophthalmoplegia complicates a spinal or cerebro-spinal affection. It will be understood that the prognosis will vary in the different forms.

Diagnosis.—Hutchinson's facies is characteristic, and cannot be confounded with the bulbar or the myopathic facies. The difficulty consists in establishing the nuclear origin of the ophthalmoplegia and in distinguishing it from the supranuclear and cortical, basal, orbital, and peripheral varieties of ophthalmoplegia. Slow and gradual abolition of the movements of the eyes, affecting progressively, without regular order, the motor muscles of the eyeballs ; special paresis less pronounced (at least at the commencement) after a night's rest ; incomplete ptosis ; absence of cerebral phenomena ; integrity of the pupil reflexes and of accommodation, are the classical characteristics of nuclear external ophthalmoplegia, and till recently nuclear ophthalmoplegia was synonymous with external ophthalmoplegia (Blanc). Nevertheless, the existence of internal ophthalmoplegia accompanying an external ophthalmoplegia must not lead us to reject the diagnosis of a nuclear lesion. On the contrary, internal ophthalmoplegia can hardly, in the present condition of our knowledge, and leaving an orbital lesion or a peripheral cause out of the question (reflex paralysis), be attributed to anything else than to a nuclear lesion of the nuclei subjacent to the third ventricle (Sauvineau).

The preceding characteristics allow us to distinguish ophthalmoplegia from paralyses which are also of nuclear origin, but are due to other causes, such as traumatism, hæmorrhage, tumour, or acute polioencephalitis.

Referring to cases of ophthalmoplegia that are independent of a lesion in the nuclei, they present special characters which generally allow them to be distinguished from cases of nuclear ophthalmoplegia.

External ophthalmoplegia has been seen with muscular atrophy and with polyneuritis. The existence of some intoxication, as a cause and the favourable course of events are in favour of polyneuritis. Ophthalmoplegia has also been found in certain forms of leprosy. Finally, external ophthalmoplegia has been met with in exophthalmic goitre (Ballet), and in hysteria (Raymond). In external ophthalmoplegia, due to neurosis, the paralysis only affects the voluntary muscles, and spares the automatic movements and the reflexes. The lesion of the nuclei of the third, fourth and sixth nerves in ophthalmoplegia consists in an atrophy of the motor cells. On microscopic examination, the cells are found to be small, rounded, and deprived of processes.

III. ACUTE AND SUBACUTE POLIOENCEPHALITIS.

The description of glosso-labio-laryngeal paralysis and of nuclear ophthalmoplegia refers to the **chronic** form of polioencephalitis. In some cases, however, the polioencephalitis runs an acute course, and generally proves fatal in a few days, while in other cases it is subacute, and most often curable.

The acute form of polioencephalitis generally appears without a definite cause. The subacute form is dependent on toxi-infectious agents (diphtheria, typhoid fever, scarlatina, influenza, measles, and pneumonia), or on toxic substances (alcohol, nicotine, lead, oxide of carbon, or poisonous food). In these cases the lesion of the nuclei is associated with the lesion of the nerves (neuritis), but the relative importance of these two factors is still obscure.

Under Glosso-labio-laryngeal Paralysis I have already described the acute fulminant forms of inferior bulbar polioencephalitis. Further reference is therefore unnecessary. The acute form of superior polioencephalitis remains to be described.

This form comes rather under the category of the hæmorrhagic lesions— hæmorrhage into the walls of Sylvius's aqueduct and into the third ventricle.

Wernicke, who in 1883 saw three cases, has called this lesion hæmorrhagic superior polioencephalitis. Since that date many other cases have been published (Thomsen, Kahler, Kojewnikoff). The symptoms of this affection reveal themselves by acute ophthalmoplegia, which is far more serious than in the chronic form. The paralysis rapidly involves the external muscles of the eye, with or without participation of the intrinsic muscles. It is often accompanied by bulbar paralysis, which may prove quickly fatal. Often, also, grave cerebral phenomena supervene, such as vertigo, intense headache, and vomiting, with invincible somnolence. This condition has nothing in common with coma, but resembles the strange disease known as **sleeping sickness.** The patient is apathetic, indifferent to every stimulus, and chained to his bed by extreme weakness, although the limbs are not paralyzed. The patient sinks into collapse, and dies in less than three weeks.

What are the lesions in this acute form? Is it a process differing in its mode of evolution, but analogous in its systematic nuclear distribution to the process of the chronic form? Wernicke, Thomsen, Kojewnikoff, and Charcot's school have adopted this view. Acute ophthalmoplegia is said to be the reproduction of acute bulbar paralysis and of acute anterior spinal paralysis, but it has not been proved that this opinion is exact. The results of post-mortem examinations published by Thomsen, by Kojewnikoff, and by Wernicke himself, show that the lesion was not seated in the nuclei of the pons and crura, or only affected them in a secondary manner. The lesion, in the shape of microscopic hæmorrhages, affected the subependymal grey matter in the walls of the third ventricle, of Sylvius's aqueduct, and of the fourth ventricle, cutting off the nuclei. Acute ophthalmoplegia in the grave form, described by Wernicke as hæmorrhagic polioencephalitis, would not then be of nuclear origin, but would belong to the obscure group of supranuclear ophthalmoplegias. It sometimes appears to be associated with alcoholism.

IV. WEBER'S SYNDROME—BONNIER'S SYNDROME.

Certain lesions of the pons and crura are due to external causes (exostoses of the base of the skull, aneurysm of the basilar artery) or to internal causes (tubercles, syphilitic gummata, hæmorrhage, and softening). The tubercles may reach the size of a pea or of a hazel-nut. The hæmorrhages arise under similar conditions to those causing cerebral hæmorrhage. The sclerosis is generally associated with insular sclerosis or with a descending sclerosis.

Description.—According as the lesion is sudden (hæmorrhage, embolism) or slow (tumours) in its evolution, the symptoms are sudden or progressive. Certain of these symptoms, such as headache, apoplexy, and convulsions, are common to many cerebral lesions, but there are others which are more especially peculiar to the lesions of the pons and crura. The latter show the following characteristics : (1) crossed paralysis (2) frequent sensory troubles.

In crossed paralysis the limbs on one side and the face on the other side are affected. To give an example, the arm and the leg are paralyzed on the left side, whilst the paralysis on the right side attacks the face (facial hemiplegia) and the external rectus (converging strabismus), or the sensory portion of the trigeminal nerve (facial hemianæsthesia).

Weber's Syndrome.—A most remarkable form of crossed paralysis is that which bears the name of Weber's syndrome. This syndrome, due to a lesion of the inferior and interior part of the cerebral peduncle, is constituted by paralysis of the common oculo-motor nerve on one side (side of the lesion), and by paralysis of the limbs and of the facial and the hypoglossal nerves on the opposite side (crossed paralysis on the side opposed to the lesion). Clinically, peduncular hæmorrhage behaves like cerebral hæmorrhage. The paralysis of the common oculo-motor nerve is either partial or total. When it is partial, the internal musculature of the eye is normal. The different partial paralyses of the eye are due to the fanlike disposition of the root fibres of the nerve in the interior of the peduncles. The paralysis is only total when the lesion is very extensive, or when it affects the trunk of the common oculo-motor nerve near its emergence from the peduncle, after it has already received the nerve fibres for the internal musculature of the eye.

In these cases of alternate paralysis, the paralysis of the limbs is on the opposite side to the lesion, whilst the paralysis of the face is direct—that is, on the same side as the lesion. This fact admits of an easy interpretation : any lesion above the neck of the bulb gives rise to crossed hemiplegia, because the motor fibres for the limbs cross in the region of the bulb, whilst a lesion of the nerves arising from the pons or from the bulb gives rise to direct paralysis. In crossed paralysis the lesion must affect at the same time the motor tracts of the limbs (they are situated in the anterior portion of the pons) and the nuclei of the sixth, seventh, and eighth nerves ; and if the tumour in the pons encroach slightly backwards into the bulb, it meets with the nuclei described under Glosso-labio-laryngeal Paralysis, and causes the symptoms due to a lesion of these nerves. A patch of sclerosis uniting the bulbar and peduncular centres might cause a variety of alternate paralysis with Weber's syndrome (paralysis of the right oculo-motor nerve and left hemiplegia), to which would be added right neuro-paralytic keratitis, with anæsthesia of the right trigeminal nerve.

Sensory troubles are fairly common in lesions of the pons. A special

hemianæsthesia, due to the lesion of the posterior bundle of the pons, which transmits sensory impressions, may be observed. The hemianæsthesia of the limbs is crossed like the hemiplegia; the hemianæsthesia of the face, of the tongue, and of hearing is direct. The preservation of sight and of smell enables us to differentiate pontine hemianæsthesia from hemianæsthesia of cerebral origin. In a case of **alternate hemianæsthesia** of embolic origin in a patient suffering from heart disease, Raymond was able to localize the lesion exactly. The focus was seated in the pons at the point where Reil's band approaches the sensory fibres of the trigeminal nerve.

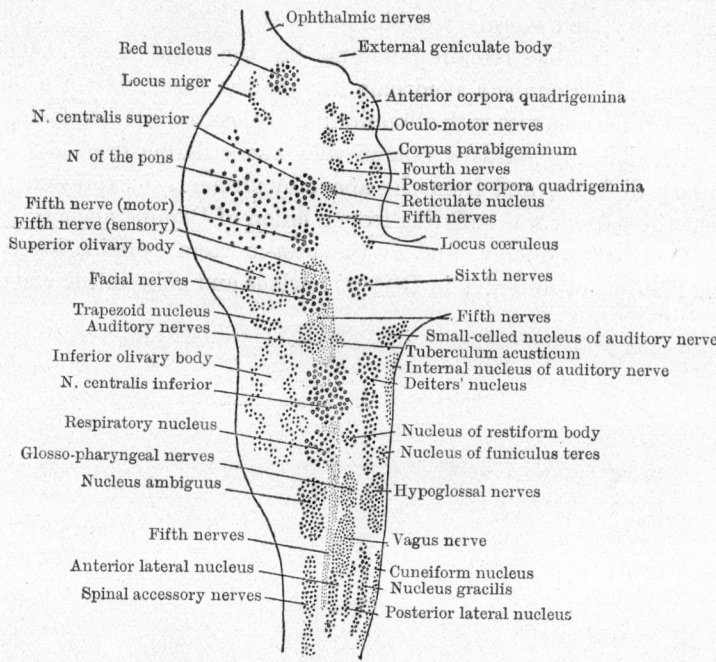

FIG. 67.—NUCLEI IN THE MEDULLA AND THE PONS.

Bonnier's Syndrome.—Bonnier has recently described a new bulbar syndrome, dependent on lesions of Deiters' nucleus, with accompanying symptoms, due to intermediate radiations. This nucleus, which is fairly large and deeply situated in the bulb, is one of the most important centres of the vestibular root of the eighth nerve. Besides its situation among the fibres and the nuclei, placed in series from the pons to the cord, it is in direct anatomical and functional relation with the nuclear systems of the auditory centres, the trigeminal nerve, the oculo-motor, glosso-pharyngeal, pneumo-gastric, and general vasomotor centres, and the neighbouring respiratory centres. It is likewise in immediate relation with the cerebellum and with the ascending parietal convolution. The cardinal symptom is vertigo, with partial or total loss of the power to maintain the vertical position. The accompanying symptoms are : (1) Oculo-motor troubles, of varying severity and duration—myosis, mydriasis, nystagmus, troubles of accommodation, diplopia, binocular and uniocular triplopia, etc. ; (2) pain in the region of the superior trigeminal branch—orbital, temporal, tympanic, or vertical neuralgia ; (3) auditory troubles—deafness and paroxysmal buzzings in the ear ; (4) nausea, thirst, and anorexia, all of which are paroxysmal ; (5) pneumogastric troubles, dyspnœa, tachycardia, or bradycardia ; or, on the contrary, a feeling that the respiration is quickened ; (6) secretory, circulatory, and thermic troubles.

Certain troubles remain unilateral, but the oculo-motor phenomena may be crossed. Bonnier's syndrome may be the first index of a bulbar affection. It may coexist with albuminuria, glycosuria, sick headache, and tabes.

I had in my wards a woman who was suffering from glycosuria, temporary diplopia, and from the above syndrome. I expressed the opinion that the patient was suffering from a lesion of Deiters' nucleus.

She died suddenly, and at the post-mortem examination we actually did find foci of softening in Deiters' nucleus and obliterating endarteritis.

CHAPTER III

DISEASES OF THE CEREBELLUM

ABSCESS, TUMOURS, AND SYPHILIS OF THE CEREBELLUM.

IN this chapter I shall especially consider abscesses of the cerebellum, quoting from my communication to the Académie de Médecine.* The other lesions of the cerebellum (tumours, hæmorrhage, and syphilis) will be considered when the diagnosis is discussed. The following case sums up the question :

On May 7 a man was admitted for violent headache and attacks of vertigo. Whilst he was walking up to the ward, he was seized with vertigo, and fell down as if in an epileptic fit. His body was thrown violently towards the left, and in his fall the left side of the head received the shock. Next day a large bruise appeared round the left eye, and spread to the eyelids, the supra-orbital region, and the right eye. The ecchymosed parts were bluish and swollen, and the left eyeball was hidden by the swollen eyelid. The patient was much depressed—not on account of his fall, but on account of his previous condition. Although his answers were slow, he could, nevertheless, give some precise details concerning his illness. He came to the hospital because for the past twelve days or so he had suffered from violent pains in the occipital region, the neck, the forehead, and the vertex. His sufferings lasted day and night. Furthermore, on making a movement, or even without appreciable cause, severe stabbing pains supervened. By pressure and percussion we discovered that the chief seat of the pain was in the occipital region. The pain was not superficial, as in neuralgia, and had not the characteristics of syphilitic osteoperiostitis. It was a deep-seated headache, with radiations and paroxysms.

Soon after the headache vertigo appeared. The sensation of giddiness occurred several times a day. Sometimes objects seemed to turn in various directions ; at other times the patient seemed to be drawn by oscillatory movements to the right and left. These attacks of vertigo were increased by standing or walking. They grew less when he sat down, and disappeared when he lay in bed. The vertigo was accompanied by a loss of equilibrium, which made his gait like that of a drunken man. He walked with his legs apart, stopping at times to gain a point of support.

A stroke occurred on May 3, the patient being thrown to the right. A fresh stroke, with a fall to the left, occurred on his admission to the Hôtel-Dieu. For the past three days he had suffered from spontaneous vomiting. The most trifling causes, such as a change of position, rising or sitting down, brought on the vomiting. Nothing was noticed so far as the limbs were concerned. The movements were free, though slow.

---

* Dieulafoy, " Les Abcès du Cervelet," communication à l'Académie de Médecine, séance du 19 Juin, 1900.

The case might have been taken for one of muscular asthenia. No paralysis, no contractures, no tremors, no epileptiform fits, and no anæsthesia. The face and the organs of the senses were, for the time being, not affected. The senses of hearing and smell were normal. Neither facial nor ocular paralysis was noticed. There was no nystagmus. The right pupil reacted well to light and to accommodation. There was neither myosis nor mydriasis. Speech was normal, though slow. It was neither stuttering nor scanning. Respiration and deglutition were not affected. The intelligence was intact. It was, however, necessary to repeat a question in order to get an answer. The patient was drowsy, and lay in the dorsal decubitus. The urinary functions were normal, the urine containing neither albumin nor sugar. The pulse-rate, which was slow at the time of his admission, in a few days increased from 56 to 108. The temperature did not rise above 101° F.

To sum up, the patient, who had been ill for about twelve days, was first seized with violent occipital headache, followed by severe vertigo, loss of equilibrium, and repeated fits of vomiting. I, therefore, had no hesitation in diagnosing a lesion of the cerebellum. Ménière's disease, meningitis, tumours of the brain and of the mesencephalon were in turn eliminated. There was no question of cerebro-spinal meningitis, Kernig's sign being absent and lumbar puncture negative. It was, therefore, logical to admit a lesion of the cerebellum, but we had still to discover its nature. In such a case abscess of the cerebellum must be first considered. It frequently follows acute or chronic otitis. The patient was asked several times whether he had ever had pains in the ears or purulent discharge. The answer was negative. Furthermore, our examination showed that his hearing was normal. Pressure on the mastoid region caused no pain. The patient had no fever. We had, therefore, to find some other cause.

It was not a case of cerebellar hæmorrhage, because the symptoms had been neither sudden nor simultaneous. They had been successive and progressive, taking twelve days to reach their maximum. It might have been tuberculosis (large tubercle of the nerve centres), which had so far been latent, although the patient was not tubercular. The probabilities were against glioma or sarcoma, because in these tumours the appearance of the symptoms is much more spaced out. Was it a syphilitic lesion of the cerebellum, gumma, or obliterating arteritis ? The patient denied syphilis, and showed no stigmata. As everything is possible in syphilis, however, I ordered a daily injection of biniodide of mercury.

During May 8, 9, and 10 the situation grew worse. The torpor became more marked, and the patient lay on his back absolutely motionless. At night he was restless and delirious, and—an important fact—the left labial commissure was paretic. As the treatment made no difference, I asked Marion to see the case.

On May 11 I requested Brissaud to give me his opinion. He at once admitted the diagnosis of a lesion in the cerebellum. In addition to the cerebellar syndrome already described, we noticed ocular symptoms which did not exist at the time of the patient's admission—nystagmus and paresis of the left external oculo-motor nerve. The paresis of the left labial commissure had also become more marked. Ophthalmoscopic examination showed, on the right side, hæmorrhage into the retina, and on the left optic neuritis. The knee-jerks were abolished. The patient, who was sunk in coma vigil, replied only with great difficulty. Everything pointed to a fatal termination, and Brissaud and myself were of opinion that the only chance of salvation lay in surgical intervention.

The operation was therefore fixed for the next morning, Saturday, and Marion asked us a question of the utmost importance : " On which side of the cerebellum was the lesion seated ?" This question required an answer, but on what were we to base the diagnosis of the localization ? As headaches, vertigo, staggering gait, vomiting, and nystagmus are symptoms common to the cerebellar lesions of both lobes and of the vermis, they were of no help in localizing the lesion either on the right or on the left side. The state of the eyes (neuritis and retinal hæmorrhages) was of no value, because both eyes were affected. The stroke and falling of the patient to the left were valueless as a few days previously a similar stroke had thrown the patient to the right. Two signs helped us in the topographical diagnosis of localization—the paresis of the left external oculo-motor nerve and of the left facial nerve. Apart from the paresis of the left labial commissure, which was three days old, Brissaud was struck by the flaccidity of the left cheek. The lesion was, therefore, in the left lobe of the cerebellum.

Under ether Marion trephined in three places—over the left fossa of the cerebellum—two below and one above, at the angles of an isosceles triangle. At this moment the respiration ceased. The heart continued to beat, but the beats soon grew weak, and then stopped. For ten minutes every means was used to restore respiration. Rhythmical traction on the tongue had no result. Marion, in the hope of lessening the intracranial pressure, opened up the inner table, incised the dura mater, and exposed the cerebellum. The pulse came back. The patient was, therefore, not quite dead, although he had not breathed for twenty minutes.

On opening the skull no lesion was seen, the meninges being normal and the cerebellum appearing to be healthy. Marion explored in every direction, and during this exploration his finger touched against the posterior surface of the bulb. Immediately, to the surprise of those present, the patient made a long and noisy inspiration. When the finger was withdrawn, the respiration at once stopped. The finger being again pushed against the posterior surface of the bulb, the inspirations reappeared and kept on, but they ceased as soon as the compression of the bulb ceased. Similar experiments were made several times following, with the same result, and in the end the respiration was definitely re-established.

The patient was dressed and taken back to bed. During the day his condition was about the same as before the operation. He replied with difficulty, the respiration was normal, and the pulse was 120. Next day his wife told us that her husband, a month before his illness, had complained of pains in the left ear, followed by discharge. The patient had, therefore, had otitis after all, although he had denied it, thus withholding valuable information. The otitis had been neither severe nor obstinate, because the patient had lost all recollection of it. It was evident that the lesion on the left side of the cerebellum, as shown by the cerebellar syndrome, was an abscess following on otitis. Although the condition of the patient had grown worse, several punctures of the cerebellum were made in the hope of striking the pus. We were not successful, and the patient died during the day.

This final result left me uneasy. I asked myself whether there had been a flaw in the diagnosis. Was the cerebellar lesion really on the left side, and had we told the surgeon correctly in pointing out to him the left lobe of the cerebellum as the sphere for action ? The post-mortem examination removed this doubt.

The abscess was of the size of a large hazel-nut, and was seated in the anterior region of the left lobe (which is the most usual place). It had developed in the white matter, not in the centre, but between the dentate nucleus and the cortical grey matter, a little upwards and outwards. The punctures had passed quite close to the abscess without reaching it.

This abscess, which was of recent formation and non-encysted, contained 2 grammes of greenish creamy pus. The pneumococcus was the only pathogenic agent, and even then the pneumococcus was not at all abundant. It had lost its virulence, for cultures remained sterile, and did not cause death when inoculated into a mouse.

The abscess was the only lesion present, the remainder of the cerebellum, the cerebrum, and the mesencephalon being healthy. There was not a trace of meningitis. The sinuses were healthy ; the petrous bone was normal. The abscess could not, therefore, be explained by the contiguity of the lesions. It was, indeed, a " remote abscess," comparable with the remote abscesses of appendicitis, and had no apparent connection with the original focus. The otitis had been cured, sections of the middle and of the internal ear revealing no lesions.

Pathogenesis.—The first point to note is : mild otitis may in a few weeks produce a fatal abscess in the cerebellum, just as mild appendicitis may in a few weeks cause suppuration in the liver* and in the pleura.† In this case the otitis had only lasted a few days, and was so slight that the patient had no recollection of it, and yet it had started the remote abscess in the cerebellum.

Otitis is rightly considered to be the most common cause of cerebellar abscesses. The cause of the otitis (angina, coryza, measles, influenza, pneumonia, etc.), and the kind of organism (pneumococcus, streptococcus, staphylococcus, etc.), as well as the duration and course, are of minor importance. When the tympanum is infected, abscess of the cerebellum or of the cerebrum may follow. In some cases, as in my patient, the otitis is recent, and the abscess forms a few weeks later. In other cases the cerebellar infection supervenes in people who have for many years been suffering from chronic otitis. In Chatelier's patient, with a cerebellar abscess at the age of twenty-six, the otitis commenced in infancy. In a case quoted by Netter and Delpeuch the cerebellar abscess appeared at the age of sixteen, while otitis had existed since the age of three years.

These quotations are sufficient to prove that any case of otitis can cause a cerebellar abscess, and that the otitis may date back a few weeks, or even thirty to forty years. The pain in the ear may be acute or moderate ; the running may be abundant, slight, or intermittent, and the hearing may be more or less affected. But when the tympanum is infected, and remains infected, cerebellar and cerebral abscesses are to be feared. It is a question of exaltation of the virulence in a closed cavity, the pathogenesis being the same as in appendicitis, as I showed in my first communication on appendicitis to the Académie.

The course of events is as follows : The middle ear is infected through the Eustachian tube. If the tube is obliterated, a closed cavity is formed, and, by a general law of pathology, exaltation of the virulence generally follows. Perforation of the membrana tympani, or removal of the obstruction in the tube, may suppress the closed cavity, and complications are warded off for a time. The antrum and the mastoid cells, however, lend themselves admirably to the formation of secondary closed cavities at a more or less distant interval ; and then the migration of organisms, with or without lesions in the petrous bone, may lead to a series of complications— phlebitis and thrombosis of the sinuses (especially of the lateral sinus), diffuse or localized meningitis, pachymeningitis, cerebro-spinal meningitis, and abscess of the cerebellum and cerebrum. In these cases, as in

* Dieulafoy, *Clinique Médicale de l'Hôtel-Dieu*, tome ii., p. 167.
† Dieulafoy. Communication à l'Académie de Médecine, 10 Avril, 1900.

appendicitis, the lesions may be brought about by contiguity, or may be remote.

The otic infection, elaborated in the closed cavity, may spread in various directions. Spread of infection downwards and outwards through the external table of the mastoid process and through the inferior wall of the mastoid cells may lead to an abscess of the neck (De Quervain). Spread of infection through the roof of the tympanum and backwards along the groove of the transverse sinus may end in multiple intracranial lesions.

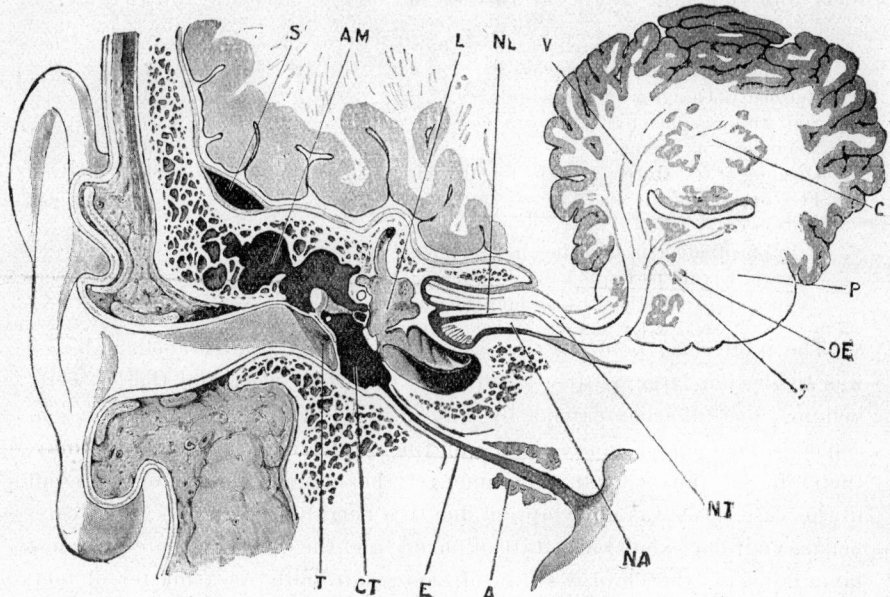

FIG. 68.—SECTION THROUGH THE EAR.

T, Membrana tympani; CT, cavity of tympanum; E, Eustachian tube; A, adenoid tissue around the tube; NA, cochlear nerve; NT and NL, vestibular nerves; F and OE, fibres communicating with the nucleus of the facial nerve (F) and the sixth nerve (OE); P, pons; C, cerebellum; V, expansion of the vestibular nerve in the cerebellum; L, labyrinth; AM, mastoid antrum; S, lateral sinus.

The organisms passing through the roof of the tympanum cause abscesses of the brain, whilst the organisms passing through the posterior surface of the petrous bone and of the mastoid process cause abscesses of the cerebellum.

These routes of migration are, however, not always followed when the suppuration takes place by continuity, and, according to the judicious remark of Picqué and Mauclaire, the germs may take any direction, no matter what is the initial point of departure.

In most cases the cerebellar abscess does not exist as an isolated lesion, but is associated with other intracranial lesions which precede or follow it. Amongst these lesions I shall especially mention caries and necrosis of the bones, pachymeningitis, and phlebitis of the sinuses, especially of the lateral sinus, which is attacked in half of the number of cases (Picqué and Mauclaire).

Abscess of the cerebellum often provokes neighbouring lesions. The more marked these lesions are, the less chance of success has surgical intervention. The following statistical table of Paul Koch, in sixty-four cases of abscess of the cerebellum, verified by post-mortem examination, shows that forty-four times the cerebellar abscess had caused lesions in the vicinity.

Purulent meningitis, consequent on perforation of the abscess into the arachnoid membranes	7 times.
Purulent meningitis by infiltration	3 ,,
Sero-fibrinous meningitis, continuous with the abscess	5 ,,
Meningeal hyperæmia	3 ,,
Opening of the abscess into the fourth ventricle	3 ,,
Free opening of the abscess	4 ,,
Diffuse encephalitis	2 ,,
Area of softening around the abscess	7 ,,
Abscess, having perforated the dura mater	9 ,,
Tissues apparently healthy around the abscess	21 ,,

The interesting point in the case quoted is that the cerebellar abscess was single, not large, clearly localized in the white matter of the left cerebellum, and unaccompanied by any other lesion. Cerebrum, mesencephalon, meninges, sinuses, bones, and nerves were all healthy. We may, therefore, be quite certain that amongst the numerous symptoms present in this case there was no symptom due to a neighbouring lesion. The cerebellar syndrome existed in a state of purity, and the case was, therefore, most favourable for the clinical study of this syndrome. As a matter of fact, when a lesion of the cerebellum tends to become external (this is very common in the case of glioma, gliosarcoma, tuberculoma, or parasitic tumour), the proper symptoms of the lesion of the cerebellum are often masked by other symptoms (crossed paralysis, spasms, etc.), due to the lesions or to the irritation of the neighbouring organs, and the result is that the cerebellar syndrome is rendered obscure. This remark also holds good if the cerebellar abscess is associated with other neighbouring lesions (abscess of the brain, pachymeningitis, abscess of the dura mater, phlebitis, and thrombosis of the lateral sinus). In such a case the cerebellar syndrome is also defaced.

In my patient, on the contrary, the cerebellar syndrome, I repeat, remained in a condition of purity. A small abscess in the white matter of one lobe of the cerebellum was sufficient to cause headache, loss of equilibrium, vomiting, vertigo, stroke, nystagmus, bilateral optic neuritis, homologous paresis of the left external oculo-motor nerve and of the left facial nerve, somnolence, and coma vigil. These symptoms may all exist, no matter whether the abscess is in the right lobe, the left lobe, or the vermis. It is only paresis of the sixth and seventh nerves which indicates the side of the lesion.

Diagnosis.—It might be supposed that the diagnosis of cerebellar abscess is an easy matter. As a matter of fact, the difficulties are often great. Let us suppose that a man has been suffering from recent or old otitis. At a given moment the complete cerebellar syndrome appears, and we find headache, vertigo, loss of equilibrium, vomiting, and nystagmus. An abscess of the cerebellum consequent on otitis will be immediately thought of, and the idea of surgical intervention will present itself. And yet the man is not suffering from an abscess of the cerebellum : the syndrome arises from the ear, and not from the cerebellum.

Certain lesions of the ear cause symptoms (auditory troubles, buzzings, vertigo, and ictus) grouped under the name of Ménière's vertigo. Other symptoms (headache, vomiting, and nystagmus) may also be present, and the auricular lesion gives rise to the cerebellar syndrome. A case of this kind is published in Raymond's " Leçons Cliniques " :

A man who had gone to bed feeling well, and who had committed no excesses during the previous day, awoke during the night with intense malaise, vomiting, vertigo, buzzing in the ears, and cold sweats. He got up, but he was seized with such severe vertigo that he fell down, and could hardly get back to bed. He suffered from headache, which lasted for two days. A week later the vertigo became less severe. The patient, reeling like a drunken man, came to the out-patient department of the Salpêtrière, where his drunken gait, nystagmus, trembling of the eyelids, and mydriasis were noticed. Examination of the ears revealed a " sclerotic constriction of the tympanum, incomplete obstruction of the Eustachian tube, and extreme mobility of the stapes, causing relative deafness and compression of the labyrinth." Raymond discusses the pathogenic diagnosis, rejecting the hypothesis of a lesion in the cerebellum, and mentions the labyrinthine lesion as the cause of all the symptoms.

I have seen a patient suffering in a similar manner. It is, moreover, an admitted fact that the cerebellar and labyrinthine syndromes are identical. This is very natural, because a part of the cerebellum may be considered as a centre of the labyrinthine nerve. These ideas are of recent date, and are largely due to the remarkable work of Bonnier, who has elucidated this question in numerous publications. In both syndromes it is, therefore, the labyrinthine nerve which is affected, either in its terminal expansions (vestibular branch of the eighth pair) or at its cerebellar origin.

In spite of the analogy between the cerebellar and the labyrinthine syndrome, it is possible to distinguish between them, and hence to avoid an operation for a non-existent cerebellar abscess. The following are the distinctive signs : headache of labyrinthine origin has neither the intensity, the persistence, nor the localization of the headache of cerebellar origin.

Furthermore, in the case of abscess of the cerebellum fever is frequent. When the symptoms have shown themselves, they do not become less marked. The somnolence becomes more severe every day. This feature is absent in the labyrinthine syndrome. It is also difficult to distinguish abscess of the cerebellum from an abscess of the brain (temporo-sphenoidal and occipital lobes). These abscesses of the brain consequent on otitis are as common as abscesses of the cerebellum. How are we to arrive at the diagnosis, an essential factor in the surgical intervention ? A patient with otitis complains of headache, vomiting, vertigo, and paralytic troubles, with or without contractures and convulsive movements. We notice, in short, symptoms of cerebral origin, and we have every reason to believe that a cerebral abscess is forming. The question is : How are we to know the seat of the abscess ? Is it in the cerebellum, or in the temporo-sphenoidal or the occipital lobe ? In the case of cerebral abscess we may find some of the symptoms of cerebellar abscess, but they are less marked : the vertigo is less pronounced, the gait is less reeling, the headache has its maximum of intensity in the temporal, and not in the occipital, region. The motor troubles are on the side opposite to the cerebral lesion, and consequently on the opposite side to the otitis. The motor troubles do not reach the stage of complete paralysis. It is a case of hemiplegic paresis, with or without spasms and with or without contractures. Finally, two signs are of great value — word-blindness and hemianopia. Word-blindness and crossed hemianopia are considered to be valuable signs of cerebral abscess by Lannois and Jaboulay.

The diagnosis must still be made between abscesses and tumours of the cerebellum. Gliomata, gliosarcomata, tuberculomata, and parasitic tumours may also cause the cerebellar syndrome. Tumours of the cerebellum, however, run a much slower course than abscess. The symptoms are further separated as regards time. Furthermore, the tumours have a tendency to grow externally, compressing and irritating the organs and the nerves in the neighbourhood. We, therefore, find borrowed symptoms which have nothing to do with a lesion limited to the cerebellum. Finally, the existence of otitis is in favour of abscess.

Although syphilis of the cerebellum is still an obscure matter, we must not forget that syphilitic arteritis occurs in the vessels of the cerebellum, and gives rise to softening, with the cerebellar syndrome. Zuber has reported the following case :

A man who had syphilis was taken ill sixteen and twenty years later with apoplectiform strokes, accompanied by headache and amnesia. Later the cerebellar symptoms supervened—vertigo and reeling gait. The patient, whether lying down or standing, suffered from continual vertigo. He walked like a drunken man, spreading his legs apart to increase his base of support. He suffered from slight facial paralysis on the left side. After a temporary improvement under antisyphilitic treatment, the situation became worse, hemiplegia of the right side being followed by contractures and partial paralysis. The patient died in coma. At the post-mortem examination an old focus of yellow softening was found, which had destroyed the inferior part of the right hemisphere of the cerebellum. This focus corresponded to the area supplied by the inferior artery of the cerebellum, which showed obliterating arteritis. The left cerebellar hemisphere showed a focus of softening and obliterating arteritis of the inferior cerebellar artery. In this case the cerebellar syndrome was defaced, because cortical and central softening were present in the cerebrum. Syphilitic lesions of the cerebellum are amenable to specific treatment. They must, therefore, be distinguished from the other lesions of the cerebellum.

The **treatment** of the tumours and of the abscesses of the cerebellum is purely surgical. It is necessary to operate before the secondary lesions have had time to arise. Prophylactic treatment consists in curing the otitis. Any individual who suffers from otitis should know the danger to which he is exposed.

CHAPTER IV

DISEASES OF THE BRAIN

I. CEREBRAL CONGESTION.

Ætiology.—Cerebral congestion may be active or passive. Active congestion may accompany the rigor of intermittent fevers and acute rheumatism. It is caused by insolation, by the sudden suppression of a habitual flux (hæmorrhoids, menstruation), by prolonged cold, by alcoholic beverages, by the presence of tumours and other brain lesions. Passive congestion arises from any cause which interferes directly or remotely with the venous circulation of the brain—compression of the cerebral sinuses and of the veins of the neck, tumours of the neck and of the mediastinum, prolonged efforts, and valvular lesions of the heart.

Description.—Jaccoud describes three forms of cerebral congestion. The slight form is characterized by pains in the head, with pulsation of the carotid and temporal arteries, and injection of the face and of the eyes. In the grave form there are also added psychical troubles, with insomnia, restlessness, and delirium. Elderly persons are subject to a variety of cerebral congestion which betrays itself by delirium followed by coma (Durand-Fardel). In children convulsions replace the delirium. The apoplectic form of cerebral congestion lasts for one or two days, and may then disappear, without leaving any traces. It is sometimes followed by a temporary hemiplegia, or is only the prelude of the delirious form. Apoplectiform congestion, sometimes associated with epileptiform convulsions, is not rare in certain diseases of the nerve centres, such as insular sclerosis, general paralysis, and descending scleroses of the mesencephalon.

The **diagnosis** of cerebral congestion must be made with regard to its particular form. The mild form must not be confounded with gastric vertigo ; and apoplectiform congestion must be differentiated from vertigo *ab aure læsa*, from cerebral hæmorrhage, and from epilepsy. Furthermore, cerebral congestion, formerly looked upon as frequent, has become much less common, since we know better the differences between it and the diseases with which it was confounded.

The **prognosis** may be grave. Apoplectiform congestion from insolation

1310

or from cold is often accompanied by pulmonary congestion. The delirious form may cause rapid death (Andral). The **treatment** consists in general or local bleeding, revulsives, purgatives, and cold applications to the head.

II. CEREBRAL ANÆMIA.

Cerebral anæmia may be limited to the brain or may be associated with general anæmia, the brain, more than the other organs, experiencing the effects thereof. Cerebral anæmia is due to a change in the quantity or in the quality of the blood. The quantitative changes have as their cause hæmorrhages, rapid or excessive evacuation of abdominal fluid, and changes in the cerebral circulation under the direct or reflex influence of the vaso-motor nerves. The qualitative changes are due to long and grave diseases, to inanition, to cachexia, etc.

The **symptoms** of cerebral anæmia vary according to the cause. When the quantity of blood withdrawn from the system is considerable, or when the loss has been rapid, the patient has attacks of vertigo and noises in the ears. He becomes cold and loses consciousness, his pallor is extreme, the pulse grows small and irregular, the respiratory movements become slower, and we sometimes meet with general convulsions and fatal syncope. When the cerebral anæmia comes on slowly, the principal symptoms are vertigo, palpitation, insomnia, and general depression, joined to an exaggerated excitability of the senses. Total anæmia of an area due to obliteration of a vessel (thrombosis or embolism) will be described under Cerebral Softening.

When the anæmia is sudden (loss of blood), the head should be lowered, the patient lying down. The treatment of the other forms is that of the general anæmia.

III. CEREBRAL HÆMORRHAGE.

The description of cerebral hæmorrhage deserves special notice—first, on account of its importance, and, secondly, because several of its primary symptoms (apoplexy, hemiplegia), and also of its secondary symptoms, (contractures, tremors) are common to other cerebral diseases, and require a thorough knowledge of the anatomy of the brain and of the circulation in its various territories.

Pathological Anatomy.—The blood extravasated into the brain tissue collects in foci, and does not retract. On coagulating, it assumes the look of gooseberry jelly. These characters vary according as the hæmorrhagic focus is recent or old. If the hæmorrhage is recent and abundant, the walls of the focus are irregular and formed of shreds of the cerebral matter ; bloodvessels and miliary aneurysms are sometimes found. When the hæmorrhage is several months old, the clot and the walls of the focus become changed. The blood is deprived of its serous portion; the solid elements (corpuscles and fibrin) are transformed, and the granulo-fatty degeneration facilitates their absorption, but the hæmatoidin remains indefinitely, and the cicatrices, even after ten to fifteen years, still preserve an ochre-like colour. In the long run the walls of the focus are transformed into sclerotic tissue. If these walls do not unite, a cyst results ; in the contrary case, a cicatrix is formed.

The hæmorrhagic foci vary much in size. They are sometimes symmetrical. They may burst into the ventricles and through the meninges. By the side of a focus as large as an egg we sometimes meet with capillary foci (Cruveilhier's capillary apoplexy) smaller than a pin's head. The brain tissue is studded with red points, presenting at the centre a capillary vessel, the lymphatic sheath of which is distended by blood and torn at some point which cannot always be discovered. These capillary hæmorrhages are often the first stage of a focal hæmorrhage.

Topography of the Hæmorrhage.—The hæmorrhages do not occur in an indiscriminate manner, but they select the grey more often than the white matter, and the convolutions are rarely attacked, as compared with the central ganglia. In order to form an exact idea of the topography of the focus, of the possible inundation of the lateral ventricles, of the invasion of the internal capsule, of the lesions of the pyramidal tract, of the secondary sclerotic degenerations that may be the result of the hæmorrhage, and of the muscular atrophy which complicates this degeneration, it is first necessary to understand the anatomical conformation of this central region.

If we separate the two lips of the fissure of Sylvius, we find a group of four or five short convolutions covered by the branches of the Sylvian artery. This is the island of Reil. If the brain is hardened, and if the convolutions of the island of Reil are carefully scraped away, we meet with a lamina of white matter, 2 millimetres in thickness, called the external capsule, and surrounding a tract of grey matter called the claustrum. If we remove the external capsule, we find a large mass of grey matter, known as the lenticular nucleus, and divided into several segments. If we next remove the nucleus, we meet with a thick tract of white matter—the internal capsule—which is of supreme importance. The internal capsule being detached, we find the grey caudate nucleus, and finally a mass of grey matter—the optic thalamus—which projects into the lateral ventricle. It is to be noted that, according to this disposition, the three masses of grey matter, the optic thalamus, and the nuclei of the striate body are fixed to the internal capsule, like cotyledons (Foville).

Internal Capsule.—The internal capsule (Burdach) plays such an important part in this region that I do not hesitate to give full details. In order to study the internal capsule properly, a horizontal section of the brain must be made, either from without inwards, a little above the fissure of Sylvius (Flechsig), or from within outwards, by directing the knife a little downwards and backwards (Brissaud). The internal capsule shows—(1) an anterior segment (lenticulo-striate) directed inwards and backwards, and bounded internally by the caudate nucleus, and externally by the lenticular nucleus ; (2) a genu, or bend, situated between the optic thalamus and the striated body ; (3) a posterior segment (lenticulo-optic), directed outwards and backwards, and bounded externally by the lenticular nucleus, and internally by the optic thalamus. The fibres of the internal capsule, after having passed the region between the central nuclei, enter the centrum ovale, form the corona radiata, and disperse in all directions towards the

Plate VII.

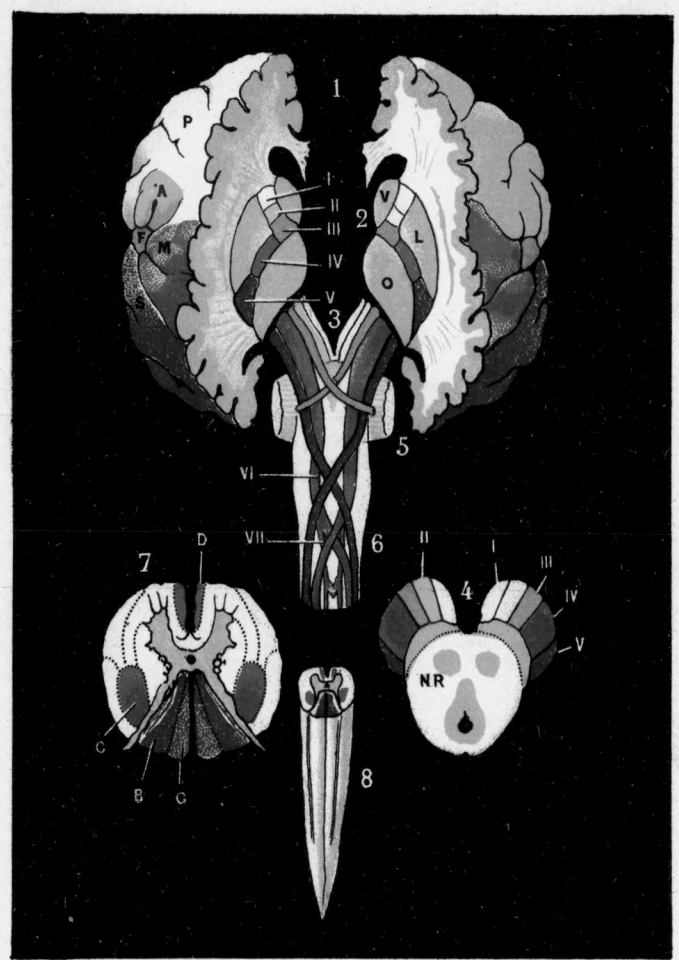

FIG. 69. — Diagram of the cerebro-spinal and Sensory tracts.

To face p. 1312

peripheral parts of the brain. The internal capsule contains the centrifugal and centripetal nerve fibres of various origins. Some, coming from the peripheral portions of the brain, end in the lenticular nucleus, the caudate nucleus, and in the optic thalamus ; others do not end in the central ganglia, but form commissures between the cerebrum on the one hand and the mesencephalon and the spinal cord on the other, constituting the pyramidal tract, the geniculate tract, and the sensory tract.

The pyramidal tract, thus named on account of the importance which it has in the anterior pyramids of the bulb, might also be called the voluntary tract (Ferrier), because it transmits voluntary impulses from the motor areas of the brain to the various segments of the spinal cord. The nerve fibres, arising in the large cells of the motor convolutions (ascending frontal and parietal convolutions and paracentral lobule), descend through the centrum ovale, and occupy the posterior segment of the internal capsule. The tract, then, passes through the middle portion of the peduncles, forms the anterior pyramid of the bulb, giving off fibres to the motor centres of the bulb, and decussates in the neck of the bulb with the other pyramidal tract, in order to pass over to the opposite side of the spinal cord. The decussation of the fibres is more or less complete, but the most important part of the pyramidal bundle (that which has undergone decussation) occupies in the opposite side of the spinal cord the portion farthest away from the lateral cord in the neighbourhood of the posterior roots. This tract, which is large in the cervical region, diminishes in size as it approaches the lumbar region. The nerve fibres of which it is composed enter into direct relation in the various levels of the spinal cord with the motor cells in the anterior cornua. The latter, in their turn, enter into relation with the muscles by the prolongations which they send into the peripheral nerves. The other portion of the pyramidal tract (Turck's direct pyramidal tract) occupies the internal portion of the anterior columns of the spinal cord, and does not descend below the lumbar region.

The geniculate tract of the internal capsule (Brissaud) is of small size. It also starts from the motor area of the brain, and is situated in the genu of the internal capsule. It is composed of motor fibres, which go to the nuclei of the bulb, and it governs the voluntary movements of the head and face.

The sensory bundle, coming from the posterior tracts of the spinal cord, crosses at the neck of the bulb, passes through the anterior pyramid, the pons, the posterior bundle of the cerebral peduncle, and reaches the internal capsule. It occupies the posterior third of the posterior segment of the internal capsule, and passes into the grey cortex of the cerebral convolutions.

Bloodvessels.—The regions of the brain just described are supplied by branches of the middle cerebral or Sylvian artery.

This vessel enters the fissure of Sylvius, and gives out branches which diverge between the convolutions of the insula. These branches are cortical and central. The former, destined for the peripheral parts of the brain, will be described in the next section, on Softening of the Brain. The latter arise from the Sylvian artery before the cortical branches enter the foramina of the anterior perforated space, and take the name of striate arteries. These striate arteries are internal and external. The internal ones, which are less important, give out branches to the two first segments of the lenticular nucleus and to the corresponding part of the internal capsule ; the external striate arteries, which are much more important, spread out on the surface of the lenticular nucleus, and divide into two groups—an anterior group, or lenticulo-striate arteries, and a posterior group, or lenticulo-optic arteries. The lenticulo-striate artery (anterior group) plunges into the third segment of the lenticular nucleus, traverses the internal capsule, and terminates in the caudate nucleus. It is so often the origin of the hæmorrhage that it has been called the **artery of cerebral hæmorrhage** (Charcot). The lenticulo-optic artery (posterior group) traverses the part farthest from the internal capsule, and enters the optic thalamus. It supplies the sensory portion of the internal capsule.

The importance of these vessels will be understood, because the central ganglia of the brain are supplied by them—not in an absolute manner, however, because the anterior cerebral artery sometimes sends a branch to the caudate nucleus, and the posterior cerebral artery gives off a branch to the internal part of the optic thalamus.

These anatomical facts will help us to grasp the **topography** of hæmorrhages in the central regions of the brain.

1. The hæmorrhage occurs most frequently in the area of the lenticulo-striate artery, where this vessel ascends over the external surface of the lenticular nucleus, so that the initial focus arises, not in the thickness of the grey matter, but on its surface between the nucleus and the external capsule. The resulting hemiplegia is curable, because the lesions of the external capsule, like the lesions of the grey nuclei, are not followed by sclerosis. If, however, the hæmorrhagic focus is large, it pushes the external capsule, with the convolutions, outwards, and displaces inwards the lenticular nucleus, the internal capsule, and the other central ganglia, and it may, by compressing these parts, diminish or destroy their functional activity.

2. The hæmorrhage takes place into the corpus striatum (the lenticulo-striate artery) or into the optic thalamus (region of the lenticulo-optic artery). In such a

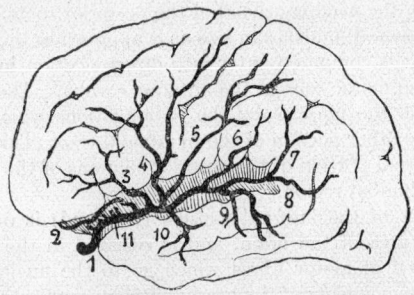

FIG. 70.—DISTRIBUTION OF THE SYLVIAN ARTERY.

1, Sylvian artery; 2, orbital artery; 3, inferior frontal artery; 4, ascending frontal artery; 5, ascending parietal artery; 6, inferior parietal artery; 7, artery of the angular gyrus; 8, 9, 10, temporal arteries; 11, perforating arteries.

case, the focus, if of small size, remains confined to the grey matter, and only causes a slight hemiplegia; if it is of large size, it invades the neighbouring parts, or at least it compresses them *en masse*, and causes grave phenomena.

3. The hæmorrhage takes place in the caudate nucleus (lenticulo-striate artery, and sometimes the anterior cerebral artery). This condition is serious, because the focus fairly frequently opens into the lateral ventricle.

4. The hæmorrhage takes place in the internal portion of the optic thalamus (the internal posterior optic artery, from the posterior cerebral). The hæmorrhage is very grave, because it is often followed by inundation of the ventricle.

Secondary Sclerotic Degeneration.—Hæmorrhage, softening, encephalitis, and in some cases tumours, may cause descending sclerosis through the brain, the mesencephalon, and the spinal cord. Descending sclerosis does not occur if the cerebral lesion is limited to the grey matter of the corpus striatum and to the optic thalamus, or to the grey matter of the motor convolutions; but if the lesion attacks the pyramidal tract in any part of its course, the tract below the lesion may become the seat of descending sclerosis.

The sclerotic tract can be made out with the naked eye, and under the microscope it corresponds exactly to the pyramidal tract. Its consistency is firm, and its colour is sometimes greyish. It occupies the anterior two-thirds of the posterior segment of the internal capsule, the median part of the inferior stage of the cerebral peduncle, and the anterior pyramid of the bulb. It decussates at the neck of the bulb, and descends into the spinal cord, diminishing progressively in size. In transverse sections of the spinal cord it is seen to occupy the posterior part of the lateral column.

Under the microscope the nerve fibres are in part atrophied, or have disappeared. The connective tissue is abundant and fibrillary. The destructive cerebral lesion causes a change comparable with Waller's degeneration. The nerve fibre becomes degenerated, and the connective proliferation is a secondary production.

In some cases the secondary degeneration does not stop in the fibres of the spinal cord, but is carried by these fibres as far as the anterior cornua of the spinal cord, with which they are in connection. The anterior cornu diminishes in size; the nerve cells are granular, and lose their nuclei and their prolongations. Muscular atrophy is the result.

Ætiology—Pathogenesis.—Many people who suffer from cerebral hæmorrhage have the so-called apoplectic constitution (short neck and congested face). The ætiology of cerebral hæmorrhage is complex, but

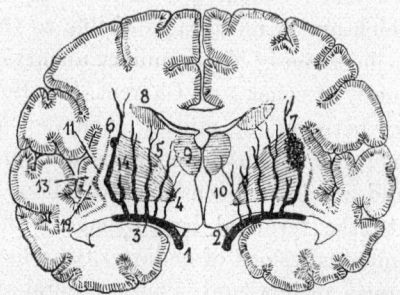

FIG. 71.—TRANSVERSE SECTION OF THE BRAIN.

1, Internal carotid artery; 2, anterior cerebral artery; 3, Sylvian artery; 4, internal striate arteries; 5, external striate arteries; 6, lenticulo-striate artery, with miliary aneurysm; 7, cerebral hæmorrhage; 8, caudate nucleus; 9, optic thalamus; 10, internal capsule; 11, claustrum; 12, external capsule; 13, insula; 14, lenticular nucleus.

side by side with secondary or rare causes, such as blood-changes, purpura, icterus gravis, leucocythæmia, etc., there exists one cause which dominates the pathogenesis of cerebral hæmorrhage—I mean the change in the blood-vessels. The diseased artery becomes ruptured; this is the initial fact, and the hæmorrhage is only the consequence. What, however, is this change in the vessel? Is it a fatty degeneration of the walls, an endarteritis with atheroma, or a periarteritis?

Certain writers (Paget) supposed that the hæmorrhage depends on fatty degeneration of the arterioles, but this so-called degeneration is only an accumulation of fatty granulations in the lymphatic sheath of the vessel, an accumulation consequent on the necrobiosis of the cerebral matter by softening, hæmorrhage, etc. (Billroth). The whole interest in the question is centred in the vascular lesions of endarteritis and periarteritis. But what share belongs to each of these lesions in the causation of hæmorrhage ? Are endarteritis and atheroma sufficient to cause rupture of the vessel (Bouillaud, Rokitansky), or are they only concomitants of the periarteritis, which is said to be the real cause of the miliary aneurysms, which rupture and give rise to the hæmorrhage ?

We know that the vascular system of the brain may be attacked by diffuse periarteritis or endoperiarteritis of slow course, and leading to a change in the vessel walls. The arterioles are invaded by sclerotic tissue. The lesion commences in the tunica externa and in the tunica intima (endoarteritis), whilst the contractile elements of the tunica media become atrophied and disappear without fatty substitution. These partial losses of substance diminish the resistance of the vessels, and are the cause of miliary aneurysms.

These small aneurysms, which, on an average, have a diameter of $\frac{1}{2}$ millimetre, and which are in most cases visible to the naked eye, finally rupture and cause hæmorrhage. These miliary aneurysms had been noticed by Cruveilhier, Meynert, Heschel, and Charcot, but Bouchard was the first to show the relations between the miliary aneurysm and cerebral hæmorrhage. We know how the miliary aneurysms are formed, and how they become ruptured, and we have been able to follow the lesion from the initial periarteritis to the terminal hæmorrhage. These changes do not resemble the atheromatous lesions of endarteritis, which are limited to the deep layers of the tunica intima, and, whilst cerebral atheroma is especially connected with thrombosis and softening, sclerotic periarteritis provokes the hæmorrhage. Does this mean that atheroma is to be banished from the pathogenesis of cerebral hæmorrhage ? The answer is negative, because we find both the lesions of endarteritis and those of periarteritis. The lacunæ of cerebral disintegration, which are frequent in old people, may be the cause of the hæmorrhage. We must not forget injury.

The vascular changes that lead to miliary aneurysms are often associated with certain morbid conditions, such as Bright's disease (arteriosclerosis), alcoholism, gout, and diabetes. Let me add that cerebral congestion from any cause tends to produce hæmorrhage in a predisposed individual (high tension, cardiac hypertrophy, sudden action of cold).

The pathogenic rôle of syphilis is evident. Syphilitic arteritis, which shows a preference for the cerebral arteries, causes either the obliteration of the vessel and consequent thrombosis and softening, or aneurysm, rupture of the bloodvessel, and hæmorrhage. I shall refer to this question under Cerebral Syphilis.

Although cerebral hæmorrhage may be the appanage of advanced age, it

shows itself also during various periods of life. It is essentially **hereditary,** *
as I have shown in a previous monograph—more hereditary, even, than
phthisis and cancer. In the same family it causes apoplexy and hemiplegia. The gravity of the case, recovery, and rapid death or survival, are
subordinate only to the localization of the cerebral lesion. It strikes several
members of the same family, and it sometimes happens that, in the same
progeny, a younger generation is attacked before an older one.

Description.—Cerebral hæmorrhage shows itself—(1) by primary symptoms, which supervene at the time of the hæmorrhage, or shortly afterwards ;
(2) by secondary symptoms, which only appear some weeks or months
later. In some cases cerebral hæmorrhage is preceded by prodromata
(headache, hot flushes, and temporary congestion of the head), which may
last for weeks or months. As a rule, prodromata are absent, and
apoplexy or hemiplegia comes on suddenly while the individual is in good
health.

1. **Primary Symptoms.**—Apoplexy is not a frequent symptom in cerebral hæmorrhage ; we might almost say that it is rare. Apoplexy means
total loss of movement and of sensation, according to the ancient definition
of Galen—a definition, unfortunately, changed by Rochoux, and turned by
him from its true sense. Rochoux was so convinced that apoplexy is
always the result of cerebral hæmorrhage that he made a synonym of it,
and from that time the word **apoplexy,** carelessly used, serves to designate
the lesion (that is to say, the hæmorrhage) or the symptom (that is to
say, the loss of movement and of sensation). The custom having once been
acquired, " capillary apoplexy " (Cruveilhier) was written for capillary
hæmorrhage, " apoplexy of the lung " for hæmorrhage from the lung—faulty
terms which must be abandoned. The word " apoplexy " usually awakens
the idea of suddenness. Let me explain. Fulminant apoplexy is very rare
(bulbar hæmorrhage) ; most frequently the apoplexy comes on slowly,
taking ten minutes, half an hour, or even longer, to develop (Trousseau).

The patient is in a condition of complete unconsciousness. His face is
congested and his features are drawn towards the healthy side, whilst the
lips and the cheek of the paralyzed side are flaccid and puffed out at each
expiration. The head is most frequently turned to the non-paralyzed side,
and the eyes are turned towards the same side (Vulpian and Prevost). This
conjugate deviation of the head and eyes generally ceases when the apoplexy
disappears.

During the apoplectic period, or after the unconsciousness, convulsions
and contractures may appear. They have been called " early " to distinguish them from the late contractures, and must be considered, says

* Dieulafoy. Communication à l'Académie de Médecine (see *Gazette Hebdomadaire*,
1876).

Straus, "rather as tonic convulsions than as real contractures." These convulsions and contractures, which may be limited to the paralyzed side or may invade both sides and the face, are phenomena of excitation, and generally indicate that the hæmorrhage affects the ventricles, the meninges, or the mesencephalon. They are hardly ever seen in apoplexy from cerebral softening. In the apoplectic patient most of the reflex movements are abolished; micturition and defæcation are affected (incontinence or retention). The respiration is noisy, irregular, slowed, and then accelerated. The temperature falls in the initial period, and rises later as high as 106° F. The patient may recover, but the gradual acceleration of the respiration and of the pulse, the constant rise of the temperature, and the appearance of general convulsions, are fatal signs.

Lumbar puncture yields limpid yellowish or bloody fluid (Sicard). It is probable that the red tint only exists when there is diffusion of the blood by ventricular inundation, consequent on cerebral hæmorrhage, or else hæmorrhage into the posterior part of the spinal pia mater, consequent on cerebral hæmorrhage.

The pathogenesis of apoplexy in cerebral hæmorrhage has been variously interpreted. The irruption of the blood into the interior of the ventricles or on the surface of the brain realizes the most favourable conditions for the production of apoplexy, often accompanied in such a case by convulsions and contractures. How are we to explain apoplexy produced by hæmorrhage limited to the opto-striate bodies? Congestion of the encephalon, pressure produced by the focus and cerebral anæmia, have in turn been suggested (Niemayer). I prefer the more rational interpretation of **reflex apoplexy** to these hypotheses (Jaccoud).

Hemiplegia.—Hemiplegia means paralysis of one side of the body. It is on the opposite side to the cerebral lesion: hæmorrhage on the left side, hemiplegia on the right side, and *vice versa*. The hemiplegia may be total or partial. When it is total, it involves the leg, the arm, and one side of the face; when it is partial, it spares one or other of these parts. Hemiplegia follows sometimes on an attack of apoplexy, but it more often appears from the outset, without apoplexy and without any loss of consciousness. A patient wakes up with hemiplegia, having been stricken with cerebral hæmorrhage during sleep. Another patient witnesses his hemiplegia; he experiences a sensation of tingling in his hand, he drags his leg, his mouth is twisted, he sputters, and the hemiplegia takes a quarter of an hour, half an hour, or even a few hours, to become complete, without any intellectual failing.

In the **face** the paralysis, unlike the peripheral paralysis of the facial nerve, does not attack, or attacks but slightly, the orbicularis palpebrarum. Facial hemiplegia betrays itself by deviation of the mouth, the healthy muscles drawing the angle of the mouth upwards and outwards towards the healthy side. When the tongue is put out, its tip is directed towards the paralyzed side of the face (action of the genio-glossus muscle).

In the **limbs** the hemiplegia is more marked in the arm than in the leg. All forms are seen, from absolute loss of movement to simple paresis. The temperature is generally higher on the paralyzed side; the muscular contractility is preserved.

The symmetrical muscles, the movements of which are associated with those of the opposite side, escape paralysis; they are the muscles of the thorax and abdomen and the motor muscles of the eyes.

In some cases the hemiplegia is crossed (Gubler), the limbs being paralyzed on the left side, and the face on the right. These paralyses, resulting from a lesion in the pons or in the bulb, have been described in one of the preceding sections.

The **duration** of hemiplegia is variable. After some days or weeks movement reappears in the leg, and then in the arm. Persons have been known to have two or three attacks and recover. Some remain hemiplegic, the paralyzed limbs being flaccid; but flaccid hemiplegia is extremely rare. Finally, others—and they are numerous—have a progressive contracture, which is permanent and localized in the paralyzed limbs.

Hemianœsthesia.—Hemianæsthesia means the loss of sensation in one-half of the body. When it is general, it affects the skin, the mucosæ, and the sense organs (sensitivo-sensorial). It is rare in hæmorrhage, and more frequent in softening. It appears when the posterior third of the posterior segment of the internal capsule is affected, this region being traversed by the sensory fibres. These fibres are said to be the general sensory conductors, and a lesion in their cerebral course is said to cause sensitivo-sensorial hemianæsthesia, whereas a lesion in the mesencephalon is said to cause incomplete hemianæsthesia (sight and smell being normal). There are, however, cases in which a lesion of the lenticular nucleus may attack only a part of the sensory fibres in the internal capsule. In this case general sensibility is abolished, the special senses being unaffected, because their nerve fibres occupy the innermost part of the sensory tract (Ballet). The territory which forms the sensory tract is supplied by the lenticulo-optic artery, so that hæmorrhage, embolism, softening, and tumours cause hemianæsthesia.

Vascular and Trophic Troubles.—Vascular and trophic troubles belong to the initial period of cerebral hæmorrhage. In apoplexy the patient is exposed to such grave troubles as bastard pneumonia, pulmonary congestion, with emphysema and hæmorrhage, lesions recalling the broncho-pulmonary changes that follow experimental section of the pneumogastric nerves (Charcot). We must also mention polyuria, albuminuria (Ollivier), ecchymoses of the pleura, of the endocardium, of the pericardium, of the stomach, and of the kidneys. The various joint troubles generally belong to the secondary period, but the gluteal bedsore appears in the initial period. This bedsore develops in the centre of the gluteal region on the paralyzed side, whereas the bedsore of acute myelitis develops in the middle of the sacral region. The bedsore begins with diffuse redness, which appears a day or two after the attack; a pustule then forms, breaks, and ends in ulceration. The gluteal bedsore is of very grave significance (Charcot).

2. **Secondary Symptoms.**—These symptoms supervene some weeks or months after the hæmorrhage.

Secondary Contracture.—In some patients with hemiplegia we notice, two or three months after the hæmorrhage, in the paralyzed limbs more or less pronounced contracture, which is at times permanent and incurable. This contracture is due to descending sclerosis in the pyramidal tract. The sclerosis is consecutive to a destructive lesion of the cerebral expansion of the pyramidal tract.

Pathological anatomy has proved, in fact, that, when cerebral hæmorrhage or softening remains confined to the optic thalamus or the claustrum, descending sclerosis does not occur, and the patient may recover from the hemiplegia ; but when the lesion involves the pyramidal tract, either in the corona radiata or in the internal capsule, secondary sclerosis is seen in the inferior part of the cerebral peduncle, the pons, the bulb, and the opposite lateral column of the spinal cord. This sclerosis is accompanied by contracture.

Descending sclerosis and contracture are not provoked by cortical lesions when the lesion only involves the grey matter of the convolutions. When the subjacent white matter is attacked—and it is always attacked in embolism of the branches of the Sylvian artery which supply the motor territories of the cortex—we meet with descending sclerosis and contracture. I may add that outside the motor regions the cortical white matter of the other regions may be affected without giving rise to secondary sclerosis.

The irritative lesion of the fibres of the lateral columns, by communicating an abnormal excitability to the anterior grey matter of the spinal cord (motor cornua), leads to an exaggerated tonus, which by its severity or permanence constitutes contracture, with exaggeration of the reflexes.

Secondary contracture in patients suffering from hemiplegia is announced by a feeling of stiffness and by an exaggeration of the tendon reflexes. When, two or three weeks after the attack, a patient suffering from hemiplegia presents exaggerated tendon reflexes on the paralyzed side, contracture may be foretold. The contracture is generally painful, and is localized at first in one of the upper limbs, more frequently in the flexor than in the extensor muscles. The fingers, the wrist, and the forearm are forcibly flexed, and the arm is adducted against the trunk. The contracture only attacks the upper limb when the sclerosis of the lateral columns does not extend beyond the superior regions of the spinal cord, but it affects the lower limb if the sclerosis attacks the lumbar region. It is less pronounced in the lower limb, and the extensor type predominates. The leg is forcibly extended, but the toes are flexed, and chloroform cannot overcome the contracture of hemiplegia, as it overcomes the contracture of hysterical patients. Babinski's sign and Strümpell's phenomenon are noticed at this period. The muscles of the face which are affected in hemiplegia sometimes show contracture. The deviation of the features, then, changes sides, and simulates crossed paralysis.

Contracture in patients with hemiplegia varies. It is sometimes so slight that it may at first be taken for flaccid hemiplegia. In other cases it is so marked that it constitutes an incurable deformity. In some patients with hemiplegia the contracture finally disappears, but as a rule the cure is incomplete. The patient can, it is true, move the limbs which have been paralyzed and contracted ; but if he wishes to apply his attention, and to make use of his hand for a specific purpose, the muscular rigidity immediately reappears. In other patients a contracture of old standing disappears in a fairly rapid manner, but this disappearance coincides with the muscular atrophy of the primarily contracted muscles.

The atrophy commences in the thenar eminence or in the shoulder, and becomes general. The tendon reflexes become sluggish or disappear. This muscular atrophy is due to the change in the anterior cornua of the spinal cord, a change carried to them by the degenerated nerve fibres of the pyramidal tract with which they are connected. When the limb is attacked by atrophy, the infirmity is incurable. People attacked by hemiplegia with contracture present the phenomenon known as syncinesia (Vulpian). When a patient is told to close the healthy hand, a similar but imperfect movement is seen in the affected hand.

Tremor—Hemichorea—Athetosis.—People who have long been suffering from hemiplegia, and who have been stricken with secondary contracture, are sometimes attacked by a tremor which only supervenes at the time of a voluntary movement. As soon as the patient tries to raise the contracted arm to the head, the entire arm and the hand are seized with a tremor, made up of regular, vertical, and rapid oscillations. This tremor disappears when the arm is at rest, but recommences as soon as the muscles are contracted. When the foot is suddenly raised in paralysis, with contracture of the lower limb, the same phenomenon is produced. This tremor must not be confounded with other motor troubles, such as epileptiform convulsions, which are sometimes seen in patients suffering from hemiplegia. The convulsions are, without doubt, dependent on the descending sclerosis and on the secondary irritation of the bulb.

Other sufferers from hemiplegia show choreiform movements in the paralyzed limbs. This symptomatic hemichorea has all the characteristics of true chorea, showing similar disorder in the voluntary and involuntary movements, whether the limbs are at rest or whether there is voluntary movement.

Hemichorea generally shows itself in hemiplegia, accompanied by hemianæsthesia. It appears progressively after several weeks or months, at a time when the hemiplegia shows a tendency to improve, and although there is a certain degree of contracture in the affected limbs. This hemichorea, which is called "post-paralytic" because it supervenes after the hemiplegia, may last indefinitely. In some cases the hemiplegia does not declare itself after, but before, the hemiplegia ; it is called " preparalytic " (Grasset), a term which is preferable to " prehæmorrhagic." This preparalytic hemichorea may develop at the moment of an attack of apoplexy, even before the stage of confirmed hemiplegia, and apart from any symptom of hemianæsthesia and of contracture. It is temporary, and lasts only a few days, even when the patient survives the apoplexy ; the choreiform movements are then replaced by hemiplegia.

Hemichorea, like contracture and tremor, may be provoked by hæmorrhage, softening, tumour, or congenital atrophy of the brain. It is therefore not the nature, but the seat, of the lesion which must be sought for in order to discover the cause of the symptom. Hemichorea is most frequently associated with hemianæsthesia. The respective sites of the lesions must be very close, but it is not a single one, because the two symptoms may be isolated. Raymond places the lesions in the posterior portion of the internal capsule. The bundles which are said to be more especially associated with hemichorea are those covering the posterior extremity of the optic thalamus. They are situated outside and in front of the bundles, wherein a lesion produces hemianæsthesia. According to the correct remark of Grasset, these two regions have practically an independent circulation. The lenticulo-optic artery, arising from the Sylvian, supplies the region wherein a lesion produces hemianæsthesia, and the posterior optic artery, arising from the posterior cerebral, supplies the territory wherein a lesion produces hemichorea.

According to some authors, hemichorea is said to supervene when the provoking lesion is seated at some point in the pyramidal tract, and the loss of equilibrium in the muscular system is said to be due to the contracture (Brissaud) or to the paralysis. According to other writers, the provoking lesion is said to be situated in the pyramidal tract, but in the neighbourhood of the optic thalamus, the optic thalami containing reflex centres which are important for the nerve supply of the co-ordinate muscles of the body.

Athetosis (Hammond) is a motor trouble, characterized by incessant movements of the fingers and of the toes. These movements are slow, and are not always limited to the fingers and the toes ; they sometimes invade the hand and the foot. It has been suggested that athetosis is a special affection of the nervous system, but as certain patients have also shown choreiform movements, it is probable that athetosis which supervenes in patients who have long been suffering from hemiplegia is only a variety of post-hemiplegic chorea.

Secondary Trophic Troubles.—Arthropathy in patients suffering from hemiplegia may supervene a fortnight, a month, or much longer after the attack. The arm is chiefly affected. The trouble is accompanied by exudative synovitis, with swelling and pain. Muscular atrophy is not rare, but it has neither the regularity nor the course of progressive muscular atrophy. On the contrary, the atrophy affects irregularly a muscle or a group of muscles ; it ends by causing incurable infirmity. The atrophy is sometimes masked by adiposis of the subcutaneous connective tissue. This adiposis, which is rare in primary muscular atrophy, is common in secondary atrophy. We must not forget hemiœdema.

Course—Duration—Prognosis.—The symptoms of cerebral hæmorrhage sometimes commence with apoplexy, but more often with hemiplegia. **Aphasia,** which is fairly frequent in softening, is here excessively rare, and the differences in the seat and in the extension of the hæmorrhagic focus give rise to various clinical types.

1. If the hæmorrhage originates in one of the nuclei or on its surface, and if it remains limited there, without bursting into the ventricles and damaging the internal capsule, the hemiplegia is very frequently curable without subsequent contracture.

2. If the hæmorrhage occurs in the lateral ventricles or on the surface of the brain, it is almost always fatal, and, in general, accompanied by apoplexy, epileptiform convulsions, early contractures, coma, and rise in temperature, which continue till death.

3. If the hæmorrhage involves the pyramidal tract in the internal capsule, or if this tract is compressed by a neighbouring focus, irritation is the result, with descending sclerosis, traceable through the corresponding peduncle, the pons, the bulb, and the spinal cord. This sclerosis becomes the starting-point of late contractures, tremors, and even of muscular atrophy, if the irritative and destructive process spreads to the anterior cornua of the spinal cord. This form of hemiplegia is incurable.

4. Another incurable, though much rarer, form is hemiplegia which persists indefinitely in the flaccid condition (Bouchard), without secondary contracture of the paralyzed limbs. It is probable that this flaccid hemiplegia is due to a lesion of the motor tracts which has not been followed by descending sclerosis.

5. If the hæmorrhage, by the extension of the initial focus or by compression, directly or indirectly destroys the sensory tract in the posterior segment of the internal capsule, hemianæsthesia accompanies the hemiplegia. In such a case we may also notice another symptom—viz., hemichorea and athetosis. Hemianæsthesia and hemichorea are exceptional, because the hæmorrhage rarely attacks this part of the capsule.

6. When the hæmorrhage remains confined to one of the striate or optic nuclei, clinical medicine has not yet shown which is the nucleus involved, and what is the value of this localization from the point of view of the course and of the prognosis of the disease.

7. Hæmorrhages into the cortical matter of the brain are very rare, and their symptoms will be better studied under Cerebral Softening and Cerebral Localization.

Diagnosis.—Meningeal hæmorrhage, acute hydrocephalus, cerebral congestion, intracranial neoplasms (tumours of various kinds, gummata, etc.), injuries to the skull, and epilepsy, are often accompanied by apoplexy. I may say as much for uræmia and plumbism, diabetes (diabetic coma), and certain intoxications (opium, belladonna, henbane). Besides the conjugate deviation of the head and of the eyes, which is a diagnostic sign of great value, a rise in temperature will eliminate toxic coma. Next, in these various cases the apoplectic condition is more rarely accompanied by **symptoms of hemiplegia,** which are met with in cerebral hæmorrhage. The apoplexy due to cerebral embolism is almost identical with the apoplexy due to hæmorrhage.

Chromo-diagnosis, based on the colour of the cerebro-spinal fluid, allows us to make the diagnosis of hæmorrhage when the colour of this liquid is blood-stained, or even yellowish (Sicard).

Hemiplegia due to cerebral hæmorrhage differs from hemiplegia due to other lesions of the brain in the course of events. In cerebral tumours the hemiplegia is incomplete, slow rather than sudden, and almost always announced by precursory phenomena, such as headache, vomiting, epileptiform convulsions, ocular troubles, and paralyses which, according to the seat of the tumour, attack one or other of the cranial nerves.

When the hemiplegia is due to thrombosis of the cerebral arteries, the patient shows the usual causes of arteritis and atheroma (old age, gout, syphilis, alcoholism). In some cases the peripheral arteries are converted into hard tortuous cords. The hemiplegia is variable,* slow, and progressive ; it is less often sudden and complete from the outset.

Hysteria may cause apoplexy and hemiplegia, with or without contracture, but hysterical hemiplegia rarely attacks the face. It is rarely accom-

---

* In variable hemiplegia the alternate progressive and retrograde march points to a lesion which at the first blow does not destroy the functions of the invaded area.

panied by contracture of the facial muscles on the side opposite to the hemiplegia. It is almost always accompanied by hemianæsthesia. Furthermore, the motor troubles in hysteria are in general associated with other manifestations of this neurosis, such as ovarian hyperæsthesia, globus hystericus, abdominal tympanism, anorexia, ocular troubles, hysterogenous zones, etc.

The diagnosis is sometimes difficult because hystero-organic associations are not rare (Babinski). Fever, incontinence of fæces, and acute bedsores are in favour of organic hemiplegia. The diagnosis of organic hemiplegia is also based on the following signs : *Signe du peaucier*, exaggerated flexion of the forearm, combined flexion of the thigh and of the trunk (Babinski). The *signe du peaucier* is as follows : when a patient with organic hemiplegia is asked to yawn, blow, or whistle, the platysma contracts better on the healthy side than on the diseased side. When the forearm is placed in the position of supination and flexed on the arm, the flexion on the paralyzed side is greater than on the healthy side. Finally, if the patient lies flat on a resisting horizontal plane, and is asked to assume a sitting position, it will be noticed that the thigh of the paralyzed side flexes on the pelvis. This movement of flexion is much less marked on the healthy side. These facts point to relaxation of the muscles in the case of organic hemiplegia. We must also inquire into the cutaneous plantar reflex (Babinski's sign). If the plantar surface of the foot is pricked, we see flexion of the toes on the healthy side and extension of the toes, especially of the big toe, on the affected side. This extension never exists in hysterical hemiplegia, where flexion is the rule. Babinski's sign has, then, a diagnostic value, which has been confirmed by several observers (Létienne, Cestan, and Le Sourd). Such are the chief factors in the diagnosis between hysterical and organic hemiplegia.

Hemiplegia of **syphilitic** origin (gummata, sclero-gummatous meningitis, obliterating arteritis, rupture of an aneurysm) is often preceded by prodromata (headache, paresis of the third and seventh nerves, etc.). It may nevertheless resemble in all points hemiplegia due to cerebral hæmorrhage. Although it is more frequent in the tertiary stage, it sometimes appears, with or without apoplexy, in the secondary stage. The history of the patient must be carefully inquired into, and we must look on the skin or elsewhere for the marks of syphilis, in order to institute treatment without delay (*vide* Cerebral Syphilis).

Treatment.—Apoplexy is treated by bleeding, leeches behind the ears, enemata, purgatives, and counter-irritation of the lower extremities. Hemiplegia may be alleviated by means of the continuous current. The early movement of the joints is of great use. By moving the joints of the shoulder, of the fingers, of the wrist, or of the elbow, etc., and massaging the muscles,

we can obtain remarkable results (Gilles de la Tourette).   The patient should
be advised to go to the seaside or to a saline watering-place.   Balaruc seems
to enjoy a well-merited reputation (Grasset).   The cure at La Malou is
also of service.   We must always remember the possible existence of syphilis,
in order to have recourse to mercurial preparations and to large doses of
iodide of potassium.

IV. CEREBRAL SOFTENING—EMBOLISM—ATHEROMA.

The expression " cerebral softening " does not answer to a morbid entity. Softening of the brain does not constitute a disease, but is the result of various pathological
conditions, such as encephalitis, atheroma, arteritis, thrombosis, and embolism of the
cerebral vessels. Encephalitis will be described separately. I shall here describe
cerebral softening due to vascular lesions (atheroma, arteritis, and embolism).

Rostan (1820) was the first to fix the clinical history of softening, and, clever observer
that he was, he took care to assign various causes for it, having remarked that in some
cases cerebral softening is the product of an inflammation, and that in other circumstances it is secondary to vascular changes due to senility or other causes. The writers,
however, who continued the study of softening after Rostan (Lallemand, Bouillaud,
Durand-Fardel) were so imbued with the teaching of Broussais, and the idea of inflammation was then so dominant, that cerebral softening was made synonymous with
encephalitis, acute softening being looked upon as an acute encephalitis, and chronic
softening as a chronic encephalitis. In 1847 Virchow produced his first monograph on
embolism and thrombosis, and though others had previously indicated or foreseen the
troubles consequent on the vascular lesions of the brain, it is just to recognize that
Virchow originated the anatomical and experimental researches (Prévost and Costard)
which have shed light on the pathogenic history of cerebral softening.

Pathological Anatomy.—When the circulation is arrested in an area
of the brain by obliteration of the arteries, veins or capillaries, by an obliterating body arising *in situ* (thrombus and thrombosis), or by a migratory body
(embolus and embolism), and the collateral circulation does not come to the
help of the anæmic area, this area degenerates (necrobiosis) and softens.
Such is, in a few words, the principle of softening from vascular lesions, but
these lesions do not all produce cerebral softening for the same reason.

Thus obliteration of the capillary vessels, simple or specific capillary
emboli, pigmentary emboli, which are said to be one of the results of melanæmia (Frerichs), calcareous emboli (Virchow), and putrid emboli (Panum),
may cause small foci of softening, but their history is too obscure for exact
details.

Thrombosis of the **venous sinuses** is a rare cause of softening, and in this
case the softening is superficial, and generally associated with other brain
lesions—œdema, hydrocephalus, and changes in the meninges.

Thrombosis and **embolism of the arteries** are the most frequent
sources of cerebral softening, and if the collateral circulation is ofter.
powerless to re-establish the course of the blood in an affected vessel, it
is because this collateral circulation is little developed in the brain.   The

central and cortical arteries of the brain are **terminal** arteries (Cohnheim)—that is to say, arteries which from their origin to their termination receive hardly any anastomotic vessels. Accordingly, obliteration of these vessels is readily followed by necrobiosis of the region supplied by them, and the result is a focus of softening.

In the post-mortem examination of an individual who has died during the first period of acute softening of the brain, or in that of an animal in which artificial embolism has been produced (Prévost and Cotard), the embolized region forms a focus which is more deeply coloured at the circumference than in the centre, and which is often stippled red; this is red softening. Embolism of the small vessels usually causes an infarct in the embolized region. The word **infarct** means infiltration of the parenchyma by the extravasated blood (Hirtz and Straus). The process is as follows: When the obliteration attacks an arteriole, the embolized region is rendered ischæmic in the centre and hyperæmic at the circumference. The ischæmia of the centre is explained by the arrest of the circulation in the vessel, and the peripheral hyperæmia arises, no doubt, from the collateral congestion of the arterioles in the neighbourhood of the obstruction. This collateral congestion raises the tension in the capillaries, causing œdema, diapedesis of the blood-corpuscles, and even hæmorrhage into the lymphatic sheath of the vessels. The nerve tissue now becomes affected; its elements, deprived of nutrition, become dissociated; the myeline breaks up, and we have red softening. Later the broken up myeline undergoes fatty degeneration, the fatty granules infiltrate the leucocytes and the sheath of the vessels, the colouring matter of the blood is altered, and the softening assumes a yellowish tint (yellow softening). Finally, in the last stage the cerebral pulp assumes the characteristics of a milky liquid, and we have white softening. These successive phases, which have been produced experimentally, do not always occur in man, and in certain large foci the initial congestion is absent, and white softening takes place from the outset.

The foci vary in size from a pin's head (Parrot) to an orange. They are often irregular, and attack especially the **cerebral convolutions**—unlike hæmorrhage, which is most common in the central portions. When the softening is very extensive, the cerebral convolutions which form the wall of the focus are depressed, and even before opening the brain we may, by the external conformation, judge where the focus of softening is seated. In old cases of softening chronic encephalitis occurs, and the sclerosed neuroglia affects the walls of the focus. If the walls do not become adherent, a cyst results; in the contrary case, a cicatrix is formed. These cicatrices have a yellowish colour (Durand-Fardel); they are indurated, and formed of connective tissue, of fatty matter, and of hæmatoidin. At these points the convolutions are deformed and atrophied.

As secondary degenerations occur under the same conditions as in hæmorrhage, I refer the reader to the preceding section for details concerning **descending sclerosis.**

Besides the cerebral lesions which I have just described, we find, post mortem, vascular lesions, which are the cause of the softening—arterial embolism, atheroma, and obliterating arteritis.

Pathogenesis.—Let us now consider the pathogenesis of (1) softening by embolism and (2) softening by thrombosis.

1. Softening by Embolism.—We have to consider the origin, course, and termination of the embolism.

Chronic diseases of the left side of the heart, especially mitral stenosis (Duroziez), acute endocarditis, especially the emboligenous and infective forms, fibrinous coagula in the auricle in the aged (Vulpian), and lesions of the aorta, are the most common sources of cerebral embolism. The embolus rarely enters the innominate trunk, which opens obliquely into the aorta. It nearly always follows the left carotid, which is the more direct prolongation of the aortic trunk. The embolus passes into the internal carotid, and almost always enters the middle cerebral artery. It then obliterates, according to its size, the trunk of the vessel before or after the origin of the perforating arteries. It may also block a secondary arteriole, producing symptoms and paralyses, which vary according to the region involved. As the history of these symptoms and paralyses is inseparable from a knowledge of the cerebral circulation, and especially of the distribution of the Sylvian artery, I shall briefly mention these anatomical points.

The middle cerebral artery in the fissure of Sylvius gives off branches which diverge between the convolutions of the insula. These branches are of two kinds—central and cortical. The central or perforating branches, described under Cerebral Hæmorrhage, are destined for the corpus striatum, the optic thalamus, the internal capsule, and the corona radiata, and one of them acquires a great importance from the lenticulo-optic branch, which it furnishes to that portion of the internal capsule in which a lesion causes hemianæsthesia.

The cortical branches, which arise from the middle cerebral artery after the central branches, are : the artery of the inferior frontal convolution (a lesion in this region produces aphasia) ; the arteries of the **motor centres**—that is to say, the artery of the ascending frontal convolution—which sends a branch to the middle frontal convolution ; and the artery of the ascending parietal convolution. Then come the parieto-sphenoidal and the sphenoidal arteries.

Accordingly, an embolus which obliterates the Sylvian artery before the origin of the perforating arteries causes softening, which extends both to the central portions of the brain and also to the cortical regions just enumerated. We find, therefore, hemiplegia, hemianæsthesia, and aphasia. If the embolus blocks the artery beyond the origin of the perforating vessels, we find hemiplegia and aphasia without hemianæsthesia, because the lenticulo-optic artery remains patent. Isolated softening of the third left convolution has often caused aphasia without paralysis, so that aphasia and paralysis of the arm, of the leg, and of the face may be, according to circumstances, isolated or associated. The localization of the softening depends, therefore, on the situation of the embolus, which abolishes the circulation in a given region, as we shall see under Cerebral Localization.

2. **Softening by Thrombosis.**—Atheroma of the arteries of the brain plays a part in the ætiology and in the progress of atheroma in general. Old age, alcoholism, gout, diabetes, and the infectious diseases are the most potent causes of obliterating arteritis and of atheroma. Chronic arteritis and atheroma narrow the lumen of the vessel. Fibrin is deposited on the granulations, due to the endarteritis and on the patches of atheroma. An obliterating clot is formed, and when the thrombosis is complete, the area supplied by the obliterated vessel undergoes necrobiosis, unless the collateral circulation is established.

Syphilitic Arteritis.—Amongst the vascular lesions capable of causing cerebral softening, syphilitic arteritis is of the highest importance ; it shows a marked predilection for the cerebral arteries. Syphilitic arteritis and its results will be discussed under Cerebral Syphilis.

Symptoms.—According to circumstances, the commencement of cerebral softening is sudden or gradual.

1. **Softening of Sudden Onset.**—The sudden appearance of symptoms (apoplexy, hemiplegia, aphasia) is especially caused by embolism, because the embolus at once blocks the vessel which was permeable, whereas the slow and gradual appearance of symptoms is rather reserved for thrombosis, which gradually obliterates the lumen of the vessel. This rule is not absolute, and although thrombosis is slow to cause complete obliteration of the artery, yet there are cases, especially in syphilitic lesions (arteritis, sclerogummatous lesions, tumour) where the symptoms **appear almost as brusquely** as in vascular obliteration by embolism.

Softening of sudden onset and cerebral hæmorrhage have many symptoms in common. Softening, however, especially when it is dependent on syphilitic lesions, is more often preceded by **prodromata** (headache). In both cases apoplexy may open the scene, with its visceral congestions (pulmonary congestion) and its trophic troubles (gluteal bedsores).

Apoplexy is often absent, and the softening commences with hemiplegia. The hemiplegia has all the characteristics described under Cerebral Hæmorrhage. It is peculiar in that it attacks the right side, and in this case it is frequently associated with aphasia. This association of right hemiplegia and of aphasia is due to the predilection of the lesions for the left Sylvian artery—a predilection especially marked in embolism.

As apoplexy and hemiplegia have been described in detail under Cerebral

II. 85

Hæmorrhage, further reference is unnecessary. Amongst the troubles produced by cerebral softening, one of the most important is aphasia (loss of speech), which may exist alone or may be associated with right hemiplegia and with hemianæsthesia. For the description of aphasia I refer the reader to the next section.

We may also observe homonymous lateral hemianopia (loss of half of the visual field) in softening of the cuneus of the occipital lobe or of the gyrus supramarginalis.

2. **Softening of Gradual Onset.**—When softening of the brain is not due to embolism, the early symptoms are slow and progressive : the patient complains of headache, vertigo, twitchings of the fingers, and numbness in the foot ; the hand becomes awkward, the speech is embarrassed, and the mouth is crooked. This course of events occurs in syphilitic obliterating arteritis. Sometimes, and especially in the case of atheroma, the troubles may be dissociated, and so slight that the patient, especially if he is an old man, is scarcely conscious of them. They grow better or worse under the influence of various causes (digestive troubles), and the hemiplegia, which is rarely complete, is called **variable.**

In some cases an acute phase follows this slow onset, and the symptoms, which are at first mild, speedily reach their maximum. More frequently a chronic phase succeeds the slow phase of the onset ; this is the typical form of chronic softening.

Sometimes **intellectual troubles** precede or overshadow the paralytic troubles. The patient loses his memory, especially the recollection of recent events. His ideas are incoherent, his speech is embarrassed ; he laughs and cries without reason, and is subject to a kind of wandering, prone to end in delirium. These complications are slow and progressive, lasting for months and years. They are sometimes interrupted by apoplectiform or epileptiform attacks, by phases of excitation (restlessness, delirium, or mania), and by periods of depression (somnolence and coma). In addition to these motor and psychical troubles, which succeed one another or appear together, we find in rare instances obstinate vomiting, and contractures, which may assume a capital importance.

Secondary Symptoms.—Softening, like cerebral hæmorrhage, may be followed by secondary symptoms—progressive and permanent contracture, tremor, post-hemiplegic hemichorea, and muscular atrophy, proving that the descending sclerosis of the pyramidal tract depends on the situation of the invaded region, and not upon the nature of the lesion.

In describing cerebral softening, I have confined my attention to the most common varieties, which correspond anatomically with a fairly extensive lesion ; but there are cases in which the lesion is limited to a restricted area of the brain, with or without implication of the meninges. It occupies only one convolution of the brain, or a part of the convolution, attacking the grey matter or the subjacent white matter. Isolated symptoms are then noticed, and depend on the localization of the lesion. These symptoms are paralysis of the arm, paralysis of the leg, with or without contracture and epileptiform movements. These various symptoms will be discussed in detail under Cerebral Localization and Cerebral Syphilis.

Diagnosis—Prognosis.—Cerebral softening of **sudden onset** has many symptoms in common with cerebral hæmorrhage (apoplexy, hemiplegia). Certain signs are, however, in favour of softening. If the patient has right hemiplegia and also **aphasia,** softening may be diagnosed, for aphasia is very seldom due to hæmorrhage. If the patient has mitral or aortic disease, embolism is the probable cause of the softening. If he has atheromatous arteries, softening by thrombosis is naturally suspected; and if the patient is **syphilitic,** it is probable that the softening has its origin in the compression of an artery by a syphiloma, or more often in **obliterating arteritis.**

Softening is sometimes difficult to distinguish from the clinical syndrome caused by **lacunæ of the brain.** A patient suffering from **lacuna** is one who has been attacked by a sudden but slight stroke, without loss of consciousness, followed by partial and incomplete hemiplegia. The gait is somewhat affected, and is known under the name of the *marche à petits pas.* We also find troubles of pronunciation and of deglutition, as well as spasmodic laughing and crying. Softening of **slow onset,** due to cerebral atheroma, is difficult to diagnose, because its manifestations are often incomplete and insidious. It must be remembered that the aged are subject to apoplectiform or epileptiform symptoms and to intellectual troubles dependent on cerebral atheroma. When a patient shows at the same time signs of general atheromasia, it is probable that his cerebral troubles are due to cerebral softening of atheromatous origin.

The gravity of the **prognosis** is readily understood. Softening by embolism is serious on account of the extent of the lesion. Softening by thrombosis is formidable, because it is often associated with general arteriosclerosis.

Treatment is generally useless, except in **syphilitic** cases. If syphilis is even suspected, active specific treatment must be employed without delay. Mercurial injections and iodide of potassium in large doses are especially indicated.

V. APHASIA.

Description.—In the preceding section I pointed out that obliteration of the left Sylvian artery by embolism or by thrombosis may be followed by right hemiplegia and by aphasia.

85—2

What, then, is **aphasia**? It is the loss of speech. It is even more. Aphasia, when complete, includes not only loss of speech, but also loss of the power of writing, of making gestures, and of mimicry. In a word, it is the loss of **language,** the word " language " being taken in the widest acceptation of the term. This question of language has been well put by Gratiolet. There is a natural language by which the internal condition of the individual is revealed, in spite of himself ; and there is an artificial language, in which thought, clothed in a certain form, is expressed, this form being, according to circumstances, speech, writing, or gesture. In aphasia, then, the person preserves natural language ; if he has a feeling of gladness, of sadness, or of anger, this feeling betrays itself in his whole person, in spite of himself. But artificial language is absent, and, if you ask him to express this same sentiment by means of speech, writing, or mimicry, he is absolutely incapable of telling you the name of an object, the use of which he knows perfectly, and he is conscious of this incapacity, which betrays itself by gestures of impatience.

When the aphasia declares itself, the patient usually has some intellectual troubles (loss of memory, hebetude). These troubles are generally temporary ; volition and understanding are preserved, and the patient can conceive and associate ideas, but he has lost the means of communicating them to others, and when he wishes to transform his ideas into signs, to adapt the proper words to them, or to reproduce them in writing, he is incapable of so doing.

The person suffering from aphasia has at his command only a few mono-syllables or a single word, which he articulates perfectly, and invariably repeats apropos of everything. One man can only say " yes "; another only the word " tan." One of Trousseau's patients could only say the word " cousisi." If the patient is shown a knife or a pencil, although he knows the object and its use, he cannot clothe the idea with the proper word. Ask him the name of the object, and his gestures will immediately manifest his satisfaction at finding this word again ; but ask him to repeat the word " knife " or " pencil," and he is quite unable to do so, or else after an effort he utters some word or other. The phonatory apparatus is intact, but the apparatus which puts the conceived idea into words is broken. In the long run the patient regains this function, but when the lesion is deeply seated the patient suffering from aphasia does not completely recover ; he is **lame in his brain** (Trousseau). It will, therefore, be understood that the capacity of patients suffering from aphasia to make a will should be raised.

In some cases, as we have said, the trouble of language, joined to a defect of transmission, is revealed by **agraphia.** The patient can no longer write. Paralysis of the right arm, which is often associated with aphasia, may prevent our noticing this symptom, but even if the paralysis is slight or absent, the patient attacked by agraphia can no more write (either with the right hand or the left) than the patient suffering from aphasia can speak. Agraphia may exist alone or may coincide with aphasia.

In addition to the variety of aphasia which I have just described, and which represents the most common case, we find other varieties. In certain subjects the intellectual faculties are affected on account of the extent of the cerebral lesion ; in others the aphasia is incomplete, and the patient **substitutes** in the midst of a word or of a phrase letters or syllables which make the word or phrase unintelligible. This is called **paraphasia.** The patient also makes this substitution when he writes. Sometimes the various modes of expression are alone attacked. Lassègue speaks of a musician suffering from aphasia who could neither read nor write, but who jotted down a musical phrase which he had heard sung. The power of mimicry is not always lost in aphasia. It is at times exaggerated. The form of aphasia just described has received the name of **motor** aphasia, in order to distinguish it from **sensory** aphasia, which we shall now consider.

Certain individuals are not, properly speaking, suffering from aphasia because they can speak and write, but they are affected, according to Kussmaul's expression, with word-blindness or word-deafness. In word-deafness the sense of hearing has preserved its delicacy, since the ticking of a watch is readily perceived ; the intelligence is intact, and the subject replies clearly and aloud to the questions addressed to him in writing. If he is spoken to, he understands nothing, hearing only a succession of noises, which do not convey to him the form of words, and have no signification to his mind.

In word-blindness the patient is able to speak and to write, but he is unable to read. The letters only represent to his mind a succession of lines, just as in the case of word-deafness the words only represent a succession of noises. In such cases the association is broken between the conventional sign (the spoken or written word) and the idea. In motor aphasia the patient is incapable of transforming his ideas into external signs, but he perceives these external signs (speech, writing) perfectly. In word-blindness and word-deafness the apparatus of reception which is to receive these signs in the brain and give them their value is destroyed. In the first case there is trouble in the transmitting apparatus ; in the second case there is trouble in the receiving apparatus.

Pathogenesis.—All spoken language is made up of a series of conventional sounds which form speech, just as written language is formed by a series of conventional signs which form writing. These conventional sounds and signs are learnt and retained by the memory, which plays the greatest part in the first act of language. The sense of hearing perceives the sounds; the arrangement of these sounds produces the word, and the impression of the words, with the idea attached thereto, is stored up in the first left temporal convolution. This is called **auditory memory**—that is to say, the memory of the conventional sounds, perceived by the sense of hearing, and forming the spoken language.

Let us suppose the destruction of the first temporal convolution by softening. What will be the condition of the patient? The patient will be able to speak, write, read, and understand what he reads, but he can no longer understand anything of what is said to him. The words represent only sounds to him. In losing the temporal convolution he has lost the memory of the value and of the order of those sounds which form spoken language; he is affected with **word-deafness.** This is a case of sensory aphasia.

The same remark applies to written language. Writing, as we have said, is but the conventional union of a certain number of signs. The eye perceives these signs, as the sense of hearing perceives the sounds, and then the value and the order of these signs impress the cerebral centre in the inferior parietal lobule on the left side, where visual memory stores up the impression of the conventional signs called writing.

Let us suppose the destruction of this inferior parietal lobule, the centre for visual memory. The patient can speak, write, and understand what is said to him, but he can no longer read writing. The writing, as far as he is concerned, only represents a series of signs, without value. In losing the function of the left inferior parietal lobule, he has lost the memory of written signs; he has **word-blindness.**

The cerebral regions, in which the auditory and verbal recollections are stored, form the apparatus for the reception of language. By this cerebral process the teaching of language commences in the little child whose brain is undergoing evolution, or in the individual learning a new language. A child or an adult is supplied with the necessary apparatus for understanding the language of others, but before they can communicate with others, either by speech or writing, they must clothe their ideas with the conventional signs, which constitute speech and writing. The education of a new cerebral region, Broca's convolution, or the third left frontal convolution, now intervenes. It has so far been a question of the centres of sensory elaboration; it now becomes a question of the centre of motor elaboration. After a long apprenticeship the child learns to educate this motor centre of co-ordination, in order to speak or to read. This region of motor co-ordination is developed parallel with the regions of sensory elaboration. Broca's convolution preserves the memory of the co-ordination of the movements necessary for speech and writing. The order to execute these movements, properly co-ordinated, is transmitted to the cerebral cells of the neighbouring regions (motor zone), and thence to the nerves and muscles ; and the organs which transmit spoken, written, or mimic language, enter into action.

Let us suppose softening of Broca's convolution. The patient can understand what is said and what he reads, but he cannot put his thoughts either into speech or writing. He has lost the cerebral region in which thought clothes the exterior signs by which man communicates with his fellows. He is attacked by motor aphasia and agraphia.

An attempt has been made to dissociate aphasia from agraphia by making agraphia dependent on lesions of the left middle frontal convolution. It is hardly probable that there is a special centre for agraphia. Aphasia and agraphia are a part of the same whole. As we advance in the study of agraphia, says Dejerine, we see that Trousseau spoke correctly, in his clinical lectures on Aphasia, of agraphia occurring in patients suffering from aphasia. He said regarding patients suffering from cortical motor aphasia, the only form known in his day : " Under ordinary circumstances, the patient suffering from aphasia is no more fit to express his thoughts in words than in writing ; and though he can use his hands with as much precision as formerly, he is as powerless to write a word with his pen as he is powerless to utter a spoken word."

The examples that I have chosen to demonstrate sensory and motor aphasia are typical cases. In many circumstances, however, these types do not appear in a pure condition. I quote examples :

Motor and sensory aphasia may exist in the same subject, or either may be present alone.

Aphasia may exist with complete preservation of the mental faculties, or may be accompanied by intellectual troubles ; it is a matter of localization.

Word-blindness and word-deafness are sometimes accompanied by pronounced paraphasia.

Word-blindness shows two distinct clinical forms : in the one, agraphia is accompanied by word-blindness ; in the other, the power of writing is preserved.

Localizations.—As I have already remarked, motor aphasia is due to cerebral lesions in the posterior third of the third **left** frontal convolution (Dax, Broca). It is also caused by lesions of the white fibres which arise from this cortical centre, and which Pitres, in his description of the centrum ovale, has described under the name of inferior pediculo-frontal bundles.

The lesions which attack the anterior segment of the internal capsule and the internal bundle of the foot of the peduncle, must provoke aphasia because the bundles which constitute it degenerate when the third convolution is affected (Charcot and Féré).

The inferior frontal artery, which arises from the middle cerebral artery, may be considered as the **artery of aphasia** or of Broca's convolution. Charcot has seen a case in which obliteration of this arteriole had caused aphasia without hemiplegia.

Agraphia is said to follow when the lesion attacks the second left frontal convolution (Exner).

Word-deafness coincides with lesions of the first left temporal convolution, especially in its postero-superior extremity, and **word-blindness** is due to the lesions of the left inferior parietal lobule.

The cerebral lesions which produce aphasia are almost always situated on the left side. This law, though not absolute, is the rule. Why is aphasia associated with lesions on the left side ? The probable reason is that we are accustomed to speak with our left brain, just as we acquire the

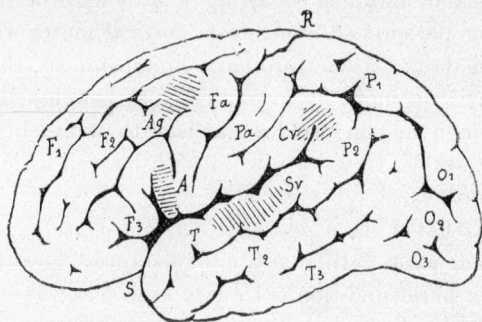

FIG. 72.—CEREBRAL HEMISPHERE.

F$_1$, F$_2$, F$_3$, frontal convolutions ; Fa, ascending frontal convolution ; Pa, ascending parietal convolution ; P$_1$, P$_2$, parietal convolutions ; T$_1$, T$_2$, T$_3$, temporal convolutions ; O$_1$, O$_2$, O$_3$, occipital convolutions ; A, centre for motor aphasia ; Ag, centre for agraphia ; Cv, word blindness ; Sv, word deafness.

habit of using our right hands. Aphasia is rarely caused by hæmorrhage. In most cases it is due to softening, and consequently to various causes— embolism, thrombosis, obliterating arteritis, or tumour.

I have already remarked that aphasia is usually associated with right hemiplegia, the explanation being that the lesion involves the neighbouring motor convolutions. The paralysis is generally slight in the face, and the more marked the paralysis of the lower limb, the less marked the aphasia. Aphasia is often associated with hemianæsthesia of the right side (Grasset)— a fact explained by the seat of the lesion, because the lenticulo-optic portion of the internal capsule is very close to the convolutions of the insula.

New Doctrine of Aphasia.—The classical conception of the mechanism and of the cerebral localization of aphasia has been modified by recent researches. Pierre Marie, from a careful examination of the brain in some

fifty cases, has met with several instances of aphasia in which Broca's convolution showed no lesion. On the other hand, he has found lesions in the
third left frontal convolution which had caused no disorder of speech.

In his historical survey he has shown that the examination of the two
brains on which Broca built up his theory was incomplete, no section being
made. Broca was content to examine only the superficial lesions. As the
specimens were preserved in the Dupuytren Museum, it was easy to prove
that in one brain the lesions were external to the third frontal convolution,
and that the other brain had no lesion in the third frontal convolution.
It may, therefore, be said that Broca's dictum regarding the localization
was based on an error, and, further, the perusal of numerous later cases
furnishes an array of facts opposed to Broca's erroneous teaching.

Marie, in consequence of these fresh facts and observations, thinks that
the lesions producing aphasia occupy a so-called lenticular zone, bounded
in front by a transverse line through the anterior sulcus of the insula to the
corresponding point of the lateral ventricle, and behind by a similar line
from the posterior sulcus of the insula to the corresponding point of the
lateral ventricle. This quadrilateral area contains the lenticular and
caudate nuclei and the internal and external capsules. The region whose
lesions contribute to the production of aphasia also contains the zone of
Wernicke, formed by the gyrus supramarginalis, the angular gyrus, and the
foot of the two first temporal convolutions. Particular disorders follow,
according as the lesion is in the lenticular zone or in Wernicke's zone. If
the lesion only affects the lenticular zone, we have classical motor aphasia—
that is, disorder of articulate speech, called " anarthria " by Marie. If the
lesion only affects the zone of Wernicke, we find Wernicke's aphasia. The
patient can speak—in some cases he speaks too much—but the words,
though well articulated, are often incomprehensible, or, at the very least,
incomplete. The power of reading and writing is abolished or is imperfect
(classical word-blindness). The patient cannot understand spoken language
(classical word-deafness). These symptoms, as a whole, constitute sensory
aphasia ; but Marie does not admit the existence of special centres for the
images of words heard and for the visual images of language. He considers
these disorders as troubles of internal expression, as opposed to the disorders
of external or articulate expression, and he thinks that Wernicke's zone is
the centre for the intellectual elaboration of language, just as the lenticular
zone is the centre for the articulation of words.

Many questions relative to aphasia are obscure, and will long remain so ;
at present, however, the important fact is that Marie has upset Broca's
dictum regarding the frontal centre. We shall see later that cerebral
localization has lost some of the accuracy formerly attributed to it by
certain writers.

Transitory Aphasia.—Besides the aphasia just described, and provoked by evident cerebral lesions, we find in patients suffering from rheumatism, gout, syphilis, typhoid fever, hysteria, ophthalmic migraine, etc., a more or less transitory aphasia, which is not accompanied by paralysis, and which disappears without leaving any trace. This transitory aphasia is not uncommon in patients suffering from diabetes. It is an isolated aphasia, without any trace of hemiplegia. It does not occur only in patients with abundant glycosuria, but it is also met with in people who pass but a few grains of sugar. I have often seen this variety of aphasia. It may last only a few days, but, though transitory, it may be total.

How are we to explain these cases of transitory aphasia, and what happens in such a case to the third left convolution ? Probably an alteration in the circulation takes place, such as transient hyperæmia or anæmia, or a dynamic trouble of the nerve cells. A certain fact of importance in prognosis is that aphasia may exist without a material lesion, just as hemianæsthesia in hysterical patients is not accompanied by any lesion of the sensory tract in the brain, and just as the permanent contractures of hysteria exist without sclerosis of the lateral cords of the spinal cord, and, finally, just as ordinary chorea and post-hemiplegic hemichorea, though almost alike, are in the one case due to transitory functional trouble, and in the other to a lesion of the brain. Identical nervous symptoms may, therefore, be caused by deep and persistent lesions or by transitory changes of an unknown nature.

Treatment.—The treatment of aphasia depends on the cause. We must always think of syphilis, especially in a young man. Re-education may give excellent results in patients suffering from aphasia. It will be much facilitated by the perfected methods employed in the education of deaf-mutes (Féré).

VI. ENCEPHALITIS—ABSCESS OF THE BRAIN.

Encephalitis is inflammation of the brain. It is a disease which was formerly considered frequent, at a period when it was confounded with softening due to embolism or to thrombosis. We know that encephalitis is rare, in striking contrast to myelitis, which is relatively frequent.

Pathogenesis.—Leaving traumatism and surgical lesions out of the question, encephalitis and abscesses of the brain are always the result of toxi-infectious agents. Nearly all the infectious diseases—ulcerative endocarditis, pyæmia, septicæmia, suppurative pneumonia, acute tuberculosis, bronchiectasis, appendicitis, etc.—may cause acute encephalitis and abscesses of the brain. The staphylococcus, the pneumococcus, the coli bacillus, Koch's bacillus, and especially the streptococcus, are the most common organisms. Amongst the causes above enumerated, some demand our attention for a moment.

The tubercle bacillus can cause cerebral abscesses. Fraenkel, Rendu, and Boulloche have reported cases. In such cases it is a question of patients being attacked by miliary tuberculosis, and the tubercle bacillus, without other microbes, may form colonies in the brain tissue, and cause abscesses.

Fœtid chronic bronchitis is a fairly frequent cause of cerebral abscesses (Biermer), and I may say the same of suppuration and gangrene of the lung. It seems that in these various cases it is necessary for the expectoration to be fœtid. Putrefaction appears to be an essential condition.

Lesions of the petrous bone, of the frontal sinuses, and of the orbit, are the chief causes of suppurative encephalitis, suppuration in the ear being the most common. At the post-mortem examination of people who have died of affections of the petrous bone it is not uncommon to find latent cerebral abscesses. Chronic disease of the ear is far more likely than acute disease to cause abscesses. An individual who has, for ten or twenty years, had suppurating otitis media, and who has not troubled himself about this painless and apparently trifling lesion, may at a given moment be taken ill with acute meningo-encephalitis or with cerebral abscess, as was one of my patients who had had chronic otitis for many years, and who died in three days from meningo-encephalitis.

Suppurative meningo-encephalitis and cerebral abscess consequent on otitis may be favoured by a fissure in the bone, which leads to the gradual formation of the abscess; but in many cases there is no direct communication between the cranial cavity and the ear, and we meet with remote abscesses in the opposite cerebral hemisphere. The mechanism which I have employed to explain the remote abscesses of appendicitis (closed cavity) may explain the pathogenesis of the remote abscesses in the brain, "the swelling of the auditory mucosa opposing the exit of the liquid" (Brissaud). To complete this question, I would ask the reader to refer to the section on Abscess of the Cerebellum.

Pathological Anatomy.—The pus in acute encephalitis may infiltrate or may be collected into an abscess. On opening the skull we sometimes find the pia mater adherent, and the subjacent convolutions depressed. The number, the seat, and the dimension of the abscesses vary. We may find only one large abscess or a series of small abscesses. A temporo-sphenoidal abscess is generally secondary to lesions of the middle or of the internal ear; an abscess of the frontal lobe follows caries of the ethmoid; an abscess of the occipital or of the temporal lobe is especially met with in caries of the petrous bone. The encysted pus is sometimes creamy and yellow, sometimes greenish and sanious, and of a fœtid odour. The abscesses become encysted by a membrane formed of sclerotic neuroglia, which commences to form about the twelfth day. The cerebral tissue around the abscess shows yellow softening.

Description.—It is customary to describe three stages in acute encephalitis. The first stage, or phase of excitation, somewhat resembles meningitis : fever, headache, vertigo, uncertainty in walking, visual troubles, delirium, contractures, convulsions, vomiting, and constipation. Headache is the chief symptom, and lasts from four to eight days ; it is sometimes limited to one-half of the brain. If the encephalitis is due to a lesion of the ear, the catarrh generally disappears as soon as the brain is invaded.

The second stage, or phase of remission, is characterized by a fictitious improvement, the patient being in a condition of torpor ; it may last for several weeks, or may give place to the paralytic, hemiplegic, apoplectic, and comatose stage. This last stage may, indeed, appear suddenly, and cause death in two or three days, without being preceded by the initial phases of excitation and depression. Acute encephalitis sometimes passes into the chronic condition, but the prognosis is none the less fatal. Fever is the principal symptom on which we must rely to distinguish encephalitis from softening. Examination of the ear must never be neglected, for this examination is often sufficient to give a clue to the diagnosis.

Two symptoms are to be noted in abscess of the brain—viz., aphasia and hemianopsia. The aphasia is very rarely true motor aphasia ; it is rather a case of sensory partial aphasia. In certain patients the examination of the eye shows the existence of hemianopsia. In the case of a patient reported by Lannois and Jaboulay there was sensory aphasia and right lateral homonymous hemianopsia, with preservation of Wernicke's reflex.

Chronic Encephalitis.—Sclerosis of the brain often coincides with sclerotic lesions of the spinal cord (insular sclerosis). Sclerosis limited to the brain (syphilis) is very rare. In general paralysis of the insane diffuse interstitial encephalitis is associated with chronic myelitis of a like nature.

VII.—CHRONIC ENCEPHALITIS OF CHILDHOOD—HÆMORRHAGE —SOFTENING—PORENCEPHALIA—LOBAR SCLEROSIS— LITTLE'S DISEASE.

General Conditions.—The forms of chronic encephalitis in children from birth to the period of the second dentition are often described under different names, according as they are designated by their anatomical lesion (hæmorrhage, softening, porencephaly, lobar sclerosis), or by their major clinical syndrome (athetosis, hemiplegia, paraplegia, spasmodic diplegia, or Little's disease). They deserve to be studied as a whole, because, even though they present, as in the adult, varying symptoms according to the localization of the lesions, their course is marked by a common clinical basis. Paralyses with contractures, and intellectual troubles that may be slight or may end in idiocy, are the elements of the syndrome common to almost all forms of chronic infantile encephalitis.

The fact that the brain of the child is incompletely developed at the time when the lesion makes its appearance accounts for this special clinical process. Let me add that the after-effects of infantile sclerosis may appear in youth in the form of epilepsy. The writings of Bourneville and of Strümpell have helped to elucidate these forms of infantile encephalitis. Their natural history has been accurately classified by Brissaud.

Ætiology.—There are two special ætiological reasons for infantile encephalopathies—premature accouchement, and especially dystocia—which explains how the disease may arise even before birth ; and infection (measles, scarlatina, whooping-cough, etc.).

Pathological Anatomy.—Infantile encephalopathy may be characterized by hæmorrhage, softening, meningo-encephalitis, sclerosis, and cavities (porencephaly), but of all these lesions two are peculiar to infancy, and demand our attention—porencephaly and lobar sclerosis.

Porencephaly. — This term does not refer to a particular lesion ; it denotes the ultimate result of a series of lesions, characterized by the presence of cavities (*porus*), opening like craters on the surface of the hemispheres ; it is the superlative degree of cicatricial retraction (Brissaud).

Following Bourneville and Sollier, we have to consider two forms of porencephaly, true and false. The conclusions of these authors are : " True porencephaly is the result of arrested development, and is consequently congenital. In true porencephaly there is a communication between the depression and the lateral ventricle. In false porencephaly this communication does not exist. This want of communication is not, however, of an absolute value, because we may readily suppose that the necrobiotic process may completely destroy the cerebral matter as far as the lateral ventricle, and thus establish a wide communication with it. The disposition of the convolutions has, on the contrary, a greater importance. In true porencephaly the latter are disposed in rays around the porus into which they plunge. In pseudo-porencephaly, on the other hand, the convolutions are cut irregularly.

" The shape of the depression is very different in the two cases. In true porencephaly we see a kind of infundibulum, sometimes a simple slit or an almost circular orifice. In pseudo-porencephaly we see a gaping excavation, the walls of which, instead of being formed by convolutions, are formed by the white matter covered by the membrane of a pseudo-cyst, which intimately adheres to it. In spite of the relatively much larger extent of the pseudo-porencephaly, the psychic phenomena may be less marked than in true porencephaly, which is almost always accompanied by complete idiocy."

The porencephalic lesion, whether congenital or acquired, is always the result of an arterial lesion. In true porencephaly we have congenital absence of an artery, and the region which it ought to have nourished has never been properly developed. In acquired porencephaly the arterial lesion results in the *porus* through the intermediary of a hæmorrhagic focus, or of softening. The chasm is filled with gliomatous tissue.

Primary Lobar Sclerosis.—This lesion occurs in earliest infancy or in intra-uterine life. It may occupy both hemispheres or be limited to one of them ; it may even restrict itself to one lobe, such as the occipital or frontal lobe, whence the name " lobar sclerosis." In some cases the sclerosis limits itself to a group of convolutions, such as the convolutions of Rolando. In the case of bilateral sclerosis the lesions are always symmetrical (Richardière) ; they are perhaps brought about by circulatory troubles (Marie).

The cerebral matter is indurated, and the convolutions appear to be retracted. The general topography remains recognizable in spite of the marked atrophy of the diseased part. This atrophy may affect all the constituent parts of the brain—convolutions, peduncles, corpora striata, etc.

The fundamental histological lesions consist in a diffuse proliferation of the neuroglia, and in vascular and perivascular changes. The neuroglia is filled with branching cells, with dense and opaque nuclei, and the diseased parts are furrowed by large wavy bundles of connective tissue, visible when slightly magnified. The vascular changes produce thickening of the walls of the capillaries. The perivascular lymphatic sheaths are enlarged, and filled with leucocytes and granular bodies. The lesion in the neuroglia commences close to the capillaries. The cells of the cortex are atrophied, and lose their pyramidal form, becoming fusiform, and even disappearing in certain lobes. The lesion is slowly invading, and there are some points at which it is more advanced. This progressive course explains the appearance of certain late symptoms (Brissaud).

Secondary Lesions.—In the infant the secondary lesions are always much more marked than in the adult. They do not only consist of a secondary degeneration, but also of an arrested development of the neuron. In the brain the atrophy and the degeneration reach the capsule, the pons, and the bulb. The striate bodies are also attacked secondarily. The lobe of the cerebellum on the opposite side (Vulpian, Charcot, Cottard) is generally much atrophied and sclerosed.

The spinal cord on the side opposite to the lesion does not only show lesions of descending sclerosis, but also a peculiar atrophy, which extends even to the bones, cartilages, ligaments, tendons, and muscles of the same side. The same arrest of development is observed in the skull, face, and eyeball of the paralyzed side, whence the formation of the keel-like skull and the Olympian brow. If the lesion is bilateral, the secondary degeneration is bilateral, and we have diplegia instead of hemiplegia.

Symptoms.—Chronic encephalitis of infancy may show several clinical forms. They end almost always in paralysis, in the form of spasmodic hemiplegia, hemiathetosis, choreic hemiplegia, double athetosis, or spasmodic chorea, and they may be complicated with idiocy.

Whatever the pathological form of the encephalopathy, says Brissaud, the general evolution of the symptoms is always much the same—appearance of acute troubles, such as restlessness, fever, vomiting, and convulsions from birth, or during earliest infancy. A phase of apparent cure follows, lasting for some days or weeks, and then paralysis supervenes, sometimes limited, at other times affecting the whole of one side or the whole musculature of the body. The acute febrile stage may be absent, especially in the new-born, and the paralysis which exists in the latent stage from birth only reveals itself when the child attempts to take its first steps. All the above types of paralysis have a tendency to become blended with one another. I shall follow the description given by Brissaud.

Spasmodic Hemiplegia of Infancy.—We find three successive phases : A phase of epileptiform movements, localized to the side which later becomes paralyzed, and showing a preference for the limbs. A phase of hemiplegia, which immediately follows the epileptiform movements ; the hemiplegia being generally flaccid and total ; affecting the limbs and the face, and generally lasting about a fortnight. At the end of this time the patient enters on the third stage, the hemiplegia becoming spasmodic, incurable, and almost like that of the adult. It differs from it at times by certain special attitudes. The hand is flexed on the forearm in exaggerated pronation. " The fingers are flexed on the palm, or strongly extended in attitudes which absolutely recall those of the hands of the Javanese dancers." The particular characteristic is a general atrophy of the limbs and face on the paralyzed side.

Hemiathetosis.—It may exist in a condition of purity, quite apart from paralysis or contracture. Most frequently it is only a symptom superadded to the hemiplegia. The contracture is much less pronounced in spasmodic hemiplegia ; otherwise the athetotic movements could not be produced. The symptomatology and the character of these athetotic movements are the same in the child as in the adult. The localization of the lesions producing them is identical. In exceptional cases hemichorea has been met with.

Double Athetosis.—All the muscles make slow, incessant, and stiff movements. The face grimaces continually. This double athetosis is caused by a symmetrical lesion affecting the neighbourhood of the pyramidal tract. Chronic double chorea, admitted as identical with double athetosis by most authors who have studied the question (Richardière, Audry), is produced by an analogous lesion with a different localization.

Spasmodic Diplegia.—Bilateral paralysis, with contracture, appearing at birth or in the earliest days of life, has been very carefully studied during the past few years. It is dependent on a bilateral lesion of Rolando's area or of the paracentral lobule. Little, in 1862, showed that its causes were

difficult labour, premature accouchement, asphyxia of the newborn, superficial meningeal hæmorrhage, and described the various clinical forms.
Little pointed out that the contracture may be general, or that it may show
itself in the paraplegic form.

Generalized Contractures.—All four limbs are in a state of contracture.
The foot clonus is very marked, and the reflexes are exaggerated. The limbs
are less paralyzed than they appear to be, and this is one of the most interesting points in this form of the disease. The rigidity lessens with age, and
when the child reaches the walking age we see that he does not take to it
partially on account of cerebral dullness, as Little well remarked. The child
is backward in speech, intelligence, and walking. The disease improves
with time, but is never completely cured ; the legs always preserve some
degree of contracture.

Paraplegic Contracture.—This contracture, localized in the lower limbs,
presents the picture of spasmodic tabes dorsalis. Children thus affected do not
begin to walk till they are about four or five years old. " Their walk is spasmodic, with double club-foot, adduction, flexion and inward rotation of the
thighs. The tendon reflexes are much exaggerated, and in the sitting posture
the legs have a tendency to raise themselves spontaneously from the ground "
(Brissaud). The little sufferers appear to be devoid of intelligence, but often
they are not so. As Marie has pointed out, the spasmodic condition of the
muscles of the face paralyzes the expression, and gives them a stupid look.
The contracture of the leg is always less curable than that of the arms.
Spasmodic encephalopathy, especially the congenital form, is often called
Little's disease. For the purposes of description I have, following Brissaud,
given clinical types which can frequently be isolated ; but these types often
combine, and in their ensemble form a single disease.

Intellectual Troubles—Idiocy.—The intellectual development is arrested
when the lesion involves the frontal lobe ; it is specially delayed in the case of
a bilateral lesion.

No matter which side of the brain is attacked by the lesions, persons who
are hemiplegic from infancy **never show aphasia,** a fact already remarked by
Cottard. As this writer observes, the functional substitution is no doubt
established by means of the zones which have been spared in those brains
that are as yet incompletely developed.

Infantile encephalopathy is one of the most frequent causes of idiocy
(Bourneville). Cerebral scleroses may, like hydrocephalus, microcephalus,
chronic meningitis, tumours of the brain, and pachydermic cachexia, cause
imbecility and mental weakness. The congenital idiot has an asymmetrical
face, unequal frontal bosses, projecting superior maxillæ, striated and unequally set teeth. He generally presents the most marked stigmata of
degeneration. In acquired idiocy the skull is regular, the expression less

dolt-like, but the disease is in general more hopeless. Feebleness, want of equilibrium, and perversion of the faculties, may be observed in all degrees in the idiot, and this condition of mental weakness may be recognized before the age of two years. The child does not sleep, and cries continually ; the sight is imperfect, and taste and smell are hardly developed. The sense of hearing is the least rudimentary of all the senses. The cutaneous sensibility is blunted, and the voluntary movements are retarded ; the speech is much affected, and may be reduced to unintelligible mumbling. The idiot often does not commence to pronounce his first words until between the ages of three and eight years.

Epilepsy.—Many individuals stricken with spasmodic hemiplegia during infancy become epileptic in adolescence. " Many cases of so-called essential epilepsy are simply the late manifestation of an infantile encephalopathy which has arrived at its definite anatomical stage " (Brissaud). Epilepsy consequent on spasmodic infantile hemiplegia is said in most cases to recover about the age of thirty (Bourneville and Wuillaumier). Infantile encephalopathy is always grave. Whatever its evolution may be, it always makes a weakling of the patient.

Diagnosis.—When the lesion is congenital, the diagnosis is generally obvious, but when the paralytic and spasmodic phenomena supervene during early infancy the diagnosis is often more difficult.

The acute onset may simulate meningitis, but doubts are dispelled by the later evolution of the disease. The acute onset may also simulate atrophic spinal paralysis of infancy, but in this myelopathy hemiplegia is rare, and the paralysis is always flaccid, with abolition of the tendon reflexes.

Crepitus of the articular surfaces and cutaneous eruptions are in general sufficient to distinguish it from the syphilitic pseudo-paralysis of Parrot and Troisier.

Obstetrical paralysis is due to the compression of a motor nerve in instrumental delivery ; it remains limited to circumscribed groups of muscles.

Spasmodic tabes dorsalis and certain kinds of spasmodic paraplegia— Pott's disease, for instance—are distinguished by their mode of appearance, by sensory troubles, and by the vesical and rectal disturbances.

Treatment.—According to Pinard, the best measure in certain cases is to prevent grave disturbance in the fœtal circulation by performing symphysiotomy in order to hasten delivery.

When the disease has developed, the future of the child depends on the surgeon, who can by orthopædic measures improve the atrophic deformities. It will also depend on the child's teacher, who may be able to improve the mental condition by following Bourneville's rules.

VIII. CEREBRAL TUMOURS.

Pathological Anatomy.—In the cerebrum we meet with tumours of every kind and of divers origin ; they develop at the expense of the meninges, of the vessels, and of the cerebral tissue. Some tumours arise on the exterior, and penetrate into the skull (orbital tumours) ; others arise in the skull, and make their way outwards.

Cancer arises in the brain or in the neighbouring parts (bones, meninges, orbital cavity). The encephaloid variety is the most frequent ; the tumour may assume the size of a fist, perforate the cranial walls, and appear externally as an erectile, nodular tumour. The soft sarcoma is much less common than cancer ; its course is much slower and less prone to invasion ; it occurs chiefly in young persons. It is formed of pure embryonic tissue, or of the same tissue in course of transformation. In the glioma, which is a variety of sarcoma, hæmorrhage sometimes occurs. The tubercle usually attacks the cerebellum, the mesencephalon, and the surface of the cerebral hemispheres. It sometimes forms large tumours, which are due to an agglomeration of granulations. The centre of the tumour passes into the caseous condition, and we often find calcification.

Syphilis gives rise to osseous and periosteal gummata, which will be described later.

Parasites are rare in the brain. We find especially the echinococcus and the cysticercus. Aneurysms are found in the arteries at the base, and especially in the basilar trunk. One of my patients had an aneurysm as large as a walnut on the left anterior cerebral artery. Cerebral tumours, by compressing the veins and the arteries of the neighbourhood, cause secondary lesions, such as thrombosis of the sinuses, œdema, hydrocephalus, softening, etc. Numerous varieties result therefrom in the history of the symptoms.

Description.—In the first place, some cerebral tumours remain latent for a long time, provided they develop slowly in the so-called tolerant regions (Jaccoud), such as the white hemispherical mass of the posterior lobes and the striated bodies. This tolerance is, however, far from being constant, and besides, a certain region which is tolerant when slowly invaded by a tumour is no longer so when the hæmorrhagic lesion or the softening supervenes suddenly.

It is customary in treatises on pathology to devote a chapter to the description of cerebral tumours. I must confess that this description, when confined to a general survey, seems to me impossible ; the situation of the tumour modifies the description of the symptoms to such a degree, and, on the other hand, the physiology of certain cerebral operations is still so obscure, that a methodical study of this question cannot be attempted for the time being. We can, however, group the symptoms and divide them into two classes : the one class under the name of diffuse symptoms, which are not exclusively dependent on the seat of the lesion, and which are the result of a direct or reflex excitation ; the other class under the name of focal symptoms, which are related to the localization of the lesion, and which assist in its topographical diagnosis.

1. **Diffuse Symptoms.**—The diffuse symptoms are generally the first to appear, and they may have no constant relation with the seat of the tumour. The most important are headache, vertigo, vomiting, twitchings in the limbs, and mental troubles. Headache met with in half of the cases (Ball and Krishaber) may be general or partial ; it is sometimes paroxysmal. It may last for weeks, and may be most severe. Violent **nocturnal** exacerbations often point to syphilis. Vomiting of cerebral origin takes place without effort, without nausea, and without gastric troubles ; the vomit may consist of food or simply of liquid.

The attacks of vertigo and giddiness assume various forms : the patient complains of feeling empty-headed, of continuous giddiness, or of fits of vertigo, which recur several times a day. Occipital headache, vomiting, and attacks of vertigo are very common in tumours of the cerebellum.

2. **Focal Symptoms.**—The various paralyses are focal symptoms ; their appearance is sometimes slow and gradual, at other times rapid ; their character is dependent on the seat and extent of the tumour. They may be grouped as follows :

1. **Hemiplegia.**—(i.) Total hemiplegia of the limbs and of the face, analogous to the hemiplegia of cerebral hæmorrhage, is a very rare variety. The hemiplegia of cerebral tumours is less complete, " less pure, less exactly circumscribed, and less systematic than common hemiplegia " (Fournier).

(ii.) Partial hemiplegia of one leg, of one arm (monoplegia), or of an arm and of the face, is fairly frequent. It results in nearly every case from a lesion seated at a fixed point of the cortical motor zone. These cases of monoplegia are almost always associated with contractures, or attacks of Jacksonian epilepsy. This question will be studied in detail under Jacksonian Epilepsy.

(iii.) Crossed hemiplegia, which affects the limbs on one side, and one or more cranial nerves on the other, is the result of a tumour in the mesencephalon, or of several tumours variously situated, or of a tumour sufficiently large to compress the cerebral hemisphere and one of the cranial nerves at the same time.

(iv.) Hemiplegia, accompanied by hemianæsthesia or by hemichorea, indicates that the tumour is attacking the sensory bundle in the internal capsule. Permanent contracture following the paraylsis proves that the tumour has injured the pyramidal tract at some point of its course, or in the anterior two-thirds of the posterior segment of the internal capsule.

These varieties of hemiplegia rarely have the sudden onset of the hemiplegia of cerebral hæmorrhage and of cerebral embolism ; they are usually preceded by headache, twitchings in the foot and in the hand, giddiness, and weakness. Amongst the tumours which give rise to them we must place in the front rank gummata of the meninges or of the brain. Hemiplegia is, we know, a frequent complication of the tertiary period, but it is by no means uncommon even within two years of the date of infection. Syphilis may cause hemiplegia, with or without apoplexy, with or without aphasia ; the paralysis may be due to gummata, sclero-gummatous meningitis, vascular compression, obliterating arteritis, and consequent softening.

2. **Paralysis of the Cranial Nerves.**—The paralysis may strike one nerve or several nerves at the same time, or it may be limited to one of the branches of a cranial nerve. Two hypotheses are given to explain paralysis limited to a part of a nerve. In the one, the lesion attacks one of the branches arising from the common trunk—it is a peripheral paralysis ; in the other, the lesion attacks the nerve branch at its origin before it joins the common bundle—it is a central paralysis. Thus, incomplete facial paralysis may be due to a cortical tumour of the motor convolutions ; the paralysis of the common oculo-motor nerve, which reveals itself by ptosis, may point to a tumour in the posterior part of the opposite parietal lobe, the ptosis of cerebral origin being crossed.

Cerebral syphilis often causes paralysis of the cranial nerves ; the nerves invaded are in order of frequency : the third nerve, the sixth nerve, the fourth nerve, the facial, etc. These syphilitic paralyses are generally rapid in their development ; they become confirmed within the space of a few hours.

3. **Disorders of vision** are frequent and early. Their importance leads me to describe them in detail. In the first place I shall mention amblyopia and amaurosis, due to lesions of the optic nerves. These lesions are generally bilateral and rapid in their evolution. The ophthalmoscope reveals optic neuritis. The optic disc is hyperæmic, and the central veins are enlarged and tortuous. The arteries, on the contrary, are diminished in size, and are partially covered by exudate.

The disc has lost its clear outline, being enlarged and prominent. Later it is swollen, and surrounded by small hæmorrhages, which are elongated so that the radial disposition of the nerve fibres appears prominently. The process may extend beyond the disc to the retina (neuro-retinitis). At this stage the optic neuritis may be cured. If the lesion progresses, it ends in atrophy; the papilla is flattened, and the red tint gives place to a whitish-grey. The arteries become atrophied. Several theories have been propounded to explain the pathogenesis of optic neuritis of intracranial origin. It has been attributed to vascular stasis (De Graefe) ; to infection (Leber) ;

to excess of intracranial tension, with a pressing backwards of the cerebro-spinal fluid into the intervaginal space of the optic nerve (Schmidt) : to lymphatic œdema, analogous to the œdema of the cerebral tissue, of which the optic nerve is the prolongation (Parinaud). The fibrous ring through which the optic nerve passes is said to favour strangulation and œdema in the same manner as a ligature placed on the limbs ; whence the name " œdematous neuritis " (Parinaud).

Optic neuritis, especially when associated with other symptoms, is of great diagnostic value as to the existence of an intracranial tumour ; but it gives no indication regarding the situation of the tumour. It is quite other-wise with primary atrophy of the optic nerves, which is, besides, very much rarer in the case of cerebral tumours. This atrophy, which generally is partial, gives rise to various kinds of hemianopia.

Homonymous hemianopia is the loss of the left or right half of the visual field in both eyes. It is related to the destruction of one of the cortical visual centres or of one of the quadrigeminal tubercles, or of one optic tract. The tumour is seated on the opposite side to the affected half of the visual field. **Temporal hemianopia** is the loss of the external half of the field of vision of each eye ; it follows a lesion of the anterior or posterior angle of the chiasma —that is to say, a lesion affecting both crossed bundles of the optic nerves at the same time (tumours of the pituitary region). **Nasal hemianopia** is the loss of the two internal halves of the field of vision ; it is the index of a lesion of the two direct bundles, affecting the two lateral angles of the chiasma at the same time.

Homonymous hemianopia, generally due to a central lesion, has well-defined symptoms : sudden or rapid evolution ; loss of both corresponding halves of the field of vision, without peripheral constriction ; preservation of the central keenness of sight on account of the integrity of the macular bundle ; whilst the other varieties of hemianopia, temporal or nasal, present variable characters. Given the seat of the lesions causing hemianopia, it will be understood that the ocular troubles are often associated with troubles resulting from lesions of the neighbouring cranial nerves—anosmia (lesion of the olfactory lobes), diplopia (lesion of the motor nerves of the eye).

The ocular paralyses which may be noticed in cerebral tumour show constant symptoms—paralytic strabismus, diplopia, etc. These symptoms themselves present variable characteristics according as the lesion is seated in the nerve trunks, in their roots, in the nuclei of origin, or, higher still, in the cerebral cortex.

4. **Epileptiform convulsions** are common in cerebral tumours. They take two distinct forms : in the one form the convulsions have all the character-istics of a true attack of epilepsy ; in the other the convulsions are dis-sociated and partial, being limited to one limb or to one side of the body.

This form of epilepsy was well described in 1827 by Bravais, and later by Jackson (Jacksonian epilepsy). In this form of partial epilepsy the patient does not lose consciousness. The convulsions commence in the arm, and extend thence to the head and to the leg, or they may commence in the face, and extend to the arm and the leg ; in rarer cases they commence in the leg, and then attack the arm and the face. Certain sudden movements, such as the forced flexion of the wrist or of the foot, may bring on the convulsive attack, and the same manœuvre at the commencement of the convulsions may sometimes stop them. General epilepsy, a variety of symptomatic epilepsy, is valueless in localizing the seat of the tumour, whilst partial epilepsy, or monospasm in the arm or in the leg, is always the index of a tumour seated at a fixed point of the **cortical motor zone.** This question will be discussed under Cerebral Localization and Jacksonian Epilepsy.

Large tubercles of the brain, exostoses of the cranial vault, syphilitic gummata of the dura-mater and of the cortical regions, are the most common causes of epileptiform convulsions. This syphilitic epilepsy will be studied later.

I have just enumerated the most common symptoms of cerebral tumours ; there are others which, though more rare, are none the less of great importance : these are aphasia, exaggerated slowing of the pulse, syncope, apoplectiform attacks, coma, and mania.

The aphasia may be transitory or permanent ; it appears alone, or is associated with hemiplegia. It may even show itself as an isolated phenomenon at the commencement of cerebral syphilis. Aphasia in cerebral tumour is generally due to the compression of the nutrient artery of the third frontal convolution.

Coma is one of the most curious manifestations of cerebral tumours, and I am speaking not only of coma following epileptiform and apoplectiform attacks, or of coma associated with the gradual and increasing troubles of cerebral œdema and hydrocephalus : but I also allude to **early coma,** which sometimes supervenes suddenly, especially in syphilitic lesions of the brain, and which is, as it were, an isolated manifestation of them, calculated, when we are not forewarned, to upset the diagnosis.

Diagnosis—Prognosis—Treatment.—After what we have said concerning the evolution of cerebral tumours, and the many complications which they produce, we see that they are generally announced by prodromata, such as vertigo, headache, and vomiting, and confirmed by paralytic and convulsive troubles : incomplete hemiplegia, monoplegia, Jacksonian epilepsy ; amaurosis, retinitis, and paralysis of the cranial nerves. There are cases, however, in which the onset of the symptoms (aphasia, coma) gives no warning, and the diagnosis then presents serious difficulties.

The conditions usual to the development of tumours are not realized in hæmorrhage or in cerebral embolism ; they are more like the symptoms of cerebral softening due to obliterating arteritis and atheroma. There is, nevertheless, this difference—that the symptoms of the prodromal period are less frequent and less pronounced, whilst the intellectual troubles are more marked in atheromatous softening than in cerebral tumour. Furthermore, cerebral atheroma is at times associated with general atheroma (aorta, radial artery, femoral artery, etc.), a fact of some value in diagnosis. In every case the patient's history must be carefully examined in order to discover whether the tumour is syphilitic or tubercular.

The **prognosis** of cerebral tumours is very grave, cancer being the worst, and a syphilitic tumour the least serious, because it often gives way to energetic treatment. I cannot here discuss surgical treatment, which has made considerable progress during the past few years. Recovery often depends on timely operation.

IX. CEREBRAL SYPHILIS—SYPHILITIC ARTERITIS— GUMMATA AND SCLERO-GUMMATOUS LESIONS—SYPHILITIC GENERAL PSEUDO-PARALYSIS.

In order to simplify the question of cerebral syphilis, I shall divide it into three parts, as I did in my lectures at the Faculté in 1892. In the first part I shall study **syphilitic cerebral arteritis,** which appears to me to be one of the most frequent forms of cerebro-meningeal syphilis. In the second part I shall deal with the **sclero-gummatous** lesions of the brain and of the meninges. In the third part the mental forms of syphilis, general pseudo-paralysis, and parasyphilitic general paralysis will be described.

Syphilitic Cerebro-Meningeal Arteritis—Obliterating Arteritis, and Arteritis followed by Aneurysm.

Pathological Anatomy.—Syphilis shows a well-marked preference for the arteries of the brain, and amongst these arteries it selects especially those forming the circle of Willis and its branches. Anatomically speaking, these cases of syphilitic arteritis do not present lesions which are absolutely peculiar to them ; they have, nevertheless, a family likeness which sometimes allows them to be recognized, either with the naked eye or under the microscope. They are often symmetrical, and sometimes limited to a segment of the vessel ; in other instances they may be multiple, and more or less generalized.

Syphilitic arteritis, said Heubner in his work published in 1864, commences as a granulation on the tunica intima. It is an obliterating endarteritis which ends in the obstruction of the vessel by growth of granulations and by thrombosis. According to Lancereaux, syphilitic arteritis is primarily a periarteritis. According to other writers it consists in a sclero-gummatous change in the walls of the artery ; the lesion commences in the tunica externa, which it sometimes envelops like a cuff, and spreads into the middle and internal coats. The cellular proliferation may be so great that the lumen of the vessel is obstructed. In these various cases the obliteration of the vessel is completed by the occurrence of thrombosis, and cerebral softening is the consequence. There is some truth in these views of the question, but Heubner's opinion deserves to be preserved. As proof thereof I would mention the lesions, described by Joffroy, in a case of syphilitic cerebral arteritis.

It has been maintained that syphilitic arteritis is caused by an active and not by a degenerative process, and that it does not end in atheroma (Heubner). This view is erroneous. Cornil has shown that syphilitic arteritis may end in atheroma ; indeed, atheroma is not uncommon. This rapid review of the arterial lesions of syphilis shows that syphilitic arteritis has many points in common with other forms of arteritis, and I will add that, like them, it may end in obliteration of the vessel, or in dilatation, aneurysm, and rupture.

Moreover, syphilis causes arteritis, with obliteration or dilatation in the superficial arteries of the limbs and of the face, so that we can account *de visu* for what takes place in the brain. In order to avoid repetition, I would ask the reader to refer to the section on Syphilitic Arteritis. This chapter is the complement of syphilitic cerebral arteritis.

Let us next consider syphilitic arteritis with dilatation, aneurysm, and rupture of the vessel; and arteritis with thrombosis and obstruction of the vessel.

1. **Syphilitic Aneurysm.**—This group includes cases of syphilitic arteritis ending in aneurysm, rupture, and meningeal hæmorrhage. To quote examples :

Spillmann : A young man suffering from syphilis was taken ill, eleven months after infection, with headache, somnolence, vertigo, and vomiting. He died from a stroke of apoplexy in a few hours. The post-mortem examination revealed a large subarachnoid hæmorrhage, caused by a ruptured aneurysm of the basilar artery. At various points the arteries of the base of the brain were the seat of syphilitic lesions. The patient was not alcoholic. In another of Spillmann's cases a young woman, ten months after infection, was seized with headache and torpor ; a little later convulsions appeared, and an apoplectiform condition declared itself. The patient died a few hours later. At the post-mortem examination a vast subarachnoid hæmorrhagic effusion was discovered, caused by the rupture of an aneurysm, at the junction of the left internal carotid and Sylvian arteries. The right carotid artery, at a symmetrical point, was attacked by syphilitic arteritis.

Lancereaux : A woman was taken ill, six years after the primary infection, with headache, vertigo, and right hemiplegia, without apoplexy. After transient improvement, the cerebral symptoms reappeared, and the patient died of apoplexy. The post-mortem examination showed subarachnoid hæmorrhage, due to the rupture of an aneurysm of the right Sylvian artery, before the origin of the perforating arteries. Several branches given off by the right Sylvian artery showed endarteritis, with an obliterating tendency.

Brault : A young woman was taken ill with early cerebral symptoms ten months after being infected with syphilis : headache, amnesia, aphasia. The patient rapidly became cachectic, and died suddenly from apoplexy. At the post-mortem examination considerable meningeal hæmorrhage was discovered. It was caused by a ruptured aneurysm of the left internal carotid at its point of entry into the cranium. The right internal carotid was attacked by arteritis at a corresponding point. Histological examination showed that the three coats of the diseased segment had lost their proper structure. They were uniformly composed of embryonic tissue. The internal elastic lamina alone remained. At another point, near the aneurysm, the lumen of the artery was almost obliterated by the thickening of its walls and by a large bud on the endarterium.

These cases show that aneurysm is not rare when syphilis affects the cerebral arteries. These aneurysms are situated, in order of frequency, in the basilar trunk, the Sylvian arteries, and the internal carotid arteries. In many cases we find multiple lesions in the same subject: a ruptured aneurysm, an aneurysm in process of formation, endarteritis with an obliterating tendency, and arteries with complete transformation of their walls. It must be remarked that these arterial lesions do not occur only in the tertiary stage ; we also meet with them soon after infection—eleventh month (Spillmann), tenth month (Brault), and eighth month (Spillmann).

2. **Obliterating Endarteritis.**—The second group comprises cases of arteritis which block the vessel, and which may cause death with or without cerebral softening, according to the intensity and the duration of the process.

Geffrier : A patient suffering from syphilis was admitted to hospital for severe headache, which persisted in spite of large doses of iodide of potassium. A few months later the pains, which had improved for a time, became much worse ; they were accompanied by giddiness, vertigo, and mental torpor. The patient could not walk without losing his balance. Delirium set in, and was soon followed by coma and death in the sixth month after the primary infection. The post-mortem examination revealed syphilitic lesions of the basilar trunk, of both Sylvian arteries, of the anterior cerebral, and of the posterior communicating arteries. The basilar trunk was filled with a very adherent clot, which commenced in the vertebral arteries. The cerebral matter nowhere showed either softening or hæmorrhage. The histological examination showed that in certain places the normal elements of the arterial coats had almost disappeared, and were replaced by embryonic tissue. At certain points aneurysmal pockets had formed. In the Sylvian artery granulations projected into the lumen of the vessel. Elsewhere the endarteritis presented the characters of typical atheroma. It is important to remember that this patient was not an alcoholic. In this case death was caused by the complete obliteration of the basilar trunk before cerebral softening had time to develop.

Mauriac : A patient, six months after infection, was seized with severe headache, weakening of memory, embarrassment of speech, awkwardness of the hands, unsteady gait. A few days later the patient lost consciousness. Complete hemiplegia of the left side declared itself and, after some improvement, death from coma eight months after infection. At the post-mortem examination scattered lesions were found in the arteries at the base of the brain. The carotid arteries were whitish and thickened. The right Sylvian artery was attacked with arteritis, and its principal branches were completely obliterated by clots. An obliterating clot also existed in the right anterior cerebral artery. Methodical sections of the brain and of the mesencephalon showed no focus of softening. Here, also, the obliteration of the vessels was so rapid that death supervened before necrobiosis had time to develop.

I shall next give some cases of syphilitic obliterating arteritis in which death was preceded by cerebral softening.

Joffroy : A man was taken ill seven years after infection with headache, transient aphasia, and numbness of the right arm. A month later right facial hemiplegia and temporary paralysis of the right arm made their appearance ; during the next few months inability to work, giddiness, and vomiting ; a short time after this, loss of consciousness, coma, and death. At the post-mortem examination the basilar trunk was found to be thickened, indurated, and contained an adherent clot, ½ inch in length. The left Sylvian artery and both posterior cerebral arteries were the seat of arteritis. The histological examination revealed lesions of endarteritis with the projecting buds, described by Heubner ; the lesions of periarteritis were less advanced. In the brain there were three foci of softening on the left side : in the internal frontal convolution in front of the paracentral lobe, and in the foot of the third frontal convolution.

In a case quoted by Mauriac a youth, eight years after infection, was taken ill with cerebral symptoms and paralysis of the right arm. He improved under treatment, but, four years later, hemiplegia occurred on the right side, and was followed by secondary contracture of the right arm, albuminuria, cachexia, and death. The post-mortem examination showed arteritis of the arteries of the base, with softening of the left corpus striatum and secondary degeneration of the pyramidal tract.

In some cases, then, we can follow step by step the process of syphilitic obliterating arteritis, terminating in death, with or without cerebral softening, dependent on the severity, the extent, and the duration of the obliterating process.

3. **Cerebral Hæmorrhage.**—The third group includes the less common cases in which syphilis does not attack the large arteries at the base of the brain, or the branches given off directly from them, but the superficial or deep arterioles of smaller calibre. In the cortical or central portions of the brain it may thus cause small foci of softening, consequent on obliteration of the arterioles, or miliary aneurysms that cause cerebral hæmorrhage, comparable at all points with ordinary cerebral hæmorrhage. Schwostek's case is a remarkable instance.

In a young man of twenty-four years of age the secondary complications were slight, but three years later very grave cerebral symptoms appeared : acute pains in the fore-head and nape of the neck, vertigo, and uncertainty in walking. These symptoms were soon followed by hemiplegia of the left side, with coma and an apoplectiform condition. Death was the consequence thereof. At the post-mortem examination syphilitic arteritis had affected the arteries at the base of the brain, and, on examining the brain, it was found that a hæmorrhage had partially invaded the lenticular nucleus, the external capsule, the claustrum, and the ventricles.

The **cerebellum** may be the seat of hæmorrhage or of softening, consequent on syphilitic disease of the cerebellar arteries. In such a case the patient suffers from the symptoms given in the section on the Diseases of the Cerebellum.

In order to simplify the description, I have divided the arterial lesions of cerebral syphilis into several categories. There are, as a matter of fact, cases in which these lesions are independent, and affect the types which I have just described ; but in other cases the lesions are associated, and the resulting clinical type is less distinct. As we know the various forms of the pathological process in syphilitic arteritis of the cerebral vessels, we shall find it easier to describe the clinical picture.

Symptoms—Apoplexy.—The attack of apoplexy may be the consequence of syphilitic cerebral arteritis. The cases already quoted prove that apoplexy and death have been caused by the rupture of an aneurysm, or by the more or less extensive obliteration of a large artery. In the former case the apoplexy is due to a meningeal hæmorrhage ; it is lightning-like in its action. In the latter case it is due to more or less extensive cerebral ischæmia, and it is not so rapid. The apoplexy may even be due to true cerebral hæmorrhage. Syphilitic apoplexy differs little, as far as the immediate symptoms are concerned, from the attack of ordinary apoplexy, but it is widely differentiated therefrom by its precursory signs. The attack of ordinary apoplexy, in fact, generally takes the individual during apparently excellent health. He is struck down during his sleep, or in the midst of his work, without any warning. It is not so in syphilitic apoplexy. The latter is generally the result of more or less intense and varied cerebral symptoms, which date back to a more or less distant period. Headache, so to say, is never absent. Vertigo, giddiness, transient sight troubles, obnubilation, temporary disorders of speech and intelligence, mental weakness, paresis of a monoplegic or hemiplegic nature, are the signs, and by their union and their idiosyncrasy are the index of the cerebral disorder which is going on, and which is too often the herald of multiple complications, the most dangerous of which is the attack of apoplexy.

Hemiplegia.—Hemiplegia is one of the most frequent complications, not only of syphilitic obliterating arteritis, but also of cerebral syphilis in general. For the time being we have only to consider hemiplegia consequent on obliterating arteritis. Syphilitic arteritis having for its seat of election the Sylvian artery, the symptoms of hemiplegia following on this arteritis vary according to the degree and extent of this obliteration. As, however, the obliteration of the artery is most often gradual, it is quite exceptional for the resulting hemiplegia to strike the patient as rapidly as in hemiplegia consequent on ordinary cerebral hæmorrhage.

In order to give an idea of this syphilitic hemiplegia, I cannot do better than quote a case in my ward.

A man who had suffered from syphilis for about twelve years had been troubled for some time with severe headache at night. On November 27, 1891, he felt a slight paresis in the right leg, but he nevertheless continued his work. Next day the paresis became worse, and was followed by paresis of the right arm. During the afternoon of the same day his speech was less distinct, and on the morning of the next day facial hemiplegia appeared. During the next few days these troubles became more marked, and the hemiplegia was quite definite on December 1. On December 2 I noticed total hemiplegia of the right side, with deviation of the tongue and incomplete aphasia. During the following days the symptoms grew worse. On December 5 the hemiplegia and the aphasia became total. There was neither hemianæsthesia nor epileptiform convulsions. We could, therefore, assert that the patient was suffering from end-arteritis of the left Sylvian artery, the obliterating process having invaded the vessel beyond the origin of the perforating arteries ; and as the obliteration was gradual, the hemiplegia and the aphasia did not become complete until the ninth day. These symptoms proved that the branches from the trunk of the Sylvian artery, going to the foot of the third convolution, and to the ascending frontal and parietal convolutions, no longer furnished a proper supply of blood to these regions. The question as regards prognosis was whether these regions were or were not in a state of necrobiosis. In any case, active treatment was instituted from the moment of the patient's admission.

Whilst the right hemiplegia commenced to improve, however, we witnessed the commencement of left hemiplegia. This left hemiplegia also ran a slow course. It commenced in the left arm and invaded the left leg. The facial paralysis being double, the patient experienced such difficulty in mastication and deglutition that alimentation became very difficult. This left hemiplegia proved that the Sylvian artery on the right side, like its fellow on the left, was attacked at a symmetrical point by obliterating endarteritis. Symmetry of the lesions is, by the way, common in the history of syphilitic disease of the cerebral arteries. The active treatment, and the chance of intervening before the ischæmia of the cerebral regions ended in necrobiosis, gave us the satisfaction of witnessing progressive improvement in the double hemiplegia. Ability to write, which was absolutely impossible at the time of the patient's admission, not only on account of intellectual troubles but on account of true motor agraphia, gradually reappeared. The difficulty in deglutition likewise improved ; the aphasia, which had been absolute for twenty-four hours, gradually disappeared. At the end of a few weeks the movements in both hands reappeared, the patient commenced to walk, and after two months very marked improvement in this double syphilitic arteritis was obtained.

The example above quoted might serve as a type, but all cases are far from being alike. According to the localization of the obliterating arteritis the symptoms may vary and reveal themselves by complete hemiplegia, with or without aphasia; by incomplete hemiplegia; by monoplegia; and, finally, by aphasia, which may be isolated or associated with paralytic troubles. Each one of these kinds exists. I might quote several cases in which they are found complete in every detail. In one case we find that the hemiplegia has remained incomplete ; in another case we may find total hemiplegia, unamenable to treatment and followed by secondary contractures, which proves that the arterial obliteration has been complete, and of such a duration as to allow necrobiosis of the corresponding region, with secondary degenerative lesions.

Aphasia.—Amongst the symptoms of which I have just spoken there is one to which I desire to refer—aphasia, the complete history of which has been given in one of the preceding sections. Syphilitic aphasia often opens the scene of the cerebral complications. It may or may not be associated with hemiplegia of the right side ; it may appear as an isolated, initial, and transitory symptom. It may supervene in the shape of a fit, which lasts for some minutes or for some hours ; it may be subject to recurrences. As a type of syphilitic aphasia without hemiplegia, I recall the case of Tarnowski, which is quoted in the admirable treatise of Fournier on cerebral syphilis. Other cases, referring to the various types of syphilitic aphasia, will be found in the same work. Charcot has published a most interesting case of syphilitic aphasia. The patient was seized with progressive hemiplegia on the right side, motor aphasia, and word-blindness. The motor aphasia disappeared later, but the word-blindness persisted. The cerebral lesion, consequent on syphilitic arteritis of the left Sylvian artery, was localized by Charcot in the psychomotor region, in Broca's convolution, and in the lobule of the angular gyrus.

Diagnosis.—I must now deal with the differential diagnosis of hemiplegia and aphasia consequent on the syphilitic obliteration of the Sylvian arteries. Apart from some exceptional cases, this form of hemiplegia is never sudden and complete from the outset; it is preceded, sometimes at a remote period, by more or less obstinate and severe headache, vertigo, obnubilation, amnesia, transitory aphasia, and twitchings or heaviness in one foot or in one hand; these symptoms may be associated with one another or may follow on one another, improving and reappearing in infinite variety. Such a condition of things does not exist in ordinary cerebral hæmorrhage, or in obliteration of the cerebral arteries by embolism. The syphilitic process resembles, though with more marked shades, the lesions of cerebral atheroma in patients suffering from alcoholism and gout, and in old people. When a patient is taken ill with hemiplegia which has required two or three days to become complete, and when for some weeks or months he has complained of violent headache (worse at night), of transient aphasia, of vertigo, etc., we must immediately think of syphilitic hemiplegia. If this general or dissociated hemiplegia has been preceded, or if it is accompanied, by more or less limited Jacksonian epilepsy, or by partial contractures, it is very probable that the syphilitic hemiplegia is caused by a cortical lesion of the motor centres. If, however, these hemiplegic or aphasic symptoms have neither been preceded nor accompanied by localized contractures, or by Jacksonian epilepsy, and, *a fortiori*, if the hemiplegia invades, though unequally, both sides of the body, it may almost certainly be said that syphilitic obliterating arteritis is the cause.

Sometimes, however, the diagnosis remains uncertain. It is then that lumbar puncture, by revealing marked lymphocytosis (twelve times out of thirteen cases—Widal and Lemierre) turns the balance in favour of the syphilitic nature of the hemiplegia, and induces us to commence active treatment (Widal and Lemierre). In other patients the presence of Argyll-Robertson's sign will remove all doubts. It will also allow us to affirm the specific nature of the disease (Babinski). Besides, even in non-hemiplegic patients who show only Argyll-Robertson's sign, the cerebro-spinal fluid is rich in lymphocytes, as the researches of Babinski, and Widal and Lemierre have shown.

The existence of lymphocytosis in syphilitic hemiplegia shows once more the importance of the meningeal irritation in the nervous manifestations of syphilis.

The **prognosis** of syphilitic cerebral arteritis is very grave. It is more easy to treat a sclero-gummatous cerebro-meningeal lesion than arteritis. To begin with, the gumma or the sclero-gummatous lesion is more clearly localized, invading only a relatively restricted region, and the tissue is easily modified by mercury and iodide of potassium, whereas arteritis is by nature more diffuse, and invades several arteries or several segments of arteries. These lesions are obstinate, and less accessible to treatment. Relapse in arteritis is frequent, and a patient whose condition has been improved or apparently cured is seized a few months later with fresh cerebral troubles. Sometimes even when the patient appears to be so much better that recovery may be hoped for, the improvement stops, and persistent troubles appear (secondary contractures, embarrassment of speech, and weakening of the intellect).

Finally, let us remark that syphilitic cerebral arteritis does not always exist in a state of purity ; in too many cases it is accompanied or followed by complications which are due to rupture of an aneurysm, to sclero-gummatous lesions, or, finally, to symptoms of general pseudo-paralysis. It would be wrong to consider syphilitic cerebral arteritis as the appanage of late syphilis. The cases previously quoted prove that fairly often syphilitic arteritis, with all its consequences, appears early, within one or two years of the primary infection.

Treatment.—In every case of syphilitic cerebral arteritis antisyphilitic treatment must be immediately adopted. The mercurial preparations and iodide of potassium must be administered in large doses, and without delay. I say without delay, because a delay of a few days may allow the necrobiosis of the brain to become irremediable. We must act as soon as the first precursory symptoms appear. As regards mercurial treatment, sub-cutaneous injections of biniodide and inunction of mercurial ointment seem to me the most certain means. About a drachm of mercurial ointment is rubbed in daily, and at the same time chlorate of potassium is given. The patient must be most careful to cleanse the mouth, so as to prevent the appearance of gingivitis or of mercurial stomatitis, which interferes with the exhibition of mercury.

The undoubted superiority of injections of biniodide leads me to recommend them in preference to all others. This method is, moreover, applicable in all cases of cerebral, spinal, laryngeal, pulmonary, naso-buccal, and cutaneous syphilis. The reader will find full details in the appendix on Therapeutics.

With the mercury we give iodide of potassium in increasing doses. Rigorous treatment is an indispensable condition of success. It is better to give large doses, although they may have to be suspended from time to time, than to give small doses. Instead of giving mercury and iodide at the same time, they may be given alternately, mercury being administered for a fortnight, and then iodide for another fortnight; but **mercury is very much better than iodide.** Brilliant success sometimes rewards our efforts, but a favourable prognosis must not be too readily given, because we might run the risk of a mistake. The arterial lesions of syphilis are amongst those which sometimes resist the best directed specific treatment, as I have already remarked and as I once more point out; and even when they appear cured, or almost cured, a relapse of the disease is to be feared.

Cerebral Gummata—Sclero-Gummatous Syphilis of the Brain and of the Meninges.

Pathological Anatomy.—Let us examine separately the lesions of the meninges and those of the brain. In the meninges, as elsewhere, we find circumscribed gummata, or diffuse, sclerotic gummatous tissue. The gummata vary in size from a millet-seed to a hazel-nut. They are usually found on the base of the brain and on the hemispheres, and especially the motor regions. Sclero-gummatous meningitis is very common. The patches of meningitis have the look of yellowish fibro-caseous tracts covering one or two convolutions; they are sometimes thick enough to form a tumour. They bind the meninges together and the meninges to the brain. The adhesion is such that the cerebral matter is torn on attempting to decorticate the brain. The sclero-gummatous lesions have the same seats of election as the gummata.

In the brain the gummatous tissue likewise presents itself in the form of diffuse infiltration, or of a circumscribed gumma. Diffuse gummatous encephalitis penetrates into the nerve tissue as an interstitial infiltration. Circumscribed gummata are not common; they vary in number and size; they occupy the central ganglia, the peripheral portions and the base of the brain in the neighbourhood of the sella turcica. It is interesting to know that the cerebral gummata are much more frequent in the frontal lobe than in the area of Rolando. In Herber's figures we find ten cases of gummata in the frontal lobe, whereas we find only two in the motor convolutions (Rolando's zone and the paracentral lobule), whence we may conclude *a priori* that Jacksonian epilepsy, following on lesions of Rolando's area, is due to tuberculoma, glioma, etc., much more often than to syphiloma.

From the anatomical and histological point of view it would seem that confusion could hardly be possible between the gumma and other tumours, such as glioma, tuberculoma, or a cyst undergoing degeneration, and yet there are cases where this confusion has occurred, as in the following case from Herber's thesis.

A man suffered from violent headache, especially at night. He had nausea, strabismus, and diplopia. Chauffard found paralysis of the external rectus of the right eye. The ophthalmoscope revealed double hæmoretinitis, having all the characteristics of syphilis. Though the patient denied syphilis, mercury and iodide of potassium were given, notable improvement resulting. The man left the hospital, but returned a fortnight later, the headache being worse than ever. The same treatment was again administered. Shortly afterwards fits of dizziness and violent delirium supervened. Two attacks of epilepsy soon occurred, and the patient was carried off by a third attack, more severe than the first.

The diagnosis of cerebral syphilis appearing certain (and everything pointed to it being correct), the following were the results of the post-mortem examination : (1) A soft gumma was found in the white matter, at the foot of the first frontal convolution. Its contents were caseous and yellowish in its upper part ; its lower part was cystic ; the peripheral zone was transparent and vitreous. (2) At the junction of the anterior and the middle third of the first frontal convolution, under the grey matter, a small, soft, transparent tumour was discovered, having the look of vitreous degeneration, and surrounded by a zone of white indurated matter. The two tumours looked like gummata.

The histological examination showed that the diagnosis made during life and at the post-mortem examination was erroneous. It was not a question of syphiloma, but of glioma. "The histological characters," says Philippe, "left no doubt as to the nature of these tumours. They were gliomata of the mixed type in which the fibrillæ and the cells had developed in equal proportions. In all the sections examined the glioma had invaded the cortex and the white matter, though to a greater extent in the latter."

In a patient at the Hôtel-Dieu who died from a syphilitic gumma of the frontal lobe the following was the result of the histological examination made by Jolly : The sections of the tumour showed that the cerebral tissue was almost completely replaced by connective tissue of new formation, fairly homogeneous, and containing but few cells. In places there were masses of rounded cells with a large nucleus. These masses most often surrounded the vessels. They were elongated or ramified, dividing the newly-formed tissue into lobules. In the vertical sections of the meninges the dura mater was but little altered. Below there was a thick adherent and vascular connective layer, which corresponded to the thickened pia mater. Numerous dilated vessels were surrounded by a mass of rounded cells with deeply stained nuclei. These vessels, surrounded by lymphatic hyaline tissue, passed down at right angles from the surface into the midst of the pathological tissue. At certain points the tissue of the tumour was homogeneous, necrosed, and lacking in cells. It did not take the stain. These points corresponded to the caseous islets visible to the naked eye. It was, therefore, not a question of a glioma, an epithelioma, a small-celled sarcoma, or a tuberculoma, which is more limited and caseous. It was a gummatous tumour.

The gummatous lesions in the brain and its membranes give rise to meningeal sclerosis, with obstruction of the small vessels in the cortex, and to more or less extensive cerebral softening from compression and thrombosis of the vessels. It is even probable that the process commences with a lesion of the arterioles (syphilitic arterio-sclerosis), and extends from them to the connective elements and to the tissue of the organ.

Symptoms.—A gumma may be present for a long while in certain regions of the brain without causing any symptom. In my clinical lectures* I have quoted the case of a patient who during the long evolution of a gumma of the frontal lobe felt nothing. The lesion suddenly revealed itself by an attack of Jacksonian epilepsy, and at that time the lesion had advanced so far that in a few days it was fatal, in spite of all treatment. How are we to explain that a cerebral lesion may remain latent for so long a time? It depends on the situation of the lesion. In the brain some regions are more tolerant than others. This toleration is not to be envied, because the patient, unaware of the danger, lives in false security, without following any treatment.

Nothing is more common than paralyses of the third and sixth nerves, because these nerves, before entering the orbit, run for a long way at the base of the skull in contact with the meninges. This region is precisely a seat of election of gummatous cerebro-meningeal lesions (Fournier). I do not say that all the syphilitic palsies which affect the oculo-motor and facial nerves are due to a lesion at the base of the brain. In some cases these paralyses, especially when they are partial, may be due to a lesion of the cortex; but, in proportion as the question is better understood, it will be found that many of these cases of paralysis are due to **peripheral neuritis,** and have nothing to do with central lesions.

Syphilitic paralysis of peripheral origin, and probably of a toxic nature, deserves recognition. It supervenes rapidly, is usually transient, and some-times dissociated; it may occur in the second, or even in the first year of the infection. Accordingly, in a syphilitic patient suffering from deviation of the mouth, facial hemiplegia, ptosis, strabismus, and diplopia, we must not be in a hurry to make the grave diagnosis of a syphilitic lesion at the base of the brain, because the paralysis may be due to peripheral neuritis; but if the third nerve is paralyzed as a whole, and *a fortiori* if the other motor nerves of the eye are also affected, and if these symptoms have gradually become more marked, and have been accompanied by vertigo and headache, with or without direct or crossed hemiplegia, a sclero-gummatous lesion of the base of the brain can be diagnosed. Syphilitic new growths are common in the interpeduncular space, whence the third pair of nerves emerge; it is also not an uncommon thing to find double paralysis of the common oculo-motor nerves. We may likewise be certain of a sclero-gummatous lesion at the base of the brain if a syphilitic patient has diminution or loss of sight, **optic neuritis** with nocturnal headache, which may or may not be accompanied by vomiting and epileptiform attacks.

Here, as in all cerebral tumours, the different varieties of **hemianopia** described under Polioencephalitis may be observed. Often, in conclusion, the examination with the ophthalmoscope reveals a chorio-retinitis, which

* Dieulafoy, *Clinique Médicale de l'Hôtel-Dieu,* 1903, 7me leçon.

has considerable value in establishing the diagnosis of syphilis. As regards the examination of the fundus oculi, the condition of the ophthalmic artery may give an idea of the condition of the cerebral arteries from which it arises.

We have said that the sclero-gummatous lesions have as their seat of election the **cortical motor zone.** Hemiplegia and partial epilepsy are the two great symptoms accompanying these localizations. The paralysis takes the form of hemiplegia or of monoplegia on the side opposite to the lesion. The face, arm, and leg may be paralyzed, as in ordinary hemiplegia. More often the arm only is attacked, or the arm and the face, or the leg alone. These paralyses are rarely complete, the power of movement not being absolutely lost; in many cases we find paresis rather than paralysis. Hemiplegia is hardly ever present from the outset; the paralysis sets in slowly and progressively. It is, for a longer or shorter period, preceded by weakness, numbness of the hand, twitchings, and heaviness of the foot and leg; for some time the patient complains of being unable to grasp objects, and of being awkward. He notices that his leg gives way; he stumbles against the steps when going upstairs, or he finds some hesitation in his speech. These prodromata are the herald of paralysis. If severe nocturnal headache is added to these prodromata, it is evident that the hemiplegic troubles resulting from a syphilitic lesion of the motor area do not resemble the hemiplegia which accompanies cerebral hæmorrhage; it is even slower, more dissociated, and more incomplete than the hemiplegia consequent on the obliteration of the Sylvian artery by syphilitic endarteritis. Finally, as we shall see, this hemiplegia, by virtue of the cortical lesion, is often associated with partial epilepsy.

Jacksonian epilepsy constitutes one of the most frequent symptoms of gummatous lesions in the motor area. This partial epilepsy appears on the side opposite to the lesion, and presents several types.

(1) In the **facial** type the convulsions are limited to the face and to the neck. They attack the commissures of the lips, the orbicularis palpebrarum, the motor muscles of the eye and of the tongue, and the sterno-mastoid. Jerking of the arm may also be present. (2) In the **brachial** type, which is more common, the aura commences in one of the fingers. The convulsions involve the hand, arm, and shoulder, and sometimes the face and the neck. (3) In the **crural** type, which is the least common, the aura commences in the foot, and the convulsions stop at the hip.

The topography of the cerebro-meningeal lesion may be diagnosed by the type of the epilepsy : facial type—lesion of the lower extremity of the cortex of the two ascending convolutions; brachial type—lesion of the middle portion of the ascending frontal convolution; crural type—lesion of the upper part of the ascending convolutions and of the paracentral lobule ;

lingual type—lesion of the lower part of the ascending convolution in the neighbourhood of the foot of the third frontal convolution.

In Jacksonian epilepsy loss of consciousness may be absent or incomplete, or it may only supervene when the convulsive attack has commenced. After the attack the patient may suffer from diplopia, dysphasia, amnesia, or vertigo. Under some circumstances the attack of partial epilepsy may be stopped by placing a ligature above the seat of the aura.

Partial epilepsy is often preceded or followed by transient paralysis (hemiplegia, monoplegia); in some cases the convulsive attack lays hold of the limbs, which are almost completely paralyzed. The fits of Jacksonian epilepsy may be isolated, or may be repeated several times a day.

A patient who had been suffering from syphilis for several years came into my ward at the Necker Hospital for hemiplegia of the right side without aphasia. The hemiplegia affected the limbs, the lower part of the face, and the tongue. It supervened gradually, and was accompanied by violent headache and intellectual torpor. From the time of his admission into the hospital the patient had fits of partial epilepsy. These fits consisted of a tonic stage, lasting some seconds, and of a clonic stage, lasting half a minute. The whole fit did not last a minute. It supervened suddenly, without any initial cry, pallor of the face, or any aura. It commenced in the right hand, spread to the face, to the neck, and sometimes to the leg on the same side, and then terminated. During the fit the patient never had stertorous respiration, the saliva was not bloody, and the tongue was not bitten. In a few days as many as 400 fits could be counted in the twenty-four hours. They were often subintrant, as in the status epilepticus, but they were never accompanied by a rise in temperature. The fit sometimes supervened when the patient had his mouth full of food. Mastication was stopped for a few seconds, and the fit having passed over, the patient continued eating. Further details are given under Jacksonian Epilepsy.

Under some circumstances the sclero-gummatous lesions produce, not partial epilepsy, but temporary or permanent contractures, which are at times very painful. The cortical lesions of syphilis which cause the troubles just described may be the origin of secondary degeneration, with late contracture, hemichorea, and athetosis.

In some cases the sclero-gummatous lesions cause paraphasia or aphasia by their localization in Broca's convolution. The aphasia may occur alone, or may be associated with monoplegia or hemiplegia of the right side.

Finally, there are some cases in which the sclero-gummatous lesions produce the syndrome described under the name of glosso-labio-laryngeal pseudo-paralysis. Incessant flow of the saliva through the half-open lips, difficulty in mastication and deglutition, paralysis of the tongue, increasing difficulty in the articulation of words, are the symptoms present. For further details as to the topography of the lesions, I refer the reader to the section dealing with glosso-labio-laryngeal paralysis.

In short, the cerebro-meningeal sclero-gummatous lesions may provoke paralysis of the cranial nerves, including disturbances of hearing and of sight (amblyopia, amaurosis); their most common symptoms are special forms of paralysis, hemiplegia, monoplegia, contractures, epileptiform fits. The epileptiform fit assists most in the cortical topographical diagnosis of the lesion, and allows us to eliminate the hypothesis of hemiplegia, or of monoplegia, consequent on obliterating endarteritis of the Sylvian artery.

These symptoms, which depend solely on the situation of the lesion, are accompanied by others which are common to all forms of cerebral syphilis, such as headache, which is worse at night, vertigo, intellectual torpor, etc.

The **prognosis** in cerebro-meningeal sclero-gummatous lesions is not as grave as in the other forms of cerebral syphilis. The lesions are cortical, and do not, like endarteritis of the large trunks, cause large foci of softening; and, again, they are more accessible to treatment than the interstitial and diffuse lesions which lead to the mental forms of cerebral syphilis. The epileptic or epilepto-paralytic form has not therefore a very grave prognosis. "It is," says Fournier, "one of the forms which yields best to treatment, and is most easily cured when attacked in time by the specific treatment."

Treatment.—The treatment has been described under Syphilitic Cerebral Arteritis.

Intellectual Troubles—Syphilitic General Pseudo-Paralysis.

We now come to one of the most delicate and most controversial questions. Is or is not cerebral syphilis capable of causing general paralysis? Before replying to this question let us proceed methodically. It is well known that cerebral syphilis is often the cause and the origin of the most varied intellectual troubles. These troubles may arise from deep foci of softening due to obliterating arteritis, and spreading to the frontal convolutions which preside over the mental faculties. They may likewise arise from the cortical lesions ending in sclero-gummatous meningo-encephalitis. Finally, they may be caused by the lesions of diffuse interstitial sclerous encephalitis.

Following Fournier's example, I shall divide the intellectual troubles of cerebral syphilis into two groups. In the first group I include the phenomena of exaltation and cerebral excitation, with relatively acute conditions of delirium or mania. The patients are excited, loquacious, and restless. They sleep, but they have hallucinations. Some of them commit acts of violence, and utter expressions significant of mental trouble, but they are conscious of it, because they are not incoherent, like patients suffering from general paralysis.

The patients of the second group, instead of being excited, are depressed. Their intelligence is weak and their memory fails. They are less fit for work, and suffer from "intellectual asthenia," which may be accompanied neither by incoherence nor by delirium. They certainly have some idea of their condition, being aware of their intellectual weakness, but they do not trouble about it, and the tranquil apathy with which they accept their condition sufficiently proves their mental decay. In some patients these symptoms are very marked; the intellectual depression is associated with incoherence, and the disease ends in dementia.

In certain circumstances the symptoms are **cerebro-spinal.** Within a few weeks or days an individual who has had syphilis is taken ill with headache, vertigo, embarrassment of speech, ptosis, numbness and heaviness in the legs, anæsthetic patches on the buttock or on the thighs, and difficulty in micturition. Walking soon becomes difficult; the patellar reflex is abolished; the sexual functions are lost, and the patient suffers from cerebral excitation or depression—in a word, the disease is cerebro-spinal, and in part resembles the picture of the slow and progressive invasion of tabes dorsalis. These cases led Fournier to assign to syphilis a large ætiological share in the pathogenesis of **tabes dorsalis** and of **cerebral tabes.**

The cerebral or cerebro-spinal symptoms just described do not give rise to a well-defined type. In another type, however, the nature and course of the symptoms recall the picture of general paralysis. It is to this form of cerebral syphilis that Fournier has given the name of **syphilitic general pseudo-paralysis.**

The symptoms of this form are described in the article on General Paralysis. It is certain that cerebral syphilis causes an affection which simulates idiopathic, progressive, chronic peri-encephalitis. The clinical manifestations are similar, and the anatomical lesion consists in a diffuse syphiloma of the cerebral cortex and of the meninges. Fournier has given the excellent name of **cerebral tabes** to the depressing form of this general pseudo-paralysis.

It has been asked whether syphilis is capable of producing true general paralysis. It would then have an important part in the ætiology of tabes dorsalis, of cerebral tabes, and of cerebro-spinal tabes.

This opinion, of which Fournier was almost the only defender, and which was for a long time contested, is now held in Germany, as well as in France, and it appears certain that syphilis is one of the most important factors in the production of general paralysis and of general pseudo-paralysis. . This does not mean, of course, that syphilis may not be much assisted by other factors : heredity, sexual or alcoholic excesses, worry, grief, and brain fag play some part. It may be the syphilitic factor alone would have remained indefinitely in the latent condition. Nevertheless its ætiological part is considerable, and at times predominant.

In any event the fact remains certain, from the point of view of the **prognosis,** that of all the forms of cerebral syphilis the **mental** one is the most serious and the most difficult to cure.

Hereditary Cerebral Syphilis.

Early or late hereditary syphilis causes the most varied pathological conditions in the nervous system. "Numerous cerebral conditions in childhood and in youth, vaguely put down to meningitis or encephalitis, are in reality nothing but the more or less late manifestations of hereditary syphilis" (Fournier). These manifestations include: intellectual torpor bordering on hebetude; repeated attacks of severe headache, labelled migraine or growing pains; vertigo, giddiness, and changes of character, wrongly looked upon as hysterical; finally and especially, the various forms of epilepsy, masked forms, nocturnal incontinence of urine, nocturnal vomiting, *petit mal*, and *grand mal*. We cannot too often think of early or late hereditary syphilis manifesting itself in childhood or in youth, because it is the cause of many ills, and is often amenable to specific treatment.

Summary.—To facilitate the description, I have divided the study of cerebral syphilis into three parts. In some clinical cases, which are fairly numerous, this somewhat artificial division holds good. Some patients, for instance, have obliterating arteritis; others have only paralysis or convulsions due to gummatous lesions; while others finally suffer from the mental form, with intellectual troubles, and more or less complete general paralysis. In other circumstances, however, these various manifestations of cerebral syphilis are associated or succeed one another. They may, indeed, spread to the spinal cord, when they become **cerebro-spinal**. Of these various forms, the one most amenable to treatment is the epileptic or epilepto-paralytic form; the one most rebellious to treatment is the mental form. In a case of cerebral syphilis mercury and iodide of potassium must be at once given in large doses. I prefer injections of biniodide of mercury. Every effort must be made to favour the tolerance of these remedies. Careful attention to the mouth will avoid or retard the appearance of mercurial gingivitis. By the intensive treatment we often succeed in limiting the disease. And yet, even in case of success we must watch, as Fournier says, for relapses. Recrudescences sometimes supervene even when recovery seems assured. Recurrences are too often met with when the cure seems definite. In spite of these disappointments, we must not be discouraged, and as long as the syphilitic process is in an active stage we must make every effort to fight it.

X. GENERAL PARALYSIS—CHRONIC MENINGO-ENCEPHALITIS.

General paralysis was for a long time regarded as a simple complication supervening during the course of madness. Such was the opinion of Esquirol, Calmeil, and Parchappe, and this explains the name of general paralysis of the insane given to this disease. Bayle, in 1826, opposed this view, but Baillarger definitely gave to general paralysis the position which it occupies to-day, by showing that it is a definite morbid entity, in which the motor disorders play at least as large a part as the psychic troubles.

Pathological Anatomy.—The lesions of general paralysis, which were at first thought to be limited to the meninges and the brain, in most cases occupy the whole extent of the nervous centres. On opening the skull the meninges are found to be thickened, especially over the frontal lobes (chronic meningitis). The dura mater is adherent to the cranium, and the pia mater to the brain. The brain matter exposed by the removal of the meninges is rough, bleeding, and ulcerated (Calmeil). The convolutions are atrophied, the brain is diminished in size, and the cavity of the ventricles is enlarged. On scraping the cortical layer with the handle of a scalpel, indurated lamellæ or ridges of the white matter are detached (Baillarger). The surface of the fourth ventricle (Joire) and of the lateral ventricles is studded with granulations (sclerotic tissue), and these various changes (ridges, lamellæ, granulations) are simply the result of a diffuse chronic encephalitis affecting chiefly the frontal lobes.

Under the microscope we see that the nerve cells are atrophied and reduced to a vitreous mass, in which neither a nucleus nor a nucleolus is any longer distinguishable; or else they are granular, pigmented, and stain badly. The cellular processes are broken, and the nerve fibres only exist in small numbers ; in their place we find numerous granular bodies.

The walls of the arteries are thickened, and the proliferated neuroglial elements seem in certain cases to smother the nerve cells. The starting-point of the lesions is the subject of controversy. The theory of cerebral sclerosis commencing around the vessels may not be true in all cases, if we accept the researches of Pierret, Friedman, Klippel, and Joffroy. According to them the theory of primary parenchymatous encephalitis is far more probable.

Interstitial encephalitis, ependymitis, and periencephalitis are represented by analogous lesions in the spinal cord, where, indeed, we find diffuse periependymal and peripheral myelitis, as well as the changes of chronic meningitis. In other cases we do not find diffuse lesions of the spinal cord, but combined scleroses (Raymond) in the posterior columns, lesions identical with those of tabes. The relation of tabes and general paralysis is discussed under Locomotor Ataxy.

The nerves themselves may be attacked by chronic neuritis. During life the symptoms noticed are patches of anæsthesia, muscular atrophy limited to a group of muscles, or, finally, one of the secondary trophic lesions common to peripheral neuritis.

The other viscera present various lesions, but not one of them seems to be in undisputed relation with the anatomical changes in the brain and in the meninges.

Symptoms.—In order to facilitate the description it is customary to divide general paralysis into three periods of indeterminate duration : the first period is called prodromal ; the second is the stationary stage ; and the third is the terminal, paralytic, and cachectic period.

At the commencement, psychic or motor troubles predominate. **Amnesia** is one of the most frequent symptoms. " Weakening of the memory is, with delirium, one of the most characteristic symptoms of general paralysis" (Luys). " Memory is the first of the faculties, sometimes the only one, which is attacked at the onset " (Ball). " The patient loses the faculty of self-control " (Dupré). According to circumstances, the patient becomes melancholy, or else irascible and violent—so much so as to strike without reason the people who are about him. One patient will be seized with an all-devouring activity. He walks the whole day long without stopping, and conceives a thousand projects, which are most often unrealizable. Another patient will indulge in reckless extravagance, and, without reason, purchase several dozen watches or a number of suits of clothes. In some subjects we meet with perversion of the moral faculties. One man obstinately refuses to pay for an article which he has just bought, or steals without a motive ; another man gives himself up to indecent acts in public, although his sexual passions are weakened. These facts are most important from a medico-legal point of view, because the patient has sometimes to appear in court, and it is the physician's duty to decide whether his patient is or is not **responsible.**

In many cases **motor troubles** open the scene. How often do we not meet with a quavering speech, awkwardness in the hand, a modification in the writing, or inequality of the pupils, in people who so far show no trace of intellectual troubles, and in whom we can foretell six months or a year in advance the appearance of other complications.

Sometimes the commencement of the disease reveals itself by apoplectiform or epileptiform attacks, loss of consciousness, or transitory hemiplegia, and the psychic troubles break out after one or more congestive attacks. The attacks are sometimes ushered in by fits of ophthalmic migraine.

Disturbances in the organs of the senses sometimes precede all the other symptoms ; amblyopia and diplopia have been noticed. Voisin has insisted on the blunting or on the abolition of the sense of smell, which often precedes the usual symptoms.

In the stationary stage the disease assumes several forms. Its most common form is characterized by delirium of grandeur. The patient lives in a condition of continual satisfaction ; he believes himself to be an Emperor, the Pope, or God. He is possessed of millions, and wishes to distribute them to those who are around him. He owns palaces built out of precious stones.

Nothing on earth equals his strength, his beauty, or his power. His ideas, however, are not, like those of the monomaniac, ambitious, connected, and well co-ordinated; they are, on the contrary, mobile and contradictory (Falret); and whilst the patient suffering from general paralysis is talking to you of his splendour, ask him his calling, and he will artlessly tell you "I am a cobbler" (Magnan).

In certain patients hypochondriasis dominates the scene. He believes himself to be dead, or fancies that he is persecuted; he refuses all food for fear of poison; he has hallucinations and ideas of suicide.

In the midst of these symptoms (exalted and hypochondriac forms) some patients have attacks of **acute mania**—their fury necessitates the application of the strait-jacket. The attack then disappears, and the general paralysis continues its progressive course (Baillarger).

Speech troubles often show themselves from the first; in some cases they are the only symptom of the onset. The change in speech is so character-istic that it alone would suffice to establish the diagnosis. When a patient suffering from paralysis wishes to speak, there is a kind of tremor in the muscles of the lips; the speech is hesitating, and participates in the tremor of the lips and tongue. The motor troubles depend on the inco-ordination and the weakening of the movements; it is a kind of ataxy mixed with paresis. The patients are less clever in manual work, and their gait becomes tottering. In certain cases the want of co-ordination predominates, and the disease assumes for a time the symptoms of locomotor ataxy (see section on Tabes).

As the disease progresses, the intellectual and paralytic troubles become more pronounced, and are sometimes complicated by epileptiform or apoplectiform attacks, with a rise in temperature and transitory hemiplegia. Contractures and paralyses may also be observed in the form of special attacks (Magnan).

The sensory nervous system is but little affected in general paralysis. Anæsthesia is more common than hyperæsthesia. Visceral pains analogous to those of locomotor ataxy have been noticed (Teissier).

Inequality of the pupils (Baillarger) is a frequent symptom often observed in the first period. It sometimes disappears during the remissions, but reappears afterwards. The pupil reflexes are sometimes sluggish or abolished, as far as light or accommodation are concerned; at times they correspond to Argyll-Robertson's sign. At the commencement of the disease the paralysis of the pupil is often associated with paralysis of the accommo-dator muscle (Parinaud, Ballet). Internal ophthalmoplegia is the result. The optic nerve is very rarely atrophied; the motor nerves of the eye are rarely affected.

Hæmatoma auris is common in general paralysis. It is situated between the cartilage and the perichondrium, and attributed by some writers to injury, by others to vascular trouble.

In women the development of general paralysis most frequently results in irregularity or suppression of menstruation, which function may return during the remissions of the disease. The terminal period of general paralysis is characterized by the mental decay of the individual. "The patients, who are constantly soiled by urine or fæces, defæcate incessantly, and plunge their hands into the excrement, with which they cover everything. They are practically isolated from the external world, merely leading a vegetative existence" (Magnan). Some reach the end of their existence, being conscious of their decay; their intelligence is weakened, but they are not insane.

Course—Duration.—General paralysis commences with motor or with psychic troubles, according as the lesion affects the motor convolutions or the psychic convolutions. In other cases, however, the lesion announces itself by spinal symptoms (inco-ordination, pains, paresis, and trophic troubles), which precede the intellectual troubles by several years; in other words, the lesions of the nervous system in general paralysis are sometimes ascending, sometimes descending, and often involve, from the outset, the major portion of the nerve centres. Sometimes the lesion is limited for a time to the optic nerves (amaurosis) and to the motor nerves of the eye (ptosis, strabismus, diplopia).

The course of the disease is slow and progressive. It is interrupted by exacerbations, and by remissions which vary from a few months to two and three years. These remissions may appear spontaneously, or may be due to an intercurrent disease, to a traumatism, to a surgical affection, or to copious suppuration. In its rapid form the disease may last less than a year. The general duration varies from one to six years; there are exceptional cases in which the remissions prolong the existence indefinitely.

Ætiology—Diagnosis.—General paralysis attacks adults from thirty to forty-five years of age. It may, however, appear at the age of fourteen years in the form of juvenile general paralysis (Charcot). Males are usually attacked, and heredity plays a considerable part in its development. Alcoholism, excess of work, prolonged grief—in a word, congested conditions of the brain—favour chronic meningo-encephalitis. The existence of a general pseudo-paralysis due to alcohol, lead, etc., has been admitted; but at present these cases of pseudo-paralysis are more usually placed under true general paralysis. According to the ætiological factor, and according to the soil in which the disease evolves, certain differences in the symptomatology and in the course are observed, but the very essence of the disease appears to be the same. The nerve elements may be damaged by toxic products of various origins, but their mode of reaction is said to be the same, no matter what agent is the cause. Furthermore, as far as syphilis is concerned, it seems that the virus of syphilis is more apt in certain cases to produce cerebral lesions. This fact would explain the cases reported by Morel-Lavallée, in which five men who had contracted syphilis from the same source all died from syphilitic general paralysis.

Syphilis is intimately associated with the history of general paralysis. The ætiological relations of these two diseases have been discussed recently at the Académie de Médecine. According to Fournier, these two affections stand to one another in the relation of cause and effect, for the following reasons : (1) Statistics show that syphilis is very common in general paralytics, the proportion, according to certain writers, being 90 per cent. (2) Many syphilitic persons become general paralytics without any other cause to be found save syphilis. (3) General paralysis is more rare in women, except in districts where syphilis is raging. (4) General paralysis is rare in the country, where syphilis is equally rare. (5) Syphilis is more common in general paralytics than in other insane persons. (6) Tabes, which is undoubtedly of syphilitic origin in many cases, is often associated with general paralysis. (7) In general paralysis, as in tabes, we find lymphocytosis of the cerebro-spinal fluid and Argyll-Robertson's pupil, which is, according to Babinski, a sign of syphilis.

In spite of these arguments, Joffroy does not think that syphilis causes general paralysis, and insists on the fact that syphilis is common among the Moors, while general paralysis is very rare. Lancereaux and Cornil oppose Fournier's opinion by pathological arguments, and deny that the lesions of general paralysis run the same course as syphilitic lesions of the nerve centres. Raymond answers this argument by a collection of cases showing the frequent coexistence of both varieties of lesion in the same individual.

I shall attempt a brief review of the pathogenesis. It is certain that general paralysis, like tabes, appears, practically speaking, only in persons who have had syphilis. Theory is not of much moment. The view I hold is that people are not exposed to the risk of paralysis or of tabes unless they are syphilitic. I readily admit that general paralysis runs a fatal course, a fact not in agreement with the usual course of syphilitic lesions. I also admit that specific treatment has no hold upon confirmed tabes or general paralysis. But, in spite of everything, I state the following aphorism—a person who is not syphilitic will have neither general paralysis nor tabes.

Fournier, in his communication to the Académie, has stated the date at which general paralysis appears ; it is between six and twelve years after the primary infection, the maximum being the tenth year. Accordingly, he advises *cures de renforcement* with mercurial treatment, beginning in the fifth year after infection, and carried out for several years.

Cases of ambitious and melancholic monomania are distinguished from general paralysis in that they have not, like it, mobile and contradictory ideas. General paralysis must be distinguished from senile dementia, insular sclerosis, alcoholism, and cerebral softening.

As in the case of tabes, lymphocytosis of the cerebro-spinal fluid is the rule in patients suffering from general paralysis (Widal, Sicard, and Ravaut). Sometimes, indeed, at the moment of certain exacerbations lymphocytosis may give place to polynucleosis (Widal and Lemierre).

Treatment.—During the prodromal period the patient must avoid fatigue, work, and excitement of every kind. A quiet country life, walks in the open air, absolute abstention from alcohol ; milk diet, together with ordinary food ; laxatives, and blisters to the nape of the neck, such are the usual methods. If syphilis is supposed to be responsible, daily injections of biniodide of mercury must be given at once ; this treatment is not, however, of much service. The periods of excitement must be controlled by the use of the douche, valerian, and bromides.

At a more advanced period it is generally necessary to place the patient in an asylum, " either because the maniacal excitement reaches an excessive degree, in which case the patient becomes dangerous to others, or because the melancholia is accompanied by refusal of food and impulse to suicide " (G. Ballet and P. Blocq).

XI. SYPHILITIC NECROSIS AND PERFORATION OF THE VAULT OF THE SKULL—DIAGNOSIS FROM TUBERCULOSIS AND FROM CANCER.

The following section is based upon two of my clinical lectures :*

Clinical case : A young woman was admitted for a perforation in the right parietal bone. The perforation formed an oval hole as large as a sixpence. The edges were clean-cut, and the external orifice was bounded by the scalp, which was neither ulcerated nor adherent. At the bottom of the hole the dura mater was exposed, and the pulsations of the brain were evident. The perforation was covered with a dressing in order to prevent infection.

About eighteen months before she had felt a boss on the bone. The tumour caused neither pain nor ill-health. Six months later it was as large as a hazel-nut, and the pain was so acute that Delannoy operated. The tumour resembled a cyst. During the exploration purulent fluid made its exit, and the surgeon found osteitis of the subjacent bone. As he concluded that the abscess was secondary to tubercular osteitis, the bone was scraped. No relief followed the operation ; the wound suppurated freely, and other tumours appeared.

The patient suffered from severe headache, insomnia, and wasting. As drugs gave no relief, a further operation was performed. The affected bone was exposed, a sequestrum was removed, and the friable edges of the bone were trimmed with forceps. The dura mater, studded with granulations, was scraped. In spite of the operation the

---

* Dieulafoy, *Clinique Médicale de l'Hôtel-Dieu*, 1906, 1re et 2me leçons.

wound continued to suppurate, and the headache was most severe, especially at night. The patient could neither eat nor sleep. Vomiting was frequent.

The fingers of the left hand now became fixed in the semi-flexed position ; a contracture of the face caused deviation of the mouth, increased at times by spasms. The picture was one of Jacksonian epilepsy.

With this knowledge it was easy to reconcile the symptom and the lesion. Stimulation of the motor cortex on the right side had caused permanent contracture of the fingers of the left hand and Jacksonian epilepsy of the face. This syndrome, including the attacks of vomiting, was not due to the sequestrum, because it had been removed months before ; it was the result of meningo-encephalitis of the Rolandic area.

Her condition was very grave, when Letulle diagnosed the lesion as syphilitic, and at once gave injections of biniodide of mercury. After the fourth injection the patient felt better than she had done for a long time, and after ten or twelve injections the symptoms yielded. The injections were alternately suspended and administered. Further destruction of the cranium was prevented, and the loss of substance began to fill up.

Syphilitic necrosis of the cranium is by no means rare. Wallet, in 1897, collected forty-six cases, and I have succeeded in finding others, making a total of eighty cases, of which I shall make use in the present discussion.

Pathological Anatomy.—Syphilis attacks the bones of the cranial vault in the following order : frontal, parietal, temporal, and occipital. This is true for the initial lesions, but untreated cranial syphilis rarely remains limited to a single bone. From the cases and specimens I have examined, I find that a large part of, or even the entire, cranial vault may be invaded by syphilis in the absence of proper treatment. The lesions are at first confined to a single bone, usually the frontal or the parietal, but untreated syphilis of long duration may affect both surfaces of the vault in various regions. When the cranial vault falls a victim, syphilis gains a firm hold, and as a rule grants no truce unless effective treatment steps in. And when we see the destruction wrought by syphilis upon the cranial vault, we ask how life could have been compatible with such lesions.

On examination of the two tables of the skull we find the bone eaten away and perforated ; in some parts the bone is destroyed, in others exostoses are present. Some skulls resemble old plates of ivory carved in relief, others have a worm-eaten appearance ; some resemble a row of teeth, in others the bone is hollowed out and tunnelled ; some skulls are full of holes like a sieve, while others resemble a macaroon-mill (Fournier) ; in some specimens we find sequestra of every size and shape ; some skulls have perforations with circular, polycyclical edges, others resemble a map of islands ; lastly, skulls are seen with astounding losses of substance.

The Figures 73 to 78 show some of these skulls.

We are now clear as to the different pathological varieties of necrosis and perforation of the skull due to syphilis. How are these lesions produced ? In the first place, the cranial bones are composed of a compact inner and outer table, separated by spongy tissue, called diploë. Externally, the convex surface is covered by periosteum, which takes part in the formation and nutrition of the bone ; internally, the concave surface is lined by the dura mater, which is considered to be an internal periosteum.

The gumma originates in the periosteum close to the outer table, or in the dura mater close to the inner table ; it rarely originates in the diploë. The syphiloma is at first composed of an accumulation of embryonic cells, producing a nodular tumour. The granulations are often as large as a pin's head ; they are due to an agglomeration of nodules.

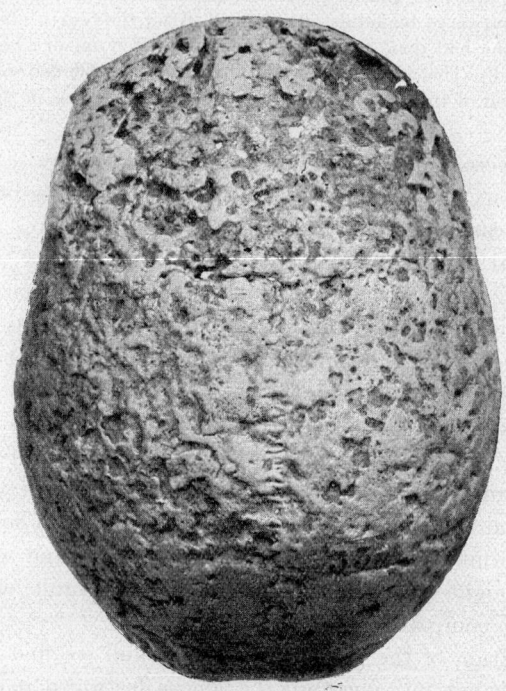

FIG. 73.—SYPHILITIC SKULL. DUPUYTREN MUSEUM (No. 593, New).

The skull-cap looks like old ivory sculptured in relief. Some parts of the skull are eaten away, while others stand out like kidneys, bridges, tunnels, arabesques, and branches of coral.

The osseous gumma, says Cornil, appears as a soft reddish vegetation, which is but little vascular, semitransparent, and of variable size ; it penetrates the table, and forms a cavity at the expense of the bone, which is absorbed by a process of rarefying osteitis. A centre of osteitis develops in contact with the gumma; the bone appears to melt away under the attack of the specific lesion.

A characteristic figure (Fig. 77), reproduced from Ziegler's work, shows gummatous osteitis of the parietal bone. The gumma has begun in the deep layer of the periosteum : on the one side it projects towards the exterior; on the other side it has invaded the outer table, which has been absorbed, and it is beginning to eat away the diploë.

Two foci of gummatous osteitis may exist : the one starts from the periosteum, the other from the dura mater ; the two foci grow to meet each other in the form of a cone, and perforation of the bone may result.

The syphiloma in its course nearly always provokes exuberant and rarefying osteitis. While one portion of the bone disappears, other parts of the bone become thickened and condensed, so that we see side by side bone in process of disappearing and hypertrophied eburnated bone. In a section

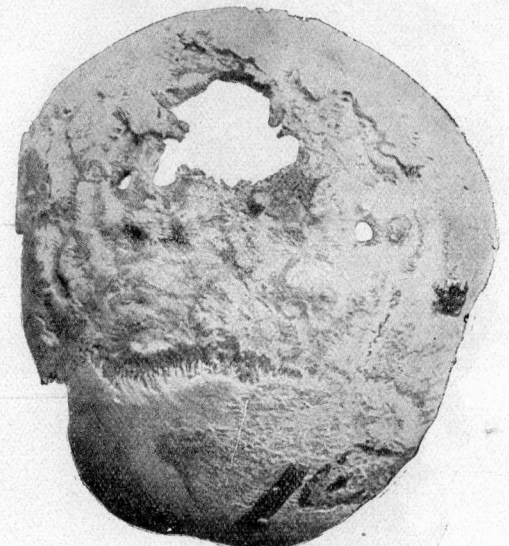

FIG. 74.—SYPHILITIC SKULL. DUPUYTREN MUSEUM (No. 339, A).

The whole skull-cap is affected. In front much loss of substance ; in other parts small circular perforations. The outer table is destroyed to a large extent. Eburnated projections are seen at certain spots.

" we are struck by the contrast between condensation and rarefaction ; numerous small holes, as large as a pin's head, are surrounded by a zone of condensing osteitis as hard as ivory " (Poulet). Whether the bony lesion is small or large we find these inverse processes—rarefaction of the bone and ivory exostoses.

Syphilitic osteitis has been said to describe a kind of spiral. " The gummatous bud, arising in the periosteum, penetrates the bone through a narrow aperture, which is not larger than a pin's head ; it, then, describes a helix in the spongy tissue " (Poulet).

We have seen how the bones of the skull-cap are eaten away and hypertrophied by gummatous osteitis, which causes both condensation and rare-faction. We have now to see how the osteitis results in perforation of the bone. It does so by the various processes just enumerated. Foci of osteitis hollow out pits in the bone, and lead to gradual perforation by molecular necrosis. In other cases the perforation is produced through the meeting of two foci, the one superficial and the other deep.

I think that the perforation usually results from the falling out of small or large sequestra. Foci of osteitis gradually isolate a portion of the bone,

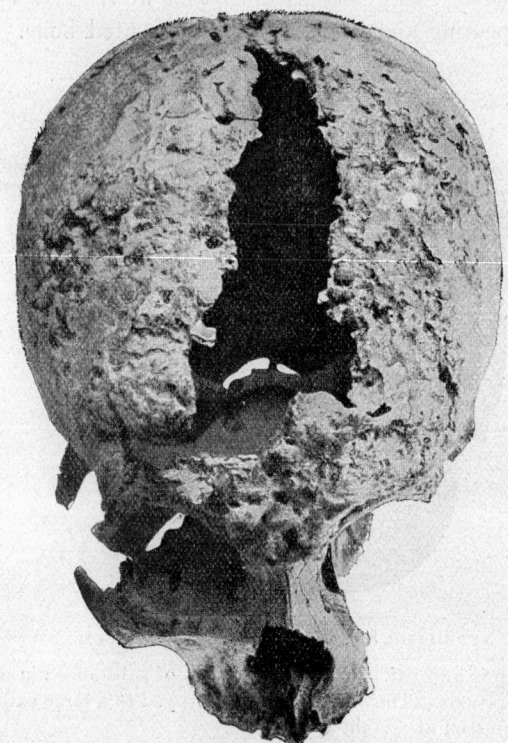

FIG. 75.—SYPHILITIC SKULL. VAL-DE-GRACE MUSEUM.

Very extensive loss of substance, affecting the anterior and middle portion of the skull as far as the occipital bones. The bones are everywhere eaten away and surmounted here and there by bosses of eburnated bone.

which necroses; the sequestrum is finally detached in one or in several pieces, and a perforation in the bone results. Accordingly, the sequestra and the perforations show great variety in size and shape. The preceding plates show skulls with incredible losses of substance.

Laqueau relates the case of a man who had necrosis of nearly the whole of the skull. A crucial incision was made from the frontal eminence to the upper angle of the occipital bone, and from one parietal eminence to the other.   The operator removed in three weeks both parietal bones, the greater part of the upper angle of the occipital and the upper two-thirds of the frontal bone.   The patient survived for some months.

I should like to mention one mode of perforation.   We find circinate and polycyclical foci of gummatous osteitis, exactly similar in shape to certain syphilides of the skin.   While I was examining a skull from Fournier's collection, I discovered this circinate osteitis in the act of causing sequestration and perforation of the bone.   In order to appreciate the specimen, it is necessary to hold up the skull and examine its inner surface while the outer

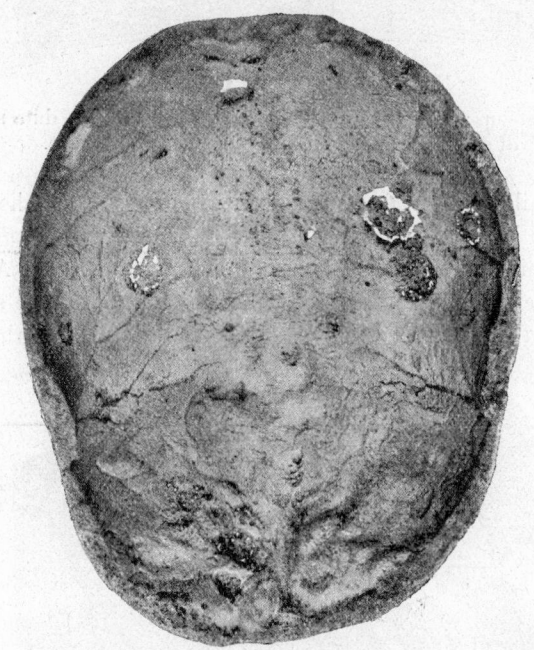

FIG. 76.—SYPHILITIC SKULL : FROM PROFESSOR FOURNIER'S COLLECTION.

The lesions are situated on the concave aspect of the skull. The centres of osteitis have a circinate and polycyclical form, which we shall study later.

surface is in a good light ; the rays of light passing through the minute pores of the gummatous foci, which have perforated or are in process of perforation, show the details of the necrotic process.

At several points on this skull I have found annular or circinate foci of osteitis.   The centre of the focus is somewhat opaque ; this is the portion of the bone which is destined to form the sequestrum, and around the sequestrum we find several small holes in the form of a ring, and not larger than the point of a needle, which allow the rays of light to pass through them.   We might well speak of it as an opaque stone surrounded by a circle

II.   88

of small diamonds ; the central sequestrum is kept in place merely by some bony filaments. The picture is even more clear if we examine the circinate focus with a lens, the skull being held in the same position as regards the light.

At another point in this skull we see a loss of substance due to gummatous osteitis ; the polycyclical edges resemble the polycyclical edges of certain

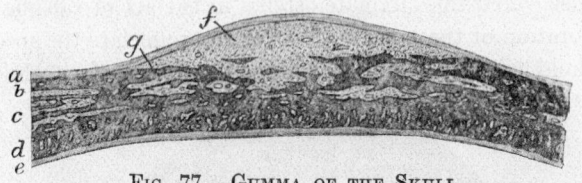

FIG. 77.—GUMMA OF THE SKULL.

a, External periosteum ; *b*, outer table ; *c*, diploë ; *d*, inner table ; *e*, dura mater ; *f*, centre of syphilitic infection ; *g*, carious bony trabeculæ.

cutaneous syphilides. In the centre of the focus we see a toothed sequestrum which has been isolated by peripheral osteitis, and which is connected somewhat like a peninsula to the bank of bone by a thin pedicle. At other parts of the skull the osteitis has taken a semilunar form, and the sequestrum is in part isolated in the loss of substance. And, lastly, at other points the

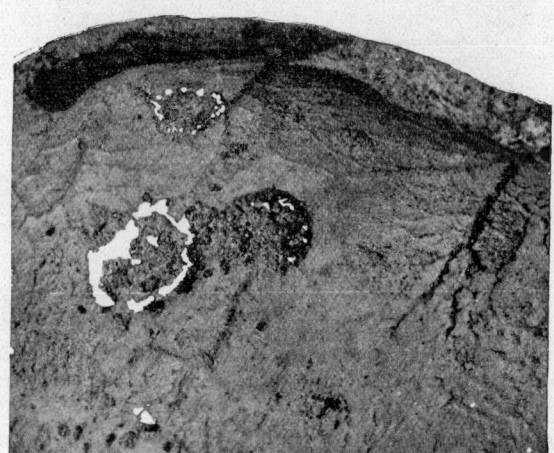

FIG. 78.—SYPHILITIC OSTEITIS OF THE SKULL.

sequestrum has disappeared, leaving an oval or irregular perforation, with toothed edges.

These various lesions are seen in the above photograph, which, however, does not do justice to the delicate points of the specimen.

In the foregoing varieties I have only considered the cranial syphiloma which starts in the bone and the periosteum ; there are, however, cases, says Mauriac, in which the lesion commences in the scalp. "Cutaneous tubercles and subcutaneous gummata break down, ulcerate, and reach the periosteum; the affection then spreads like the perforating or serpiginous process seen in certain syphilides."

A case of this nature has been published by Hobbs and Broustet. A woman was suffering from ulcerated gummata of the scalp, the process running a rapid course, somewhat like phagedæna; the gummata spread from the skin to the bones, from the bones to the meninges, and the patient died. The autopsy showed that the disease had, in a short space of time, destroyed the outer table and eaten through the whole thickness of the skull. This case proves that gummata of the scalp and of the forehead must be watched for and treated, because they may be the starting-points of a most serious osteosyphiloma.

Cranial sequestra present interesting features: the outer table disappears by exfoliation, and the inner table opposes a marked resistance. Some sequestra are surrounded by a line of demarcation, which finally frees the necrosed fragment of bone. This process of elimination lasts for months; it may last indefinitely if the sequestrum is set in a wide circle of hypertrophied bone; the surgeon is, then, obliged to remove it with the aid of the gouge and mallet. The sequestrum, when exposed to the air, becomes of a blackish-green colour. The surface of the syphilitic sequestra often has a worm-eaten appearance, while the tubercular sequestra are rather smooth and polished.

The cranial syphiloma may become infected and suppurate. Sometimes the abscess projects under the scalp; at other times it burrows between the skull and the dura mater, forming the so-called button-hole abscess. The sequestra keep up abundant fœtid suppuration.

The meninges and the brain may participate in the specific process; the dura mater is sometimes the seat of a gummatous infiltration. Pachymeningitis, with granulations, is often seen. In the case of Hobbs and Broustet the thickened dura mater was converted into fibrous tissue, composed of large parallel fibres, in the midst of which nodular gummata were present. Abscess of the brain and lesions between the cerebrum and the meninges have been noted in several cases.

A specimen in the Saint-Louis Museum shows the surface of the dura mater exposed by the falling out of a sequestrum, and covered with a circinate eruption. Mauriac quotes similar cases. It is indeed remarkable that cranial syphilis shows this circinate form in the skin, the bone, and the dura mater.

Cicatrization of the bony lesions takes place in the following manner: If the external table only has been destroyed, a simple depression is left; if, however, the whole thickness of the skull has been destroyed, the scar mats together the scalp, the bone, and the dura mater.

Brief mention must be made of the cranial lesions of hereditary syphilis.

Some are the result of deformities which commence shortly after birth, and give rise to the natiform skull, to the forehead with lateral bosses, to the keel-like forehead, and to the Olympian brow (Fournier). Others supervene, as the first manifestation of syphilis, at a more or less advanced period of life, and comprise rarefying osteitis and overgrowth of bone.

I shall now give a short summary of the lesions of cranial syphilis. Syphilis of the cranial vault, unless arrested by timely treatment, has a tendency to perforate the skull. The lesions may predominate either on the exterior or on the interior of the skull. Whether these lesions are small or large, we nearly always find, side by side, a double process, ending, on the one hand, in absorption and destruction of the bone, and, on the other hand, in overgrowth and eburnation of the neighbouring bony tissue. The cranial syphiloma starts in gummatous granulations, which originate in the periosteum near the outer table, or in the dura mater near the inner table. In some cases the syphiloma commences in the skin, and then spreads to the bone. The perforations are produced in different ways : sometimes the gummatous buds perforate the bone right through; at other times two gummata, one on the inner table, the other on the outer table, meet one another, and establish the perforation. In many cases, whether the focus of osteitis is or is not circinate, a certain number of gummata isolate a fragment of bone ; this fragment forms one or several sequestra, and more or less considerable loss of substance results. The meninges and the brain may participate in the syphilitic process.

Symptoms.—For the sake of clearness in description let us separate the cases in which the gumma arises in the outer table, thus forming a visible tumour, from the cases in which the syphiloma arises in the inner table, thus escaping observation. In the first stage of the external syphiloma pain and swelling are the only indications of the lesion, and even the pain is not a constant symptom. Absence of pain is not enough to exclude the diagnosis of gummatous osteosyphiloma. In the presence of an indurated or softened cranial tumour we should be wrong to exclude syphilis on the ground that the lesion, if syphilitic, must be painful. And yet it must be said that the absence of pain is exceptional ; the pericranial syphiloma causes pain, which is sometimes excessive, especially at night, and the headache commonly extends over the whole of the cranium.

As the syphiloma projects externally, it forms a tumour, which is not movable, because it starts from the bone. The tumour is hard at first and somewhat spread out ; later it softens at the centre, and an abscess may result. This condition lasts for months. Nevertheless, the osteosyphiloma, even though it is fluctuating, may, under proper treatment, end neither in ulceration nor in abscess. I may quote a case from Fournier :

A young woman who suffered from severe headache had a frontal osteo-syphiloma, which was fluctuating in the centre. In spite of this advanced lesion there was no ulceration, and recovery followed mixed treatment.

The syphiloma adheres to the skin, which grows thin; an opening then forms, through which purulent liquid makes its exit. An oval or circular ulceration, with clean-cut edges, sanious floor, and purulent secretion, results. The edges are sometimes limited by indurated bone. The bottom of the ulcer is filled in by the bone, which is attacked by osteitis or necrosis. The ulcerations may be smaller than a sixpence or larger than a crown-piece. It is not uncommon to see several ulcerated osteosyphilomata.

Galtier-Boissière has reported the case of a patient who had on the left side of the frontal bone an ulcerated osteosyphiloma as large as a pigeon's egg. Two years later (the first ulceration being still unhealed) an osteosyphiloma, which ulcerated, appeared on the right side of the forehead. Intense headache was present. Later another osteosyphiloma appeared in the middle of the forehead. Finally two other growths appeared above the right and left orbits, and perforated the bone so that the pulsations of the brain could be seen. These lesions were much improved by mixed treatment.

In this destructive process the necrosis is sometimes limited to the outer table of the bone, which is eliminated by exfoliation, the inner table forming a rampart; or the whole thickness of the bone is necrosed, with the formation of a sequestrum, which may be movable, or may be set in a ring of hypertrophied bone. When the sequestrum is eliminated spontaneously, or when it is removed by the surgeon, the thickened dura mater is exposed, and the brain is seen pulsating at the bottom of the wound.

I have just said that the pericranial gumma usually begins as a small painful tumour. We must not, however, confound this formidable tertiary lesion with the benign tumour of the periosteum seen in the secondary stage. Some patients suffer early in the secondary stage from periostitis of the skull, tibia, clavicle, etc. The cranium is one of the seats of election ; this periostitis is circumscribed and very painful ; slight pressure may cause the patient to cry out from pain. The patches of periostitis at times project slightly; at other times they form hard nodes, about as large as a shilling. These nodes resolve in two or three weeks under appropriate treatment. They differ, therefore, in several points from the gummatous osteosyphiloma.

I have so far considered the pericranial osteosyphiloma which reveals itself by pain and swelling. When the tumour is endocranial, swelling is absent, or, if it does occur, it is after a long period, when the lesion has extended through the bone to the surface. In the endocranial syphiloma we have no swelling to help us, and we must rely on the pain alone.

A patient complains of headache, which has been growing worse for some

weeks ; the whole head is painful, and yet the pain is more severe at certain
points. Methodical percussion of the head reveals the most painful region,
but the most exact examination does not show any swelling. An important
point is that the pain is worse at night, and prevents sleep in spite of every
remedy, such as aspirin, veronal, antipyrin, pyramidon, or morphia. Inquiry
justifies the exclusion of Bright's disease as the cause of the headache. In
answer to questions the patient admits syphilis ; he also shows some stigmata.
Examination of the mouth may reveal a patch of leucoplasia on the cheeks.
The increase of the pain at night and the failure of non-specific drugs
complete the diagnosis, and show that the patient is suffering from a syphilitic
lesion of the cranium. As, however, no sign of meningeal or cerebral
mischief has so far appeared, it is probable that the lesion is still limited to
the bone. In any case an injection of biniodide of mercury is given daily.
After six or seven injections improvement sets in, the headache disappears,
sleep returns, and the success of the treatment proves the correctness of
the diagnosis. I am quite convinced that many syphilitic headaches are
the result of an endocranial osteosyphiloma, of which the only symptom for
the time being is pain, cerebral symptoms and pericranial tumour being
absent. We must be on the watch for this endocranial syphiloma, because
mercurial treatment is necessary before the patient is exposed to grave
dangers.

   We must not, however, ascribe to osteosyphiloma every pain in the head
which a syphilitic patient may have sooner or later after infection. I do
not refer to painful periostitis in the secondary stage. I merely mention the
early headache which accompanies the secondary fever and syphilides.
I wish, however, to insist on certain intracranial lesions of which headache
is so often the forerunner.

   Syphilitic arteritis of the cerebral vessels, occurring at an early or remote
date after the primary infection, is often ushered in by acute headache.
In some cases patients have suffered from severe headache without other
signs, and have died suddenly from rupture of a syphilitic aneurysm of the
circle of Willis. In other cases patients have suffered from severe headache
without other signs, and have been stricken with hemiplegia due to obliterating arteritis of the Sylvian artery. Intracranial arteritis is, then, the
cause of intense headache, which may be the herald of an approaching
catastrophe. In gummatous lesions of the meninges and of the brain headache may be the chief feature ; its importance is very great. In short, headache, especially when it is paroxysmal and more severe at night, is a sign
which must always disturb the patient and his physician. It is often
accompanied by important signs, such as vertigo, vomiting, tingling in the
fingers, paralysis, contractures, etc. ; but in some cases the headache remains
for a time the chief feature, and overshadows the other signs. Gummatous

osteitis of the deep surface of the skull-cap may cause transient or intense headache. I admit that it is often difficult to say whether the headache is due to a bony lesion, to arteritis, or to meningitis, but the therapeutic indication in each case is to give promptly injections of mercury.

Our description has so far been confined to osteosyphiloma which does not encroach upon the meninges or the cerebral convolutions. The meninges and the brain, however, may be affected by the osteosyphiloma ; sometimes these organs are compressed by an exostosis, a sequestrum, or an abscess ; at other times they are the seat of pachymeningitis or encephalitis. In order to simplify the description, let us take the cases in which the lesion is limited to one lobe of the brain.

Let us begin with the frontal lobe, which is most frequently affected. We should naturally expect lesions of the frontal lobe to excite troubles having a definite relation to the functions of this lobe, such as weakening of the memory, loss of mental power, etc. Observation shows that such is not always the case.

For example, Fournier has published a case of osteosyphiloma with encephalitis of the right frontal lobe.

A woman who had had syphilis many years before suffered from headache and swelling of the frontal bone. The tumour became painful ; its diameter measured 3½ inches. The intellect was but little affected ; memory and speech were intact. Mercury and iodides produced marked improvement, and recovery seemed probable, when the patient died of hæmorrhagic smallpox. At the autopsy the antero-lateral fossa of the frontal bone was found to be riddled with hollows ; the surface of the bone was worm-eaten ; the dura mater was much thickened, and showed two patches of gummatous infiltration ; the brain was adherent to the meninges.

In some cases with lesions in the frontal lobes intellectual troubles are absent, and motor disturbances predominate.

The following case is quoted by Wallet:

A man, six years after the chancre, was seized with violent frontal headache, which became worse at night. For a year the headache was the only symptom. At intervals of some weeks the patient had three attacks of epilepsy, followed by incomplete paralysis on the left side. Later a large frontal tumour appeared ; it opened and gave exit to a quantity of pus. Mauclaire removed some sequestra. The aperture in the bone was as large as a crown piece, and the brain could be seen pulsating at the bottom of the wound. Inunction of mercury and iodide of potassium were ordered. The troubles ceased, and the aperture began to fill up. In this case the frontal lobe was attacked by a syphilitic lesion, but yet intellectual disturbance was absent. It was simply a question of epilepsy and paralysis.

Verchère's case also deserves mention :

A woman who had had gummatous osteitis in different regions of the body suffered from an osteosyphiloma to the right of the median line of the frontal bone. A sequestrum formed and was removed by the patient. Later another osteosyphiloma appeared in the frontal region. When Verchère saw the patient, he found two deep holes, the edges of which were clean cut and blended with the thickened bones. One aperture was situated near the eyebrow; the other was close to the roots of the hair. The end of a black sequestrum could be seen between the dura mater and the thickened frontal bone. It was bathed in foul-smelling pus. One night the patient was seized with hemiplegia. She could not raise her heel from the bed; the arm hung helpless. Verchère performed craniectomy, and removed a sequestrum as large as a crown-piece. Next day the headache and the paralysis had disappeared, and recovery set in.

In this case the frontal lobe was affected, and yet no intellectual troubles were seen; motor disorders were alone present. Therefore, hemiplegia and epilepsy, including Jacksonian epilepsy, may be caused by lesions of the frontal lobes. I have given further proofs of this point in a paper read at the Académie de Médecine (October 22, 1901).

Let us now consider the symptoms present when the parietal lobe is involved. Invasion of the Rolandic area determines contractures, paralysis, and Jacksonian epilepsy on the side opposite to the lesion. In the case quoted at the beginning of this section contractures affected the left hand, and partial epilepsy attacked the face.

A patient of Troisier had had on the scalp early nodes, cured by treatment with mercury. Later, attacks of Jacksonian epilepsy involved the right arm and the right side of the face. There was severe headache on the left side of the cranium. One day the patient had a right hemiplegia, without loss of consciousness. The hemiplegia only lasted twenty minutes, and was accompanied by some disturbance of speech. The headache was continuous, and worse at night. The attacks of hemiplegia returned several days in succession. Mercurial treatment was given, and the cerebral troubles finally disappeared. Troisier expressed the opinion (which I endorse) that these cerebral troubles were due to intracranial syphilitic exostoses, compressing the parietal lobe.

Lancereaux has published the following case:

A woman had on the right frontal bone an osteosyphiloma, which ulcerated and exposed a sequestrum. Convulsions, followed by left hemiplegia, appeared a little later. The frontal bone presented three large apertures, from which thick fœtid pus escaped. The convulsions recurred and the patient died. The autopsy revealed a sequestrum 3 inches by 4 inches. The underlying dura mater was ulcerated. The ascending frontal and parietal convolutions were destroyed by gangrene.

In short, contractures, hemiplegia, and Jacksonian epilepsy are the usual symptoms when lesions of the Rolandic area are associated with osteo-syphiloma of the parietal bone.

Many cases do not conform to a set description; these cases concern osteosyphilomata starting from the outer or inner table, spreading in various directions, and causing necrosis of the cranial vault without perforating it. Headache, vertigo, dizziness, mental weakness, disorders of speech, amnesia, vomiting, contractures, paralysis, and epileptiform convulsions occur in succession or in combination, inducing cachexia.

Evolution.—The gummatous osteosyphiloma of the cranium is a tertiary lesion. In a general way the term " tertiary " awakens the idea of syphilitic lesions appearing many years after infection. In the majority of cases the tertiary troubles appear five, ten, twenty, or even thirty years after the chancre. This rule is, however, far from being absolute, and it is liable to numerous exceptions. Many so-called tertiary lesions appear within a year of infection ; so-called malignant syphilis may prematurely engender gummata and phagedænic lesions. A case in point is the cerebral arteritis which in the first year may end in an aneurysm, or in obliteration of an artery, with all its consequences.

Syphilitic necrosis, as considered in this section, is also essentially a tertiary manifestation ; it may, however, occur early in the first or second year after the infection. The following case, related to me by Critzman and Nattan-Larrier, is a proof :

A man, forty-five years of age, suffered in January, 1901, from a chancre of the tongue, followed by typical roseola. In February syphilitic iritis made its appearance. In April papular syphilides appeared on the scrotum, and were soon followed by epididymitis. Injections of benzoate of mercury relieved these troubles. In May the face and the neck were invaded by an eruption of papulo-squamous syphilides. In spite of continuous treatment, the patient noticed in April, 1902, a swelling in the right parietal region. The tumour broke down and gave exit to a putty-like substance while the patient was in Portugal, where he took no medicine. On his return to Paris a deep suppurating ulcer was present. In spite of treatment with grey oil, the necrosis went on, and several small sequestra were removed. In January, 1903, the inner table necrosed, and a large sequestrum formed. The patient begged for operation. Legueu, on February 26, removed a sequestrum as large as a florin. Daily injections of biniodide of mercury arrested the necrosis, and a scar formed over the dura mater. In this case perforation of the skull took place within fourteen months from the appearance of the chancre.

In a case of Vedrennes' the osteosyphiloma appeared six weeks after the chancre. An abscess symptomatic of necrosis of the frontal bone appeared on the forehead. The headache was intense, ulceration set in, and seven months later sequestra from the outer table were removed. The following year aphasia came on, with paralysis on the right side, delirium, and convulsions. The patient was unconscious, the respiration was jerky, the pulse-rate 140, the limbs flaccid, and the only hope lay in trephining. A disc of bone was removed over the necrosed area. The patient came to and answered questions. Several sequestra were removed. The patient recovered, and his intelligence appeared to be intact, since he could play chess ; but the aphasia and the paralysis persisted.

Diagnosis.—Two cases may present themselves. In the first case the osteosyphiloma may be on the inner table, and escape observation because no tumour is present. In this event progressive headache, paroxysms of pain at night, and a definite area of pain on percussion are important signs in a case of syphilis ; they lead to a suspicion of the existence of deep osteosyphiloma, and furnish good reason for prompt injection of mercury.

Let us now pass on to the differential diagnosis of osteosyphiloma forming a tumour on the surface of the cranium. Sebaceous cysts and lipomata present but little resemblance to osteosyphiloma. The distinction between osteosyphiloma and osteotuberculoma, however, demands attention.

The osteotuberculoma is ushered in by more or less acute pain ; fever is absent ; the headache is sometimes very severe, and may be worse at night. After some weeks a swelling appears and rapidly grows to the size of a hazel-nut, of a walnut, or of an egg. The tumour breaks down in the centre, and an abscess forms. The pus contains clots, and is sometimes fœtid. Fungoid growths are common. Exploration with the probe reveals bare bone. A sequestrum is separated by the line of demarcation which occurs between the dead and the living tissue. The removal of the sequestrum exposes the dura mater, thickened and covered by tubercular granulations. The tubercular sequestrum is smooth, and usually comprises the whole thickness of the bone.

The tubercular skull differs anatomically from the syphilitic skull, as we can readily see from the figures shown in this section. The syphilitic skull is

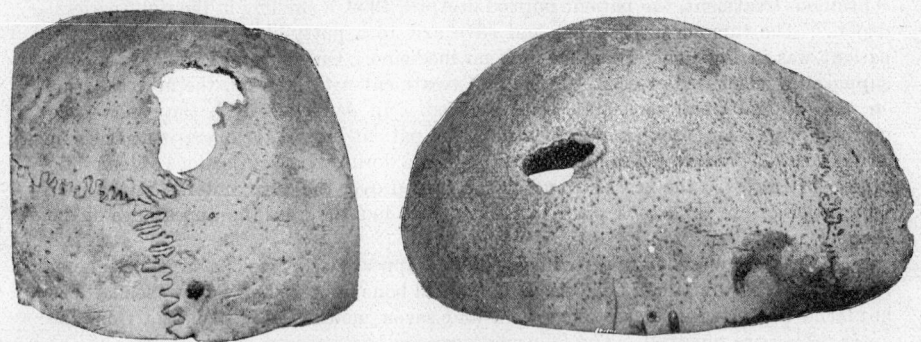

FIGS. 79 AND 80.—TUBERCULAR SKULLS. VAL-DE-GRACE MUSEUM.

These two crania show tubercular perforations with much loss of substance. Around the perforations, and also over the whole skull-cap, the bone is as smooth as in a normal skull. No roughness, no projections, and no eburnated bosses are seen.

more or less rugged ; the tubercular skull is smooth and uniform. In the tubercular skull the loss of substance is often more marked on the inner than on the outer table, and the edge is bevelled. The bone around the tubercular perforation is smooth ; we do not see rarefying osteitis, eburnated bosses, and osteophytes, as in the syphilitic skull.

The foregoing considerations give the anatomical diagnosis when we have the specimen. How are we to decide clinically whether an ulcerated tumour of the skull is syphilitic or tubercular ?

Headache, growing worse at night, is present in both cases. Pulmonary tuberculosis is in favour of osteotuberculoma, but mischief in the lungs is absent in most cases. Osteosyphiloma is probable if the patient has recently shown other manifestations of syphilis. Pus containing clots and fungous growths are in favour of a tubercular lesion. In doubtful cases, however, we must examine for Koch's bacillus, and make inoculations in the guinea-pig. On the other hand, injections of biniodide of mercury will speedily clear up the diagnosis, because a syphilitic lesion is almost certain to show prompt improvement.

Cranial osteosyphiloma should not be mistaken for osteomyelitis of the bones of the skull-cap. The latter occurs in young persons. The temperature is high, 103° to 104° F. ; the course of the disease is very rapid ; in a few days the skin becomes red and ulcerates, the wound suppurates, and the bone necroses. This acute process, which may speedily induce delirium and coma, differs absolutely from the evolution of the osteosyphiloma.

Hydatid cyst of the cranial bones somewhat resembles cranial osteo-syphiloma. Keate reports the following case :

A girl, eighteen years of age, had a tumour as large as a small orange on the fore-head. The operation showed that it was due to a hydatid ; the cavity in the bone was roughened. The patient recovered.

Cases of this kind are common in foreign countries, especially in the Argentine Republic. The hydatid develops in the frontal sinuses, between the dura mater and the temporal or parietal bone, or at other parts of the skull. The cyst, as it grows, affects both the bones and the brain. The bone in contact with the cyst is rough, and reduced through the loss of the inner table to a thin parchment-like layer. Vegas and Cranwell have found small perforations. Bony projections have also been met with. In Antonin's case the right parietal bone presented, at the insertion of the tumour, a firm crust of a circular shape ; on the inner surface of the crust there were small stalactites of bone, the bone between them being composed solely of the outer table. The right cerebral hemisphere was compressed, and showed a depression at the fissure of Rolando ; the convolutions were flattened, but softening was absent.

What are the symptoms of hydatid cysts of the skull, and how can we distinguish them from osteosyphiloma ? After a latent period the disease is ushered in by certain indefinite symptoms, such as headache, loss of appetite, and wasting ; deformity of the skull and cerebral symptoms then appear. A swelling in the frontal, parietal, or other region indicates the appearance of a cranial lesion, but gives no information as to the nature of the tumour. Contractures, paralysis, and epileptiform convulsions prove that the brain is involved, but they do not indicate the nature of the lesion. Owing to this incomplete information, the diagnosis of hydatid cyst is very difficult, because the same symptoms may exist in the case of osteosyphiloma. I know only of two ways of making a diagnosis : the first is the use of injections of biniodide of mercury, which, in the case of syphilis, will bring about rapid improvement, showing the nature of the mischief; the second is surgical intervention.

There is another disease which, like osteosyphiloma, may show itself by tumour and perforation of the skull. I mean fungus of the dura mater. The growth arises in the dura mater; the bone over the tumour is slowly absorbed, and finally perforated.

When perforation has occurred, the growth raises the skin in the form of a rounded or nodular tumour, which is hard at first, but which softens later. The skin then perforates, and the tumour expands outwards like a mushroom. In this stage the diagnosis is easy, but at a less advanced stage, when the tumour is covered by the skin, the diagnosis is very difficult, and we are the more likely to think of osteosyphiloma, because headache, vertigo, vomiting, etc., occur in both cases. In case of doubt mercurial treatment will decide the point.

Treatment.—The treatment of cranial osteosyphiloma is essentially medical, although surgical intervention is at times necessary. As a general rule, whether the growth is large or small, and is or is not accompanied by meningeal and cerebral complications, mercurial treatment is imperative.

Of the mercurial preparations, I prefer an aqueous solution of the biniodide. While the injection need not be intramuscular, it should be deep; a fold of the skin in the lumbar or gluteal regions is pinched up, and the needle is inserted deeply at right angles to the surface. The susceptibility of the patient is tested for a day or two by an injection of $\frac{1}{13}$ grain, and an injection of $\frac{1}{6}$ grain is given daily for twelve days. The injections are then stopped for a week, when a fresh series is given. The interval between the injections should be gradually increased. If the whole thickness of the bone is not destroyed, or if the lesion consists only of gummatous ulceration, with superficial osteitis, the pus dries up, the ulceration fills up, and recovery follows. If, however, the bony lesion is deep, if a fragment of bone has necrosed, if a sequestrum is in process of formation, or if the suppuration is extending between the cranium and the dura mater, surgical intervention is essential.

Some people will say that, before resorting to an operation, we may wait and attempt a cure by medical measures. I do not hold this view; in my opinion, medical and surgical treatment should be associated in certain cases. We know that the sequestrum may be fixed by osteophytes and bridges of bone, so resistant that the surgeon is obliged to use a chisel and mallet to free it. Under these conditions the sequestrum may remain *in situ* for an indefinite period in spite of medical measures; valuable time is lost by postponing surgical intervention.

In every case of ulcerated osteosyphiloma the physician should, I think, appeal to the surgeon in order to verify the exact condition of the subjacent bone, and to ascertain the possible presence of a sequestrum. The sequestrum induces suppuration, prevents healing, and favours the onset of intracranial complications ; it must be promptly removed, so that mercurial treatment may be efficacious.

In some cases the dura mater is thickened and covered with granulations, for which curetting has often been performed. Although this operation is practically painless, it is unnecessary, because the pachymeningitis will improve under mercurial treatment.

Medical and surgical treatment together yield remarkable results even in very grave cases. To the cases already quoted in this section I would add the following :

In a woman who had had syphilis a tumour appeared on the right side of the forehead. Some months later the tumour ulcerated, and a year later the patient was admitted under Besnier. A large ulcer, 2 inches in diameter, was present on the forehead. The centre was occupied by a blackish sequestrum ; the pus was abundant and foetid. Exploration with the probe showed another sequestrum. Richelet removed the sequestra and freed the adhesions. The wound measured 4 inches in length and 3 inches in breadth. The exposed dura mater was covered with granulations. The result was excellent.

I have said that it is essential to begin treatment as early as possible, but it is also essential to keep on with this treatment in spite of apparent cure. We must not forget that, in addition to the visible lesion, the skull is frequently affected by deep lesions which may run a latent course.

XII. CEREBRAL LOCALIZATION.

The question of cerebral localization has taken such an important place in the pathology of the brain as to deserve a special section, in order to give a general survey.

The study of cerebral localization has during the past few years received a considerable impulse. Physiology opened the way, and pathology followed it. Experiments have been made on animals, the brains of dogs and of monkeys being subjected to galvanic and faradic currents (Hitzig, Ferrier, Carville, and Duret), and most of the experimenters, after certain contradictory results, are, however, agreed on these two points : (1) That the grey matter of the cerebral convolutions is experimentally excitable ; (2) that excitation, limited to a convolution, or to a still more restricted portion, determines movements which are always localized in a certain part of the body (Ferrier).

It must be said, however, that the experimenters did not all obtain the same result as regards the exact localization of the **motor centres.** Pathological anatomy, however, furnished facts agreeing with physiological experiments ; the **topographical** diagnosis made during life was frequently verified at the post-mortem examination, and the cortical motor centres have since been gradually mapped out.

These positive ideas gave to cerebral pathology an accuracy previously unknown. If a patient was attacked by paralysis, contracture, or convulsions limited to the arm, the leg, or the face, the cerebral origin of the lesion being admitted, it became possible to make the exact **topographical** diagnosis of this lesion. Surgery profited thereby, and the application of the trephine was no longer a matter of chance. In the following pages we shall see that these ideas are not as correct as we have been wont to think.

The question of cerebral localization includes not only the localization of the tumours (syphiloma, glioma, tubercle), but also the localization of the **vascular lesions** which may produce cerebral softening by thrombosis or by embolism. Given an arterial obliteration, can the seat of the embolism or of the thrombosis be diagnosed, and can we state precisely the area of the consequent softening? We may feel the more correct in so doing since researches regarding the cerebral circulation in France (Duret) and in other countries (Cohnheim, Heubner) have given the following conclusions :

1. The arteries of the brain are not anastomotic ; there are no anastomoses either between the peripheral arteries and the central ones; in other words, these arteries are terminal (Cohnheim).

2. Certain regions in the brain are supplied by only one artery, and when this artery is obliterated, death follows in the area supplied by it, because the artery does not anastomose.

These data being given, the morbid localization could not then fail to be precise ; the question, however, on further examination, has been modified. In the first place, the cerebral arteries are not deprived of anastomoses at this point (Cadiat), and it is not uncommon to see the small arterioles anastomose (Lucas). These anastomoses may establish in certain cases a collateral circulation that prevents the death of the affected area. In the second place, further researches have shown that an area supposed to possess only one artery receives its blood from various sources. Contrary to the opinion of Duret, Hallopeau has discovered that the Sylvian artery is not the only vessel which supplies the corpus striatum ; he found, moreover, either a branch of the anterior cerebral, which reached the lenticular nucleus after having traversed the perforated space, or a branch of the anterior choroidal ; this explains why the internal segment of the corpus striatum is generally spared in lesions dependent on the Sylvian artery. The " arterial territories " lose, therefore, some importance, but the question of localization has none the less acquired great accuracy. With regard to this we may say that in most cases the topographical diagnosis made during life has been proved to be correct at the post-mortem examination or at the operation. In the following paragraphs I shall give our actual knowledge with regard to this question :

1. Localization in the Cortex.

Aphasia.—Until the recent work of Marie the lesion which produces ordinary aphasia was placed in the posterior third of the third left frontal convolution (Broca's convolution), and in the white fibres (inferior pediculo-frontal bundles) which arise in this cortical centre.

Agraphia appears to be due to lesions of the foot of the second left frontal convolution.

Word-deafness appears to coincide with the lesions of the first left temporal convolution, especially in its postero-superior extremity, and **word-blindness** appears to be due to the lesions of the left inferior parietal lobule in the neighbourhood of the angular gyrus (see Section V.).

Paralysis. — The following account concerning the localization of paralyses is largely taken from the monograph of Charcot and Pitres, and from the writings of Grasset :

1. All cortical lesions of the cerebral hemispheres in man do not give rise to motor disorders. From this point of view the cortex of the brain may be divided into two distinct parts—the **non-motor zone,** in which destructive lesions never cause permanent paralysis; and the **motor zone,** in which destructive lesions cause permanent paralysis of the opposite side of the body.

2. The non-motor zone comprises :

(*a*) The prefrontal region of the brain (orbital lobe, first, second, and third frontal convolutions).

(*b*) The occipito-parietal region (occipital lobe, superior and inferior parietal lobules).

(*c*) The entire temporo-sphenoidal lobe.

3. The motor zone comprises only the ascending frontal and parietal convolutions and the paracentral lobe ; perhaps also the foot of the frontal convolutions.

4. Paralyses caused by destructive lesions of the cortex affect various forms, according to the seat and to the extent of the lesions. Total hemiplegia of cortical origin is produced by extensive lesions of the ascending convolutions. Partial paralysis is produced by limited lesions of the same convolutions.

Amongst the varieties of partial paralysis we may distinguish :

(*a*) Brachio-facial monoplegia, due to lesions of the inferior half of the ascending convolutions.

(*b*) Brachio-crural monoplegia, due to the lesions of the superior half of the ascending convolutions.

(c) Facial and lingual monoplegia, depending on very limited lesions of the inferior extremity of the motor zone, and particularly of the ascending frontal convolution.

(d) Brachial monoplegia, dependent on very limited lesions of the middle portion of the motor zone, and particularly on the middle third of the ascending frontal convolution.

(e) Crural monoplegia, due to lesions of the paracentral lobule.

(f) Paralysis of the levator palpebræ superioris, which appears to depend on a limited lesion of the lobule of the angular gyrus (Grasset, Landouzy).

5. Total or partial paralysis, provoked by destructive lesions of the cortex, is permanent, and is accompanied after a certain time by secondary contracture of the paralyzed muscles and descending degeneration of the pyramidal tract.

Contractures.—I need not dwell on contractures and spasms limited to the arm and to the leg. They have the same localization as the paralyses, only in one case we have to deal with irritative lesions (contractures), in the other with destructive lesions (paralysis).

Convulsions.—The cortical lesions which produce convulsions cannot be localized as clearly as the lesions which produce paralysis. On this subject Charcot and Pitres are of the following opinion: Irritative lesions of the cortex may give rise to epileptiform convulsions (partial, Jacksonian, or cortical epilepsy). These convulsions are as a rule quite distinct from the convulsions of true epilepsy. They commence with a motor aura, and may become general, or may remain limited to one half of the body (hemispasm), or to a single group (monospasm).

Lesions capable of causing epileptiform troubles are seated in the motor zone itself or in its neighbourhood, and between the variety of partial epilepsy and the topography of the provoking cortical lesion there is not always the constant relation that is found between paralyses of cortical origin and the seat of the destructive lesions which give rise to them.

Numerous observations show that in many cases partial epilepsy assumes the following types, depending on clearly defined lesions: (1) In the facial type the convulsions are limited to the face and the neck; they involve the commissure of the lips, the orbicularis palpebrarum, the motor muscles of the eye and tongue, and the sterno-mastoid; jerky movements of the arm are sometimes present. (2) In the brachial type, which is more common, the aura commences in one of the fingers; the convulsions attack the hand, the arm, the shoulder, and sometimes the face and the neck. (3) In the crural type, which is the rarest, the aura commences in the foot, and the convulsions stop at the hip.

The topography of the cerebro-meningeal lesion may be diagnosed by the type of the epilepsy: facial type—inferior extremity of the two ascending convolutions ; brachial type—middle region of the ascending frontal convolution ; crural type—superior region of the ascending convolutions and of the paracentral lobule ; lingual type—inferior region of the ascending frontal convolution in the neighbourhood of the foot of the third frontal convolution.

For further details I would refer the reader to the section on Jacksonian Epilepsy.

2. Localization of the Central Lesions.

Localization in certain central parts of the brain is extremely precise : thus the lesions producing hemianæsthesia, accompanied or not by hemiplegia, hemichorea, etc., may be placed with certainty in the posterior portion of the posterior segment of the internal capsule. These localizations have been described under Cerebral Hæmorrhage.

XIII. DISCUSSION ON MEDICO-SURGICAL ERRORS REGARDING CEREBRAL LOCALIZATION.

In the previous section I remarked that the current doctrines of cerebral localization had induced physicians and surgeons to localize in the area of Rolando the lesions (syphiloma, tuberculoma, glioma, etc.) which cause certain types of partial epilepsy, with or without paralysis of the convulsed parts. Physicians and surgeons confident in this doctrine have been able to operate on the region of the skull corresponding to Rolando's area.

We should be wrong, however, to rely too much on these localizations, because certain mistakes have been made, and the trephine has been applied, but the expected lesion has not been found. I wish to point out these mistakes, as I have already done at the Académie.

On January 10 a man was sent into the Hôtel-Dieu. He was unable to give us any information. He had been seen by Dr. Maynau on the night of January 5, when he answered questions with difficulty. The previous day he had done his work and had eaten well. He had gone to bed, and since that time he had lost consciousness. His wife stated that about midnight she was awakened by his snoring. She shook her husband, who was unconscious. It was impossible to awake him from his torpor. She called in a doctor, who noticed that the patient had bitten his tongue, and that he had passed his urine under him. He immediately thought of the possibility of an attack of epilepsy, possibly due to syphilis, and prescribed Gibert's syrup and iodide of potassium.

Next morning, January 6, the man's brother confirmed the hypothesis of syphilis, contracted ten years previously. The patient was prostrate, and spoke with difficulty. He, nevertheless, showed by signs that he understood what was going on around him.

On the night of January 6 the doctor was again called : the patient had just had an attack "to which there was no ending." He was in a comatose condition, the breathing was stertorous, and the rectal temperature was 104° F. Suddenly a noisy inspiration supervened ; the head and the eyes were turned to the right, and immediately the right arm, and then the right leg, were thrown into convulsions. It was an attack of

II.   89

Jacksonian epilepsy. About ten similar attacks took place, one after the other, and the comatose condition persisted from one o'clock to five o'clock in the morning. On Wednesday, the 9th, the patient partially regained consciousness, but he declined to submit to the prescribed treatment, and he was sent to the Hôtel-Dieu in a semi-comatose condition, his temperature reaching 102° F.

When I saw the patient on Friday morning, the fifth day of the disease, I could not obtain any precise answers from him, and yet he made attempts at understanding, replying by gestures, or by monosyllables. His tongue showed traces of having been bitten. The limbs on the right side, the arm particularly, were flaccid, but not completely paralyzed. Sensibility seemed to be diminished on the right side of the body. From the previous evening nine convulsions had been counted, and just as I was examining him an attack of partial epilepsy came on. He suddenly uttered a muffled growl. His face and lips were deflected to the right, the right hand became contracted, the fingers were flexed, and in a few moments convulsions appeared in the upper limb. The attack did not remain limited to the right arm, but soon invaded the right leg (brachio-crural type). On the left side slight communicated movements were noticeable. During the crisis the patient did not seem to have lost consciousness completely. In forty seconds the convulsions ceased ; the patient remained cyanosed, and the breathing was laboured.

In this case we had to make a topographical and a pathogenic diagnosis. The former seemed obvious. The limitation of the attack to the right side of the body, with marked predominance in the right arm, indicated a lesion of the motor cortex on the left side. This localization was the more probable because paralysis was also present. According to current ideas, the lesion should attack the ascending frontal and parietal convolutions, and as the leg was affected after the arm, it was probable that the lesion was in the middle part of these convolutions, the upper region and the paracentral lobule being immune.

In case of surgical intervention I should have indicated the left motor convolutions to the surgeon : the trephine would have been applied over this part of the skull. There was not, however, any question of operation. As the patient had had syphilis, everything pointed to the lesion of Rolando's area being gummatous or sclero-gummatous. Injections of biniodide of mercury were given, but, in spite of the treatment, the Jacksonian attacks continued day and night. In twenty-four hours he had forty or fifty attacks.

On Saturday, the 12th, the temperature was 103·5° F. The attacks followed one on another, and the patient died on Sunday night. The cranial cavity was opened, and the Rolandic area on the left side was examined. Nothing appreciable was found— no tumour, no depression, no adhesions. When we tried to remove the brain, we noticed that the dura mater was adherent to the pia mater over the anterior portion of the left frontal lobe. The pia mater was severed, and the cerebrum, cerebellum, and bulb were removed.

The examination of the brain gave the following information : Rolando's convolutions were healthy, as were the parietal, occipital, and temporal lobes. The only apparent lesion was limited to the left frontal lobe. At this point the tissue was softer than the grey matter of the convolutions. The lesion was gummatous.

The gumma, seen from the external surface of the frontal lobe, occupied the anterior third of the first, second, and third frontal convolutions. On the inferior surface of the brain the lesion occupied the outer part of the olfactory convolutions over an area of 3 centimetres. On making a median horizontal section of the brain we found that the lesion extended to within $1\frac{1}{2}$ centimetres of the anterior horn of the lateral ventricle. Its limits were clearly defined. The brain tissue around the tumour was in no wise changed. The tumour was of the size of a small egg. On section, its tissue presented the following aspect : the dura mater adhering to the pia mater had a thickness of 1 to 2 millimetres. The newly-formed subjacent tissue had invaded and replaced the white and the grey matter. This tissue was yellowish-brown, fairly soft and friable, and somewhat resembling œdematous connective tissue. It was traversed by whiter and more resisting filaments, and in several places there were small islets of caseous aspect and consistency.

We had now to decide as to this strange case. The patient had suffered from cerebral gumma, and so far the pathogenic diagnosis was correct ; but we had localized the lesion in Rolando's area, and in that respect the topographical diagnosis was wrong, because the lesion occupied the frontal lobe. I then asked myself whether this case was an isolated one. I looked the question up, and found some identical cases. Seeing the importance of the subject, I shall quote them :

Lépine has published a case entitled " Jacksonian Epilepsy ending in Death. Autopsy : old abscess of the anterior lobe of the brain." An old woman was admitted for Jacksonian epilepsy of the limbs on the left side, the face remaining immune. Besides the attacks, which were complicated by loss of consciousness, he noticed slight jerks in the fingers and in the forearm, and rigidity of the arm, but no loss of consciousness. Did not these convulsions point to a lesion in the middle portion of the right motor convolutions ? The patient died. At the post-mortem examination Rolando's area was healthy. An old encysted abscess was found in the first right frontal con-

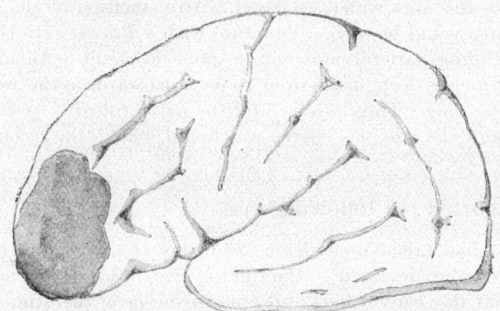

FIG. 81.—TUMOUR IN FRONTAL LOBE.

volution. As Lépine remarks, if trephining had been carried out, it would not have exposed the lesion, " because, relying on the symptoms in the attack, we should have opened the skull far back in a region intermediate to the centre for the upper limb and to that for the lower limb." Lépine and myself, in our respective cases, arrived at the same erroneous conclusion.

In another case Lépine had to deal with a syphilitic patient who was suffering from cerebral symptoms : ambitious ideas, amnesia, with strangeness of manner, and attacks of Jacksonian epilepsy limited to both arms. This limitation of the convulsive attacks would lead us to place the cerebral lesion at a symmetrical point in the Rolandic area. The patient died, and at the post-mortem examination two gummata were found placed symmetrically, not in the convolutions of Rolando, but in the first convolution of the two frontal lobes.

Faguet and Lowitz have published the following case :

A woman who had had syphilis was seized with Jacksonian epilepsy, limited to the left side of the body. The convulsions commenced in the hand, spread to the arm, attacked the mouth and the upper eyelid, and ended in the lower limb, always on the left side. The convulsions disappeared in the following order : they ceased first in the face, then in the arm, then in the leg, and finally in the hand During the attacks

89—2

the patient did not lose consciousness. Memory, intelligence, and speech were normal. Percussion of the skull over the psycho-motor zone caused fairly acute pain.

As antisyphilitic treatment gave no result, and as the symptoms pointed to a lesion in the right motor convolutions, Lannelongue trephined over the lower part of the fissure of Rolando. The dura mater was laid bare, but the suspected lesion was not found. The convulsions continued, and the patient died. The post-mortem examination showed that the motor zone was healthy. The lesion, a gumma of the size of a nut, was seated in the posterior third of the second right frontal convolution.

The following case is taken from Chipault :

A man who had already had some cerebral symptoms was seized with Jacksonian epilepsy, localized in the left arm and left leg. The convulsions were followed by paralytic symptoms. Nevertheless, nearly every morning on rising the patient experienced an involuntary extension of the paralyzed arm, which raised the coverlet of the bed. The forearm and the hand were straight, the fingers were extended and separated. The condition lasted a moment. When the patient was excited, the paralyzed hand showed rapid tremor, which could be lessened or arrested by supporting the hand. As these symptoms indicated a lesion of the right Rolandic area, the trephine was applied, and this area was widely exposed. After incision of the dura mater no lesion of the motor area could be seen. Puncture with a Pravaz syringe in the frontal and then in the ascending parietal convolution gave no result. An incision 1 centimetre long and 2 centimetres deep, made from above downwards in the ascending frontal convolution, showed nothing. Three weeks later the patient died. At the post-mortem examination a glioma of the size of a cherry was found, but in the second right frontal convolution.

Crouzon has reported the following case :

A coachman, who had fallen unconscious from his box, was brought to hospital. The head and the eyes were deviated to the right. The limbs showed neither paralysis nor contracture. Next day convulsions appeared in the face, the arm, and the leg, on the left side. The cutaneous and tendon reflexes were normal. Two days later Jacksonian epilepsy was typical in the face and in the left arm (facio-brachial type). The patient was in a condition of coma. Lumbar puncture gave a clear liquid, rich in lymphocytes.

The clinical evidence pointed to a lesion in the right motor area, and an operation was performed. After incision of the meninges, which were healthy, Rolando's area and the neighbourhood were explored, but, contrary to all expectations, no change was found. The patient died, and the post-mortem examination showed that Rolando's area was normal. The lesion which had caused the Jacksonian epilepsy was seated at the apex of the right temporal lobe. This lesion, in the shape of an adherent fibrous patch, was probably tubercular. The remainder of the brain was healthy.

Lucas-Championnière showed at the Société de Chirurgie a tumour of the right frontal lobe. It was as large as a tangerine orange, and had been removed from a patient suffering from Jacksonian epilepsy in the left arm (brachial type). This localization pointed to a lesion in the ascending frontal and parietal convolutions. Nothing of the kind was present. These convolutions were absolutely healthy, and the lesion was seated in the frontal convolutions.

These cases furnish valuable information. In my patient suffering from Jacksonian epilepsy (brachio-crural type) I had made the natural diagnosis of a cerebral lesion in the area of Rolando. In the event of an operation the surgeon would have trephined at this spot, but he would have found nothing, because the post-mortem examination showed that the lesion was seated in the frontal lobe. The same remark applies to the other cases just quoted. Jacksonian epilepsy in Lépine's patient induced him to diagnose a lesion in Rolando's area, and at the post-mortem examination it was seen that the lesion was seated in the first frontal convolution. Jacksonian epilepsy in the patient of Faguet and Lowitz pointed to a lesion in the area of Rolando. The trephine was applied, and nothing was found ; the post-mortem examination showed that the lesion was localized in the second frontal convolution. In Chipault's patient the lesion was thought to be in the motor area ; at the post-mortem examination it was discovered that the lesion was in the second frontal convolution.

Jacksonian epilepsy in Crouzon's patient (facio-brachial type) led to the diagnosis of a lesion in Rolando's area. An operation was performed, and it was found that this region was absolutely healthy ; at the post-mortem examination it was seen that the lesion was seated at the apex of the temporal lobe. Jacksonian epilepsy in the patient of Lucas-Championnière (brachial type) led to the diagnosis of a lesion in Rolando's area, but the operation showed that this region was healthy, and the post-mortem examination proved that the lesion was in the temporal lobe.

Accordingly, a lesion (glioma, syphiloma, tuberculoma, etc.) in the frontal lobe, remote from Rolando's area, may cause Jacksonian epilepsy, such as we are accustomed to see when the lesions are localized in Rolando's convolutions. Physicians and surgeons have been deceived thereby. It must be admitted that cases of this kind, which are relatively numerous, leave some uncertainty as to the accuracy of the topographical diagnosis of the cerebral lesions, and cause legitimate difficulty when the question arises of indicating the area of the brain to be exposed.

Is there no symptom by which we can say that in one case Jacksonian epilepsy is caused by a lesion of Rolando's area, and in another case by a lesion in the frontal lobe ? It would seem a priori that a lesion of the frontal lobe would produce mental troubles, which are not caused by lesions in the convolutions of Rolando ; but this hypothesis, though rational in itself, does not always correspond with the actual facts. My patient, who had a lesion in the frontal lobe, had shown neither psychical nor intellectual troubles when he was attacked with Jacksonian epilepsy ; on the previous evening he was in good health, and carried out his duties as telegraph operator without any failing of his mental faculties. In the case of Faguet and Lowitz it is recorded that the patient, who was suffering from Jacksonian epilepsy caused by a lesion of the frontal lobe, " had no intellectual trouble. His memory was perfect, and his speech was normal." In Chipault's case we see that the patient, who was suffering from Jacksonian epilepsy caused by a lesion of the frontal lobe, " had no intellectual troubles."

The absence of psychical and intellectual troubles cannot therefore serve to differentiate between Jacksonian epilepsy caused by a Rolandic lesion and Jacksonian epilepsy due to a frontal lesion.

Are the paralytic symptoms of help in making a diagnosis ? We know, as a matter of fact, that the lesions of Rolando's convolutions cause convulsions, and also give rise to special paralysis ; paralysis or paresis of the arm and of the leg may precede the attacks of Jacksonian epilepsy, may coexist with them, or may survive them. Many patients suffering from Jacksonian epilepsy of the upper or of the lower limb suffer after a convulsive attack, or in the interval between the attacks, from more or less lasting paralysis of the limbs which have been convulsed. If the addition of paralytic troubles were peculiar to Jacksonian epilepsy of Rolandic origin, and if it were absent in Jacksonian epilepsy of frontal origin, we should have a valuable aid to the topographical diagnosis.

This aid, however, is wanting, since paralysis may be associated with Jacksonian epilepsy of frontal origin. Thus, my patient had partial paralysis in his arm and in his leg, and we noticed in his case the coexistence of paretic symptoms and of convulsions ; the convulsive attack having ended, the paralytic symptoms became the chief feature. In one of Lépine's patients the arm and the left leg were paralyzed after the convulsions, and the paralysis persisted until death. The patient of Faguet and Lowitz had flaccid hemiplegia in the interval between the convulsive attacks, and the paralysis persisted in an absolute manner. Chipault's patient had paresis of the limbs affected by Jacksonian epilepsy, and the arm remained paralyzed.

The presence of paralysis cannot assist us in differentiating with certainty between Jacksonian epilepsy caused by a Rolandic lesion and Jacksonian epilepsy caused by a frontal lesion.

Therefore, we must admit Rolandic and frontal Jacksonian epilepsy, and also temporal Jacksonian epilepsy, which are absolutely identical. Jacksonian epilepsy, caused by a Rolandic lesion, is much more common than Jacksonian epilepsy due to a frontal lesion ; nevertheless the latter form is met with fairly frequently, as the cases quoted prove.

At present we have no sign and no symptom which enable us to differentiate between Rolandic and frontal epilepsy. We should be much embarrassed if we were asked to point out precisely the cranial region to which the trephine ought to be applied. We should be liable to give an incorrect answer, as witness my own case and the cases of Faguet and Lowitz, of Lépine, of Chipault, of Cruzon, and of Lucas-Championnière. Were such a case to occur, we should not dare to express an opinion.

I must make a remark, if only in the nature of a simple reflection. Amongst the types of Jacksonian epilepsy due to a Rolandic lesion there is one which I have not seen reproduced in Jacksonian epilepsy of frontal origin—viz., the crural type, where the convulsive attack commences in the leg.

In such a case the cerebral lesion which causes the attack of epilepsy is localized in the paracentral lobule, or in the highest part of the motor convolutions which unite to form the paracentral lobule. Does the crural type of Jacksonian epilepsy escape the similitude which we have just pointed out in the other types, and may it not be produced by a frontal lesion? I do not know.

XIV. TUBERCULAR MENINGITIS.

The word "meningitis" includes the inflammation of the arachnoid, of the subarachnoid tissue, and of the pia mater; but it does not apply to inflammation of the dura mater, which will be described later.

Acute meningitis may be divided into two large classes : (a) non-tubercular meningitis ; (b) tubercular meningitis. I shall first describe tubercular meningitis.

Ætiology.—The designation tubercular meningitis does not apply indiscriminately to all cases of meningeal tuberculosis ; the tubercles may become agglomerated so as to form a large tumour, which causes symptoms of cerebral tumour, but not of meningitis. Tubercular meningitis varies in its appearance. Sometimes it forms a part of the general invasion of the system by acute tuberculosis, and in this case it is of secondary importance ; sometimes it appears to be the entire disease : the latter form is generally described under the name of tubercular meningitis.

Tubercular meningitis is almost always accompanied by pulmonary or abdominal tuberculosis. It is seen at all ages, but it is most common in children between the ages of two and seven years. It is hereditary, like all the manifestations of tuberculosis, and it is not rare for several children of the same family to be carried off at about the same age by meningitis. Head injuries have an undoubted influence on the development of tubercular meningitis, just as traumatism has an undoubted influence on the development of pulmonary tuberculosis.

Martin, Vaudremer and Martin, and Sicard have produced tubercular meningitis experimentally by injecting bacilli into the bloodvessels or into the cerebro-spinal fluid. The toxines secreted by the bacillus play an important part in the evolution of the meningitic process. Armand Delille, by means of the caseifying and sclerosing poisons of Auclair, has been able experimentally to reproduce the lesions of tubercular meningitis. The lymphatic system does not seem to serve as a means of transport in this experimental infection, except when the leucocytes emigrate from adjacent cavities (nasal, ocular, or auricular cavities). Tubercular meningitis may be secondary to more or less latent infection of the naso-pharyngeal cavity, adenoid and tubercular lesions, described under Masked Tuberculosis of the Three Tonsils. Once *in situ*, Koch's bacillus and its toxines seem to make use of the cerebro-spinal fluid as their means of transport.

Pathological Anatomy.—Acute tubercular meningitis is generally more marked at the base than at the convexity of the brain ; it affects the fissure of Sylvius. The exudation is more or less abundant, greyish, purulent, and sometimes almost lardaceous. The meningitis is generally diffuse, but in some cases it is localized (see the section on Jacksonian Epilepsy). The grey semi-transparent granulations are usually found on the lymphatic sheath of the vessels of the pia mater ; they tend to be confluent at the base of the brain, and if the Sylvian artery, with its branches, is carefully removed and floated in water, it is easy to observe the disposition of these tubercular granulations. Under the influence of the granulations, and of the obliterating arteritis which accompanies them, the blood coagulates in the interior of the vessels and causes arterial thrombosis, which produces superficial or deep centres of softening (Rendu).

Bacilli are found in the tubercular granulations around the vessels, in their walls, and in their contents. Other pathogenic agents—streptococci, pneumococci, etc.—are sometimes associated with the tubercle bacillus.

The meninges are often adherent to the cortical substance, which at this point presents a superficial encephalitis (Hayem). The pia mater is thickened, and its small vessels (venules and arterioles) are often obliterated by fibrinous coagula. The central parts of the brain, commissures and walls of the ventricles are softened, and the ventricular cavities often contain so much effusion that the disease formerly received the name of acute hydrocephalus.

The choroid plexuses often show tubercular granulations ; in some cases the trouble in the choroid plexuses may be the only tubercular lesion present, so that Loeper has described a choroidal form of tubercular meningitis.

The choroid is almost always the seat of tubercles. According to circumstances, more or less generalized tubercular lesions are met with, especially in the thoracic and abdominal organs. Changes analogous to those of the brain may exist in the spinal cord (see the section on Cerebrospinal Meningitis).

Description.—As tubercular meningitis is much more frequent in children than in adults, I shall lay most stress on the meningitis of childhood in the present description. The disease generally commences with a prodromal period, varying from a few days to three months. This period is characterized by various phenomena : there are general symptoms, such as change of character, loss of flesh, attacks of fever, partially attributable to pulmonary, or abdominal tuberculization which precedes or accompanies the tubercular meningitis; and there are local symptoms, such as visual troubles, diplopia, headache, and vomiting, depending on the invasion of the brain by tuberculosis.

Period of Excitation.—Three symptoms open the scene : **headache,** which may be most intense ; **vomiting** of greenish bilious matter ; and **constipation.** The fever is of a remittent character, being higher at night and showing oscillations during the day. The temperature rarely exceeds 103° F. The little patient suffers at times from generalized hyperæsthesia ; he has convulsive jerks, contractures of the nuchal muscles, strabismus, and constriction of the pupils. Patients who are older at times suffer from delirium.

At this period appears the hydrocephalic cry (Coindet). It is a short and plaintive scream, repeated at varying intervals.

Period of Depression.—The period of excitation, lasting from a few days to two weeks, is followed by a period of depression. The headache and the vomiting disappear; somnolence follows the insomnia, and the child seems to enjoy rest, which might, wrongly, lead us to believe in an improvement which is fictitious. The little sufferer, indifferent to everything and plunged in torpor, replies with difficulty to questions. Anæsthesia replaces hyperæsthesia, and the hydrocephalic cries become less frequent. The temperature, though lower, still remains above normal. The pulse is irregular, and falls to 60 per minute. The belly is retracted, the face is red and pale in turn, and the *tache cérébrale* is very pronounced (Trousseau). The respiration is irregular. Thus the patient, after a few deep and hurried inspirations, stops suddenly for a few moments, as though he had forgotten to breathe. At this period we see convulsions, which may be general or limited to a leg, to an arm, or to the face ; transitory contractures may affect the hands, the muscles of the neck and of the jaws (trismus), and the muscles of the eye (strabismus).

This period of depression, sometimes complicated by transitory phenomena of excitation, lasts a few days, and gives place to the paralytic period. The paralyses of tubercular meningitis have special characters. They generally follow on a convulsive attack ; they often assume the hemiplegic form, involving an arm and then a leg, and are successive rather than simultaneous. They rarely attack the face (Rendu).

In the last period the fever reappears. The pulse goes up to 130 to 150 beats a minute, the belly becomes ballooned, the breathing is distressed, and the little sufferer, who has lost consciousness, dies in coma or in convulsions, or is carried off by progressive asphyxia.

The **ocular troubles** of tubercular meningitis are of divers kinds. At the commencement of the disease the pupil and the motor nerves of the eye show irritative phenomena—myosis, nystagmus, and strabismus. Later the paralytic phenomena predominate—mydriasis, ptosis, and paralytic strabismus.

The ophthalmoscope reveals multiple lesions of the fundus. The tubercles of the choroid generally occupy both eyes in the neighbourhood of the optic nerve and of the macula ; they form rounded, greyish protuber-ances, variable in number ; they emanate directly from the spreading of the meningitis, along the sheath of the optic nerve or the vessels of the eye. When tubercles exist in the choroid, they are of value in the diagnosis of tubercular meningitis, but they are often absent. Œdema of the optic papilla is frequently met with as a consequence of the hydrocephalus and cerebral œdema (Parinaud). This œdematous neuritis, which is sometimes accompanied by hæmorrhage into the retina, often ends in more or less complete atrophy of the optic nerve.

The convulsions, contractures, and paralyses met with in tubercular meningitis deserve notice. The paralyses appear to be due to foci of softening in the corpora striata, the cerebral peduncles (Rendu), and the motor zones of the fronto-parietal convolutions. These foci of softening are caused by thrombi, induced by the tubercular granulations in the vessels. The pathogenesis of the convulsions and of the contractures differs, according as they are general or partial. When they are general, remote cerebral excitation may be invoked ; when they are partial, they result from the direct excitation of the fronto-parietal motor zones (Landouzy).

Tubercular Meningitis in the Adult.—Meningitis in the adult does not always resemble the meningitis of childhood. Its abnormal forms, which are fairly frequent, have been described by Chantemesse. In some cases the meningitis, after being latent for some time, appears suddenly with an apoplectiform attack, epileptiform convulsions, or an attack of acute delirium. These various forms rapidly end in coma and death ; and the delirious form presents this peculiarity—that the disease may run its course without any rise of temperature.

A comatose form of tubercular meningitis may be seen. The first, and sometimes the only, symptom is an invincible desire to sleep. The following case occurred in the Hôtel-Dieu :

A young man was seized with rapid coma ; vomiting, headache, and delirium were absent. Lumbar puncture showed numerous lymphocytes. At the autopsy the meninges showed no tubercles ; the ventricles were distended by fluid ; the walls of the ventricles had a characteristic washed appearance, while the choroid plexuses were granular, swollen, and filled with tubercular granulations—some young, others in process of caseation.

Our knowledge of the troubles consequent on exaggerated distension of the ventricles allows us to consider the comatose form of tubercular meningitis as dependent upon changes in the choroid plexuses and in the ventricles, with marked hydrops ventriculorum (Loeper).

In other cases the spinal symptoms open the scene; the disease simulates a meningo-myelitis, and then the symptoms of cerebral meningitis declare themselves. Tubercular cerebro-spinal meningitis will be studied in one of the following sections.

In some patients cerebral meningitis concentrates its action on the motor convolutions of the brain. Patches of tubercular meningo-encephalitis are found over the ascending frontal and parietal convolutions and the paracentral lobule. These patches are announced by contracture or paralysis, limited to the arm or to the leg. Dissociated paralysis of the third pair of nerves (**ptosis**) has been seen in cases of meningitis of the angular gyrus.

The other symptoms of meningitis—headache and vomiting—are wanting; but restlessness, delirium, somnolence, and coma soon carry off the patient, if he does not succumb to the rapid progress of the pulmonary tuberculosis.

Diagnosis.—The diagnosis between meningitis and typhoid fever is given under the latter disease. *À propos* of the diagnosis, apoplectiform meningitis in the adult must not be forgotten. Tubercular meningitis does not give **Kernig's sign** as long as the spinal meninges are not affected. The bacteriological examination of the fluid obtained by lumbar puncture gives valuable information. I shall give full details in the chapter dealing with cerebrospinal meningitis, when we shall see that we can make the diagnosis of tubercular meningitis by laboratory methods (Widal, Griffon).

The **prognosis** is always grave, and death is the natural result of tubercular meningitis. There is said to be only one undoubted case of cure, that of Freyhan. The **treatment** is very limited. It consists in the application of ice to the head and of leeches behind the ears. Inunctions and intravenous injections of collargol have been recommended. The object of the palliative treatment is to maintain the nourishment of the child, and to prevent, as far as possible, any cause of cerebral excitation. With regard to the treatment, we must bear in mind the possibility of meningeal complications due to **hereditary syphilis**, and apply specific treatment if necessary.

XV. NON-TUBERCULAR MENINGITIS.

Pathogenesis.—A few years ago the pathogenesis of non-tubercular meningitis was almost unknown. A patient died of meningitis, and the postmortem examination revealed more or less purulent exudate. As tuberculosis was not found, the meningitis was called primary or idiopathic. The study of non-tubercular meningitis is the outcome of bacteriology. We know that most of the microbes which cause pleurisy, peritonitis, pericarditis, etc., are also capable of causing meningitis. Meningitis may be pneumococcal, streptococcal, or staphylococcal. Some cases of meningitis are due to Eberth's bacillus, to the *Bacillus septicus putridus* (Roger), or to the *Bacillus coli*, while other cases are due to the associations of these various agents. In some circumstances the entrance gateway of these agents remains unknown, and we then speak of auto-infection. In the greatest number of cases these agents enter the system or reach the meninges by reason of traumatic causes or of infectious diseases. Traumatism, insolation, osseous lesions, otitis, rhinitis, amygdalitis, influenza, pneumonia, erysipelas, pyæmia, typhoid fever, the eruptive fevers, rheumatism, and syphilis are the most common causes of non-tubercular meningitis.

Meningitis following on Otitis.—Suppurative meningitis is fairly common in acute or chronic otitis media. It may likewise result from lesions of the internal and of the external ear, polypi, boils, abscesses (Duplay). Netter found that in young children the middle ear is almost always affected. Post-mortem examinations performed between the ages of nine months and two years have, in a large number of cases, shown that the middle ear contained muco-pus, with streptococci, staphylococci, or pneumococci. It is probable that these agents enter through the Eustachian tube. The propagation of the lesions from the ear to the meninges is easy, whether it occurs by contiguity or by way of the bloodvessels. As a matter of fact, the veins of the tympanum empty themselves into the middle meningeal vein, and anastomoses exist between the veins of the tympanum and the superior petrosal sinus (Troeltsch). The infectious diseases which are accompanied by otitis—namely, syphilis, pneumonia, measles, scarlatina, or influenza—may cause meningitis preceded by otitis, or meningitis without previous otitis.

The variety of the pathogenic agents in meningitis consequent on otitis explains the equal variety of the symptoms. These cases of meningitis may be fulminant, rapid, acute, subacute, or chronic (Jaccoud). The fulminant form kills in twenty-four hours, with convulsions, intense headache, and coma. One form simulates typhoid fever, except for the period of onset, which commences suddenly with vomiting and headache. In another form we find the symptoms of pyæmia—febrile attacks, rigors, and sweating. Finally there is the common form of classical meningitis.

Pneumococcal Meningitis.—This is the most frequent form of non-tubercular meningitis. It supervenes in the decline or in the course of pneumonia ; it may be independent of pneumonia. Pneumococcal meningitis is often associated with endocarditis, and in many cases it becomes generalized in the spinal meninges, so that there is pneumococcal cerebrospinal meningitis. The fœtus may suffer from this form. Netter found that a pregnant woman attacked by pneumonia may transmit both pneumonia and meningitis to the fœtus.

In pneumococcal meningitis the lesions are most marked over the convexity of the brain. The exudate is incorporated in the pia mater, and it may be detached without injuring the cerebral cortex. The exudate is of a soft consistency, and differs from the greyish lardaceous exudate of tubercular meningitis, as well as from the creamy pus seen in meningitis due to caries of the petrous bone (Netter). The spinal meninges are frequently attacked. Sometimes the lesions are less extensive ; they are localized in various regions of the cerebro-spinal axis in the form of milky tracts or in the shape of islets of variable dimensions. In the spinal meninges the pus is more abundant at the cervical and lumbar swellings. The character of the pneumococcal pus is evident when other microbes are associated with the pneumococcus.

Pneumococcal meningitis at times presents special symptoms. Sometimes, in a patient suffering from pneumonia in process of resolution, a sudden and considerable rise in the temperature is the only symptom pointing to the presence of meningitis (Jaccoud). A prominent and almost constant symptom is the rigidity of the nape of the neck : the rigidity often attacks the muscles of the face, and descends, in the shape of painful contracture, to the muscles of the dorsal and of the sacro-lumbar regions.

Our knowledge of the frequent generalization of the pneumococcus in the cerebro-spinal meninges explains the rigidity and the more or less general contractures. In young children the abundance of the purulent effusion sometimes causes excessive intracranial pressure (Vaudremer), with bulging of the anterior fontanelle. Pneumococcal meningitis runs a very variable course. Sometimes the disease is fulminant, and kills in twenty-four hours ; in some cases the onset is apoplectiform (Netter).

Meningitis caused by the Bacillus Coli.—The *Bacillus coli* may produce suppurative meningitis, as well as pseudo-puerperal fever and pseudo-enteric fever, when it spreads through the system by changes in the organs which normally contain it. Most cases of suppurative meningitis which have been published during the past few years, and in which a pseudo-typhoid bacillus was incriminated, are due to the *Bacillus coli* (Chantemesse, Widal and Legry).

Conclusions.—I have just reviewed the principal forms of non-tubercular meningitis ; this question is still under discussion. In many cases non-tubercular meningitis shows all the symptoms described under tubercular meningitis. On what, then, are we to base the diagnosis ? Non-tubercular meningitis generally differs from tubercular meningitis in the absence of a prodromal period, which is especially met with in children. Furthermore, in young children with tubercular meningitis or with latent tuberculosis, it is very rare not to find enlargement of the inguinal, axillary, cervical, or submaxillary glands. The diagnosis of the pathogenic agents is simplified by lumbar puncture, which allows bacteriological examination of the liquid. The method will be described under Cerebro-spinal Meningitis. We must not forget that early hereditary syphilis may reveal itself by symptoms of meningitis which yield to specific treatment.

XVI. CEREBRO-SPINAL MENINGITIS.

History.—I have devoted two clinical lectures* to cerebro-spinal meningitis, and I shall make use of them in this section.

In 1837 a severe epidemic of cerebro-spinal meningitis broke out at Bayonne and in the department of the Landes. Two regiments paid a heavy tribute to the disease. The regiments were removed from their initial station, but in their changes of quarters they transported the disease with them, and sowed it as they went. Epidemics then broke out in Perigueux, Auch, Rochefort, Versailles, Metz, Strasbourg, etc.—so much so that during a period of four years many garrisons were afflicted by the scourge. Furthermore, the 26th Regiment, which embarked at Port Vendres, took meningitis to Constantine. From this period originate the remarkable works of Lalanne, Forget, Tourdes, etc., to which publications from abroad were added, because cerebro-spinal meningitis made its appearance in several European countries.

Since then the clinical and pathological history of cerebro-spinal meningitis has been written. We must notice, in fact, the scrupulous exactness with which our predecessors described cerebro-spinal meningitis : fulminant forms which kill in twelve hours ; slower forms which last four or five days ; drawn-out forms, with or without remission, which last for weeks ; and attenuated forms. They have left us an almost complete picture of the disease : its sudden commencement with rigors, fever, terrible headache, vomiting, pains and contractures in the muscles of the nape of the neck and of the back; trismus and opisthotonos, contractures and convulsive movements of the limbs, ocular troubles (strabismus and photophobia), delirium, torpor, somnolence, and coma. They noticed facial herpes, morbillous, papular, and peteohial eruptions. Their anatomo-patho-logical description is as complete as it could be at that period : dissemination of the lesions throughout the cerebro-spinal axis ; turbid and sero-puruelnt fluid ; purulent tracts, thin or thick, and discrete or confluent, spread unequally over the surface of the brain and of the spinal cord, etc.

Relying on these descriptions, it seemed that the morbid entity of cerebro-spinal meningitis was definitely settled. Many points were, however, still obscure, and the pathogenic agent had to be discovered. This want has been supplied. The researches of the past few years have completed the clinical picture of the disease, and bacteriology has revealed the nature of the micro-organisms. The discovery of the meningococcus (*Diplococcus intracellularis meningitidis*), made by Weichselbaum in 1887, seemed to settle the specific nature of cerebro-spinal meningitis, just as the discovery of Eberth's bacillus settled the specific nature of typhoid fever ; but, whereas typhoid fever is a morbid entity, due solely to Eberth's bacillus, cerebro-spinal meningitis is not a clearly-defined morbid entity. In other words, there is no such thing as " a cerebro-spinal meningitis " due to Weichselbaum's meningococcus ; there are pneumococcal, strepto-coccal, staphylococcal forms of cerebro-spinal meningitis, and also cases due to Koch's bacillus, to mixed infections, including Eberth's bacillus, etc.

---

* *Clinique Médicale de l'Hôtel-Dieu*, 1899, 16ᵉ et 17ᵉ leçons.

From the pathogenic point of view it is sufficient if the micro-organism (meningo-coccus or other microbe), endowed with sufficient virulence, invades the cerebro-spinal axis, and by diffusion produces the lesions and the complications of cerebro-spinal meningitis. The pneumococcal, streptococcal, staphylococcal forms of cerebro-spinal meningitis are clinically identical with the meningococcal form ; they may have the same onset, the same symptoms, the same course, and the same termination by death or by recovery.

From the ætiological point of view cerebro-spinal meningitis may be primary or secondary—primary, as is customary during an epidemic, when the patient has pre-viously shown no pathological defect capable of being the starting-point of the infection ; secondary when the patient, by reason of some pathological defect, such as otitis, pneumonia, Pott's disease, etc., presents an opening for the infectious agent.

Clinical Cases.—A healthy man, thirty years of age, was suddenly taken ill on Wednesday with rigors and profuse epistaxis. At the same time the headache rendered sleep impossible. Next day fresh epistaxis, fever, and continuous headache. On Thursday night diarrhœa, persistence of the fever and of the headache. The onset thus far resembled that of typhoid fever. On Friday morning the man was admitted to my wards, and whilst he was being undressed he was seized with vomiting, and brought up, without any effort, greenish fluid. The respiration was normal, the pulse was 100, and the temperature 102° F. During the day the patient complained of violent headache, and frequently carried his hand to his forehead, crying : " My head, my head !" There was, however, no photophobia, and pressure on the eyeballs did not cause pain. The intelligence was intact, and the patient replied clearly to questions, but he was so fatigued that the examination had to be stopped repeatedly.

The left tonsil was enlarged and covered with a pulpy exudate. The heart and the lungs were normal. The belly was not painful ; it was neither tympanitic nor re-tracted. On the outer and back part of the thighs there was an erythematous eruption, formed of non-prominent rosy patches, which almost disappeared on pressure. During the day this eruption spread over the whole body, the head excepted. The headache, the epistaxis, and the diarrhœa at the onset were rather in favour of typhoid fever. On the other hand, the greenish vomit and the terrible headache on his admission were in favour of meningitis. It was true that several meningitic symptoms—photophobia, pain in the back of the neck, and muscular contractures—were for the moment absent.

On Saturday morning I found the patient lying in the position called *chien de fusil*. The pains in the head had lasted all night, the delirium had been violent, the muscles of the nape of the neck and of the vertebral column were contracted, the photophobia was intense, the belly was slightly retracted, constipation had taken the place of the diarrhœa, and Kernig's sign was present. Although tubercular meningitis may in the adult assume the most varied forms, as Chantemesse has shown, we could hardly admit the hypothesis of a tubercular lesion. Griffon obtained by lumbar puncture 3 c.c. of turbid cerebro-spinal fluid, which became clear on standing and formed a deposit in the tube. This puncture caused transient im-provement. The cyanotic tint disappeared, the respiration improved, and the paralysis of the limbs became less complete. The coma, nevertheless, persisted, and death occurred on the fifth day. The autopsy confirmed the diagnosis of cerebro-spinal meningitis and revealed the following lesions : the lower lobe of the right lung was much congested ; it was not granular on section, and the tissue was only slightly friable and did not sink in water. The examination of the brain showed neither the granulations of tubercular meningitis nor the thick and purulent exudate of pneumococcal menin-gitis. At the junction of the vessels we found some tracts of pus so firm that it was difficult to remove sufficient for examination. The pus was more abundant in the fissures of Sylvius and over the superior vermis of the brain. In the cerebro-spinal fluid Griffon found Weichselbaum's meningococcus.

Another patient was admitted to the same ward for cerebro-spinal meningitis —on a Saturday morning. On admission he sank down on a chair, incapable of replying to our questions, which he did not seem to understand. The policeman who brought him to the Hôtel-Dieu had no information to give. He had been found on the second story of a mansion, which he had entered without being known. The patient's brother-in-law could not tell us anything except that the patient, who sometimes drank to excess, had been in good health during the previous days, and that on Saturday morning he had left home early to go to his work.

When the patient was put to bed, he turned on his side, his legs bent in the so-called *chien de fusil* position. The mouth was slightly drawn to the left, and the right half of the face was immovable and paretic. The eyes were wide open. The hands were constantly moving. Pressure on the eyeball produced reflex contraction of the jaws. The nape of the neck and the vertebral region were rigid and contracted. This rigidity made auscultation difficult, on account of the difficulty in moving the patient and making him sit up. Kernig's sign was present. The heart and the lungs appeared to be healthy ; the respiration was normal. The urine contained much albumin, but not any sugar. The fever was high—pulse 90, temperature 102° F.

The unconscious patient did not seem to be suffering ; he had no photophobia and did not carry his hand to his head. He neither groaned nor complained. Nevertheless, in spite of the absence of pain, the rigidity of the nape of the neck and of the trunk, the muscular contractures, Kernig's sign, the rapid and febrile onset of the disease, and the prostration of the patient, led me to diagnose cerebro-spinal meningitis.

The following night the patient became delirious and very restless ; his motions were passed under him. On Sunday morning, the second day of the disease, the contracture was still more pronounced. The *tache cérébrale* (Trousseau's sign) was clear, and the patient uttered a few groans. I prescribed antispasmodic treatment, as well as very hot baths (102° F.), with cold compresses to the head. On Monday the condition was the same—contractures, plaintive cries, lateral decubitus, and Kernig's sign. Griffon performed lumbar puncture, and withdrew 3 c.c. of cerebro-spinal fluid. In the evening an epileptiform attack appeared.

On Tuesday, the fourth day of the disease, the body was stiff and so contracted that the trunk seemed to form only one piece. The respiration was noisy and hurried— 80 respirations to the minute ; pulse 112. During the morning there was a fresh epileptiform attack, similar to that of the previous evening. The patient died about eight o'clock in the evening.

The post-mortem examination confirmed the diagnosis of cerebro-spinal meningitis. On examining the brain, tracts of firm pus were found at the confluence of the principal sulci. The exudate was firm and difficult to remove ; it occupied the arachnoid space and was plastered over the brain. Many purulent patches were found on the inferior surface of the cerebellum; they were less spread out and more consistent over the anterior perforated space. Throughout the whole length of the spinal cord this same firm pus covered the posterior surface of the spinal cord. The cerebro-spinal fluid was turbid and scanty. The lungs were congested at their bases. The spleen was enlarged. Nothing was noticeable in the other organs.

The cerebro-spinal fluid, which was very turbid at the time of its evacuation, grew clearer on standing, and deposited a slightly rose-coloured coagulum. The microscopic examination of the turbid liquid showed numerous polynuclear leucocytes and meningococci—some intracellular, others encapsuled and extracellular and unstained by Gram, a fact which eliminated any question of the pneumococcus. The pus, on various media (broth, agar, rabbit serum, jellified ox serum), gave rise to colonies of Weichselbaum's meningococcus. Some blood taken during life by an aseptic puncture from a vein, and sown on agar and rabbit serum, did not give a positive culture of the meningococcus ; the tubes remained sterile.

In conclusion, these two patients succumbed—the former in five days, the latter in three days—to classic meningococcal cerebro-spinal meningitis. In these cases it was not a question of cerebro-spinal meningitis consecutive to pre-existing lesions, such as pneumonia, otitis, etc. The disease here certainly had the appearance of primary cerebro-spinal meningitis, with its microbe, which is considered as the specific agent: Weichselbaum's meningococcus.

If we were to rely only on this type of cerebro-spinal meningitis, we might make a specific disease of it, having its own pathogenic agent. But, as I have said, the question deserves to be examined from another aspect. Other pathogenic agents—pneumococcus, streptococcus, staphylococcus, etc.—with or without pre-existing organic lesions, may, in times of an epidemic or not, cause the complete syndrome of cerebro-spinal meningitis.

I shall first describe cerebro-spinal meningitis consecutive to **pneumonia**. We know that in many cases the pneumococcal infection does not remain limited to the lung. It is not rare to find otitis, endocarditis, pericarditis, or meningitis in patients suffering from pneumonia. In the case of meningeal complications the cerebral meninges are generally affected. Sometimes, however, the pneumococcal infection spreads to the spinal meninges, and gives rise to cerebro-spinal meningitis. The following case was published by Rendu:

In a certain family three little girls were successively attacked. One of the sisters was taken ill with a rigor, temperature of 104° F., intense angina, otitis, and perforation of the tympanum. A week later the elder sister was taken with severe apical pneumonia, which ran a regular course, the crisis occurring on the seventh day. The third sister, a little girl of five years of age, was taken ill during the night of February 18 with a violent rigor, high fever, restlessness, and delirium. Rendu, thinking that the delirium was pneumonic, placed the child in a bath at 90° F., and prescribed an enema of antipyrine. On Monday the situation remained about the same. On Tuesday, February 21, the third day of the disease, auscultation revealed for the first time some signs of pneumonia. On Wednesday the signs of pneumonia were evident. The child was restless and delirious; the respiration-rate was 60.

On Saturday, the seventh day of the pneumonia, the crisis showed itself, but, contrary to expectation, a sudden change took place. On Sunday morning, February 25, the temperature rose to 104° F.; the pulse was 140. The pupils were widely dilated, and the jaws were fixed; the head was retracted. The nuchal muscles were contracted. The upper limbs were rigid, and it was almost impossible to flex them. The thighs were flexed on the pelvis; Kernig's sign was evident. The legs were readily extended when the child was lying down, but with difficulty when she was seated. Moreover, the sitting position was very difficult on account of the opisthotonos. It was noticed that the tubular breathing had reappeared, the pneumonia having undergone a recrudescence when the cerebro-spinal meningitis declared itself. In three days the signs of cerebro-spinal meningitis reached their maximum, and the prognosis was most grave. The child, who was unconscious, could neither see nor hear. The rigidity of the nape of the neck became more marked; the contracture of the limbs was permanent; the passage of urine was involuntary; the fever was high, and the pulse was 140. Boils covered the occipital region, and a fairly large bedsore appeared over the buttocks.

On Thursday, the fifth day of the meningitis, the meningeal symptoms improved. On Friday the pneumonia entered the defervescent stage. On Sunday, the fifteenth day of the disease, the rigidity of the nape of the neck had disappeared. The contracture was no longer present in the right arm, but it persisted in the left arm and in the lower limbs. These symptoms gradually disappeared, and recovery followed.

I quote two fatal cases of the same kind, also from Rendu :

A man was admitted into hospital with symptoms of adynamic pneumonia. After an incomplete crisis, he was taken ill on the twelfth day with delirium and contracture of the nape of the neck. He succumbed in forty-eight hours, and the post-mortem examination revealed suppurative cerebro-spinal meningitis. The pneumococcus was the cause. The second case refers to a man admitted into hospital with severe pneumonia. Contrary to all expectation, the pulmonary complications improved, and the crisis was normal. After the temperature had been normal for six days, the fever reappeared, and lasted for a week without definite local symptoms. The patient then had an apoplectiform attack, with rigidity of the nape of the neck, contraction of the pupils, and coma. Death supervened in thirty-six hours. The autopsy showed cerebro-spinal meningitis. The brain, the bulb, and the spinal cord were covered with purulent exudate. The bacteriological examination showed a pneumococcal infection.

These cases prove beyond a doubt that cerebro-spinal meningitis may supervene with all the classic symptoms during the course of pneumonia, or after the crisis, when the patient is on the high-road to convalescence. The **pneumococcus** is the pathogenic agent. Up to what point can epidemic influence be invoked here ? I do not know. One thing is certain—viz., that, in the cases just quoted, the cerebro-spinal meningitis was consecutive to pneumonia, and it is probable that it would not have appeared if pneumonia had not been present.

Let us now study the relations which may exist between suppurative otitis media and cerebro-spinal meningitis. Abscesses of the cerebrum and of the cerebellum, phlebitis of the sinuses and cerebral meningitis, may follow on otitis, whether it is in active progress or apparently cured. This question is discussed in detail under Abscesses of the Cerebellum. Besides these complications, however, otitis may be the starting-point of cerebro-spinal meningitis.

A youth, nineteen years of age, was admitted into Rendu's ward on the fourth day of an acute infectious disease of an ataxo-adynamic nature. The patient, whilst in a state of good health, had been taken ill with lassitude and heaviness in the head. On the third day he had epistaxis, pains in the nape of the neck, and headache, followed by insomnia and delirium. On his admission, the patient seemed to be suffering from severe ataxo-adynamic typhoid fever. The tongue was dry, the nostrils were caked, the lips were covered with sordes, and the breath was foetid. The motions were serous, abundant, and passed under him. The belly was slightly distended, and the ileo-cæcal gurgling very clear. No rose spots were noticed, which is not surprising on the fifth day of the disease. The spleen was enlarged, and showed a dullness of 5 inches. The urine was scanty, turbid, and albuminous. The lungs were absolutely normal. The thermometer registered 105° F., and the pulse-rate varied between 120 and 130.

The chief symptoms were cerebral. The patient was in a condition of stupor, having restless dreams and uttering incoherent words. It was hardly possible to rouse him from his condition of somnolence by questioning him. He seemed, besides, to be rather deaf. This deafness, as we found out, arose from a former otitis of the right ear, an otitis which seemed to be extinct, because there was no actual running from the ear. The patient complained chiefly of headache. The movements of the head and of the neck were very painful. The act of sitting him up for auscultation caused him to complain, and he instinctively kept his head fixed, without daring to touch or move it.

These symptoms led Rendu to think of typhoid fever of the cerebral form. Some blood was removed to examine for Widal's reaction. Before the result was known the disorder suddenly entered on a new phase, which proved the diagnosis of cerebro-spinal meningitis. The patient took on a marked cerebral look ; his physiognomy was expressionless ; the right pupil was contracted, the left one was dilated ; the belly was retracted. Large cyanotic patches appeared on the skin of the limbs and of the abdomen. The patient, instead of being stretched on his bed, lay bent in the *chien de fusil* position, the knees and the thighs flexed on the abdomen. The nape of the neck was more rigid than during the previous days, and opisthotonos was present. Straightening of the legs was painful. Kernig's sign was manifest. The patient remained delirious, and mumbled incoherent words. No convulsions, no paralysis, no Jacksonian epilepsy. The urine was passed involuntarily. The respiration assumed the bulbar type. The patient died on the ninth day of the disease

At the post-mortem examination the lesions confirmed the diagnosis of cerebro-spinal meningitis. Under the pia mater, over the surface of the hemispheres, there was thick purulent exudate, which occupied the frontal region, the interhemispherical fissure, and the Sylvian fissures, following the anatomical distribution of the middle and anterior cerebral arteries on each side. Similar but less confluent exudate was seen on the upper surface of the cerebellum, in the anterior subarachnoidal space, on the optic chiasma, and on the anterior surface of the bulb and of the pons. These exudates were of a yellowish colour, and not as green as the pus of pneumococcal meningitis. They resembled butter or cooked albumin ; in some places they were ½ centimetre in thickness. Their consistency was elastic, and they did not tear to pieces. The cerebro-spinal fluid was turbid and moderate in amount. The convolutions were fairly difficult to decorticate, adhering to the pia mater, from which they could not be separated without leaving behind some brain tissue. They were injected, and manifestly hyperæmic, but not softened.

In the spinal cord the lesions were less confluent. A fibrino-purulent exudate formed a continuous layer under the pia mater of the posterior spinal region from the bulb to the cauda equina. The arachnoid was distended, and at the lumbar swelling it was easy to collect, before the removal of the meninges, a considerable amount of pus in sterilized pipettes for subsequent bacteriological examination. The other organs presented some accessory lesions, pointing to the presence of an infectious agent. The liver was enlarged, soft, and yellowish-brown ; the kidneys were fatty ; the spleen was enlarged and soft. The alimentary canal showed no ulcerations and no folliculitis—in a word, not one of the lesions of typhoid fever.

The right ear contained some muco-purulent exudate. Therefore, it is probable that the otitis was the starting-point of the cerebro-spinal infection. Bacteriological examination of the pus showed the presence of the streptococcus.

This case is a type of streptococcal cerebro-spinal meningitis, consequent on a partially extinct, but still virulent, focus of otitis media. The signs and symptoms observed in the course of this case are quite comparable with those of epidemic or non-epidemic meningococcal cerebro-spinal meningitis.

Netter, at the Société Médicale des Hôpitaux, showed the anatomical specimens from a child in Josias's ward, which proved that, in this child, suppurating otitis had been the entrance gateway of the cerebro-spinal infection.

Traumatism may cause cerebro-spinal meningitis, having the classical signs and symptoms of epidemic cerebro-spinal meningitis. As an example :

Stadelmann saw a man who, several weeks after a severe injury to the skull, was seized with symptoms of cerebro-spinal meningitis : rigors, headache, vomiting, rigidity of the nape of the neck, convulsions, and obnubilation. Lumbar puncture gave issue to 50 grammes of a purulent liquid. A second puncture, a few days later, gave issue to 15 grammes of similar liquid. In spite of the punctures the muscular spasms became general. A third puncture was made, and 15 grammes of less turbid liquid were withdrawn. After various ups and downs improvement supervened. A fourth puncture yielded only 5 grammes of limpid fluid. The bacteriological examination of the spinal fluid revealed the presence of large and very mobile bacteria.

With regard to Stadelmann's case, Frankel states that he has seen a boy of six years of age in whom meningococcal cerebro-spinal meningitis immediately followed on an injury. In order to explain the pathogenesis, Frankel admits that the meningococcus, which was present in the upper air passages, had emigrated after the injury into the cranial cavities. Whatever may be the explanation of these facts, and whatever opinion may be adopted with regard to the migration and the exaltation of virulence of the pathogenic microbes, it is none the less true that, clinically, we may see cerebro-spinal meningitis following on traumatism.

Guibal has published a case of streptococcal and staphylococcal cerebro-spinal meningitis following on Pott's Disease :

A little girl had dorsal curvature, with spasmodic paraplegia and paralysis of the sphincters. One day the child was taken ill with high fever, vomiting, headache, and general hyperæsthesia. The belly was hard and retracted. During the next few days, rigidity of the nape of the neck, paralysis of the left half of the face and of the left arm, somnolence and coma, terminating in death. At the autopsy purulent cerebro-spinal meningitis was discovered. The bacteriological investigations revealed the presence of the streptococcus and of the staphylococcus. It is probable that the infection was due to a fistulous abscess in contact with the spinal dura mater.

Pneumococcal, streptococcal, and staphylococcal cerebro-spinal meningitis are not only secondary to pre-existing lesions (pneumonia, otitis, osseous suppurations, etc.); they may be primary, like meningococcal meningitis. As an example :

A child of eleven years of age was admitted into Josias's ward with pains in the head ; fever, and constipation. During the following days fresh symptoms appeared : vomiting, pains in the nape of the neck, paralysis of the limbs on the right side, and inferior facial paralysis. These symptoms were followed by rigidity of the nape of the neck and of the trunk (opisthotonos), by convergent strabismus, and by retention of urine. An eruption of herpes was noticed around the lips. The patient grew emaciated, and the eyes became hollow. Netter made a lumbar puncture, and obtained some purulent liquid. The child died in coma. At the post-mortem examination the case was found to be one of cerebro-spinal meningitis. The bacteriological examination was carried out by Netter. "The culture, on various media (broth, agar, serum, and gelatine), revealed the *Staphylococcus pyogenes aureus* in a condition of purity, with its normal characters.

At the same meeting of the Société Médicale des Hôpitaux Antony reported two cases of cerebro-spinal meningitis, caused by the *Staphylococcus aureus*, " though it was impossible to find on the patient a suppurating spot which might have been considered the origin of the infection." It was, then, a case, like the cases of Netter and Josias, of primary staphylococcal cerebro-spinal meningitis.

Ætiology—Pathogenesis.—In its epidemic form cerebro-spinal meningitis affects the military more than the civil population. It may be imported, and it is contagious. The history of former epidemics shows that it changed its quarters with our regiments in Rome, in Algeria, etc. The epidemics develop gradually, attacking, first, a certain barracks, a few houses, or a certain quarter, " the third storey of the North building and the second storey of the South Block " (Lemoine), and radiating thence in the shape of secondary foci.

It is an important fact that epidemic cerebro-spinal meningitis is often associated with some other epidemic disease. Thus, in 1848, Michel Lévy noticed the coexistence of meningitis and influenza ; in the Rastadt epidemic of 1864 meningitis coexisted with typhoid fever ; its coexistence has been noted with typhus (Boudin), with mumps (Massonaud), with measles (Vallin), and with scarlatina (Laveran). Lemoine's monograph dealing with the subject is most interesting. In the epidemic which he observed at Orléans, in 1886, cerebro-spinal meningitis appeared at the same time as a double epidemic of scarlatina and pneumonia. The patients suffering from meningitis suffered from throat troubles, recalling scarlatina, and at the post-mortem examination of the patients in whom the meningitis proved fatal (in the proportion of 50 per cent.) the pneumococcus was found.

During a slight epidemic in Paris, in twenty-one cases of cerebro-spinal meningitis observed in 1899, Netter's figures are as follows : Seven cases, the pneumococcus ; six cases, Weichselbaum's diplococcus (meningococcus) ; four cases, a streptococcus ; three cases, the streptococcus pyogenes ; one case, a staphylococcus. If we also add cases of cerebro-spinal meningitis, due to Koch's bacillus, to Eberth's bacillus, and to associated infections, it is clear that the question is singularly broadened.

This proves, then, as I remarked at the commencement of this section, that cerebro-spinal meningitis does not form a definite morbid entity. It must be divided into several varieties. In one of its varieties, the most important one, especially in time of an epidemic, Weichselbaum's meningococcus appears to be the specific agent, as was the case in two of my patients.

In the other varieties, leaving epidemics out of the question, the lesions and symptoms are dependent on various micro-organisms—pneumococcus, streptococcus, staphylococcus, Koch's bacillus, Eberth's bacillus, etc. Several varieties of cerebro-spinal meningitis may be primary, like the meningococcal type. They may be secondary—that is to say, dependent on pre-existing lesions. Whatever the entrance-point of the infective agent, its diffusion to the cerebro-spinal axis causes cerebro-spinal meningitis. A single pathogenic agent may, according to circumstances, limit its action to the brain, or invade the entire cerebro-spinal axis. A single pre-existing lesion may be the origin of an infection which limits itself to the brain, or which becomes diffused through the entire cerebro-spinal axis. Thus, side by side with cases in which suppurative otitis produces only cerebral complications, there are others in which it causes general cerebro-spinal infection. Side by side with cases in which Pott's disease causes only spinal complications, there are others in which it is the origin of an infection of the entire cerebro-spinal axis, just as a tubercular lesion, visible or latent, sometimes causes cerebral meningitis. At other times tubercular infection of the entire cerebro-spinal axis. If, however, the varieties of cerebro-spinal meningitis are distinct as to their pathogenesis, it may be said that, clinically, they resemble one another—similar symptoms, similar course, fulminant, ambulatory, rapid, or slow; similar anomalies; similar masked or attenuated forms.

Description.—The onset of cerebro-spinal meningitis is generally sudden and febrile, with or without rigors. There are few or no prodromata. Patients are sometimes attacked in the midst of good health. An individual who was in excellent health on the previous day is suddenly struck by the disease, especially during an epidemic. In a few hours the temperature rises to 104° F. Headache is almost always the first signal; it may be either frontal or occipito-frontal, and dull or lancinating. The headache becomes so severe as to provoke the hydrocephalic cry. The patient complains of pains in the nape of the neck, in the back, in the limbs, and in the joints. In some cases the articular pains somewhat resemble those of acute rheumatism.

Vomiting of food and of bile generally appears during the first stage of meningitis; the attacks follow one after the other, and the fluid is brought up without effort. Diarrhœa is exceptional, constipation being the rule; the belly is hard and retracted. On the first day painful contracture of the muscles of the nape of the neck, with retraction of the head, supervenes. " This cramp in the nape of the neck " is rarely absent. It was, however, absent in some of Netter's cases. The painful contracture likewise attacks the muscles of the back, and the trunk is bent backwards in the position of opisthotonos. The painful contractures may extend to the muscles of the arms and of the legs.

From the commencement of the disease, or during the first few days, paralysis sometimes supervenes ; hemiplegia of the face, or of the limbs, paralysis af the muscles of the eye (strabismus), of the sphincters (incontinence of urine) ; photophobia, and hyperæsthesia have been noted in several cases. The *tache cérébrale* (Trousseau's sign) is easily obtained. Kernig's sign is almost always present.

Sometimes, in the first phase of cerebro-spinal meningitis, the patient, who is prostrated, replies with difficulty to the questions put to him. He looks like a patient suffering from enteric fever. The respiration is often panting, irregular, and of the Cheyne-Stokes type, and auscultation is made very difficult, because the rigidity produced by the contractures prevents easy movement of the patient. The heart-beats are often irregular. Erythematous eruptions, accompanied at times by purpura and by petechiæ, are seen fairly frequently. Herpes is present in a fair number of cases. It may be seen on the lips, on the tonsils, and on the trunk.

The symptoms of excitation (delirium, restlessness, cries, and groans) are often followed by depression, the patient remaining in the dorsal or lateral decubitus in a state of prostration bordering on coma. Cerebro-spinal meningitis, though very grave, sometimes ends in recovery. We had such a case at the Hôtel-Dieu. When death occurs it supervenes on coma, as in my first patient, or after epileptiform convulsions, as in my second one.

I must now refer to " **Kernig's sign**," a diagnostic sign of the first importance, discovered in 1882 by Kernig, and studied in France by Netter. Kernig's sign is as follows : As long as the patient is in the dorsal decubitus, his legs can be extended and can be kept so, without meeting any muscular resistance. If the patient is seated (which is sometimes difficult on account of the painful rigidity of the muscles of the nape of the neck and of the back), the legs are at once flexed on the thighs and the thighs on the trunk ; it is a contracture of flexion. In other words, the patient, whilst seated, by an involuntary movement, draws the legs and the thighs towards himself, and the knees are raised. Firm pressure on the knees is required to overcome this movement and to keep the limbs extended. If the patient is replaced in dorsal decubitus, the contracture of flexion ceases immediately, and the legs are extended. Although we are unable to explain the mechanism of this sign, it certainly indicates the participation of the spinal meninges.

Kernig's sign is rarely absent in cerebro-spinal meningitis. It has been verified by Bull of Christiania, Henoch of Berlin, Friis of Copenhagen, Widal, and Merklen. Netter, who has collected their papers, met with it in twenty-three cases—epidemic cerebro-spinal meningitis in twelve cases (six in the stationary stage), four defaced forms (two on the road to convalescence), eight cases of tubercular meningitis, three cases of mixed meningitis (association of the meningococcus and of the tubercle bacillus). " Kernig's sign persists in convalescents for a longer or shorter time. Kernig and Henoch have seen it after two months and a half. We have also seen it in convalescent or cured patients. It, therefore, enables a retrospective diagnosis to be made, and has no less a value in revealing the defaced forms of the disease " (Netter).

A method of investigation very useful in the diagnosis of cerebro-spinal meningitis is lumbar puncture, first advised by Quincke, and employed in France by Netter. In 1890 Quincke proposed to puncture the subarachnoid space in the lower portion of the lumbar column. His idea was to diminish the excess of tension of the cerebro-spinal fluid by giving an issue to the liquid contained in the large subarachnoid space of the cauda equina. The therapeutic value of lumbar puncture has declined to-day; not so, however, its diagnostic value.

The method is as follows : The patient is placed on his right or left side. The thighs are flexed on the pelvis, and the legs are flexed on the thighs, so as to separate the vertebral laminæ to their utmost. The landmarks are as follows : First the base of the sacrum, then the space between the fifth lumbar and the first sacral vertebra (the selected point for lumbo-sacral puncture (Chipault), which is preferable to Quincke's true lumbar puncture), and, finally, the spinous process of the fifth lumbar vertebra. The trocar, or the needle, is then inserted about half a centimetre external to the median line (Sicard). The depth should be from 4 to 6 centimetres in the adult, and from 1 to 3 centimetres in a child. The instrument is directed forwards, slightly upwards and inwards, towards the median line. The cerebro-spinal fluid then flows out, but it should be evacuated slowly, drop by drop. It is collected in sterilized tubes, centrifugalized, and examined bacteriologically. The amount of fluid withdrawn should not exceed 15 to 20 grammes, since paralysis and death may result from the removal of too much fluid.

The liquid may be limpid or turbid. It may be limpid and yet contain micro-organisms. When the liquid is turbid, it suffices to leave it standing in the tube, and it becomes clear, whilst a small clot forms at the bottom of the tube. Cultures made with the fluid obtained by puncture enable us to ascertain the nature of the pathogenic microbes.

In short, the recent study of cerebro-spinal meningitis has been enriched by two new signs : Kernig's sign, and lumbar puncture (Quincke), which allows histological and bacteriological examination of the liquid. These two signs are of supreme importance when the diagnosis is uncertain.

Diagnosis.—The diagnosis of cerebro-spinal meningitis is at times very difficult. In fact, this disease presents many points of analogy with influenza and with typhoid fever of an ataxo-adynamic type. In other cases, rare it is true, the joint troubles are of unusual importance. To quote examples :

A man, forty-two years of age, who had previously had two attacks of acute articular rheumatism, was admitted under Galliard for very sharp pains in the left sacro-lumbar muscles and in the sacro-iliac joint. The temperature was close on 104° F. The case was diagnosed as rheumatism of the left sacro-iliac articulation. There was no blenorrhagia. Salicylate of soda was prescribed. Eight days later symptoms of meningitis appeared : headache, delirium, strabismus, and rigidity of the muscles of the nape of the neck. The course was rapid, and the patient succumbed. The post-mortem examination showed the case to be pneumococcal meningitis. Netter saw a patient who, during the course of cerebro-spinal meningitis, had pains in the right elbow. At the post-mortem examination a turbid liquid, containing the meningo-coccus, was withdrawn from the joint. In one of Frentz's patients meningococci were found in the purulent fluid from an inflamed ankle-joint. In the recent Bayonne epidemic " articular complications were frequently noted " (Camiade).

The diagnosis must be made between cerebro-spinal meningitis and certain forms of influenza of an ataxo-adynamic type. In such cases, it must be admitted, we think of influenza rather than of meningitis. Kernig's sign and lumbar puncture will clear up the diagnosis.

Cerebro-spinal meningitis often resembles ataxo-adynamic typhoid fever—headache, photophobia, restlessness, delirium, depression, somno-lence, torpor, coma, are all symptoms common to both conditions—and we have to decide whether the patient is suffering from cerebro-spinal menin gitis of a typhoid form or from typhoid fever of a meningeal type. Th duration of the disease is of value in diagnosis, because the ataxo-adynamic symptoms appear much earlier in meningitis ; furthermore, they are accom-panied by Kernig's sign, which is not present in typhoid fever. Finally, Widal's reaction is in favour of typhoid fever. These means, to which the lumbar puncture may be added, will give the diagnosis. We must, however, reckon with cases in which the sero-diagnosis is delayed in its appearance. Account must also be taken of the cases in which meningitis supervenes in an individual who has had typhoid fever and whose serum has preserved the agglutinative power. Finally, it must not be forgotten that typhoid fever and cerebro-spinal meningitis may coexist in the same patient.

In this connection the following cases are instructive :

One of my colleagues was taken ill with symptoms which might have been due to influenza, to typhoid fever, or to meningitis. After an indefinite phase, the late appear-ance of rose-spots and sero-diagnosis proved the presence of typhoid fever, but the patient also had symptoms of cerebro-spinal meningitis, including Kernig's sign. I had the happiness of seeing him recover. In this case, however, must we admit that Kernig's sign was due to typhoid fever alone, or must we suppose that the typhoid fever was complicated with cerebro-spinal meningitis ? This latter hypothesis is not admissible, because this association has been verified, as the following case will prove.

A boy was admitted under Netter with the symptoms of typhoid fever in the second week : typhoid look, dry tongue, tympanitic abdomen, diarrhœa, enlarged spleen, rose-spots, sibilant râles in both lungs, urine albuminous and rich in indican, and temperature 104° F.   Widal's reaction gave a positive result.   The patient showed no meningeal symptoms (delirium, painful contractures, paralysis, and convulsions being absent), and yet Kernig's sign was present.   It was thought that Kernig's sign might be due to the typhoid fever.   The patient, who was treated with cold baths, died suddenly after a week's treatment.

The post-mortem examination showed the lesions of typhoid fever : intestinal per-foration, ulcerations of Peyer's patches, softening of the mesenteric glands, swelling of the spleen.   Cultures revealed the presence of Eberth's bacillus in the spleen and in the glands.   The patient, therefore, had had typhoid fever, **but he had also had typhoid cerebro-spinal meningitis.**   Purulent tracts were, in fact, discovered in the brain and in the spinal cord, with accumulation of serous fluid at the cauda equina.   The cultures showed the presence of *Staphylococcus pyogenes aureus* at these points, together with Eberth's bacillus.   The presence of Kernig's sign was thus explained, the typhoid fever having caused cerebro-spinal meningitis.

It is not sufficient to diagnose cerebro-spinal meningitis ; we must also decide whether it **is, or is not, tubercular.**   The diagnosis is sometimes beset with difficulties, but it is of great importance, because tubercular meningitis is fatal, whilst the non-tubercular infections are fairly often curable.   If we confine ourselves to the classical descriptions, the difference is great between tubercular and non-tubercular meningitis.   The former, it is said, is generally preceded by prodromata, whilst the other forms have a sudden commence-ment.   This statement is generally true.   There are, nevertheless, cases (I have had some in my wards) in which tubercular meningitis breaks out suddenly, and, on the other hand, cases have been cited (Netter) in which non-tubercular cerebro-spinal meningitis is preceded by prodromata, and is characterized by several outbursts, with periods of calm, which lead to the hope of recovery.   Non-tubercular meningitis, it is asserted, is often limited to the convexity of the brain, and causes contractures, paralyses, and localized convulsions, which show the nature of the disease.   This is true, but similar localizations (hemiplegia of the face or of a limb—partial epilepsy) exist likewise in the case of tubercular meningitis.

Kernig's sign, it is said, does not occur in tubercular meningitis ; this is true when the meningitis is purely cerebral.   Marfan told me that in two years he had not once met with Kernig's sign in young children with cerebral tubercular meningitis.   If, however, tubercular meningitis spreads to the spinal meninges, the medullary symptoms are added to the cerebral symp-toms, and Kernig's sign appears (Netter).   The presence, or the absence, of Kernig's sign cannot, therefore, settle the question as to whether a case of cerebro-spinal meningitis is, or is not, tubercular.

It has been thought that the bacteriological examination of the nasal muco-pus might throw light on the diagnosis in difficult cases.   Scherer, who has found Weichselbaum's diplococcus in eighteen cases of epidemic cerebro-spinal meningitis, attributes great diagnostic value to this examination. The importance of this fact must not be exaggerated, first, because cerebro-spinal meningitis may be produced by organisms other than the meningococcus, and, secondly, because the meningococcus is often absent from the nasal fossæ in meningococcal meningitis. It is, therefore, not the presence or the absence of the meningococcus in the nasal muco-pus which will prove that meningitis is, or is not, tubercular.

The bacteriological examination of the blood may be of help in making a diagnosis. Netter found the meningococcus three times in the broth sown with blood from patients with cerebro-spinal meningitis ; but the absence of the meningococcus is not sufficient to prove that the meningitis is tubercular.

These methods of diagnosis have their importance, but they are insufficient, because they often leave us undecided as to the tubercular or non-tubercular nature of the meningitis. There remains lumbar puncture. The cerebro-spinal fluid obtained by lumbar puncture can be analysed for the pathogenic agent, either by direct examination or by culture. When the presence of the meningococcus, of the pneumococcus, or of the streptococcus has been observed, we are almost certain as to the nature of the disease— I say " almost " certain as to the nature of the disease, but not quite, because cerebro-spinal meningitis may be tubercular, although the culture remains sterile. These two hypotheses have been verified by Netter, who, in ten cases of tubercular meningitis which were punctured during life, found that six times the sown liquid remained sterile, and that three times staphylococci developed. " The presence of these latter microbes," adds Netter, " does not exclude the diagnosis of tubercular meningitis."

The presence of Koch's bacillus in the liquid withdrawn by lumbar puncture proves the tubercular nature of the meningitis. In seventy-nine cases of tubercular meningitis lumbar puncture showed Koch's bacilli in the cerebro-spinal fluid on fifty-two occasions (Fürbringer). That is an important result, but it is inconstant, and, consequently, insufficient, because, in a third of the cases, the diagnosis remained doubtful.

In conclusion, the above means of control render much service, but they are insufficient, because they often leave a doubt as to the tubercular, or non-tubercular, nature of the meningitis. Can this doubt be removed ?

Bezançon and Griffon have obtained cultures of Koch's bacillus on blood agar. The first application of this method in the diagnosis of tubercular meningitis was made on a patient in my ward by my house-physician, Griffon. The subjoined account was made to the Société de Biologie :

The results obtained by cultivating the tubercle bacillus on blood agar, a medium of which we have given the mode of preparation, have led us to cultivate on this favourable medium various pathological liquids, which appear clinically to be tubercular in nature. By cultivating the sero-fibrinous effusion of acute pleurisy with success, we have been able to realize this desideratum. It was interesting to apply the same method of bacteriological examination to other serous fluids, and in particular to the cerebro-spinal fluid of patients with meningitis. We were able to put this project into practice in a case of tubercular meningitis in an adult under Dieulafoy's care. By lumbar puncture we collected transparent liquid, the last drops of which were slightly yellow. The sown tubes, which were put into the oven at 39° C., showed, at the end of four weeks, colonies smaller than pin's heads, and containing Koch's bacillus. They were much more numerous than in liquid cultivated under similar conditions from a case of pleurisy. Each colony was well developed, and the spherical form, the mulberry-like aspect, and the chocolate colour were characteristic. A guinea-pig, weighing 260 grammes, which had received an intraperitoneal injection of 5 c.c. of this same liquid, was alive two months later. We killed it. The post-mortem examination revealed the lesions of experimental tuberclosis predominating in the lymphatic organs.

These interesting researches have been continued, but when we have to deal with cerebro-spinal meningitis—a disease of rapid course—we cannot wait a month in order to confirm the diagnosis. Widal, Sicard, and Ravaut have proposed more expeditious methods (cryoscopy of the cerebro-spinal fluid). The freezing-point of the cerebro-spinal fluid is, in the normal condition, lower than that of blood serum; it varies between 0·56° and 0·75° C., being generally above 0·60° C. It is, therefore, hypertonic with regard to blood serum, the freezing-point of which is 0·56° C. Widal, Sicard, and Ravaut have shown that in four out of five cases of tubercular meningitis the cerebro-spinal fluid is, on the contrary, hypotonic with regard to blood serum, the freezing-point varying, then, between 0·48° and 0·55° C. We have here a new method, of easy clinical application. Hypertonia of the cerebro-spinal fluid is in favour of tubercular meningitis.

Some information may also be gathered from the meningeal permeability. The ingestion of 3 to 5 grammes of iodide of potassium is, in the normal condition, not followed by the passage of the iodide into the cerebro-spinal fluid. In tubercular meningitis, on the contrary, the iodide may be found in the liquid by ordinary reagents. Meningeal permeability, however, exists only in 54·7 per cent. of the cases (Widal, Sicard, and Lutier).

The method of cyto-diagnosis proposed by Widal and Ravaut in sero-fibrinous pleurisy is applicable to tubercular meningitis. Widal, Sicard, and Ravaut have shown that in tubercular meningitis the liquid withdrawn by lumbar puncture, even when it is limpid, contains lymphocytes, which are readily brought into evidence by centrifugalization and by staining. If, in certain cases, some polynuclears are found, a simple count shows that they are always much fewer in number than the lymphocytes. In non-tubercular cerebro-spinal meningitis, on the contrary, the cerebro-spinal fluid contains almost solely polynuclears, and the number of the lymphocytes is always restricted. The diagnosis of the tubercular form may be made by Nattan-Larrier's method of injecting 1 c.c. of the cerebro-spinal fluid into the breast of a nursing guinea-pig ; a few days later the milk contains Koch's bacilli.

Acute syphilitic meningitis is also characterized by the presence of lymphocytes (Widal and Le Sourd, Brissaud and Brecy), but this variety of meningitis is exceptional. From the point of view of the lymphocytic formula of meningitis in general, it must be remembered, in order to avoid a mistake, that the cytological examination, made at a period remote from the commencement of bacterial meningitis, will show only the lymphocytes. The polynuclears have disappeared. The observations of Labbé and Castaigné, Sicard, Widal, Griffon, and Apert show clearly the pathogenic interpretation of such cases. When the disease tends towards recovery, the polynuclear, the element of severe infection *en masse*, gives place to the lymphocyte, the element of organization.

The diagnosis of cerebro-spinal meningitis, therefore, comprises two stages. It is not sufficient to distinguish cerebro-spinal meningitis from influenza or from typhoid fever ; we must also make a pathogenic diagnosis, and ascertain whether the lesion is, or is not, tubercular. It is not always easy to avoid a mistake. Clinical observation must be supplemented by laboratory methods.

Prognosis.—Every variety of cerebro-spinal meningitis, except the tubercular, may end in recovery ; the cures vary from 15 to 40 per cent. In Netter's statistics " the proportion of cures is about two in three—a very encouraging number—which shows how important it is to distinguish nontubercular from tubercular meningitis by accurate diagnosis."

Incomplete recovery may also occur, the cerebro-spinal meningitis leaving sequelæ behind. Military physicians (Vincent, Simonin) have noted persistent disturbance of sight and of hearing, intellectual troubles, and hydrocephalus. Raymond and Sicard have described a special type— cerebro-spinal meningitis of the infantile paralytic type. They have shown the relations which may exist between cerebro-spinal meningitis and infantile paralysis. During the course of certain epidemics (the Vermont epidemic of 1894) some children were stricken with cerebro-spinal meningitis, others with infantile paralysis. Certain cases of poliomyelitis may be considered as the ineffaceable relics of cerebro-spinal meningitis.

Bacteriology.—In 1887 Weichselbaum described a microbe which he called the *Diplococcus intracellularis meningitidis*, and which has been considered the specific agent of cerebro-spinal meningitis. This microbe is an immobile coccus, occurring in pairs, never in chains, but sometimes in masses. Each element of the diplococcus possesses a plane surface, which faces an analogous surface of the opposite element. This form, which is that of the coffee-bean, recalls the aspect of the gonococcus. The meningococcus is often enclosed in the protoplasm of a leucocyte. It deserves, therefore, the name of intracellular, but it would be wrong to suppose that it is always enclosed in a cell. It is sometimes extracellular and encapsuled. These two varieties existed in the spinal fluid of our two patients.

The meningococcus on rabbit serum shows a perfect capsule. Some elements may show but a single coccus, and, in the common two-grained form we often meet with a small grain opposite to a grain two or three times as large.

The meningococcus is decolourised by Gram's reaction, and therefore differs from the pneumoccocus. " It differs radically from the common pneumococcus by its culture characters on serums and on gelatine." Griffon made the following communication to the Société de Biologie concerning Weichselbaum's meningococcus, found in a state of purity in the cerebrospinal fluid of my first patient :

The meningococcus grows with difficulty on the usual media ; it does not develop on gelatine. Even on favourable media it grows slowly, and the colonies are not well formed until after an incubation of forty-eight hours in the oven at 37° C. The broth is slightly turbid, or remains sterile. On agar, no apparent colonies are at first developed on the surface of the solid medium ; nevertheless, the condensed liquid in the lower part of the tube is turbid and rich in diplococci. At the end of three or four days an isolated colony may appear on the surface of the agar where it reaches maturity—a large, flat colony, opaque in the centre, with translucent and somewhat irregular edges, remarkably viscous. In proportion to the number of stabs, the microbe becomes acclimatized to the artificial media, and the growth on agar is then more rapid, more certain, and more abundant. To the naked eye it may present the look of a culture of Eberth's bacillus.

The microbe does not grow abundantly in milk. Only a few diplococci are seen in the preparations. The culture medium does not coagulate, even at the end of ten days. Non-coagulated rabbit serum gives a culture which, at the end of forty-eight hours, is fairly abundant, though less rich than in the case of the pneumococcus. Blood agar, so valuable for growing Koch's bacillus, is also a good medium for the meningococcus. The colonies are abundant, close to the stabs, and early in their appearance. They are flat, macular, of a brownish-yellow, translucent, and, if several colonies coalesce, they look like a plaque with polycyclical edges.

Experimentally, the action of the microbe on the mouse was such as Weichselbaum described it. Subcutaneous inoculations gave no result, whether the pus was injected or whether a culture was employed. On the other hand, intrapleural injection caused the death of the animal in three days, and the post-mortem examination revealed double pleurisy with sero-hæmorrhagic effusion, more abundant on the side of the puncture, and generalization of the microbe in the blood and in the organs. A rabbit was taken, and a small dose of the culture was injected into a vein. It did not die, even at the end of twelve days ; but it became cachectic, and examination of the blood showed intense leucocytosis and the presence of free meningococci between the white and red corpuscles. It was interesting to examine the agglutinating property in the blood of the patient. The serum did not agglutinate the meningococcus, whether we employed a broth culture, as in Widal's method, for Eberth's bacillus, or whether we tried to cultivate the microbe in pure serum. The meningococcus did not develop in undiluted serum.

At the same meeting of the Société de Biologie Netter gave a description of Weichselbaum's meningococcus, which he had previously considered

" as a variety of the pneumococcus." Chantemesse, speaking on these communications, summed up the question by remarking : " Everybody knows that cases of cerebro-spinal meningitis are produced by Weichselbaum's meningococcus, which has no connection with Talamon's pneumococcus."

Treatment.—The treatment of cerebro-spinal meningitis is the more important, in that we are dealing with a disease which is often curable. It was hoped that a therapeutic means had been found in lumbar puncture. Quincke expected to obtain favourable decompression of the nerve centres by means of the puncture, but experience proves that the withdrawal of too large a quantity of the cerebro-spinal fluid may cause grave complications. The puncture is an excellent means of diagnosis, but it is not a means of treatment. In some subjects, as in the case of my first patient, the puncture caused a slight and transient improvement in the disease, but that was all. Therefore, lumbar puncture cannot be called a therapeutic measure.

Hot baths have been rightly advised. Baths at 102° F., lasting from five to ten minutes, and repeated several times in twenty-four hours, produce a certain remission, and give a good result. During the bath it is necessary to apply cold compresses to the patient's head. The painful contractures of the limbs, of the nape of the neck, and of the loins makes the administration of these baths difficult. It is difficult enough to sit the patient up in his bed to auscultate him, and *a fortiori* it is more difficult to keep him in a bath.

The headache and the delirium must be treated by bleeding, leeches behind the ears and on the nape of the neck, and wet cupping to the spine. The bleeding may be repeated daily, some 5 ounces of blood being withdrawn. The bleeding may be followed by the injection of artificial serum. Intravenous injections of collargol have been advised. Antispasmodic remedies find here a perfect application—bromides, in doses of 40 to 60 grains a day ; musk, antipyrine, chloral, hypnal, sulphonal, syrup of ether, and small injections of morphia.

XVII. CHRONIC MENINGITIS—PACHYMENINGITIS— HÆMATOMA OF THE DURA MATER.

Of the different varieties of chronic meningitis two deserve special attention : the one comprises cases of partial meningitis at the base of the brain, the other refers to meningitis, which is often hæmorrhagic ; it is known under the name of " pachymeningitis," and usually affects the convexity of the hemispheres.

1. **Basal Meningitis.**—This form is usually secondary ; it often accompanies tumours at the base of the brain, and is frequently of syphilitic

origin (Fournier). Circumscribed sclero-gummatous meningitis has a well marked predilection for the base of the brain. I have described it under Cerebral Syphilis.

2. **Pachymeningitis—Hæmatoma.**—Pachymeningitis means chronic inflammation of the dura mater, the inflammation being especially limited to the parietal surface when it follows on changes in the bones of the skull. Inflammation of the visceral layer of the dura mater forms a part of the history of hæmatoma. Pachymeningitis is frequent at the two extremes of life. Its causes may be grouped thus : mania, diffuse periencephalitis, injury, alcoholism, rheumatism, and fevers (Jaccoud).

Pathological Anatomy.—In pachymeningitis we find thin superposed neomembranes, which arise on the inner surface of the dura mater ; as many as twenty stratified layers may be counted (Virchow). These false membranes, which are often symmetrical, are usually situated on the cranial vault, on both sides of the falciform process of the dura mater ; the most recently-formed membranes are next to the dura mater. As they grow older they become thick and vascular. The vessels in these membranes are friable, and their rupture causes a **hæmatoma of the dura mater.**

The pathogenesis of the clot and of its encystment has given rise to much discussion. The membrane around the clot is not formed at the expense of the clot. The hæmatoma is formed as the result of the pachymeningitis and the hæmorrhage arises, not between the dura mater and the false layer of the arachnoid, but in the thickness of the neomembrane itself. This theory, however, does not apply to all cases. Most often the hæmorrhage is consequent on the pachymeningitis, just as, in other regions, hæmorrhage is consequent on neomembranes of the pleura and of the tunica vaginalis ; but this mode of formation of the meningeal hæmatoma must not be looked upon as exclusive. In 1837 Baillarger asserted that the meningeal hæmorrhage is primary, and that its enveloping membrane is secondary. Recent experiments (Vulpian, Laborde) prove the correctness of this view, and are in favour of the existence of primary supra-arachnoid hæmorrhages, which later become encysted ; but their envelope is not formed of organized fibrin as Baillarger had supposed, it is formed of a membrane due to the irritation of the neighbouring tissue.

The hæmatoma of pachymeningitis is not always encysted ; the blood may tear the membranes and inundate the arachnoid cavity, but, most frequently, the hæmorrhage collects in the shape of a cyst, the clot retracts, a part is absorbed, and the remainder assumes the yellow aspect of old hæmorrhagic foci in the brain. The cerebral matter is generally depressed and softened at the site of the hæmatoma.

Description.—Pachymeningitis may at first pass unnoticed, or may reveal itself by headache, vertigo, and contraction of the pupils. This first period, which, in the adult, lasts for several months, is followed by a phase of depression, generally provoked by the formation of the hæmatoma. If the hæmorrhage is slight, acute symptoms are absent ; if it is sudden and abundant, it causes apoplexy and coma. It usually induces incomplete hemiplegia, and in some cases contractures and convulsions. In grave cases the pulse is slow and irregular, the pupil is contracted on the side of the lesion, the sphincters are paralyzed, and death is the usual termination.

The paralytic phenomena may exist alone, without any previous apoplexy ; they differ materially from hemiplegia due to cerebral hæmorrhage. Facial paralysis is rare, and the hemiplegia is generally incomplete or dissociated. The **diagnosis** of hæmatoma in certain cerebral lesions (softening, tumour) is sometimes impossible.

XVIII. MENINGEAL HÆMORRHAGE.

Pathological Anatomy.—I have just described hæmorrhage of the dura mater (hæmorrhagic pachymeningitis). Therefore, the question of meningeal hæmorrhage remains limited to the supra- and subarachnoid hæmorrhages. In the new-born child the hæmorrhage is almost always supra-arachnoid, whilst it is subarachnoid in the adult. In supra-arachnoid effusion, the more or less coagulated blood accumulates at the base of the skull, and, in the previous section, we saw that it may become encysted by the formation of an enveloping membrane. When the effusion is subarachnoid, the pia-mater is infiltrated, the choroïd plexuses are injected, the ventricles may be inundated, and clots are frequently found, but the blood is not encysted. Below the coagulum the cerebral convolutions are flattened, and if the hæmorrhage has been considerable the brain is anæmic.

Ætiology—Description.—The differences of the symptoms caused by meningeal hæmorrhage in adults and in children leads me to divide this question.

1. **In the adult** the hæmorrhage is almost always subarachnoid. It is due to the rupture of a vessel, to degeneration of the arterioles, to peri-arteritis with or without miliary aneurysms (heredity, alcoholism), to interstitial nephritis, and to the arterio-sclerosis (Sutton), which accompanies it. It is caused by diseases of the liver and by the hæmorrhagic diathesis. As regards **syphilis,** full details are given in the chapter on Cerebral Syphilis.

Meningeal hæmorrhage is sometimes ushered in by prodromata, such as headache, vomiting, and pain limited to the area of the trifacial nerve. The onset is sometimes sudden, and the comatose phenomena appear first.

The prodromata are almost constant in the case of syphilitic lesions. For several weeks, or several months, the patients suffer from more or less violent headache (which may be worse at night), dimness of sight, giddiness, vertigo, intellectual torpor, nausea and vomiting, speech troubles, unsteady gait, tendency to torpor, contractures, and convulsions.

When the hæmorrhage comes on, the apoplexy may be fatal in a few minutes. Sometimes it is slower in establishing itself; the patient is seized with somnolence, from which he can be roused with difficulty. He scarcely understands what is said to him, his movements are slow and difficult, and in a few hours, or in a few days, according to the progress of the hæmorrhage, he passes into a state of coma.

The compression of the brain by the effused blood is the cause of these complications. Apoplexy and coma are slower to appear than in certain cases of cerebral hæmorrhage, and, except in rare instances (Lépine), we do not find hemiplegia.

The course of the temperature is the same as in cerebral hæmorrhage. Rapidly spreading bed-sores have been found on the buttocks. The disease rarely lasts longer than a week.

2. **In the child,** especially in the new-born, the hæmorrhage is generally supra-arachnoid. It is met with in children who are still-born, or born apparently dead; in the new-born; and during the first year of life. The hæmorrhage is due to difficult labour, to compression of the cord, and to diffuse steatosis (Parrot). In the new-born the symptoms show themselves immediately after birth, or a few days later. The child is seized with convulsions, and dies in coma.

Diagnosis.—Meningeal hæmorrhage was, until a few years ago, one of the most difficult diseases to recognize; its existence, though often suspected, could never be affirmed with certainty.

The diagnosis can now be established with certainty by means of Kernig's sign and lumbar puncture. I have already described Kernig's sign under Cerebro-spinal Meningitis. I have also discussed lumbar puncture (see Meningitis), but only from the cytological point of view. Here lumbar puncture will give us information as to the colour of the cerebro-spinal fluid. The amber-yellow tint (Bard, Sicard), or bloody tint, when we know how to interpret it, has almost an element of certainty.

XIX. HYDROCEPHALUS.

Division—Ætiology.—Hydrocephalus is dropsy of the brain. The fluid may be ventricular or extraventricular, a matter of great difference as regards the pathology and the symptoms. Extraventricular hydrocephalus includes subarachnoidal dropsy, œdema of the pia mater, and of the brain. " According as the effusion is subsequent to the definite occlusion of the cranial cavity, hydrocephalus is called acquired or congenital" (Jaccoud).

Acquired hydrocephalus is due to mechanical causes and to diathetic conditions. The mechanical causes are those which interfere with the venous circulation in the brain—cerebral tumours, meningeal exudates, tumours of the neck and of the mediastinum, and lesions of the right side of the heart.

The diathetic causes include Bright's disease and cachexia, especially tubercular and cancerous cachexia. Congenital hydrocephalus is due to arrested development of the brain, to a slow inflammation of the ependyma, and to obliteration of the sinuses. It may be a manifestation of hereditary syphilis, which is, indeed, the most common cause of hydrocephalus, as appears from the interesting publications of Fournier. I have had the opportunity of seeing two cases of hydrocephalus which were certainly the result of hereditary syphilis.

Pathological Anatomy.—Œdema of the brain and of the pia mater is easily recognized. On making a section of the organ, we notice the oozing of a few drops of liquid, and the œdematous brain retains the imprint of the finger. Ventricular hydrocephalus is not very abundant when it is acute (2 to 3 ounces). It may amount to 12 ounces when it is chronic, and may exceed several pints in congenital cases. The cerebral tissue is softened, the ventricles are dilated, the choroid plexuses are œdematous and hypertrophied (Claisse and Lévi), and, in the case of congenital hydrocephalus, the cerebral convolutions are flattened and, as it were, unrolled. Congenital hydrocephalus is sometimes limited to a portion of the ventricle, to the anterior or posterior cornu, which gives a peculiar shape to the child's head.

Symptoms.—Acquired hydrocephalus may cause no deformity of the skull. If the accumulation of the fluid is rapid, serous apoplexy results, and if the cerebral liquid is of slow formation, the patient often passes through a phase of excitation (delirium, convulsions, and contractures), followed by a phase of depression (coma, resolution, asphyxia). As fever and limited paralyses are not seen, we can from the first eliminate inflammation of the brain and focal tumours. Hydrocephalus also affects a slow form, in which the symptoms of depression show themselves from the first, and become gradually worse.

Congenital hydrocephalus deforms the skull: the head becomes enormous, the orbits are sunken under the protuberance of the frontal bones, the vertical diameter of the face is diminished, whilst the transverse diameter of the forehead is considerably increased by the separation of the frontal bones. The bones of the skull, which are united at their bases, separate like the petals of a flower (Trousseau). Convulsions are frequent, the

91—2

appetite is voracious, the power of movement is deficient, and the intelligence is lacking.

Acquired hydrocephalus, though very serious, is not absolutely fatal. It should be treated with drastic purgatives and local and general bleeding. Congenital hydrocephalus may be compatible with life for ten or fifteen years, and even more. Operations for the removal of the fluid do not give definite results. I have several times performed aspiration of the cerebral fluid with a No. 1 needle. I have been surprised at the harmlessness of the operation. Although I have often obtained a transient improvement, I have never seen a case of cure.

CHAPTER V

NEURITIS

POLYNEURITIS.

SINCE the researches of Duménil, which date from the year 1864, a share, formerly given to lesions of the nerve centres, has been given to the peripheral lesions of the nerves. Duménil endowed the peripheral nervous system with a morbid entity which it did not previously possess. Since that time numberless anatomical, clinical, and experimental researches have been published, pruning the pathology of the central nervous system to the advantage of the peripheral nervous system.

If a patient is attacked by rapid and progressive paralysis, invading the lower and the upper limbs, and speedily followed by muscular atrophy, we are very careful before making *a priori* a diagnosis of poliomyelitis. On closer scrutiny we often make the more correct diagnosis of peripheral polyneuritis.

If a patient is attacked by lancinating pains of the lower limbs, with ocular troubles, and imperfect co-ordination of movements, we are very careful about making *a priori* a diagnosis of tabes. We examine more carefully, and we often make the more exact diagnosis of alcoholic peripheral polyneuritis or pseudo-tabes.

If a patient is attacked with bulbar symptoms, oculo-motor troubles, ophthalmoplegia, etc., we are very careful about making *a priori* a diagnosis of disease in the medulla and the pons. We look closer, and we often make a diagnosis of peripheral polyneuritis, which is less serious.

There are, then, two morbid conditions, which at first sight present great analogies—in the one case, grave troubles, depending on lesions of the nerve-centres ; in the other case, benign troubles, depending on peripheral lesions of the nerves. Paralyses, amyotrophies, trophic troubles, pain, and sensory troubles, anæsthesia, secretory and vasomotor troubles are common to both morbid conditions.

In what, then, does the lesion of peripheral neuritis consist, which may up to a certain point simulate a lesion of the nerve-centres ? As Ettlinger in his excellent work says, the lesion of polyneuritis may be summed up as follows : The small muscular and cutaneous nerve-trunks are degenerated in the regions where the paralysis, the atrophy, and the sensory troubles are observed. This degeneration consists in destructive changes of the axis-cylinder and of their myeline sheath. Its peculiarity consists in the fact that it attains its **maximum in the smallest nerves.** The number of the fibres remaining healthy becomes greater and greater as we reach the large

1429

nerve branches ; for instance, whilst the nerve branches to the muscles of the antero-external region of the leg have hardly any healthy fibres, the external popliteal and the sciatic nerve show hardly any diseased fibres—or, at least, they diminish in number as we reach a higher point of the nerve trunk. The same feature holds good in the cutaneous branches ; their lesions diminish from the periphery towards the centre.

Pathogenesis.—The causes of polyneuritis are the same as those of myelitis. On referring to the section on Myelitis in general, the reader will find in part the pathogenesis which governs the development of neuritis. It may be said that polyneuritis is due to two great causes : (1) to infective or toxi-infective agents ; (2) to toxic substances. Amongst infective agents, I would mention almost all the infective diseases which act directly by means of their microbes, or indirectly by means of the toxines : tuberculosis, typhoid fever, influenza, diphtheria, small-pox, syphilis, malaria, leprosy, streptococcia, coli bacillosis, etc. Amongst the toxic substances, I would mention lead, alcohol, arsenic, and carbonic oxide. To these must be added the autointoxications of diabetes, uremia, gout, and cancer. Finally, there is an essential factor which must not be neglected—cold (polyneuritis *a frigore*)—which plays an undoubted, though obscure, part in the causation of neuritis.

Is it, however, really true that the infective, toxic or toxi-infective agents can limit their noxious action to the periphery of the nerves, just as they limit it to a certain part of the nerve-centres ? It is undeniable that there are more or less isolated peripheral nervous lesions which seem to be independent of any central lesion, but can we say that the lesion of general polyneuritis, seeing that it is wholly peripheral, is not governed by some visible or invisible change of the cells of the nerve-centres ? For example, do we not find diphtheria and influenza (toxi-infectious diseases), causing peripheral lesions (neuritis) and central lesions (myelitis) ? And, again, diabetes may cause peripheral and central lesions. The same pathogenic agent, therefore, may separately or simultaneously cause peripheral lesions (neuritis) and central lesions (poliomyelitis) in the same individual. It is easy, I repeat, to admit the autonomy of certain isolated cases of neuritis, but it is more difficult to admit the autonomy of polyneuritis of a systematically ascending and progressive form. These cases of polyneuritis may be due to central lesions (Marie, Babinski), but little appreciable by our present means of investigation (Raymond), though Renaut has pleaded the cause of the nutritive independence of the cylinder as regards the ganglion cell.

In any case, it is certain that we can clinically describe neuritis and polyneuritis, which in the course of their symptoms and in their mode of termination behave differently from spinal lesions ; and, supposing that the morbid condition of the bulbo-spinal cells escape our observations, the evolution of the symptomatology of what we are agreed to call " peripheral neurites " allows us to describe them as a distinct morbid group, whilst making a few restrictions.

I have remarked that it is necessary to make some restrictions, because it is evident that some authors have gone too far in trying to cut out certain morbid conditions of spinal origin in order to swell the list of polyneuritis. I understand the warning given by Grasset, and no more than he have I ever doubted the autonomy of certain definite spinal types : acute spinal paralysis in the adult, and subacute anterior spinal general paralysis.

Description.—The troubles caused by peripheral neuritis vary according as the lesion chiefly affects the motor, sensory, or trophic nerves ; according as the lesion attacks an isolated nerve or a group of nerves ; and according as the nerves attacked are spinal, cranial, or sympathetic.

The causes of peripheral neuritis sometimes undertake of themselves to make a selection ; thus, lead-poisoning selects the motor and the muscular trophic nerves, producing only paralysis and amyotrophy ; it passes over the sensory nerves. On the other hand, alcohol especially affects the peripheral sensory nerves, but it also produces paralytic and amyotrophic troubles ; it is generally confined to the lower limbs. Peripheral neuritis sometimes attacks special nerves, the optic nerves (alcoholism), the nerves of the external musculature of the eye, strabismus, diplopia, external ophthalmoplegia (diabetes) ; the nerves which preside over accommodation (diphtheria) ; the nerves of the larynx (tuberculosis, plumbism) ; the pneumogastric nerve, with dyspnœa and tachycardia, etc.

These varieties of polyneuritis may exist alone, or may be associated with more general forms. Amongst these general forms, that generally described under the name of polyneuritis, without other qualification, must detain us longer.

Polyneuritis is a fairly frequent type, which may sometimes supervene without apparent cause, or may follow on some infectious disease (influenza), though it more often results from cold. Its course is as follows : An individual, otherwise well, experiences twitchings, shooting pains, cramps, and heaviness in the feet or the legs. Movement and walking become difficult (paresis) ; the steppage gait is seen, and in a few days, if the evolution of the disease is rapid, the paraplegia is complete. The paralysis is symmetrical ; it is generally more pronounced in the extensor muscles, and an important feature is that it commences in the muscles of the extremities of the limbs, diminishing in severity as it ascends upwards. Thus, in the legs the muscles most affected are the small muscles of the foot, the extensor muscles of the toes, and the peroneal muscles. The attitude of the foot is also characteristic ; the foot drops, and the toes are flexed, as if the flexor muscles were contracted ; but there is no real contraction, because the foot shows neither rigidity nor resistance ; it is flaccid and swinging.

The paralysis rarely remains limited to the leg ; in a few days the arms are attacked in their turn. The disease announces itself by tingling, shooting pains and numbness, and the paresis, or the paralysis, spreads from the hands to the shoulder, selecting the extensors, and diminishing in intensity as it ascends. The wrist-drop recalls the attitude seen in lead palsy ; the patient can neither raise the arm nor execute any movement, and in certain cases, as in a patient whom I saw with Raymond, the paralysis of the four limbs is absolute, or nearly so. The sphincters, however, are normal.

Sensory troubles precede and accompany the paralysis. I have already spoken of tingling and painful twitchings in the limbs ; in this variety of polyneuritis the pains are not, as a rule, as acute as they are in alcoholic neuritis. On the other hand, pain is rarely absent, as in saturnine neuritis. Areas of hyperæsthesia or of anæsthesia may be observed, and we may find dissociation of sensibility to pain, to touch, and to temperature, but the usual fact in the variety of polyneuritis under discussion is that the spontaneous pain is not acute ; whilst the pains caused by pressure on the muscles or on the nerves, at their points of exit, and in the sciatic nerve by forcible extension and abduction of the leg show clearly that the disease is situated in the branches and in the nerve-trunks.

The tendon reflexes are abolished ; this abolition of the reflexes is one of the chief symptoms of polyneuritis.

The electrical changes follow the motor and the reflex changes. Electrical examination has the twofold advantage of assisting in the diagnosis of polyneuritis and of gauging its importance and its severity. In a general manner, the electrical contractility is much affected in the paralyzed regions ; the reaction to the faradic current is weak or absent ; the action of the galvanic current is inverted in the regions which are severely affected. The reaction of degeneration is observed. Between the extremes we find intermediate stages, which enable us to form an idea of the severity and of the probable duration of the lesions.

Muscular atrophy is a constant symptom of polyneuritis. The atrophy appears at the same time as the paralysis ; but it runs a much slower course than the paralysis. The coexistence of paralysis and amyotrophy in polyneuritis is explained by the fact that the branches of the nerves which supply the muscles govern both the motor and the trophic functions.

The muscular atrophy causes deformity of the paralyzed regions. The bones stand out, and the masses of muscle are replaced by flattening. The muscular pads in the feet are flattened, whilst the interosseous spaces become hollowed ; in the leg, the bulging of the muscles of the calf is replaced by flaccid skin, and the antero-external surface is excavated like a furrow.

In the thigh there is a similar disappearance of the muscles. In the upper limbs the hand somewhat resembles the hand of progressive muscular atrophy; the thenar and hypothenar eminences disappear. The back of the hand becomes hollowed out in the interosseous spaces, and the forearm is flat.

In spite of the extensive decay, which gives to the limbs the appearance of a skeleton, the general condition remains excellent, the appetite does not diminish, all the functions are performed regularly, and it is only after weeks and months that reparation commences. The muscular atrophy and the paralysis disappear, and in the majority of cases recovery is complete.

Some cases of polyneuritis are subject to relapses or to recurrences. Fatal cases of polyneuritis are quite exceptional; the danger, then, arises from neuritis of the bulbar nerves, or from bulbo-medullary lesions which complicate the peripheral lesions. In a few rare cases multiple neuritis is accompanied by mental troubles—**polyneuritic pyschosis** (Korsakoff). The condition, then, is most frequently one of mental confusion, associated with lesions of the cerebral cortex, changes being seen in the pyramidal cells and in Betz's giant cells—swelling and chromatolysis (Ballet and Faure).

As polyneuritis is relatively benign, it is very important, from the point of view of prognosis, not to confound polyneuritis with other grave diseases which may simulate it. In its painful form, which is generally of alcoholic origin, polyneuritis simulates tabes. This pseudo-tabetic form is far from being rare.

The most remarkable case which I have met with refers to a young man of twenty-five years of age, who for several months drank a bottle of cognac a day without getting drunk. He came from America, where he had been considered to be suffering from tabes. The diagnosis of polyneuritis, however, seemed to me to be obvious. Lacaille gave him electrical treatment, and in six months he was completely cured.

In its paralytic, amyotrophic, and rapidly progressive form polyneuritis simulates acute poliomyelitis. I saw a most remarkable case with Raymond:

A young officer, who had taken a chill during the manœuvres, was seized in a few days with paralysis, commencing in the lower limb, and then spreading to the upper limbs. The paralysis was soon followed by rapid amyotrophy. I have described this case in detail under Acute Spinal Paralysis in the Adult.

Treatment.—I shall not discuss here the prophylactic treatment peculiar to each variety of polyneuritis (removal of the cause, alcohol, lead, etc.), but I shall merely say a few words concerning the indications for electrotherapy. Babinski expresses the following opinion, which I quote verbatim: " Electricity is one of the agents most commonly used in the treatment of peripheral neuritis. It must, however, be used with circumspection, and under certain determined circumstances. It may be said, in a general manner, that electrotherapy must not be prescribed at the commencement of the disease, when the case is one of sensory or of mixed neuritis, but that its use is clearly indicated when the morbid process seems to have spent its action, and when we are only dealing with the sequelæ of the lesions which it has provoked. In the former case, the electrical stimulation of the muscles would have no other result than to exaggerate the pains, and it might even increase the lesions ; whilst in the second case this mode of treatment is effective, and favours, at least, the restoration of the atrophied muscles."

CHAPTER VI

NEUROSES

I. ESSENTIAL EPILEPSY—SECONDARY EPILEPSY.

FORMERLY, only one kind of epilepsy was admitted—primary or idiopathic epilepsy. Secondary epilepsy, symptomatic epilepsy, and partial or Jacksonian epilepsy formed a group of epileptiform conditions. The more we study, the more extensive becomes this group of epileptiform conditions. The result is that true idiopathic epilepsy is less common than was formerly believed to be the case. Moreover, this true epilepsy might not absolutely be a case of neurosis. It might be associated with cerebral lesions which had previously been latent. But then, if it is no longer the disease *sine materia*, it enters into the group of secondary epilepsies, and there is no longer such a thing as idiopathic epilepsy. I shall refer to this question again under the pathogenesis of epilepsy, but I am of the opinion in any case that the time has not come to include everything in a single description, and in the present section I shall first describe essential or idiopathic epilepsy, and I shall then review the various forms of secondary epilepsy.

Description.—In true epilepsy two chief forms occur—the one convulsive, *grand mal ;* the other non-convulsive, *petit mal.*

1. *Grand Mal—the Attack of Epilepsy.*—The attack is sometimes preceded some hours or some days in advance by prodromata, such as psychical troubles, genital excitation, insomnia, palpitations, or heaviness in the head, and at the moment of the outburst it is frequently preceded by a sudden and rapid warning which is called the aura (*aura*, vapour). The *aura epileptica* assumes various forms ; sometimes it is a strange sensation of cold or hot vapour, or of sharp pain, starting in the hand, the foot, or some other part of the body, and ascending to the head ; sometimes there is flushing of these same parts, sudden functional trouble may occur, such as a fit of vomiting, palpitation, pain in the chest, constriction of the throat, an irresistible impulse to run or to turn round, hallucinations of sight and of hearing (flashes of lightning, whistling noises, and streaks of light), or some psychical perversion (fear of a mad dog or of a terrifying object). The aura, then, is sensory, motor, vasomotor, and psychic ; in all cases it is a phenomenon of central origin. The **aura** lasts a few seconds or a few minutes ; in some cases it constitutes in itself an outline of the epileptic attack.

Whether there is or is not an aura, the attack is as follows : The patient

1435

utters a cry, loses consciousness, and falls down, as if struck by lightning. The suddenness of the fall explains the bruises which are often seen on the face ; and the loss of consciousness accounts for the terrible burns in epileptic patients who, at the time of the attack, fall into the fire. At the commencement of the attack the face is deathly pale, all sensibility is abolished, the coma is complete, and the convulsive period commences. At first the convulsions are tonic, and all the muscles participate in the tetanic rigidity. The muscles of the eyes, of the face, of the neck, of the thorax, of the abdomen, and of the limbs are in a state of tetanus ; the eyeball is convulsed under the eyelid ; the face is drawn ; the teeth are firmly clenched ; the head is drawn backwards and to one side ; the limbs are contracted ; the hand is turned backwards ; the thumb is in the position of forced adduction, and flexed under the fingers, and momentary arrest of the respiratory movements occurs. The face, which was pale at the commencement of the attack, becomes congested. The arterial tension is raised, and the pulse-rate reaches 120 or 150.

The tonic stage lasts twenty or thirty seconds, and then the clonic stage commences. The convulsions at first recur every second ; they soon become much more rapid, and their amplitude gradually increases. The limbs are jerked about ; the face grimaces ; the eyeballs roll in their sockets ; bloody froth bathes the lips ; the respiration is noisy, jerky, and sometimes stertorous ; involuntary emission of urine and of fæces is common.

The convulsive stage lasts for a minute or two ; the patient utters a deep sigh, and the third stage of the attack then commences : this is an apoplectiform condition, which lasts for a variable period, and which is often followed by sleep. The attack being over, the patient, unconscious of what has happened, gradually comes round ; but for some time he suffers from confusion of ideas, profound lassitude, pains in the head, and transitory aphasia or hemiplegia.

Such is the *grand mal*, and it must be remembered that attacks of epilepsy, especially at first, take place during the night, and unknown to the patient, who falls out of bed, and is quite surprised to wake up on the floor. The physician must bear these nocturnal attacks in mind. " An individual will tell you that he awoke in the morning with a headache. He will tell you that, during the night, he passed his urine in the bed. He has a certain embarrassment in his speech, due to painful swelling of the tongue, which he has bitten. You notice on the skin of the forehead and of the neck ecchymotic patches (purpura). You may then state positively that the patient has had a nocturnal attack of epilepsy " (Trousseau).

In some cases the nocturnal attack comprises convulsive movements, preceded or accompanied by snoring and by vomiting, put down to indigestion.

The attacks of epilepsy have no fixed time for their appearance. Days, weeks, and months pass without an attack, or else the attacks recur frequently—in some cases, so frequently as to constitute the *status epilepticus*. This name is given to the incessant repetition of the fits, which may, indeed, become subintrant, a new fit appearing before the preceding one is finished. The status epilepticus is characterized by collapse and by coma, which are prolonged indefinitely; the respiration is embarrassed, the temperature may exceed 104° F., and remain high in the intervals of the attacks. The sphincters are paralyzed, and the situation becomes so grave that Delasiauve reported six cases where death supervened during the status epilepticus. The condition may last for several days.

In some epileptic patients their sleep is disturbed by dreams, which are the picture of the attacks. These *rêves d'accès* have an important semeiological value; they may constitute a precursory symptom of a subsequent attack (Féré).

2. *Petit Mal.*—Petit mal is non-convulsive epilepsy, characterized by attacks of vertigo, by mental aberration, and by delirium of various kinds. The individual, attacked by epileptic vertigo, suddenly experiences a kind of stupor; he loses consciousness, and falls down stunned, but gets up immediately, without any other manifestation. The patient attacked by mental aberration experiences, unknown to himself, a sudden suspension of thought. He stops in his reading or his conversation, grows pale, and makes some mumbling movements. His look is fixed and empty; two or three seconds afterwards he resumes his conversation, quite unconscious of what has happened. The seizures may occur several times during the same day. The attacks of vertigo and mental aberration are sometimes followed by fits of somnambulism (Voisin).

In other individuals the petit mal consists in a more or less violent delirium; one patient will utter incoherent words in a loud voice, another will indulge in fits of laughter, or in strange or obscene gesticulations. Some patients only experience the various sensations of the aura epileptica, not followed by convulsions. The petit mal is the most frequent form of epilepsy. It often changes to the grand mal, whilst the converse is very rare. In some cases the epilepsy assumes the so-called "procursive" form: the patient commences to run, sometimes in a straight direction, sometimes in circles, jumping over obstacles, and unconscious of his condition. This unconscious procursion may constitute the whole attack; in other cases the procursion is a sort of aura, and the epileptic attack appears subsequently. Finally, in other patients, the epileptic attack opens the scene, and the procursion is postepileptic.

The relation of epilepsy to **mental alienation** is most important from a medico-legal point of view. Intellectual troubles may manifest themselves either during the attack of epilepsy, as an epiphenomenon, or apart from the attacks, and in an independent manner. The patient is generally irritable and morose; he is often inclined to vicious habits, and sometimes subject to true delirium. The character of epileptic delirium is essentially **impulsive and instantaneous** (Falret). Its invasion is much more rapid than that of the other varieties of mania, and it ceases as suddenly as it appears. Under the influence of irresistible impulses the patient with epileptic delirium leaves his home and wanders about; he fancies himself persecuted, suffers from terrifying hallucinations, and in the most unexpected and sudden manner gives himself up to suicide, manslaughter, theft, or incendiarism, having hardly any recollection of what has happened when he comes round. These attacks of mania may last for some hours or for some days; they vary in severity, from passing dimness of the intelligence to the most acute mania. In such cases the **responsibility** of the individual is absolutely lost, and it is the duty of medical jurist to solve this often difficult problem. The petit mal, as well as the grand mal, may lead to epileptic mania.

Ætiology.—True idiopathic epilepsy is often hereditary, the parents suffering from epilepsy or from general paralysis, alienation, hysteria, or tabes. Epilepsy appears most frequently about the age of puberty; it rarely declares itself after twenty years of age. Fright, moral impressions, alcoholic excesses, and onanism are, according to certain authors, the usual determining causes. Congenital malformation of the skull has been given as a cause. Lasègue has upheld an analogous theory, by pointing out the relation between epilepsy and facial asymmetry. This facial asymmetry is said to result from a defect in the conformation, or from a vicious consolidation of the bones at the base of the skull.

The determining cause of the attack of epilepsy seems to be due to abnormal excitation of the bulb (Schröder, van der Kolk). This excitation, whether primary or reflex, and the cerebral radiations which accompany it in part explain the convulsions, the loss of consciousness, and the initial pallor of the face (spasmodic contraction of the vessels of the pia mater and of the face).

According to Chaslin, epilepsy is said to depend on more or less appreciable changes in the brain. His description of the lesions in the brains of several epileptic patients is as follows : " In the first three brains the lesions were visible to the naked eye. The meninges were not adherent, nor were they appreciably changed. The convolutions, which in certain places appeared completely normal, were in other places reduced in size, hard to the touch like cartilage—some being shagreened, others smooth. The cornua of Ammon and the bulb were also affected to a more or less marked extent." The microscopic examination showed sclerosis of the neuroglia, which he considers is the result of an hereditary process.

Diagnosis.—In a subsequent section I shall give the distinctions between epilepsy and hysteria. True epilepsy must not be mistaken for the epileptiform conditions which I shall describe in a moment. Given an attack of epilepsy, it is not sufficient to differentiate it from the other convulsive neuroses (hysteria) ; we must also ascertain whether we are dealing with a case of true epilepsy or with convulsions symptomatic of intoxication (plumbism, uræmia), of cerebral tumour (syphilis, cancer), of cerebro-bulbar sclerosis or with epilepsy of reflex origin (foreign bodies in the intestine, tænia, worms).

The diagnosis must also be made in the case of the petit mal, which must not be confounded with vertigo *ab aure læsa* or with laryngeal vertigo. Furthermore, we must not forget that epilepsy may assume a defaced form limited to the aura, and that many cases of so-called apoplectiform cerebral congestion, and of angina pectoris, are simply cases of disguised epilepsy (Trousseau).

The prognosis of epilepsy is extremely grave, because it often induces weakening of the faculties and different forms of mental alienation.

Treatment.—The treatment of the fits of epilepsy is almost nil. Certain patients, in whom the aura commences in the hand or the foot, can arrest the attack by compression of the parts above the seat of the aura. The most efficacious measure in epilepsy appears to me to be the association of bromide of potassium and belladonna, continued for a long time. The bromide of potassium must be taken in doses of 30 to 120 grains daily during the first and third weeks of each month, while the belladonna is administered in doses of $\frac{1}{2}$ to 1 grain daily during the second and fourth weeks. The bromide of potassium may be replaced by bromide of camphor or of sodium, and by Yvon's polybromide. The elimination of salt from the diet renders the patient more susceptible to the action of the bromide (Richet and Toulouse).

This treatment must be continued for years, with periods of intermission. The bromides may be administered in large doses as enemata. Physical and mental depression, dilatation of the pupils, and paresis of accommodation indicate that the bromide must not be pushed.

In a recent work De Fleury has shown that most epileptic patients suffer from physiological distress ; tonics should then be given with the bromide. Nerve stimulants are unsuitable (alcohol, coffee). On the other hand, they benefit from douches, massage, static electricity, and especially saline injections, which lessen the mental dullness, whilst increasing the absorption and the elimination of the bromide. In this manner most of the patients may be kept free from attacks, on the limits of bromide saturation, with much smaller doses than are usually given. The same writer has pointed out the importance of diet in the treatment of the haut mal. It suffices, in fact, to put a fair number of epileptics on an easily digested diet, and to give them water or milk to drink in order to render the attacks less frequent and less severe, the doses of bromide being unchanged. **Surgery** has a place in the treatment of epilepsy. Championnière has obtained encouraging results from trephining, not only in symptomatic (exostoses, tumours), but also in true epilepsy.

Secondary Epilepsy—Epileptiform Conditions.

We may place in one class cases of secondary epilepsy with more or less coarse lesions of the brain. In the first place, I would mention epilepsy associated with infantile cerebral hemiplegia, consequent on porencephalia, cerebral lacunæ, and lobar sclerosis. In such a case the course of events is : Some months after birth a child is taken ill with fever, convulsions, and hemiplegia. The storm then disappears, the hemiplegia gradually improves, and the intelligence remains practically normal, but a few years later, or at the onset of puberty, the attacks of epilepsy appear. Perhaps the epilepsy develops as the result of a secondary infection. Epilepsy, consequent on cerebral tumours (glioma, sarcoma, cysts, tuberculosis, syphilis), on general paralysis, or on descending sclerosis of the mesencephalon, belongs to the same category.

To a second class belongs secondary epilepsy of toxic origin (saturnine encephalopathy, uræmia). Under convulsive uræmia we saw that the epileptic attacks of Bright's disease very closely simulated true epilepsy.

To a third class belongs secondary epilepsy of reflex origin (foreign bodies in the intestine, worms, tænia). I have, with Krishaber, published the case of a young boy who had swallowed prune-stones. He was seized with epileptiform convulsions, and died. At the post-mortem examination we found the stones in the lower portion of the ileum.

The varieties of secondary epilepsy just enumerated differ somewhat from true epilepsy. The initial cry is often absent, the pallor of the face is less pronounced, the convulsions are not so markedly unilateral, and the comatose condition which follows the attack is less prolonged, but the clinical resemblance between secondary epilepsy and true epilepsy is absolute (Trousseau).

Acquired or hereditary syphilis claims the largest share in symptomatic epilepsy ; according to circumstances, it produces partial or true epilepsy. The crises which at first occur far apart appear closer together, and are often accompanied by paralyses. " If a healthy adult, over thirty years of age, is attacked for the first time with epilepsy, the chances are that the epilepsy is of syphilitic origin " (Fournier), and the reason is that essential epilepsy always shows itself in childhood or youth. There is, however, a form of syphilitic epilepsy which may show itself in childhood or in youth—viz., epilepsy consequent on hereditary syphilis. This question is discussed under Cerebral Syphilis.

II. PARTIAL EPILEPSY—JACKSONIAN EPILEPSY.

Partial epilepsy was named by Charcot **Jacksonian** epilepsy, because Jackson gave an excellent description of it. To give an idea of it, I shall quote a case from one of my clinical lectures :*

A man was send into my ward at the Hôtel-Dieu. On the evening of his admission, and during the next morning, he had two attacks, which I saw. At the moment of the attack the patient uttered a cry, without losing consciousness, the head and the eyes were turned to the right, the right arm became contracted, the fingers were flexed on the forearm, the forearm was flexed on the arm, and the arm was abducted over the chest. Immediately after this phase of contraction, which lasted but a few seconds, the upper limb showed jerky movements, as in the clonic convulsions of epilepsy. Two minutes later the convulsions became less severe, and were replaced by fibrillary contractions, followed by convulsive movements of the right side of the face and of the neck. The face had a grimacing look, the angle of the mouth twitched, the alæ nasi were raised, but the tongue was neither bitten nor pushed forward between the teeth, and we noticed no foaming at the mouth.

The whole attack lasted from three to four minutes, during which time the head and the eyes remained in a condition of conjugate deviation. The patient, who remained conscious, was an alarmed witness of the seizure, but was incapable of uttering a word. The attack was not followed by incontinence of urine, intellectual torpor, or stertorous breathing; in short, none of the symptoms which follow the major attack of epilepsy (but which may, nevertheless, exist after Jacksonian epilepsy) were present. In my patient this partial epilepsy invariably commenced in the right arm, and remained limited to the arm and to the right side of the face. There was, therefore, no possible doubt as to the diagnosis of Jacksonian epilepsy of the brachio-facial type.

The affected region was paretic, the face was slightly deviated to the left, the arm had lost some of its power, as was shown by the dynamometer, and the patient could only write with difficulty. This paresis was not simply a sequela of the epileptic attack, since it preceded the attacks. Speech was embarrassed, and a certain degree of paraphasia was present. Sensation was quite normal. The reflexes were slightly exaggerated on the right side.

The patient, about a fortnight prior to his admission into the hospital, had suffered from vertigo and heaviness in the head ; he was less able to carry out his duties as an accountant. His arm grew heavy, and writing became more difficult every day. In the meantime, a couple of days prior to his admission, the patient happened to be in a shop, when he felt a painful twitching in the index-finger of his right hand. This **aura** was followed by the first attack of brachio-facial epilepsy. During this attack, although he did not lose consciousness, there was slight mental confusion, because, after having witnessed the first period of the attack, he did not perceive that he had been taken from the shop to a neighbouring chemist.

What was the precise seat of the lesion, and what was its nature ? The precise seat of the lesion must be in the middle portion of the frontal and ascending parietal convolutions, without encroachment on the paracentral region. As to the nature of the lesion—the man was not syphilitic—I diagnosed a patch of chronic tubercular

---

* " Épilepsie Jacksonienne " (*Clinique Médicale de l'Hôtel-Dieu*, 1897, 9me leçon).

II. 92

meningitis. As a matter of fact, our patient had an abscess of the ribs, and a cold abscess in the neck, the pus of which was tubercular. It was, therefore, reasonable to admit three tubercular lesions in his case, two abscesses, and a patch of meningo-encephalitis.

Description.—Jacksonian or partial epilepsy is characterized by convulsive attacks, commencing in a definite group of muscles. The attack may be limited to the region attacked, or may extend to other regions. Following Bravais's example, we may describe three principal varieties of partial epilepsy : epilepsy commencing in the arm (brachial), in the face (facial), and in the leg (crural).

The brachial type is the most common. In this variety the various parts of the upper limb are flexed on one another by contraction of the flexor muscles, and the convulsive attack limited to the arm at once follows. In the facial or cervico-facial type the head and the eyes are deviated (conjugate deviation) ; the convulsions are limited to the face and to the neck, affecting the angle of the mouth, the orbicularis palpebrarum, the motor muscles of the eye and of the tongue, and the sterno-mastoid muscle. In the crural type the lower limb is extended ; the attack commences in the big toe, and extends to the entire limb.

In some cases Jacksonian epilepsy is partial, in the true sense of the word—that is to say, that it does not go beyond its original limits ; it remains confined to the arm, the face, or the leg, without extending to other regions. Most frequently, however, it commences, for example, in the arm, and extends to the face, thus realizing the mixed brachio-facial type. Or, again, after commencing in the arm and in the face it invades the leg, thus realizing the brachio-cervico-crural type ; it may commence in the face, and then invade the upper limb and the lower limb, thus realizing the mixed facio-brachio-crural type ; or, finally, it may commence in the lower limb, subsequently attacking the arm and the face, thus realizing the mixed cruro-brachio-facial type. Jacksonian epilepsy may not remain confined to one side of the body, but may cross to the opposite side.

The onset of the attack is not always identical ; the aura, the initial cry, and the loss of consciousness may be present or absent. My patient had an aura which commenced in his right index-finger in his first attack. In the two attacks which I saw he uttered the initial cry, but did not lose consciousness. The duration of the attack varies from a few moments to an hour ; on an average it lasts for a few minutes. The attack is sometimes followed by stertorous breathing, delirium, amnesia, vertigo, vomiting, and headache.

The regions which have been convulsed during the fit are generally paretic after the attack ; the condition may go as far as complete paralysis. These paralyses are of the same type as the convulsive attack, being facial, brachial, or crural ; they may be slight and transitory, or severe and permanent; they may follow or precede the convulsive symptoms. In my patient the paralysis had preceded the convulsions, since the arm and the face remained paretic.

It is to be noticed that the limbs which are contracted and convulsed during the attack are, apart from the attack, in a condition of flaccid hemiplegia. This proves that a muscle may be alternately paralyzed and convulsed by the same nervous lesion; it is paralyzed as long as it is deprived of normal stimulus, but it may nevertheless become convulsed or contracted when the stimulus is very much increased. This condition must be compared with that of the glottis in lesions of the recurrent nerve. I have given details under Aneurysm of the Aorta: A lesion of the left recurrent nerve causes paralysis of the left vocal cord, which does not prevent severe spasms of the glottis from supervening—that is to say, contracture of the two vocal cords.

The frequency with which the Jacksonian attacks may be repeated is most variable; they are sometimes separated by intervals of several weeks or months; at other times they recur at close intervals. In some cases, which are fortunately very rare, they become subintrant, cause a considerable rise in temperature, and the subject dies in a condition of status epilepticus.

Some years ago I had in my ward at the Necker Hospital a patient with Jacksonian epilepsy on the right side, of the brachio-facial type. The attacks increased in number and in severity. We counted as many as 380 attacks in the same day, and the patient succumbed in a condition of status epilepticus, with general epileptiform convulsions, the temperature reaching 104° F. At the autopsy, I found a glioma in the left ascending frontal and parietal region. Last year, at the Hôtel-Dieu, I had a patient suffering from Jacksonian epilepsy operated on by Marion. This patient had as many as 300 attacks daily.

Diagnosis of the Site of the Lesion.—It is not difficult to recognize partial epilepsy, but this is only the first step in the diagnosis. There are two other steps, the topographical diagnosis and the pathogenic nature of the original lesion. These facts are indispensable in treatment.

In general, attacks of Jacksonian epilepsy have their origin in a cortical lesion of the ascending frontal and parietal convolutions, separated by the fissure of Rolando.

This motor area may be divided into three chief motor centres: one for the face and the tongue, another for the arm, and a third for the leg. The motor centre of the face and of the tongue corresponds to the lower extremity of the convolutions, and more particularly to the ascending frontal convolution. The motor centre of the arm is placed higher in the ascending, frontal, and parietal convolutions. The motor centre of the leg corresponds to the upper portion of the ascending convolutions, which, on the internal surface of the hemisphere, form the paracentral lobule. The paracentral lobule is a narrow and circumscribed area of the internal surface of the cerebral hemispheres. It is bounded in front by the first frontal convolution, and behind by the quadrate lobe, below by the convolution of the corpus callosum, and above by the upper edge of the hemisphere.

As Charcot has pointed out, we must extend, at least above, the classic limits of the paracentral lobule, and join to it the terminal extremity of the

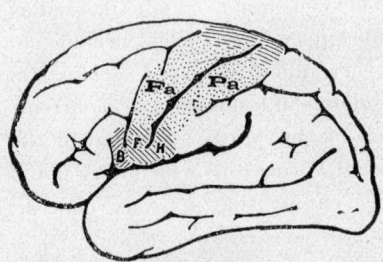

FIG. 82.—MOTOR AREA OF BRAIN.

Fa, Ascending frontal convolution; *Pa,* ascending parietal convolution; *F, H,* centres for face and tongue; *B,* centre for speech.

ascending, frontal, and parietal convolutions which form a part of the external surface of the hemispheres. In other words, the region of the paracentral lobule, or the crural centre, must comprise, on the one hand, the paracentral lobule, and, on the other hand, the upper extremity of the ascending frontal and parietal convolutions which bend over the upper edge of the hemisphere prior to entering the paracentral lobule, properly

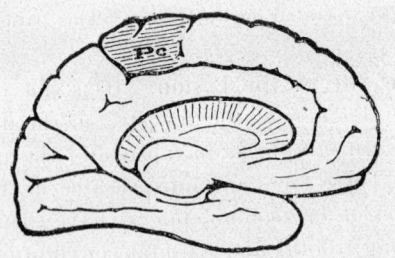

FIG. 83.—INNER ASPECT OF HEMISPHERE.

PcL, Paracentral lobule.

so called. " In this circumscribed crural region arise the anatomo-physiological changes which govern the execution of the usual movements of the lower limb " (Charcot).

The lesions, limited to each of these motor regions, may give rise to symptoms which are also limited to the face, to the arm, and to the leg. According to the degree of destruction, or of irritation of the affected region, the corresponding symptoms assume the form of paralysis, of contractures, or, finally, of attacks of Jacksonian epilepsy. It is, indeed, not rare to find these different forms appearing together or in succession.

In order to be thoroughly convinced of the value of these cerebral localizations, I shall quote cases in which the Jacksonian epilepsy and the cerebral localization are, so to say, superposed. Let us first deal with lesions of the paracentral lobule.

Potain: A carman, walking beside his cart, suddenly felt a sharp pain in his right foot. He gripped a neighbouring trelliswork to prevent himself from falling, and after his boot had been taken off by a friend, he noticed that the muscles of the calf were hard, as in cramp, that the foot was extended, and that the muscles of the leg were affected with painful jerks. This attack of Jacksonian epilepsy lasted for ten minutes. Four days later, at ten o'clock in the morning, a similar attack occurred, and the patient was admitted under Potain. The convulsive attack reappeared on his admission into hospital; it was strictly confined to the left leg. When the attack was over, it was noticed that the leg was paralyzed, the sensibility was diminished, and the reflexes were sluggish. After this time the Jacksonian epilepsy did not reappear, but erysipelas invaded the buttocks, and a bed-sore developed on the sacrum. Signs of tuberculosis were found in both lungs, and the patient soon died in coma.

At the post-mortem examination the lungs were found to be infiltrated with tubercles, but the interest was centred in the cerebral lesion. This lesion, except for some tubercular granulations over the convexity of the hemispheres, was clearly localized in the left paracentral lobule, which was capped by a patch of meningitis as hard as cartilage. This patch not only covered the paracentral lobule, properly speaking, but almost the whole paracentral region—that is to say, the upper portion of the parietal convolution.

This case is an example of a tubercular lesion of the paracentral region, followed by Jacksonian epilepsy of the lower limb.

Charcot: A patient suffering from pulmonary tuberculosis was admitted under Charcot. Three months previously she had felt numbness in the left leg, which made walking difficult. A fortnight later an attack of Jacksonian epilepsy suddenly supervened; it commenced in the left leg, and extended to the arm and to the face on the same side. A second attack occurred a week later, followed in four days' time by a third attack, and the left arm became paralyzed. Charcot diagnosed meningeal tuberculosis of the paracentral lobule. The patient died a fortnight later.

At the post-mortem examination pulmonary tuberculosis was found. The paracentral region only was attacked. On the paracentral lobule and on the upper part of the ascending frontal and parietal convolutions of the right hemisphere a patch of thick, yellowish meningitis was found, infiltrated with tubercular granulations and with pus. This patch, clearly limited to the paracentral region, was firmly adherent to the brain tissue, which also showed tubercular infiltration.

This case proves that tubercular meningitis may occur as a circumscribed patch. It shows, furthermore, the relation of crural Jacksonian epilepsy to lesions of the paracentral region.

Rendu: The patch of tubercular meningitis may be bilateral, affecting the paracentral region of both hemispheres. The symptoms then affect both lower limbs in the same manner as an attack of paraplegia, caused by a lesion of the spinal cord. Rendu has published a case of this kind. He had in his wards a patient with paraplegic symptoms simulating a disease of the spinal cord. The patient died, and " instead of the supposed spinal meningitis, we found circumscribed and symmetrical tubercular meningitis strictly confined to the area supplied by the anterior cerebral arteries. The progressive and simultaneous destruction of the paracentral lobule on both sides had caused the special symptomatology in this case."

Charcot: A physician requested Charcot to give him his opinion. While he was dining two evenings previously at a friend's house, he had been acutely troubled with headache, from which he had suffered for several days. He started to walk home, but he had only taken a few steps when his right leg became suddenly rigid, and was at the same time shaken by violent rhythmical convulsions. Almost immediately the arm of the same side was invaded in a similar manner, and the patient fell senseless. He was carried home, the loss of consciousness lasting for an hour. During the night and the next morning more epileptiform attacks occurred.

These attacks were not accompanied by loss of consciousness, and the patient was able to witness, not without alarm, the progressive and regular invasion of the convulsions, which always started in the left leg, and then spread to the arm and to the corresponding side of the face. He had had syphilis, and as his attack of Jacksonian epilepsy always commenced in the leg, Charcot diagnosed a syphilitic lesion of the right paracentral lobule, and consequently prescribed treatment with mercury and iodide. Speedy recovery followed.

Personal case: A man was brought into my ward on November 6, 1899. He had hardly got there when he had an attack of Jacksonian epilepsy. The head was turned to the left, the left leg and the arm were extended, and were almost immediately affected by slight convulsions; the right leg was also affected by convulsions. The crisis lasted for half a minute without the patient losing consciousness, and without the face participating. The man had always been well. For the past year he had only been troubled with slight headache, which had recently increased in severity. Partial epilepsy had suddenly made its appearance on the previous evening. The patient had had since that time about 300 crises in twenty-four hours. In spite of all, he remained quite conscious, but his anxiety was extreme. Although the arm seemed to be attacked at the same time as the leg, I placed the lesion at the top of the right paracentral lobule, thinking, too, that, convulsions being present in the right leg, the left paracentral lobule was also affected. It was impossible for me to state the nature of this lesion. As mercurial treatment gave no result, I asked Marion to operate, and the topographical diagnosis was absolutely verified. In the highest portion of the motor convolutions, near the upper extremity of the fissure of Rolando, in the right paracentral lobule, on the surface of the cortex, there was a hard tumour of the size of a cherry. Its removal was easy. The microscopic examination of this tumour had nothing characteristic. The absence of adhesions to the dura mater, the seat, the size, the mulberry-like appearance, and the delimitation found in my case are seen in the most varied cases. The histological examination did not reveal the exact nature of this tumour. It was markedly fibromatous.

We are now clear, I think, as to the relations between Jacksonian epilepsy of the crural type and the lesions of the paracentral lobule. When the attack commences in the leg, whether it remains there, or whether it extends, the cerebral lesion (tuberculoma, syphiloma, glioma, osteoma, fibroma, or parasitic tumour) is localized in the paracentral region.

Let us next study the localization of the motor convolutions in which a lesion causes brachial epilepsy. The following case gives a very clear idea of it:

Chantemesse: A woman, twenty-eight years of age, in good health, said that one day, on rising, she felt twitchings and jerks in the left arm. The jerks then invaded the leg on the same side, and the patient became unconscious. Next day a similar attack of Jacksonian epilepsy commenced in the left arm, and was followed by paralysis. On her admission, we noticed paralysis of the left arm, with contracture and flexion of the elbow. These symptoms were much less marked in the leg. The face and tongue were slightly deviated to the right. A few days later the patient died in coma.

At the post-mortem examination we found tubercular meningo-encephalitis over the right ascending frontal and parietal convolutions; the paracentral region was healthy. This localization was in close relation with the appearance of the symptoms, the epilepsy always commencing in the left arm.

Charcot has published the case of a man of fifty years of age suffering from Jacksonian epilepsy beginning in the right arm, and accompanied by paresis. The post-mortem examination showed a sarcoma in the left upper portion of the fissure of Rolando, invading the upper two-thirds of the ascending frontal convolution and the anterior half of the upper two-thirds of the ascending parietal convolution. The paracentral lobule was healthy.

These cases and many others which I might quote show the relations between Jacksonian epilepsy of the brachial type and lesions in the ascending frontal and parietal convolutions. When the epilepsy commences in the arm, the cerebral lesion (syphilis, tuberculosis, glioma, sarcoma, etc.) may be localized in this portion of the motor zone.

In conclusion, there are cases in which Jacksonian epilepsy commences in the face.

Milion has published a case of Jacksonian epilepsy commencing on the left side of the face. The post-mortem examination revealed a large subcortical tumour, seated on the right side at the junction of the foot of the ascending frontal with the foot of the ascending parietal convolutions, the cortical centre of the movements of the face.

All that I have just said with regard to the relations between the varieties of partial epilepsy and the localizations of the lesions in Rolando's region is applicable to the great majority of cases. **Unfortunately this topographical diagnosis has often been found at fault,** as will be seen in the section dealing with these errors.

Pathogenic Diagnosis.—Let us now study the diagnosis of the cause, which has provoked the Jacksonian epilepsy. We must always think of syphilis (bony, gummatous, or sclero-gummatous lesions), and this diagnosis must not be abandoned until it has been absolutely proved by rigorous treatment that the patient is not syphilitic. Patches of chronic tubercular meningitis often give rise to partial epilepsy. If we are not acquainted with this question, we are surprised to hear of such limited tubercular meningitis. Syphilis at first sight seems more likely to be so limited; periostosis, gumma, and sclero-gummatous meningitis are more limited than tubercular meningitis, which in its nature is more diffuse. This argument is true, but, after all, such arguments are of little value. We must remember that local tuberculosis of the brain may confine itself, as elsewhere, to a certain region (Ballet, Chantemesse).

Charcot dwells on these cases of localized meningitis: " When we consider tuberculosis of the brain in general, we notice that diffuse granular meningitis, with its seat of election at the base of the brain and in the fissure of Sylvius, is the most common form. Next comes patchy meningitis, which is usually localized in the psychomotor zone, and especially in the paracentral region. This patchy meningitis, which is clearly circumscribed, is much more frequent in adults than in children. Remember, too, that here everything seems made to lead the observer astray if he is not forewarned as to the diagnosis of this localized meningitis. In fact, it is the rule that in this form of meningitis headache, vomiting, delirium, and fever are wanting, and if, in some rare cases, the evolution is rapid and febrile, and ends in coma, there are other and more common cases in which the disease runs a chronic course lasting for months and even for years." And as a proof of this assertion, Charcot quotes the case of a patient in whom localized tubercular meningitis lasted for fourteen months, without provoking any other symptom, except attacks of Jacksonian epilepsy. Pulmonary tuberculosis caused death.

When the provoking lesion of the Jacksonian epilepsy is neither syphilitic nor tubercular, it is a question of one of the numerous tumours—sarcoma, glioma, fibroma, parasitic tumour, etc.—which are really difficult to diagnose.

Treatment.—In a case of Jacksonian epilepsy, we must always think of syphilis. Mercury and iodides (especially mercury) must be immediately given. If the cerebral lesion is tubercular in nature, surgery has little chance of successful intervention. In other cases (parasitic tumours, glioma, sarcoma, etc.) an operation is indicated; it must be performed without delay. The precision of the topographical diagnosis made by the physician will enable the surgeon to direct his attention with certainty to the proper cerebral region.

III. TRAUMATIC EPILEPSY.

Description.—Epilepsy may follow any head injury, such as blows, bruises, depressed fractures, and wounds caused by sabres or by firearms. Splinters, sequestra, exostoses, abscesses, subcranial adhesions, cortical lesions, and thickenings of the dura mater may induce cerebral irritation expressed as epilepsy.

An individual may become epileptic as the result of a lesion affecting the parietal, frontal, or occipital regions. The time at which the epilepsy appears is very variable; it may set in a short while after the injury, or it may not appear until months and years later. Nevertheless, the patient usually suffers from cerebral troubles, such as headache or vertigo, during the period between the injury and the appearance of the epilepsy. Traumatic epilepsy is often partial, but this is by no means the only form; injury may give rise to the grand mal, to the petit mal with vertigo and mental aberration, to intellectual troubles, mania, delirium, and irresistible impulses. Traumatic epilepsy, says Echeverria, may lead to madness; in his statistics we find eight men and four women with homicidal impulses; one man and one woman kleptomaniacs, and three women pyromaniacs.

Many cases of so-called essential epilepsy are doubtless due to a cranial injury which has escaped notice. It is therefore necessary in every case to make a minute examination for a cicatrix, caused by a recent or an old injury, which may have produced the epilepsy. Epilepsy may also recur or appear after trephining—a proof that the cause, either cicatrix or adhesions, still persists in spite of the operation.

Treatment.—Medical measures are at times insufficient in traumatic epilepsy. Surgical intervention must then be employed. In the following cases surgical measures were successful :

A child, six years of age, fell and cut himself over the left side of the occipital protuberance. Ten years later he suffered every morning from spasms and shocks in the arms. An attack of grand mal appeared thirteen years after the injury. The attacks recurred every three or four days, and then twice daily. The frequency of the attacks made the patient irritable and impulsive; he lost his memory. An exostosis, due to the former injury, was found on the occiput, and was held to be the cause of the attacks. The exostosis, which was pressing on the dura mater and the brain, was removed. Recovery followed.

A girl was struck on the head by a shutter, and fell down unconscious. A depression of the right parietal bone was found. The injury was followed by headache, vertigo, nocturnal epilepsy, rapid mental decay, and suppression of menstruation. The depressed fragment of bone was removed by trephining. The attacks of epilepsy ceased, and complete restoration of the mental faculties followed.

Operations on the cranial bones and the dura mater are not always successful, and epilepsy often persists in spite of more than one operation. Horsley has proposed the more radical operation of removing the cerebral centre producing the attacks. Removal of a portion of the motor cortex is especially indicated in Jacksonian epilepsy, and electrical excitation of the ascending parietal and frontal convolutions is employed in order to ascertain the part to be removed. The objection has been made that removal of a portion of the motor area would produce paralysis on the opposite side of the body. Experience has shown that the removal may be accomplished without inducing paralysis as a necessary result; substitution takes place, and the movements soon reappear; they may be marked by inco-ordination, known as cortical ataxy, but paralysis is not present. Although this operation has given some good results, its true worth cannot yet be stated. Operations upon the cranial bones and the dura mater alone, and also operations for removal of a portion of the brain, have been successful, and the reverse. A factor to be reckoned with is the presence and the extent of histological lesions in the cerebral focus. Thus, in a case of extirpation of the motor centre for the upper limb, histological examination of the fragment removed shows degeneration of the large pyramidal cells and condensation of the neuroglia.

IV. HYSTERIA.

Hysteria is a neurosis more frequent in women than in men, and appearing in two principal forms—the one convulsive, the other non-convulsive. In some women, in a third of the cases, according to Briquet, convulsive hysteria appears without having been announced by other symptoms; but often, especially at an early age, hysteria is most often announced a long time in advance—the little girl becomes impressionable and nervous; she is subject to attacks of suffocation, palpitation, headache; her character changes, her appetite becomes capricious, and she gradually goes on to confirmed hysteria.

The convulsive attack is often preceded by certain stigmata of hysteria, such as the clavus hystericus and the globus hystericus. Sometimes, on the contrary, hysteria, whether it is or is not convulsive, occurs in persons free from any nervous taint, and in men who were apparently quite unlikely to suffer from hysteria. Careful investigation, however, into the antecedents of these people generally reveals some precursory signs.

According to Babinski, " hysteria is a psychical condition, rendering the patient capable of auto-suggestion. It manifests itself principally by primary troubles, and to a minor degree by secondary symptoms. The characteristic feature of these primary troubles is the possibility of reproducing them by suggestion in certain subjects, and of causing their disappearance by the sole influence of persuasion. The secondary troubles are characterized by the fact that they are strictly subordinate to the primary troubles."

According to Babinski, suggestion is the act by which we seek to make others accept an idea that is obviously unreasonable, while persuasion is the act by which we seek to make others accept an idea that is eminently reasonable.

The hysterical symptoms are therefore said to be the result of suggestion or of auto-suggestion; they are phenomena which the will can reproduce. In the same way they will disappear under the exclusive influence of persuasion, and this character is practically essential to hysteria, since the other psychical troubles, insanity of doubt and neurasthenia, may be improved by persuasion, while they cannot be cured by it.

Convulsive Hysteria.—This form comes on in attacks. The hysterical attacks behave differently, according to the case, and two varieties may be described : the one is ordinary hysteria (*petite hystérie*) ; the other, which is more rare, is *grande hystérie* or *épileptiforme hystérie*.

1. *Ordinary Hysteria.*—The attack is almost always announced some hours or some days in advance by prodromata, such as palpitation, yawning, lassitude, malaise, unreasonable crying or laughter, constriction of the thorax and of the neck (globus hystericus). The attack commences in most cases with an aura. The aura may be complete or incomplete. The complete aura is characterized by a painful sensation, which starts from the ovary, reaches the pit of the stomach, ascends along the sternum, reaches the pharynx and the larynx (*strangulation*), and ends in cerebral phenomena (whistlings in the ears, dimness of the sight), which are more marked on the side where the aura commenced. The attack then commences, and the patient falls down ; but, unlike the epileptic patient, she has time to select the place where she is going to fall, and she does not lose consciousness—at least, at the commencement of the attack. She utters cries, and feels as though she were being suffocated. Her face is congested, and the cervical veins are distended. She puts her hand on her throat as if to tear away something which is impeding respiration, and the convulsions are accompanied by sighs and hiccough.

The convulsive movements are essentially clonic. They are very extensive and disordered ; contortions sometimes agitate the limbs, and move the body as a whole ; sometimes the convulsive movements are more rhythmical, and affect chiefly the muscles of the pelvis (libidinous hysteria). The trunk shows a kind of rocking movement. Sometimes the head is jerked violently, and hits neighbouring objects. The face is not grimacing as in epilepsy, the abdomen is distended with gas, and the loss of consciousness is generally absolute. After a duration of some minutes to several hours, according to the number of fits, the movements calm down, the physiognomy betrays the various expressions of fear, anger, or voluptuousness, and the attack ends in copious tears, and in the emission of colourless urine.

The attacks of hysteria are not always so acute and so complete. In some cases the patients hear what is said, and understand what is going on round about them. In hysteria, as in epilepsy, the attacks may follow one after the other for several days ; the evacuations which mark the termination of the attack are absent, and the patient feels that the attack will recur. The attacks of hysteria do not take place at night. It is often possible to provoke or arrest at will an attack of hysteria ; it is sufficient to press firmly on the ovaries, the left ovary principally, or else over a hysterogenous zone. The attack of hysteria is not always complete ; it is sometimes preceded by a tonic stage, with spasms of the œsophagus, of the glottis, or of the masseters, and this stage may *per se* constitute the whole attack.

2. *Epileptiform Hysteria.*—Ordinary hysteria, as above described, may be considered as a mild kind of epileptiform hysteria. The latter, which is

very uncommon, differs from the slight attack, in that it commences with an epileptiform phase. The crisis, preceded by an aura and by the prodromata already described, consists of four periods, which occur in the following order :

(*a*) The first, or epileptoid, period simulates an attack of epilepsy, with tonic and clonic convulsions and resolution.

(*b*) After this epileptoid period, which lasts three or four minutes, the other periods are pure hysteria. There is at first a phase of contortions or clownism (Charcot). The patient rests on her head and on her feet in the form of a bridge, or performs a rhythmical rocking motion with the upper part of her body, a sort of salutation, etc.

(*c*) Then the phase of passionate attitudes supervenes ; they manifest themselves under the influence of sad or gay hallucinations (fear, love, voluptuousness).

(*d*) The terminal period comprises hallucinations with terrifying visions (rats, snakes, black animals).

The succession of these attacks constitutes a *status hystericus*, which may last for several weeks, with a hundred attacks a day ; there is no rise of temperature, such as occurs in the status epilepticus, and compression of the ovary may arrest a severe, as well as a mild, attack of hysteria.

Epileptiform hysteria assumes other less common forms ; these are the syncopal form (Briquet), syncope constituting the entire attack, the cataleptic form (Lasègue), and the lethargic form, coma and lethargy supervening at the termination of the attack.

Non-convulsive Hysteria.—The manifestations of this form are many : paralyses, trophic troubles, muscular atrophy, contractures, tremors, anæsthesia, neuralgia, congestion with or without hæmorrhage, respiratory, digestive, and urinary troubles, disorders of the genital organs and of the organs of the senses, and intellectual troubles. All these are met with in hysteria.

Paralysis.—The involuntary and the voluntary muscles were involved 139 times in 430 patients (Briquet). Hemiplegia and paraplegia are the most frequent forms. Sometimes only one limb is attacked (monoplegia), especially the upper limb. The paralyses either follow an attack or supervene apart from any convulsive manifestation ; slight injury, emotion, and fright are often the determining cause. According to circumstances, their appearance is sudden or gradual; they are mobile, appearing and disappearing with equal facility ; they may persist indefinitely, or may recover suddenly. Paralyses, accompanied by anæsthesia, the anæsthesia taking the form of outlines perpendicular to the longitudinal axis of the limb, with normal electrical contractility, and exaggerated, normal, or diminished reflexes, are the characteristics of hysterical paralysis.

Amongst other distinctive characteristics hysterical hemiplegia differs from hemiplegia, caused by cerebral lesions, in that it rarely attacks the face. This distinctive sign is of great importance, although it is not absolute, because in some cases of hysterical hemiplegia the face was slightly deviated. "But," says Charcot, " a mistake has been made, facial hemiplegia having been mistaken for hemispasm." In hysterical hemiplegia the inferior facial nerve is never affected, as it is in ordinary hemiplegia. The deviations of the face associated with hysterical hemiplegia are the consequence of hemi-lateral glossolabial spasm on the opposite side to the hemiplegia, or on the same side. In this glossolabial spasm the angle of the lips and the tongue are drawn over to the convulsed side ; the cheek is sometimes affected by convulsive jerks." Charcot, later, withdrew this statement, and hysterical facial hemiplegia is now proved. It seems only to supervene in the grave forms of hysteria.

Contractures.—Nearly all the voluntary and involuntary muscles may be attacked. We find monoplegic, hemiplegic, and paraplegic forms ; they may involve the four limbs, the lumbar muscles, the muscles of the neck, of the jaws, of the tongue, of the eyeballs, etc. ; at other times they are limited to a muscle or a group of muscles. The contractures are permanent. They are generally very painful, and last for months and years, appearing gradually or suddenly, and disappear in some cases with equal suddenness. They may follow the paralyses, or may set in apart from any paralytic condition. They do not relax during sleep, although they yield for the time being to chloroform. Intermission of the contractures is exceptional ; it was well marked in one of Rénon's cases, with total facial hemispasm : the crises occurred seventy or eighty times during the day.

These features distinguish hysterical contractures from those due to sclerosis of the lateral columns of the spinal cord. The latter establish themselves slowly and progressively, and are not modified by chloroform. It appears nevertheless that the hysterical contracture may, in the long run and in very exceptional cases, be associated with a lesion of the lateral columns of the spinal cord (Charcot). This condition must be very exceptional, for in a remarkable case seen by Vulpian no spinal lesions were found in a hysterical patient, who for five years had suffered from general contractures, with trophic troubles, muscular atrophy, and fibrillary contractions of the muscles (Klumpke).

The arm is in the position of forced flexion, the leg is in extension with talipes equino-varus. Every attempt to overcome the contracture is accompanied by severe pains. If, during contracture of the lower limb, the point of the foot is forcibly straightened, an epileptoid tremor is provoked in the limb ; the tremor lasts for some time, and may be arrested by sudden flexion of the foot. The application of a magnet sometimes causes the transfer of the contracture to the opposite side. I shall next enumerate certain hysterical contractures : contracture of the extremities (tetanus); periarticular contractures of the knee and of the shoulder, which are often very painful (Brodie) ; contractures of the muscles of the hip, which simulate coxalgia ; contracture of the muscles of the neck (torticollis) ; of the masticator muscles (trismus) ; of the motor muscles of the eye (strabismus) ; of the muscles of the tongue, without counting contracture of the sphincters (retention of urine), spasms of the œsophagus, which may last for weeks and months (spasmodic stricture) ; spasms of the glottis, with consequent dyspnœa, etc., which will be studied under each of these organs.

The hysterical contractures sometimes supervene spontaneously ; at other times they are occasioned by insignificant causes, by a slight injury (fall, contusion, sprain, prick with a needle), and it is remarkable that the contracture caused by traumatism is often the first manifestation of hitherto latent hysteria.

Tremors. — Hysterical tremors generally supervene suddenly in consequence of emotion, fright, or of a complete or incomplete attack of hysteria. According to circumstances, the tremor is partial or general ; it assumes the hemiplegic, paraplegic, or monoplegic form. The tremor may improve and disappear after a few hours or a few days, but it may be continuous, interrupted only during sleep, and lasting for months. The excitation of a hysterogenous zone may sometimes cause the tremor to reappear. The intensity varies from the least tremor to such violent agitation as to interfere with walking and with the grasping of objects. The rhythm of the tremor is regular. Dutil has divided them into three groups : (1) Tremors with rapid or vibratory oscillations, numbering eight to twelve per second, and resembling the tremor of Basedow's disease, of general paralysis, and of alcoholic poisoning ; (2) tremors of five to seven oscillations per second, resembling the tremor of mercurialism and of spasmodic paraplegia, and more rarely, when they are intentional, imitating the tremor of insular sclerosis ; (3) slow tremors of four to five oscillations per second, resembling the senile tremor and paralysis agitans.

Hemianæsthesia.—The anæsthesia of hysterical patients may be general and disseminated ; it is more often local in the form of hemianæsthesia. It is especially frequent on the left side, and has been noted 93 times in 400 cases by Briquet. The insensibility affects the whole of one side of the body as far as the median line, and invades the superficial and deep planes, the skin, the mucosæ, the muscles (loss of muscular sensation), and the joints. It is a strange fact that many hysterical patients are not aware of this anæsthesia. Total hemianæsthesia not only affects tactile sensibility, but also the sensations of pain and of temperature, and the special senses (taste, smell, hearing, sight). Pharyngeal anæsthesia is very common. The anæsthetic skin is pale, cold, and bloodless, and may be pricked without the loss of a drop of blood. The muscles of the paralyzed side are much weaker (amyosthenia) than those of the healthy side. This hemianæsthesia is quite analogous with that described in diseases of the brain, caused by a lesion of the posterior part of the internal capsule.

Burcq's researches on hysterical hemianæsthesia have brought to light some very interesting facts (metalloscopy and metallotherapy). If discs of gold, tin, or copper are applied to the anæsthetic skin, the anesthesia disappears after an application, ranging in duration from a few seconds to fifteen minutes. As the sensation reappears in the anæsthetic regions, the skin regains its colour, the circulation is re-established, and the amyosthenia disappears : a patient who only registered 30 pounds on the dynamometer actually registers double. Whilst these changes are taking place on the anæsthetic side, the other side, which was healthy, becomes anæsthetic in the symmetrical regions : a phenomenon of transference takes place.

The results obtained with discs of copper in one patient are not obtained in another one, except by the application of discs of gold or of tin. One patient is " sensitive to gold, another to copper." These metals develop a current, and only act when impurities are present. A similar result is obtained by the application of a galvanic current or of a magnet.

These various means are not limited to the hemianæsthesia of hysterical patients ; they act also on the hemianæsthesia which accompanies intoxications (alcoholism and plumbism) and cerebral lesions. It must also be noted that the improvement which is generally transient in hysterical hemianæsthesia may be permanent in the other varieties.

Hyperæsthesia—Neuralgia.—Hysterical patients are subject to various pains affecting the skin, the muscles, the joints, and the viscera. The **clavus hystericus** is a lancinating pain, situated at the sagittal suture. The headache of hysterical patients is said to be a muscular hyperæsthesia (Briquet), a neuralgia, or a migraine. It is sometimes characterized by a painful spot on the temple ; but whatever the variety of this headache, its appearance, as an obstinate symptom in young girls near the age of puberty, is a frequent index of hysteria. The backache is due to hyperæsthesia of the muscles of the back and of the spine ; it may extend to the whole mass of the sacro-lumbar muscles and to the longissimus dorsi, or it may be limited to one of the regions of the back ; the pain is readily provoked by pressure on the spinous processes, or on the muscles.

In hysterical patients we find **hysterogenous zones**—that is to say, regions endowed with a special and permanent sensibility. Prior to the attack, these points are the seat of increased pain, which forms a part of the aura. The aura may also be provoked by pressure, or by rubbing of the hysterogenous patches, and, if we keep on, the attack of hysteria may be as certainly provoked as by exerting pressure on the ovary. Conversely, the hysterical attack may be arrested by firm pressure on the hysterogenous zones. These zones are very numerous ; they are found at the bregma, the xiphoid cartilage, under the breasts, at the angle of the scapula, in the lumbar region, in the ovarian region, in the testicle, in the arms, in the legs, etc.

Ideogenous zones have also been described ; as a rule, they are only active in the **hypnotic** condition. The excitation of the zone of ecstasy, situated on both sides of the vertex, places the patient in an attitude of ecstasy. The excitation of the zones of chattering, situated over the mastoid processes, causes the patient to talk volubly. The excitation of the zone of laughter over the external occipital protuberance causes convulsive and noisy laughter, which it is impossible to interrupt.

Hysterical women are subject to attacks of intercostal neuralgia, and to visceral pains, gastralgia, hepatalgia, ovaria, hysteralgia. They have painful crises comparable with angina pectoris, abdominal pains due to hyperæsthesia of the ovary, and neuralgia of the abdominal wall. These symptoms, joined to exaggerated meteorism of the belly, are called false peritonitis. Care must be taken not to confound this condition with appendicitis.

Aphonia—Mutism—Aphasia.—I have grouped hysterical aphonia, mutism, and aphasia in the same paragraph, in order the better to oppose these various troubles, and to show their differences. This description is taken from Charcot's lectures. **Hysterical aphonia,** like all other forms of aphonia, is characterized by loss of voice ; the larynx can no longer emit the sounds necessary for the voice. The patient can still speak in a whisper, which is produced by the tongue and the lips, and has nothing to do with the larynx. The aphonia is due to the paralysis of the vocal muscles ; the sound is absolutely lost, but this, however, does not prevent the cough from being noisy. Hysterical aphonia supervenes suddenly as the result of some moral cause, or after a convulsive attack ; it lasts for several days or weeks, and disappears as it came, sometimes as the result of a moral emotion. Patients suffering from hysterical aphonia often have a cutaneous patch of anæsthesia in the supra- and subhyoid regions. Hysterical aphonia may be cured by almost any measure (electricity, magnetization, or metallotherapy), or it may resist all means.

Hysterical mutism commences suddenly in consequence of a fright, an emotion, or a convulsive attack, or even without apparent cause. It may last for weeks, for months, or for years. It is always cured, and suddenly, but it is subject to recurrences. Like all the manifestations of hysteria, it is more frequent in women, but it is also met with in men. The hysterical mute is aphonic and mute at the same time ; aphonic, that is to say, her larynx can produce no sound ; mute, that is to say, she is absolutely deprived of speech, being unable to articulate a single word even in a low voice ; she cannot whisper, and yet she has not lost any of the movements of the tongue and of the lips ; she can whistle and blow, but she can neither co-ordinate nor imitate the movements necessary for the articulation of words. In this respect hysterical mutism resembles organic motor aphasia, but it differs from organic aphasia in many respects, and without speaking of other troubles, such as agraphia, word-deafness, and word-blindness, which enter more or less into the domain of aphasia, a patient with complete organic aphasia can utter cries or even a few words.

The hysterical mute retains his intelligence, writes with facility, and contrives to make himself understood by gestures—two things which are rare in a person suffering from organic aphasia. Accordingly, the preservation of writing, of mimicry, and of intelligence in a man or woman who has suddenly become mute shows the hysterical nature of the mutism. This diagnosis is almost always confirmed by other stigmata of hysteria, hemianæsthesia, pharyngeal anæsthesia, sensory troubles, ocular troubles, hysterogenous zones, facility of provoking contracture in a limb by the application of a circular ligature. On the other hand, the union or the absence of these various signs allows us to recognize cases of simulation. Mutism may be readily provoked in hypnotizable hysterical patients ; this artificial syndrome, produced during the period of somnambulism, persists when the subject is awakened. " We must look in the grey cortex of the cerebral hemispheres for the dynamic lesion from which the symptoms in question are derived, and the mechanism which must be here invoked is none other than that which accounts, in my opinion, for the production of so-called cases of psychic or mental paralysis " (Charcot).

Typical aphasia has sometimes been observed in hysterical patients ; it is generally associated with hysterical apoplexy.

Hysterical Apoplexy.—Hysterical apoplexy has all the clinical characters of apoplexy of organic origin (Debove) ; apoplexy with or without aphasia, with hemiplegia, and almost always with hemianæsthesia. Hemianæsthesia is a prominent symptom, whilst the hemiplegia is not so marked. The sequelæ of the attack—hemianæsthesia, hemiplegia, hemichorea, and contracture—are readily curable by esthesiogenic measures.

Psychic Troubles.—The hysterical woman always exaggerates, and loves to make an exhibition of herself in order to excite interest ; she indulges in every kind of simulation, and is capable of the most repugnant acts. Hysterical women are often malicious and untruthful ; some of them lie with unheard-of effrontery ; they sow disagreement and discord everywhere ; they are at a loss what to invent in order that they may be talked about. They threaten suicide, and worry their family by announcing that they intend to make away with themselves. They accuse themselves of acts which they have never committed, and bear false witness against others of theft and murder. They profess to be the victims of assaults and of rape, and they cause innocent people to be arraigned before a court of justice, when they do not succeed in having them burnt at the stake, as was that unfortunate man, Urbain Grandier, whom the Ursuline sisters of Loudun accused of imaginary crimes. Most hysterical women have hallucinations during the convulsive attack; in some women these hallucinations persist outside the attack; thus, a woman who is quietly reading or working rises suddenly, and utters cries, fancying that she sees fantastic animals on the wall or on the floor. Erotic and religious delirium is common to them, and sometimes leads to dementia.

Hysteria renders patients particularly liable to neurasthenia, and makes them good subjects for hypnotism.

A rabid form of hysteria has been described by Grasset.

An important medico-legal question is associated with the mental condition of hysterical patients, and hysteria has been more than once a prominent feature in certain *causes célèbres*. With regard to this subject, Grasset's interesting case, published under the title "Roman d'une hystérique," should be read.

Trophic Troubles. — Numerous trophic troubles are associated with hysteria. The cutaneous troubles include zona, falling out of the hair, shedding of the nails, spontaneous ecchymoses, and sweating of blood. To the troubles of the cellular tissue belongs œdema, which is sometimes cyanotic. In hysterical œdema we find a hard swelling of the skin, which does not pit on pressure. The skin is cyanosed, whence the name of blue œdema. This œdema may be limited to a hand or to a limb; it is almost always associated with contracture, or with paralysis of the invaded limb.

In some patients we find painful swelling of the breasts, with secretion of milk. Chipault has seen a case of hæmorrhage from the breast, and he has succeeded in collecting several similar cases. I must add that the foregoing trophic troubles are no longer admitted as being functional of hysteria.

The muscular atrophies belong to the trophic disorders of hysteria. The atrophy is usually present in the regions attacked by paralysis, contracture, and anæsthesia; it is very rarely independent. The atrophy attacks the hand, the arm, or the leg. In some cases it has an ascending course, commencing in the hand and spreading to the arm. Hysterical muscular atrophy differs considerably from myelopathic amyotrophy. It does not attain the degree of wasting seen in progressive muscular atrophy, and is not, as a rule, accompanied by fibrillary tremors. The electrical contractility is diminished in proportion to the atrophy, and there is in most cases no reaction of degeneration. These distinctive signs are, however, not absolute, because in some cases fibrillary contractures and slight reaction of degeneration have been noted. The onset is rapid, and as soon as an improvement supervenes recovery speedily follows. The pathogenesis of this atrophy is obscure; it may perhaps be due to a dynamic change in the nerve centres, and it is said to be comparable with the amyotrophy which follows joint injuries (Vulpian).

Viscera.—The respiratory system shows various disorders. Spasms of the glottis provoke attacks of dyspnœa. Paralysis of the posterior crico-arytenoid muscles is accompanied by dyspnœa, with inspiratory stridor. Convulsions of the laryngeal muscles and spasms of the diaphragm provoke barking and grumbling noises, which may occur in attacks, or may follow one another incessantly. The spasmodic movements of the diaphragm cause uncontrollable fits of yawning, hiccough, and laughter. Some hysterical women suffer from broncho-pulmonary congestion, with hæmop-tysis; others, especially young girls, have an incessant, dry cough, which tires the family more than the patient. This cough diminishes or disappears at night; it is very obstinate, lasting for weeks and months.

Digestive Troubles.—Gastralgia, dyspepsia, and perverted appetite are of common occurrence; hysterical patients frequently vomit water or food; they may have attacks of hæmatemeses. The vomiting of food is painless; it may last for several months without injuring health, and without causing marked loss of flesh. Constipation is the rule; intestinal pneuma-tosis is frequent, and abdominal meteorism consequently results. This abdominal swelling and the abdominal pains constitute the false peritonitis of hysteria.

Some patients lose their appetite completely. A young girl with anorexia delights in fasting, and the phenomena of disassimilation are so slow that she can fast for a long time, and apparently without losing flesh. Grave complications may, however, result.

I saw with Lafont of Bayonne a young girl who, by deceiving her family, had managed to reach a stage in which she was literally dying of hunger. She looked like a skeleton. The extremities were cold and blue. The voice was reduced to a whisper, and her breath was cold. We set to work with gavage. When she saw that she was van-quished, she commenced to eat, and her health returned.

Tuberculosis may attack hysterical patients with anorexia. The alimentary canal is frequently the seat of spasms—spasms of the pharynx, of the œsophagus (spasmodic stricture), of the stomach (cramps), of the intestine, which may lead to fæcal vomiting.

Eructations and borborygmi are very frequent in hysterical patients. The sounds may be irregular or regular, and coincident with the respiratory movements. The noises provoked by these eructations and borborygmi are audible at a distance; they may come on in fits, and alternate with fits of hiccough. Pitres attributes the rhythmic borborygmus in hysterical patients to a spasmodic contraction of the respiratory muscles.

Urinary System.—The urinary troubles may be excretory or secretory. The former (retention of urine) are due to a contraction of the sphincter of the bladder, or to paralysis of the viscus. The latter, oliguria or anuria, are more difficult to explain. Hysterical patients may go for several weeks without passing water, not from retention, but because the kidneys do not act. And in spite of this suppression we find no uræmic symptoms, doubtless because the processes of metabolism are almost at a standstill.

Hysterical polyuria has long been recognized. At the present time nearly every case of simple or nervous polyuria is said to be hysterical; the polyuria would then be the only symptom of the hysteria. To make a diagnosis Babinski advises hypnotic suggestion; by this means the polyuria can be made to appear and to disappear at will. Hysterical polyuria is only seen in men; it is exceedingly rare in women. It usually begins with excessive thirst.

On cryoscopic examination the freezing-point of the urine may be lower than that of the blood (0·56° C.). Souques and Balthazard have seen it fall to 0·40°, 0·30°, and even to 0·17° C.

Organs of the Senses.—I have already spoken of cutaneous anæsthesia, and of hemianæsthesia affecting the senses of hearing, of smell, and of sight. The organs of the senses may be attacked separately by hyperæsthesia, anæsthesia, paralysis, or contracture. Hardness of hearing is frequent, but deafness is rare. I have seen a young girl with such marked hyperæsthesia of the lingual mucosa that everything tasted like vinegar. A woman who was in Vulpian's ward had contracture of the tongue for several months. A case has been reported of a hysterical patient who showed such marked vasomotor disturbance in the skin that characters drawn on the surface of the body remained in relief for several hours, and Mesnet in 1890 made an interesting communication to the Académie de Médecine on hysterical autographism.

The ocular troubles of hysteria are so characteristic that it is customary to unite them under the term " hysterical eye." The amblyopia is characterized by anæsthesia of the retina, and by contracture of the ciliary muscle (Parinaud).

Anæsthesia of the retina is revealed by two symptoms : constriction of the field of vision and dyschromatopy. The contracture shows itself by monocular polyopia, micropsia, and megalopia. The constriction of the field of vision commences at the circumference, and becomes regularly concentric ; it may reduce the sight to central vision alone. The constriction of the field of vision is often complicated by disturbance of colour vision. The perception of colours disappears in the following order : violet, green, blue, yellow, and finally red. As in the normal condition, it is the blue field which is the most extended (white being excluded), so, on the other hand, in hysteria the perception of red is the last one affected. The following paradox results—viz., the red field becomes, from the outset, more extended than the blue (Parinaud). This phenomenon has received the name of change in the relative extent of the fields of the different colours. If a magnet or a plate of gold, copper, or tin be applied to the temple of the patient, the colours reappear in the inverse order of their disappearance, according to the metallic idiosyncrasy of the hysterical patient.

These symptoms are most important ; they belong especially to hysteria, and they allow us to distinguish hysterical amblyopia from tabetic and alcoholic amblyopia. In alcoholic amblyopia the red and the green disappear first, whilst a central scotoma develops. In tabetic amblyopia the red also disappears first ; the constriction of the field of vision is peripheral, but it is notched and not regularly concentric. Finally, the ophthalmoscope reveals atrophy of the optic nerve, whereas the fundus is always normal in hysteria.

Monocular diplopia and polyopia are very curious symptoms. If an object is held vertically in front of the hysterical eye (the other eye being closed), the object is distinct only at a certain distance. Within this distance, or beyond it, the object becomes blurred, and at the same time it appears double or triple, although seen with only one eye. This variety of diplopia is due to defective accommodation, which varies in hysterical patients in the three segments of the crystalline lens, and therefore reproduces a separate image for each of the three segments (Parinaud). Defective accommodation also produces micropsy and megalopsy—symptoms which often accompany monocular diplopia. This monocular diplopia, in which two images are perceived by one eye (the other eye being closed) must be distinguished from the diplopia due to paralysis of the motor muscles of the eye, in which case each of the two images is perceived by the eye of the corresponding side, or by the eye of the opposite side (homonymous, or crossed diplopia).

Hysterical amblyopia may be limited to one eye ; it is, however, almost always double, and more marked on the side of the hemianæsthesia. Amaurosis may follow amblyopia, or may appear suddenly.

I have already said that the fundus always remains normal in hysteria. Let me add, while the pupil reflex is absent in tabes and in the other cases of amblyopia due to an organic lesion, it remains present in hysterical amaurosis, because the impression, although it is not perceived by the subject, nevertheless reaches the brain.

We may also find motor troubles of the eye ; they are, however, of minor importance. Spasm of the eyelids (blepharospasm) betrays itself by a drooping of the eyelid, which simulates ptosis (pseudo-paralytic ptosis), or by clonic movements, with continual winking of the half-closed lids. This symptom is associated with a zone of anæsthesia or of hyperæsthesia, which affects the eyelid and the conjunctiva, but respects the cornea. On the side of the blepharospasm the eyebrow is lowered. We must also notice contractures of the recti muscles, especially of the internal rectus, causing strabismus and diplopia which at first sight simulate paralysis. Paralysis of the motor muscles of the eye has yet to be proved.

Blindness.—I have given two clinical lectures * on hysterical blindness; I shall give a résumé of them.

I have collected over sixty cases of hysterical blindness. In five instances it was the only symptom of hysteria present, the patients being apparently free from any stigmata of hysteria. The blindness is usually associated with other manifestations of hysteria. It sometimes follows an attack of hysteria. Hemianæsthesia, anæsthesia of the cornea and of the pharynx, hemiplegia, loss of the senses of taste and smell, deafness, mutism, œsophagism, contractures, etc., are often satellites of the blindness. One patient is blind and hemiplegic; a second is blind and deaf; and a third is blind, mute, deaf, and paralyzed.

One of the features of hysterical blindness is its sudden onset without warning. In one of my patients the loss of sight came on in less than a quarter of an hour; another patient became suddenly blind. Abadie's patient went to bed, and woke up next day quite blind; a young man, of whom Marlow speaks, became suddenly blind as he was entering his house. A rapid or sudden onset is therefore characteristic of hysterical blindness. In some patients the amaurosis may not become complete for several hours, and in exceptional instances it affects one eye before the other.

Hysterical blindness is absolute. Cases in which the patient retains some perception of light are very rare; the patient is in total darkness, no matter how bright a light is placed in front of the eyes.

A special feature of hysterical blindness is the preservation of the light reflex both to natural and artificial light, even though the patient has no perception of light.

A fundamental characteristic of hysterical blindness is the integrity of the media and of the retina. The information yielded by the ophthalmoscope is of capital importance.

I have said that prodromata are usually absent in hysterical blindness. Headache is, however, an important precursory symptom. One of my patients had severe headache before he became blind, and as he had had syphilis it was not unnatural to consider the headache as syphilitic. In a

* Dieulafoy, "La Cécité Hystérique" (*Clinique Médicale de l'Hôtel-Dieu,* 1907, 5me et 6me leçons).

woman under my care the blindness was accompanied by intense headache, lasting ten months.

Headache has been noticed repeatedly in cases of hysterical blindness. It has no fixed seat; we must be careful not to put it down to a cerebral tumour or to meningitis, when it accompanies hysterical blindness.

Contracture of the oculo-motor muscles frequently accompanies hysterical blindness. Many patients keep their eyes tightly closed, like persons who suffer from keratitis and keep their eyes shut because they dread the light.

My patient in the Sainte-Jeanne Ward was a typical case. Not only did she keep her eyes closed, but the eyelids were contracted from spasm of the orbicularis. When she was told to open her eyes, she tried to overcome the contracture of the orbicularis, and the eyelids were raised to a slight extent. The eyes did not open completely. During this effort a well-marked frown was noticeable. At the same time the eyeballs were deviated to the right side by the jerky contraction of the right external rectus and the left internal rectus. This deviation was accompanied by a jerky contracture of the muscles of the neck, which drew the head to the right. Her position and her appearance were so characteristic that I at once diagnosed hysterical blindness.

The blindness has a duration varying from some days to several months. Relapses are common, and we may see several attacks of blindness at variable intervals.

The poor sufferers ask anxiously as to the probable duration of the blindness; an answer is impossible, because we have no means of telling whether recovery will be prompt or tardy. It appears to be a question of chance. The blindness sometimes disappears suddenly without apparent cause; at other times it ceases after an attack of hysteria. In some patients the sight gradually returns.

The prognosis is good in hysterical blindness; the duration may vary, but recovery finally ensues. It is important, therefore, to make a diagnosis. In some cases the diagnosis is easy. When an individual, whose vision has previously been normal, becomes blind after an attack of hysteria, the blindness is obviously hysterical. This diagnosis also holds good if we find sensitivo-sensory hemianæsthesia, hysterogenic zones, contractures, etc.

The question is by no means so simple in every case. The blindness may supervene in persons, showing but few stigmata of hysteria; it may appear as the only symptom of hysteria. On the other hand, a patient with hysteria may also be suffering from syphilis, alcoholism, or lead-poisoning, conditions in which visual troubles are common.

Under the name of " symptomatic triad of hysterical blindness," I have collected the symptoms by which a diagnosis may be made. These symptoms are sudden onset of the blindness, preservation of the light reflex, and integrity of the media and of the retina. When a blind patient presents this triad, we can state that the blindness in hysterical, although the patient appears to be free from any trace of hysteria.

Is it possible to find this triad in blindness due to other causes ? Let us examine the question. Blindness due to tumours and lesions of the brain, including syphilis, is far from presenting the fundamental characters of the triad ; the loss of sight is not so sudden, the light reflex is lost, and the media show abnormalities, apart from the fact that other symptoms (paralysis of the cranial nerves, hemiplegia) often accompany a brain lesion.

Some lesions of the brain, however, may cause blindness, which resembles in character the triad of hysterical blindness ; they are combined lesions (hæmorrhage, softening, etc.) of both occipital lobes at the cortical origin, or in the course of the two optic tracts. Chauffard has employed the term " cortical anopsia." Hemianopia appears suddenly on one side without the patient's knowledge, and is followed by hemianopia on the other side. This bilateral hemianopia gives rise to anopsia—that is to say, sudden blindness, with normal light reflex and normal media. Cortical anopsia occurs in elderly persons and in general paralytics ; they may suffer from other cerebral lesions (foci of softening), with organic hemiplegia, aphasia, epileptiform attacks, and rapid cachexia—a striking contrast to the person with hysterical blindness.

I need not discuss the diagnosis of hysterical blindness and of blindness in tabes, because the latter shows totally different characteristics. Alcoholism and tobacco-poisoning may give rise to amaurosis. The amaurosis, however, comes on slowly, and lesions of the optic nerve are constant—a condition quite opposite to that found in hysterical blindness. Lead-poisoning may lead to blindness, but in this event optic neuritis is found.

Uræmic amaurosis may resemble hysterical blindness. In hysteria we find signs from which we can deduce the nature of the disease, and yet these signs may be absent. In uræmia we find albuminuria and œdema, the two great symptoms of nephritis ; they may, however, be absent, at any rate for a time, in Bright's disease, as I have already pointed out. On what facts, then, are we to base a diagnosis ? We must inquire carefully into the patient's history. If the blindness is uræmic, the patient will have shown some of the symptoms of Brightism : the arterial tension is high, a *bruit de galop* is heard on examining the heart, the uræmic poisoning has already been shown by dyspnœa, etc.—in short, uræmic blindness appears in a patient already sick, and subject for some time past to symptoms of Brightism or of uræmia. Hysterical blindness appears in a healthy individual, or in one who has so far shown only the nervous stigmata of hysteria. We have a diagnostic method of supreme importance. Even after the disappearance of hysterical blindness the perimeter shows narrowing of the visual field and overriding of the coloured circles.

What is the treatment of hysterical blindness ? In some cases it defies every method : magnetization, static electricity, metallotherapy, blisters, collyria, hydrotherapy, douches to the eyes, suggestion, isolation, bromides, and injection of ovarian extract. In other cases it disappears without any treatment after an attack of hysteria, or after some violent emotion, for no reason at all.

Genital Functions. — Besides false peritonitis, which I have already mentioned, hysterical patients may suffer from spontaneous or provoked pain in the iliac region : the pain is due to hyperæsthesia of the ovary. Compression of the painful ovary may cut short or bring on an attack. The genital troubles also include vaginismus and hyperæsthesia of the breast (mastodynia).

Troubles of the Circulation—Fever.—The vasomotor nerves play a large part in the circulatory troubles. At the present time, however, we do not admit that the congestions may go as far as hæmorrhage, hæmoptysis, hæmatemesis, hæmaturia, tears of blood, and sweating of blood.

Is there such a thing as **hysterical fever ?** Certain cases tend to prove that hysterical patients may suffer from fever which is continuous, like typhoid fever, and which may last for several weeks. I have seen several cases of this kind ; the temperature may exceed 106° F.

Diagnosis.—The diagnosis must include (1) convulsive hysteria, (2) non-convulsive hysteria.

Convulsive hysteria (*petite hystérie*) differs from epilepsy in the characters I have enumerated. In certain cases epilepsy is associated with hysteria, but the association of these two neuroses is **sometimes real, sometimes apparent.** It is real when the attacks of hysteria and of epilepsy remain distinct. Thus, a young epileptic girl, who becomes hysterical at puberty, may have definite attacks of hysteria or of epilepsy. In other cases the association of the two neuroses is only apparent : this is *grande hystérie*, or the **epileptoid attack,** but it is not true epilepsy (Charcot). In fact, the attack of hystero-epilepsy may be stopped by the compression of the ovary ; the temperature does not rise after a series of attacks, as it does in epilepsy. Babinski's sign is not met with in hysteria, while it exists in epilepsy as well as in hemiplegia of organic origin. Hysteria differs from **catalepsy**—a neurosis characterized by momentary loss of intellect and by exaggeration of the muscular contractions, the limbs remaining immovable in the position in which they have been placed. Catalepsy is, however, frequently associated with hysteria.

The diagnosis of local (non-convulsive) hysteria comprises the diagnosis of the innumerable symptoms which I have mentioned. Hysterical hemiplegia must not be confounded with the hemiplegia due to cerebral lesions ; the diagnosis is discussed under Cerebral Hæmorrhage. Hysterical contractures must be distinguished from the contractures due to lateral scleroses of the spinal cord. Certain hysterical syndromes may simulate insular sclerosis, syringomyelia, tabes, and paraplegia.   The diagnosis is, in general, possible even when there are hystero-organic associations (Souques).

We must distinguish hysterical gastralgia and hæmatemesis from similar symptoms, due to a lesion of the stomach.   Cough and hæmoptysis due to hysteria must be differentiated from pulmonary lesions of a tubercular nature. In these difficult cases we must try to find out if the patient has not had attacks of convulsive hysteria, or if in her condition there is not some suspicious stigma, such as the globus hystericus, hemianæsthesia, ovarian hyperæsthesia, pharyngeal anæsthesia, hysterogenous zones, ocular troubles, etc.   Finally, the special characters of the symptom in question must be carefully analyzed.   We shall not then look upon ovarian hyperæsthesia in a hysterical patient as appendicitis.

Ætiology—Prognosis—Treatment.—Hysteria may occur in children, but it generally makes its appearance about the age of puberty, and it becomes much less frequent at the menopause.   Heredity prepares the soil.   According to certain writers, it is said to be intimately connected with tuberculosis (Grasset).   Emotions, grief, unfortunate love-affairs, imitation, and chlorosis are the usual causes.   It often coexists with exophthalmic goitre, with neurasthenia, with astasia-abasia, and with Sydenham's chorea.

The great predisposing cause of hysteria is nervous heredity, and the provoking agents are numerous.   Amongst the latter I would mention the infectious fevers (typhoid, pneumonia, malaria, acquired and hereditary syphilis, rheumatism), the chronic intoxications (lead, mercury, alcohol), genital diseases, pregnancy, accouchement, and trauma.

With respect to **trauma,** I must make some restrictions.   Trauma is no doubt the occasional cause of many hysterical complications—but are not these complications sometimes hysteriform ?   The proof is that auto-suggestion, which has such a happy influence on certain hysterical complications—for example, on flaccid paralysis—has no effect on hysteriform paralysis of traumatic origin.   Many of these cases might be described as cases of **secondary** or **symptomatic** hysteria, just as, side by side with epilepsy, we find secondary or symptomatic epilepsy.   The syndrome of hysteria may be realized, with some of its most marked characteristics, in poisoning by lead, mercury, alcohol, and sulphide of carbon.

Hysteria is far from being as serious as epilepsy.   It may, however, lead to dementia, and to suicide ; it may cause paralyses and contractures, the results of which we can never foresee ; and, in conclusion, it is a source of torment to the patient, a source of constant worry to the family.   In some exceptional cases death supervenes during an attack of hysteria.

Male Hysteria.—Hysteria is more frequent in men than was at first supposed ; it is frequently observed in the Army.   It does not only develop in men who have the characteristics of feminism, but it is also seen in robust adult men, who are not of an effeminate type ; maternal heredity plays a great part in its development. In men, as in women, hysteria may be non-convulsive or convulsive, and the attacks assume the forms of *petite* or of *grande hystérie*. Paralysis (monoplegia, hemiplegia, paraplegia), hemianæsthesia, anæsthesia of the pharynx, and constriction of the field of vision are frequent symptoms. Contractures, with or without muscular atrophy, aphonia, and mutism, are also met with in male hysteria. Hysterogenous and hypnogenous zones are also met with ; the patients are susceptible to suggestion and to hypnotism. Ovarian hyperæsthesia is replaced by irritation of the testicle ; pressure may provoke or arrest the attack of hysteria.

In men, as in women, hysteria may simulate Sydenham's chorea and every disease of the spinal cord. Many complications, such as hysterical apoplexy, which simulates true apoplexy, tympanites with acute pain, which simulates peritonitis, insomnia, and trophic troubles, are seen not only in women, but also in the most robust men, who from their previous life and social position would not seem, at first sight, to be in the least predisposed to hysteria. In men, as in women, hysteria may be associated with astasia-abasia.

The **treatment** of hysteria must be palliative and curative. In a predisposed child education plays a large part ; every cause of excitation and of emotion must be avoided. A country life and somewhat vigorous exercise are to be recommended. Marriage has no drawbacks, when it takes place under favourable circumstances ; in certain cases it is beneficial. When hysteria has declared itself, use is made of anti-spasmodics ; isolation is an excellent remedy. Hydrotherapy, change of air, and a sea-voyage should be prescribed, and any causes which may assist its development should be carefully looked for.

Hydrotherapy is certainly one of the most powerful remedies against certain manifestations of hysteria. The paralysis, the contractures, and the anæsthesia generally yield to the application of electricity, but the disappearance of these disorders is often only temporary.

Suggestion may render great service, and in several cases attacks of hystero-epilepsy, paralyses, and contractures of many months' duration, which had resisted every measure, have been completely cured by suggestion.

V. HYPNOTISM—LETHARGY—CATALEPSY—SOMNAMBULISM.

Braid has defined **hypnotism** ($\H{u}\pi\nu\sigma\varsigma$, sleep) as " a peculiar condition of the nervous system, brought about by artificial manœuvres." This condition is also called **nervous sleep**, in order to distinguish it from **natural sleep**, with which it has only the most coarse resemblance. According to Babinski, " hypnotism is a psychical condition, rendering the subject capable of submitting to external suggestion. It manifests itself by phenomena, which suggestion calls into being. These phenomena disappear as the result of persuasion, and are identical with hysterical symptoms. Hypnotism was for a long time practised by quacks under the name of animal magnetism; it was placed on a scientific basis by Braid (1843). It may show itself in three different forms (Charcot)—lethargy, catalepsy, and somnambulism.

Ætiology.—Nervous, impressionable women and boys are more readily hypnotized than men. Hysterical people are hypnotized even more easily ; and yet all hysterical people cannot be hypnotized, and all hypnotizable subjects are not hysterical. Grief, deep emotions, and convalescence from acute diseases predispose towards it.

The will-power of the subject is of great importance. In order to be put to sleep rapidly and deeply, the subject's whole attention must be given to the operator. The patient must will to be put to sleep. Certain subjects can only be sent to sleep when they resist mentally, and they then succeed, on the contrary, in hypnotizing themselves when they wish to do so.

When we try to put a person to sleep for the first time, sleep has often to be waited for. If the patient is submitted to further experiments, the hypnosis will be produced much more rapidly. Education (Richet) is, therefore, of great importance.

Contrary to the generally accepted opinion, any person can be put to sleep. There is, in this case, no fluid or divining influence. We merely acquire, by habit, more authority over the persons who are to be put to sleep, and more still over those who have been already put to sleep.

The artificial means used to provoke nervous sleep are numerous (Chambard). The most simple one consists in seating the subject face to face with the operator, in taking hold of his hands so as to keep him quiet still, and in making him fix his eyes on the latter. After three or four minutes the eyelids move, slight convulsive jerks appear in the muscles of the face and of the limbs, the respiration is sighing, the head falls on the shoulder, and the result is obtained. The act of looking at a shining object held 12 to 15 inches from the root of the nose, so as to make the eyeballs converge at the same time as they look upwards, may lead to the same result, provided the subject fixes the object and devotes all his attention to it (Braid). Subjects accustomed to hypnotic séances often put themselves to sleep by compressing the eyeballs, by closing of the eyes, or by looking at a shining object. Others are easily influenced by auditory sensations—an unexpected noise, the sound of the diapason, the tick of a watch, music, etc. Hypnosis is sometimes produced under the influence of psychical phenomena—faith, expectation, emotion, and intellectual fatigue ; or is consequent on the action of certain substances—ether, chloroform, alcohol, and Indian hemp. Cutaneous friction and touching of the so-called **hypnogenous** zones (Pitres)—

vertex, angle of the scapula, etc.—also lead to nervous sleep. Finally, an experienced subject can go to sleep by merely thinking of the fact that he or she is about to be put to sleep. It is sufficient to say to some of them, " In an hour, or to-morrow at such-and-such an hour, you will go to sleep," for them to be soundly asleep at the time named, even in the absence of the operator (Bernheim).

Symptoms.—The process of hypnotization just described does not produce the same phenomena in all subjects ; but the condition provoked may always be classified in one of the three forms described by Charcot.

Lethargy.—In the condition of **lethargy** the patient appears to be in a deep sleep : the eyes are closed, the muscles are relaxed, and the uplifted arm falls down inert ; the general sensibility is abolished ; the tendon reflexes are exaggerated, and every effort to rouse the patient by shaking him fails. Charcot has shown that, in this condition, there is very marked muscular hyperexcitability. If we touch the cutaneous points corresponding to the course of the superficial nerves (ulnar or facial) with the point of a pencil, the muscles supplied by these nerves contract, just as they do with the electric current. By continuing the excitation, we cause contractures, which persist even when the subject is awakened. Gentle friction to the skin over the antagonistic muscles makes them cease. Richet and Brissaud have shown that in the limbs rendered anæmic by Esmarch's bandage, the muscular hyperexcitability disappears. Certain excitants may, on the contrary, act at a distance ; thus, the application of an electrical current to one side of the skull may cause muscular contractions on the opposite side of the body— a phenomenon not seen in the waking condition. If the light falls on one eye, the whole of the corresponding side is seen to become cataleptic, so that the subject is at the same time hemilethargic and hemicataleptic. If the right eye has been open, aphasia may be met with. As soon as the eyelid is closed, the limbs again relax.

Catalepsy.—If both eyes are opened in the presence of a bright light, lethargy is replaced by catalepsy. The same result may be obtained directly by one of the procedures mentioned above, especially those which act suddenly, such as an unexpected noise. The eyes are then open, and the limbs are not contracted, but keep the position in which they have been placed. If the arm is raised, it remains so for a long time. Through this peculiar condition of the muscles, the subject may be placed in the most extraordinary positions. The general anæsthesia is complete, the tendon reflexes are diminished or abolished, and the pulse is accelerated, but the respiration is not altered ; whereas in the malingerer the effort necessary to maintain the arm in the given position increases the respiration rate, while the muscles concerned show fatigue tremors. By placing the limbs in a position which corresponds to a passionate attitude, we excite or suggest an expression of the face corresponding to a similar sentiment or a similar passion. The muscular system is in a condition which is the counterpart of that seen in lethargy. Gentle friction of a muscle produces paralysis which may persist when the experiment is finished.

Somnambulism. — Somnambulism is the condition most often seen in hypnotic séances, and is produced most readily in certain subjects. It consists in a kind of intellectual torpor, with preservation of the muscular activity. The patient, in a condition of provoked somnambulism (Barth), can therefore walk and talk as in the waking condition ; he often replies only to questions put by the operator. The general sensibility is abolished, but cutaneous hyperæsthesia is often present to such a degree that contact with certain metals may cause a burn. The special senses are usually rendered more acute. A patient of Azam heard the ticking of a watch at a distance of nine metres.

In somnambulists there is often a cataleptoid condition of the muscles ; in this case the hyperexcitability is as marked as in the lethargic patient. When the somnambulist or the cataleptic patient is told to fix an object, and when he cannot turn his eyes away from it, he is said to be in an ecstasy.

A similar phenomenon is produced when a person is concerned, the somnambulist imitating all his or her movements. From the intellectual point of view, the somnambulist is an automaton. We can suggest to him a certain act which we wish to see him perform. He often resists, but if we insist, he ends by giving way. We can, at will, provoke illusions, hallucinations, and memory troubles ; by means of suggestion we can even cause paralyses and contractures. The suggestion, instead of referring to something which has to be accomplished immediately, may refer to something which has to be performed some time hence ; thus arise hallucinations, or irresistible impulses which appear long after the order, and unknown to the subject. The question of suggestion is being studied to-day ; it has only entered the sphere of science during the last few years (Bernheim, Pitres, Charcot, Dumontpallier, etc.). From the medico-legal point of view, it is pregnant with consequences ; the question arises how far hypnotizable subjects are responsible, especially if, as Bernheim asserts, we can make suggestions to certain trained individuals, even in the waking condition.

Whatever the hypnotic condition produced, it suffices to open the eyes of the patient, and to blow vigorously on them in order to awaken him. When he has come round, he loses the recollection of what has happened, and of the orders which he has received to carry out at a specified date. Certain cataleptic patients, however, remember the séances at which they were present, but maintain that they were unable to prevent them or to withdraw from them.

Much has been written during the past few years on the advantages of hypnotism from a therapeutic point of view. Broca, Verneuil, and Pozzi have made use of the anæsthesia of lethargy in order to perform operations of short duration, but this means is uncertain. Certain hysterical paralyses, or contractures, and hystero-epileptic attacks have been cured by these means. We must, however, be guarded in our practice, because the **inconveniences** might be greater than the advantages. The repetition of the séances causes great excitability of the nervous system, and the latter often brings about hysterical complications.

VI. NEURASTHENIA.

In 1869 Beard gave the name of neurasthenia to a peculiar condition which had received many denominations—spinal irritation (Frank), general neuralgia (Valleix), neurosism (Bouchut), general hyperæsthesia (Monneret), etc. Krishaber's cerebro-cardiac neuropathy, with a few exceptions, comes under this heading. Attention has for some years been directed to this disease, and the tendency is to include under it many ill-defined morbid conditions, due to hysteria according to some, and to simulation according to others. These indefinite limits must not astonish us when we remember the varied troubles which neurasthenia may provoke in most of the systems, and consequently the many aspects which it assumes according to the patients concerned.

Ætiology.—The affection usually develops between the ages of twenty-five and fifty years of age, affecting men and women in equal proportions. Uterine affections play a great part as provoking agent. Intellectual efforts, mental overwork, prolonged watchings, and emotions favour its appearance, and explain its frequency in authors, scientists, doctors, speculators, etc. ; hence the frequency of neurasthenia in the Jewish and the Anglo-Saxon races, whose intellectual life is very active. The Slavs are predisposed to it, as they are to all kinds of neuropathic affections. Grief, emotion, and moral preoccupations (love, gambling, ambition, etc.) lead to a similar result. Charcot has laid especial stress on injuries, and principally on those accompanied by shock, by excessive emotion (railway accidents, explosions). Sexual excesses, masturbation, and diseases of the genital organs are also a frequent cause of neurasthenia. Digestive troubles have been regarded as the result and also the cause of neurasthenia ; such is said to be the mode of action of dilatation of the stomach and of the resulting auto-intoxication (Bouchard), of enteroptosis (Glissard), and of chronic gastritis (Hayem). It is certain that neurasthenia develops especially in people of neurotic stock and in arthritic subjects (Huchard). This fact explains its frequency in hysterical and diabetic patients ; its coexistence with gravel, gall-stones, rheumatism, gout ; and its association with tabes, exophthalmic goitre, general paralysis, etc.

De Fleury, who has published some interesting work on this question, thus states his conception of neurasthenia. The gastro-intestinal theory

does not appear to him to be admissible. The digestive troubles so frequent
in neuropathic patients undoubtedly have a secondary action on the brain;
but they themselves arise from a faulty innervation. Neither is neurasthenia
a disease of the imagination; its symptoms are not comparable with those
of hysteria, which result from a fixed idea, and gradually disappear under
the influence of suggestion. According to De Fleury, neurasthenia is
primarily a fatigue of the nerve centres, producing in all the organs a diminution of the muscular tonicity and of the glandular secretion. As each part
of the economy performs its functions sluggishly, the sensory nerves carry
to the brain the continuous idea of poor vitality, and it is the consciousness
of this physical condition which constitutes the mental state of neurasthenia.

Symptoms.—Neurasthenia shows certain fixed symptoms or **stigmata**
by analogy with the equivalent symptoms of hysteria (Bouveret).

In this group must be included **headache,** the most constant of all
the stigmata. It is generally frontal and occipital, and is comparable with
the pressure of a heavy and narrow helmet (Charcot's neurasthenic helmet);
it follows a circular line passing round the temples. In other cases it is
limited to the occiput, is seated between the eyebrows, or is hemilateral.
It manifests itself on awakening, and continues the whole day, with slight
diminution after meals. It ceases at night, even though the patient is troubled
with insomnia. It is increased by sensory stimuli—noises, strong odours,
and by intellectual fatigue. It is sometimes accompanied by hyperæsthesia
of the scalp and by creaking in the occipital articulations. Rachialgia is
often associated with neurasthenia. At times the rachialgia exists alone;
it may be limited to the sacrum or to the coccyx. It betrays itself by a sensation of pressure or of heat, brought on by percussion of the vertebral column.

Mental depression is never wanting. The patient has no longer the
same faculty of attention nor the same will-power. The least work becomes
difficult; the memory fails, especially for proper names. The neurasthenic
patient becomes depressed, seeks isolation, and often passes his time in
reading works on medicine, or in writing long monographs intended for his
physician. In the morning he feels fatigued, and this fatigue is often real,
because it betrays itself by a diminution of the muscular force appreciable
with the dynamometer.

The gastric troubles are also constant. Flatulent dyspepsia, distension
after food, hot flushes, somnolence, constipation, and pseudo-membranous
colic may cause us to think of cancer of the rectum, or of dilatation of the
stomach. These gastric manifestations are generally accompanied by loss
of flesh and by decoloration of the skin.

We also find numerous morbid manifestations, varying according to the
subject, and involving all the systems; such are insomnia, vertigo, agoraphobia, claustrophobia, disturbance of the cutaneous sensibility, neuralgic

pains, sensations of heat and of cold, heaviness of the eyelids, accommodation asthenopia, hyperacousia, buzzing and whistling in the ears, muscular jerks, and giving way of the legs.

In the circulatory system we find periodic attacks of pseudo-angina pectoris, with restlessness and dyspnœa. Tachycardia, palpitation, and coldness and pallor of the extremities are also common.

Profuse sweatings, or, on the contrary, dryness of the skin and of the mucosæ, seminal emissions, impotence, and increase of the urates and of the uric acid in the urine must also be mentioned.

Pitres describes six forms of neurasthenia, according to the system, most affected : (1) Cerebral form ; (2) spinal form ; (3) neuralgic form ; (4) cardialgic form ; (5) gastro-intestinal form ; (6) general form. Blocq describes in addition a local form, often characterized by painful zones, without organic lesions. It is needless to say that these forms are often combined. Neurasthenia rarely occurs in an acute form ; it generally assumes " a circular form," even when it is due to injury. It lasts for months and years, but it is susceptible to complete cure, excepting in hereditary cases ; it then leads to hypochondria, which is often irremediable.

Diagnosis.—The diversity of the forms and of the symptoms of neurasthenia cause it to resemble many diseases. It may simulate general paralysis, but it is not accompanied by pupillary troubles, embarrassment of speech and tremors ; the diagnosis may be in doubt until the case is far advanced. Cerebral tumours, and in particular cerebral syphilis, lead to confusion. Neurasthenic pseudo-tabes is distinguished from true tabes by the presence of the reflexes, by the absence of pupillary troubles, and by the less intensity of the pains.

The gastro-intestinal form is at times most difficult to diagnose. Not only may cancer of the stomach or of the intestine, in the absence of a tumour. be confounded with neurasthenia, but chronic gastritis and dyspepsia have many symptoms in common with neurasthenia, thus explaining why a case is regarded by one physician as gastric, and by another physician as nervous. The examination of the gastric juice does not always settle the question.

Treatment.—Tonics, kola, coca, injections of cacodylate of sodium, the glycero-phosphates, absolute rest, isolation, massage, electrical methods, and hydrotherapy, together with the use of iron and of bromide of potassium, are the means generally employed in neurasthenia. The bowels should be regulated by the daily use of a laxative. The hours of meals should be regulated, and the diet should be carefully selected in every case. When the lost flesh and strength are being regained, moderate exercise and subcutaneous injections of organic extracts (Brown-Séquard) and of artificial serum should be prescribed.

" Neurasthenic patients, properly so called, are not amenable to suggestion. Their condition may be almost always improved, and they are at times cured by a diet from which alcohol and indigestible foods are eliminated, and by systematic mechanical stimulation of the nervous system (douches, change of air, massage, saline injections, static electricity). Drugs should be used as little as possible. After a period of rest, permitting the restoration of the energy in the nerve centres, the lost habit of physical and intellectual work must be gradually resumed. Isolation in an asylum is only necessary in the most serious cases " (De Fleury).

VII. ASTASIA-ABASIA.

Description.—These terms were applied by Blocq to a syndrome, characterized by impossibility, or difficulty in standing erect (ἄστασις) and in walking (ἄβασις), while the muscular power, the sensibility and co-ordination of the other movements of the lower limbs are perfect. In 1864 Jaccoud had given to this condition the name of " ataxy from want of automatic co-ordination."

Apart from the difficulty in standing erect and walking normally, the patient when lying down can execute all the movements he is asked to perform without hesitation, weakness, or want of co-ordination. He has an exact idea of the position of his legs, and when he has risen he sometimes succeeds in walking by means of certain subterfuges ; thus some patients manage to walk on all fours, or with their legs crossed, or with very small steps, or, on the contrary, with large steps (actor's walk) ; some can even run.

In some patients the trouble appears as soon as they try to stand up, and they sink down unless they are held up. Others have recourse to crutches, and drag their seemingly inert legs after them.

In most cases the abasia predominates ; it may be divided into three varieties :

1. *Paretic Abasia*, characterized especially by the diminution in the muscular force. Walking is difficult ; it is only possible by means of the greatest efforts, and it very rapidly becomes impossible.

2. *Choreiform Abasia* (Grasset).—When the patient stands up, the legs are seized with sudden movements of flexion and extension ; at the same time the trunk is flexed or extended on the pelvis, and the movements are thus propagated to the arms. It seems as though the contortions would throw the patient down, but nothing of the kind happens ; on the other hand, normal progression forwards is rendered absolutely impossible.

3. *Trembling Abasia*.—In this form the contradictory movements predominate ; the legs become entangled just as in certain forms of incomplete spasmodic paraplegia.

As astasia-abasia is almost always of an hysterical nature, the strange forms which it may assume will be readily understood. In general, it is a syndrome of long duration, persisting for months or years, and subject to relapses; it disappears and reappears suddenly. Patients suffering from abasia sometimes show hysterical stigmata: ovarian or testicular pains, various hysterogenic zones, anæsthesia in patches, convulsive attacks, etc. Séglas is of opinion that it is connected with insanity, and Charcot with an indeterminate lesion of the brain. As a rule, however, astasia-abasia must be attributed to some dynamic trouble in the brain or in the spinal cord, either because the cerebral cells which transmit to the spinal cells the stimuli necessary for the performance of normal walking have lost their power, or because the spinal cells, receiving a normal stimulus from the brain, are no longer capable of transmitting it properly to the nerves of the lower limbs. Stasobasophobia is abasia accompanied by emotional troubles.

Diagnosis.—Astasia-abasia was for a long time confounded with paraplegia and ataxy. It differs from the former in the preservation of the muscular force when the patient is lying down, in the integrity of the sphincters, and in the possibility of walking other than normal walking. It must not be confounded with ataxy, because the co-ordination of the movements is intact when the patient is lying down, and the muscular sense is preserved. Chorea, and especially rhythmical chorea, show some analogy with astasia-abasia, but here the upper limbs and the face show their own proper movements, and not the propagated movements found in astasia-abasia. Furthermore, we have to deal with extensive movements, either forwards or backwards, and but little comparable with the movements of sudden flexion and extension of the legs.

The giving way of the legs in cases of neurasthenia and of ataxy might also lead to confusion, but in patients suffering from ataxy the want of co-ordination exists when they are in bed, and the neurasthenic patient often refuses to stand erect or to leave the room. Every attempt to overcome the resistance of the patient is accompanied by a characteristic agony.

In **Thomsen's disease** the rapidity with which the spasms produced on attempting to walk disappear is an excellent means of diagnosis; besides, the upper limbs, the neck, the jaw, and the tongue are sometimes attacked.

Paramyoclonus multiplex is accompanied by jerks, which extend to the whole body, or to a great part of the body, and which supervene as the result of very slight stimuli. Nothing of this kind occurs in astasia-abasia.

VIII. CEREBRO-CARDIAC NEUROPATHY—KRISHABER'S DISEASE.

Description.—Under the name of **cerebro-cardiac neuropathy,** Krishaber has described a neurosis with such definite symptoms and characters that it may be looked upon as a morbid entity.

The onset may be slow or rapid, and the slowness of the onset is generally a favourable sign. The rapid onset is very rare. The disease supervenes almost without prodromata. The subject has a distressing sensation of a **cerebral void.** He complains of vertigo, insomnia, nightmares, photopsia, palpitation, and tightness in the chest ; he is liable to attacks of syncope.

These troubles, instead of appearing suddenly, supervene gradually in the slow form of this neuropathy ; they follow and replace one another until the disease is completely established. Whether the symptoms come on slowly or suddenly, a time comes when the descriptions of the two forms of the disease may be blended together. **Vertigo** is one of the earliest and also the most obstinate symptom ; it lasts for months and for years. The organs of the senses are affected, especially those of sight and hearing, which become very acute ; a bright light is intolerable, and the sense of hearing is increased to such a degree that the slightest noise causes genuine distress. The tactile sensibility is increased.

The patient lives in a world of dreams : the aspect of the exterior world seems changed to him ; his own voice is strange to him. He finds himself so changed that he hardly recognizes himself, and would readily take himself for somebody else if reason did not rectify the aberration of his senses. Insanity is never present, and the patient is conscious that "his senses are perverted, and give him incorrect ideas of the external world" (Krishaber).

The heart troubles consist in palpitation, angina pectoris, and syncope ; they are often accompanied by sensations of strangulation.

The neuralgia is multiple, and affects the head, the face, the ear, and the sciatic nerve.

Insomnia is one of the most painful symptoms in the grave form. The patient cannot enjoy a moment's rest, and if he goes to sleep, it is only to be awakened by nightmares, accompanied by angina and palpitations. The duration of cerebro-cardiac neuropathy varies from a few months to several years. It is almost always cured ; it never ends in mental alienation, but the nature and the persistence of the symptoms render the disease most distressing. It is provoked by all kinds of excesses, especially in a predisposed person. The intimate cause of the symptoms seems to be cerebral anæmia, produced by a permanent contraction of the vessels of the brain (Krishaber's experiments).

Diagnosis.—Cerebro-cardiac neuropathy differs from the nervous conditions known as general neuralgia, spinal irritation, and nervosism.

In **general neuralgia** (Valleix) the principal phenomenon is pain, disseminated throughout the whole surface of the body, and complicated by neuralgia of various nerves. Dizziness, dimness of sight, and more or less marked weakness, feebleness, and depression complete the picture of this morbid condition.

Spinal irritation is characterized by a general nervous condition, in which rachialgia is the chief feature. This rachialgia, which is, according to circumstance, most marked in the cervical, dorsal, or lumbar regions, is accompanied by muscular weakness, by spermatorrhœa, and by hypochondria. This nervous condition is said by Hammond to be due to an anæmia of the posterior columns of the spinal cord.

IX. PARALYSIS AGITANS—PARKINSON'S DISEASE.

Paralysis agitans is a neurosis characterized by a special tremor, which is absent in some cases, by a peculiar rigidity of the muscular system, and by a paralytic condition which appears late, and is simply an accessory element in the disease.

Description.—In some cases the disease appears suddenly after fright, emotion, or trauma, and the tremor at once declares itself ; but this is the exception. As a rule, the onset is insidious, and the course is slowly progressive. The tremor first affects the hand, the thumb, the foot, but this tremor is so slight that the patient hardly notices it. It disappears, and then returns with renewed intensity. It becomes general, or else in certain subjects it assumes the hemiplegic and paraplegic forms.

The tremor of paralysis agitans has characteristics distinguishing it from other tremors. The hand looks as if it were holding a pen. The fingers are stretched out and tremble as a whole, while the thumb moves on them with isochronic and rhythmical tremors, though the hand as a whole seems to be spinning wool or crumbling bread (Gubler). The tremor of the wrist on the forearm is produced by movements of flexion and extension, and sometimes extends to the whole of the upper limb. The writing shows the effect of these tremors ; the down-strokes are sinuous. In the lower limbs the tremor of the toes and of the feet is produced by successive movements of flexion and extension.

All the tremors occur when the muscles are at rest ; they cease during sleep ; they diminish and may cease under the influence of the will—an essential difference from the tremor of insular sclerosis, which only takes place during voluntary movements. The head is at times affected by the movements of the body : there is a borrowed tremor ; but the head may also be affected by spontaneous tremors. Amongst the muscles which participate in the tremor, I would especially mention those of the jaw, of the tongue, and of the eyelids.

Muscular rigidity is an essential element in paralysis agitans, and it may be the chief element ; it commences with transient cramps, and gradually becomes permanent. As the result of this muscular rigidity, the head, the trunk, and the limbs assume special attitudes. The patient's head is stretched forward and fixed in this position ; the eye is fixed, the features lose their mobility, and the physiognomy has a dull look.

In the erect position the trunk is bent ; the elbows are slightly separated from the body ; the hands rest on the waist, and show tremors ; the legs are slightly bent on the thighs ; the movements are slow and occur together, the patient looking as though he were soldered together. When the patient commences to walk, he starts with his head and his trunk forward, taking small steps and hopping, as though he were running after his centre of gravity (Trousseau), and he quickens his pace, as if he were moved by some irresistible impulse. Certain patients, impelled by a backward movement (retropulsion), would fall down if they were not prevented.

At a later period the muscular rigidity causes abduction of the thighs, but we observe neither the true contracture nor the epileptoid tremor of lateral sclerosis. The rigidity of the muscles may in the long run cause deformity of the hands, analogous to those of chronic rheumatism, but without the bony swellings, and also without the characteristic deformity of the thumb, which in Parkinson's disease presents both in front and behind a flattening, due to its permanent application to the index-finger.

Besides the above symptoms, the patient experiences painful cramps, and has to change his position constantly ; he complains of a sensation of excessive heat. In some cases the tremor is absent, and the muscular rigidity constitutes the chief symptom of the disease. At times symmetrical spontaneous ecchymoses, probably of myelopathic origin, are noticed (Carrière).

The disease makes incessant progress, and ends in a kind of paresis, which has been called the paralytic period, although there is no paralysis, in the true sense of the word, and the tremor disappears in proportion as the muscular weakness increases. This incomplete and disseminated paralysis has been variously interpreted : Charcot thinks that it is a question of muscular rigidity rather than a true weakness of the muscles ; there are, however, cases in which the paresis is evident. Trousseau admits that the paralysis is due to the continual loss of nervous stimulus in the muscles, which no longer store the force necessary to produce true contractions.

The terminal period of the disease supervenes after ten, twenty, or thirty years. This cachectic period is characterized by disorders of nutrition, and by psychic troubles. The patient loses flesh and falls into marasmus, with anasarca, diarrhœa, incontinence of urine, and weakening of the intellectual faculties. Prior to this period death is often brought about by some intercurrent disease (pneumonia).

Diagnosis—Ætiology.—The co-ordinated tremor of the hands in paralysis agitans in no way resembles the short and isochronic oscillations of the so-called senile tremor. It also differs from the toxic tremors (alcohol, mercury, lead), and from the tremor of insular sclerosis, which appears only on the occasion of voluntary movement. Finally, in no other disease do we find the special attitudes of the face and trunk which characterize paralysis agitans. There are defaced cases in which the tremor is slight, and the diagnosis is made by means of the rigidity of the muscles and the special attitude of the patients. Paralysis agitans is rare before the age of forty. Its causes are most frequently unknown : great emotions, terror, cold, and traumatism of a nerve have at times caused it ; heredity has played a part in some cases.

Pathological Anatomy.—The lesion of paralysis agitans has still to be found, and the disease at present deserves to be placed amongst the **neuroses,** although various changes have been noted, such as : diffuse sclerosis in the bulb, the pons, and the lateral columns of the spinal cord ; obliteration of the central canal of the spinal cord ; fragility of the protoplasm of the cells in the posterior cornua (Ballet) ; and lesions of the peduncle, or of the suboptic region.

X. SYDENHAM'S CHOREA—ST. VITUS'S DANCE.

Description.—**Chorea** (Bouteille), which has been called by Sydenham **St. Vitus's dance** (χορεία, dance), is a disease especially frequent at an early age, and more common in the female sex. This disease has derived its name from the remarkable intervention which St. Vitus seemed to have in conjuring certain epidemic affections of the Middle Ages—affections which were evidently hysterical, and characterized, among other symptoms, by frenzied dancing.

Chorea may commence suddenly as the result of a deep emotion, but it is more often announced by precursory signs, such as changes of character, symptoms of spinal irritation, pains in the limbs, and continual restlessness ; the subject becomes capricious, impressionable, forgetful, and inattentive. At times motor troubles open the scene, the voluntary movements being affected before the involuntary movements. The child is scolded because he has dropped his food or spilt his milk. He is scolded because he has broken a certain object, and it is not seen that this awkwardness, for which he is not responsible, must be ascribed to the want of co-ordination of the voluntary movements which so often precedes confirmed chorea (Jaccoud). The choreic movements commence in the face with grimaces, in the arm, or in the hand. At the same time, involuntary jerks in the shoulders, neck, and face supervene, and the patient tries to hide these jerks by various voluntary movements. The choreic movements soon increase in intensity, and become general, affecting more especially the left side.

In the choreic patient the muscular system shows arrhythmical movements, quite different from the rhythmical movements of hysterical chorea, and having nothing in common with the short oscillatory tremors of paralysis agitans. The choreic patient rises suddenly, stumbles, and sometimes falls ; the gait is strange and hopping, because he throws out his legs in different directions. He finds a difficulty in grasping an object, because the arms execute the most varied movements of flexion, extension, rotation, etc., without order, and one after the other. There are incessant contortions of the trunk and of the head. The muscles of the face work in a thousand different ways : the forehead is wrinkled and unwrinkled ; the eyebrows are drawn and separated ; the eyes turn in their sockets ; the tongue is suddenly protruded from the mouth, or smacks against the palate ; the lips are pulled in every direction, so that the subject shows almost at the same instant " the contradictory expressions of joy, grief, or anger " (Simon). The muscles of the tongue, of the larynx, and of the pharynx participate in the want of muscular co-ordination ; the result is a kind of stuttering and barking. Mastication and deglutition are difficult, and the speech is jerky. The restlessness is incessant, whether the patient is seated or is lying down, whether he wish to perform some movement or not. It is a case of **muscular madness** (Bouillaud), and, notwithstanding these continual movements, the patient is but little fatigued.

Every voluntary movement exaggerates the chorea, and yet the object is always gained ; thus the patient at last succeeds in lifting a glass of water to his mouth, but it is only after " a thousand gestures and a thousand contortions " (Sydenham), which bear no relation to the object in view. When the chorea is violent, sleep is impossible. When it is of moderate severity, the restlessness ceases during sleep, provided the patient does not dream (Marshall Hall).

The muscular force diminishes during the disease, and reappears immediately. In some cases the paretic or paralytic troubles predominate, the choreic movements being of minor importance, and passing unnoticed in the absence of a careful examination. This variety has received the name of chorea mollis. The paresis may be limited to an arm or a leg, or may become general. It may invade the muscles of the upper and lower limbs, of the neck, of mastication, of deglutition, and of phonation. The patient lies motionless in bed, incapable of making the slightest movement. The tendon reflexes are generally preserved; there is neither muscular atrophy nor loss of sensation. Chorea mollis may recover directly, or may end in ordinary chorea. Chorea is sometimes accompanied by anæsthesia or hyperæsthesia; hemianæsthesia is frequent in hemichorea, symptomatic of a cerebral lesion. In women chorea is often associated with chloro-anæmia and dyspeptic troubles (gastralgia, constipation).

Psychical disorders are frequent. In a general way it may be said that the intellectual faculties are more or less affected in most patients. The mental condition in chorea has been very carefully studied by many writers (Trousseau, Marcé, Ball). Raymond and Joffroy have reviewed all its phases. In the choreic patient the psychic troubles vary from the slightest symptoms to the most pronounced mental disorders. In children the character becomes changed several weeks prior to the appearance of the chorea. These children become irascible, wilful, disobedient, lazy, taciturn, or emotional. A child who was studious and diligent becomes absent-minded, and falls to the lowest place in his class. Another child is moved by a trifle, and cries without a motive. A child who was fond of his family becomes indifferent to all around him. One child loses his memory, and no longer remembers his lessons; another is restless and excited: his sleep is disturbed by dreams and nightmare. The face may have a dull look, the eye grows haggard, and the intellectual faculties become weak. Some choreic patients have speech troubles, due to chorea, properly so called (stuttering, want of co-ordination between the tongue and the lips); others suffer from a sort of mutism due to mental idleness.

Marcé has well described this intellectual condition in choreic patients: " In most choreic patients we meet with that nervous instability which accompanies all the neuroses. The subjects are impressionable; their sleep is light; they are troubled with vertigo, fits of suffocation, and other hysteriform symptoms. . . . We may observe, especially in children, sometimes an unusual gaiety or a silly laugh, brought on by the most futile causes; sometimes sadness, tendency to cry, or else alternate excitation and depression. At the same time the character is changed, and the most docile children become irascible, impatient, and wrangling; they lie about everything, and strike those who approach them. Adults suffer from these changes, but in a less degree; some become extravagant, strange in their manner, and intolerant of any contradiction." We shall see in the next section, referring to fatal chorea, the importance of the mental condition of choreic patients.

Duration—Complications.—Chorea in youth recovers after an average duration of two to three months; it often leaves tics behind, and it is subject to recurrences, which break out on the occasion of emotion, at the approach of puberty, or in pregnancy. An intercurrent febrile disease (pneumonia, eruptive fever) may modify or arrest the chorea (*febris accedens spasmos solvit*).

St. Vitus's dance has its complications. Some patients suffer from such severe movements that they are compelled to keep their bed, and in their incessant movements they literally wear away their skin. The result is excoriations, ulcerations, sores, and abscesses. Others suffer from terrible insomnia, from nightmare, from hallucinations, accompanied by delirium, and from attacks of acute mania, which may cause death in a few days.

The cardiac complications, and especially endocarditis, will be discussed under the Ætiology.

Chronic chorea is especially met with in adults and old persons; the motor troubles are those of ordinary chorea, but they are, however, slower, less extensive, and more subordinated to the influence of the will. Chronic chorea has a slow and progressive course, does not recover, and it is often accompanied by mental decay. Nervous heredity is the most common cause of chronic chorea. It must not be confounded with symptomatic chorea, with the convulsive tics, or with double athetosis. Here, as in acute chorea, pathological anatomy is still silent.

Ætiology.—St. Vitus's dance is especially a disease of early age, and is more common in the feminine sex. It supervenes at the period of dentition, during the course of second infancy, and at puberty; it has, nevertheless, been observed in old people. Chorea in the aged presents some special characteristics. The onset is fairly sudden; it leaves the intellectual faculties intact; but it persists in the condition of infirmity, and does not recover like chorea in early age. **Heredity** has a manifest influence on the development of chorea. Epileptic or hysterical parents beget choreic children. This transformation of neuroses by heredity is seen every day (Trousseau). The most common determining causes are emotions, fright, anger, anæmia, pregnancy, imitation, and rheumatism. Imitation, which is frequent in children's hospitals, accounts for epidemics of chorea.

The relations between chorea and rheumatism must detain us longer. These relations were clearly established by Botrel in 1850. According to Sée, the rheumatic diathesis causes chorea, in the same manner as it causes the articular pains or the endocarditis. The chorea may directly attack the heart without the patient showing the phase of articular pains. In other words, chorea, endocarditis, and articular rheumatism are manifestations of the rheumatic diathesis. In a lecture on St. Vitus's dance, Trousseau reports a series of cases, showing the association of rheumatism, chorea, and endocarditis. " In many circumstances," says he, " I have been able to predict that St. Vitus's dance would affect children whom I attended for rheumatism. Furthermore, I have been able to predict conversely that children who were brought to me with St. Vitus's dance would sooner or later have rheumatism. You will, however, rarely see chorea preceding rheumatism, whilst it often follows it, and that in the proportion of a third of the cases."

Broadbent has opposed another theory to the preceding conclusions. He holds that the relations of chorea and of the affections of the heart follow quite a different course. Rheumatic endocarditis is the first, as far as date is concerned ; this endocarditis gives rise to capillary emboli, which lodge in the brain and cause chorea. This theory cannot be accepted, because in most cases chorea appears without previous endocarditis.

According to some writers, rheumatism does not play in chorea the predominant part which has been attributed to it. In many choreic patients the rheumatic diathesis is absent, and besides, whatever may be the causes contributing to the development of the chorea, it is especially a cerebro-spinal neurosis of growth, having this feature in common with chlorosis, which also appears in most cases at the time of puberty (Joffroy). Marie is of opinion that chorea is most intimately allied with hysteria. Marfan replies to this statement : " I have attended a large number of children, and I have never met with hysteria, or with a single stigma of hysteria." According to Marfan, chorea almost always follows some other disease. It is generally preceded by an acute infectious disease : typhoid fever, measles, influenza, mumps, or more often by rheumatism.

The question may, I think, be thus stated : It is undeniable that the association of chorea with rheumatism, with or without endocarditis, is very common, but I would point out that in this association we are dealing especially with rheumatism in children or in youths. This clause seems to me to be important. I do not believe that an adult attacked by rheumatism is on that account a candidate for chorea. He is suffering from endocarditis, but not from chorea. I have attended many patients of twenty, thirty, or forty years of age for acute articular rheumatism, and I have scarcely ever seen the rheumatism followed by chorea. Nevertheless, some had had chorea in their infancy. In short, the choreigenic rheumatism is the rheumatism of childhood. When I see a child with articular rheumatism, I think of the chorea which may come later. This idea does not occur to me in the case of an adult.

The cardiac complications of chorea consist in mitral and in aortic endocarditis ; the endocarditis is often vegetative. An attack of articular rheumatism is not the indispensable intermediary between chorea and endocarditis ; we meet with choreic patients who have never had rheumatism, chorea alone having brought on the endocarditis. It is, therefore, necessary to auscultate the chest in patients with chorea, so that we may not miss any cardiac complications.

Pregnancy has a marked influence on the development of chorea (*chorea gravidarum*), but some determining cause, such as fright, emotion, imitation or traumatism, is frequently present as well. The disease makes its appearance during the first four months of gestation, though it may not appear until lactation, and it is not rare for it to reappear at each subsequent pregnancy. Primiparæ are particularly predisposed to it. Chorea generally disappears after delivery ; nevertheless, the prognosis in a pregnant woman with chorea must be reserved, in view of the possibility of a miscarriage or of a premature birth. We must also remember that mental troubles are frequent.

Diagnosis.—Chorea must be distinguished from symptomatic hemichorea. This hemichorea, which is generally associated with hemiplegia and hemianæsthesia, appears to result from a lesion in the foot of the corona radiata, close to the region where a lesion produces hemianæsthesia.

Athetosis (Hammond) is characterized by continuous movement of the fingers and the toes, and by the impossibility of keeping them at rest ; it is a variety of post-hemiplegic hemichorea.

Hysterical chorea must claim our attention for a moment, because the association of chorea and hysteria may take place in various ways. Sometimes a patient with ordinary chorea is clearly hysterical ; at other times the hysteria is less manifest, but undeniable stigmata are found, such as painful hysterogenous points, constriction of the field of vision, and hemianæsthesia (Marie). In these various cases the morbid association takes place between hysteria and ordinary chorea, and the patient is attacked by arrhythmic chorea, with contradictory and illogical movements. "But in opposition to this variety of chorea, complicated by hysteria, we must place another variety of hysterical chorea in which hysteria has the largest part, because it gives to the choreic movements their signification. This variety, also called hysterical rhythmic chorea, is characterized by systematic, rhythmical movements. One patient shows movements of the shoulder, movements of flexion and extension of the trunk. We must speak of it as a deep and repeated salutation, rendered ridiculous by its very repetition and by its exaggeration" (Charcot). This form of chorea may last for months and years ; in some cases, on the contrary, it ceases suddenly.

Under the name of **electrical chorea,** Dubini has described an affection, characterized by rapid shocks, accompanied by acceleration of the pulse and rise in temperature, and generally ending in an attack of apoplexy. "It may be asked whether it is a special form of cerebro-spinal typhus, or an abnormal meningitis, but it certainly is not chorea" (Jaccoud).

The name of electrical chorea has also been given to a rhythmical convulsive neurosis, differing from chorea, and especially frequent in children.

Several times a minute the little sufferer is seized with sudden and rapid muscular spasms, like an electrical discharge ; the head is suddenly jerked forwards or backwards. In another patient the spasm consists in a sudden elevation of the shoulders, or in a jerking forward of an arm. Tartar emetic sometimes causes the immediate disappearance of the choreiform movements.

Under the name of **variable chorea** (Brissaud) a kind of chorea has been described, which in its initial period resembles true chorea, and which later becomes modified, and is accompanied by complex, polymorphous movements. After remissions and sudden recurrences, the movements become more rare, more sudden, and more limited, reappearing almost always under the same form, and resembling a tic. Variable chorea is essentially degenerative ; it appears in most cases at the age of puberty.

Chorea must be distinguished from cramps, tics, and "systematic locomotor impulses" (Jaccoud), which have nothing in common with true chorea. Most of these morbid conditions, *chorea saltatoria et festinans* and *chorea rotatrix*, differ from true chorea, in that the abnormal movements are not continuous ; they may even be suspended by an energetic effort of the will. Volition never suspends the movements of chorea ; on the contrary, it increases them.

The convulsive condition described by Friedrich under the name of *paramyoclonus multiplex* must be distinguished from Sydenham's chorea. This disease is characterized by sudden involuntary clonic convulsions, generally without displacement of the affected limb. The convulsions are repeated at unequal intervals, and generally affect a certain number of symmetrical muscles of the limbs. The movements may be diminished by an effort of will. Psychical, secretory, and vaso-motor troubles are generally absent. The disease may appear suddenly, last for months or years, and then recover.

Various methods of treatment have been praised in chorea. The ether spray to the vertebral column, arsenical preparations, bromide of potassium, chloral, cold douches, sulphur baths, gymnastic exercises, have all given some results. Antipyrin gives remarkable results ; salicylate of soda may be given with it. In hypnotizable subjects suggestion has sometimes cut short the attacks of chorea.

The **pathological anatomy** of chorea is still obscure, and side by side with absolutely negative post-mortem examinations dissimilar lesions of the nerve centres have been found, but they have no pathogenic value. I shall return to this subject in the following section.

XI. CHOREA GRAVIS—CHOREIC PSYCHOSES.

Although chorea is generally a benign disease, especially in children, there are, nevertheless, cases in which it is followed by death. The relative gravity of chorea is shown by the following statistics : In 158 cases of Sydenham's chorea Sée quotes nine deaths. In 235 cases in children Bonnaud quotes only one death. In 327 cases of chorea in childhood Triboulet collected eight fatal cases. After adding up these various statistical tables, we find that chorea is fatal on an average in 2 to 3 per cent. of the cases. These statistics agree with Trousseau's assertion : " Although St. Vitus's dance generally ends in recovery, this disease may be fatal. However rare these cases may be, they are none the less too frequent."

The point, however, is to know why and how chorea is fatal, because the prognosis is especially affected by the answer. I shall follow Leudet, Sturges, and Charcot, and divide the cases of fatal chorea into two classes. The first group includes those cases of chorea in which death results from the complications ; the second group includes those cases of chorea which are fatal *per se*.

Death from Complications.—Let me mention first the cardiac lesions— endocarditis, especially vegetative endocarditis, which is a frequent complication of chorea in the adult. The choreic patient may die during an attack of chorea, from endopericarditis or myocarditis, but he is more likely to die later, when he is no longer choreic, the cardiac lesion giving rise to cerebral embolism, apoplexy, or softening.

Amongst the complications which may cause death in the choreic patient cerebral hæmorrhage has been noticed.

In Buchanan-Baxter's case—a young girl, eight years of age, who suffered from recurrent chorea, and who died from apoplexy—the post-mortem examination showed a cerebral hæmorrhage, which had invaded the left ventricle.

Chorea is sometimes fatal, in consequence of purulent infection. In Thompson's case a child nine years of age suffered during the decline of its chorea from pustules on the index-finger, on the sacrum, on the occiput, with abscesses in the scapular region, and consecutive gangrene. At the post-mortem examination lobular pneumonia was found. Trousseau speaks of a young girl who, during an attack of chorea, suffered from a whitlow, with cellulitis of the hand, wrist, and forearm. Cellulitis soon appeared in the lower limbs, and the patient succumbed. Guinon has published a case of chorea which proved fatal in consequence of complications of a similar nature. The patient had a diffuse cellulitis of the left arm, purulent infiltration of the right arm, foci of lobular pneumonia in both lungs, and, further, the patient was four months pregnant. Pregnancy generally makes the prognosis of chorea worse ; the pregnant condition, when associated with chorea, aggravates the latter (Jaccoud).

We have, then, in the first group a certain number of dissimilar cases, which prove that cardiac lesions, cerebral lesions, purulent infection, bronchopneumonia, and pregnancy may, for various reasons, render the prognosis of chorea more grave, and may cause death.

Death in Consequence of Chorea.—In the other group, however, the chorea is fatal *per se*. The following case is taken from one of my clinical lectures :*

A young man, nineteen years of age, was admitted for Sydenham's chorea. The diagnosis presented no difficulty. From the first I was struck with the severity of the attack, which was only five days old. The movements never stopped day nor night; he performed thousands of involuntary gesticulations. He sat down on his bed, as if moved by a spring. He turned round suddenly, and would have hurt himself had it not been for the attendants who were looking after him. His head beat the pillows; his face made the most various grimaces. The muscles of the tongue and of the pharynx participated in these disorderly movements, so that deglutition was extremely difficult, and speech was reduced to an unintelligible mumbling. The skin over the elbows, the hips, and the heels was erythematous.

As the patient was incapable of giving any information, we questioned his parents. They told us that the chorea had commenced five days previously on the left side of the body, and had speedily become general. They also told us (and this is of the utmost importance) that about ten days prior to the appearance of the chorea their son had shown some intellectual disorder. He commenced to make incoherent speeches, talking to himself, rambling in his speech, and showing extreme irritation. He suddenly broke the thread of his conversation, and turned to another subject. He complained bitterly of imaginary wrongs. Several times he was seized with hallucinations of sight and hearing. He came home one day looking very worried, and saying that he had just seen his father fighting with several strange men. As he was telling his tale, his father arrived, and he had the greatest difficulty in convincing the boy that the fight existed only in his imagination. This mental condition lasted four or five days, and then gave place to stupor and to profound melancholia. The chorea then made its appearance. Whilst in this state the patient was admitted. He had a dull look, and was incapable of making any intellectual effort. The pulse was quick, the insomnia was complete; there was incontinence of fæces. The urine contained neither albumin nor sugar. The patient had not had rheumatism, and the heart was healthy. I gave a very bad prognosis, stating that I feared the youth would only live a few days. I did not take this view because of the severity of the choreic movements, because the most violent chorea may recover; but it was suggested to me by the association of the mental condition with the chorea, an association which is nearly always of fatal augury. I recalled to my mind a young girl who suffered from chorea, associated with acute mania, and whom I had seen die in about a fortnight in Trousseau's ward. I prescribed cold douches, wet packs, bromides, and antipyrin—treatment which succeeds well in cases of simple chorea. The treatment proved futile. In a few days grave complications appeared: the temperature rose, the pulse-rate was 150, the heart was irregular, and, as it were, delirious. The choreic movements were followed by a relative calm. The patient lay stupefied, and uttering inarticulate cries. The loss of flesh was so rapid that the muscles seemed to melt away before our eyes; an ecthymatous eruption appeared on the face, the trunk, and the limbs. The temperature rose to 104° F., and the patient died six days after his admission into my ward, and twenty-one days after the commencement of the illness. The family refused a post-mortem examination.

Charcot: A youth of eighteen had been suffering for three weeks with Sydenham's chorea. On his admission to the Salpêtrière the choreic movements had reached their maximum, being present day and night without intermission. The patient, whether in bed or in an arm-chair, was a prey to the most extensive movements. The elbows

---

* " Un Cas de Chorée mortelle " (*Clinique Médicale de l'Hôtel-Dieu*, 1897, 8me leçon).

and the bony points became red, in consequence of the violent and incessant rubbing. Immediately after his admission he created a scene, saying that he could not stand the smell in the ward, and that he could not remain with such common persons as his fellow-patients. Next day he complained that he was being persecuted by the nurses. He said that they accused him of suffering from syphilis. He maintained that his scrotum had been removed. During the following days the chorea and the mental condition remained the same. He had complete insomnia and involuntary emission of urine.

The patient, who had lost much flesh, did not recognize the people around him. The pulse was irregular, and the rate was 140 a minute, and the temperature was over 104° F. His hands and nose became cyanosed; his face was expressionless. Subsultus appeared, and death supervened on the twenty-seventh day of the disease. The autopsy only revealed some scattered adhesions between the pia mater and the cerebral cortex. The results of the post-mortem examination were, says Charcot, purely negative. The complications causing death were evidently not due to an appreciable organic lesion, and the comparison made by Charcot between the status epilepticus and the status choreicus is perfectly justified. Some old vegetations were present on the mitral valve. The patient had not suffered from rheumatism.

De Beauvais: A little girl, fourteen years of age, was taken ill with Sydenham's chorea, and almost at the same time with cerebral disorder. When the chorea appeared, she experienced a sudden distaste for study and for music, of which she was fond. She almost lost her memory; her character became capricious and violent without any reason. She struck her little sister, aged eighteen months. She had gloomy forebodings, and on seeing a hearse, she cried excitedly : "That is the carriage which is soon going to take me away." In a few days her condition became most grave. The spasm of the laryngeal and thoracic muscles brought on fits of suffocation ; deglutition was almost impossible. The patient seemed to be suffering from aphasia. The fever was high ; the pulse was 120. There was continual insomnia and incontinence of urine. The restlessness became extreme. The elbows became excoriated ; the ears, the nape of the neck, the sacrum, and the heels were raw from the incessant rubbing of the skin on the sheets. During the next few days the fever increased ; the pulse-rate rose to 150. The patient fell into a state of coma, and died about twenty days after the commencement of the chorea.

Mitchinson : A woman, twenty-one years of age, who had had four previous attacks of chorea of increasing gravity, was admitted into hospital for a severe attack of chorea. The temperature was 104° F. The patient was very noisy and restless. During the next few days the insomnia was absolute. The mental phase became complete ; delirium set in. The pulse-rate was 144, and the temperature ran up to 107° F. The face was livid, the respiration irregular. The pulse became almost imperceptible and the extremities grew cyanosed. The patient died on the twelfth day. At the post-mortem examination the cerebral lesions were unimportant ; the brain was hyperæmic. Vegetations were found on the mitral valve. The patient had not had rheumatism.

Another case of Mitchinson refers to a youth of sixteen years of age with chorea consequent on an attack of rheumatism. The mental phase soon appeared. The patient became noisy, calling out and throwing himself in every direction. No treatment succeeded in calming him. The choreic movements continued. The pulse-rate rose to 130 ; the respiration became quick ; the temperature reached 105° F. ; and the patient died. At the post-mortem examination cerebral hyperæmia was found. There were a few vegetations on the mitral valve.

Donkin and Hebb : A young girl, twenty years of age, was admitted into the Westminster Hospital for generalized chorea. The patient was also suffering from violent mania. She struck the attendants, and rushed about the staircases, uttering piercing shrieks. The insomnia was absolute ; the delirium continued night and day. She suffered from hallucinations, thinking that her mother was dead, and that she saw her in the next ward. Under the influence of morphia the patient went to sleep for a short time, but on awakening, it was impossible to keep her quiet. She drove the nurse out of the ward, locked herself in, and broke the furniture. She was at last overcome, but only with much difficulty. The patient gradually wore herself out. She began to get drowsy; the respiration became halting, and she died. Nothing was discovered at the post-mortem examination.

Powell has reported two similar cases. A youth, nineteen years of age, was taken ill with generalized chorea six weeks after rheumatism. At the time the chorea was most violent; the pulse-rate was 170. Deglutition was almost impossible. The patient, who was violent and suspicious, had delusions of persecution, and believed that his food was poisoned. The restlessness and delirium gave place to a phase of calm. The appetite and thirst were so excessive that the patient gained 22 pounds in less than a fortnight. The disease then resumed its course. The choreic and delirious symptoms reappeared, and would not yield either to chloral or to other sedatives. The patient became comatose, and died six weeks after the onset of his illness. Hyperæmia of the brain and of the meninges was found at the autopsy. A few vegetations were present on the mitral valve.

In another case of Powell a woman of twenty years of age had violent generalized chorea. A fortnight after the commencement of the chorea, the patient showed symptoms of mental alienation, with hallucinations of sight and hearing. The pulse-rate was 140; there was nystagmus of both eyes; the temperature rose above 120° F. After alternating amelioration and aggravation, the patient fell into a condition of exhaustion, which gradually became more marked. The choreic movements ceased almost completely, and the mental faculties grew clear. Coma then set in, and the patient died. The autopsy revealed acute congestion of the meninges and of the brain.

Cook and Clifford have reported a case in which a little girl of nine years of age was taken ill with hemichorea on the right side. It soon became generalized, and was complicated with delirium. On her admission into hospital, violent choreic movements were present. The pulse stood at 160 pulsations a minute. The face expressed terror. During the following days the little sufferer uttered cries, and passed her motions and her urine under her. The heart beat quickly, and the pulse grew imperceptible. The respiration was irregular and jerky, and the patient died on the sixth day. The post-mortem examination showed that the brain and the upper part of the spinal cord were healthy. There were a few vegetations on the mitral valve.

Rousseau: A youth, nineteen years of age, was taken ill on the third day of an attack of chorea with furious delirium. He was taken to Beaujon Hospital, where they had the greatest difficulty in putting him to bed. His agitation increased; his eyes were haggard; he talked incessantly; and deglutition was most difficult. Hydrotherapy did not quiet the patient. He suffered from paroxysms, in which the choreic movements and the maniacal condition became more severe. He also had hallucinations of sight and hearing. He refused his draught, saying it was poisoned. He died, and at the autopsy no especial lesion was discovered.

Discussion.—These cases give us an exact idea of fatal chorea. In the first place, I would point out that all the cases of fatal chorea which I have just described (cases of chorea fatal of themselves) refer to young people or to adults. One single case, that of Cook and Clifford, refers to a little girl of nine years of age. The other patients were at least fourteen years of age.

It is, therefore, very rare for this variety of chorea to be fatal before the age of fourteen, which explains the absence of fatal cases in the statistics referring to young children. The gravity of the disease coincides especially with the age of puberty. Thus, as Charcot has pointed out, under the age of twelve to fourteen years, although the choreic convulsions may be most severe, a fatal issue is not to be expected as long as there is no rheumatic, cardiac, pulmonary, or other complication. " But after this a remarkable change takes place in the clinical history of chorea ; and we may then witness, contrary to the rule in the previous periods of life, the onset of grave symptoms, whether the disease remains in the chronic condition, or whether it takes the more or less rapid form, and, without the aid of any visceral complication, leads to a fatal termination " (Charcot).

If we look carefully for danger-signals, we shall find them in the **mental condition** of the patients. We have seen in the previous chapter that chorea is almost always accompanied by some intellectual troubles. They are so frequent that they may be considered as epiphenomena. They are more or less lasting and more or less marked, but they do not affect the prognosis. The symptoms which constitute the mental condition present in each of the preceding cases are very different. These symptoms— hallucination of sight and of hearing, acute delirium, delusions of persecution, melancholia—comprise the mental troubles, or **choreic psychoses**, which, when associated with chorea, point to a fatal issue. If we take these cases separately, we find in each one similar cerebral troubles.

In my patient at the Hôtel-Dieu the mental phase appeared a fortnight before the choreic phase, with hallucinations of sight and hearing, incoherent speech, great restlessness, stupor, and melancholia. In Charcot's patient the choreic phase preceded the mental phase, and the principal symptoms of the latter were maniacal excitement, delusions of persecution, and melancholia. In Beauvais' patient the choreic phase and the cerebral condition appeared at the same time. The principal symptoms of the latter were violent delirium and lipemania. In the two patients of Mitchinson the choreic phase preceded the onset of delirium. In the patient of Donkin and Hebb the choreic phase was immediately followed by a mental phase, characterized by most violent delirium, with hallucinations of sight and hearing. One of Powell's patients suffered during the course of the chorea from delirium of persecution. In the other patient the choreic phase preceded the phase of mental alienation by a fortnight. In Rousseau's patient the choreic phase preceded the mental phase by three days. It was characterized by most violent delirium, with hallucinations of sight and of hearing.

I shall not attempt to discuss the pathogenesis of choreic psychosis, because it is still a matter of theory. That it may be a question of heredity, of predisposed subjects, of degenerates, and of a soil being favourable to the production of psychoses, is absolutely true. This, however, does not prevent our seeing cases in which heredity is not in evidence, and the patient is not a degenerate, but yet the mental condition associated with chorea appears in a most marked degree.

Whenever we find grave mental troubles (hallucinations of sight and of hearing, mania, and delirium) in a young adult, especially if there is also any hereditary taint, we must be on our guard. I do not say that the prognosis must necessarily be fatal, but in any case it is most serious. The imminent gravity of the prognosis rests on certain signs which Charcot has described : rise of temperature, cardiac arrhythmia, unusual acceleration of the pulse, paralysis of the sphincters, cyanosis, rapid loss of flesh, diminution or cessation of the choreic movements, which are replaced by subsultus tendinum, fictitious improvement, and sudden disappearance of the delirium, replaced by stupor. These signs, which point to death within a short time, were all present in the case of Charcot's patient, and I found them in my patient.

Such is the picture of chorea gravis. The mental condition dominates the situation and regulates the gravity of the prognosis, and the patient dies, according to Charcot's comparison, in a status choreicus, resembling the status epilepticus, without our being able to find the reason of this excessive gravity at the post-mortem examination.

Unfortunately, treatment is very unsuccessful in this variety of chorea. It would seem at first sight that we might obtain good results from chloroform, administered in large doses ; but in one of Mitchinson's patients, who took so much chloroform that he slept for nearly forty-eight hours, the symptoms reappeared, and terminated in death. Another of Mitchinson's patients was treated with large injections of morphia, but neither the injections of morphia nor the inhalations of chloroform which were also given affected the disease.. I may say the same for the administration of chloral and of bromides, which Charcot employed without result. Hydrotherapy has been recommended. While a douche can be given, baths are absolutely impracticable. It might, perhaps, be rational in such a case to use the ether spray along the vertebral column, to apply leeches behind the ears, and to blister the scalp ; but I am afraid that these remedies would have no more success than the others.

XII. TETANY.

Description. — Tetany, described by Dance under the name of "intermittent tetanus," is generally announced by a sensation of tingling and of numbness in the parts which are about to be affected by spasms. Rigidity then appears, followed by painful contraction analogous to cramp. The cramps occur in a constant order, first affecting the upper limbs. The thumb is adducted, the fingers are pressed against one another, slightly bent on the metacarpus, and the hand has been compared with the hand of a beggar asking for alms, or with the hand of the accoucheur which he is about to insert into the vagina (Trousseau). Flexion and extension of the fingers are less common. In a case reported by Hérard the flexion of the fingers was so great that the nails penetrated the flesh. The wrist is nearly always in the position of flexion. When the contraction reaches the lower limbs, the toes are flexed and pressed together, the heel is drawn upwards, and the foot is strongly arched. The contracted muscles are painful, and resist attempts to alter the position of the tetanized parts.

The contraction may last for several hours in the shape of a fit. It disappears, and then returns during the day, or during the following day, and the series of fits constitutes the attack, which lasts for several weeks. It is easy to reproduce the fit artificially. It is sufficient " to exercise a compression on the affected limbs, either along the nerve trunks or on the bloodvessels " (Trousseau).

The tetany just described is the benign form of the disease. It is sometimes accompanied by anæsthesia, paresis, and œdema of the invaded parts. It is generally bilateral, affects the upper extremities more often than the lower ones, and recovers without other complications. More severe forms, however, occur. The contraction, instead of remaining limited to the extremities, attacks the muscles of the trunk and of the face. It causes spasms of the muscles of the eyes, of the pharynx, and of the larynx (spasms of the glottis), and it may attack the muscles of respiration, causing attacks of dyspnœa similar to those of tetanus and threatening the life of the patient.

Ætiology.—The disease is most frequent about the age of twenty, and from the first to the third year (Rilliet and Barthez). We find a primary form, provoked by cold, and more or less associated with rheumatism, and a secondary form, determined by typhoid fever, cholera, dentition, diarrhœa. Pregnancy and lactation are such frequent causes that the disease was called " rheumatic contracture of wet-nurses." Tetany is met with in hysteria, and imitation provokes it. An epidemic form has been described (Simon).

Albarran and Caussade are of opinion that the same origin may be ascribed to tetany and to tetanus when it is consequent on lesions and on intestinal troubles. Clinically, it is difficult to define the absolute limit between tetanus and tetany, and in some cases doubt has persisted (Guinon, Bouveret, and Devic). Experimentally, Albarran and Caussade have been able to provoke convulsions and transitory contractions in the hind-legs of a dog by injecting Nicolaiev's bacillus into the intestine after having ligatured it. Furthermore, these authors, by causing acute intestinal obstruction, found in the intestines of dogs which had died with more or less localized convulsions a drum-stick-like bacillus, that differed from Bienstock's bacillus. These facts would seem to indicate that tetany may be due to Nicolaiev's bacillus.

XIII. OCCUPATION NEUROSES.

The immoderate use of certain muscles ends by causing such an irritability in these muscles that they pass into a condition of contracture.
Cramps and spasms are the result.   These spasms are met with in many
professions—writers (writer's cramp is the most common), pianists, com-
positors, etc., are liable to this neurosis, and it must be remarked that a
special predisposition of the patient is also present in most instances.

In **writers** the cramp appears as soon as the individual tries to write.
It attacks the flexor and extensor muscles of the fingers, and may extend
to the muscles of the forearm.   Before arriving so far the troubles have
been transient and gradual.   The subject at first has a feeling of stiffness
and of numbness in the fingers.   This sensation is produced after writing
for some considerable time, and the disease gradually declares itself.   The
very idea of holding a pen then brings on the functional spasm, and if
the patient learns to write with his left hand, the spasm sometimes appears
in it.   The spasm may be replaced by choreiform movements.

Duchenne has quoted many cases of occupation neuroses.   In a tailor the hand
turned inwards as soon as he tried to make a few stitches.   In a fencing-master the
sword-arm turned inwards as soon as he stood on guard.   A turner could not work
his lathe without the flexor muscles of his foot becoming contracted.   In a pavior the
sterno-cleido-mastoid muscles were contracted.   In a country parson who played the
serpent the inspiratory muscles on the right side became contracted at each violent
inspiration.

Cramps have been noted in the left hand of violinists, in the right hand
of telegraph operators who used the Morse instrument (Onimus); in the
fingers of milkers (Eulenberg); in the legs of dancers, etc.

These various spasms have an indefinite duration, and are rebellious to
all forms of treatment.

CHAPTER VII

NEURALGIA

I. MIGRAINE.

Description. — Migraine is a disease of attacks. "Every person who suffers from continuous headache is therefore excluded." The fits recur every week or every month, or at more distant intervals, and it is exceptional for a patient to have two fits in one week. The attack of migraine lasts at least six hours, and not more than forty-eight hours.

The initial or prodromal period is characterized by symptoms of depression—inaptitude for work and loss of appetite ; or by symptoms of excitation—alacrity and intellectual vivacity. The disease then pursues its incubation, and after a night of heavy and prolonged sleep the fit appears.

In the second period the headache appears. There is at first a sensation of pressure, which is most severe in the orbital, supra-orbital, or temporal regions, and the pain then makes its appearance. It becomes diffuse, without limiting itself, like neuralgia, to the course of a nerve trunk, and without encroaching on the suborbital region. The pain of migraine may be unbearable (sensation of crushing, of perforation, or of dislocation of the bones of the skull). It is rather dull than lancinating, and is increased by walking and by movement. The face is pale or injected ; the temporal artery is hard and prominent, and beats forcibly on the side of the hemicrania. The bloodvessels of the retina are dilated. The senses become very acute, the least noise or the least ray of light increasing the pains. Sudden displacement of the pain during the attack is a curious fact, hemicrania of the right side passing to the left side, and *vice versa*. From the commencement of the attack the patient suffers from nausea, which increases as the day wears on. The fits of yawning, the attacks of nausea, the eructations and the vomiting, are not accompanied by pain in the stomach or by diarrhœa. Constipation is the rule. Vomiting in the first period is not an index of recovery. In the second period it sometimes shortens the attack. During the period of decline the headache and the nausea become less severe, but the sufferer remains in a condition of mental torpor, which only disappears with sleep. The sufferer is not cured until he has eaten.

Ophthalmic Migraine.—The predominance of ocular troubles has led to the description of an ophthalmic form of migraine. In the simple forms, eye symptoms of a nervous character form the most important part of the attack. The patient experiences a kind of obnubilation, of monocular or binocular hemiopia, or of scintillating scotoma. He sees a sheaf of stars, balls of fire, or fortification figures. Frontal headache, nausea, and vomiting then appear. In the severe forms ophthalmic migraine is accompanied by transient aphasia, and by numbness, formication, jerks, and paresis of one side of the body. Epileptiform convulsions have been noted. Although ophthalmic migraine is not grave, we must remember that in some cases it has been the precursor of locomotor ataxy and of general paralysis (Charcot).

Ætiology—Diagnosis.—Whether considered as a neurosis or as a neuralgia, migraine is rarely an isolated disease. It is almost always associated with the gouty diathesis, of which it is only a manifestation. It is hereditary, like the diathetic diseases. An individual who in his youth suffers from migraine will later be liable to eczema, asthma, gravel, or gout (Trousseau). Rheumatism, chorea, and migraine are closely related. Migraine generally makes its appearance at an early age. If a person has not had migraine at the age of twenty-five years, he is almost certain to escape it. The attacks of migraine often return without appreciable cause. At other times they are brought on by late hours, digestive disorders, certain odours, bright lights, menstruation, excess of work, or change of weather.

The anatomical cause of migraine has been variously interpreted. It has been attributed to excitation (Dubois-Raymond), or to paralysis of the sympathetic nerves (Mollendorff), and to neuralgia of the meningeal branches of the trifacial nerve.

The characteristics of migraine are so clearly defined that it is impossible to confound the headache of migraine with any other headache (headache due to cerebral tumours, growing headache, syphilitic and hysterical headache, pains of meningitis). Errors of diagnosis are, however, made for want of sufficient attention. Headache is too readily called migraine when it does not possess the true character of migraine. Mistakes are often made in the case of growing headaches and of paroxysmal headaches, caused in children or in youths by late hereditary syphilis. The headache of uræmia is often called migraine.

The methods of treatment advised in migraine are numerous. During the attack subcutaneous injections of morphia, antipyrin in solution or in cachets, pyramidon (5 grains), spraying with ether and with chloride of ethyl to the cilio-spinal region, the application of electricity to the forehead, massage, etc., have been recommended.

As a general treatment, hydrotherapy and the bromides constitute the

most efficacious means. To these may be added alkalis, arsenic, and iron.
In certain cases (gouty alternation) the salicylic preparations give good
results.

II. NEURALGIA OF THE TRIFACIAL NERVE—
TIC DOULOUREUX.

The trifacial nerve emerges from the Gasserian ganglion, which is situated
on the internal portion of the anterior surface of the petrous bone. From
the ganglion which has received the root of the trifacial nerve three branches
arise—the ophthalmic, the superior maxillary, and the inferior maxillary
nerves.

Description.—Neuralgia of the trifacial nerve (facial neuralgia)
rarely attacks all three branches of the nerve at the same time. The
ophthalmic branch is more often affected than the superior and inferior
maxillary branches. In some cases the neuralgia confines itself to a single
filament, to the dental nerve, or to the lingual nerve.

The neuralgia reveals itself (1) by continuous pains ; (2) by paroxysmal
pains. The continuous pains are not acute. There is a kind of
numbness in the invaded region. The paroxysmal pains constitute the
attack, which arises as the result of a slight stimulus, and the subject experiences a series of painful shocks, which increase in intensity until the attack
reaches its maximum. The painful shocks, which may be very acute,
recur at more or less close intervals. They sometimes run along a nerve
branch, like a flash of lightning ; at other times they arise at various points,
and rush in various directions. The attack may last for an hour, or even
longer, if the neuralgia is of long standing. It recurs every day, or several
times a day, and often at a fixed hour, with a periodicity which is also met
with in almost every case of idiopathic or symptomatic neuralgia. Pulsation of the arteries, redness of the face, and rise of temperature often
accompany the neuralgia.

Apart from the attack, the skin of the face preserves a hyperæsthesia
which may later give place to anæsthesia. The teeth, the lingual and buccal
mucosæ, and the hair, are also hyperæsthetic. Pressure on the skin is particularly painful : (1) at the exit of the nerve trunks ; (2) at the points where
a nerve filament leaves a muscle to enter the skin ; (3) at the expansion
of the nerve in the skin. Those are Valleix's painful points, which present
the same characteristics in most cases of peripheral neuralgia. To these
painful points the apophysial point must be added (Trousseau). It is
seated over the external occipital protuberance and the second and third
cervical spines. Such are the general characteristics of facial neuralgia,
but, according to the branches invaded, the neuralgia reveals itself by the
following symptoms :

1. *Neuralgia of the Ophthalmic Nerve.*—The ophthalmic nerve enters the orbit by the sphenoidal fissure, and breaks up into three nerves : the lachrymal, which emerges at the outer side of the upper eyelid (palpebral point) ; the frontal, the external branch of which leaves the orbit by the supra-orbital foramen (supra-orbital point) ; the nasal, the external branch of which leaves the orbit near the nose, below the inner canthus of the eye (nasal point), and the internal branch of which enters the nasal fossæ, and furnishes a filament, which traverses the lateral cartilage of the nose, and spreads over the lobule of the nose (naso-lobar point). According to the anatomical distribution of this nerve, we see which are the regions invaded by the neuralgia. During the attack the eye is red, injected, and painful, and cannot bear the light. Lachrymation is profuse. Chemosis, mydriasis, and transitory amaurosis have been met with (Notta).

2. *Neuralgia of the Superior Maxillary Nerve.*—The superior maxillary nerve, after having traversed the supra-orbital canal, emerges through the supra-orbital foramen (supra-orbital point). Amongst the number of its numerous branches are : the orbital nerve, a filament of which—the temporo-malar—traverses the cheek-bone, and spreads over the cheek (malar point) ; the dental nerves, each dental root possibly becoming a centre of pain (dental points). The spheno-palatine ganglion, which is connected to this branch, perhaps explains the secretion from the nasal mucosa during the attack (Vulpian).

3. *Neuralgia of the Inferior Maxillary Nerve.*—From the inferior maxillary nerve arise the branches frequently affected by neuralgia. These are : the auriculo-temporal nerve, which passes through the parotid gland, winds round the neck of the condyle, and distributes itself to the temple and the auricle (auriculo-temporal point) ; the lingual nerve, which supplies the edges of the tongue (lingual point) ; the inferior dental nerve, which supplies the teeth in the lower jaw (dental points), and which makes its exit through the mental foramen (mental point). At the time of the attack the movements of the tongue, speech, mastication, and deglutition are excessively painful, and the saliva, secreted in abundance (reflex action of the lingual nerve on the chorda tympani), flows from the mouth.

Trophic Troubles.—Consequent on violent or inveterate facial neuralgia, the nerve being probably attacked by neuritis, we see various trophic troubles.

Herpes is frequent on the skin and on the mucosæ. It affects, according to circumstances, the lips, the tongue, the forehead, and the face. Herpes of the eye, or ophthalmic zona, has been specially described. It may invade the eyelids, the conjunctiva, and the cornea.

Atrophy, induration (sclerodermia), and hypertrophy of the skin have been noted. The hair and the beard are sometimes attacked. The hair falls out and loses its colour, becoming white throughout its entire length, or only wanting in pigment in sections, this alternation coinciding with the paroxysms of neuralgia. It was at first supposed that the trophic troubles only existed when the Gasserian ganglion was involved. This interpretation, though true in many cases, is not absolute, because similar troubles may be produced when the lesion goes beyond the ganglion to the bulbar root of the trifacial nerve (Duval).

Tic Douloureux of the Face—Epileptiform Neuralgia.—In certain individuals facial neuralgia assumes special characters. The patient is suddenly seized with acute pain ; he presses his face in his hands or rubs it violently, hoping thereby to lessen the pain, and after a few seconds—a minute at the most—the attack ends. Most frequently at the moment of the attack the muscles of the face, especially on the side of the neuralgia, show rapid convulsive movements, which produce the most varied grimaces, so that

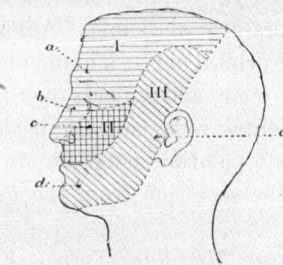

Fig. 84.—Branches of the Trigeminal Nerve.

i, Ophthalmic branch ; ii, superior maxillary branch ; iii, inferior maxillary branch ; *a*, supra-orbital point ; *b*, nasal point ; *c*, infra-orbital point ; *d*, mental point ; *e*, auriculo-temporal point.

the disease has been called **tic douloureux of the face.** These two forms of facial neuralgia—the one non-convulsive, the other convulsive—were called epileptiform by Trousseau, because they resembled the vertigo and the aura of epilepsy. They have its suddenness and its duration. Nevertheless, says Trousseau, they are merely analogous, and not identical with epilepsy.

Tic douloureux does not always establish itself from the outset, but is at times the transformation of a non-convulsive facial neuralgia. In certain patients the attacks follow one another almost without respite. In others there is a longer interval between the attacks. The attack is sometimes produced without apparent cause ; at other times it is produced by the most varied and trifling causes. A simple scratch, the act of mastication, the contact of food and drink, the movements undertaken for the purpose of speaking or of expectorating, may bring on the spasm, so that the patient suffers agony. The question is thoroughly discussed in the lecture given by Trousseau. From this lecture I borrow the following case :

" An old lady," says Trousseau, " came under my care in 1845. She had been suffering from epileptiform neuralgia of the face for the past ten years. The attacks lasted from a few seconds to three minutes. They sometimes commenced in the sub-orbital nerve, sometimes in the mental, and at other times in the supra-orbital nerve. The trouble rapidly spread to the three branches, and when the paroxysm was at its height the muscles of the face worked convulsively. The poor woman had sometimes twenty attacks in an hour ; they returned on the least movement. She could not speak, cough, eat, or drink without having a most severe paroxysm. To moderate the pain, she rapidly carried her hand to her face, which she pressed violently, making the skin move over the bones. When the pain was more acute, she started up and walked about the room, stamping her foot and uttering dull groans. At times the attacks did not appear for a week, a fortnight, a month, or even longer. They then returned with renewed vigour.

" The most remarkable thing was that the pain disappeared completely after each paroxysm, except for a feeling of numbness. I ordered morphia internally, commencing with fairly large doses of 3 to 5 grains a day, and being resolved to increase the doses if the drug was well borne. In less than a fortnight I was giving 60 grains each day. The improvement was great. During the course of the day she had only slight shocks of dull pain in the branches of the trifacial nerve. The digestive functions were but little disturbed, and the intellectual faculties were in good condition ; but the patient having a limited fortune, the enormous price of morphia almost ruined her. I therefore had recourse to opium. She began to suffer as soon as she ceased using the remedy. I found a chemist who consented to sell her raw opium at the market-price, and she was able to obtain raw opium, which she made up into 15-grain pills, and took five, ten, or twenty a day, as occasion arose.

" It is remarkable that these enormous doses of opium did not notably disturb her digestion. There was no somnolence, and she obtained her usual rest at night. For six years I saw the patient from time to time, and I was able to notice the following therapeutic effects : She sometimes had no attack for two or three months. She then suspended the use of the opium, after having gradually diminished the quantity in proportion as the pains diminished. The epileptiform neuralgia then returned suddenly with renewed violence. She took from the first about $\frac{1}{2}$ ounce of raw opium, and kept up this dose until the attack had calmed down. The opium, therefore, gave her immense relief, but did not completely cure her, and I repeat, especially since my attention has been especially called to this kind of neuralgia, I have never met with a case that was curable."

Ætiology.—Every neuralgia presupposes a change in a sensory nerve at some point of its origin, course, or termination. The change in the nerve may betray itself by more or less gross lesions, by neuritis, congestion, œdema, or abnormal condition of the blood ; or the change may be purely dynamic, then escaping our means of investigation. Dynamic troubles are met with in all the manifestations of the nervous system, whether we have to deal with the nerve centres (neuroses) or with the sensory or motor nerves. The nervous organ the functions of which are disturbed is evidently in an abnormal condition, but this abnormal condition may reveal itself by material lesions, or by a purely dynamic change, without alteration of structure or of texture.

With regard to this subject certain correct comparisons have been made. A Leyden jar charged with electricity and one not so charged, a piece of soft iron which is magnetized and a piece which is not magnetized differ in their properties, and yet there is no change in the texture or in the structure of the anatomical elements ; there is only a modification in the **transmission of the forces.** Analogous comparisons are applicable to the disorders of the nervous system.

Facial neuralgia is often the result of an infection (malaria, syphilis). It is associated with rheumatism and with gout. The local causes act at some point of the nerve : at its periphery (trauma, foreign bodies, dental caries, coryza) ; along its course (lesions of the bone and of the periosteum, tumours, aneurysm of the internal carotid artery) ; in the Gasserian ganglion (cancer, exostosis of the petrous bone) ; at the bulbar origin (locomotor ataxy). Cold, a frequent cause of facial neuralgia, attacks the terminal expansion of the nerves, or causes swelling of the nerve-trunk and its strangulation in the bony canal of the petrous bone. Neuralgia is sometimes the result of a reflex action (intestinal worms).

Amongst these causes malaria is frequent, and deserves to arrest our attention. The malarial infection has a predilection for the ophthalmic nerve. Many people infected with malaria one or two years previously are seized, without warning and without fever, with facial neuralgia, which is really an attack of larval malaria. The neuralgia reappears every day or every other day. It may be very severe, and accompanied by intolerable pains, vomiting, prostration, and sweating.

The **diagnosis** of facial neuralgia is simple. Its pathogenic diagnosis is important, because it decides the treatment. The duration of the disease, its course, and its gravity are dependent on the cause. We see benign cases which readily yield to therapeutic means, and obstinate cases which resist all remedies.

The **treatment** differs according to the cause of the neuralgia. Quinine is absolutely indicated in cases of malarial origin. It must be given in large doses, 15 grains in two doses, repeated every day for a week. From this period a longer interval is allowed between the doses of quinine. In the other varieties of facial neuralgia we may employ the following remedies : Opium in large doses ; aconitine, in doses of $\frac{1}{2}$ milligramme daily, and gradually increased to 4 to 5 milligrammes, has been praised by Gubler.

Subcutaneous injections of morphia diminish the attacks, and may be curative. We may inject daily a grain of hydrochlorate of morphia, and in certain individuals the toleration is such that we may use enormous doses. I have several times had a patient suffering from epileptiform facial neuralgia, which I could only relieve by injecting daily from 10 to 15 grains of hydrochlorate of morphia.

The methyl chloride spray (Debove) has been advised. Antipyrin may be given in doses of 30 to 60 grains a day. Bromide of potassium in large doses gives good results. The application of electricity must be tried (Lacaille). A continuous current of from ten to twelve units is passed for a few minutes, the negative pole being placed at the exit of the nerve, and the positive pole at the periphery of the nerve (Onimus). We must never forget that syphilis, as we shall see in the next section, may in various ways cause facial neuralgia.

Surgical treatment has given good results. The first measure is resection of the affected branch. If this is not sufficient, the Gasserian ganglion may be removed.

III. SYPHILITIC NEURALGIA OF THE TRIFACIAL NERVE.

Let me first quote a case from a clinical lecture which I gave on this subject :*

A man, forty-one years of age, came to me "as a last resource," being unable to bear the terrible pains which "had tortured him for the last fourteen years." He had facial neuralgia of the right side, the three branches of the trifacial being affected, but to an unequal degree. As regards the ophthalmic nerve, the frontal branch was chiefly affected, the lachrymal branch to a slight extent, and the nasal branch hardly at all. The orbital and suborbital branches of the superior maxillary nerve were affected, the dental nerves to a slight degree. The inferior maxillary nerve was chiefly affected in its auriculo-temporal and mental branches ; the dental branch was slightly involved, and the lingual branch was unaffected. The patient was admitted into my wards during an attack. The pains were especially severe at night. During the day the pain was bearable. The pain at night prevented any rest, and led him to think of suicide.

The course of the disease had been as follows : The facial neuralgia had commenced, without any apparent cause fourteen years before, in the year 1884. At this period the patient felt some pain in the right side of his face. From the outset the ophthalmic nerve was most affected, whilst the other branches of the trifacial nerve were hardly involved. From the commencement of the disease the nature of the attacks had varied but little. The acute stage of the attack lasted from a fortnight to a month. During this period the pains, which were paroxysmal at night, were accompanied by lachrymation. The patient compared them "with grinding of the bones and tearing of the flesh." There was not in this case, as in tic douloureux, any complete remission, and the pain lasted for hours at a stretch without diminishing.

After a period of suffering, extending over a fortnight or three weeks, the patient experienced relative relief. The sharp pains ceased, and sleep returned, but the region remained painful, and slight shooting-pains proved that the disease was always ready to be awakened. In fact, after a few days or weeks of comparative rest, the attacks reappeared.

The patient had consulted physicians, surgeons, pharmacists, herbalists, and quacks, begging for a relief from his pains, without result.

---

* " Névralgie Syphilitique du Nerf Trijumeau," (*Clinique Médicale de l'Hôtel-Dieu*, 1899, 15me leçon).

Feeling that an operation might help, he went into a private hospital under the care of Schwartz. The pains at this time were so severe and so obstinate that morphia was given in increasing doses. The pains were relieved for the time being, but if the doses of morphia were insufficient, they reappeared. The result was that the patient left the hospital a morphomaniac, and continued the injections of morphia at home. For some time the facial neuralgia was kept in check by injecting large doses of morphia. As soon as the doses of morphia became insufficient, the pains reappeared.

The time came, however, when the injections of morphia had to be abandoned, the punctures having caused numerous abscesses. In 1895—that is to say, after treatment with morphia for over two years—he entered the Saint-Louis Hospital, in order to be treated for morphinomania. The morphia was suppressed, but the facial neuralgia reappeared, and the patient, on the advice of a physician, had recourse to opium. He obtained some relief by increasing the doses progressively.

It was under these conditions that the unfortunate man came into my wards in the hope that I would advise an operation. Whilst I was examining the patient, my attention was directed to the deformity of his nose and to the fœtid odour of his breath. His nose had the appearance of one deformed by syphilis. The rhinoscopic examination proved the existence of tertiary syphilitic rhinitis, with exostoses in both nostrils, and almost complete destruction of the septum and of the inferior meatus. The patient told us that the rhinitis had made its appearance some little time after the facial neuralgia. In 1885 he had symptoms of syphilitic coryza—swelling of the nose, muco-purulent discharge, thick crusts, and fœtor of the breath. The rhinitis did not recede, sequestra came out from the nose, and the ozæna was most distressing.

As the rhinitis had run a parallel course with the facial neuralgia, was it not likely that the neuralgia was also syphilitic ? And this hypothesis granted, was there an exostosis compressing the trifacial nerve at its exit from the Gasserian ganglion, or was there a sclero-gummatous neuritis ? I cannot answer this question, because the examination gave no help in the matter. The point was to decide whether the neuralgia was or was not syphilitic.

The fact that the facial neuralgia had persisted for fourteen years without other symptoms was no reason for eliminating the hypothesis of syphilis. I have quoted elsewhere (Syphilis of the Palate, Syphilitic Sciatica) examples in which syphilis had been limited for ten or twelve years to a special point. An injection of the oily solution of biniodide was administered daily, and I permitted the patient to continue for the time being the daily dose of opium (3 grains) to which he had been accustomed for a long time.

After the eighth injection the relief was so marked that he abandoned the opium. At the same time the rhinitis improved. The ozæna diminished. After fourteen injections the patient slept well, ate with a good appetite, and had put on flesh. The nasal syphilis improved, nasal respiration was almost free, the muco-purulent secretion was slight, and the ozæna had disappeared. Examination of the nose showed that the lesions were rapidly healing.

After the eighteenth injection the patient left the hospital on urgent business. He returned twelve days later, still quite satisfied with his condition, the pains being slight and of short duration. I gave five injections, and he left the hospital cured. He was now able to work from three o'clock in the morning till six o'clock in the evening. To sum up : By means of twenty-six injections of biniodide of mercury we were able to cure one of the most painful diseases which it is possible to see—a disease which had lasted for fourteen years, and which had resisted all remedies. Mercury alone, without the addition of iodide of potassium, brought about this result.

I had a woman in the Hôtel-Dieu under my care for severe syphilitic neuralgia of the trifacial nerve and syphilitic retinitis. Injections of mercury cured the neuralgia, and at the same time considerably relieved the retinitis.

Although syphilitic neuralgia of the trifacial nerve has not been the object of a monograph, it has still received attention. Fournier ("Traité de la Syphilis") devotes a chapter to syphilitic neuralgia. He looks upon secondary facial neuralgia as fairly common. "This secondary facial neuralgia," says he, "is peculiar, in that it does not affect, save in exceptional cases, the inferior branch of the trifacial nerve and the middle branch in rare cases; while the supra-orbital branches are often attacked. Supra-orbital neuralgia certainly occupies the front rank as regards frequency of appearance." Fournier, with regard to this subject, quotes the following case:

"I was called some years ago to see a young married woman who had suffered for four or five months from acute facial neuralgia. All imaginable treatment (sulphate of quinine, opium, belladonna, chloral, bromide, hypodermic injections, blisters, etc.) had been tried, and had little or no result. This want of success with the most rational and most energetic remedies in a young woman whose general health was good, and who had so far been free from any nervous affection, seemed to me somewhat suspicious.

"I sought for the cause of the neuralgia for a long time, and I did not find it. I then examined the patient for any sign of syphilis, and discovered nothing suspicious. I questioned her in this respect, and only obtained a formal denial. As the colleagues who had preceded me had left me nothing to do if it were a case of ordinary neuralgia, I decided to prescribe mercury. The result was dramatic. After two days the patient, who had not slept for several months, was able to rest a little. A week later she was cured. I had, therefore, hit the nail on the head." The patient subsequently confessed that she had had syphilis.

IV. CERVICO-OCCIPITAL AND CERVICO-BRACHIAL NEURALGIA.

Description. — 1. Cervico - occipital neuralgia affects the posterior branches of the first four cervical nerves (cervical plexus), and especially the suboccipital nerve, which arises from the second cervical pair. The pains are analogous to those of facial neuralgia, being continuous or paroxysmal. The pains are seated in the occipital and in the posterior cervical regions. Certain painful points are found. The most frequent one is the **occipital point**, at the exit of the occipital nerve, about midway between the mastoid process and the first cervical vertebra. Apart from the usual causes of neuralgia (cold must be placed in the front rank), there are local causes, such as Pott's disease, periostitis, and caries of the cervical vertebræ, hypertrophic cervical pachymeningitis, adenitis, and cancer of the spine. These lesions give rise to neuralgia, which is almost always bilateral, thus differing from primary cervico-occipital neuralgia, which is unilateral.

2. Cervico-brachial neuralgia attacks most of the sensory branches of the brachial plexus, and especially the ulnar nerve. Neuralgia of the circumflex nerve is sometimes complicated by paresis and atrophy of the deltoid muscle. In neuralgia of the ulnar nerve several painful points are found : the epitrochlear point, where the nerve lies in the epitrochlear groove ; and the ulno-carpal point, where the nerve grooves the carpus before reaching the palm of the hand. Hypertrophy of the heart has been met with in cases of this kind of neuralgia (Potain).

Injury has a large share in the ætiology of this form of neuralgia (dislocations, fractures, burns). I must also mention syphilis. I have seen a case of ulnar neuralgia of syphilitic origin, where the intense pain ceased after a few days of treatment. The treatment of these neuralgias is analogous with that of facial neuralgia. Do not let us forget that syphilis may be a cause, in which case specific treatment must be at once given.

V. NEURALGIA OF THE PHRENIC NERVE.

Although the phrenic nerve is more motor than sensory, its sensory filaments acquire in the pathological condition an exquisite sensibility. The phrenic nerve arises from the third, fourth, and fifth pairs of cervical nerves. It is one of the most important branches of the cervical plexus. It runs along the front of the scalene muscle, enters into the thorax, and spreads out over the diaphragm. The left phrenic nerve passes between the pleura and the pericardium. It may therefore be affected in pericarditis.

Description.—The causes of phrenic neuralgia are those of all forms of neuralgia (cold, rheumatism), to which must be added the causes peculiar to this nerve—diaphragmatic pleurisy, lesions of the organs in the neighbourhood of the diaphragm (liver, spleen), pericarditis, and lesions of the aorta, which act through the pericardium (Peter).

The pain is seated at the base of the thorax, on a level with the insertion of the diaphragm, and by pressure we can determine painful points over the lower ribs at the points of insertion of the diaphragm, and over the lateral part of the neck, in front of the scalenus anticus. The pains often radiate to the branches of the cervical and brachial plexuses and to the circumflex nerve, which explains the pain in the shoulder and the formication and numbness in the hand. The pain in the diaphragm makes the act of respiration painful. It is increased by any movement of the diaphragm, by cough, by yawning, by sighing, and by sneezing. Neuralgia of the phrenic nerve is associated with certain forms of angina pectoris, and forms a part of the symptom-complex in diaphragmatic pleurisy.

VI. INTERCOSTAL NEURALGIA—ZONA.

The twelve dorsal nerves give off posterior and anterior branches. The posterior branches perforate the muscles along the costo-vertebral groove, and spread out over the skin as the posterior perforating nerves. The anterior branches form the intercostal nerves. Each intercostal nerve is placed in the groove of the rib; between the muscles and at about the middle of its course it gives off the lateral perforating branch. The lateral branch of the first two intercostal nerves supplies the skin of the arm ; the others supply the skin of the thorax and of the abdomen. The intercostal nerve continues its course, becomes superficial, and makes its exit just external to the sternum and to the rectus abdominis as the anterior perforating branch.

Description.—Intercostal neuralgia is most frequent on the left side, and more common in women. Chlorosis and hysteria are the most common causes. As regards local causes I may mention pulmonary tuberculosis, caries, necrosis of the ribs and of the vertebræ, Pott's disease, and aneurysm of the aorta. The pain in the side which accompanies pneumonia and pleurisy has been variously interpreted, but it is generally attributed to neuritis or to intercostal neuralgia.

The neuralgia generally attacks several nerves at the same time, and the attacks are not as clearly defined as those of facial neuralgia. The pain, which is more or less continuous, is increased by pressure, by the contact of the clothes, and by deep inspirations. The most constant painful points are the spinal point (Trousseau) and the anterior perforating point. Hyperæsthesia is constant. It is easy to provoke hyperæsthesia by gently rubbing the skin, and thus to define the limit of the neuralgia, which stops just on the median line.

The pains of intercostal neuralgia often cause patients much alarm. Some patients attribute the thoracic pains to an affection of the chest ; others fear a lesion of the heart, because the præcordial pains are brought on by the palpitation that accompanies chlorosis. One patient will speak of gastralgia, when the condition is really epigastralgia (pressure of the corset) ; another talks about disease of the liver, when the skin of the hypochondrium is affected by the neuralgia.

Treatment must include both the general and the local condition of the subject. Antipyrin, tonics, iron, quinine, and hydrotherapy, are of use in the former condition. Locally, injections of pure water or injections of morphia may be given (Potain and Dieulafoy). An ointment of methyl salicylate, one or two leeches, wet-cupping the actual cautery, or a small blister, may be used over the painful area.

Zona—Herpes Zoster.

Zona belongs to the trophic troubles of intercostal neuralgia. The name "zona" (herpes zoster) is given to the groups of vesicles of herpes which develop along the track of one or more intercostal nerves, and form a half-circle around the trunk (ζώνη, girdle). This name "zona," originally reserved for the eruptions of herpes in intercostal neuralgia, is now applied to similar eruptions in the other forms of neuralgia, and we speak of ophthalmic (neuralgia of the trifacial nerve), cervical, brachial, sciatic, lumbo-abdominal, and plantar zona. The vesicular eruption which characterizes zona shows itself in two different conditions. Zona exists as a primary disease ; zoster fever, analogous to the eruptive fevers, is sometimes epidemic, and was considered by Trousseau as being contagious. It has been placed among the infectious diseases by Landouzy. On the other hand, we find **zosteroid eruptions,** symptomatic of grave lesions of the nerve centres or of the peripheral nerves. Such is the zosteroid eruption accompanying the lightning pains of tabes and the zosteroid eruption of syphilis. I shall here deal with **zona.**

Symptoms.—Every case of zona is generally composed of two elements— pain and eruption. The eruption may be limited to one or two small groups of vesicles ; at other times large areas are invaded, the vesicles appearing along the track of the pain. A characteristic eruption may, however, exist without any pain being present. The description of zona applies to all the localizations of the disease, but I shall here confine my description chiefly to intercostal zona, which is the most frequent form. The neuralgia precedes the eruption, and often persists after the eruption has disappeared. The eruption appears at first in the form of erythematous patches, separated by intervals of healthy skin. Transparent vesicles of herpes appear on these patches. In three or four days the development of these vesicles is complete, and the erythematous patch extends about an inch beyond the vesicles. After five or six days the fluid in the vesicles becomes turbid, the vesicle shrivels and becomes covered with a dark crust, and about the twelfth day the eruption ends. The vesicles may unite and form bullæ. The eruption may be accompanied by fever and by enlargement of the glands (Barthélemy). The existence of aberrant vesicles (Tenneson, Jeanselme, Leredde, Giraudeau) is a further plea in favour of the infectious nature of zona.

The intensity of the eruption is not in proportion with the severity of the pains, because pain may be almost absent. Furthermore, the eruption does not always follow the anatomical course of a nerve. Thus, in the thorax the half-circle formed by the eruption is almost perpendicular to the axis of the body, whilst the ribs and the intercostal nerve run an oblique course from above downwards. The same remark applies to the other varieties of zona.

Zona is often followed by painful neuralgia, which may last for months and years. Painful facial paralysis is sometimes accompanied by zona. I shall discuss this question under Facial Paralysis. Raymond, Klippel, and Aynaud have quoted some examples. Zona presents special features, according to the age of the patient. Thus in children at the breast zona is generally benign and painless. In old people, on the contrary, the pain is very severe and obstinate. In some cases zona is chronic, and may persist for many months, whether it recurs *in situ* or in a neighbouring region, or whether the vesicles give place to ulcerations, which sometimes end in keloid (Leudet).

Pathogenesis—Metamerism.—Zona was formerly considered as a trophic trouble due to changes in the sensory nerves, and has been explained in an ingenious manner by Brissaud. He has emphasized the discord between the topography of zona and the nerve supply of the peripheral nerves, the vesicles not corresponding in all cases to the sensory distribution of these nerves. He considers that zona has a spinal origin. The topography of zona can be explained by the embryological relation between each segment of the skin and a metameric segment of the spinal cord. These segments comprise a series of superposed metameres. The metameres are readily seen in the embryo of the chicken from the sixty-eighth hour, and even in the human embryo in the shape of lateral protuberances of the primitive nerve axis—Houssay's neurotomes. The limbs are composed of metameric stages of the second order. This metameric disposition accounts for certain facts which are apparently inexplicable, such as the girdles of anæsthesia in syringomyelia, the symmetrical disposition of the tropho-neuroses, the strange colouring of the coat in certain mammals—in the Belgian hare, for example. The metameric segmentation of the spinal cord, which supervenes in the embryonic period, is alone capable of explaining zona (Brissaud).

The examination of the cerebro-spinal fluid often shows lymphocytosis, pointing to meningeal irritation. In some cases the fluid contains micro-organisms (infective zona).

Pathological Anatomy.—Zona (atrophic trouble) recognizes as its anatomical origin either a lesion of the intervertebral ganglia or of the Gasserian ganglia, or a lesion of the nerves or of their peripheral branches. This ætiology includes all the local or general causes capable of provoking neuritis and peripheral neuritis—tuberculosis, tabes, syphilis, chills, certain forms of poisoning (carbonic oxide); but the condition is generally one of zosteroid eruption rather than of true zona.

Treatment.—The pain may be relieved by injections of morphia or by the application of compresses soaked in a solution of cocaine, 1 in 100. The following powder is applied locally :

Powdered starch	..	..	..	..	40 parts.
Oxide of zinc	..	..	..	..	18 „

This powder is kept in place by means of a layer of oil (Hardy).

VII. LUMBAR NEURALGIA.

The lumbar nerves are the analogues of the dorsal nerves. They give off the sensory posterior branches which perforate the muscles of the vertebral groove, in order to spread out in the skin and the anterior branches which form the lumbar plexus. The lumbar plexus furnishes collateral branches, the seat of lumbo-abdominal neuralgia, and terminal branches, the most important of which—the crural nerve—is the seat of crural neuralgia.

1. In lumbo-abdominal neuralgia the collateral branches of the lumbar plexus are affected. Shooting-pains, pain on pressure, and hyperæsthesia are met with here, as in all forms of neuralgia. Neuralgia of the ilio-scrotal branch has its painful points about the middle of the iliac crest (iliac point), at the exit of the inguinal canal (inguinal point), and at the termination of the nerve in the scrotum or in the labia majora. Neuralgia of this nerve comprises the affection described under the name of " irritable testicle " (Cooper), or testicular neuralgia, often accompanied by a sensation of syncope, which might lead us to suppose the participation of the great sympathetic nerve.

In neuralgia of the femoro-cutaneous nerve we find a painful point near the antero-superior iliac spine.

2. Crural neuralgia affects the antero-internal part of the thigh and of the knee and the inner side of the leg and of the foot. The principal painful points are the inguinal point, where the nerve leaves the Fallopian ligament, outside the crural ring, the points where the branches of the musculo-cutaneous nerve perforate the fascia, and a point on the level of the internal condyle. In crural neuralgia walking is often painful.

VIII. SCIATIC NEURALGIA—SCOLIOSIS.

Sciatic neuralgia, which is more common than facial and intercostal neuralgia, is most important. The sciatic nerve is the only terminal branch of the sacral plexus. It leaves the pelvis by the great sciatic notch, and the gluteal point which corresponds to this level is affected in neuralgia of the small sciatic nerve, which is often associated with sciatica. The great sciatic nerve passes between the ischium and the great trochanter (trochanteric point), and reaches the popliteal space. It then divides (popliteal point) into the internal and external popliteal, the latter passing round the head of the fibula (peroneal point). The terminal cutaneous branches of the sciatic supply the skin of the leg and of the foot, excepting the inner side (external malleolar and plantar points).

Description.—The pain of sciatic neuralgia is both continuous and paroxysmal. It breaks out in the form of attacks, which are caused by walking, or by the heat of the bed. Shooting-pains start from various points, and run through the limb in various places (foot, leg, knee, thigh, and buttock). During the attack radiation of the pain is frequent. It follows the collateral branches of the sacral plexus, the branches of the lumbar plexus, and the intercostal nerves. Apart from the attack, the patient experiences a sensation of pain, numbness, formication, or burning. There is cutaneous hyperæsthesia, or anæsthesia if the neuralgia is of long standing. The pain may be provoked by pressure on the points already indicated, or in the course of the nerve along the posterior portion of the thigh. If the leg, in a case of sciatica, is lifted and bent at the same time, the patient only experiences slight pain ; but if the leg is lifted while in the extended position, he utters a cry of pain (Lasègue).

The patient often complains of cramps or of painful shocks in the muscles of the leg and of the thigh. Some patients have zona ; others suffer from muscular weakness in the same regions.

Atrophic lesions are sometimes seen in the limb affected with sciatica. It is not a simple loss of flesh, due to the inertia of the muscles, but a muscular atrophy, which may be masked by hypertrophy of the skin and by development of the subcutaneous tissue. These trophic troubles are said to depend on the anatomical condition of the nerve. They are absent or only slight in the case of simple neuralgia, and very marked in the case of neuritis. The gradual increase of the pain, the numbness and formication preceding the acute attacks, the pain spreading along the trunk of the nerve itself, are said to be symptoms in favour of neuritis.

Scoliosis.—In the case of severe or inveterate sciatica the attitude of the patient when stripped and in the erect position is characteristic. We often meet with crossed scoliosis, and sometimes with homologous scoliosis. In crossed scoliosis, which is the more frequent, the lateral curvature of the spine and of the trunk and the lowering of the shoulder occur on the side opposite to the sciatica. Let us take a patient suffering from sciatica on the left side. The body is bent to the right ; the lumbar column describes a curve, with its concavity towards the right ; the right hand is lower than the left one ; the left leg is semiflexed, and the fold of the left buttock is pulled upwards.

It is " the position which the patient suffering from sciatica instinctively takes to relieve the painful limb. He takes the weight off it by displacing the centre of gravity, and the hip of the diseased side stands out " (Phulpin).

When the scoliosis is very marked, the costal margin comes in contact with the pelvis. Furthermore, the degree of the scoliosis is generally in proportion to the severity of the pain. In the long run this crossed scoliosis, which at the commencement is an instinctive attitude assumed to relieve the pain, becomes a permanent attitude, and may persist for weeks and for months after the disappearance of the sciatica, as though the muscles had acquired the habit of remaining contracted.

In some cases the scoliosis is homologous—homologous meaning that the scoliosis is on the same side as the sciatica. In a case of syphilitic sciatica of the right side, with homologous scoliosis, we see flexion of the diseased leg, lowering of the fold of the buttock, bending of the spine and of the body to the right, while the left hip stands out.

At first sight this fact seems paradoxical, because in such a case the weight of the body rests on the painful limb. It is true that the patient partially remedies this by bending the healthy hip out by means of a compensatory curvature. " In such a case," says Brissaud, " the patient has the attitude of a person who is carrying a pail of water at the end of his arm, and who is trying to avoid wetting himself."

In order that a patient with sciatica should not allow himself to assume the instinctive attitude of crossed scoliosis, and in order that, in spite of himself, he should adopt the paradoxical attitude of homologous scoliosis, there must be a reason, because homologous scoliosis, the compensatory curvature notwithstanding, makes walking more difficult and more painful. What, then, is the cause of homologous scoliosis ? According to Brissaud, the reason is : " Whilst crossed scoliosis is produced by the contraction of the muscles of the healthy side, homologous scoliosis is produced by the contraction of the muscles of the diseased side. The contraction is not limited to the muscles supplied by the sciatic nerve, but extends in the lateral region of the trunk to the muscles supplied by the branches of the lumbar plexus." It is therefore a lumbo-sacral neuralgia, with contraction and painful points in the flank and along the course of the crural nerve, with exaggeration of the patellar reflex and epileptoid tremor. Brissaud in one of his cases which is identical with one of mine—a case labelled " sciatic neuritis "—speaks of a patient who had sciatica of the left side, with homologous scoliosis, exaggeration of the patellar reflexes on both sides, and epileptoid tremor as soon as the foot was straightened. Lumbo-sacral neuralgia, with homologous scoliosis, or Brissaud's spasmodic sciatica, with painful contraction and epileptcid tremor, has also been studied by Lami, who has published two cases. In some cases the leg of the healthy side is attacked by paresis or by spasmodic symptoms. I shall describe in the next section (Syphilitic Sciatica) a remarkable example of this condition.

Ætiology.—Cold and rheumatism are frequent causes of sciatic neuralgia. Many people have got sciatica in consequence of having gone to sleep on the grass, or of having had their feet in cold water. Sciatica is brought on by injury, by lesions of the vertebral column, of the meninges, and of the spinal cord, and by compression of the nerve (pelvic tumours, exostoses, or cancer), whence the necessity of rectal and vaginal examination, when it becomes necessary to establish the pathogenic diagnosis of sciatica. Gout and gonorrhœa deserve, as regards ætiology, special mention. Syphilitic sciatica will be dealt with in the following section. Double sciatica is often dependent on diabetes (Worms).

The sciatic nerve, like all the nerves, may be attacked by neuralgia during the course of tuberculosis. According to Peter, sciatica is sometimes the initial sign of tuberculosis. We have seen, as a matter of fact, under Pulmonary Phthisis that sensory troubles of all kinds are very frequent in patients suffering from tuberculosis, and are often due to peripheral neuritis.

The **diagnosis** of sciatica is easy. It is not, however, sufficient to diagnose sciatica ; we must also find its cause, because the treatment must be varied according to this cause. The sciatica of diabetes and of syphilis requires the treatment for diabetes and syphilis. Sciatica associated with tumour in the neighbourhood demands surgical treatment.

Certain remedies are of service in sciatica. Prolonged baths (Krishaber) give excellent results. The patient must remain in his bath for several hours. Antipyrin may be prescribed in doses of from 15 to 45 grains. Injections of morphia and inunction of an ointment of methyl salicylate may give relief. Blisters, the actual cautery, injections of sterilized water (Potain and Dieulafoy), injections of air, and epidural injections by the sacro-coccygeal route, have their indications. Bleeding, leeches, and cupping are useful. Local freezing gives good results. A spray of ethyl chloride is played over the painful area, so as to reduce the temperature to 76° F. The spray is directed by means of a special siphon (Debove). Electricity has achieved many successes. I have often noticed the good results of massage and of nerve-stretching. Mercury and iodide accomplish marvels in the case of syphilitic neuralgia.

IX. SYPHILITIC SCIATICA—HOMOLOGOUS SCOLIOSIS.

Description.—A young man was admitted one day into my wards in great distress. The left hip stood out, the body was bent to the right side. He took short steps, supported by an attendant, leaning to the right side on a stick, dragging his bent right leg, and seeking by means of this position to lessen his sufferings. I had him put to bed, and then examined him. The right leg, buttock, hip, and lumbar region showed marks of blisters and scars, with cicatrices, due to spraying with ethyl chloride. He gave us the following history of his case :

Three years ago, without apparent cause, he felt increasing pain in the right buttock, the thigh, and the leg. In spite of his sufferings, he continued his work as a carter as well as he could. This condition continued to grow worse all the time until the month of November. At this period, six months before his admission to the hospital, the pains became extreme. They were most marked in the thigh or in the calf, and sometimes radiated into the groin, the front of the thigh, the penis, and the scrotum, after the manner of lumbo-sacral neuralgia. At night the suffering was much increased, and he was unable to lie down and sleep. In six months he had lost 18 pounds in weight.

During these three years of suffering, and especially during the last six months, he had consulted several physicians, and had taken many forms of treatment, without obtaining the slightest relief.

He obtained admission into the annexe of the Hôtel-Dieu, where sciatica was diagnosed, and the ethyl chloride spray was used without success. He was discharged unrelieved. He then came to the out-patients' department at the Hôtel-Dieu, and was at once admitted under my care.

Questioned as to the nature of his pains, he told us that they never ceased. He described them as dragging and crushing. He could bear them during the day-time when at rest, but at night they were terrible, no matter what position he assumed. Sometimes he felt himself becoming "as stiff as a poker." The leg was affected by a painful contraction, in which the lumbar region participated. On pressure, we found the painful points of sciatic neuralgia—over the right buttock, the sciatic notch, along the ischio-trochanteric groove, in the popliteal space, in the antero-external region of the leg, and on the dorsal surface of the foot. Furthermore, the pain ascended into the lumbar region, and extended to the gluteal muscles. The patient even stated that in severe attacks the pain radiated into the scrotum (genito-crural sphere) and into the left leg.

Lasègue's sign was present. When the right leg was lifted and bent, the patient felt but slight pain; but when the extended leg was lifted, he uttered a cry of pain. In short, there was no doubt that the patient was suffering from sciatica, but from a somewhat special form.

When in bed, the patient kept his leg slightly flexed. He could only sit on a chair at the cost of great suffering. Even then he sat down in a peculiar manner, resting the left buttock on the edge of the chair, and keeping the right buttock from it. As soon as he sat down, he was seized with the epileptoid tremors in the right leg and shooting pains, which made him get up. When he wished to unlace his boots, he did not lean forward, as any other person would do, but, standing up, he lifted his foot backwards, bent his body sideways, and with his extended arm reached his boot, without having bent his leg. At meal-times he assumed the most varied positions, standing with one knee on a chair, or with his body bent.

The right leg had got thinner and less firm than the left leg, but the sensation was normal, and the electrical examination did not show any degeneration. The cremasteric and plantar cutaneous reflexes were intact. The patellar reflexes were exaggerated, especially on the right. Both legs showed the epileptoid tremor, although it was very slight in the healthy leg.

In view of these latter symptoms, which had a tendency to be bilateral, it might be asked whether the diagnosis of sciatic neuralgia was sufficient, and whether the lesion ought not to be placed higher, and meningo-myelitis thought of.

The patient on admission had the appearance of a man suffering from **sciatica with homologous scoliosis.** The trunk was bent, forming a concavity towards the affected side. The left hip stood out; the right shoulder was inclined to the right; the interval between the costal margin and the iliac crest was much diminished; and the fold of he buttock was lowered. In an individual with sciatica, homologous scoliosis—that is to say, scoliosis on the same side as the sciatica—is rare. The scoliosis is almost always crossed ; in other words, the lateral curve of the backbone and of the trunk and the lowering of the shoulder are on the side opposite to the sciatica. ɟ This crossed scoliosis " is the position instinctively taken by the patient to relieve the painful limb. He does this by displacing the centre of gravity, and the hip on the diseased side stands out." (I refer the reader to the preceding section for the description of scoliosis in sciatica.) The patient, therefore, had spasmodic sciatica, with homologous scoliosis.

We had next to think of the treatment, but seeing that attempts as numerous as they had been unsuccessful had been made for the past three years, the task was not an easy one ; and yet, in order to succeed, it was only necessary to go back to the cause of the disease.

My first care, after having made the diagnosis, was to seek for the cause of this severe sciatica. The patient was not suffering from malaria, tuberculosis, diabetes, or rheumatism ; he was syphilitic. In 1889, ten years previously, he had had a chancre, roseola, and headache. It was, therefore, logical to think that the sciatica was of syphilitic origin. I could not say whether the nerve itself was affected (sclero-gummatous neuritis), or whether it suffered from the contact of a neighbouring lesion (gumma or exostosis). I ordered a daily injection of 1 gramme of oily solution of biniodide of mercury, which represents 4 milligrammes of the active principle. I purposely did not order any other remedy, so as to note the effect produced by the mercury. For about a week the effect of the treatment was unnoticeable, but from that time forward it was possible to follow day by day the rapid improvement. After the twelfth injection the patient passed a better night than he had done for the past six months. After the fourteenth injection he slept the whole night through. He sat down on his bed, got up, and took a few steps without much difficulty.

In the next few days the patient walked from one end of the ward to the other without a stick. He walked almost erect. The scoliosis had considerably diminished. The left hip was much less prominent. The fold in the right buttock was not so low. The right leg was hardly flexed, and movements impossible a fortnight ago on account of the pain were now performed by the patient, who seemed quite surprised. His appetite was good, and he regained his strength. He was now able to "run like a hare," as he expressed it. This marvellous result was obtained after eighteen mercurial injections. From this date all the symptoms disappeared. The patient could sit down without difficulty. The reflexes were normal, and the sudden straightening of the foot no longer provoked an epileptoid tremor. The muscular contraction causing the homologous scoliosis had, however, not completely disappeared, the trunk being slightly bent towards the right side. A few days later I ordered a new series of injections to be commenced, and the cure was definite. In this case, as in many others, I obtained a cure of the syphilitic mischief by means of mercury alone. Iodide of potassium was not associated with it.

I quote other cases of syphilitic sciatica. De Lavarenne communicated the following case to me :

A man, forty-six years of age, was taken ill with sciatica, and sent to him at Luchon in July, 1888. The pains had commenced sixteen months previously in the left lumbar region. They then attacked the left leg in the form of sciatica. A noteworthy feature was that the pains were more severe at night, and the patient, blaming the heat of the bedclothes, always slept with his left leg outside the bed. In the past eight months the sciatica had become much worse. De Lavarenne noticed that the patient bent over to the left side, the side of the sciatica (homologous scoliosis). The left leg was soft, and commenced to atrophy. The measurement through the middle of the thighs showed that the left side was 2 inches smaller than the right side.

The patient had so far been treated for rheumatic sciatica. As sulphate of quinine in large doses, salicylate of soda, injections of morphia, the cautery, blisters, and inunctions had failed, it was proposed to stretch the nerve—an operation to which the patient would only consent after having tried the thermal cure. The sulphur treatment was then prescribed : baths and sitz baths at a temperature of 110° F. In spite of the sulphur baths, the pains became still more severe. Injections of morphia were given.

On account of certain indications, De Lavarenne got an idea that the patient might be syphilitic. He ordered inunctions of mercurial ointment. The result was surprising. After the third inunction the disease began to yield. In a week the pains had diminished, so that the patient could sleep without the aid of morphia. He walked without a stick, and could put on his boots. The mercurial inunctions, and then iodide of potassium, were continued for a month, and the patient left Luchon perfectly cured. A year later he was in good health.

The following cases are taken from Dubois's paper :

A lady, twenty-three years of age, suffered intense pains in the left thigh. The painful points extended along the sciatic nerve, and descended as far as the foot. Several methods of treatment had been tried without success, when Gérard found gumma, flat pustules, and vegetations. Antisyphilitic treatment cured the sciatica in a fortnight.

Zambacco speaks of a man who had had syphilis eighteen months previously. He came to the Hôpital du Midi for syphilitic sciatica. The painful points were situated over the sacrum, the left buttock, and the posterior portion of the thigh and of the leg. Walking caused intense pain. Pills of proto-iodide of mercury were prescribed. Ten days later the patient left, completely cured.

Another case of Zambacco referred to a syphilitic patient. Two years after the chancre he was taken ill with sciatica on the left side, thought to be rheumatic. The pains, which were very severe at night, were, for the time being, relieved by cold compresses, but they reappeared as soon as the compresses got warm. The patient came to Paris and consulted Zambacco, who found sciatica on the left side. The pains were intense, especially at night. Pressure over the left sciatic nerve from the lower portion of the buttock as far as the popliteal space caused extreme pain. The most careful exploration revealed no tumour along the sciatic nerve. As the patient had the stigmata of syphilis on his legs, mercury and iodide of potassium were immediately prescribed. By the fourth day the improvement was noticeable, and six weeks later the patient returned to London, completely rid of his pains.

Taylor quotes the case of a man who contracted syphilis, and was several months later seized with intense neuralgic pains in the sciatic and crural nerves on the right side. The sciatic pain extended from the ischium to the knee. It was continuous, with violent exacerbations at night. It was at first thought to be a case of malarial neuralgia, and sulphate of quinine was prescribed in large doses. The result was nil. Taylor then suspected the syphilitic origin of the neuralgia, and ordered inunctions of mercury and iodide of potassium. The pains quickly subsided. Next summer a slight relapse was cured by similar means, and the sciatica did not reappear.

I will conclude with a case of Oettinger :

A young woman, twenty-one years of age, who had had syphilis the year before, came to the hospital in 1883 for extremely acute sciatica on the left side. The pains were particularly severe at night. The warmth of the bed and pressure of the bedclothes were so painful that the patient got up and vainly tried to get some relief by moving about. When she did succeed in getting a few moments' rest, she woke up with a start, thinking of the pain. On pressure, the sciatic nerve was painful from the thigh to the leg. Near the big toe the pressure made the patient cry out. Injections of morphia gave but little relief. An injection of ammonio-mercury peptonate was given every other day (1 centigramme). After the first injections the patient felt a marked improvement. A few days later she was able to get up and to put her foot on to the ground. The treatment was continued for six weeks, and she left the hospital completely cured.

Discussion. — The foregoing cases give a fair picture of syphilitic sciatica. The sciatic nerve, as well as the trifacial, facial, oculo-motor, ulnar, and other nerves, may be attacked by syphilis. Whether syphilis is localized directly in the sciatic nerve in the form of sclero-gum-matous neuritis, or whether the neuralgia is provoked by a neighbouring syphilitic lesion, such as gumma, osteo-periostitis, etc., matters little. The result is the existence of sciatica, which may be most severe, and which resists all therapeutic remedies other than antisyphilitic treatment.

Syphilitic sciatica in nowise differs from the other kinds of sciatica. Continuous and paroxysmal pains, localization of the painful points, Lasègue's sign, zones of anæsthesia, wasting of the limb, exaggeration of the reflexes, spasm of the muscles, epileptoid tremor, and crossed or homologous scoliosis, may be met with in any of the varieties of sciatica.

As regards the evolution of the sciatica, there is no sign or symptom which allows us to say that the sciatica is or is not syphilitic. A point in favour of syphilis is the nocturnal recrudescence of the pains. My patient dreaded the approach of night-time, because it was during the night that the pains were so severe. Zambacco's patient suffered more at night than in the day ; Oettinger's patient also had the most severe pains during the night. The nocturnal exaggeration of the pains is here, as in all cases of pain with nocturnal recrudescence, an index in favour of syphilis. In deciding the pathogenic diagnosis, we have particularly the information which the patient is able to give, and the presence of stigmata (cicatrices) or of syphilitic lesions (eruption, gummata, periostitis, etc.) contemporary with the sciatica.

Sciatica may appear in the early secondary stage as well as in the tertiary stage. " Sciatica," says Fournier, " is not a rare symptom of secondary syphilis. If it appears to be less frequent than it really is, it is because its real cause remains unknown." I am quite disposed to consider it at least as frequent as in the tertiary stage. It is our duty to find it out. In a case of severe sciatica, which is worse at night, and which has resisted all treat-ment, we must think of syphilis. Let us inquire into the previous history : question your patient ; search his past life, and examine for old or recent marks of syphilis (cicatrices, nodes on the tibia) ; and if it is certain that the patient has had syphilis, let us prescribe immediate treatment. Give mercury, which may be combined with iodide of potassium. Of all the mercurial preparations, I know of none which acts with greater efficacy than the aqueous injection of biniodide of mercury, which is described in detail in the Appendix on Therapeutics. If the sciatica is syphilitic, we shall soon know the result. After eight or ten injections the patient experiences considerable relief, and the progress is then rapid.

X. PARÆSTHETIC MERALGIA—NEURITIS OF THE EXTERNAL CUTANEOUS NERVE.

Description.—This affection is constituted by " disturbance of the cutaneous sensibility of the thigh, due to a change in the superficial nerves, and, in particular, to the crural branch of the external cutaneous nerve " (Claisse).

The first symptom is numbness, soon followed by formication in the antero-external region of the thigh. The pains are frequent. They have the rapidity and the severity of lightning pains (Dopter). They have been compared to the stabs of a knife (Lop), or to pinchings. The skin is red, cyanotic, hot, and stiff. Anæsthesia is the rule, and takes the shape of a racket, with the handle uppermost. Pricks are not felt. Sensibility to cold is much decreased, and a difference of several degrees of temperature cannot be felt. The reflexes are never abolished. Walking is difficult, sometimes impos ible.

The course of paræsthetic meralgia is very slow. Recurrences are not rare. It may disappear after some years, or may persist for a lifetime. The prognosis is not serious. The diagnosis is based on the symptoms above described.

The ætiology of paræsthetic meralgia is very obscure. It occurs in adults, and in men more often than in women. Injury seems to have some action by reason of the superficial course of the nerve filaments. It has been attributed to the infectious diseases, to alcoholism, to lead-poisoning, to arthritism, and to obesity (the paræsthetic troubles disappear during a cure for obesity) (Florand). Cold may play some part (Dopter). The pathogenesis is still in doubt. A varicose condition of the limbs has been blamed, because meralgia has some analogy with varicose sciatica (Dopter) ; but, after all, we have probably to deal with peripheral neuritis, which owes to the composition of the nerve a clinical physiognomy exempt from motor and trophic troubles. The local treatment by massage, rubbing with alcohol or turpentine, gives good results. In fat or gouty persons strict hygiene is imperative.

CHAPTER VIII

PARALYSES

I. FACIAL PARALYSIS.

PARALYSIS of the facial nerve does not lend itself to a general description, because the symptoms vary according to the part of the nerve affected. It is therefore customary to describe central and peripheral paralysis. As this division is, in my opinion, insufficient, I shall describe the following varieties : (1) Paralysis of peripheral origin ; (2) paralysis of intra-temporal origin ; (3) paralysis of bulbar origin; (4) paralysis of cerebral origin.

1. Paralysis of Peripheral Origin.—This variety is the most common. It attacks the terminal branches of the nerve after its exit from the Fallopian aqueduct. The facial nerve emerges from the Fallopian aqueduct through the stylo - mastoid foramen, traverses the parotid gland, and supplies two branches—temporo-facial and cervico-facial. These two branches anastomose to form the subparotid plexus. From this plexus branches are distributed to the muscles of the skin, of the neck, of the face, and of the anterior portion of the scalp. The facial nerve, therefore, supplies all the muscles of the face, with the exception of the muscles of the eyeball (third, fourth, sixth nerves), of the upper eyelid (third pair), and of the lower jaw (the motor portion of the fifth pair). Below the stylo-mastoid foramen the facial nerve gives off the posterior auricular nerve to the occipitalis muscle, and to the posterior and superior auricular muscles.

Cold is the most common cause of this paralysis, especially in subjects with the gouty diathesis. A draught of air, an open window in a train, cold rain, and living in a damp locality, are responsible in many cases. In a patient of Trousseau facial hemiplegia showed itself after a severe fright. Injury, parotid tumours, compression of the nerve by the forceps during delivery, are less common causes.

Syphilis often causes facial paralysis. I shall devote a special section to it later.

Facial paralysis appears suddenly or gradually, according to the pro-voking cause. It is almost always unilateral (facial hemiplegia).

The paralysis is often preceded or accompanied by pains in or behind the ear, in the cheek, and in the temporal and frontal regions. According to Weber, these pains are present in more than half the cases of facial paralysis. I have met with them several times, and I have had in my wards

1517

a young patient in whom painful paralysis of the facial nerve was accompanied by zona, while in another patient very severe pain preceded the onset of paralysis by several days. The pathogenesis of these pains (painful facial paralysis) will be discussed in the following section on Syphilitic Facial Paralysis.

The paralysis reveals itself by signs which become more marked if the patient is made to laugh or to speak, because the contraction of the muscles on the healthy side pulls the paralyzed muscles over. As the facial nerve presides over the facial mimicry, all expression on the paralyzed side is abolished. The result is deviation of the features and deformity of the face. When we look straight at a person with facial hemiplegia, the paralyzed side looks as if it were pushed forwards by the healthy side, which hides itself behind it. The paralyzed side is immobile, and presents a strange contrast with the animation of the other side of the face. The muscles no longer contract, the skin of the forehead is smooth, and the wrinkles are effaced on the paralyzed side. Facial hemiplegia is accompanied by paralysis of the muscles which co-operate in the working of the sense organs.

(1) *Organ of Vision.*—The eye of the paralyzed side appears larger and more widely open, on account of the paralysis of the orbicularis muscle. Two muscles govern the movements of the eyelids. The one serving to close them is the orbicularis muscle, supplied by the facial nerve ; the other, serving to open them, is the levator palpebræ superioris, supplied by the third nerve. When the orbicularis is paralyzed, complete closing of the eye is impossible, and the elevator then keeps the upper eyelid raised ; winking is imperfect, and the eyeball remains partially uncovered, even during sleep. The lower eyelid undergoes commencing ectropion ; the palpebral aperture is deformed ; the inner canthus of the eye becomes narrow ; the tears do not flow uniformly, and the conjunctiva becomes injected, dry, and inflamed.

Paralysis of the facial nerve gives rise to epiphora, or flowing of the tears on to the cheek, from paralysis of Horner's muscle, which makes the punctæ lachrymales stand out, by carrying them towards the lachrymal gland, whence they draw the tears.

Bell, in 1823, first drew attention to the upward and outward displacement of the eyeball when a person with peripheral facial paralysis attempts to close his eye. Palpebral occlusion and elevation of the eyeball are two associated phenomena. When vertigo, syncope, or sleep suppresses the oculo-motor act which presides over the function of looking, the eyeball is raised upwards and outwards. If we prevent the occlusion of the eyelid with the finger, or when the want of occlusion is due to peripheral facial paralysis, the second part of the synergic action takes place of its own accord—that is to say, the eye is raised as though the eyelid really closed.

This phenomenon, variously interpreted by Romberg, Erb, Bonnier, is, after all, normal. Bonnier has shown that in cases where the facial paralysis is accompanied by labyrinthine irritation the movement of the eye may assume the spasmodic character of an " eye on springs," as in one of my patients suffering from facial paralysis of otitic origin. This fact is due to the action of the labyrinthine apparatus on the nuclei of the oculo-motor nerve.

(2) *Organ of Smell.*—The facial nerve moves the nostrils. Accordingly, in facial hemiplegia the tip of the nose is slightly turned to the healthy side, the nostril is constricted, the ala nasi is no longer uplifted at each inspiration, and the sense of smell is less acute, on account of the constriction of the nostril. In man, whose nostrils are rigid, facial paralysis has little influence on respiration; but in the horse, in the case of double paralysis of the facial nerve, the nostrils fall in at each inspiration, and as the larynx is drawn up to the posterior nares, grave respiratory troubles result.

(3) *Speech and Mastication.*—The movements of the lips are abolished on the paralyzed side. The patient can neither whistle nor blow, and the pronunciation of the labial letters is almost impossible. The mouth is twisted. The angle on the healthy side is drawn upwards, the deformity being increased when the patient laughs or speaks. The occlusion of the lips being incomplete, the saliva sometimes flows from the mouth. The paralyzed cheek is flaccid on account of the inertia of the buccinator muscle, and the food accumulates between the dental arch and the paralyzed cheek. Mastication is imperfect. The cheek, having become flaccid, presents no resistance to the expired air. It is raised like a sail at each expiration, and the patient is said to be " smoking a pipe."

(4) *The Disorders of Taste and Hearing* will be described under Intra-temporal Paralysis.

In facial paralysis *a frigore* the electrical contractility undergoes notable modifications. When the paralysis is slight, the contractility is almost normal (Erb). In this benign form recovery follows in two to three weeks, but in the grave forms the galvanic and faradic excitability of the nerves is lost, as well as the faradic excitability of the muscles—an indication that the paralysis will last for some months. It is not uncommon for the move ments to remain affected for several years, and certain muscles may become contracted.

Injections of pilocarpin on the healthy side and on the paralyzed side show a delay of one to three minutes in the appearance of the perspiration on the paralyzed side. This phenomenon is peculiar to peripheral facial paralysis of a grave type. It does not exist in facial paralysis of cerebral origin. In the latter case " the sweating reaction " to pilocarpin is equal on both sides of the face (Strauss).

2. Paralysis of Intratemporal Origin.—The facial nerve, after entering the internal auditory canal, with the auditory nerve and Wrisberg's nerve, takes a long course through the temporal bone. It enters the Fallopian aqueduct, where it presents the geniculate ganglion, in which Wrisberg's nerve loses itself. From the ganglion there arise the large and small superficial petrosal nerves. The facial nerve continues its course, gives off the nerve to the stapedius, the chorda tympani, and a few nervous branches, and leaves the aqueduct by the stylo-mastoid foramen.

Paralysis of intratemporal or petrous origin reveals itself by the symptoms already mentioned under Peripheral Paralysis, to which are added symptoms dependent on the paralysis of the various branches just enumerated. These symptoms are:

(1) *Organ of Taste.*—(a) In certain patients the sense of taste is perverted. If we place a sapid substance alternately on the healthy and on the paralyzed side of the tongue, the sensation is obscure, and is slow in being produced on the paralyzed side. The sensation of taste in the posterior third of the tongue, due to the glosso-pharyngeal nerve, remains intact, and the general sensibility, due to the trifacial nerve, also remains intact throughout the whole extent of the tongue, but the sensation of taste is absent in the anterior two-thirds of the paralyzed half. This loss of taste is due to the paralysis of the chorda tympani, paralysis of this nerve being said to produce the loss, either by modifying the circulation of the lingual mucosa (Brown-Séquard), or by producing in the contractile elements of the papillæ certain changes which affect their relations with sapid substances (Bernard).

(b) The deviation of the tongue met with in some cases and the difficulty of turning the tip of the tongue upwards are due to the paralysis of the nerves supplying the digastric and stylo-glossus muscles. It is not uncommon to meet with deviation of the uvula and with slight dysphagia, because the palatine nerves come from the spheno-palatine ganglion.

(c) Dryness of the mouth and diminished secretion of saliva are sometimes observed. These symptoms are caused by paralysis of the chorda tympani, which governs the secretion of the parotid gland (Bernard), and by paralysis of the small petrosal nerve, which regulates the secretion of the submaxillary gland.

(2) *Organ of Hearing.*—The facial nerve supplies the pinna of the ear. In long-eared animals, such as the rabbit, the ear falls as soon as the nerve is cut. Certain persons with facial paralysis show increased power of hearing on the paralyzed side. This phenomenon may be thus explained: The tensor tympani supplied by the small superficial petrosal nerve and the stapedius muscle, which also receives a twig from the facial nerve, constitute the motor apparatus of the chain of ossicles. The tensor tympani has as its function the stretching of the membrana tympani—that is to say, to diminish the amplitude of the vibrations, and consequently to moderate

PARALYSES 1521

the intensity of the sound-waves. These conditions are no longer fulfilled when the muscle is paralyzed and the sense of hearing becomes more acute (Landouzy).

Facial paralysis of intratemporal origin is produced by many lesions—fractures, otitis, syphilitic lesions, tubercular caries of the petrous bone. Cold, which so often causes peripheral paralysis, may also cause this variety. The nerve affected by cold undergoes an inflammatory swelling (Berard, Erb), and is then compressed in different points of its course or at its exit from the Fallopian aqueduct. This explanation of paralysis *a frigore*, which has also been given for peripheral paralysis, must not be applied to all cases of paralysis from cold.

3. **Paralysis of Bulbar Origin.**—The facial nerve has two nuclei in the bulb : (1) an upper nucleus, in common with the sixth nerve, and situated in the floor of the fourth ventricle, at the lower border of the pons ; (2) an inferior nucleus, in common with the motor-root of the fifth nerve (Pierret), and situated between the nucleus of the hypoglossal and spinal accessory nerves. It is easy to follow the fibres of the facial nerve, which start from these nuclei, in order to go from the bulb to the periphery. The cerebral fibres of the inferior facial nerve arise at the foot of the ascending frontal convolution, descend with the geniculate bundle, and, after passing through the lower part of the cerebral peduncle, enter the pons, where they cross, in order to join lower down the fibres arising from the bulbar nuclei. This intercrossing of the fibres of the facial nerve takes place about the middle of the pons.

The region which extends from the crossing of the cerebral fibres of the facial nerve to the bulbar nuclei comprises the inferior half of the pons, a region which also comprises the tract of the motor fibres destined for the limbs, with this difference—that these fibres cross lower at the decussation of the pyramids. The result is that a lesion (tumour, hæmorrhage, softening) in this part of the pons may attack both the fibres which have crossed and the motor fibres of the limbs prior to their crossing. In this way a crossed paralysis results (Gubler). The paralysis, as far as the face is concerned, is on the same side as the lesion, whilst it is on the opposite side as far as the limbs are concerned.

Facial hemiplegia of bulbar origin is, therefore, associated with crossed hemiplegia of the limbs. Furthermore, it is complete—that is to say, it attacks the orbicularis palpebrarum, as well as the orbicularis oris—and the muscles lose their electrical contractility, as in the peripheral paralysis, previously described.

4. **Paralysis of Cerebral Origin.**—Facial paralysis of cerebral origin must be divided into two varieties, according as the cerebral lesion is **central** or **cortical.**

(1) The central lesions of the brain (hæmorrhage, softening, tumour) are accompanied by ordinary hemiplegia, whether the lesion occupies the opto-striate nuclei, the internal capsule, or the fronto-parietal bundles of the centrum ovale. The facial hemiplegia is on the same side as the hemiplegia of the limbs, and presents the following characters : The face is paralyzed in the lower portion only ; the orbicularis palpebrarum is almost

II.   97

always spared ; the paralysis is rarely as marked as in cases of peripheral origin ; the faradic contractility is preserved, and the sweating reaction to pilocarpin is equal on both sides (Strauss).

The absence of paralysis in the orbicularis palpebrarum in facial hemiplegia of cerebral origin has been variously interpreted. In the first place, the integrity of the muscle is not always absolute ; it is latent, and requires to be sought for. In order to explain the majority of the cases—that is to say, the apparent integrity of the orbicularis palpebrarum—we might adopt Broadbent's opinion. In hemiplegia of cerebral origin the immunity is not limited to the orbicularis, but is common to all the muscles performing associated movements. Such are the muscles of the eyes, of the trunk, and of the larynx. It is probable that the nuclei of the nerves of these muscles are united together by commissures, which allow the healthy nucleus, in a certain measure, to supplement the destroyed nucleus.

Three cases of hemiplegia have been collected (Huguenin, Chwostek, Hallopeau) in which, contrary to the general rule, there was complete paralysis of the orbicularis. In these cases a hæmorrhage involved the lenticular nucleus. It is, therefore, probable that the upper fibres of the facial nerve, arising in a part of the cerebral cortex as yet undefined, traverse the lenticular nucleus, and continue their course to the internal part of the cerebral peduncle. In order to go from the lenticular nucleus to the cerebral peduncle, they certainly do not follow the internal capsule, because the lesions of this tract do not paralyze the orbicularis. It is probable that they follow the ansa lenticularis. In the cerebral peduncle they meet with the lower fibres of the facial nerve, which passes down in the geniculate bundle of the internal capsule, and the two united bundles cross in the middle of the pons, and continue their course through the bulb. An objection has been raised to the hypothesis that a lesion of the lenticular nucleus had been in these cases the cause of the paralysis of the superior facial nerve. If it were so, it has been argued, we ought to find paralysis of the orbicularis in cases of obliteration of the Sylvian artery, because the arteries of the corpus striatum come exclusively from the Sylvian artery (Duret), and the superior facial nerve might well have its origin, not in the lenticular nucleus, but in the ansa lenticularis (Mathias Duval). The answer is (Hallopeau) that the distribution of the Sylvian artery varies, that in many cases other arterioles from the anterior cerebral artery or from the anterior choroidal artery enter the lenticular nucleus, and that, consequently, obliteration of the Sylvian artery does not necessarily cause softening of the lenticular nucleus.

(2) Cerebral lesions of **cortical** origin may cause facial hemiplegia similar to the facial hemiplegia of central origin. The inferior facial nerve alone is paralyzed. The electro-muscular contractility is preserved, and the facial paralysis is associated with hemiplegia of the limbs on the same

side. Nevertheless, this association is less complete than in the central lesions. The facial paralysis is the chief feature, and to it is added monoplegia or aphasia, according to the site and to the extent of the cortical focus.

Atheroma, softening, meningitis, and tumours are the most common causes of facial paralysis of cortical origin. The lesion is situated at the base of the ascending frontal convolution, the supposed origin of the inferior facial nerve, and when hemiplegia of the limbs is also present, the lesion occupies the upper two-thirds of the ascending frontal and parietal convolutions or the paracentral lobule.

Prognosis — Termination.—According to Erb, three forms of facial paralysis must be distinguished—slight, grave, and moderate, the symptoms of which are summed up by Grasset in the following manner :

1. In the slight form there is no change in galvanic or faradic reactions in the muscles or in the nerves. In these cases the prognosis is very favourable. Recovery generally takes place in two to three weeks.

2. In the grave form we find complete reaction of degeneration ; diminution and, later, abolition of the galvanic and faradic excitability of the nerves ; loss of the faradic excitability of the muscles ; quantitative increase and qualitative alteration of the galvanic excitability of the muscles ; increase of their mechanical excitability. The prognosis is essentially unfavourable. The duration varies from three to six months. Contractures often appear.

3. Between these two extreme types every intermediate type exists.

Contracture is the worst complication of facial hemiplegia, and must be studied in detail. When the facial paralysis forms part of an ordinary hemiplegia (cerebral lesions), the secondary contracture, so frequent in the muscles of the limbs, is very rare, and is but little marked in the muscles of the face. When the facial hemiplegia is of peripheral origin, permanent contractures of the muscles of the face are to be feared. These contractures were most accurately described by Duchenne in his " Traité de l'Électrisation Localisée." They may attack all the paralyzed muscles or only some of them. They appear three or four months, or even longer, after the onset of the paralysis. They are often announced by premonitory signs : spasms supervening in the paralyzed muscles under the influence of their natural excitability, too rapid return of the tonic force in the paralyzed muscles (Duchenne), and spontaneous shocks analogous to the convulsive tic of the face, are the precursory signs of contracture.

" The return of the tonicity to the normal condition usually takes place in a certain order. It generally requires two or three weeks in paralysis of the facial nerves of the second degree for the first tonic movement to become manifest. The buccinator muscle seems to be the first to recover its tonic power, and then come, in the following order, the zygomaticus major, the zygomaticus minor, the levator communis alæ nasi et labii superioris, the muscles of the pinna, the depressor labii inferioris, the depressor anguli oris, the levator menti, the orbicularis oris, the orbicularis palpebrarum, the frontalis, the corrugator supercilii, the compressor naris, and the dilator alæ nasi. These details are of importance, because if one of these muscles recovers its tonicity more rapidly than usual (during the first week), especially when the muscle recovers its tonicity out of its turn, it means the commencement of a contracture which will accentuate the features more than in the normal condition, and which will become gradually worse " (Duchenne).

The contracture rarely affects all the paralyzed muscles. Certain muscles —the zygomatic muscles and the buccinator—are more often attacked than the others. In proportion as the contracture becomes marked, the features of the face which were defective and weakened during the paralysis first become regular and then deformed in an opposite direction, the face assuming the most strange expressions.

The contracted muscles are often affected by convulsive movements. In the long run they may retract and greatly impair the various movements. The causes of these contractures are numerous, but it is certain that the improper use of electrical currents plays an important part.

Diagnosis—Treatment.—The diagnosis of facial hemiplegia is easy. One cause of error, however, deserves notice. We must not attribute the deviation caused by a contracture of the left side to a paralysis of the right side. This error is easily avoided when the contracture is well marked ; but this is not always the case, and if the reader will refer to the section on Hysteria, he will find that several authors have wrongly described a contracture as facial hemiplegia, because facial paralysis is rare in hysteria.

The treatment of facial paralysis varies according to the cause. We must always think of **syphilis,** which may in all its stages be the cause of facial paralysis. Faradization is the best treatment for facial paralysis. The treatment is the same in the case of contracture, but faradization must be used with the greatest care, because it may lead to the development of contractures.

Summary.—1. Facial paralysis of peripheral origin presents the following characteristics : The hemiplegia is generally total—that is to say, the inferior and the superior facial nerves are affected. It is often preceded or accompanied by pain in the paralyzed regions. It completely abolishes mimicry and expression on the paralyzed side. The reflex movements are lost, and various changes are noticed in the electrical excitability. According to circumstances, the paralysis is slight and easily curable, or severe, of long duration, and sometimes followed by contractures. In the case of severe paralysis the sweating reaction caused by pilocarpin is delayed on the paralyzed side.

2. Facial hemiplegia of intratemporal origin presents the same paralytic symptoms as the preceding variety, but it also presents change of taste, deviation of the uvula, and excessive acuteness of the sense of hearing, due to the paralysis of the nerve branches arising in the interior of the Fallopian aqueduct.

3. Facial paralysis of bulbar origin resembles paralysis of peripheral origin in many symptoms, but it differs in that the facial hemiplegia is accompanied by crossed hemiplegia of the limbs.

4. Facial paralysis of central origin differs from the preceding varieties in many ways. It is this variety which accompanies common hemiplegia. The paralysis spares the superior facial nerve and the orbicularis palpebrarum, and only attacks the inferior facial nerve. The reflex movements are preserved ; the faradic contractions are normal ; the sweating reaction with pilocarpin is identical on both sides ; the facial paralysis is on the same side as the hemiplegia of the limbs ; secondary contractures are extremely rare.

5. Facial paralysis of cortical origin closely resembles facial hemiplegia of central origin. The inferior facial nerve alone is paralyzed. The electromuscular contractility is preserved, and the facial hemiplegia is associated with paralysis of the limbs on the same side. Nevertheless, this association is less complete than in the central form. The facial paralysis is the chief feature, and monoplegia or aphasia is joined to it, according to the site and to the extent of the cortical focus.

II. SYPHILITIC FACIAL PARALYSIS.

Syphilitic paralysis of the facial nerve may be early or late : early when it appears during the secondary stage ; late when it supervenes years after the infection during the tertiary stage. Between these two extremes every intermediate variety is met with.

1. Early Paralysis.

Clinical Cases.—A young woman under my care had been suffering from syphilis for three months ; she had a maculo-papulous roseola, mucous patches in the throat, and enlarged glands in the groin. Since the appearance of these secondary symptoms the patient complained of pain in the ear and in the right side of the face ; the headache was so severe that she could not sleep. She had lost her appetite, and was so tired that she was often compelled to keep her bed—symptoms frequent in a woman at the commencement of syphilis, as Fournier has pointed out. One morning the patient perceived that her mouth was slightly drawn to the left ; she could not close her left eye, and the tears flowed on to her cheek. The earache grew worse. When I examined the patient (eight days after the commencement of the paralysis), I found right facial

" presented a strange expression of immobility and sottishness." The difficulty in mastication was so great that the food accumulated between the teeth and the lips, and then fell out of the mouth. The mercurial and iodide treatment was prescribed as soon as the paralysis appeared. In thirteen days the effect was noticeable : the patient could close his eyes almost completely, the movements of the lips were easier, and food was better retained in the mouth. After twenty-three days' treatment the improvement was very apparent : the eyes closed completely, the patient ate with much greater ease. In two months " there was not a trace of the double facial paralysis with which the patient had been affected."

Bouveret : A man had on the dorsal surface of his prepuce the indurated cicatrix of a chancre and enlarged glands in both groins. Over the whole of the body there was a fading roseola. During the course of the secondary troubles, probably in the second or third month after infection, facial paralysis of the left side appeared. When the patient was admitted to hospital, the paralysis had existed for about a fortnight : inability to close the eye and marked epiphora ; great deviation of the right angle of the mouth ; immobility and pulling down of the left angle ; inability to whistle. Specific treatment was at once prescribed. The facial hemiplegia on the left side was improving, when paralysis of the right side set in. The improvement was gradual, and the patient left the hospital before the complete cure of this double facial paralysis.

I have quoted several cases in order to convince the reader that early syphilitic facial paralysis is not rare. We can count by dozens the cases of unilateral or of bilateral facial paralysis supervening within a few months of the syphilitic infection. Many years ago Fournier expressed this opinion, which has since been absolutely justified. " Of the paralyses in secondary syphilis," said he, " the most common is facial hemiplegia. Let me add that it is also the earliest." The precocity of this syphilitic complication is, in fact, remarkable. In looking over fifteen cases in which the onset of the paralysis is clearly stated, I find the following distribution :

The facial paralysis appeared once in the seventh month of the syphilitic infection, once in the sixth month, once in the fourth month, four times in the third month, seven times in the second month, and once in the first month.

The name of " early " is, therefore, well applied to this kind of paralysis, as its most common time of appearance is two or three months after the infection. Even the most severe syphilitic troubles may appear a few months after the infection. It is important to remember this fact, as I never fail to point out whenever the opportunity presents itself. In my lectures* on syphilitic nephritis I have quoted cases in which acute syphilitic nephritis appeared in the second, third, and fourth months of the infection. In the section on Cerebral Syphilis I have reported several examples of early cerebral arteritis, supervening only a few months after the chancre, and ending in apoplexy and in death by the rupture of an aneurysm, or in hemiplegia, by obliteration of the vessel (obliterating endarteritis). I

* " Néphrite Syphilitique et Syphilis du Rien " (Clin. Med. de l'Hôtel-Dieu, Paris, 1898, p. 242).

have repeatedly met with early syphilitic myelitis supervening during the
first year of the infection, and ending fatally in some cases.

I repeat, then, that, with regard to events in syphilis, "time has nothing
to do with the case," because grave troubles may appear very soon after
the infection. We must finish, once and for always, with the narrow
classification, "secondary troubles and tertiary troubles." It has been
the custom to consider the secondary (or early) troubles as being much
less formidable than the tertiary (or late) ones. In many cases this is
true, but the exceptions are so numerous that they have been classified
under the rubric of "early tertiarism" (Fournier).

Description.—Let us consider the history of early syphilitic facial
paralysis. The onset is sudden, and from the outset the facial nerve is
paralyzed throughout its entire extent. The paralysis does not instal itself
in a slow and progressive manner. We do not see it commencing in the
mouth and spreading in a few days to the cheek and the eyelid. From
its appearance, or thereabouts, the paralysis attacks the whole of one side
of the face. The patient notices that his mouth is twisted, and at the
same time he finds some difficulty in closing his eye. The saliva drools
from the angle of the mouth and the tears fall on to the cheek. From the
outset the paralysis is general, like the peripheral form due to cold. The
superficial branches of the facial nerve may be alone attacked, or the deep
branches (intratemporal) may be also affected. Loss of taste in the anterior
two-thirds of the tongue on the paralyzed side (chorda tympani), deviation
of the uvula (palatine nerves), changes in the power of hearing (nerves
supplying the motor system of the ossicles), are seen in the intratemporal
form of facial paralysis.

The interpretation of these early paralyses is difficult. Are they due
to an osseous or a meningeal lesion compressing the facial nerve at its
entrance into, or during its course through, the aqueductus Fallopii ? While
it is not impossible, it is not probable. Are they due to a central lesion of
the nuclei of origin of the facial nerve ? This is hardly likely, because the
whole nerve is affected from the outset, whilst the nuclei of the superior
and inferior facial branches are distinct in the bulb. It is more rational
to admit a toxic peripheral neuritis.

This theory, applicable to unilateral facial paralysis, is less admissible
when the paralysis is double. In the latter case, is the paralysis due to a
central lesion instead of peripheral neuritis ? I do not think so. In the
first place, the paralysis is not double at first. In two-thirds of the cases
which I have quoted the second paralysis supervened some days after the
first, and it is therefore reasonable to suppose in such a case that syphilis
determines two symmetrical paralyses, symmetry being fairly common
in syphilis. When the Sylvian artery or some other artery at the base of

the skull is attacked by syphilitic arteritis, it is common to find a symmetrical lesion in the artery of the opposite side. When a patient has syphilitic hemiplegia, due to obliterating endarteritis of one Sylvian artery, we sometimes see a second hemiplegia (I have met with such a case) caused by a symmetrical lesion. In a case in which Leudet was able to observe closely syphilitic obliterating arteritis of the left superficial temporal artery, he found later a symmetrical arteritis of the right superficial temporal artery. We have, then, numerous examples of syphilitic symmetry. I am, therefore, of opinion that facial paralysis, becoming double within a few days, is a question of symmetry.

Diagnosis.—Let us next consider the question from another point of view. Facial paralysis in a syphilitic patient does not make its appearance without causing some trouble to the patient and to the physician. We ask whether the paralysis is not an indication of more or less grave cerebral lesions (early syphilitic hemiplegia being common). An individual who has had a syphilitic chancre and secondary symptoms for some months wakes up with his mouth twisted. He fancies that he is threatened with apoplexy. If we examine him carefully, we find immediately that we have to deal, not with paralysis of the inferior facial nerve associated with symptoms of hemiplegia, but with paralysis of the entire facial nerve. Whether the paralysis is slight or severe, all the superficial branches of the facial nerve are involved, and sometimes also the deep branches. The mouth and the face are drawn over to the healthy side (region supplied by the inferior facial nerve); the eye on the paralyzed side remains wide open, the patient being unable to close it; the act of winking is affected (region supplied by the superior facial nerve), and a few tears flow on to the cheek. Electrical examination often reveals a more or less marked reaction of degeneration. Under such circumstances we can give a favourable prognosis as to the localization of the lesion. The patient need not fear hemiplegia or apoplexy. The facial paralysis is not the result of a cerebral lesion, because it affects the superior and inferior facial nerves. It is peripheral, and though it may last for some time, it is not of evil omen. Moreover, the most minute examination of the patient fails to reveal any trace of brachial or of crural hemiplegia. The hand shows no loss of power; the arm is not heavy, and easily executes all movements; the gait is natural, and the patient does not drag his leg or trip when going upstairs.

Syphilitic facial paralysis, limited to the inferior facial nerve, is very different. In such a case only the lower part of the face is paralyzed. The mouth is deviated, the angle is drawn over by the muscles of the healthy side, the cheek is flaccid, and the act of whistling or of blowing is difficult or impossible; but the muscles supplied by the superior facial nerve have apparently lost none of their functions. The eye closes as well as the one on the opposite side ; the act of winking is normal ; there is no epiphora. In such a case the lesion is of cerebral origin. The electro-muscular contractility of the paralyzed muscle is preserved.

Moreover, we find that the paralysis is not limited to the lower part of the face. The arm and the leg on the same side are also paralyzed— in short, there is hemiplegia. The symptoms of this hemiplegia may be slight or severe, but, however slight they are, they nevertheless exist. If we question the patient, he will say that he has less power in the hand, that the arm appears to be heavy, and that his walk is defective. " All these things came on," says he, " at the same time as the deviation of the mouth, with or without some speech troubles."

This last variety of facial paralysis (affecting only the inferior facial nerve) comes under the **early syphilitic hemiplegia,** which may supervene during the first months after infection. The dominating factor is not the paralysis of the face ; it is the more or less marked hemiplegia which strikes the whole of one side of the body, and which is irrefutable evidence of a cerebral lesion, the prognosis of which may be very grave.

Early syphilitic facial paralysis may, therefore, show two very different forms. In the first form, which is the more frequent, the paralysis affects the superior and the inferior facial nerves at the same time ; the nerve only is in evidence ; the brain is spared ; the limbs are not paralyzed ; the prognosis is benign, and the disease ought to be called " facial paralysis, or paralysis of the facial nerve." In the second form the disease ought to be called " hemiplegia." The facial paralysis attacks only the inferior facial nerve. On the other hand, we find a more or less marked paralysis of the arm and of the leg. The lesion is cerebral, and the prognosis is doubtful, being at times very grave.

2. Late Syphilitic Paralysis.

In these cases the paralysis appears many years after the infection. The pathogenic criterion may not be as conclusive as in the early form, because paralysis supervening in an old syphilitic patient may not be syphilitic. Nevertheless, the following cases appear to me to be conclusive :

A man admitted into the Hôtel-Dieu said that he had been ill for the last five weeks. At first he felt very sharp pains in the face, followed about a week afterwards by general facial paralysis of the left side. His mouth was drawn over to the right, the left cheek was flaccid and immovable, the left eye remained open, and winking was impossible. On admission I found all the symptoms of facial paralysis : asymmetry between the two sides of the face ; immobility of the features on the left side, contrasting with the animation of the features on the right side. The cheek was flaccid and blown out like an empty sail at each expiration, and the mouth was strongly pulled over to the right. When he took a deep breath the left nostril did not expand. The left eye was open more widely than the right eye ; it did not close perfectly, and the tears flowed on to the cheek. Mastication was impeded by the food, which collected between the jaw and the left cheek.

The sense of taste was affected. A sapid substance, placed on the anterior two-thirds of the left half of the tongue, caused no sensation of taste. The mouth was dry, and the patient noticed a diminution in the salivary secretion. The sense of hearing on the left side was blunted. Lacaille found that the reaction of degeneration was very marked. The patient was therefore suffering from peripheral facial paralysis of the left side (intratemporal variety), attacking most of the superficial and deep branches of the facial nerve. This facial paralysis was not accompanied by any weakness in the arm or in the leg. There was therefore no question of any cerebral lesion.

I have remarked that in this case the paralysis had been preceded by very intense pains in the face, which still continued at the time of his admission into hospital. I think it well to discuss the nature of these pains which constitute " the painful paralysis of the seventh pair." The pains had commenced about eight days prior to the paralysis ; they involved the entire left half of the face. It was evident, however, that their distribution over the face coincided, not with the distribution of the trifacial nerve (sensory nerve), but with that of the facial (motor) nerve. The pains had commenced in the ear, and had reached their maximum in the auricular region. On the cheek and on the temple the patient compared them to a strong pressure ; elsewhere, especially in front of and behind the ear, they had a shooting character. Although they were continuous, they also took the form of repeated paroxysms during the twenty-four hours. During the night they were severe enough to keep the patient awake. These pains are far from rare in facial paralysis (whether the paralysis is or is not syphilitic). They were very acute in the ear and in the face on the right side in one of my patients. One of Mauriac's patients " experienced very severe pains behind the left ear and in the mastoid region." I saw formerly, with Vulpian, a lady in whom the pains preceded the facial paralysis, and persisted for six months. I once had in my ward a young patient in whom the painful paralysis of the facial nerve was accompanied by zona. According to Weber, the pains are said to exist in more than half the cases of facial paralysis. The pains sometimes precede the paralysis, sometimes they appear with it, and they may survive it. They are usually situated in or behind the ear, in the cheek, in the temple, and in the forehead.

What is the meaning of these pains ? Are they due to neuralgia of the trifacial nerve running parallel with the paralysis of the facial nerve ? Are they due to a reaction on the nervous filaments, amongst others the auricular branch of the pneumogastric, which anastomoses with the facial nerve ? The explanation of these pains is fairly simple, since we know that the facial nerve is both sensory and motor. Wrisberg's nerve appears to be the sensory portion of the seventh pair. This nerve, intermediate as regards its situation between the facial and the auditory nerves, extends from the bulbar exit of these two nerves to the geniculate ganglion of the facial nerve. " Its signification remained doubtful for a long time. Anatomists and physiologists looked upon it as the sensory portion of the facial nerve, but without positive proof, until Duval, by virtue of its central origin, showed that it was the detached or aberrant portion of the glosso-pharyngeal nerve. Numerous researches have definitely proved that it is the equivalent of a posterior spinal root ; it is the posterior root of the facial nerve, and its ganglion is the geniculate ganglion " (Poirier).

Painful paralysis of the facial nerve is thus explained. This painful type only exists in paralysis of peripheral or intratemporal origin ; it does not occur when the paralysis is limited to the inferior facial nerve, and forms part of a hemiplegia of cerebral origin.

Let us now return to the patient who was suffering from painful paralysis of the facial nerve. We had to ascertain the cause of his paralysis. There was no evidence in favour of cold. On the contrary, we had to think of syphilis, for which he had formerly been treated in Algeria during his term of military service. Relying on this hypothesis, I prescribed injections of biniodide of mercury, and the result was remarkable. We must not forget that in this case the pains were so severe that sleep was impossible. After the fifth injection the pains disappeared and the insomnia ceased. At the same time the paralytic symptoms improved rapidly, the deviation of the mouth grew less, closure of the eye became possible, and the sense of taste returned in the tongue. After the fifteenth injection recovery was complete. The reaction of degeneration, very pronounced before the treatment, had disappeared six weeks later.

The rapid effect of the mercurial treatment would be sufficient to show in this case the syphilitic nature of the paralysis, but I have other arguments to adduce in favour of this opinion. Three months later the man came back completely cured of the facial paralysis, but this time he had paralysis of the third pair, with headache. We know how frequent syphilitic paralysis of the common oculo-motor nerve is. The patient was again submitted to mercurial injections, and the paralysis of the third nerve was cured, just as the facial paralysis had been. He left the hospital, and came back two months later with severe headache. There was not the slightest trace of any paralysis being left. The mercurial treatment was again given, and the headache disappeared.

What do we know about late syphilitic facial paralysis ? We must divide it also into two varieties. To the first variety belongs facial paralysis, properly so called, affecting the entire nerve, the limbs being absolutely free from any paralysis. To the second variety belongs the paralysis of the inferior facial, associated with a more or less complete paralysis of the limbs.

The late form of this facial paralysis rarely affects the entire facial nerve, and therefore differs from the early form. The late form " is only, to speak the truth, the previous expression of a total hemiplegia. It is, in technical terms, **a segment of dissociated hemiplegia** " (Fournier). It is a hemiplegia in which the inferior facial nerve participates, but the superior facial nerve remains free. The eye closes well, the act of winking is normal, and the tears do not flow on to the cheek. On the other hand, symptoms of hemiplegia are seen in the limbs : the hand is awkward, the arm is heavy, the leg is dragged—in a word, there is hemiplegia, and the lesion is cerebral. In such circumstances the prognosis must be reserved. It always has a certain gravity, whereas peripheral facial paralysis is practically benign.

III. PARALYSIS OF THE MOTOR NERVES OF THE EYE.

The motor muscles of the eye are supplied by three cranial nerves—the common oculo-motor (third pair), the pathetic (fourth pair), the external oculo-motor (sixth pair).

I shall describe isolated paralysis of these three nerves, next their associated paralysis, and, finally, ophthalmoplegia.

1. Paralysis of the Common Oculo-Motor Nerve.

Anatomy and Physiology.—This nerve arises in the motor cells, below the floor of the aqueduct of Sylvius. From these cells (nucleus of origin) there arise certain distinct root filaments, which pass through the cerebral peduncles, and emerge outside the nerve centres in the interpeduncular space, where they unite into a single trunk, which, after a short course along the base of the skull, lies against the external wall of the cavernous sinus, and then enters the orbit, where it separates into two branches : an upper branch, which supplies a twig to the levator palpebræ, and another to the rectus superior ; and a lower branch, which supplies three branches to the internal rectus, the inferior rectus, and the inferior oblique muscle. Furthermore, the branch to the oblique muscle gives off the motor root of the ophthalmic ganglion, and consequently furnishes the nerve supply of the iris and the ciliary muscle. The nerve therefore divides in the orbit into as many branches as there are muscles to supply.

If the reader will refer to the anatomical points mentioned in the section on Polio-encephalitis, he will see that the nucleus of the third pair, a grey column situated under the floor of the aqueduct of Sylvius, is in reality formed of a series of five small nuclei for the principal portion of the nucleus, and two in number for the other portion of the nucleus, situated in the third ventricle. The result is that the nucleus of origin of the third nerve is divided into exactly as many small secondary nuclei as the muscles to be supplied. Each one of these secondary nuclei is, in fact, the nucleus of origin of the fibres which go to each of the muscles of the eye (Hensen and Voelkers, Kahler and Pick). The root filaments which issue from each of these nuclei are clearly defined in the cerebral peduncle, but soon unite to form the common trunk of the third nerve.

It will now be understood that the paralysis of a certain muscle of the eye may be isolated, the lesion attacking the terminal network of the nerve, or its nucleus of origin. We can thus explain the partial paralyses of the third pair of nerves, which in that respect differ from the paralyses of the sixth and of the fourth pair ; the latter are of necessity always total, because each of these nerves supplies only a single muscle, and has only one nucleus of origin.

The nuclei of origin of the nerves and the muscles of the eye which these nerves supply are situated on the same side, the only exception being the pathetic nerve. This nerve undergoes total decussation in the valve of Vieussens, so that the right nucleus supplies the left superior oblique muscle, and *vice versa.* Let us add that there are between certain nuclei very important connections for the purpose of associating the muscles that perform the same movement in both eyes.

Summary.—The common oculo-motor nerve, by virtue of its distribution, presides over the movements of raising the upper eyelid, over all the movements of elevation and of convergence, over almost all the movements of lowering and rotating the eye beyond its antero-posterior axis. We see that abduction belongs rather to the other nerves of the eye. The oculo-motor nerves also govern the movements of the sphincter of the iris, and the function of accommodation.

This brief description shows the importance of the total paralysis of the common oculo-motor nerve, and the disturbance which it causes in the external and in the internal movements of the eyeball.

Ætiology.—In proportion as the domain of neuropathology extends, the ætiology of ocular paralysis becomes more exact, and we are led to abandon almost entirely the old denominations of essential and of reflex paralyses—terms greatly abused, especially with reference to the oculo-motor nerve. It is better, then, to mention cold, rheumatism, gout, etc., as causes often invoked, although it is not possible to give a satisfactory explanation of their action. Diabetes deserves special mention.

The common oculo-motor nerve is sometimes affected in the intoxications. The paralyzing action of lead on this nerve seems to be fairly well established, and Mallet has collected a considerable number of cases of paralysis due to the ingestion of black-puddings and of "high" sausages. In these cases the action of the ptomaines is clearly established. Mydriasis is one of the first symptoms of belladonna-poisoning. We may compare the toxic paralysis of the third nerve with the paralysis of the accommodation so often met with in diphtheria.

Syphilis often affects the nerve, either directly in the form of neuritis (peripheral neuritis), or indirectly by lesions, such as exostoses, periostitis, sclerotic and gummatous meningitis, arterial lesions, gummata, and cerebral sclerosis. Meningeal exudates, tubercles, and orbital suppuration may compress the third nerve ; it may be bruised or torn by traumatism or by fracture of the skull. In the new-born infant paralysis of the levator palpebræ is fairly frequent, whether it is a case of accidental and transient ptosis, due to the action of the forceps on the branch to the levator, or another variety, which really deserves the name of "congenital ptosis," and which seems to be dependent on an arrest in the development of the nucleus of origin of the nerve. The most common causes of paralysis of the third nerves are **affections of the nerve centres**—lesions of the peduncles, such as gummata, tubercles, hæmorrhage, or softening ; changes in the corpora quadrigemina, in the grey matter below the aqueduct of Sylvius, and in the nuclei of the ventricles. Tabes, especially at the commencement, brings on various dissociated transient and mobile paralyses, due either to peripheral neuritis or to lesions of the nuclei of origin.

The paralysis of the upper eyelid may depend on a cerebral lesion of cortical origin. In several cases the blepharoptosis has been associated with a lesion in the posterior region of the parietal lobe, as though the levator palpebræ had a motor centre in the angular gyrus. In such a case the ptosis is isolated, or is associated with hemiplegia. The blepharoptosis is situated on the same side as the hemiplegia. It is on the side opposite to the cerebral lesion.

In some cases the paralysis of the oculo-motor nerve alternates with the hemiplegia of the limbs. This alternate paralysis generally points to a lesion in the cerebral peduncle. As a matter of fact, the cerebral peduncle contains the motor and sensory conductors which unite the brain to the periphery. The motor bundles are said to be situated in the internal portion of the peduncle and the sensory bundles in its external portion (Maynert). The common oculo-motor nerve emerges from the internal surface of the peduncle, the fibres having traversed the peduncle without decussating. The result of this disposition is that a lesion of the peduncle may attack at the same time the oculo-motor nerve and the motor tracts for the limb muscles prior to their decussation. The paralysis will then be crossed— direct as far as the motor nerve of the eye is concerned, and crossed in reference to the hemiplegia of the limbs.

Symptoms.—The paralysis may be complete or incomplete (dissociated). Let us take a case of complete paralysis. The first thing to strike us is ptosis of the upper eyelid. The levator palpebræ being paralyzed, the eye remains more or less closed by the contraction of the orbicularis supplied by the facial nerve. The patient, in spite of every effort, cannot open the eye ; in order to see, he throws his head backwards, and lowers the eyeball as much as possible by means of the superior oblique muscle. This attitude is characteristic.

The globe of the eye is motionless, except for certain movements downwards and outwards. There is divergent strabismus from the contraction of the external rectus (sixth nerve), and the globe is turned downwards by the contraction of the superior oblique muscle (fourth pair). This deviation causes diplopia. The subject sees two crossed images, with consequent vertigo and erroneous projection of objects in space. When the ptosis is complete, as the patient sees with the healthy eye alone, there is neither diplopia nor vertigo.

The pupil is dilated and fixed. This mydriasis is explained in the following manner : The muscular fibres of the iris, which co-operate in the dilatation of the pupil, are supplied by the great sympathetic nerve, and the muscular fibres which co-operate in the contraction of the pupil come from the third nerve, and reach the iris through the medium of the ophthalmic ganglion. The paralysis of the constrictor fibres permits free action to the dilator fibres of the great sympathetic.

The power of accommodation may be paralyzed, because the third nerve supplies the ciliary muscle, which plays an important rôle in the act of accommodation (Brücke).

Incomplete Paralysis.—The paralysis of the third nerve may be partial, affecting a single branch. In this case we may notice only one isolated symptom — for instance, ptosis in paralysis of the levator, mydriasis in paralysis of the sphincter iridis.

Paralysis of the internal rectus is the most frequent of the partial paralyses of the third nerve. Its principal characteristics are defective movement of the eye inwards, divergent strabismus, deviation of the head away from the paralyzed eye, crossed diplopia, with separation of the images, increasing in proportion as the object is moved in the direction of the paralyzed muscle.

Paralysis of the superior rectus is characterized by inferior and external strabismus, by crossed diplopia, with the false image higher than the true one, and inclined towards the latter, which is only seen when the patient looks upwards.

In paralysis of the inferior oblique the strabismus is inferior and internal, the diplopia is homonymous, and only exists in the upward look. The images are inclined in such a manner that they are separated above, and approach one another below.

When the inferior rectus is paralyzed, there is superior and slightly divergent strabismus, then upward diplopia, crossed on looking downwards. The difference of level in the two images increases in proportion as the object is lowered and abducted.

In paralysis of accommodation mydriasis is nearly always present. Near vision is indistinct, and the object is smaller than normal (micropsia).

Diagnosis.—In complete paralysis of the third nerve the diagnosis is obvious, and there is no need to look for diplopia and for the respective position of the images. This examination is, on the other hand, indispensable when the paralysis is incomplete, and especially when there is simple paresis, in order to ascertain which branch is attacked, or in order not to confound paralysis of the third nerve with that of a neighbouring nerve. I cannot discuss here the differential character of the varieties of diplopia, already described under the symptoms of the various paralyses. It will suffice to compare them in order to avoid mistakes. I must, however, explain how we examine for diplopia. The patient is seated in front of the observer, both eyes open, and one of them covered with a piece of red glass. The physician, who stands with a lighted candle in his hand, places himself some distance from the patient, moves the candle to all the points of the field of vision, and ascertains in the various situations the respective position of the two images, an easy task, because, on account of the piece of coloured glass, the patient, who sees a red and a white image, can state precisely their respective positions. The diagnosis is incomplete if we only rely on the memory, the interrogation, and the general condition of the patient. In paralysis of the third nerve the attention of the physician must be directed to the condition of the central nervous system. For example, in a patient previously considered to be suffering from rheumatism (because he has complained of various pains), or from neuropathy, partial paralysis of one of the muscles, we may find slight ptosis, paresis of the pupil, or some disturbance of accommodation, appearing suddenly, and disappearing in the same manner. We must think of tabes, in which these transient paralyses are often the first symptom.

I would point out that syphilis is one of the most frequent causes of paralysis of the third nerve. If the origin of the disease remains obscure, antisyphilitic treatment should always be employed.

I have already shown under the ætiology the great importance of certain paralyses of the oculo-motor nerve as regards cerebral localizations (cortical paralysis, crossed paralysis).

Course—Duration.—The commencement of the paralysis may be sudden or gradual. The duration and the course depend on the cause. In patients suffering from ataxia, if the paralysis of the onset is transient, appearing and disappearing several times, the paralysis of the terminal period often becomes definite. The paralysis of cerebral origin is more obstinate than the peripheral paralysis. Paralysis of a syphilitic origin is easily cured, especially if treatment is inaugurated from the commencement—inunction of mercury and iodide of potassium. A duration of two to three months is not, however, exceptional.

2. Paralysis of the Fourth Nerve.

This nerve supplies the superior oblique muscle, which moves the eye downwards, and at the same time rotates the vertical meridian inwards. It assists to a slight extent the external rectus in the movements of divergence, and to a greater extent the inferior rectus in movement downwards.

Description.—The objective symptoms are less pronounced than in the other varieties of paralysis. The movements of the eye are hardly affected. Strabismus upwards and inwards is but little marked. The head is, however, inclined downwards and towards the paralyzed muscle.

Diplopia is noticed as soon as the patient looks downwards. It is very troublesome, because it interferes with walking and often causes dangerous falls. The images are homonymous.

The false image is the lower one. The difference of height increases in adduction in proportion as the object is lowered. It diminishes in abduction. The false image is inclined in such a manner that its upper end is near to the true image. The false image appears nearer than the true image.

3. Paralysis of the Sixth Nerve.

Anatomy.—The sixth nerve arises in the floor of the fourth ventricle, on either side of the median raphe, from nuclei which are very close together ; this origin explains the fact that the paralysis is so often double. The nerve has a long course in the cranial cavity, approaching the base of the skull, and coming in relation with the apex of the petrous bone. These anatomical facts show why the sixth nerve, which is very slender, is often ruptured in fractures of the base of the skull (Chevallereau).

The sixth nerve supplies the external rectus, which moves the eye outwards without having any influence on the height or on the vertical meridian of the pupil ; it is therefore a pure abductor.

Description.—This paralysis, which is the most frequent of the diabetic paralyses, presents very exact characters—diminished mobility of the eye outwards ; convergent strabismus, due to the contraction of the internal rectus ; inclination of the head towards the side of the paralyzed muscle ; homonymous diplopia, in which the separation of the two images increases in proporton as the object is moved towards the side of the affected muscle.

II.

98

Graux and Féréol have pointed out a rare form of this paralysis, which supervenes when the lesion occupies the nucleus of origin of the sixth nerve, and which is accompanied by conjugate deviation of the other eye.

4. Paralysis of Associated Movements.

These paralyses consist in the abolition of a movement common to both eyes—the movement of raising or of lowering, movement of convergence or divergence, lateral movement to the right or to the left. Here we have not to deal with paralysis of a certain nerve or of a certain muscle. As Parinaud has correctly said : " We have to deal essentially with the **paralysis of a function** relating to the nerve supply of several muscles taking part in this function, whilst respecting the innervation of these same muscles for other acts."

Description.—The paralyses of the horizontal and lateral movements are the most frequent and the most interesting. Their explanation gives rise to many controversies. In order to explain how two muscles opposed in function (internal rectus on one side and external rectus on the other one), and supplied by different nerves, become associated in order to perform the same movement, we must remember that the internal rectus may contract in order to execute two totally different movements : (1) It may produce a converging movement, both eyes being directed towards the median line. In this case the right internal rectus has as its associated muscle the left internal rectus. (2) It may produce lateral movements, both eyes being directed to the same side of the body. In looking to the left, the right internal rectus has as its associated muscle the left external rectus, and *vice versa*. In order to produce these varieties of movements the internal rectus receives a double nerve supply. It receives a nerve filament from its special nucleus (nucleus of the third pair) on the corresponding side. This filament governs convergence, but for the lateral movement the nucleus of the internal rectus receives a nerve filament from the nucleus for the external rectus of the opposite side. The existence of this anastomotic filament explains the various types of associated paralysis for lateral movements.

As a matter of fact, the nucleus of the sixth nerve on the left side, for instance, supplies the left external rectus, and by its anastomotic branch it also supplies the right internal rectus. It results therefrom that a central lesion, destroying the nucleus of the sixth nerve on the left side, produces paralysis of the conjugate movements to the left—that is to say, the left external rectus and the right internal rectus, which move the eyes to the left, are paralyzed.

If the lesion is peripheral, and if, instead of affecting the nucleus, it affects the trunk of the sixth nerve or the anastomotic branch to the internal rectus of the opposite side, two very different clinical types result therefrom. In the first type the external rectus of one side is paralyzed, and the internal rectus of the other side is in a condition of spasm. The eye to which the paralyzed external rectus belongs can no longer turn outwards. The other eye, however, is strongly drawn in that direction by the spasm, and consequently turns inwards (Parinaud). In the second type there is paralysis of the internal rectus on the one side, with spasm of the external rectus of the opposite side. In this case the eye to which the internal rectus belongs can no longer move inwards, whilst the other eye is turned outwards. Diplopia is often absent in these paralyses of the associated horizontal movements, and, when it exists, it is of only secondary importance. Paralyses of this kind are especially recognizable by objective examination of the ocular movements.

Let us next consider the associated paralyses of the vertical movements. They involve in both eyes at the same time the movement of elevation or the movement of lowering, or both these movements together. In the three cases paralysis of the movement of convergence coexists. The horizontal movements are preserved in a lateral direction.

Paralysis of convergence is characterized by the abolition of the three muscular acts which determine the fixing of a near object—convergence, accommodation, and contraction of the pupil (Parinaud). The symptoms are as follows : Lack of convergence in the eyes ; crossed diplopia persisting throughout the whole extent of the field of vision, without noticeable separation of the images ; double paralysis of accommodation, without mydriasis ; absence of the pupil reflex of accommodation. We find side by side with this typical form of paralysis of convergence another form, in which the paralysis coexists with associated paralysis of the vertical movements. As regards the so-called paralysis of divergence—a trouble characterized by inability to bring the visual axes parallel, with only slightly pronounced homonymous diplopia—it seems that it is rather a contracture of convergence than a paralysis of the opposite movement.

Pathogenesis.—The cause of paralysis of the associated movements is still obscure. Paralysis of the horizontal movements, accompanied by deviation of the head (conjugate deviation), is met with in some cerebral lesions (hæmorrhage, softening, etc.). The pure forms of this affection have been noticed in certain cerebro-spinal affections—insular sclerosis, cerebral syphilis. They may follow a stroke, and may be accompanied by various kinds of paralysis. Essential paralysis of convergence has been met with in neurasthenia, in hysteria (Borel), in certain cases of intoxication by morphia, or by alcohol (D. Graefe), in locomotor ataxy (Hübscher), and in exophthalmic goitre (Mobius).

Where are the lesions situated in paralysis of the associated move-
98—2

ments ?   Are the nuclei of the muscles which co-operate in the same movement joined together by anastomotic filaments, or are there, below these
nuclei, centres for co-ordinating the movements ?   The question is far from
being solved.   Paralysis of the horizontal movements is readily explained
by the existence of the anastomotic filament, which is said to pass from the
nucleus of the sixth nerve to the opposite internal rectus ; but it must be
added that the very existence of this filament has been doubted, and that
this explanation, besides, is opposed to what we know concerning the
other forms of associated paralysis, which appear to be due to lesions
of the co-ordinating centres — corpora quadrigemina, vermis inferior
(Henoch).

The **treatment** is that of the cerebral affection which has caused the
paralysis.   In a case of syphilis at the Necker Hospital rapid recovery
took place.

IV. OPHTHALMOPLEGIA.

Description.—**External ophthalmoplegia** is a clinical type due to the
paralysis of all the extrinsic muscles of the eye, or at least to the paralysis
of all the muscles supplied in the same eye by two different nerves, one of
them always being the third nerve.   The aspect of the patient is most
characteristic.   The eyelids droop, the forehead is wrinkled, the eyebrows
are arched (to remedy the blepharoptosis caused by the contraction of the
frontalis muscle), the eyes are immovable, and when the eyelids are lifted
up by the fingers the eyeball looks as though it were made of wax (Bénédikt).
Finally, the patient is obliged to supplement the defective movements of
the eyes by moving the head and the neck.

Internal ophthalmoplegia is the paralysis of the entire intrinsic musculature of the eye (sphincter of the iris and the ciliary muscle).   These two
forms together constitute **total ophthalmoplegia.**   Each form may be
unilateral or bilateral.   Ophthalmoplegia may be divided, according to
the site of the lesion, into cortical, supranuclear, nuclear, or radicular, the
cortex, the co-ordinating centres of the muscles of the eyes, and the nuclei,
the nerve roots being respectively affected.   The nerve trunks may be
affected at the base of the skull or in the orbit, thus producing basilar or
orbital ophthalmoplegia.   Ophthalmoplegia may also be caused by peripheral neuritis.

I have previously described nuclear ophthalmoplegia.

Supranuclear ophthalmoplegia (Sauvineau) is always bilateral, and is
due to lesions affecting the co-ordinating centres above the nuclei (corpora
quadrigemina, subependymal grey matter).   The lesions of these centres
provoke paralyses of the associated and conjugate movements of the eye.
When these paralyses affect at once the different associated movements they

constitute ophthalmoplegia. Supranuclear ophthalmoplegia usually takes an acute form, and is accompanied by the most grave cerebral phenomena.

Cortical ophthalmoplegia exclusively affects the voluntary movements which are abolished, whilst the automatic reflex movements are preserved. This dissociation appears to be peculiar to hysteria. It has been met with in exophthalmic goitre (Ballet), but it is likely that it is here due to hysteria, which in the cases quoted accompanied Basedow's disease.

Radicular ophthalmoplegia affecting the roots of the motor nerves of the eye at their exit from the nuclei does not exist, and cannot exist. The fourth nerve, in fact, does not traverse the peduncles, and, on the other hand, the radicular filaments of the third nerve and those of the sixth nerve are at a considerable distance from one another. It is simply a question of paralysis of the sixth nerve or of paralysis of the third nerve, with hemiplegia of the opposite side.

Ophthalmoplegia of basilar origin is generally unilateral. The paralysis is always mixed and total, because a lesion of the base of the skull can hardly injure in the trunk of the third nerve all the filaments which go to the motor muscles of the eye without affecting the filaments which go to the internal muscles. It may be laid down as an axiom that every case of ophthalmoplegia which is external alone, is not of basilar origin.

It is often difficult to distinguish orbital ophthalmoplegia from nuclear ophthalmoplegia. We must look for the cerebral symptoms, such as headache, vomiting, etc., which are caused by a lesion of the base of the skull, and we must rely on the lesions of the optic nerve (amblyopia, optic neuritis of the paralyzed eye), of the olfactory nerve (unilateral olfactory paralysis), or of the trifacial nerve. Hemianopia is not characteristic of a lesion at the base of the skull.

The usual causes of basilar ophthalmoplegia are basal meningitis (tubercular and syphilitic), meningeal hæmorrhage, lesions of the bloodvessels and neoplasms.

Orbital ophthalmoplegia, due, perhaps, to a primary lesion of the retrobulbar cellular tissue, or to a lesion of the extrinsic muscles, is generally caused by a change in the nerves themselves or in their terminal branches. These cases of ophthalmoplegia are generally unilateral, mixed, and accompanied by more or less pronounced exophthalmos and pain.

Peripheral ophthalmoplegia, though very rare in the infectious diseases and in the intoxications, is sometimes due to injury (Morel). It has been noticed particularly in tabes, in the form of an early and transient paralysis. The principal characteristics are curability (Dejerine), and the existence of spasms in the associated muscles—retraction of the levator palpebræ of the diseased eye, spasms of the associated muscles of the healthy eye (Parinaud).

V. PARALYSIS OF THE MUSCULO-SPIRAL NERVE.

Description.—Of the branches of the brachial plexus the musculo-spiral nerve is the one most often paralyzed. The paralysis generally announces itself by formication and numbness, and the loss of movement gradually becomes complete.

In paralysis of the musculo-spiral nerve the attitude of the hand is characteristic. If the patient raises the arm, the hand drops on to the fore-arm, and it is impossible to lift it, because the extensor muscles of the wrist, the two radial extensors, and the extensor ulnaris are paralyzed. A more careful study shows the following symptoms :

The dorsal surface of the hand is slightly rounded, and the palmar surface is hollowed, because the muscles of the thenar and hypothenar eminences are no longer opposed by the extensor muscles.

When the hand and the forearm are placed on a horizontal surface, the patient cannot execute any lateral movement of the wrist, because the extensor muscles are also paralyzed—the extensor ulnaris muscle being an adductor muscle, and the extensor radialis longior being an abductor muscle (Duchenne).

The fingers are bent on the metacarpus, and the patient cannot extend them, on account of the paralysis of the common extensor.

The extension of the last two phalanges is possible because this movement is performed by the interosseous muscles (Duchenne); this extension of the last two phalanges is only possible if care be taken to make up for the deficiency in the action of the common extensor by previously lifting the metacarpal phalanges.

The movements of flexion of the fingers are also affected, and, in spite of every effort, the patient cannot bring the extremities of the fingers in contact with the thenar and hypothenar regions. This weakness of the flexor muscles is only apparent. It is due to the shortening of these muscles by the paralysis of the extensors (Duchenne), and the movements of flexion regain their power if care is taken to raise the patient's wrist.

The long and short supinator muscles are paralyzed, which **is never the case in lead palsy.** The paralysis of the long supinator is readily discovered. The patient is asked to flex and to pronate the forearm, whilst the movement is being opposed by drawing the forearm into the position of supination. It is then seen that the long supinator does not stand out in relief. It does not contract.

Condition of Sensation. — In musculo-spiral paralysis there is no anæsthesia of the posterior and external half of the forearm and of the hand, parts which receive their sensory innervation from the musculo-spiral nerve. This fact is peculiar, and we may ask how the same cause acting on a mixed nerve spares the sensory filaments of this nerve when it affects the motor filaments. Several explanations have been given. The sensation is said to be preserved, not because the sensory filaments of the nerve are spared, but because the deficiency is supplied by other nerve branches. The physiological researches of Arloing, Tripier, and Vulpian, and the clinical observations of Weir Mitchell, Richet, etc., prove that the cutaneous sensibility may be preserved in a region deprived of its ordinary cutaneous nerve. This phenomenon is based on the following anatomical conditions : If the motor root of a mixed nerve is cut, it will be seen that the peripheral end of the cut nerve is still sensitive on account of the recurrent sensory fibres which come from the posterior roots and go to the anterior roots. When a cutaneous nerve of the paw is cut in a dog (Arloing and Tripier), it is seen that the peripheral end of the cut nerve contains some fibres which do not degenerate. They are, consequently, in relation with the spinal cord, and probably come from the anastomoses of the collateral nerves of the digits (Sappey) or from the plexuses formed by their terminal ramifications. These peripheral recurrent fibres do not go as far as the centres with the nerve which they accompany. They lose themselves on the road in order to enter the skin. It is, therefore, by this means of supplying the deficiency that the sensation is re-established after the section of the cutaneous nerve of the hand, and this explanation has been given to explain the conservation of the sensation in paralysis of the musculo-spiral nerve.

Nevertheless, certain writers (Onimus), though recognizing the possibility of supplementing the deficiency by recurrent means, have looked elsewhere for the cause of this phenomenon. When the musculo-spiral nerve is attacked at its seat of election, either by compression or by cold, it cannot for a moment be admitted that the motor fibres only are affected, the sensory fibres being spared ; but what can be admitted is that the resistance of the sensory fibre is greater than that of the motor fibre. It may be still further admitted that the functions of sensation are more difficult to abolish than those of motion. We meet with an analogous case in the spinal cord. We know (Vulpian) that sensation does not follow in the spinal cord a path marked out in advance ; it passes, according to circumstances, through the grey matter or through the posterior columns. When one of these parts is compromised, the other may supply the deficiency, and these parts must be destroyed over a large extent in order that the anæsthesia of the corresponding regions may be complete. In other words, the conductors of sensory impressions easily make up for mutual deficiencies, and the preservation of a small number of them explains the persistence of the sensation when an analogous lesion of the motor conductors would produce paralysis.

Faradic Contractility.—The electro-muscular contractility is preserved in paralysis of the musculo-spiral nerve, whilst it is lost in paralysis of the facial nerve (I am speaking of what takes place in severe cases of facial paralysis). These differences in the condition of the electro-muscular excitability have been variously interpreted. Duchenne says : " If it be true that cold causes swelling of the nerve, the Fallopian aqueduct, which is traversed by the facial nerve, must oppose this increase in size, and, consequently, compress the nerve, so as to diminish the irritability of the muscles to which it is distributed. As this cause of compression does not exist in the case of the musculo-spiral nerve, it is clear that the paralysis of this nerve may exist without the electro-muscular contractility being weakened." The explanation given by Duchenne is not sufficient. It rests on two hypotheses, which mutually destroy one another. The first is that the facial nerve is always compressed in the Fallopian aqueduct, which is not proved, and the second that musculo-spiral paralysis is always due to cold, whereas it is often due to compression ; and if, according to Duchenne, the compression of the facial nerve in the Fallopian aqueduct suffices to abolish the electro-muscular contractility, compression of the musculo-spiral nerve ought to bring about a similar result ; but this does not take place. We must, therefore, look for other explanations. According to Onimus, the apparent difference in the electro-muscular reactions in cases of musculo-spiral and of facial paralysis is only a question of degree.

Ætiology—Pathogenesis.—The pathogenesis of musculo-spiral paralysis is obscure, and its mode of production is in dispute. Without speaking of rare cases, such as compression of the nerve by the use of crutches, by wounds, tumours, fractures, dislocations, and occupation paralysis (water-carriers), it may be said that the usual ætiology of musculo-spiral paralysis can be summed up in two words—cold and compression.

According to Duchenne, the paralysis is always due to the action of cold, and is improperly named rheumatic paralysis. We find in the works of Duchenne great stress laid on cold as the cause. If the patient has lain down on the grass or on the damp ground, if he has gone to sleep in a chair with his arms crossed, or if he has left them outside the bedclothes, Duchenne speaks of the action of cold.

In opposition to the exclusive opinion of Duchenne, another equally exclusive opinion attributes the paralysis to the compression of the nerve. Panas denies the action of cold, and declares that " in the immense majority of cases, not to say in all, the paralysis is due to compression of the nerve trunk. " This compression is favoured by the superficial situation of the nerve, which becomes subcutaneous as it winds round the outer border of the humerus, to descend into the muscular interspace between the supinator longus and the brachialis anticus. The compression of the nerve at this point may be accomplished by various mechanisms. In some cases the patient goes to sleep with his arm under his head ; at other times he goes to sleep with his arm leaning on a hard surface (bed, table, back of a chair, step), which compresses the nerve.

Paralysis of the musculo-spiral nerve by compression is accepted by everybody. Panas deserves credit for having brought it into relief. But why reject absolutely paralysis *a frigore?* Why should not cold, which causes paralysis of the facial nerve and of the external laryngeal nerve (paralysis of the crico-thyroid muscle) also cause paralysis of the musculo-spiral nerve ?

One of the principal reasons leading Panas to reject musculo-spiral paralysis *a frigore* is its localization. Thus, the triceps never participates in the paralysis, whilst the supinator longus is always paralyzed ; and this localization, easily explained in the case of compression, cannot be explained by cold.

This argument does not appear to me to be sufficient, because as far as localization is concerned, we find at every turn examples which, though inexplicable, are nevertheless positive. Why, for instance, is lead palsy, which so closely resembles musculo-spiral paralysis, localized in the extensor muscles, whilst it spares the supinator longus ? Why does progressive muscular atrophy always commence in the abductor brevis muscle of the thenar eminence ? Why does glosso-labio-laryngeal paralysis at first and above all attack the superior lingual muscle ? These facts are undeniable, and, as far as the localization of musculo-spiral paralysis is concerned, if cold spares the nerve in its superior parts and abolishes its functions in the region of the supinator longus, it is no doubt because it attacks it at the point where the superficial position renders the nerve more accessible to external agents. Besides, there are undeniable cases of musculo-spiral paralysis *a frigore* (Chapoy, Vicente, Duplay). It is true that it has been asserted (Richet) that even in the case of cold the paralysis is due to compression, because the nerve, swollen in the interior of its osteo-fibrous canal, undergoes a kind of strangulation. This hypothesis, advanced by Erb, with regard to paralysis of the facial nerve *a frigore*, appears to me to be only applicable in some cases, because other motor or mixed nerves are paralyzed as the result of cold, although it is not possible to invoke the strangulation or the compression of the nerve in a rigid canal.

The **diagnosis** is simple. I have already said that paralysis of the musculo-spiral nerve differs from lead palsy of the extensors in that the latter is not accompanied by paralysis of the supinator longus.

The **course** and **duration** of musculo-spiral paralysis vary according to its causes and to its varieties. The paralysis recovers after a longer or shorter time. Faradization is absolutely indicated.

hemiplegia : the mouth was drawn over to the left, the lines of the face and of the forehead were effaced on the right side, and the right nostril was partially closed : the right eye was wide open, and could not be completely closed ; epiphora was present ; the sense of taste in the right half of the tongue was blunted ; no deviation of the uvula and no auditory troubles were present. I prescribed mercury and iodide of potassium. The first result of the treatment was to diminish the headache, and to relieve the insomnia. In ten days noticeable amelioration of the facial paralysis was evident : the mouth was less twisted, the eye closed better, and the epiphora was insignificant. In three weeks recovery was complete.

Bahuaud : A man had a chancre and glands in the left groin. Eighteen days later a roseola appeared, and eight days later—that is to say, twenty-six days after the chancre—the patient perceived that the left side of his face was paralyzed. He consulted Bahuaud, who found facial hemiplegia. The left side of the face was expressionless ; the cheek was flaccid and pendulous, and was often nipped between the teeth during the movements of speech ; the food collected between the jaw and the cheek ; and the mouth was drawn upwards and outwards. The patient could neither whistle nor retain the air in his mouth during the efforts of expiration. The left eye did not close, and the movement of winking was impossible. No other cause except syphilis could be discovered to explain the facial paralysis. Mercurial treatment was immediately commenced. In a week the patient was better. The deviation of the mouth was less marked ; expectoration was more easy. In three weeks recovery was complete.

The following cases are taken from Dargaud's thesis :

Marty : A man, aged twenty-five years, with chancre and glands in the groin, was seized, five weeks later, with roseola and paralysis of the right side of the face. The eye could not be closed ; the right nostril could not be dilated ; the mouth was drawn over to the left ; the saliva escaped continually from the right angle of the mouth ; the cheek was flaccid, and the food accumulated behind the dental arch. Vidal de Cassis : A man had a syphilitic chancre in February. The roseola appeared soon afterwards, and in April—that is to say, two months after the syphilitic infection—facial hemiplegia of the left side declared itself, with loss of taste in the left half of the tongue. After eight days of mercurial treatment the paralysis had disappeared.

In all these cases of early syphilitic paralysis the paralysis was unilateral. In other cases the paralysis is double, and attacks both facial nerves. To quote an example :

A man was admitted to the Necker Hospital with a papular roseola, mucous patches in the throat, and facial paralysis on the left side. The infection was of two months' duration. The paralysis was classical. The patient was put on specific treatment (pills of proto-iodide of mercury and iodide of potassium). A week later facial paralysis of the right side (facial diplegia) appeared. The face then assumed the strange aspect of an expressionless mask. The improvement was gradual, and the cure supervened in two months.

Double syphilitic facial paralysis has been known for a long time. In 1836 Bell reported a case seen by Dupuytren in 1828.

Fournier : In a man who had two syphilitic chancres facial paralysis of the left side declared itself three months after the infection. The mouth was drawn over to the right ; the right cheek was flaccid, and was slightly puffed out during expiration. The patient could neither whistle nor blow ; he could only half close the right eye. Two days later facial paralysis appeared on the right side. " The face," said Fournier,

tion of dislocations, gun-shot wounds, compression by the forceps (Duchenne), vicious callus (fracture of the clavicle), abscess (Pott's disease), and glandular tumours. They may be the result of cold, or they may be of reflex origin (Rendu), being then dependent on a gastro-hepatic affection. Finally, in some cases the cause is unknown.

Symptoms.—The paralysis may be total or partial.

1. When total, it affects all the roots of the plexus : the arm falls lifeless, the point of the shoulder is lowered and flattened, and the patient cannot bend the forearm or move the fingers. The anæsthesia is complete in the hand and in the forearm, and ascends more or less high to the arm and the shoulder. The reflexes are abolished. The muscles present the reaction of degeneration, and stimulation at Erb's point produces no contraction. Muscular atrophy occurs early. The trophic troubles commonly met with in peripheral nerve lesions are very complete—atrophied and glossy skin, malformation of the nails, cyanosis, suppression of the sweat, and fall in the temperature, at times amounting to 2° or 3° F. (Giraudeau), sub-cutaneous adiposis, fibrous ankylosis, etc.

Oculo-pupillary phenomena may also be noticed, with myosis (paralysis of the radiating fibres of the iris, supplied by the sympathetic), with con-striction of the space between the eyelids (paralysis of the orbito-palpebral muscle), and at times smallness and retraction of the eyeball (Hutchinson, Le Bret). The retracted pupil still reacts to the light, but less so than the pupil of the healthy side. These disorders of innervation are connected with the destruction of the communicating branch from the first dorsal nerve, as the experimental researches of Klumpke have shown.

We must distinguish two kinds of total paralysis (Raymond). The lesion, according to its seat, may attack the plexus at the very exit of the roots (tearing, Pott's disease, etc.), or in its cervico-axillary course (fracture of the clavicle, interstitial hæmorrhage of the plexus, exostosis, etc.). In the first case (radicular paralysis) there are oculo-pupillary troubles. The anterior and posterior roots may be unevenly affected, whence a purely motor or purely sensory paralysis (Raymond). Finally, the anæsthesia reaches the deltoid region. In the second case no oculo-pupillary troubles are observed, and the anæsthesia of the arm does not ascend higher than an oblique line drawn from the epitrochlear process to the humeral insertion of the deltoid (paralysis of the brachial plexus, properly speaking).

2. *Partial Paralysis.*—In partial paralysis we find two principal types :

(*a*) The **superior type** comprises the paralysis of the deltoid, of the biceps, of the brachial anticus, and of the supinator longus. It corresponds with the distribution of the fifth and sixth cervical nerves. This form attracted the attention of Duchenne. The muscles of the point of the shoulder may be involved. Thus, in Giraudeau's case the supraspinatus and infraspinatus were paralyzed. These muscles are supplied by the sub-scapular nerve, which arises in the angle of union between the fifth and sixth nerves before their entry into the plexus, so that we have another proof in favour of the radicular theory enunciated by Erb. Sensory and trophic disturbances are wanting, as well as the oculo-pupillary troubles. Secrétan has collected twenty-eight cases. Guillain and Crouzon have published a case of radicular paralysis (superior type), with osseous atrophy and diminution of the arterial tension.

(b) The **inferior type** is much rarer. I had a particularly interesting case of this kind at the Hôtel-Dieu.

A child of four and a half years was knocked down by a heavily-laden cart. Several injuries resulted therefrom, in particular a large contused wound of the right side of the head and the neck, followed by cicatricial torticollis, which a physician reduced by main force. The right arm became paralyzed, and .the child grew up with its arm paralyzed and atrophied. The years went by, and at the age of thirty-three the patient was admitted under my care for phthisis. The findings were : The right arm showed muscular atrophy ; the radio-carpal articulation was flail-like ; the forearm, semiflexed on to the arm, was in the position of forced supination ; the fingers were flexed, and deprived of all movement ; the elbow-joint was fixed by fibrous adhesions in semiflexion, thus forming a kind of hook, on which the patient could suspend heavy objects. The deltoid, the supraspinatus, and infraspinatus appeared to be as large as their fellows of the opposite side. The biceps was still apparent, but powerless to flex the forearm. The epicondylar muscles formed an appreciable mass, especially in their superior portion, but the epitrochlear muscles had disappeared, as well as the extensors. Finally, both pectoral muscles were atrophied. In the hand the thenar eminence had almost disappeared. There were no sensory troubles. We found, furthermore, one of the characteristic signs of a lesion of the inferior brachial roots—viz., the oculo-pupillary phenomena (myosis, diminution of the pupil reflex, constriction of the palpebral aperture). The diagnosis of inferior radicular paralysis was therefore obvious.

Some time later the patient died from phthisis. At the post-mortem examination we found avulsion of the eighth cervical and of the first dorsal nerves. The dissection of the arm revealed the integrity of the supraspinatus and infraspinatus, of the subscapularis, teres minor, subclavius, deltoid, biceps, supinator longus, and supinator brevis, and the radial extensors. All the other muscles of the arm were completely atrophied and degenerated. The pectoral muscles (including the clavicular head), the teres major, the latissimus dorsi, the coraco-brachialis, the triceps, the epitrochlear muscles, the flexors and extensors of the fingers, and the muscles of the hand had disappeared. Their tendons, though still recognizable, were lost in a mass of greyish fibrous tissue, in which it was impossible to find any semblance of muscle. The localization of the muscular atrophies, as will be seen, does not correspond to the muscles supplied by any of the nerves of the arm.   In fact, amongst the atrophied muscles, some received their nerve supply from the ulnar nerve (hypothenar, flexors, etc.), others from the median (thenar, epitrochlear), others from the musculo-spiral (triceps, extensors), and others from their special nerves (pectorals, teres major). The musculo-spiral nerve supplied at the same time the muscles which had remained healthy (the supinator longus, and the radial extensors) and those which were atrophied (triceps, extensors). There was therefore no proper relation between the atrophied muscles and the distribution of a nerve trunk. On the contrary, there was an intimate relation between the atrophied muscles and the distribution of one or more roots of the brachial plexus.

The atrophied territory corresponded exactly to the zone of distribution, which the researches of Féré and of Ferrier have attributed to the two inferior roots of the brachial plexus.

Course.—According to Rendu, the radicular paralyses commence with more or less marked pain, which in certain cases passes unnoticed. The motor troubles are then said to appear, and to be accompanied by atrophy at the end of a few days. The paralysis is often total at the commencement. It then becomes localized, and assumes either the superior type or the inferior type. In their evolution they present similar characters to those of peripheral paralysis. In slight cases they last from three to six weeks. In grave cases they are often persistent.

Diagnosis.—They may be confounded with paralyses, consequent on injuries of the shoulder (dislocation or fracture), but in the latter case the muscles of the scapulo-humeral zone are alone affected, and the shoulder-joint becomes ankylosed. **Hystero-traumatic** paralysis (Charcot) generally supervenes six, eight, or ten days after the accident. It is accompanied by complete anæsthesia of the upper limb or by hemianæsthesia. It is susceptible to transference. It is not always flaccid, and is never complicated by oculo-pupillary troubles. **Myelitis** is often bilateral. The sensory troubles which accompany it do not always present the same topography. The reflexes are often exaggerated, and the electrical reactions are different. The paralyses just described are tributary to revulsives, to electricity, and to massage, in the same manner as peripheral neuritis. Duchenne has noted a case of radicular paralysis which was suspected of being due to a syphilitic exostosis. The patient recovered rapidly under the influence of specific treatment.

VII. PARALYSIS OF THE TRIGEMINAL NERVE.

This nerve is formed of two portions: one, the sensory portion, comes from the large root, to which the Gasserian ganglion is attached, and gives off three sensory nerves—the ophthalmic, the superior maxillary, and a portion of the inferior maxillary nerve; the other, or motor one, unites with the branch of the inferior maxillary, and supplies the masseter, temporal, pterygoid, and suprahyoid muscles, which preside over the act of mastication.

Complete paralysis of the fifth nerve includes, therefore, the anæsthesia of a sensory nerve and the paralysis of a motor nerve.

Description. — 1. *Paralysis of the Ophthalmic Branch.* — The ophthalmic branch is distributed to the eye, after having divided into three branches—the lachrymal, the frontal, and the nasal. The paralysis of this nerve causes anæsthesia of the skin and of the mucosæ in the area supplied by it—the forehead, the upper eyelid, the nose, the conjunctiva, and the pituitary membrane. This facial anæsthesia stops at the median line. The remarkable thing is that the whole of the eye may be insensitive, with the exception of the cornea. Bernard explains this phenomenon as follows : The nasal nerve supplies a root to the ophthalmic ganglion, but besides the indirect filaments which the nasal branch sends to the eye by way of the ophthalmic ganglion, it supplies direct ciliary filaments to this organ. The sensation which the eye receives by means of the indirect filaments of the ophthalmic ganglion differs from the sensation which it receives from the direct ciliary filaments of the nasal nerve. The iris and the conjunctiva receive both kinds of filaments—the direct ciliary nerves and the indirect filaments—whilst the transparent cornea receives only the indirect filaments.

It may, then, be supposed that a lesion may cause loss of sensation in the entire eye, with the exception of the cornea, and reciprocally that the cornea may lose sensation, while all the other parts of the eye retain it.

The starting-point of reflex action being abolished, winking is no longer performed automatically, and the movements of the iris are sluggish.

2. *Paralysis of the Superior Maxillary Nerve.*—This nerve is distributed to a portion of the nose and of the cheek in the suborbital region, to the gums, the lip, and the upper teeth. It also supplies the mucous membrane of the nose. These parts become insensitive in the paralysis of the nerve. The excitation of the mucosa no longer causes sneezing, and the sense of smell is imperfect. If the sense of smell is less acute, it is not that the maxillary nerve, like the olfactory nerve, has a special sensibility, but it appears that the integrity of the sensibility of the mucosa is necessary to the proper functional action of the sense of smell.

3. *Paralysis of the Inferior Maxillary Nerve.*—This nerve is formed of two portions, the one sensory and the other motor. In paralysis of the sensory portion the anæsthesia occupies the temporal region, part of the cheek, the mucosa of the mouth and of the velum palati, the teeth and the lower gums, the anterior two-thirds of the tongue, the lower lip, and the chin. The result of the anæsthesia of the buccal mucosa is that the saliva flows from the mouth, and that food accumulates behind the teeth. If the patient lifts a glass to his mouth, the glass appears to be broken in the middle, because the tactile sensation is limited to the lips and the teeth of the healthy side. This symptom is characteristic. The velum palati is insensitive. It may be touched without reflex movements being provoked. The act of swallowing is impeded. The lingual nerve supplies the general sensibility to the tongue, and is associated with the chorda tympani in supplying the sense of taste in the anterior two-thirds of the tongue, the glosso-pharyngeal nerve being reserved for the posterior portion. Paralysis

of the inferior maxillary nerve, therefore, seriously affects the sense of taste in the corresponding half of the tongue.

4. *Motor Branch.*—In paralysis of the motor branch of the trifacial nerve the muscles of mastication are paralyzed, and the lower jaw is pulled over towards the healthy side.

The **trophic troubles** which at times accompany paralysis of the trifacial nerve have been described under neuralgia of this nerve.

Ætiology.—Paralysis of peripheral origin is either total or partial. Cold produces both varieties. As to the various lesions which have been noticed (cancer, exostosis, chronic meningitis, contusions, and wounds), they produce partial paralysis if they affect one of the branches of the nerve, and total paralysis if they attack the nerve before it reaches the Gasserian ganglion.

Paralysis of Central Origin.—Paralysis of the trifacial nerve may depend on a change in its nuclei of origin, such as is seen in locomotor ataxy. A lesion of the pons may affect the sensory bundle of the trifacial nerve at the same time as the general sensory tract. The result is facial hemianæsthesia, with hemianæsthesia of one entire side of the body. The two cerebral senses, sight and smell, are the only ones preserved (Couty).

Complete hemianæsthesia, with loss of the senses of sight and of smell, may exist when the cerebral lesion is seated in the most posterior part of the internal capsule. Apart from hysteria, in which this hemianæsthesia may exist alone, it is rare for ordinary hemiplegia or paralysis of the cranial nerves not to exist at the same time, according to the seat of the lesion. Aphasia has been noticed.

CHAPTER IX

TROPHIC AND VASOMOTOR TROUBLES

I. TROPHIC TROUBLES IN GENERAL—DYSTROPHIES.

Description.—Lesions of the nerve centres and of the nerves sometimes cause disorders of nutrition, known as **trophic troubles.** These disorders affect the skin, the mucosæ, the cellular tissue, the muscles, the bones, the joints, and the viscera. They give rise to eruptions, losses of substance, ulcerations, atrophy, gangrene, necrosis, and arrested development: sometimes, on the contrary, they reveal themselves by excess of development.

Most of the trophic troubles have been described under the Diseases of the Nerve Centres and of the Nerves; the others will be discussed in the following sections. I shall here mention in general terms certain clinical types of dystrophic origin.

1. **Skin.**—Trophic changes in the skin are frequent. The eruptions of herpes sometimes affect the form of **zona.** Eczematous, pemphigoid, and erythematous eruptions supervene in diseases of the nerves (neuritis, peripheral neuritis, neuralgia, and wounds), and in diseases of the spinal cord (tabes dorsalis or tumours). Pustules and eschars of rapid course (decubitus acutus) are met with in lesions of the brain and of the spinal cord. Lesions of the brain (hæmorrhage, softening) are accompanied by the gluteal bedsore; acute infective or traumatic myelitis is complicated by the sacral bedsore. Eschars of slow development are met with in the perforating disease of the hands and feet and in symmetrical gangrene of the extremities. The hairs (decoloration and falling out of the hair) participate in these trophic troubles (neuralgia of the trifacial nerve, facial trophoneurosis, hysteria). The so-called glossy skin, which ends in the atrophy of the sebaceous glands, in a cracked condition of the skin, and in sclerosis, is seen in lesions of the nerves and in sclerodermia. Calcification of the skin has been noted by Rénon and Dufour in a man who had hard nodules in the skin, with pigmentation and muscular atrophy. The nodules were composed of tribasic phosphate of lime and of fibrous tissue.

1552

Vitiligo is a trophic disorder of the skin, characterized by the development of whitish patches, surrounded by a pigmented area. It occurs in the course of the most varied nervous affections, such as hysteria, insanity, tabes, and syphilis of nervous system, where it may coexist with Argyll-Robertson's sign.

2. **Cellular Tissue.**—The cellular tissue sometimes disappears, as in facial trophoneurosis. At other times adiposis occurs, as in deuteropathic muscular atrophy. In myxœdema it is swollen, œdematous, and indurated.

This adiposis may show different forms. It affects the supraclavicular regions in the shape of an elastic, painless swelling, called the supraclavicular pseudo-lipoma (Potain). It may invade the legs and the thighs (neuropathic pseudo-elephantiasis of Mathieu). Each segment of the limb may be affected alone (segmentary œdema of Debove). Symmetrical adeno-lipomatosis of the cervical region is a very curious form (Lannois and Bensaude). The description is given later. Meige has described another form of dystrophy of the cellular tissue under the name of hereditary chronic trophœdema.

3. **Mucosæ.**—Herpes of the nasal mucosæ, of the tongue, of the lips, and of the conjunctiva, and ulceration of these mucous membranes accompany lesions of the trifacial nerve and zona.

4. **Muscles.**—The muscular atrophies following on diseases of the spinal cord may be divided into two classes. In the one the anatomical and clinical evolution of the atrophy is acute (acute myelitis, hæmatomyelia, infantile paralysis). Progressive muscular atrophy is the type of the second class. The change in the muscles is variable. Sometimes it takes the form of pure muscular atrophy ; in other cases the atrophy is accompanied by fatty or fibrous degeneration. These muscular atrophies must be attributed to a change in the anterior cornua of the spinal cord.

Under the influence of the lesions of the motor nerves (especially traumatic lesions) the muscles undergo more or less rapid change, and their electrical contractility disappears completely or in part.

The atrophies seen in alcoholism and in lead-poisoning are types of neuritic atrophy. Peripheral neuritis plays a great part in these trophic disorders.

Muscular atrophy is one of the trophic troubles found in **hysteria.** In some cases the muscle, instead of being atrophied, appears to be hypertrophied, the hypertrophy being due to overgrowth of the connective tissue (pseudo-hypertrophic muscular paralysis). Finally, myopathy occurs in some patients. The trophic trouble is not in the spinal cord or in the nerves. It appears to reside in the muscle itself (Landouzy-Dejerine type).

II.   99

5. **Nerves.**—The fibrous tissue of the nerves is markedly hypertrophied in the curious affection called **general neurofibromatosis** (Recklinghausen's disease). It is characterized by a triad of symptoms (Landowski)—tumours of the skin and of the nerves, pigmentation of the skin, with slowness of the movements, cramps in the legs, and mental depression. It ends in cachexia and death.

6. **Cartilages.** — **Achondroplasia** (Parrot) betrays itself by an increase in the size of the head, and by dwarfism. The limbs are exceedingly short. " In Anatole, forty-one years of age, the leg was 3 inches shorter than that of an eight-year old child. In Claudius, eighteen years of age, the leg was 6 inches shorter than the leg of a child of eight years of age " (Marie). The hand looks like a " square." The fingers of the same hand are almost equal in size, and are separated from one another by their extremities. The hand sometimes has the shape of a trident (Marie).

7. **Bones.**—The bones show rarefying osteitis. They become fragile in **tabes dorsalis,** and are atrophied in facial trophoneurosis. They undergo an arrest of development in infantile paralysis, and they become hypertrophied in acromegaly (Marie) and in hypertrophic pulmonary osteoarthropathy. They are deformed in Paget's disease (osteitis deformans).

8. **Articulations.**—The joint changes differ in lesions of the skull and of the spinal cord. In lesions of the skull the changes develop after a few weeks, during the period of secondary contractures. The pain and the swelling of the joint simulate articular rheumatism. In the diseases of the spine the arthropathy is acute, if the myelitis is acute ; in tabes dorsalis the arthropathy is not accompanied by pain and fever, and is characterized by enormous swelling of the articulation, with rapid wearing away of the bony surfaces. Articular dystrophy accounts for the strange affection described by Marie under the name of *spondylose rhizomélique*, characterized by an almost complete ankylosis of the vertebral column and of the shoulder and hip joints. The vertebral column is welded together. The patient, in order to maintain the erect position, stands in the form of the letter Z, the upper portion of the body being carried forward, while the knees are more or less bent. In 1906 we had in the Hôtel-Dieu a case of osteo-hypertrophic vascular nævus. The clinical aspect is the same in all the published cases—a more or less extensive zoniform nævus on one limb and hypertrophy of the bone. The juxtaposition of these lesions gives the diagnosis.

Pathogenesis. —-Several theories are given in explanation of these trophic troubles. At first paralysis of the vasomotor nerves was suggested, but the numerous experiments of Bernard and of Brown-Séquard show us that the only result of the paralysis of the motor nerves is to cause congestion of the part which they supply. " Atrophy of the muscles of the head has never been met with in animals after cutting the cervical cord of the great sympathetic nerve " (Vulpian).

Another theory has been proposed—the theory of **trophic nerves** (Samuel). The trophic nerves are said " to make the exchanges which constitute anabolism and katabolism more active in the depth of the tissues." The existence of trophic nerves as distinct nerves is not admissible, but we are, nevertheless, face to face with the undeniable fact that the nerves derive their trophic properties somewhere in the nervous system, just as they derive their motor and sensory properties.

It is, therefore, not the nerve which is trophic, but the nerve centres which communicate this property to the nerve; and by nerve centres I not only refer to the collections of cells in the spinal cord or in the brain, but also to the peripheral ganglia found in the neighbourhood of the organs and in their parenchyma.

Are the trophic troubles due to a suspension or to an exaggeration of this trophic power of the nerve centres ? This question has been well put by Onimus. I will give a brief summary of it :

In a general way, the nutrition of the cells consists in an incessant interchange of materials : this is anabolism and katabolism. Some of the lower animals possess only one property, nutrition ; in them the nutrition is blended with the function. On the other hand, in highly-developed organisms the function is apparently more isolated ; it results from the activity of the elements, and from the manifestation of their properties (movement, sensation, secretion), and, chemically, it consists in a combination of the molecules present, a combination which is almost always an oxidation. **The function uses what nutrition has slowly stored up. Nutrition is a slow oxidation and a continuous act ; the function is a rapid oxidation and a more or less intermittent act.**

What is the rôle of the nervous system in the economy, and how does it act on the nutrition and on the function ? In the end it always acts like a force of discharge through the intermediary of the nerve. The nerve is a conductor which always plays the same part. It reveals and renders active the properties of the elements with which it communicates : it makes them act; or, in other words, it provokes the oxidation of the immediate principles which compose them, and the more it causes them to act, the more it uses them up, so that the nervous system is rather antitrophic than trophic (Onimus). It is said to be trophic when nutrition and function counterbalance ; antitrophic, when the income does not balance the expenditure. In this case there is autophagia of the element. Under the influence of the nervous lesions above described (irritative lesions), the elements act (or destroy one another, which comes to the same thing) more quickly than they are nourished; this rapid wear and tear provokes dystrophic or atrophic troubles.

While this theory is attractive, it is only a theory.

II. FACIAL TROPHONEUROSIS.

Description.—Facial trophoneurosis, or progressive unilateral atrophy of the face, may invade in succession the structures of the face, from the skin down to the bone. The atrophy is unilateral.

The disease commences in the skin in the shape of patches that are white at first, and then become coloured. They may be isolated or confluent, and they may or may not coincide with the anatomical course of a nerve branch. These patches are found at various points on the chin, on the cheek, or above the eyebrows. Their edges are ill-defined. Over the patch the skin grows thin, and becomes depressed. It is hard to the touch, like scar tissue. The beard, the hair, and the eyebrows lose their pigment, and fall out. As the subcutaneous tissue becomes atrophied, the side of the face affected by the trophoneurosis grows thin, wrinkled, and hollow. The sebaceous secretion disappears, the skin is dry, and the secretion of the sweat-glands is diminished.

The smooth muscles of the skin are partly atrophied. They preserve their power of contraction and often present fibrillary twitchings. Atrophy of the muscles of mastication has been noticed (nerve supply of the facial nerve). The cartilages of the nose, the superior maxilla, the inferior maxilla, and the malar bones may be attacked by atrophy. The teeth fall out. The tongue, the velum palati, and the uvula sometimes participate in the atrophy.

The arteries are not atrophied. The lachrymal and salivary secretions are not affected. The temperature remains the same on both sides of the face.

In many cases the disease commences insidiously, without prodromata. At other times it is associated with facial neuralgia, or with convulsive movements of the face. Its course is extremely slow, and it lasts from fifteen to twenty years, without endangering the patient's life. Long remissions have been met with, and in some cases the progressive course of the atrophy has been arrested.

Raymond and Sicard have described a special type of trophoneurosis —total and family hemiatrophic trophoneurosis. In their cases the atrophy affected not only the face, but also the whole of one side of the body. It was progressive, attacking the deep and superficial structures. The family feature was found in two generations.

Pathogenesis.—The ætiology of facial trophoneurosis is very obscure. The pathogenesis is no better elucidated. It is evidently the result of trophic troubles. Why do these troubles supervene ? Which are the centres and which are the nerves primarily affected ? It has been suggested (Gintrac, Lande) that the connective tissue is the initial seat of the trophic lesion. The cellulo-adipose tissue is said to disappear, with the exception of the elastic fibres. Retraction of the skin and atrophy of its elements are said to result therefrom. Several objections have been made to this theory. How are we to reconcile it with the atrophy of the deep parts of the face, with the changes in the bones, with the accurate and unilateral localization of the disease, when the lesions which commence in the interstitial tissue are essentially diffuse ? The theory which places the initial seat of the mischief in the nervous system is, in my opinion, more correct, and there is no question here of circulatory disturbance due to vasomotor troubles. It is rather a question of trophic troubles arising in the sphere of the trigeminal nerve and of the facial nerve, and also in the sphere of the cervical plexus, because facial trophoneurosis sometimes extends as far as the neck.

III. SCLERODERMIA.

Description.—Sclerodermia, or disseminated trophoneurosis (Hallopeau), is in character and nature closely allied to unilateral atrophy of the face.

First Period.—Sclerodermia usually commences with nervous troubles. Some patients experience numbness, formication, and shooting-pains, analogous to rheumatic pains, in the limbs. The pains come on in fits. They may last for several months, and may be sometimes accompanied by cutaneous eruptions (herpes, zona, pemphigus, or ecthyma). In this period we also find vasomotor troubles—excessive pallor or congestion of the skin, cramps, contractures, and hyperidrosis.

Second Period.—When the sclerema first appears, the condition is that of œdematous sclerema. Later the skin and the cellular tissue attacked by sclerema become as hard as wood and look like stone.

The patches of sclerodermia appear in various regions of the body. They are white or dark coloured, according as there is or is not an accumulation of pigment. These patches may be confluent or discrete. They are usually **symmetrical,** and present a **metameric disposition** (Raymond). The skin of the patch is thin, indurated, and analogous to scar tissue. " The characteristic feature of the disease is a special induration, affecting a more or less considerable area of the skin, and accompanied by a certain degree of immobility of the affected parts " (Thirial).

When the sclerema is situated in the fingers, they become rigid and diminished in size. The atrophy sometimes attacks the palm of the hand, and the retraction of the skin flexes the fingers and the metacarpus, and holds them fixed in this position. Ankylosis sometimes supervenes.

Sclerema of the neck impedes the movements of the head, which seems to be fixed on the shoulders. In the face the affection attacks both sides. The face resembles a wax mask, and the natural orifices undergo marked narrowing. The eyelids are retracted. The alæ nasi are thin and flattened. The lips become small, and the patient, being unable to open and close his mouth properly, cannot retain the food and the saliva. The troubles of mastication and of deglutition are the more marked because the tongue and the frænum are sometimes attacked by sclerodermia.

In the limbs the embarrassment of the movements depends on the seat and the extent of the sclerodermia. The movements of flexion of the fore-arm and of elevation of the arm are very limited. The affection is far less common in the lower limbs.

Sclerodermia does not always remain limited to the cutaneous tissue. The disease also attacks the deep tissues, and in this case the word " sclero-dermia " is no longer sufficient, and the denomination disseminated tropho-neurosis is to be preferred (Hallopeau).

In a case of Ball the disease made its appearance in the fingers, with symptoms similar to those of local asphyxia. The sclerodermia appeared later. The lower limbs were attacked, and the bones were also affected—atrophy of several phalanges and ankylosis of certain articulations. Vulpian has reported a case of sclerodermia, with atrophy and disappearance of several phalanges. These trophic troubles were not accompanied by suppuration or by the formation of sequestra. A patient seen by Hallopeau was not only attacked by sclerodermia, but she had also atrophy of the bones and arthropathy. " The lingual mucosa, the muscles of the lips and of the tongue, and probably also those of the forearm, were atrophied. Wherever the skin was deeply affected the subcutaneous fat had to a large extent disappeared."

We see, therefore, that sclerodermia closely resembles **facial hemi-atrophy.** In some cases the facial hemiatrophy was not only limited to the face, but was accompanied by sclerodermia in other parts of the body. Certain changes in the thyroid body (exophthalmic goitre, simple goitre, and atrophy of the gland) may be followed at an earlier or later date by the appearance of sclerodermia (Jeanselme). Let me also add that sclerodermia has some relation with Raynaud's disease. It has several times commenced with the same symptoms, so that some writers hold that it does not constitute a definite morbid entity. According to Favier, " sclerodermia and symmetrical gangrene of the extremities are closely related." According to Apollinario, " there is a close affinity between sclerodermia and local asphyxia." According to Grasset, local asphyxia, gangrene, sclerodermia, and leprosy are all manifestations of a general pathological condition.

According to Brissaud, every case of sclerodermia which is chronic from the outset results from a previous affection of the system of the great sympathetic nerve.

IV. LOCAL ASPHYXIA—SYMMETRICAL GANGRENE OF THE EXTREMITIES.

Under the name of " local asphyxia," or symmetrical gangrene of the extremities, Raynaud has described a form of dry symmetrical gangrene, affecting the fingers and the toes, and more rarely the nose and the ears.

Description.—The evolution of the disease may be divided into three periods (Raynaud) :

The **first period,** which is generally insidious, lasts from a few days to a month. It is characterized by local asphyxia. The ends of the fingers become pale, bloodless, and insensitive. The patient has formication, and the fingers feel dead. At other times the ends of the fingers, instead of being bloodless, become livid ; there is a venous stasis, or **local asphyxia.** The invaded parts are **symmetrical.** The thermometer shows a marked fall of temperature. These troubles are at first intermittent ; later, they become continuous. It is not uncommon to see hard œdema at the end of the affected fingers.

In the **second period,** or stationary stage, the formication gives place to sharp pain. The diseased parts assume a livid tint, and sloughing is imminent. The gangrene is sometimes preceded by the formation of pustules, which break and leave the derma exposed. As a rule, the gangrene is superficial and limited. It does not extend below the superficial layer of the derma, and the nails are not always shed. In other cases the entire phalanx is invaded, and the dead parts become as black as coal. The second period lasts about ten days.

In the **third period** we find elimination of the eschars and cicatrization. This process lasts for several months. When the gangrene has been very superficial, the pulp of the fingers shows whitish parchment-like cicatrices. The end of the finger has a tapering shape. In more severe cases a line of demarcation appears at the base of the gangrenous part. The suppuration at this line favours the throwing off of the slough.

In some exceptional cases the gangrene is not confined to the extremities of the fingers and of the toes. It also invades the ears and the tip of the nose (Fischer), and it may, indeed, be limited in these latter parts, whilst sparing the fingers (Grasset).

Ætiology — Diagnosis. — Symmetrical gangrene of the extremities usually occurs between the ages of eighteen and thirty years. Although it is rare after forty, it has, nevertheless, been met with in an old man of seventy years of age (Rénon). It is more frequent in women. It has often been apparently associated with malaria (Mourson), with sclerodermia, with leprosy, with pericarditis (Widal), with diabetes (Apert), with ergotism (Ehlers), and with tuberculosis (Rénon). At the present time it is rather a syndrome than a proper disease. Certain forms, however, appear to preserve their autonomy. It is probable that it is caused by a tetanic condition of the great sympathetic nerve, thus causing contracture of the arterioles (Raynaud).

Goldschmidt thinks that symmetrical gangrene of the extremities and sclerodermia must be placed under the same heading. He says that obliterating endarteritis appears to be the primary lesion, which depends, perhaps, on some nervous trouble.

The **diagnosis** must be made in each stage of the disease. It must not be confounded with the sensation of dead fingers met with in consequence of cold and in hysteria (Armaingaud). I have described the symptom of dead fingers in Bright's disease. Gangrene of the tips of the fingers has been met with in these cases.

The so-called senile gangrene is due to vascular lesions. It is not symmetrical, and is not limited to a single focus.

PART V

GENERAL AND INFECTIOUS DISEASES

CHAPTER I

ERUPTIVE FEVERS

I. VARIOLA.

TROUSSEAU wrote as follows on variola : " Variola, whether it is or is not modified, assumes two chief forms : it may be discrete or confluent, and whatever form it takes, it is normal or abnormal in its course. These two forms must be carefully distinguished, since discrete variola is usually free from danger, while the confluent form is nearly always fatal. Their course and termination are so different and their characteristics are so well defined that it is most important to follow Sydenham's example, and study them separately."

Discrete and Confluent Variola.

Description. — Discrete variola is characterized by an eruption of pustules, separated from one another by large areas of healthy skin. The febrile remission is well marked, the apyretic periods are clearly defined, and the prognosis is usually good.

Confluent variola is characterized by an eruption, so closely set that all trace of healthy skin disappears. The febrile remissions are incomplete or of short duration, and the prognosis is usually bad.

We find varieties which have been called **coherent-confluent.** They occupy an intermediate place between the two chief forms, and commence like discrete variola; but the pustules suppurate, and finally become **confluent** by fusion. These cases are not confluent from the outset, and are far from presenting the grave prognosis of true confluent variola ; we must therefore be careful not to confound the two forms.

Incubation. — The duration varies from seven to fourteen days, irrespective of the kind of variola. It is customary to describe four phases of the disease—invasion, eruption, suppuration, and desiccation.

1561

1. **Invasion.**—In **discrete** variola the phase of invasion is marked by one or more chills, which in children are often replaced by convulsions. By the end of the first day the thermometer shows a reading of 103° or 104° F., and the temperature remains at its maximum, with some oscillations, during the whole of this period. Perspiration is seen with the onset of suppuration, and at the same time headache, nausea, and vomiting appear. Pains in the loins are constant, and constipation is the rule. In some cases, however, these symptoms are not clearly defined.

In **confluent** variola the symptoms of invasion are practically the same, although constipation is often replaced by diarrhœa, and perspiration is absent; but at this period the difference between the symptoms is not sufficiently marked to enable us to say whether the eruption will be discrete or confluent. Indeed, we see patients in whom the symptoms of invasion are very severe, but only result in an eruption of a few papules. The backache, which is one of the symptoms of this phase, appears to be due to congestion of the spinal cord, which may be so severe as to cause pain in the limbs and paraplegia, with or without retention of urine.

The primary rash which precedes the true eruption, and which English authors have called the " variolous rash," belongs to the period of invasion. The rash assumes two chief forms. These are hyperæmic and hæmorrhagic, and develop either alone or simultaneously in the same patient. The hyperæmic rash may resemble the eruption of measles, erysipelas, erythema, or urticaria; but the hæmorrhagic rash is scarlatiniform. The former is very extensive, fades on pressure, and lasts only one or two days. The latter appears a little later, and is composed of plaques with a red base, upon which several small ecchymoses are found, which do not disappear on pressure, although the red base becomes pale for a moment. The rash is called " astacoid " (ἀστακός, boiled lobster) when the redness is intense. This rash is usually confined to the axillæ and the groins, but it may become general, lasting several days, and disappearing slowly. We must not confound the scarlatiniform rash, which is slightly hæmorrhagic, and without dangerous signification, with the **purpuric** eruption met with in hæmorrhagic variola.

The frequency of the rash varies in different epidemics, and has been noted forty-four times in 395 cases by Barthélemy. It is found in all forms of variola, and has neither the benign nor grave prognosis which has been attributed to it.

The presence of the rash may be of assistance in the diagnosis of variola in a difficult case, but we must be careful not to make the mistake of taking the morbilliform rash for measles and the scarlatiniform rash for scarlatina.

What is the duration of the invasion? The classical opinion held by

Sydenham and Trousseau has lately been criticized. According to these great observers, the period of invasion is longer in discrete than in confluent variola, and lasts three full days—that is to say, the eruption appears at the end of the third day or in the course of the fourth, but very rarely on the second day. In confluent variola the period of invasion is shorter, and the eruption appears at the end of the second or in the course of the third day. To this rule, however, there are exceptions, without speaking of abnormal cases.

2. **Eruption.**—In discrete variola at the time of the eruption the patient feels better, the symptoms of the period of invasion disappear, and the fever gradually falls in twenty-four or in thirty-six hours. The eruption first appears on the face, the neck, and the scalp (Borsieri), and is always most marked on the **face**, whatever the variety of the variola. It invades the rest of the body almost simultaneously, and is complete in thirty-six hours. The eruption at its onset is present on the face, in the form of scattered macules or of papules, which are red and slightly pointed. During the next few days these little papules change into vesicles of unequal size, in which a milky fluid begins to form. This period marks the onset of suppuration. The papules on the face are not umbilicated, but those on the trunk and limbs often show a central depression, called " umbilication." However slight the eruption on the face may be, it produces swelling, which chiefly invades the eyelids.

The eruption appears on the mucosæ at the same time as on the skin (mucous membrane of the mouth, pharynx, larynx, and conjunctiva), and produces, according to its situation, dysphagia, cough, hoarseness, or ocular symptoms.

In confluent variola the eruption shows quite a different course. While in the discrete and coherent forms we always find intervals of healthy skin between the initial papules, in this form, on the contrary, the face is invaded by a diffuse, erysipelatous redness, and the eruption occurs *nunc erysipelatis ritu, nunc morbillorum* (Sydenham). The papules become confluent, so that the skin often looks " sad," like shagreen. On the second and third day of the eruption the papules become vesicular, but the vesicles are smaller than those seen in discrete variola. They open into one another, lift up the epidermis, and commence to fill with milky serous fluid. The face is swollen, and the onset of suppuration is now seen. Similar phenomena, although they are less marked, occur on other parts of the body. The eruption on the mucosæ is more general than in the discrete forms. The pustules invade the mouth and pharynx (dysphagia), the conjunctivæ and corneæ (photophobia), and the larynx (cough and dyspnœa). They may even spread to the intestine, vagina, and urethra. Orchitis has been seen in variola.

While complete defervescence with the period of eruption is the rule in discrete variola, the fever persists in the confluent form, or, at any rate, the defervescence is slow and incomplete, and some patients become delirious.

3. **Suppuration.**—In discrete variola at the time of suppuration the pustules are surrounded by an inflammatory areola, and the umbilication disappears. On the face the pustules, which are more or less spaced, are at first soft to the touch—*leves ad tactum* (Sydenham) — but later they become rough—*asperiores*—because a sero-purulent oozing takes place on their surface, and then they dry up. On the body suppuration takes place from twenty-four to thirty-six hours later, and the pustules do not dry up as they do on the face, but burst, and allow the escape of the contained pus. On the hands and feet suppuration occurs late, and is accompanied by pain and swelling, while the pustules often resemble " bright drops of pure wax." During this period the face is swollen, there is profuse lachrymation, salivation is sometimes abundant, and the fever reappears. But this fever, which marks the onset of suppuration, and occurs about the eighth day of the disease, is generally of slight duration and moderate intensity. Delirium, when present, is slight, and is chiefly seen at night.

In confluent variola events take a different course. The swelling of the face is universal, and the angle of the jaws and the ears are almost as much swollen as in erysipelas. The epidermis is raised by the milky secretion in the confluent pustules. Opaline, greyish blisters appear, and give the skin of the face the appearance of a parchment mask (Morton). Later, these blisters become yellowish and wrinkled, and exhale a most fœtid odour. Similar symptoms, though less severe, are seen on the other parts of the body.

When suppuration occurs, the fever returns, and the temperature sometimes exceeds that of the period of invasion. The fever is continuous, with a morning remission, and lasts during the whole period of suppuration. Delirium is fairly frequent, and sometimes lasts until the end of the second week. Salivation is excessive, and viscous saliva, which soils the sheets and pillows, constantly drools away from the mouth. The salivation diminishes about the eleventh day of the disease, and the swelling of the face also decreases at this period; but the **feet and hands** now commence to swell, and this swelling of the extremities was considered by Sydenham and Trousseau as such a necessary fact that its absence meant a most gloomy prognosis.

The patient suffers excessively during the whole of this period. The swelling of the head and face render him unrecognizable. He can neither open his eyes nor move his lips or tongue. Thick mucus collects in the mouth and fauces, and the dysphagia is so great that he may find it difficult to quench his thirst. The breathing is compromised, speech is difficult, and the bed-linen becomes fœtid and soiled with pus, in spite of every care. The patient is indeed fortunate if these terrible sufferings do not result in death.

4. **Desiccation.**—In discrete variola the dry pustules become covered with crusts, which are more or less thick and yellowish, soft at first and then hard. When the crusts fall off, they leave reddish scars, which later become depressed and white, and sometimes persist indefinitely. In the confluent forms the crusts are not isolated, but assume the appearance of large dark-coloured scales, which are imbricated and foul-smelling. The resulting scars in confluent variola (pitted and scarred face) cause great deformity.

Convalescence, especially in the confluent forms, is not free from danger. An eruption of boils, lasting several months, may appear about the fourth week, when the fever has fallen to normal and the crusts have all dropped off. This tendency to suppuration is also shown by abscesses in the joints, the cellular tissue, and the muscles, and the patient often dies from prolonged suppuration.

Coherent Variola.—The differences between discrete and true confluent variola are evident from the preceding description. This description, however, only applies to typical cases, and does not include all the clinical forms. Accordingly, under the term **" coherent "** writers have described cases of variola, which begin like the discrete form, but in which the pustules are so numerous, especially on the **face,** that, although isolated when the eruption commences, and before their complete development, they become confluent when they reach their mature stage. This secondary confluence is quite different from true confluent variola. These cases are of necessity more serious than the discrete ones, and the description of the latter is not exactly applicable to them, and yet they rarely show the gravity of true confluent variola.

Varioloid.—This term does not signify benign variola, for varioloid may be very severe ; neither does it mean very discrete variola, for it may be coherent. The term " varioloid " is applied to any case of variola which does not suppurate, or which shows only slight suppuration. The distinguishing-point is that varioloid does not end in a stage of suppuration. The symptoms of invasion and eruption are like those of variola. They are generally **attenuated.** The progress of the eruption is then arrested, the secondary fever does not appear, and the vesicles dry up ; and if a few of them do suppurate, they become **horny,** without leaving scars. Although varioloid is, as a rule, quite benign, it may also be hæmorrhagic. Is varioloid variola attenuated by vaccination or by a previous attack, or is it rather a special form of variola ? In no case must it be confounded with varicella.

Hæmorrhagic Variola.—It is necessary to distinguish two forms—the one early, which precedes the eruption, and the other late, which appears during the course of the eruption. The first is far more severe than the second. It is always fatal. The early form begins like ordinary variola, but the patient sometimes suffers from restlessness, dyspnœa, and general malaise, which are of bad augury. A hæmorrhagic and purpuric rash then appears, with bluish or blackish ecchymoses in the groin, upon the neck, the face, the conjunctivæ, and the eyelids. We might say that the patient has .been plunged into a butt of wine (Trousseau). The patient suffers from epistaxis, hæmoptysis, and hæmaturia ; blood oozes from the gums ; the skin is covered with blisters, full of blackish serum ; and the restlessness and dyspnœa are extreme. The tongue is dry, the breath fœtid, the voice is reduced to a whisper, and the pulse is thready. In some cases the patient retains consciousness, but he more often sinks into an ataxo-adynamic condition, with or without convulsions, and dies on the third, fourth, or fifth day, either before the appearance of the eruption, or at any rate before the vesicles have definitely appeared.

The late form of hæmorrhagic variola appears in the course of the eruption, which is, moreover, often retarded. It is more frequent in confluent than in discrete variola. The hæmorrhagic symptoms are those which I have just described, but they are further accompanied or preceded by hæmorrhages into the pustules. This form is less severe than the preceding one, and sometimes recovers. Hæmorrhagic variola is more frequent in some **epidemics.** It was terrible during the epidemic of 1871 (during the war and the Siege of Paris). I saw a large number of cases in my capacity as house-physician to Axenfeld. The late hæmorrhages are favoured by alcoholism and the puerperal state.

Congenital Variola.—When variola is transmitted by the mother to the fœtus, it may cause different clinical varieties. The infant may be born during the stage of incubation, showing at the time no signs of variola, which appears some days later, and carries off the child. The incubation may have been intra-uterine ; the infant is born with the eruption well out, and death supervenes in a few hours. The child may be born with scars, or, indeed, without any trace of previous variola, and is immune, being refractory both to variola and to vaccination. The liquor amnii is sterile.

Anomalous Variola.—The following description will indicate the meaning of the term " anomalous variola ": An individual falls sick of discrete variola, which is apparently quite benign ; but the eruption appears in successive crops, and is not complete until the sixth or seventh day. The pustules develop in an irregular manner, or are depressed ; perspiration is absent, and cannot be induced by any means ; the urine is scanty or absent ;

VI. RADICULAR PARALYSIS—RADICULAR PARALYSIS OF THE BRACHIAL PLEXUS.

The spinal nerves sometimes present changes between their exit from the spinal cord and their entrance into the various plexuses, shown clinically by paralyses. These paralyses have received the name of **radicular paralyses.**

There exist as many varieties of radicular paralysis as there are plexuses. Those dependent on lesions of the first cervical nerves and of the sacral nerves have not yet been described. The radicular paralyses of the lumbar plexus are very obscure. They are generally met with during pregnancy, and especially after delivery, and are attributed to the compression exercised by the head of the fœtus on the nerve roots. They generally affect the lumbo-sacral nerve (fourth and fifth lumbar nerves) as it winds behind the prominence of the brim of the pelvis. They give rise to a limited paralysis in the area supplied by the external popliteal nerve, and sometimes (Vinay) in the area of the superior gluteal nerve—gluteus medius and minimus and tensor fasciæ latæ.

The radicular paralyses of the brachial plexus, on the contrary, have been during the past few years the object of much important research.

Anatomo-physiological Survey.—The brachial plexus is formed by the last four cervical and the first dorsal nerves. It supplies the muscles of the upper limb, some of the shoulder muscles, as well as the subclavius, serratus magnus, levator anguli, rhomboids, pectorals, and latissimus dorsi. It supplies sensation to the skin of the upper limb, with the exception of the internal and posterior surface of the arm, as well as a portion of the point of the shoulder. The nerves which supply this cutaneous area come from the second and third intercostal nerves. Finally, each of the nerve branches forming the brachial plexus gives off, immediately after the union of its two roots beyond the spinal ganglia, **communicating branches,** which form the trunk of the great sympathetic nerve.

The entanglement formed by the brachial plexus is at first sight inextricable, but the careful researches of Féré have shown the part taken by each pair of spinal nerves in the constitution of the various nerves emanating from the plexus. Thus, the fifth and sixth cervical nerves give rise to the musculo-cutaneous (biceps, brachialis anticus, and coraco-brachialis), to the circumflex (deltoid), to the nerves of the supraspinatus and infraspinatus, the teres major, the latissimus dorsi, the pectoralis major, and the serratus magnus, as well as to the fibres of the musculo-spiral nerve, which supplies the supinators. The experiments of Ferrier and Yeo, as well as those of Forgues, have proved that electrical stimulation of these two pairs of nerves in the monkey causes the contraction of these muscles. Finally, Erb, who first drew attention to the **radicular localizations,** has shown that in man the electrical stimulation of a point in the supra-clavicular hollow produces simultaneous contraction of the deltoid, of the biceps, of the brachialis anticus, and of the supinator longus. This point is about an inch above the clavicle, immediately external to the posterior border of the sterno-mastoid, over the anterior tubercle of the transverse process of the sixth cervical vertebra.

Ætiology.—The radicular paralyses are generally the result of injury—violent falls on the shoulder, sudden traction of the arm (Mirallie), reduc-

the tongue becomes dry ; the pulse is small and irregular, and nervous symptoms (subsultus tendinum, delirium, dyspnœa, and coma) herald the onset of danger, and death occurs from the eighth to the tenth day, because discrete variola, when it is anomalous, is much more quickly fatal than the confluent form. These anomalous or malignant cases, as Van Swieten and Borsieri called them, are most frequent in some epidemics. Sydenham had seen them, and Trousseau has described them ; while we may class them with anomalous cases of scarlet fever, which are also called malignant.

Prognosis—Complications.—According to the general law, epidemic variola is much more serious than sporadic. The prognosis of variola is benign as regards the discrete form, unless the case is an anomalous one, and it is also benign in varioloid. It is much more serious in the coherent forms, and fatal in the confluent and hæmorrhagic cases. Patients suffering from confluent variola usually succumb from the twelfth to the fourteenth day. The absence of vaccination may be considered as making the prognosis serious, even from the onset of the disease. Variola is almost always fatal in the new-born and in young infants. In women the menses generally appear early under the influence of variola, and metrorrhagia is common during the eruption (Gubler). In the pregnant woman miscarriage is frequent if the pregnancy is advanced and if the variola is severe. The child usually dies, and the mother succumbs in 60 per cent. of the cases ; but the prognosis is less serious if the pregnancy is not far advanced. Ordinary variola may become hæmorrhagic as the result of the puerperal condition and from the second day after the confinement (Raymond).

The causes of death in variola have been given as :—sideration of the nervous system ; changes in the blood resembling those caused by carbonic oxide poisoning ; suppression of the functions of the skin, causing cutaneous asphyxia ; pyæmia consecutive to the purulent collections in the skin. The local complications, such as œdema of the glottis caused by the eruption in the larynx and pleuro-pulmonary inflammation, which tends to suppurate, may be added to these causes.

Broncho-pneumonia (secondary infection) is frequent in some epidemics. It is insidious, and frequently assumes the pseudo-lobar form. Myocarditis and cardiac paresis are by no means rare.

The endocarditis of variola is slight, and usually leaves no trace. The changes in the larynx may result in necrosis and stenosis. The ophthalmia may terminate in destruction of the eye and loss of sight ; the otitis may result in deafness ; and the transient paraplegia of the period of invasion may be lasting. In the course of variola we sometimes see secondary eruptions of ecthyma and pemphigus, which become a serious complication in some cases. Dropsy, with or without albuminuria, peripheral neuritis, and gangrene of the mouth and of the parotid glands, have also been seen. The nephritis of variola, which is usually transient and curable, may pass into chronic disease.

Ætiology.—Variola is epidemic and contagious at every period, and here, as in other fevers, the contagion is direct or indirect. The agents of contagion are the blood (Fournier), the pus, and the crusts, which, in a finely divided state, preserve their virulence for a long time in rags, linen, clothes, rooms, or vehicles, and which, being light and mobile, may be carried to a distance and meet with an organism in a state of receptivity. The contagious element enters the system through the respiratory tract. The specific organism has not yet been found.

Diagnosis.—The symptoms of variola are sudden intensity of the fever, headache, vomiting, and backache. The presence of a general scarlatiniform rash may for a moment cause doubt between scarlatina and variola, but scarlatina is accompanied by angina, and not by backache. The eruption in certain vesicular cases of measles at first somewhat resembles that of variola, but the ocular, nasal, laryngeal, and bronchial catarrhs which characterize the invasion of measles are not present in variola. Pustular or varioliform acne is almost always limited to the face or to the upper parts of the back and of the chest, while the pustules present a comedo in their centre, and the general symptoms of variola are absent. The general erysipelatous tint of the face which follows the invasion in confluent variola is not likely to be confounded with the clearly defined redness and prominent edge in erysipelas.

Pathological Anatomy.—At the onset of the eruption the lesion is situated in the middle portion of the Malpighian layer, and is covered by the superficial epidermis, which shows no change, and adheres deeply to the papillary layer. The section of a ripe pustule shows the following points : At the edge of the pustule there is an accumulation of young cells arising from the Malpighian layer, and the centre of the pustule is partitioned off by threads, and contains but few cells. This disposition explains the umbilication of the pustules. Complete repair is possible when the Malpighian layer is intact. When this layer is completely destroyed, the scars are indelible.

The changes in the blood are marked The gases are diminished by one-half in the hæmorrhagic forms (Brouardel). The diminution of the hæmoglobin commences before the eruption, and continues to the end of the disease (Quinquaud). The red corpuscles are deformed, and lose their power of taking up oxygen.

The other lesions—granulo-fatty degeneration of the muscles and of the heart, changes in the cells of the liver and of the kidneys, swelling and softening of the spleen—are common to all severe fevers.

Treatment.—The patient should be placed in as large and airy a room as possible. If the disease is mild, it will suffice to prescribe cool drinks, gentle laxatives, broth, and milk. If the disease is severe, tonics must also be employed. Opium should be used for the nervous complications, and if the fever is severe and the paroxysms are marked, sulphate of quinine or salicylic acid should be given. When suppuration occurs, the most careful nursing is necessary, and two beds should be employed, so that the sheets may be frequently renewed. Cool baths and sponging with tepid water are indicated. Trousseau's custom was to place the patient in a bath and pour three or four buckets of water at a temperature of 70° F. over him, and then to put him to bed wet and wrapped in a blanket.

Ducastel has employed a mixture of ether and opium, giving the patient daily 6 spoonfuls of a draught in which opium is mixed with ether ; but as this draught is often nauseating, it may be replaced with advantage by 2 grains extract of opium in the twenty-four hours, and a subcutaneous injection, containing 30 minims of ether, morning and evening. This treatment does not appear to have much influence on the general intoxication, but in some cases it modifies the eruption favourably, and appears to lessen the degree of suppuration.

Finsen, by placing patients suffering from variola in a room into which only the red rays penetrate, has seen the eruption come out more rapidly. The suppuration diminishes, and the scars disappear almost completely. Œttinger has confirmed in France the favourable action of photo-therapy in the eruption of variola.

Prophylactic measures cannot be too rigorously observed. Patients must be isolated, and the isolation must be carried out in a thorough manner. The hospital staff who are brought into contact with patients suffering from variola should be revaccinated. The patients should be given frequent baths. We must not forget that the crusts are most contagious, and that the patients must be isolated until every crust has fallen off.

II. VACCINIA.

History.—Before the discovery of vaccinia it was customary to inoculate the patient with variola, the fluid being taken from the vesicles of as discrete a case as possible, and inoculated in the same manner as in the case of arm-to-arm vaccination. Four days later a vesicle appeared, and soon changed into a pustule, called the "mother pustule," and surrounded by secondary pustules. About the seventh day the fever of invasion made its appearance, and the variola ran its course. As a rule, the patient inoculated with discrete variola became immune, and had no longer cause to dread the terrible consequences of this epidemic scourge. Unfortunately, inoculation sometimes caused severe or fatal variola, and, in addition, the patient inoculated with variola became an epidemic centre, so that vaccination was preferred. Vaccination, however, was not accepted at first, and in England an Act of Parliament was required before vaccination was substituted for variolization.

Although Jenner did not discover the vaccine, yet he introduced its use and made it popular, so that the honour of having bequeathed this great benefit to humanity belongs to him. Jenner, who was inoculator for his own district (Gloucestershire), had remarked that, according to popular tradition, milkers who came in contact with the cows contracted a pustular disease known as **cow-pox,** but were immune during epidemics of variola. Accordingly, Jenner inoculated a child, eight years old, with the fluid from the pustules which a milkmaid had contracted while tending to her cows. In this way vaccine was discovered ; the child was vaccinated, and two months later an attempt at variolization of the same child failed. Such is the origin of vaccination, and Jenner published his first paper in 1798.

Vaccinia (*vacca*, cow) derives its origin from an eruptive disease in the bovine species which attacks cows, and especially young calves, when two or three months old. This eruptive disease, **cow-pox,** is characterized by an eruption of large umbilicated and flat pustules on the udder of the animal. The horse also suffers from an eruptive disease of the same nature, the pustules being situated around the nostrils, in the cavities of the nose and mouth, and also on the lower part of the legs, with abundant secretion. This disease, which is accompanied by marked general symptoms, has been called **horse-pox** (Jenner called it " grease ").

The virus of cow-pox, inoculated into the human species, takes the name of vaccinia, and prevents variola. Inoculation of human beings with the virus of horse-pox gives the same result. Is the vaccine virus simply the virus of variola, modified by its passage through the cow, or is it a disease special to the bovine species ? I shall answer these questions by quoting Chauveau's conclusions :

1. Vaccinia, no matter how exalted its virus, never changes into variola.

2. We may inoculate the cow with variola, but it never becomes vaccinia in passing through the bovine species. The disease is variola, remains variola, and gives rise to variola, if it is reproduced in the human race. This statement also applies to variola inoculated in the horse and transferred to man. The virus of variola and that of vaccinia are therefore of different natures. On the other hand, horse-pox and cow-pox are of the same nature, although the vaccine grows better in the cow than in the horse.

Chauveau's statements have not been accepted without dispute. Depaul was convinced of the identity of variola and vaccinia, while numerous experiments undertaken in Germany and Switzerland would also tend to identify the two diseases, but these experiments are not yet sufficiently conclusive. From the clinical point of view, the dualists have a better case than the unicists. We see clearly, say the dualists, that vaccinia and variola are different diseases, for variola is essentially contagious and epidemic, while vaccinia is never epidemic and never contagious (Bousquet, Hervieux) ; we must admit that variola and vaccinia are two different diseases, because they may run their course simultaneously in the same individual or animal. Moreover, says Chauveau, in the millions of vaccinations performed since Jenner's time we have never seen vaccinia recover its so-called virulence and reappear as variola ; all these successive passages have never been able to exalt its virulence. We have never seen those returns to the parent form which are " so characteristic of the attenuated virus, and of which examples are fairly frequent with the most perfectly prepared artificial vaccine, such as the vaccine from the anthrax pustule made by Pasteur." In short, until there is proof to the contrary, Chauveau's opinion must stand good.

Pathological Anatomy.—The structure of the pustule in vaccinia is comparable to that of variola, and we find the same vacuolar change in the cells of the epidermis and the same necrosis. The base of the pustule is indurated, the cavity is divided by septa, and the juices with which it is impregnated form the lymph. The lymph, which is clear and transparent in man up to the seventh day, and in the cow up to the fifth day, contains leucocytes, red corpuscles, granulations, and micro-organisms.

The microbe of vaccinia is still unknown. Straus followed day by day the evolution of the vaccine pustule in the calf, and by means of histological preparations showed its different phases. We see clearly in these sections colonies of microbes, which at first occupy the lips of the inoculation wound, then pass into the Malpighian layer, and reach the lymphatic tracts.

Various microbes, including the *Staphylococcus aureus*, the *Bacterium termo*, and a saccharomyces, as well as other forms, have been found in vaccine lymph (especially in the calf), but they are the microbes of secondary infection. The absence of the *Streptococcus pyogenes* would, according to Pfeiffer, explain the rarity of erysipelas in vaccination. A coccus (Voigt), to which a certain amount of importance has been assigned, has also been noted by Garré.

Vaccination.—Until lately human or Jennerian lymph was usually employed, but animal vaccination has rightly become more general, and will soon be the only method of vaccination.

If Jenner's method is employed, a healthy child should be chosen, and the lymph be taken on the seventh day. One of the pustules is punctured by a lancet, so that the lymph exudes. The point of the lancet is charged with this lymph (care being taken to avoid admixture with blood), and three or four punctures are made upon the arm of the person to be vaccinated.

If we employ animal lymph, the following are some of the previous conditions formulated by Saint-Yves Ménard as being necessary to obtain good lymph: A young heifer, which has already been weaned, is taken, because we can thus avoid diarrhœa and other diseases frequent in the animal before weaning. The heifer is inoculated with horse-pox, natural cow-pox (when obtainable), or cow-pox from other heifers. The animal is placed in the stable and tied up with a short cord, in order that it may not be able to lick the wound. The fever is absent or insignificant. The lymph which is collected on the fifth or sixth day is the best.

It may be prepared as a pulp or a powder, and every antiseptic precaution should be observed. This lymph will keep for a long while, but it is obviously less likely to be successful than vaccine taken directly from the heifer.

If the patient is vaccinated with **antiseptic precautions,** the course of events will be the same whether the lymph has been taken from a human or from an animal source. There is no invasion period, as in eruptive fevers, but there are three clearly defined stages. The **eruption** of vaccinia corresponds to the first stage, and about four days after vaccination a papule

100—2

forms. It becomes umbilicated on the fifth or sixth day, and filled with clear, transparent fluid, called " lymph." On the seventh day the pustule is formed. It is flat, umbilicated in the centre, swollen at the periphery by the lymph, and surrounded by a reddish areola. About the eighth day the mature or suppuration period begins, when fever, lassitude, headache, and gastric disturbance are sometimes seen. The corresponding lymphatic glands are painful, the pustules become of a whitish tint, the umbilication disappears, the lymph becomes turbid and sero-purulent, and the skin of the region is red and shiny. Desiccation begins about the tenth day. A brownish spot appears at the centre, and then invades the whole pustule. Desiccation ends on the fourteenth day, and we see a dry, thick, adherent brownish crust, which does not fall off until the eighteenth day, if it has not been already pulled off. Whitish scars are left by the pustules.

False vaccinia, which is abortive and confers no immunity, is characterized by vesicles that appear on the day after vaccination. They are accompanied by sharp itching, dry up rapidly, without presenting umbilication, and sometimes have the appearance of a boil.

Such is the evolution of vaccinia. Vaccination may be performed at any age, and it is remarkable that in the new-born it usually produces no fever. Jennerian and animal vaccine give the same results, and confer the same immunity against variola. How long does this immunity last? It begins about eight days after vaccination, and in some cases confers immunity and prevents variola for a lifetime; but in others the period of immunity is limited to eight or ten years, so that **revaccination** is absolutely necessary, especially during epidemics. We cannot, then, have recourse to vaccination too freely. In the German and French armies, in which vaccination has been compulsory for many years, variola may be said to exist no longer. In England the mortality from variola was minimized as long as the law prescribed compulsory vaccination, but it has increased since the law is no longer in force. Specious arguments regarding the liberty of the subject do not take into consideration the most important fact in such circumstances —namely, the safety of the majority.

In some colonies variola causes terrible ravages, and in Cambodia the proportion of deaths among children is 60 per cent. (Nogué). " In the Far East no more deadly scourge than variola exists. No one who has not seen it break out in a country where vaccination has not penetrated can form any idea of the incalculable number of its victims " (Jeanselme). Accordingly, all possible means must be employed to make vaccination compulsory.

General Vaccinia.—In some cases the eruption is not limited to the seat of inoculation, but is more or less disseminated over different parts of the body. It may result from animal or from Jennerian vaccine. It would appear chiefly to supervene after vaccination with horse-pox. Certain dermatoses (eczema, impetigo) place the skin in a state of receptivity, and favour the dissemination of the vaccine. The eruption in general vaccinia runs its course at the same time as that of inoculation, the two eruptions being contemporaneous, which proves clearly that vaccinia is not the result of auto-inoculation, but that it is distinct, and constitutes a true eruptive fever, which sometimes determines fatal infectious troubles in children.

Vaccinal Eruptions.—From the eighth to the twelfth day after vaccination, when the vaccinal eruption is at its height, we sometimes see various eruptions appear without warning, fever, or general symptoms. In some cases we find a vaccinal rash which may resemble the rash of measles, scarlet urti-fever, or erysipelas, or may be erythematous, exudative, papular, or carial; it commences around the pustules, spreading thence to the neck, the arms, and the whole of the body. Sometimes the eruption has the appearance of miliaria, being vesicular, and accompanied by pruritus and desquamation. Lastly, in very rare cases the eruption is pemphigoid or purpuric. These vaccinal eruptions are comparable to those produced by drugs, or to the rashes caused by the toxines of numerous microbes, and by injections of serum.

Complications of Vaccinia.—Vaccination is sometimes followed by complications, of which some are benign, while others are grave. There is one—vaccinal syphilis—which exclusively results from Jennerian vaccination.

Vaccinal Syphilis.—This terrible complication of vaccination (Fournier) has been proved clinically by cases seen at Coblentz (nineteen persons who became syphilitic), at Rivalta (thirty-nine children), at Algiers (fifty-eight soldiers), and at Paris (five persons). It has been proved experimentally by Cory, who voluntarily inoculated himself with syphilis by means of vaccine from a syphilitic child. The vaccino-syphilitic inoculation assumes the following forms : (1) Chancre develops alone, and vaccinia is absent ; (2) the chancre develops either on a pustule or in one of the punctures which have not taken.

Chronologically, the chancre appears several weeks after the vaccinia, and the vaccinal eruption has long since ended when the chancre commences, for syphilis has an incubation period of three to four weeks. This is one of the chief distinctive signs from ulcerative vaccinia. At first the chancre has the appearance of a papule, which becomes encrusted. Under the crust a circumscribed sore with an indurated base is found.

Contagion may occur, although the giver is not suffering from active syphilis, but only from latent syphilis (hereditary or acquired), which has not shown any traces upon the skin or elsewhere. It will, therefore, be seen that the source of the lymph is a very important matter. It has been asserted that all accidents may be avoided by taking only the lymph, and by avoiding lymph mixed with blood. To this the answer may be given that it is non-proven that the lymph may not contain at one and the same time the active principle of vaccinia and of syphilis, and, further, no matter what precautions are taken, red corpuscles are always found in vaccine lymph collected from a vaccinifer. The only safe method of preventing this accident is to employ **animal lymph.**

Ulcerated Vaccinia.—We sometimes see ulcerations instead of pustules between the eighth and twelfth days after vaccination. These ulcerations may exceed the size of a sixpence. They are deep, hollowing out and destroying the skin. The edges are straight-cut, and the base is anfractuous, pulpy, diphtheroidal, or gangreniform. They are surrounded by a large red areola, and the tissues upon which they rest show diffuse inflammatory induration. In some cases the ulcers unite, the suppuration is abundant, and the œdema is very extensive. Impetiginous and ecthymatous eruptions, lymphangitis, and lymphatic œdema, may complicate the vaccinal ulcer, which, as a rule, is not painful. These troubles cause indolent and hard inflammation of the glands, while fever is rare, and the general health does not suffer.

These ulcers do not only develop, as was at first supposed, in feeble or lymphatic patients : they occur sometimes in epidemic form in those who are in good health, as, for instance, in the epidemic at Motte-aux-Bois, in which forty-two children suffered from vaccinal ulcers.

The claim that ulcerative vaccinia is more frequent when animal lymph is employed is ill founded, since in several epidemics of ulcerative vaccinia—among others, that at Motte-aux-Bois—the lymph had been taken from a child, and, moreover, appeared to be perfectly good. This ecthymato-ulcerative vaccinia is certainly the result of secondary infection, and due to pathogenic agents developing in lymph which has been kept too long, and has become purulent. From the point of view of diagnosis the ulcerative vaccine will not be confused with vaccinal syphilis, because the chancre does not suppurate or form an ulcer, while its edges are not straight-cut. Lastly, ulcerative vaccinia appears from the eighth to the tenth day after vaccination, while the chancre does not appear until three weeks after. Accordingly, the period of incubation is totally different in the two cases.

Vaccinia in some cases, which are, fortunately, exceptional, may be followed by other complications, including erysipelas, profuse inflammation, and fatal septicæmia ; but these complications are due to secondary infection, which may easily be avoided.

The fear of vaccinal **tuberculosis** is illusory. Neither animal nor Jennerian vaccination is capable of causing tuberculosis. **There is not a**

single positive case. Koch's bacilli have never been met with in lymph taken from tubercular patients, while, if the lymph is taken from an animal, we must remember that tuberculosis in young calves (which are used as the source of the lymph) is so rare that only one case of tuberculosis has been found in 22,000 calves slaughtered in the abattoir at Augsburg.

We can, with proper precautions, avoid all complications. In the first place, vaccinal syphilis is no longer possible, if animal lymph be employed. In the second place, we can prevent any other complications by employing fresh lymph taken on the fifth day from the calf, or on the seventh day from a child, and by being careful to perform inoculation with aseptic instruments on an area of skin which has previously been rendered aseptic.

Sero-therapy.—The first experimental point to establish is that "serum of a vaccinated heifer, collected after the virulent period—*i.e.*, ten to fifty days after vaccination—possesses immunizing properties against inoculated vaccinia"; and it further exercises "*in vitro* on the vaccine an action which may be called **antivirulent,** since the vaccinal virus, after being bathed in this serum, can no longer be successfully inoculated, and produces hardly any local reaction. The attempts of sero-therapy to cure variola with serum from the vaccinated heifer have not yet given any conclusive result.

III. VARICELLA.

Varicella is an eruptive fever, contagious, epidemic, inoculable, very benign, and distinct from varioloid, from which it differs by its mode of invasion, the character of its eruption, as well as by its course and nature. It presents three periods—incubation, invasion, and eruption.

Description.—The incubation period of varicella is a fortnight when it results from contagion, but varies from three to seventeen days when it is caused by inoculation (D'Heilly). In 1895 Apert saw in a maternity hospital an epidemic of varicella which lasted five months, and attacked ten children and two wet-nurses. The cases succeeded one another with an almost mathematical regularity every fortnight, thus allowing the duration of the incubation to be fixed. The symptoms of the period of invasion are very slight. They comprise fever, malaise, and loss of appetite. In less than twenty-four hours small rose-coloured spots can be seen on the skin. Next day these spots form vesicles, filled with clear or slightly coloured fluid. By the second day the bleb is fully formed. It is sometimes umbilicated. It reaches the size of a lentil or of a small pea. On the next day it is surrounded by a painful inflammatory area, and the fluid in it becomes purulent. It then breaks and dries up, leaving a blackish crust, like that which follows a pustule of ecthyma. The evolution of the bleb is therefore complete in three days, while eight days are necessary for the pustule of variola.

The eruption in varicella often leaves some slight scars, especially in children who scratch themselves and pull off the crusts.

The eruption of varicella comes out in successive crops, which are accompanied by fever, and follow each other for four or five days, and even a week to a fortnight. The eruption shows no especial predilection for any part of the body, but commences and spreads at the same time on the face, trunk, and limbs. On the first day a dozen papules may be seen; on the following day thirty to a hundred may be counted, and so on for several days. Varicella, however, always remains more or less discrete, and the eruption, however general it may be, does not become confluent.

Varicella is sometimes accompanied by a scarlatiniform, morbilliform, or erythematous rash, which lasts about twenty-four hours. It may follow or may precede the true eruption.

The eruption of varicella may invade the mucous membranes of various regions (mouth, tongue, uvula, tonsils), as well as the conjunctivæ and corneæ (kerato-conjunctivitis), and it may also be found in the larynx, where it may cause laryngitis, with spasm of the glottis and death. In the laryngeal eruption small circular ulcers are often found on the vocal cords.

Complications are rare in the course of varicella. Nevertheless, **nephritis,** which is usually benign and transient, has been seen (Henoch). **Gangrene** is one of the most unusual complications in varicella. The disease has run a normal course, the pustules have dried up, and recovery is at hand, when, without appreciable cause, and without warning, some of the vesicles become injected with blood, necrose, and ulcerate. The gangrenous ulcers increase in extent and depth, and the disease generally ends fatally. **Arthritis,** which is very rare, may supervene during the decline of the disease. It chiefly attacks the large joints—namely, the knee, shoulder, and hip. The arthritis is always multiple, and the streptococcus is the pathogenic agent (Braquehaye and De Rouville).

Diagnosis.—The vesiculo-bullous appearance of the eruption which occurs in successive crops is diagnostic of varicella. On examination of the eruption over the whole surface of the body, it is rare that we do not find in the midst of growing vesicles and of vesico-pustules, which are more or less purulent or dried up, some adult vesicles in the form of crystalline blebs, which are transparent, rounded, and pathognomonic of varicella. The distinction, however, between varicella and modified variola is sometimes difficult. Certain diagnostic points are, however, present. Thus, the period of invasion in modified variola lasts three days at least, and the usual symptoms are fever, headache, backache, and vomiting; while in varicella the period of invasion lasts one day, and the symptoms are trifling (malaise, lassitude, and slight fever). The eruption of modified variola does not appear before the end of the third or the commencement of the fourth day, while that of varicella appears in twenty-four hours.

The eruption of modified variola commences on the face, while that of varicella commences with a primary crop on different parts of the body. The eruption in modified variola gradually passes into the umbilicated pustule, while that of varicella results within twenty-four hours in a vesicle.

This discussion upon the diagnosis of varicella and varioloid brings us to another question of primary importance—viz., are varicella and varioloid two distinct diseases, each showing its own individuality and specific nature, or is varicella an attenuated variety of varioloid ?

Trousseau was the first to separate varicella from varioloid. Varicella considered in a general manner, said Trousseau, presents clearly marked differences from varioloid, so that it is scarcely comprehensible how confusion has been possible. Indeed, the history of epidemics teaches us the fact that variola may be present alone, but that varioloid is never present in epidemic form without being accompanied by cases of true variola. Variola never attacks a child who has been vaccinated two or three years previously, and the inoculation of variola may be attempted with impunity ; but the same child readily takes varicella if he comes in contact with another child suffering from this disease. Further, if an individual who has just had varicella is placed in contact with variola, he ought not to contract the latter disease if the varicella, of which he still carries traces, is only modified variola. We know, on the contrary, that the individual may contract true variola. Lastly, these two exanthemata, varicella and varioloid, may occur simultaneously or successively in the same patient. Varicella and variola are therefore two absolutely distinct diseases.

The great authority of Trousseau had so clearly decided the question that no one in France attempted to uphold the ancient doctrine of the identity of varicella and varioloid. Abroad, on the other hand, some observers were of the opposite opinion, and proclaimed the identity of the two diseases (Kaposi, Hébra). Their opinions have recently found some partisans in their own country, who run a great risk of remaining isolated, for Trousseau's teaching is more alive than ever. The ideas which our great master, with so much reason and good sense, caused to prevail in the name of clinical medicine have been confirmed by indisputable observations, of which I give a résumé.

Senator and Tordeus have successfully vaccinated children who have had varicella, and D'Espine has seen varicella occur on the twenty-second day in a case of variola. Those who believe in the identity of the two diseases should carefully ponder over the following case :

A child, thirteen months old, in whom Œttinger found characteristic varicella, was sent by mistake to the annex for cases of variola. In a short while the child recovered from the varicella. Œttinger, having found no marks of previous vaccination, had very properly recommended immediate vaccination, which, however, was done only ten days later. Two days later the child showed symptoms of variola, which proved fatal, although the vaccinal pustules had appeared at the three inoculated points at the same time as the eruption of variola. This case is most instructive. If varicella and variola were the same disease, this child, who had just had the former, would not have contracted the latter some days later, and if varicella and vaccinia were the same disease, as some authorities have upheld, the vaccine would not have taken in the child who had just had varicella. " This case," says Œttinger, " in conjunction with one of Dr. Sharkey and many others, is another **plea in favour of the specific nature of varicella.** It is only one case, but it is irrefutable, and should prevail against all the contrary hypotheses which might be formulated."

In some cases varicella suppurates. After one or two days the fluid in the vesicle loses its limpid character, and becomes opalescent, yellowish, and purulent. It contains polynuclear leucocytes in large number, while the citron-coloured fluid of varicella, like the purulent fluid of the pustule in variola, contains chiefly mononuclear cells. The staphylococcus, with or without the streptococcus, is the organism which produces the suppuration. This suppuration lasts a few days, and ends in rupture or slow desiccation of the vesicle, with the formation of crusts and scars, like those of variola. The appearance of pus is sometimes accompanied by fever. Epidemics of suppurative varicella have been seen. The diagnosis between variola and suppurative varicella is not always free from difficulty, and yet in a case of suppurative varicella we always find clear or limpid vesicles, which permit us to make a diagnosis.

Treatment.—The treatment of varicella consists in attention to hygiene, mild purgatives, milk diet, and the application to the vesicles of an ointment, in order to avoid infection (oxide of zinc, 1 part ; powdered talc, 5 parts). A bath is given when the disease is at an end, and until then the patient should be isolated, for varicella is markedly contagious in children. Infection and dissemination take place with the greatest rapidity.

IV. SCARLATINA.

Description.—I shall choose as my type a case of scarlatina of moderate severity, and I shall then describe the malignant, hæmorrhagic, and defaced forms,* which are far more rare.

The evolution of scarlatina is usually divided into four periods—incubation, invasion, eruption, and desquamation.

Incubation.—The period comprised between the introduction of the infective agent into the economy and the appearance of the first symptoms has not been exactly determined. Certain facts would indicate that it may be very short—not longer than twenty-four hours (case reported by

* See p. 1583.

Trousseau)—but the average duration is four to seven days, while it may be more than a fortnight. During the period of incubation, which is generally latent, the patient's general health is excellent. Sometimes, however, the infective process which is going on in the economy shows itself by general malaise.

Invasion.—Scarlatina usually commences with more or less severe phenomena, including rigors, quick pulse (110 in adults and 140 in children), rise of temperature to 104° F., sore throat, and headache. Nausea, vomiting of food or of bile, and convulsions in young children, or delirium in adults, are sometimes seen in the severe forms. In some persons the vomiting at the onset of scarlatina is frequent and uncontrollable, and in some epidemics it has been the chief feature (Greifs-wald epidemic, 1826). Sore throat is the symptom noticed, almost to the exclusion of others, during the period of invasion. I may say that most cases of scarlatina in children commence with acute tonsillitis, which is set down to cold, and it is only some hours later or on the next day that we see the appearance of the exanthem in the mouth and pharynx, or of the rash upon the skin. We can then correct an erroneous diagnosis, or confirm a doubtful one. The angina causes pain on swallowing ; the throat is dry, and the tonsils are swollen, as at the onset of tonsillitis, and of a dark red colour, which extends to the throat and soft palate. The retro-maxillary glands are painful and enlarged. The tongue is coated, but red at the tip and edges. Anorexia is present, and the thirst is acute, but diarrhœa is rare. The respiratory system remains free. Absence of cough is the rule—an important and striking contrast to the invasion of measles.

Eruption.—The period of invasion usually lasts twenty-four to thirty-six hours. It may last only a few hours, and the eruption and sore throat may appear at the same time. The eruption does not show itself first on the face, as in measles and variola, but usually begins on the neck and chest, and becomes more or less general, the hands being invaded last.

At first the eruption is composed of red spots, which are small and not prominent. They quickly unite, without leaving intervals of healthy skin, and form extensive patches of a strawberry or scarlet colour ; whence the name of **red fever** formerly given to scarlatina. A large area of the body may be thus coloured by the eruption, but the tint is not absolutely uniform. A darker stippling shows on the red ground of the exanthem. The redness of the skin is most marked on the neck, the abdomen, and the inner surface of the thighs and arms. When we press on the parts invaded by the erup-tion, or trace lines with the point of a pencil, the redness gives place for a moment to a whitish colour, which contrasts with the red ground.

This classical description of the eruption does not include all cases, for there are discrete eruptions in scarlatina, formed by a multitude of little red points, rounded, isolated from one another, and somewhat like the eruption of measles.

The eruption on the face differs somewhat from that on the body, being streaky, or formed by red and white tracts, like the finger-marks seen after the ears have been boxed (Trousseau). In addition, the face is puffy and swollen, and this swelling is also noticeable in the feet and hands. The swelling begins and increases with the eruption, so that by the second or third day it hampers the movements of the fingers; but it is not painful, and must be distinguished from the rheumatic swelling, which I shall describe later. More or less acute itching accompanies the eruption, and is usually associated with the benign forms and with abundant sweating.

The eruption, though sometimes transient, usually lasts from three to five days, and if it is at all confluent, it is accompanied by a crop of miliaria on the neck and the abdomen. The miliary eruption gives to the skin the appearance called "goose-flesh." The vesicles of the miliary rash are perceptible to the touch, and are at first filled with a colourless fluid, which thirty-six hours afterwards becomes milky.

Can any relation be established between the intensity of the eruption and the gravity of the fever ? Trousseau held the following opinion : It is said that when the eruption is "well out," in vulgar parlance, the patient has less chance of being attacked by serious complications. The contrary opinion, however, holds good, for in scarlatina, as in the other eruptive fevers, the more intense the eruption, the more severe is the disease. This proposition, however, is not absolute, and in scarlatina, just as in variola, if the eruption is prevented by some grave antagonistic inflammation, by severe hæmorrhage, or by profound nervous disturbances, it does not appear in a typical form, but is ill-defined and incomplete. This occurs, then, in anomalous scarlatina, which is not always free from danger.

The angina must now occupy our attention. It forms from the onset of scarlatina the chief symptom, and increases in severity during the eruptive period. The movements of deglutition are so painful that the patient cannot swallow the saliva. He expectorates continuously; he can drink only at the risk of sharp pain, and fluids regurgitate through the nose; the voice is nasal. The swelling of the uvula and tonsils may embarrass the breathing. On examination of the throat, we find that the tonsils are large, the uvula is œdematous, the mucous membrane is swollen, and a diffuse redness (scarlatinal exanthem) invades all these regions, and at times covers the mucosa of the cheeks and lips. On the third or fourth day the angina becomes pultaceous (*puls*, *pultis*, pap), and on the tonsils, which are large and red, we see in the crypts a deposit of small whitish or greyish concretions, forming a pultaceous coating that is not adherent to the subjacent parts, and is readily removed with a tampon of wool. This pultaceous coating is formed by the products of epithelial desquamation and by the mucus secreted by the follicles of the tonsil. It is perfectly soluble, as can be proved by shaking it for a few moments in a glass of water. The angina ends in three or four days, and the concretions disappear from the tonsils, which remain red and sometimes excoriated (Trousseau).

The tongue is absolutely characteristic. After the coated condition at first seen, the epithelium is gradually laid bare, and between the third and sixth day of the disease the organ presents a scarlet surface, which is swollen and thickly set with large papillæ, giving it a strawberry-like appearance. About the seventh or eighth day the tongue, although it preserves its red colour, becomes smoother, and loses its strawberry appearance ; but it is only about the twelfth day that its appearance approaches the normal, the red tint being still marked.

The lesions of the mouth and pharynx affect the tonsils (tonsillitis) and the mucosa of the cavity (bucco-pharyngeal erythema). Berger has even insisted on the importance of the dissociation of these two local lesions (of which tonsillitis is the first) from the point of view of pathogenesis.

Adenopathy in scarlatina is constant. With the onset of angina the glands at the angle of the jaw become painful, enlarged, and indurated.

Fever persists during the whole of the eruptive period, and shows a continuous type, with a slight morning remission. It ceases when the eruption disappears.

Desquamation.—Desquamation begins from the sixth to the tenth day, sometimes even while the rash is still out. It commences on the neck and the chest, and finishes on the palms of the hands and the soles of the feet. It never assumes the branny form of measles. On the face it takes place in small scales ; on the trunk larger scales are seen. On the arms and legs, and especially on the feet, where the epidermis is thicker, patches of large size may peel off. On the fingers the epidermis is sometimes shed in strips, which may resemble the fingers of a glove. Shedding of the nails has also been seen (Graves). Desquamation lasts, on an average, from eight days to a fortnight. It may, however, be prolonged to thirty, fifty, and seventy days (Trousseau). The knowledge of these facts is of the highest importance, for scarlatinal desquamation may give a clue to such complications as albuminuria, anasarca, severe angina, endocarditis, etc.

Slight Forms.—Sydenham's dictum that " scarlatina scarcely merits the name of a disease " may be applied to these forms. After fever lasting for some hours and slight sore throat, a trifling eruption appears, but the patient only experiences slight malaise. The digestive functions are not

affected.   The desquamation is very slight, and in a few days the disease is
at an end.   **Every intermediate form** between these benign and the serious
cases is seen.

Severe Forms—Malignant Scarlet Fever.—I have preserved the
epithet malignant, because this term, given to the disease by our predecessors, is most applicable to the forms which I shall now describe.
Malignant scarlet fever runs the following course :

On the first day, says Trousseau, or during the first few hours, the
disease reaches its maximum.   It may prove fatal within twenty-four hours.
This form which kills patients, like a superacute intoxication, is characterized by extremely rapid pulse, hyperpyrexia, delirium, restlessness, convulsions, uncontrollable vomiting, diarrhœa, dryness of the skin, cyanosis,
suppression of urine, and attacks of suffocation.   And as these troubles
may be fatal before the appearance of the rash, the diagnosis would be very
difficult in the absence of an epidemic.

The following cases, quoted by Trousseau, will show better than any
description the picture of malignant scarlet fever :

" I was summoned," says Trousseau, " by my friend Dr. Bigelow to a boarding-
school in Paris to see a young American girl.   Since the morning she had been a prey
to frightful delirium, with incessant vomiting and high fever ; the pulse was so rapid
that the beats could not be counted, and there was extraordinary dryness of the skin.
These symptoms caused me to state, on seeing the patient, that the case was one of
scarlet fever, and, indeed, although no other symptoms appeared, my diagnosis was
confirmed by the presence of a characteristic rash upon another young lady at the
same school, in which an epidemic was raging. The patient died before the end of the day.

" In 1824, at the beginning of the disastrous epidemic which broke out at Tours,
and of which I have spoken, I saw, with Bretonneau, a young girl who died in less than
eleven hours with acute delirium, excessive restlessness, and extraordinary frequency
of the pulse.   Here there was nothing to indicate the nature of the disease, except that
an epidemic of scarlatina was raging, and that in the girl's family several persons had
been attacked.

" Beware, then, under such circumstances, of nervous complications marking the
onset of illness in the midst of an epidemic of scarlatina which has already attacked
members of the same family as the patient to whom you are called.   These symptoms
nearly always indicate malignant scarlet fever, which almost always kills with astonishing
rapidity those whom it attacks."

Side by side with these fulminant forms we see very similar cases, which
are, however, slower in their evolution, and which may end in recovery.
In them, too, the nervous troubles play the chief part, and the period of
invasion is characterized by extreme frequency of the pulse, by delirium, and
by insomnia, which yields to no remedies.   The temperature, which is
already very high, continues to rise.   The patient complains of præcordial
distress, and the dyspnœa is so great that the respiration-rate may be
40 or 50 per minute, although auscultation does not reveal any broncho-
pulmonary lesion.   This dyspnœa is of nervous origin—or sine materia,

as the old writers were wont to call it. It is often of evil augury in the toxi-infectious diseases. Vomiting and diarrhœa are rarely absent, and if the patient succumbs, he is usually carried off during the eruptive period.

In some cases grave complications supervene, not so much at the onset of the disease, as during its course, when the eruption is fully out. Lastly, there are cases in which the nervous troubles assume an adynamic form, and the patient dies in a typhoid state.

These terrible forms, exceptional in sporadic scarlatina, belong to the epidemic form of the disease, and are more or less frequent, according to the particular epidemic.

Hæmorrhagic Scarlatina.—This form is very rare, for scarlatina is much less prone to hæmorrhagic complications than variola and measles. The hæmorrhage generally appears at the same time as the rash. The patients experience some serious symptoms—the skin is covered with petechiæ ; hæmaturia and epistaxis are common. The prognosis in hæmorrhagic scarlatina is bad.

Defaced Scarlatina.—The word "defaced," coined by Trousseau, is an excellent one. He applied the term defaced to those cases of scarlatina in which the eruption is wanting, and which show only some one symptom by which the diagnosis can be reconstructed, just as in archæology an inscription is called defaced when a more or less considerable part is blotted out, and some words alone remain by which we can reconstruct the entire inscription. Defaced scarlatina is chiefly seen in epidemics (Graves). In one patient who has had no rash the only prominent symptom of the disease is angina. In another patient the scarlatina reveals itself by desquamation, anasarca, nephritis, albuminuria, or hæmaturia, which may or may not be preceded by angina.

I quote two cases of defaced scarlatina reported by Trousseau :

"In 1854, at Meaux, I saw, with my friend Blache, a case of defaced scarlatina. In the same house a young girl, fourteen years of age, had been taken ill with severe scarlatina, characterized by pultaceous angina, high fever, and specific rash. A few days later her sister was also taken ill with the same symptoms ; almost at the same time a housemaid fell sick ; and, two or three days later, a valet, who remained during the whole day in the house, was affected by severe sore throat, with pultaceous exudate on the tonsils, redness, and then cleaning of the tongue and acute fever, although no eruption appeared on the skin. It was clear that all these patients had scarlatina, and that the valet, remaining in such an epidemic centre, had contracted it just as the whole family did, but in another form, so that in his case the inscription was defaced, while in the others the scarlatinal phase had been complete. There was also a young boy, six years of age, who suddenly became swollen up, without having been ill for a moment. Blache and I were then called in consultation, and recognized scarlatinal anasarca, which had been the first symptom to appear ; it was considerable in amount, and was accompanied by hæmaturia. The father and mother, who were very careful about their son's health, declared that he had eaten his breakfast as usual that morning, and his schoolmaster also told us that he had played about as usual. He had neither fever nor rash ; the disease was indicated in his case by the single complication for which we were called in consultation.

" In December, 1860, I saw, with my friend Dr. Gros, a youth, fifteen years of age, who furnished another example of defaced scarlatina, and in whom the diagnosis would have been impossible if we had not had assistance from the accessory conditions. This youth had come from college with slight fever and sore throat. The illness was so slight that Dr. Gros was not called in, and the patient recovered after two days of trifling indisposition. A few days later his younger sister took scarlatina, and when she was convalescent her brother was attacked by hæmaturia, which lasted more than a month. I did not doubt for a moment that this youth had given scarlatina to his sister, and that the hæmaturia was the result of the pyrexia, the manifestation of which had been so slight."

I have several times witnessed defaced scarlatina. In a family in which five persons were attacked by true scarlatina, I saw, with Jules Simon, a remarkable example of defaced scarlatina in a child four years old. In this case the expected rash did not appear, but the sore throat which had marked the onset of the disease was followed by considerable swelling of the neck and glands ; anasarca and pyelitis, with scanty and muco-purulent urine, followed. The patient finally recovered.

I saw a child in the Avenue Montaigne with fever, rapid pulse, and sore throat ; the redness of the soft palate and of the tonsils (enanthema) was so marked that I at once diagnosed scarlatina. We watched closely for the appearance of the rash, but it did not appear ; in short, the scarlatina was absolutely defaced. About the eighth day, however, characteristic desquamation supervened. Desquamation may occur in scarlet fever without any previously appreciable rash.

I saw one of my colleagues from the provinces who, after attending a child with scarlet fever, was himself taken ill with fever and a sore throat of strawberry-like appearance. As he was certain that he had scarlatina, he watched closely for the rash, but it did not appear. Eight days after, desquamation began ; and nephritis, which was fortunately slight, appeared some days later.

In epidemics of scarlet fever we see attenuated forms, comprising a simple sore throat, so slightly marked that the disease passes unnoticed, and also apyretic forms which are not free from complications.

Complications of Scarlatina.

The conditions which we call " complications," in order to conform to custom, and which are usually the result of **secondary infections,** may supervene in the most benign cases of scarlatina. They appear during the course of the disease, or during the period of defervescence.

Scarlatinal Angina.—Scarlatina is essentially a disease accompanied by sore throat. I have already described the early erythematous angina, which may hamper deglutition and respiration, and which is often accompanied by marked glandular enlargement. This form, usually associated with the streptococcus or the staphylococcus, yields rapidly.

Membranous angina, a condition of much interest, presents quite another picture. Trousseau was the first to admit two varieties of membranous angina in scarlatina. The one which is not diphtheritic is usually early and benign, and has no tendency to spread to the larynx. It was in this connection with this form that Trousseau enunciated the celebrated aphorism, " Scarlatina does not like the larynx." The other variety, diphtheritic in nature, and more serious, may invade the respiratory tract, or run the course of malignant diphtheria. Bacteriology has demonstrated the truth of Trousseau's observation, and also of his clinical teaching. Bacteriological research has clearly elucidated the question of buffy angina in scarlatina, which was formerly so confused (*vide* p. 602).

Early and late membranous buffy angina is seen in scarlatina. The early cases usually appear from the third to the sixth day of the fever, and are hardly ever diphtheritic. They are due to a streptococcus, with which other microbes, including the *Bacillus coli* and the staphylococcus, are associated. These cases resemble diphtheria, by reason of the fibrinous false membranes, by the accompanying glandular enlargement, and by the reproduction of the membranes ; but they do not produce croup, are not followed by paralysis, and are generally benign.

Although they are not diphtheritic, they may assume a certain degree of gravity. They resemble the form described by Hénoch under the name of " necrotic inflammation." In this form the membranes in the throat may spread to the mouth and lips, and are very adherent. When they are removed, the mucosa is ulcerated and bleeding. The breath is fœtid ; the enlargement of the glands and the submaxillary œdema are very marked, and the fever is somewhat high. They usually terminate in recovery, in spite of their apparent gravity.

In other circumstances these cases of membranous angina, although not diphtheritic (I am still speaking of the early form), run a malignant course. They are characterized by the rapid spread of the membranes, by the marked swelling of the glands (Bourges), by the obstinate character of the angina, which lasts as long as three weeks, and by the persistence of the fever. Hæmorrhages and gangrene are also seen. The mucosa of the mouth and of the pharynx is œdematous, ecchymosed, bleeding, and necrotic (Hénoch). The gangrene eats away the tonsils, and causes ulceration of the base of the tongue, of the pillars of the fauces, and of the uvula. The breath is excessively fœtid, and a viscous liquid dribbles from the mouth. This process, although not diphtheritic, may affect the nasal fossæ, the eyelids, the conjunctivæ, and the larynx. Buboes, nephritis, broncho-pneumonia, and otitis are fairly often associated with it, and the patient usually dies in a condition of adynamia.

While discussing the severe non-diphtheritic angina of scarlatina, I remarked that the *Staphylococcus aureus* is often associated with the strepto-coccus. The streptococcus is the chief factor in these cases of angina, just as it is in most of the complications of scarlatina, and the angina may assume the membranous or the malignant type, although diphtheria is absent.

pseudo-membranous (non-diphtheritic), and the nasal cavities are covered with membranes, due to streptococci.

Nephritis and Urinary Troubles.—We find albuminuria, nephritis, hæmaturia, anuria, and pyelitis.

Albuminuria occurs at an early period in a half, or at least in a third, of the patients suffering from scarlatina. This early albuminuria is usually febrile, and is connected with very transient change in the renal epithelium. It is not as a rule accompanied by any other symptom of nephritis, and disappears during the course of the second week. It may, indeed, last only a few days. I have, however, seen early albuminuria last for some weeks, and be accompanied by puffiness of the face—a proof that we cannot make too clear a distinction between the early albuminuria of scarlatina and the nephritis which appears later. In both cases nephritis is present, and the severity of the process alone distinguishes them.

Apart from the cases which I have just quoted, it may be said that **scarlatinal nephritis** does not, as a rule, appear before the fifteenth day— that is to say, when the fever and rash are no longer present. It may assume every form.

Nephritis of moderate intensity is the most common form. It is characterized by albuminous urine, which is sometimes smoky or bloodstained, and by more or less general œdema, which commences in the face. In some cases, indeed, the anasarca is the first symptom. After some weeks, recovery, or at least apparent recovery, takes place, and yet the kidney may carry the mark of the lesion for a long time.

In exceptional cases the nephritis is very grave, and ends in a few days in acute uræmia. Sometimes gastro-intestinal troubles, with vomiting and diarrhœa, are the first symptoms to appear; but at other times dyspnœa, with or without pleural effusion, and œdema of the lung dominate the scene. In other cases the uræmia sets in with nervous symptoms—headache, convulsions, and coma—which prove rapidly fatal. Œdema of the glottis may appear as the initial manifestation of scarlatinal nephritis. Abundant epistaxis and visual troubles, such as amblyopia or amaurosis, are seen in some patients.

Scarlatinal nephritis may appear in an epidemic state, being sometimes associated with typical scarlatina and at other times with the defaced forms of the disease. Fiessinger has published an interesting paper, in which he quotes an epidemic of acute nephritis, where some cases were independent of scarlatina, while others were associated with it.

Scarlatina is fairly often the starting-point of Bright's disease, and it cannot easily be explained how an opposite opinion (Bartels, Charcot) was upheld a few years ago. Acute scarlatinal nephritis may not only end in chronic nephritis, but in some cases the nephritis seems to have been chronic from the first. We see adults or children in whom the initial phase of scarlatinal nephritis is so slight that it may pass practically unnoticed. We see children or adults in whom the symptoms of nephritis are reduced to albuminuria, with slight and transient œdema. These cases are too often treated lightly, being termed " early albuminuria," and no further attention is paid to them. And yet five or six months later œdema of the eyelids and puffiness of the face are seen, and the albuminuria reappears. This subacute process may pass unnoticed if the child is absent from home or a boarder at school, and the disease progresses until symptoms of greater importance sound a warning.

Scarlatina is, therefore, a frequent cause of Bright's disease, as the following cases show :

I saw, with Charrier, a child six years of age. He had suffered two years before from slight scarlatinal nephritis, but had never completely recovered, being at times troubled with albuminuria, œdema of the face, dyspepsia, and vomiting. In this case improvement was obtained only by the most rigid milk diet. Several years ago I attended a youth suffering from Bright's disease, consecutive to scarlatina seven years previously. His father, who was head-master of one of our colleges, told me that the nephritis came on during the attack of scarlatina, but was so slight that no attention was paid to it ; the later symptoms ran a very slow course, with well-marked periods of arrest, until uræmia set in. I receive from time to time a visit from a young man who has been on a milk diet for some years : he caught from his sister a very benign scarlatina, complicated by mild nephritis, albuminuria being the only symptom. When the scarlatina got better, the kidneys were not attended to ; later, œdema and headache supervened, and finally the symptoms of uræmia became threatening.

The chronic form of scarlatinal nephritis did not escape the notice of Trousseau. " Scarlatinal albuminuria may pass into the chronic state— that is, into Bright's disease." Chronic nephritis of scarlatinal origin is now admitted by nearly all authors, and Lécorché and Talamon quote absolutely characteristic cases.

Scarlatina exercises a peculiarly noxious action on the kidney, and in this regard I do not know any other disease which can be compared with it. Typhoid fever, influenza, erysipelas, etc., are far from attacking the kidney with the same frequency and severity. The scarlatinal toxine has a powerful and lasting effect on the renal epithelium. For my part, I consider that the greatest danger in scarlatina, aside from some rare complications, is to be found in present or in future renal trouble. In the statistics of scarlatina at the Hôpital des Enfants-Malades in 1895, Apert found nephritis in 20 per cent. of the cases, and in 6 per cent. the disease was serious. The clinical records of a hospital, however, give us no information as to the future of these children suffering from scarlatinal nephritis, for we lose sight of them. Many leave the hospital, although albumin is still present in the urine. Their kidneys are diseased, and many of these children are likely to develop Bright's disease. The renal lesions may remain dormant, and be revived later by a fresh infection, such as typhoid fever, influenza, mumps, or syphilis ; but in any case, when the kidney has been damaged by scarlatina, it does not lose the taint quickly.

Few lesions have been as much discussed as scarlatinal nephritis, which has been in turn described as catarrhal, interstitial, glomerular (Klebs' glomerulitis), and parenchymatous. It forms part of the group of acute diffuse nephritis. According to the case, the inflammation is slight or severe. According to the time of death and the nature of the process, we find post mortem the large white kidney, the large hæmorrhagic kidney, the red hyperæmic kidney, the soft, white, œdematous kidney, and the kidney undergoing fibrous atrophy ; but the character of the lesions is not so clearly marked that we can place scarlatinal nephritis in a separate class.

The chief lesions in scarlatinal nephritis comprise glomerulitis, glomerular and tubular hæmorrhages, and interstitial œdema—that is to say, diapedesis of a large number of white corpuscles into Bowman's capsule, between the glomeruli and the tubules (Wagner's acute lymphomatous nephritis). Cloudy swelling of the epithelium, necrosis, and granulo-fatty degeneration in the epithelium of the convoluted tubes, are the lesions found, according to the particular case.

Scarlatinal nephritis is of toxi-infectious origin. It is due to the micro-organisms which accompany the disease as a secondary infection, and which have been found in the kidneys (streptococci, micrococci, diplococci), to toxines elaborated by these microbes, and especially to the poison of scarlatina, the nature of which is as yet unknown to us.

Hæmaturia.—Hæmaturia is a frequent symptom during the decline of scarlatina. If the blood is in fairly large quantity, the urine is of a blackish or brownish colour, and a more or less thick deposit of blood is seen at the bottom of the specimen-glass. If the hæmorrhage is trifling, it may, on superficial examination, pass unnoticed. As a rule, hæmaturia is associated with other symptoms of acute nephritis, but it may precede or even accompany them, whether the case is one of classical or of defaced scarlatina, and, indeed, the frequency of hæmaturia in defaced scarlatina is very remarkable. The hæmaturia, which may be severe or slight, lasts several days. It then disappears, leaving the acute nephritis to continue its course, which may be transient or lasting. A patient of whom Trousseau speaks was taken ill with hæmaturia, lasting more than a month, and forming the prelude of nephritis, lasting nearly a year. Scarlatinal hæmaturia fairly often appears at the same time as does the œdema. One child of whom Trousseau speaks was attacked during an epidemic with defaced scarlatina, characterized by considerable dropsy and hæmaturia. The attack was very severe and affected both kidneys in the form of hæmorrhage, and the subcutaneous cellular tissue at the same time in the form of general œdema.

Scarlatinal hæmaturia, however, is not always associated with nephritis. Blood may come from the kidney without the hæmaturia being necessarily the prelude of nephritis.

Blondeau reports the case of a little boy, eight years of age, suffering from defaced scarlatina. Among other symptoms he had hæmaturia, which lasted forty-eight hours, but which was not followed by nephritis. Some days later the urine regained its normal character, and contained no albumin.

Let us note, lastly, hæmaturia as a part of the multiple hæmorrhages which occur in the hæmorrhagic form of scarlatina.

Scarlatinal Anuria.—Scarlatinal anuria has several origins. Sometimes, in the course of scarlatinal nephritis, the urine falls to a few ounces in the twenty-four hours (oliguria)—a symptom of very bad augury. In such a case, however, the urine is that of acute nephritis, and the cause of the oliguria is revealed by analysis of the urine, which is rich in albumin and cylindrical casts, while the oliguria and anuria in scarlatina at times supervene apart from any nephritis; the urine contains no albumin, and becomes scanty, or may be suppressed completely. Uræmia appears, and the prognosis is very grave.

Bartels reports two cases in which death supervened very rapidly (nine hours in one and twelve hours in the other case). The anuria came on suddenly, the urine having been normal in appearance, without the least trace of albumin. At the autopsy, Leichtenstern found large white œdematous kidneys, and facts such as these, says Bartels, led him to explain the anuria, not by glomerulo-nephritis, as Klebs believed, but by œdema of the kidney.

In 1892 I attended a child for scarlatinal anuria, which had lasted twenty-four hours without other symptoms. The scarlatina, which was of moderate severity, had up till then run a normal course. The child was put on milk diet, and the urine, which I examined daily, contained neither blood nor albumin, when the secretion of urine, which hitherto had been abundant, suddenly ceased. My satisfaction when the urinary secretion was re-established can be easily understood.

Anuria and oliguria usually supervene during the decline of the disease. Juhel-Rénoy has described anuria in the early stage of scarlatina. The patient of whom he speaks died seven days after the appearance of anuria, and the autopsy revealed embolisms and infarcts containing micro-organisms in the vessels of the glomeruli. In short, the mechanism of scarlatinal anuria is obscure; but it is certain that the scarlatinal poison may paralyze the renal function, affecting the secretion of urine, and thus provoking uræmia.

Pyelitis is also seen in scarlatina. The urine is scanty and contains pus.

Dropsy.—It is customary to consider dropsy in scarlatina as being associated with nephritis, and, indeed, dropsy and albuminuria both arise from the nephritis ; but in some cases these two symptoms are dissociated. We see cases of scarlatina in which the albuminuria is transient or slight, while the dropsy assumes unusual proportions, so that in such a case the dropsy appears to evolve on its own account. Further, even though scarlatinal dropsy is always the result of nephritis, it is none the less true that the soil upon which it develops offers conditions that do not exist in the case of non-scarlatinal nephritis. Dropsy in acute or chronic nephritis does not set in so suddenly, and does not become general with such rapidity. Accordingly, scarlatina is of considerable moment in the pathogenesis of this dropsy. Dropsy is seen more frequently in the moderate than in the severe forms of scarlatina, and has often been found in defaced scarlatina. Thus, a child during an epidemic suffers from a sore throat, without any rash, and hæmaturia, followed by dropsy, or dropsy without hæmaturia, appears twelve or fourteen days later. The dropsy is nearly always a complication of convalescence, rarely appearing during the first week of scarlatina, and more rarely still after the fifth week (Tripp). The dropsy may or may not commence with fever. The swelling generally starts in the face, and invades the trunk and limbs so rapidly that it becomes general in twenty-four to thirty-six hours. For example, a child who the evening before was thin and miserable appears next day to be fat, from the enormous swelling which has occurred. The dropsy disappears gradually, but local œdema, especially that of the face, is obstinate, and subject to recurrence.

Although dropsy is usually a benign complication, we must not forget that it is sometimes accompanied by effusion into the pleuræ or the peritoneum and by œdema of the larynx, which rapidly endangers life. Œdema of the palato-pharyngeal mucosa is the more easily understood, as this mucous membrane has been prepared by the scarlatinal angina. Trousseau reports several cases of pharyngo-laryngeal œdema in which tracheotomy became necessary.

When the dropsy appears independently of the renal lesion and of the albuminuria, we invoke, without sufficient proof, " cold as a cause. Otherwise the origin remains obscure, and we can only suspect the changes produced in the cutaneous capillaries by the exanthem, and especially by desquamation " (Jaccoud). These facts may have some bearing on the œdema studied by Potain, which supervenes apart from any cardiac or renal lesions, and appears to depend on the rheumatic diathesis. However this may be, we see on closer inspection that dropsy in scarlatinal patients is, above all, associated with nephritis.

Pseudo-Rheumatism in Scarlatina.—Joint troubles are fairly frequent in scarlatina—at any rate, in adults. " In a large number of cases," says

Graves, " I have found articular rheumatism following scarlatina." This rheumatism, says Trousseau, is generally quite slight. It must be looked for by pressure over the wrist or over the instep, where it is most often found. This pseudo-rheumatism rarely runs the same course as acute rheumatism, being more fixed, less subject to relapses, and not as a rule returning again in the joints which it has left. Sometimes, however, it may, like true rheumatism, attack the organs in the chest, without first touching the joints. It may also become general. When I was house-physician to Axenfeld, I remember seeing a patient who was attacked by acute articular rheumatism, with endocarditis, iritis, and cerebral troubles, during the decline of scarlet fever.

Hiller, Ashby, and Picot also quote cases of general articular rheumatism, with or without endocarditis, occurring during convalescence from scarlet fever. Chorea, which in children is so closely related to rheumatism, sometimes appears two or three months after scarlatina.

Is it that scarlatina only reawakens the rheumatic diathesis, as Peter thinks ? We might be tempted to think so when we see cases of general rheumatism, but as a rule they are cases of infective pseudo-rheumatism, so that the different visceral manifestations—namely, endocarditis, which may be infective, pericarditis, and pleurisy—depend less upon rheumatism than upon the scarlatinal infection.

Suppuration.—Scarlatina predisposes to suppuration, and this fact is not surprising, seeing that the streptococcus is inseparable from most scarlatinal manifestations and their secondary infections.

Pleurisy, which is of rapid course, insidious, and variable according to the particular epidemic, is sometimes sero-fibrinous, sometimes purulent. In children it may be purulent from the first, and may end in vomica.

Pericarditis may be sero-fibrinous, hæmorrhagic, or purulent, and may be associated with endocarditis and with pleurisy.

The suppurative arthritis shows various characters. In the most common form the arthritis is serous at first, and suppuration does not occur till later. Hénoch quotes cases of suppurative coxalgia and gonalgia. In another form the inflammation, which affects the joints and tendon-sheaths, is purulent from the first, and forms a true pyæmia, accompanied by delirium and coma. This pyæmia may result from septic embolisms, originating in a focus of suppuration, such as an abscess in the neck.

We must consider at some length **adeno-phlegmon of the neck.** Even the simplest scarlatinal angina is always accompanied by swelling of the glands at the angle of the jaw. This adenitis, which is generally painful, clears up in a few days. Sometimes the swelling is more marked, and the neck is more brawny ; but yet resolution occurs, and recovery follows. In other cases suppuration occurs and buboes form in the neck.

They appeared quite early in an epidemic of scarlatina observed by Guéretin; but more often they supervene during the stationary stage, or even when convalescence is fully established. They are associated with pseudo-diphtheritic angina, and the streptococcus is the pathogenic agent. The adeno-phlegmon transforms the side of the neck into a stiff, painful area, and all movement of the head and neck becomes impossible. The œdema may reach the face, and may involve the cervical region as far as the clavicle and the palato-laryngeal cavity. The patient is, as it were, fixed in a yoke. The pain is intense, deglutition is impossible, phonation is difficult, the respiration is embarrassed, and œdema of the glottis may cause death.

Suppuration in adeno-phlegmon is not always ushered in by fluctuation. The tissues are hard and brawny, the skin is pale or shiny, and the pus from the abscess is blood-stained, foul-smelling, and rarely homogeneous. These adeno-phlegmons are sometimes accompanied by gangrene, which lays bare the vessels, the muscles, and the aponeuroses. The internal jugular vein and the internal and external carotid arteries are sometimes involved in the inflammatory process, and fatal hæmorrhage is the result, the blood coming from the mouth or from the opening in the phlegmon.

The adeno-phlegmon just described, although serious, may end in recovery; but the **diffuse phlegmon,** which appears early and at once invades the cellular tissue and the glands of the neck, does not recover.

Abscesses and cellulitis may develop in different regions—in the axilla, the thigh, or the leg. They are complications seen during the decline of the disease.

Inflammation of the parotid glands is very rare.

Otitis.—Otitis is frequent in scarlatina, and this is not surprising when we consider the condition of the throat and the ease with which infections spread from the pharynx to the middle ear through the Eustachian tube. In the slight and common form of otitis, pain, noises in the ears, and diminished acuteness of hearing are the only appreciable symptoms. Resolution takes place in a few days, and recovery follows. In the more severe forms, which generally supervene towards the end of the eruption, the pain is very acute, the temperature is high, and the child is restless, and may suffer from delirium and convulsions. We find here infection in a closed cavity, which I have discussed under the Pathogenesis of Appendicitis. If the Eustachian tube recovers its permeability in time, the symptoms disappear, but the infection usually ends in perforation of the membrana tympani, and the pus escapes through the external auditory meatus. As a general rule, the perforation puts an end to the acute symptoms. The suppuration, however, is slow to dry up, and many children suffer from otorrhœa for weeks and months. The otitis, which is nearly always bilateral, may expose the patient to the most terrible complications, such as meningitis, encephalitis, cerebral abscess, caries of the petrous bone, ulceration of a large vessel, or facial paralysis. Deafness may follow scarlatinal otitis.

Streptococci and staphylococci are found in the pus from a case of otitis, just as in the pus from cases of suppurative adenitis. In some cases the diphtheria bacillus and the tubercle bacillus are also found as a secondary infection.

Sequelæ.—Scarlatina may leave indelible sequelæ. I have just spoken of **deafness.** Hæmoplegia consecutive to cerebral arteritis has been noted (Alexeff).

In some patients of lymphatic temperament scarlatina leaves glandular tumours in the neck and chronic eczema of the nose and ear (Hardy). **Endocarditis** may pass unnoticed during the course of scarlatina. Sometimes it supervenes later, at the same time as the pseudo-rheumatism or the chorea. It may persist in the chronic form. I shall not refer again to Bright's disease, which is a possible sequela.

Diagnosis.—The eruption may be confounded with the scarlatiniform eruptions which appear at the onset of variola, but the general symptoms give more assistance in diagnosis than the eruption does, and I would say the same of scarlatiniform eruptions appearing in the course of rheumatism, diphtheria, typhus, and cholera, or arising from the use of drugs (antipyrin, belladonna). Scarlatinal angina should not be confounded with simple tonsillitis. The defaced forms are distinguished in that they appear during an epidemic. In eczema rubrum we find fever and diffuse redness of the skin, but the invaded region shows vesicles rapidly replaced by fine branny scales, which do not reappear when once they have fallen off. The itching and smarting caused by eczema are more marked than the simple pruritus seen in scarlatina.

Infective scarlatiniform erythema may resemble scarlatina so closely that the diagnosis is difficult, and, among other examples, I may mention a patient who was under my care at the Necker Hospital.

A man was taken ill with fever, headache, and lassitude. The throat was red, the tonsils were large, and covered with a pulpy exudate; there was a polymorphous eruption, which had in places the diffuse redness of scarlatina. We thought of scarlatina, but fresh crops appeared, although desquamation had begun; these crops were erythematous, morbilliform, urticarial, and scarlatiniform, so that in all these points the case did not look like one of scarlatina, and yet it was necessary to await the polymorphous character of the eruption and its successive crops in order to eliminate the hypothesis of scarlatina, and to make the diagnosis of infectious scarlatiniform erythema.

Accordingly, the **dermatoses,** which are general, red in colour, and accompanied by desquamation, may simulate scarlatina in a singular manner. Brocq, in his treatise upon the treatment of diseases of the skin, gives the following description of desquamative scarlatiniform erythema, or acute exfoliative dermatitis. It is, says he, a kind of pseudo-exanthem, characterized by a febrile onset, simulating that of scarlatina. After a variable period, a more or less bright red rash supervenes, which is uniform, or punctuated by petechiæ, especially on the lower limbs. The rash tends to become general, and is more marked in the articular folds, the neck, the lateral parts of the body, and the palms of the hands or the soles of the feet. Abundant dry, flaky desquamation occurs three or four days after the appearance of this rash, although the redness is still persistent.

Ehrlich's diazo-reaction, which is constant in scarlatina, is absent in scarlatiniform erythema.

Puerperal Scarlatina.—What view should be taken of puerperal scarlatina? Does it deserve description under Scarlatina, or should it be put under the Scarlatiniform Erythemata? A woman during the puerperal period may take true scarlatina, just as she may take measles or variola; but this is not the question. I allude to those epidemics of so-called puerperal scarlatina which formerly caused such terrible ravages in lying-in hospitals or in different localities before antiseptic methods were practised, and which, as a rule, coincided with erysipelas in new-born children, so happily called by Trousseau " a manifestation of puerperal fever in the new-born." Are these cases of so-called puerperal scarlatina, whether they are epidemic or isolated, true or pseudo scarlatina?

So-called puerperal scarlatina usually begins suddenly a few days after delivery. The woman, who has so far been in good health, is suddenly seized with slight chill, followed by fever, nausea, and vomiting. Oculo-nasal catarrh, which at first sight simulates measles, may be seen. After this period of invasion, which may last only a few hours, the eruption comes out, and shows all the characters of the scarlatinal rash. The angina is perhaps less marked or less inevitable than in scarlatina, and perhaps, too, the inflammation of the submaxillary glands is slighter. Desquamation follows the eruption, large shreds of the epidermis peeling off. The lochia and the secretion of milk are suppressed or modified. Patients sometimes recover, and when death supervenes, it does so from cholera-like complications (diarrhœa, coldness of the body, and livid colour of the skin), collapse, or coma.

It is quite evident that there is here material for discussion, and the dualists and unicists have not yet come to an agreement. For my part, I accept the conclusions of Wurtz, which I have found very sensible. " There is," says he, " an important fact which throws a singular light on the true nature of puerperal scarlatina—namely, that, since the application of antiseptic methods in obstetrics, the disease has become practically unknown in maternity hospitals (Varnier). It is therefore rational to admit that these **so-called cases of scarlatina were only cases of infec-**

tious erythema, due to the toxines of the streptococcus." In my opinion a point in favour of this view is that so-called puerperal scarlatina, which is contagious from patient to patient in a lying-in ward, does not attack those who come in contact with the patients. The cases are, therefore, infectious scarlatiniform erythema.

I may say the same of wound or surgical scarlatina. Our bacteriological classifications as regards the streptococci are far from being sufficiently advanced to decide the specificity of scarlatina, because these different conditions have for their essential agent the toxine of the streptococcus, and because the streptococcus appears to be an important agent in scarlatina. In short, we find scarlatina on the one hand, and on the other hand scarlatiniform erythemata.

Prognosis.—A reserved prognosis must always be given in scarlatina, even in apparently benign cases, for many complications may supervene during convalescence (dropsy, uræmia, diphtheria, empyæma, and abscesses), or appear after the patient seems cured. The chronic sequelæ of the disease, including cardiac lesions, Bright's disease, chorea, etc., must also be reckoned. In scarlatina, just as in all epidemic diseases, the severity and the course of the disease vary, according to the epidemic. Sydenham, who saw only the most benign forms of scarlatina, hesitated to give it the name of a disease. Graves says that the epidemics of 1800 to 1804 in Ireland were terrible, while they became extremely benign for a period of thirty years, and then reappeared with exceeding severity in Dublin in 1831 and 1834. Bretonneau, who, like Sydenham, considered scarlatina as a very benign disease, because he did not lose a single patient in twenty years, changed his opinion when a terrible epidemic claimed numerous victims at Tours.

Epidemics of scarlatina may not only severely affect an entire population, but their gravity may be **circumscribed** to a small centre, to a single house, or to a single family, as the writings of Stoll and Graves clearly show. Whether the malignancy depends upon the nature of the infective agent, or whether it is some inherent peculiarity of the constitution of the individual, it is none the less true that " when scarlatina attacks a family and kills the first members attacked, it must be feared, because it will probably claim other victims " (Trousseau). I have recognized the truth of this statement. In a family at Amiens three persons—mother and two children—were taken ill with scarlatina, complicated by diphtheria, and all died in a few days.

The severity of scarlatina in the Anglo-Saxon race has been often recognized. While in France it is responsible for only one-third of the deaths that measles causes, in Belgium it kills more than the latter disease. In England it figures in the first rank among the causes of mortality : in Paris it shows an average of 100 deaths a year ; in London, 4,000 to 5,000. Scarlatina is more frequent and more severe in English people living on the Continent than among the natives.

Age is important from the point of view of prognosis. In the figures given by Marfan and Apert we find that among children in the hospitals of Paris the mortality is greater the younger the patient (50 per cent. below one year, 11 per cent. between one and two years, 2 per cent. between two and ten years, and nil above this age). Legendre has seen a mortality of 1·88 per cent. in adult patients at Aubervilliers.

Ætiology.—Scarlatina is epidemic and contagious. The inoculations which have often been made have given no positive result. It chiefly attacks children between the ages of six and ten years, and usually confers immunity. There are some cases which prove that the fœtus may receive the contagion from the mother.

While scarlatina is contagious during the eruptive period, it is especially so during desquamation, and the dust from the epidermic scales is very contagious. Contagion may be direct or indirect—direct when there is contact with the patient; indirect when the disease is transmitted by different objects, such as toys, toilet articles, and clothes which have belonged to a patient with scarlatina. Contagion may even occur at a distance through articles carrying the contagious germs. Books and letters have rightly been held guilty, and I will quote some undeniable cases.

Sanné reports that a lady and her daughter living in Brittany received from a friend in Germany a letter, in which she said that she was convalescent from scarlatina, and was peeling so freely that while writing the letter she was obliged to shake the paper several times in order to get rid of the scales which fell on it. The mother and daughter who received this letter were taken ill with scarlatina, and the former died, while the latter narrowly escaped death.

Grasset, of Riom, reports a similar case: The parents of a girl who was suffering from scarlatina collected some of the scales of skin, and sent them, as a curiosity, in a letter to her little brother, who took scarlatina. I have quoted in this article the case of a young girl suffering from a chronic scarlatinal nephritis: she, too, took the disease from her sister, who kept on sending letters which evidently contained contagious particles of skin.

How does the contagion enter the system ? Is it by the respiratory tracts, or does not the tonsil receive the virus ? The question is still a moot point.

Bacteriology.—Bacteriological researches, made in order to discover the microbe of scarlatina, are not as yet conclusive. Klebs, in 1875, described certain nomad forms in scarlatina, but did not cultivate them. Later, Edington noted in the blood and the scales eight kinds of bacteria, of which one, in the form of a rod or of a diplococcus, was capable of producing in animals, and particularly in calves, a febrile affection, accompanied by a cutaneous rash resembling that of scarlatina. The *Strepto-*

coccus conglomeratus, which Kurth considered as the pathogenic agent of scarlatina, has no specific property.

The bovine origin of scarlatina has been upheld for several years by numerous physicians and veterinary surgeons in England, and the contagion is supposed to result from ulceration of the udders of cows and from the use of milk.

In short, we do not know the pathogenic microbe of scarlatina, but we do know what agents cause **secondary infections** in patients with scarlatina (Marie, Raskin, Babès, Wurtz, Bourgès). I must, in the first place, mention the streptococcus which is present in nearly all the lesions (simple and suppurative arthritis, ulcers of the tonsils and pharynx, adenitis and adeno-phlegmon in the neck, diphtheroid exudation in the throat, pus in cases of otitis, pleuritic effusion, and nephritis).

Staphylococcus, coli bacillus, pneumococci, saprogenic bacilli (Babès), etc., are often found, in addition to the streptococcus, which in scarlatina assumes special virulence, but which is not specific *per se*. It produces suppuration and erysipelas in animals, while scarlatinal angina appears able to cause erysipelas by contagion.

Treatment.—Scarlatina, when slight or of moderate intensity, requires only careful hygiene; but the severe forms, with very high temperature and marked nervous symptoms, should be treated by cold sponging or by baths. I have witnessed the good effect of this treatment in Trousseau's clinic, and I have often followed his practice.

The patient is placed naked in an empty bath, and three or four buckets of water at 70° F. are poured over his body, the affusion lasting half a minute. Instead, he may be placed on a stretcher and sponged by two attendants with water at 70° F. to which aromatic vinegar has been added. In either case, after the bath the patient is placed, still wet, in a cotton sheet, and given an infusion of camomile tea, or peppermint-water; healthy reaction, generally followed by perspiration and reduction of the temperature, speedily takes place. The affusions may be repeated several times in the twenty-four hours. In some cases the patient may be placed in a cold bath, the method described under Typhoid Fever being employed.

Acetate of ammonia, musk, syrup of ether, and bromide of potassium, are of service in the severe nervous forms.

At the onset of scarlatina the patient should be put on milk diet (Jaccoud), in order to prevent possible nephritis, and this principle is absolutely essential. Not only do I prescribe exclusive milk diet during the disease itself, but I continue it for three or four weeks after recovery. We thus avoid—or, I believe, at least lessen—the likelihood of renal complications.

The treatment of scarlatinal angina differs according as the disease is or is not diphtheritic. In every case antiseptics should be applied to the pharynx, and for this purpose mouth-washes of a solution of chlorinated soda may be employed (Roux), and the throat may be painted with equal parts of menthol and camphor, as extolled by Roux.

When diphtheria complicates the scarlatinal angina, injections of anti-diphtheritic serum must be given ; but in these cases the combination of the streptococcus with the diphtheria bacillus produces an increase of virulence, and it is especially in such cases that the injection of serum produces morbilli-form eruptions, which Sevestre attributes principally to streptococcal infection. This fact agrees with the statistics of Marfan and Apert, who found that in scarlatinal patients suffering from non-diphtheritic mem-branous angina, and treated with injections of antidiphtheritic serum, the frequency of post-serotherapic eruptions is 28 per cent., while it is only from 10 to 15 per cent. if the angina is diphtheritic.

As the streptococcus plays the chief part in non-diphtheritic angina, ought we to make use of antistreptococcic serum ? The following con-clusions are given in an article which appeared on this subject in the *Gazette Hebdomadaire*, July 19, 1896 : Marmorek was the first to publish a series of cases favourable to the employment of his serum in scarlatina, and Dubois, who has devoted much time to researches with this serum and speaks in its favour, reports four cases in which it is said to have produced beneficial results. All authorities, however, are far from sharing this enthusiasm. Baginski did not obtain conclusive results from his experi-ments, and Josias considers that the serum has no marked influence on the course of scarlatina. The cases published by Marfan and Apert and by Comby are far from being encouraging.

Prophylactic treatment consists in isolating the patient during the whole period of the disease, and we must not forget that the shreds of epidermis detached during desquamation are endowed with contagious properties, which they preserve for a long while.

V. MEASLES.

The old writers often described measles under the name of **morbillus fever, morbilli,** or the small plague. The whole subject was in confusion until Sydenham, between 1760 and 1764 (London epidemics), clearly dis-tinguished measles from scarlatina and variola.

Description.—I shall choose for my descriptive type an ordinary case of measles of moderate severity, and I shall consider later the less common forms of abnormal and hæmorrhagic measles. The course of measles is generally divided into four periods—incubation, invasion, eruption, and desquamation.

1. **Incubation.**—The incubation is generally latent, while the economy hatches the morbid seed. In some cases, however, we see during this period elevation of temperature, malaise, cough, and coryza. In children the weight rapidly falls, and there is already an outline of the symptoms which appear during the next period. The incubation lasts from eight to eleven days.

2. **Invasion.**—The invasion of measles is not as sudden as that of variola and scarlatina. The course of the fever is worthy of study, for it is sometimes slight, and at other times reaches 104° F., with chills, headache, and sneezing. The fever often falls during the next day, and reappears with the eruption.

At the commencement of the disease the mucous membranes of the nose and eyes, and sometimes those of the Eustachian tubes, larynx, and bronchi, are attacked by catarrh. The eyes are red, swollen, and weeping. The nasal catarrh causes sneezing and abundant secretion. The laryngeal catarrh is accompanied by frequent obstinate cough, hoarseness, and sometimes by complete aphonia. Otitis appears later, and is accompanied by sharp pain. In some cases the catarrh affects one or other organ to such an extent that an error in diagnosis may result. Some children appear to have only simple or stridulous laryngitis, when the eruption appears four or five days later. Other children, again, are treated for several days for bronchitis or for intestinal catarrh, and then the eruption appears, giving the lie to the diagnosis. In consultation with Waltelet I saw a young child in whom otitis preceded the eruption, and caused us to suspend our judgment. During the period of invasion the laryngeal symptoms are the most frequent and the most important. Laryngitis (frequent spasmodic cough, hoarse and muffled voice) is a valuable factor in making an early diagnosis.

Epistaxis is frequently seen at this period, and young children are sometimes seized with **convulsions.** If the patient's throat is carefully examined in a good light, we see that the eruption (enanthem) is already out on the mucous membrane of the roof of the palate, on the anterior pillars of the fauces, and on the pharynx, in the form of a red stippling, which usually shows neither swelling nor pulpy deposits. The enanthem may precede the eruption on the skin by one or two days, marked dyspnœa resulting.

I have often seen a **submaxillary adenitis,** which I think might be included among the symptoms of invasion of measles, and which is not absolutely special to this disease.

The duration of the period of invasion is long, since it may last from four to seven days, while it is very short in scarlatina, in which disease it may last only a few hours. The fever is not continuous, and falls on the second or on the third day, but reappears with the rash. In some very mild cases fever may be practically absent. The different symptoms just described are trifling, and the eruption is practically the first symptom of the disease.

3. **Eruption.**—At the time of the eruption the symptoms of invasion do not disappear, as in the cases of discrete variola, but, on the contrary, they return with fresh severity. The cough is frequent, paroxysmal, and painful. The voice becomes hoarse, and is sometimes lost, and the fever reaches its maximum, decreasing later when the eruption disappears. The eruption may appear on the fourth, fifth, sixth, or seventh day of the disease. It commences on the face, around the lips, and on the forehead. It then invades the neck, trunk, and limbs. In its usual form, when we examine the rash on the chest or on the abdomen, we see that it is composed of little red, velvety projections, which are not as rough as those of scarlatina. The spots in measles are about as large as a grain of rice, uneven, fade for a moment on pressure, and are grouped in irregular patches of a crescentic shape, separated by intervals of healthy skin. In some cases, however, the eruption is confluent, and the redness of the skin becomes diffuse and uniform. In exceptional instances the erythema of measles may show the greatest analogy with the rash of scarlatina (Sanné, Rénon, and Follet).

The eruption becomes general in twenty-four to forty-eight hours. It fades in the same order as it appeared, commencing on the face, which becomes pale, while it is still fully out upon the limbs.

When the inflammatory exudate forming the morbillous spot is associated with the presence of colloid deposits in the Malpighian cells, the projection formed by the papule gives to the eruption the appearance known as **pimply measles.**

During this period the catarrh reaches its maximum. The cough is less dry ; the sputum in adults (children do not expectorate) becomes thick and nummular, like that of phthisis, and bronchitic râles are heard.

Diarrhœa is common in children when the rash comes out. This intestinal catarrh may last twenty-four hours, and is sometimes accompanied by true colitis, with hæmorrhage and mucous diarrhœa.

4. **Desquamation.**—The fever falls about the eighth day of the disease, and the rash tends to disappear first from the face. Desquamation begins from the fourth to the seventh day of the eruption. It is so slight that there is not really a period of desquamation, although some desquamation in the form of branny scales usually occurs on the skin of the face and forehead.

The nervous form of measles is more frequent at an early age, and is characterized during the period of invasion by convulsions, with delirium, vomiting and very high temperature. The eruption is late and incomplete, or unrecognizable ; the fever is persistent ; the skin is livid and dry ; the pulse is small and very quick ; the urine is scanty ; and death by coma ends the scene.

In exceptional cases abnormal complications supervene in the course of typical measles. I have seen the following case :

A young girl was taken ill with measles ; invasion and eruption were classical. All went well until the second day of the disease, and then the menses appeared ; the patient experienced some nausea at this time. Next morning paraphasia appeared ; her mind was less clear, and the temperature suddenly fell from 102° F. to 97° F. ; a series of epileptiform attacks, with loss of consciousness and coma, followed. In a few hours the temperature rose from 97° F. to 106° F. ; the attacks succeeded one another without interruption, and the patient died the same day in convulsions.

Writers have described, and I myself have witnessed, malignant cases with dyspnœa or delirium, the severe symptoms coming on in the course or during the decline of the eruption. Measles only becomes malignant at a later stage during the eruption, in contradistinction to scarlatina, which assumes the malignant type from the very onset.

Hæmorrhagic measles is characterized by cutaneous ecchymoses and purpuric spots, which do not disappear on pressure, and may last eight or ten days after the eruption. This form is obviously more grave than normal measles, but as long as the hæmorrhage remains limited to the skin, it does not imply a fatal prognosis. The case, however, is quite different when the hæmorrhage becomes general. If epistaxis, hæmaturia, metrorrhagia, and hæmorrhages from the mouth and bowels appear, the patient dies with adynamic and typhoid symptoms.

Complications of Measles.

I have just described the normal form and also the anomalous varieties of measles ; but at any period of the disease we may witness the onset of complications which are in some cases an exaggeration of the ordinary symptoms, but in other cases comprise unusual signs. These complications are sometimes due to the excessive virulence of the pathogenic agent ; at other times they result from secondary infection or from the association of other microbes (diphtheria, gangrene, tuberculosis), and vary in different individuals, surroundings, and epidemics.

Convulsions, epistaxis, and false croup belong to the period of invasion. The convulsions special to infancy are not of fatal omen if they are transient and solitary, though the case is not the same if they occur in the so-called nervous forms. Epistaxis is a common symptom of the disease. It may become so profuse as to threaten the life of the patient.

Laryngeal Complications.—Measles shows a predilection for the larynx, and even in the period of invasion the laryngeal symptoms are prominent, cough and vocal troubles being, so to say, constant. This laryngitis in measles comprises both erythema and catarrh. Laryngoscopic examination reveals discrete or confluent erythema, with exudation, papules, and erosion of the vocal cords.

This catarrhal laryngitis in children between the ages of two and five years may run the course of false croup, but it is not a serious accident, and it sometimes announces the onset of measles.

In short, laryngitis in measles is, as a rule, a transient and harmless phenomenon. At other times it becomes a formidable complication, and ends either in very severe catarrhal laryngitis or in an ulcerative form.

The severe form is not simply a catarrhal inflammation. The mucosa is profoundly affected, as has been shown by Coyne. The chorion is infiltrated with leucocytes, the mucous glands are much swollen, and the mucous membrane of the larynx is œdematous, so that we can understand how in children these lesions, with spasm of the glottis, may cause asphyxia. The little patients in the epidemic of 1809, reported in Campaignac's thesis, died from this cause. The mucous membrane was found to be swollen and infiltrated, but there were neither ulcers nor false membranes on post-mortem examination. This form is the severe erythematous laryngitis described by Rillet and Barthez.

In another form the laryngitis is ulcerative, and the ulcers are superficial, erosive, and anfractuous, or sometimes serpiginous and deep, so as to lay bare the cricoid and arytenoid cartilages. The ulcerations may be situated at the free border or at the posterior extremity of the vocal cords, but they are principally seen in the neighbourhood of the arytenoids. Clinically, this ulcerative laryngitis appears during or after the eruption of measles, and produces symptoms like those of croup ; but yet it differs from croup in a pain localized to the larynx, in the slower evolution of the symptoms, in the absence of false membranes, and in the lesions of the larynx, which are readily recognized with the laryngoscope. An interesting case of this kind has been noticed by Cardier in Barbier's monograph, and I have had a similar one under my care. This form of laryngitis is much less serious in adults than in children, in whom it may necessitate tracheotomy.

Membranous laryngitis may occur in measles, and the false membrane may or may not be diphtheritic. In the latter event the laryngitis was pseudo-diphtheritic, and due to the streptococcus and the staphylococcus. It is, however, exceptional, and the croup seen in measles is usually diphtheritic.

Speaking generally, measles lends itself admirably to the generalization of the diphtheria bacillus, which may be found in the pharynx, bronchi, nasal fossæ, mouth, and skin, but the larynx is its favourite seat. This primary croup, so rare in primary diphtheria, is fairly frequent in the secondary diphtheria of measles. It is a complication special to childhood, and may supervene either during or after the eruption. From the local point of view this croup is attenuated, in the sense that it provokes less dyspnœa than primary croup ; but from the general point of view it is formidable, because it assumes the toxic character of malignant diphtheria.

For this reason Trousseau advised against operation in children suffering from croup in measles. It is often difficult to diagnose diphtheria in a larynx already affected by measles. The coexistence of laryngeal diphtheria, rejection of membranes from the larynx, and bacteriological examination, will establish the diagnosis.

Sometimes, indeed, although the pharynx seems to be free from diphtheria, it is sufficient to cultivate a particle of mucus from the tonsil of a child supposed to be suffering from croup, in order to obtain cultures of the diphtheria bacillus.

Broncho-Pulmonary Complications.—*Capillary bronchitis* and *lobular pneumonia* are in adults and children, but especially in children, the most formidable complication of measles. This complication may appear as early as the third or the fourth day of the disease—that is to say, before the eruption. It may not show itself till later, during convalescence. As a rule, this complication appears about the sixth or the seventh day of the disease—that is to say, when the rash is fully out. It is ushered in by a return of the fever and by increasing dyspnœa. In addition, if about the eighth day of the disease the fever, which should have fallen, persists or becomes severe, and if the bronchitic râles become finer and more numerous, we should fear the invasion of capillary bronchitis and lobular pneumonia, to which children so often succumb. The frequency of these broncho-pulmonary complications varies according to the particular epidemic. They are chiefly seen in children's hospitals and in the army.

Capillary bronchitis and broncho-pneumonia are not only attributable to the poison of measles; they are especially the result of secondary infections caused by the pneumococcus, streptococcus, staphylococcus, and diphtheria bacillus.

In some cases, especially in adults, the chief lesion is capillary bronchitis; but it does not end in broncho-pneumonia, for it has not had time to do so, the patients being carried off in a few days by this suffocative catarrh, which may appear during the invasion and before the rash. It might be said that the entire exanthem is confined to the bronchi, while the rash upon the skin is absent or much delayed. The production of pus characterizes this capillary bronchitis. In adults the sputum is purulent, " phlegmorrhagic " (Trousseau) by the first or by the second day. Indeed, it may be said that the patient coughs up the pus from an abscess and fills the sputum mug, and, as in the last hours of life expectoration no longer takes place, the pus accumulates in the bronchi, the trachea, and the nasal fossæ, so that after death it is sufficient to lower the head of the corpse for the pus to flow out freely (Joffroy).

Pleurisy is more frequent in adults than in children. It sometimes assumes the purulent or the putrid form.

Tuberculosis.—The broncho-pulmonary complications of measles are formidable, because they are often associated with other infections, such as diphtheria, gangrene, suppuration, and tuberculosis.

Tuberculosis associated with measles may assume various forms. In young children and babies the broncho-pneumonia of measles is often tubercular, and, post mortem, rarely presents the nodular forms seen in tuberculosis of the adult lung ; but the tubercle bacillus is frequently found by curetting or by examination of cut sections after hardening. Hypertrophy of the spleen and of Peyer's patches and fatty degeneration of the heart are lesions which accompany this double infection.

Babès has described a form of morbillo-tubercular pneumonia, which he has met with in a certain number of autopsies. The lesion seems to begin in the softened peribronchial glands, which contain both tubercle bacilli and streptococci. He found around the glands pneumonic infiltration, which was hard, whitish and uniform, slightly granular, and of a sarcomatous appearance. Bacilli were found in this tissue, which was infiltrated with embryonic cells.

Acute miliary tuberculosis may occur during the course or during the convalescence of measles. In children tubercular meningitis is not rare after measles. Lastly, some patients only experience at a late date the first symptoms of tuberculosis which has commenced during measles.

Enlargement of the bronchial glands, which is sometimes tubercular, is almost constant in children suffering from measles. It may pass unnoticed, or it may assume a clearly marked character, and last for several months, with the general symptoms of dyspnœa and of spasmodic cough (Guéneau de Mussy).

Digestive System.—We must note the following complications in the digestive system :

Stomatitis. — The stomatitis of measles, really an enanthem of the mouth, is often followed by desquamation of the tongue, which bears some resemblance to the strawberry tongue of scarlatina. This stomatitis is comparable to the erythema and catarrh of the throat and larynx, and opens the door to the following secondary infections :

Aphthous stomatitis, in which the ulcers are very painful, and occur on the tongue, the lips, and the inner surfaces of the cheeks.

Ulcero-membranous stomatitis, which usually appears during the decline of the disease or during convalescence.

Diphtheritic stomatitis, or buccal diphtheria, affecting the gums, tongue, cheeks, and lips, and forming in some cases the starting-point of pharyngolaryngeal diphtheria.

Thrush, which is often seen towards the end of severe cases of measles.

Gangrene of the mouth (noma) has become infinitely more rare since antiseptic and prophylactic measures have been rigorously employed. Noma is often a late complication, which appears about the twentieth or about the thirtieth day. It is not, as might be supposed, the apanage of severe cases, since it may appear in very benign ones. Its course is so rapid that a gangrenous cavity may be produced in two days. The gravity of noma in measles is the greater in that it often coincides with gangrene of the lung, vulva, and pharynx.

Enteritis.—Diarrhœa is the natural result of the intestinal catarrh in measles. It may form a serious complication in children when it runs the course of cholera infantum. It may be asked if there is not in such cases a bacterial association analogous to that described by Baginsky at the Medical Society of Berlin.

The entero-colitis of measles may be dysenteriform, the patient suffering from tenesmus, and passing blood in the stools. In adults I have often seen this form of entero-colitis.

Organs of the Senses.—Measles may cause ocular and aural complications.

Ocular Complications.—Conjunctivitis is one of the benign and constant symptoms of the period of invasion, but several ocular complications may occur in measles. Phlyctenular conjunctivitis and kerato-conjunctivitis are seen, and are characterized by the appearance of isolated or confluent vesicles. This complication, which generally supervenes during convalescence, may occur during the onset of the disease. It may be the only manifestation of defaced measles.

These ocular complications are in some children the origin of grave and persistent lesions : Chronic blepharitis, which is obstinate and rebellious to treatment, and causes the eyelashes to fall out ; opaline spots, or leucoma of the cornea (λευκόω, to whiten) ; inflammation of the lachrymal sac, or dacryocystitis (δάκρυον, tear ; and κύστις, sac) ; ulcer and abscess of the cornea ; effusion of pus in the anterior chamber, or hypopyon (ὑπό, under ; and πῦον, pus) ; perforation of the cornea, staphyloma, and loss of sight ; disorders of refraction, strabismus, and asthenopia.

Otitis.—Otitis in measles especially affects the middle ear. It is nearly always double, and is so common that in twenty-three autopsies on patients who had died from various complications in measles Cordier found otitis media in twenty. Out of sixteen autopsies in children who had succumbed to the complications of measles, München found otitis in **every** case, even when death supervened on the third day of the disease. This frequency is explained by the fact that the Eustachian tube establishes a communication between the middle ear and the naso-pharynx, which is always invaded by catarrh. München, however, does not consider that the otitis is **always** due to the spread of infection from the pharynx. He thinks that the middle ear is infected on its own account. The otitis would, therefore, be comparable to the conjunctivitis, bronchitis, and enteritis, and would result from an enanthem, like that of the mucosæ.

Slight otitis is characterized by muco-purulent catarrh of the tympanum, with exudation and vascularization of the mucous membrane. In a more advanced degree the catarrh is purulent, affects the tympanum and Eustachian tube, and, according to the age of the patient, invades the pre-mastoid or the mastoid cells. In some cases the chain of ossicles is affected.

This otitis in its slight forms may pass almost unnoticed, because there is little or no pain. No auditory troubles are present, and the muco-purulent fluid often flows through the Eustachian tube, which has again become permeable. The severe forms are accompanied by sharp pain, auditory troubles, and painful swelling in the mastoid region. There is, however, less pain in the otitis of measles than in the other forms of infective otitis. The speculum shows that the membrana tympani has lost its pearly grey tint, and is of a rosy colour, while it bulges outwards instead of being flat, especially in its subumbilical segment. This otitis often ends in perforation of the membrane, in which case the patient obtains very great and instant relief.

The otitis of measles, when properly treated, can nearly always be cured, without leaving any trace of deafness ; but it is sometimes followed by chronic otorrhœa, which ends in irremediable lesions of the tympanum (thickening, vegetations, adhesions, and necrosis of the ossicles). The power of hearing is impaired or abolished.

In some cases very grave complications arise—suppuration in the mastoid cells, calling for operation ; invasion of the meninges (otitic meningitis) ; general purulent infection, with abscesses, jaundice (Trousseau), gangrenous broncho-pneumonia, and pleurisy (Netter). These various complications may supervene during the decline of measles, or even during convalescence.

Complete deafness is one of the saddest sequelæ of measles. In children under the age of three years it results in deaf-mutism. It may be said that of a hundred deaf-mutes in twenty-five the condition is due to otitis following the eruptive fevers, such as scarlet fever, measles, or typhoid ; and of these figures measles claims the largest share.

In the autopsies reported by München the exudation in the tympanum was nearly always purulent or sero-purulent, but in four cases fibrinous exudate was also present. Bacteriological examination of the exudate has sometimes shown the presence of streptococci alone, and at other times the presence of staphylococci. The exudate from the ear after puncture of the membrana tympani has given the same result.

Other Complications.—Gangrene of the lung, of the vulva, and of the mouth (*noma*) may supervene after measles, especially in children's hospitals. It must be said that these troubles are far less common since the rules of antisepsis have been rigorously observed.

Diphtheria, whether pharyngeal, laryngeal, cutaneous, or malignant, is a terrible complication that has become much less frequent, on account of prophylactic measures and of antiseptic treatment.

Associated Eruptive Fevers.—Measles and scarlatina may occur at the same time in the same patient. It appears to me that the association of these two eruptive fevers in the same subject may be classified in the following manner :

The two fevers **succeed** one another—that is to say, the one commences when the other ends. They are sometimes simultaneous. The clinical picture differs according to the particular type. Whooping-cough is often associated with measles.

Diagnosis.—The diagnosis of measles is often difficult in the period of invasion. If all the symptoms are present, no hesitation can be possible ; but if one of them is predominant, we may look upon the case as laryngitis, false croup, bronchitis, enteritis, or influenza, until the appearance of the eruption some days later corrects our error.

Koplik's sign (white and bluish spots on the mucous membranes of the lips and cheeks during the pre-eruptive period) is not of great value in the early diagnosis of measles, for it is sometimes absent, and, on the other hand, it may be found in other diseases (Widowitz). I may say the same of Bolognini's sign (peritoneal friction perceived by repeated pressure over the patient's abdomen), which is absent in half of the cases (Koppen).

Morbilliform eruptions simulate the rash of measles, as, for instance, that of variola (rash), diphtheria, malaria, German measles, and roseola ; but in measles the **period of invasion** is characterized by catarrh, and I have constantly made this remark to my class : In an eruptive fever the symptoms of the period of invasion rather than the eruption give the disease its specific character. Difficult cases may, however, occur, and I shall therefore mention them.

Syphilitic Roseola.—At first sight the diagnosis between measles and the roseola of syphilis appears quite simple. The latter appears from six weeks to three months after the contagion. It is the earliest and commonest of the manifestations of syphilis. It is usually apyretic and discrete. Itching is completely absent, and when the eruption occurs in successive crops, their various colours give the skin a peculiar appearance, which Petit called the trout's skin. Syphilitic roseola shows two chief forms, which are often associated. The former is macular, and characterized by flat rose-coloured spots, which disappear on pressure, while the other is papular, and composed of projecting spots. The spots are scanty on the limbs and face, and are not seen on the feet and hands. Desquamation does not occur. These characters appear sufficient to establish the diagnosis, but the roseola sometimes assumes a slightly different character. It may be confluent, morbilliform (Bazin), and accompanied by fever, erythema, and pharyngo-laryngeal catarrh, so that the diagnosis from measles then requires careful attention.

Roseola from Drugs.—Copaiba, cubebs, antipyrin, and iron sometimes produce morbilliform eruptions, which do not, as a rule, commence on the face, and are usually accompanied by itching. In a case of real difficulty inquiry as to the cause will clear up the diagnosis. Subacute poisoning by arsenic deserves notice, because it has many points in common with measles. This poisoning, as may be seen from numerous cases, may cause not only a morbilliform eruption, but also catarrh of the eyes, nose, larynx, and bronchi, simulating the catarrh seen in measles. Accordingly, in cases of doubt the nervous symptoms of arsenical poisoning (paresis, anæsthesia, and hyperæsthesia) must be carefully looked for, and the urine and the hair of the patient tested for arsenic.

Other Diseases.—The diagnosis of measles from miliaria, roseola, and rubeola will be discussed in the description of these diseases.

Prognosis—Sequelæ.—Measles is *per se* a benign disease, but the numerous complications which I have enumerated show how serious it may be. Measles may leave sequelæ, of which some constitute an infirmity, while others are dangerous. Among these sequelæ I will mention deaf-mutism, chronic otitis, visual troubles, blindness, inflammation of the mediastinal glands, and pulmonary tuberculosis. In predisposed and lymphatic subjects measles leaves behind it blepharitis, ophthalmia, and chronic eczema, by reason of the local lesions in the eyes, nose, and ears.

I have twice seen in an adult, as a sequel of measles, chronic bronchial catarrh, with cough, night-sweats, wasting, and râles in both lungs, simulating tuberculosis. The bacteriological examination showed that the case was one of false tuberculosis, Koch's bacilli and elastic fibres being absent. The microbic flora was made up of micrococci grouped in masses, in short chains, tetrads, and short and thick-set rods, which did not stain with Gram.

Ætiology. — Although measles may appear at any age, it is more common in infancy. Cases of congenital measles, transmitted to the fœtus by the mother, have been quoted. Measles is rare during the first year, and reaches its maximum in children between three and five years of age. It is epidemic and extremely contagious, and one case of measles among a number of children may cause the disease in ten, twenty, or thirty of them.

The contagiousness of measles commences during the period of invasion, and lasts until the end of the eruption. The fact that measles is chiefly contagious during the period of invasion proves that the germ in measles comes less from the skin than from the respiratory tracks (mucus from the nose, the larynx, or the bronchi). The germ shows little tendency to spread to a distance, and measles is no longer contagious a few yards away. On the other hand, indirect contagion is much more frequent than was formerly thought, and the germ may be carried by an intermediary (third person, clothes, utensil, etc.) to a distance of several miles in a very short time. The agent in measles rapidly loses its pathogenic properties, and if a child with measles has left its room, other children may enter by the next day without fear. A child suffering from another infectious disease, such as enteric fever, diphtheria, or scarlatina, is not, as was supposed, immune to measles. These affections may develop simultaneously.

The first attack of measles generally confers immunity. The disease may, however, appear several years apart, and may show relapses, as in a typical case reported by Vergely. The question of recurrences and relapses in measles is still obscure, because writers have not given sufficient details. Nevertheless, they are not frequent, and recurrence is much less common than a relapse (Vergely).

The infectious agent in measles has yet to be discovered. Klebs described in 1875 certain monad forms in measles, but was unable to cultivate them. Babès found small micrococci—single, in pairs, or in chains—in the products of secretion and in the pulmonary alveoli of a patient who died from measles. Lesage has met with an extremely small micrococcus, agglomerated into a zoogloea and decolorized by Gram, in mucus from the throat and nose during the eruptive period of measles. Culture on simple agar yields a very fine sand, which is transparent and analogous to the small cultures of the streptococcus or of Pfeiffer's bacillus. In the rabbit subcutaneous or intravenous injection causes hæmorrhagic septicæmia, which lasts from two to twenty days. It is possible to produce the same septicæmia by placing the mucus from a case of measles in the nasal fossæ of the rabbit. Blood taken from an infant during an attack of measles and injected in a rabbit also causes septicæmia. This microbe must not be confounded with the bacillus of Pfeiffer, nor with that of Wilks. It is, however, impossible to say whether the microbes are indifferent or pathogenic. Inoculation experiments have given positive results only in the monkey. Josias was able to give measles to Sajou monkeys, while the macaques were refractory. In the ape the disease runs its course in five days, with coryza, lachrymation, and fever. Measles, it is said, may appear in the monkey when it is living amidst infected surroundings.

Treatment.—In an ordinary case of measles the treatment consists in hygienic measures—antiseptic irrigation of the nose, throat, eyes, and vulva ; milk diet (with the addition of lime-water in cases of diarrhœa) ; soothing drinks, with a few drops of aconite or of syrup of opium for the cough. Otitis must be carefully looked for. As measles is very contagious, **strict isolation** and disinfection, as recommended in all contagious diseases, must be carried out. Grancher has formulated rules for isolation which have given remarkable results in his practice ; and L. Martin, at the Pasteur Hospital, has instituted a system of isolation and hygiene which has reduced the contagion and the mortality (measles, scarlatina, variola, diphtheria, etc.) to a degree previously unknown.

When measles assumes a malignant form, with the typhoid state, delirium, or hypertoxic symptoms, I have successfully used the cold-bath treatment. The reader will find in the *Bulletins de la Société Médicale des Hôpitaux*, Séances du 9 Mai et 20 Juin, 1890, an account of two young girls suffering from measles, which threatened to be speedily fatal. They were certainly cured by the cold baths which I ordered.

In one of these cases the patient was a girl sixteen years of age. The attack had run a regular course until the sixth day, when the temperature rose to 105° F. ; the pulse-rate reached 140 ; the tongue became dry and red, the urine scanty, and delirium appeared on the scene. Dyspnœa and prostration were also marked. I then ordered cold baths, six being given in the twenty-four hours, and the result, which was excellent, was soon evident. In the other case, a child ten years of age, whom I saw with Blache, was suffering from measles of a malignant character. The symptoms were restlessness, dyspnœa, the respiration-rate being 80 a minute, temperature of 104° F., pulse of 140, and almost total suppression of urine. In spite of severe bronchial catarrh, I recommended cold baths, and the treatment, which was rigorously carried out, gave a very favourable result. I think, therefore, that I may state the following conclusions :

1. As, in spite of cold baths, the eruption continues its normal course, we need not be afraid of **driving in the rash.** In my second patient, who took seven cold baths on the second day of a general and almost confluent eruption, the rash became slightly pale during the bath ; but a quarter of an hour later it reappeared, and desquamation took place in a classical manner on the proper day.

2. The secretion of urine tends to return under the influence of cold baths, so that it is customary to treat by cold baths infectious diseases of a severe type, such as scarlatina, enteric fever, or pneumonia, in which the urinary secretion is scanty.

3. The cold baths do not show any bad effect on bronchitis or on pneumonia in measles, since capillary bronchitis and broncho-pneumonia, which threatened in my second patient, yielded, in spite of the continuation of the cold baths, and perhaps as the result of them. The same remark applies to bronchitis and to pneumonia in typhoid fever, which do not form a contra-

indication to cold baths. It is injurious to apply a blister to a patient in whom the secretion of urine is already below the normal, and a blister should not be used in a case of primary or secondary pneumonia, especially when the urinary function is affected, with or without albuminuria. A severe case of pneumonia of the ataxo-dynamic form, which I treated successfully by cold baths and without drugs, induces me to refrain from the use of blisters in such cases.

In short, every infectious disease which assumes the severe type known as malignant, ataxo-adynamic, etc., whether it is a question of measles, scarlatina, or pneumonia, should (unless there is some contra-indication) be treated with cold baths. This treatment, which has been almost exclusively reserved for enteric fever, should be generally employed in infectious diseases in which the infection assumes certain characters and marked intensity. Drugs and other means of treatment, useful though they may be, appear to me of secondary importance, and cold baths in such conditions form the best method of treatment.

The temperature of the bath should be regulated according to the nature and severity of the disease. In any case, we must not be content with tepid baths, but must give them cold—that is to say, baths in which the temperature varies from 68° to 72° F. We may place the patient in a bath at 72° F., and gradually cool the water to 68° F., according to the principles stated under Typhoid Fever.

By means of phototherapy, similar to the method employed by Finsen in variola—that is to say, by placing the patient in a room lighted with red glass—Chatinière has been able to modify many of the symptoms in measles. The eruption, the hyperthermia, and the bronchitis have made progressive improvement.

VI. RUBELLA.

Rubella is an eruptive fever which is more frequent in Germany than in France. It is contagious, and sometimes breaks out in epidemics, distinct from those of scarlatina and measles. It may also attack individuals who have or have not had scarlatina and measles, and confers upon them no immunity against these two diseases. These characters compel us to admit that rubella is a distinct morbid entity.

Description.—Rubella is a disease of early life, and is extremely rare in adults. Its incubation period is imperfectly known, but a period of invasion is absent, and the disease appears to begin with the eruption. The eruption is sometimes preceded by injection of the conjunctiva, hoarseness, slight dry cough (as in measles), and enlargement of the jugular and subauricular glands, which has been given as a characteristic sign of rubella, but which I have also seen in measles. The eruption invades the face, trunk, and limbs in succession. It is **polymorphous,** being morbilliform and scarlatiniform, macular and papular, discrete or confluent, and scanty on the hands, feet, and forehead, but well marked on the cheeks and around the mouth. The eruption disappears after a duration of one to five days. It is sometimes followed by slight branny desquamation. Relapses are not rare. Although the prognosis is good, severe cases and complications have been noticed. Broncho - pneumonia, albuminuria, and œdema have been seen.

From this description we see that rubella somewhat resembles attenuated measles, or measles associated with scarlatina. Is it identical with the *roséole saisonnière* described by Trousseau? This roseola, says Trousseau, is an eruptive fever, sometimes epidemic, and probably contagious. It is really modified measles, which is not accompanied by ocular, nasal, or bronchial catarrh, and which does not expose the patient to the complications of morbillous fever. The period of invasion lasts from two to three days (chills, headache). The eruption differs from that of measles, the spots being paler and more distinct from one another. They give rise to acute itching (Vogel), do not form papules, and are of short duration.

I think that there is a *roséole saisonnière*, as Frank, Vogel, and Trousseau have described ; but there is also rubella, the distinctive characters of which are not yet clearly defined. And, lastly, there are combined forms of the eruptive fevers (scarlatina and measles), which must not be confounded with roseola and rubella.

VII. MILIARY FEVER.

Ætiology.—Miliary fever is an infectious, endemic, and epidemic disease, probably of microbic origin, which appears with abundant sweats, accompanied by a rash and nervous symptoms. It is not inoculable ; it is contagious. It confers no immunity ; it may pass from the mother to the fœtus, which may or may not be born alive. In the three cases so far observed the fœtus suffered from the disease.

Miliary fever occurs at every age and at any season of the year, in the form of epidemics, preceded by sporadic cases, which are, as it were, the seeds of the epidemic. The epidemic, therefore, arises from an endemic focus which is sometimes nearly latent, and invades countries which it has never before visited. When the disease breaks out in virgin soil, the power of diffusion is so extraordinary that hundreds of individuals are taken ill at once. The epidemic reaches its height in eight days, and then decreases. The extension of the epidemic follows no rule. In some cases the epidemic centre is localized to one region ; in others it becomes scattered, somewhat like influenza. Miliary fever has broken out several times in France, the last epidemics being at l'Hérault (1865), and Poitou (1888), Charente and Deux-Sèvres (1907).

Description.—The duration of the incubation may be less than twenty-four hours. Three periods are described—invasion, eruption, and desquamation.

Invasion.—The disease sometimes begins with prodromata, such as malaise, headache, chills, heat, dyspnœa, vomiting, epistaxis, and cough; but as a rule the sweats form the initial symptom of the disease. These sweats are so abundant that the disease is called " sweating sickness." The bedclothes and the mattresses are soaked. They have neither special odour nor critical characters, and bring the patient no relief. The thirst is excessive, the urine is scanty and thick, and constipation is the rule.

The sweats are often paroxysmal, and the attacks are especially frequent at night. An attack is ushered in by a feeling of angina or of dyspnœa, with tightness in the epigastrium and pharynx, palpitation, tendency to fainting, or a terrible sensation of approaching death. The end of the attack gives only a relative relief, because the other symptoms—headache, cramp, and subsultus tendinum—persist apart from the attacks. The day is relatively more restful, but at night the whole train of severe symptoms reappears. Insomnia, nightmare, or delirium may also be present. The period of invasion lasts from two to four days. The temperature may rise above 105° F.

Eruption.—Between the second and fourth days of the disease the eruption appears, with pricking, formication, and recrudescence of the nervous symptoms. The eruption is composed of two elements—the exanthem and the miliary rash. When the exanthem is absent, the miliary rash is white, like the vesicles of sudamina. The exanthem, however, makes the miliary rash **red**. The exanthem may be morbilliform, scarlatiniform, hæmorrhagic, or purpuric. It varies in different epidemics. The miliary rash is composed of very small transparent vesicles, which in some cases unite and form blebs (bullous miliaria).

The miliary eruption commences on the neck and the front of the body, and then spreads to the back and the limbs, especially to the wrists (miliary bracelet). It generally spares the face. It comes out in several crops, and lasts on an average from five to seven days. During this period the general symptoms become less severe, the fever falls, and the period of desquamation begins.

Desquamation.—Desquamation in sweating sickness may assume several forms. It may be furfuraceous, or it may take the form of a collarette around the dried-up vesicles. In some cases it is scarlatiniform, large shreds of epidermis being thrown off. It lasts three or four weeks. **Polyuria,** which is a sign of recovery, then appears.

The disease lasts from seven to fourteen days. Convalescence is usually long and painful, even in the benign forms of the disease. The gravity of miliary fever varies in different epidemics and in different patients, but here, as in all epidemic diseases, benign and severe cases occur. In some cases the disease is from the first so acute that death may supervene early from cerebral troubles, such as delirium and coma (early malignant form), or at a later period (late malignant form). In some cases hæmorrhages appear, and are of evil augury. Miliary fever may be associated with malaria, with the eruptive fevers, and with typhus.

The epidemics of miliary fever are often preceded or accompanied by those of measles or of scarlatina. In some instances, indeed, measles and miliary fever appear to be associated. I say " appear," for in the majority of cases it is not so much an association of the two diseases, but rather that the miliary fever takes on a morbillous form.

We must not confound miliary fever, which is a definite morbid entity, with the **sudamina** which appear as an epiphenomenon in the course of other affections.

Tonic treatment has given the best results, and the use of quinine is indicated if the fever assumes a periodic type.

I shall now give a summary of the important communications made by Chantemesse to the Academy of Medicine in 1907. It deals with the epidemic of 1907 in Charente, Charente-Inférieure, and Deux-Sèvres. Within forty-five days the disease attacked 6,000 people. From the pathogenic point of view, microscopical examination, attempts at making cultures from the blood and from the cerebro-spinal fluid, and inoculation of macaque monkeys and other animals, gave no results. The epidemic was remarkable for its rural localization. The towns in the affected districts were not attacked.

The epidemic furnished no evidence that miliary fever is directly contagious. Thus, at the fair of Rouillac, 226 people from Angoulême remained all day in an infected centre, and yet they did not take the disease back to Angoulême. The virus of the miliary fever especially attacked those who lay on the ground, and houses without floors furnished most of the cases.

Chantemesse believes that the disease may be communicated to man by fleas from the field-rat. The arguments for this view are : the area invaded in 1907 by sweating sickness had been overrun two years previously by field-rats. " When we visited the houses in Genac, where the fever first appeared, we found innumerable flea-bites on the bodies of the inhabitants. Many of them had noticed the increase in the number of fleas, which they attributed to the invasion of their houses by water-rats driven away from a stream in flood." If this theory is proved, the destruction of field-rats is essential as a prophylactic measure in miliary fever.

VIII. DENGUE.

Ætiology.—"Dengue is a contagious or transmissible epidemic febrile disease, characterized by a polymorphous and diffuse cutaneous eruption, severe pains in the joints and muscles, and a cyclical course, comprising four periods, of which the last, or convalescent, is often tedious" (Mahé).

This affection arises in the tropics, and affects two chief centres—the former, in America, bounded on the one side by a line passing through the United States to the south of Boston, and, on the other hand, by a line through Brazil and Peru. The second is on the shores of the Indian Ocean and the Red Sea (India, Southern China, Tonkin, Mozambique, Arabia, and Egypt). Apart from these two centres, dengue has existed in an endemic or epidemic condition since 1845 in Tripoli, and since 1861 in Syria (De Brun). In 1889 the whole of Asia Minor, Turkey, and Greece were visited by the disease. Each of these epidemics is remarkable for the large number of persons affected, for the suddenness of its appearance, and the ease with which the disease has assumed an endemic form in a country recently invaded.

Dengue shows no distinction of sex, race, age, or of social condition. Animals also are said to suffer from it. The contagion is spread by the air, but the micro-organism which gives rise to it is at present unknown. Laughlin has found in the blood small spherical elements to which he assigns a pathogenic influence, but the benign nature of this disease has not given us an opportunity to examine the viscera.

Symptoms.—In tropical countries dengue has often a sudden onset, which roots the patient to the spot where he is, and compels him to be carried home. In the Temperate Zone the onset is less sudden. For some hours the patient feels out of sorts, complains of headache or of insomnia, and is unwilling to move about. Then the characteristic pains of the disease appear. They are unbearable, and affect the head, the trunk, and the limbs, either separately or together. The headache, which is often the chief symptom, occupies the forehead, the superciliary ridges, and the temples. It is sometimes accompanied by painful aching of the scalp, and pains in the orbit or in the motor muscles of the eye, and in the levator palpebrarum. The lumbar pains are increased by walking, and diminished by rest in bed. The pain in the limbs chiefly affects the knees. It may affect the muscles more than the joints (De Brun).

These muscular pains may invade every part of the body, and form the chief symptom in some epidemics. In others the chief symptom is swelling of the joints, of the tendon-sheaths, of the hands, and of the feet.

As regards the digestive system, we find loss of appetite, nausea, vomiting, and unquenchable thirst. The belly is slightly distended, but supple;

constipation is the rule; the spleen is not swollen, but the liver is sometimes congested, and the skin then assumes a subicteric tinge.

The helplessness is very pronounced, and compels the patient to take to his bed on the first day. Any movement or mental effort is painful or impossible.

At the end of from twenty-four to forty-eight hours, sometimes earlier, the eruption, which varies in appearance and in distribution, comes out. It may resemble that of measles, rubella, scarlatina, or urticaria, or it may be papular. The eruption, while often of a vivid red, is never ecchymotic. It usually lasts three or four days, but it may disappear at the end of twenty-four hours. It rarely lasts a week. At the onset of some cases writers have seen a vegetative eruption, followed after a few days by the characteristic rash. These eruptions give place to **desquamation,** which may resemble that seen in measles or in scarlatina, and which is accompanied by sharp itching.

Fever is practically constant (the thermometer registers about 104° F.), but falls at the end of two or three days, and this fall is often accompanied by crises (diaphoresis, diarrhœa, epistaxis). Apart from boils and abscesses and delirium or convulsions in children, the complications of dengue, such as epistaxis, adenitis, or orchitis, are exceptional and transient. De Brun rejects the cardiac forms which are said to occur by Zuelzer, Dunkby, etc.

This affection is essentially proteiform (gastric, rheumatic, cerebral, eruptive, febrile, or apyretic), and is followed by convalescence, which is always very long, and at variance with the shortness of the febrile period. Moreover, it may be interrupted by relapses. Recurrences are not uncommon in dengue.

Diagnosis.—The many forms of dengue explain the large number of diseases with which it may be confounded. **Influenza** forms the most frequent source of error. The absence of respiratory symptoms, the frequency of eruptions compared with their rarity in influenza, the desquamation and the subsequent itching, and the benign character of the disease, will, as a rule, prevent errors.

The epidemic character, the marked contagiousness, the suddenness of onset, and the rapid recovery in dengue, are features found neither in **typhoid fever** nor in **febrile gastritis.**

The pains in the muscles, joints, and lumbar region may suggest rheumatic trouble (lumbago, sciatica, or acute rheumatism), and yet the rapid helplessness, the eruptions, the desquamation, and the other symptoms present in dengue, are not found in these diseases.

The intense headache may suggest **acute meningitis,** especially if fever, constipation, and vomiting are also present ; but the eruption and the rapid recovery quickly decide the point.

The febrile form is distinguished from **scarlatina** by the absence or by the slight importance of the palato-pharyngeal symptoms; from **measles** by the sudden onset and absence of symptoms in the chest; from **rubella** by the absence of enlargement in the jugular and subauricular glands, and by the infrequency of angina. The error of mistaking the disease for variola may be committed at first, but it is, in general, of short duration, and the same holds good in the case of typhus.

Treatment.—Rest in bed, diet, and purgatives are generally sufficient in a slight case. If the disease is severe, we should prescribe acidulated and effervescing drinks, or hot toddy, and if vomiting occurs, ice. Sulphate of quinine does not reduce the temperature, and has the further inconvenience of causing noises in the ears. For the insomnia chloral should be prescribed, and during convalescence bitters, quinine, and iron will assist in promoting recovery.

CHAPTER II

TYPHOID DISEASES

I. TYPHOID FEVER.

History.—At the present time we include under the term **typhoid fever** the various forms of a disease which the old writers had described under the name of putrid fever (Stoll), malignant nervous fever (Huxham), putrid hæmorrhagic fever, ataxic and ataxo-adynamic fever.

The progress of pathological anatomy at the commencement of the century has united under one heading these different varieties, which were previously considered as distinct species. Since that period the classification of fevers has entered upon a new path.

In 1804 Prost, in a work entitled "Médecine Éclairée par l'Ouverture des Corps," had noted the inflammation and the ulcers found post mortem in those who had died with ataxic, putrid, or malignant fever; but he thought that these fevers were only an excess of intestinal phlogosis, causing death. Broussais' teaching arose from this false interpretation.

In 1811 Petit and Serres, in their treatise on "Fièvre Entéro-mésentérique," came nearer the truth by establishing the specific nature of the intestinal lesions, but they committed two errors; firstly, in thinking that there were three varieties of entero-mesenteric fever—namely, simple, granular, and ulcerative—without seeing that the appearance of the lesion varied with the stage of the disease; secondly, they also thought that the intestinal lesion comprised the whole malady.

Bretonneau, in 1820, first described the intestinal lesion, and clearly established the relations existing between the disease and the lesion. He settled the question of its specific nature, and united in one morbid species, which he called **dothiénentérie** (δοτιήν, button; ἔντερον, intestine), all the scattered varieties previously described. Next, appeared the work of Trousseau, Andral, and Bouillaud, who threw such a vivid light on medicine in France, and typhoid fever definitely took the place which it now occupies in medical nosology.

The discovery of the typhoid bacillus (Eberth) has proved the specific nature of this disease, and has given a striking confirmation of the teaching of Bretonneau and of Trousseau.

Symptoms.—I shall first describe a typical case of typhoid fever, and I shall then discuss the special forms and the many complications of this disease.

1. **Onset—Period of Ascension.**—As a rule, the invasion of typhoid fever is preceded by a period which lasts from a few days to two weeks, and which some authors describe as being prodromal. The patient complains of lassitude, muscular pains, loss of appetite, giddiness, and sometimes of

1619

epistaxis. In other cases, however, this prodromal period is absent, and the disease commences suddenly with rigors and high temperature. In some cases the morbid localization is marked at a particular point, even from the outset, and therefore in rare instances typhoid fever has begun with lobar pneumonia. " These cases of initial pneumonia, which run the course of simple primary inflammation, mark, however, the invasion of enteric fever. During the first week, while the symptoms proper to pneumonia improve, the signs of typhoid fever (swelling of the spleen, rose-spots, and pain in the iliac region) show themselves. In certain patients dyspeptic or intestinal troubles open the scene, so we may take the onset of enteric fever for appendicitis, if due care is not exercised. In other cases a catarrhal angina especially attracts our attention.

Normal typhoid fever shows three stages—ascending, stationary, and descending. The first two stages have been included by Jaccoud under the term " period of invasion," while the descending stage, in his opinion, coincides with the period of repair. The course of the fever is practically parallel with these three stages, and is represented on the temperature chart by oscillations which in succession ascend, remain stationary, and descend (Jaccoud). These divisions, though convenient for descriptive purposes, are clinically not so clearly marked, and the periods often follow one another by such an insensible transition that it is difficult to say where the one begins and the other ends.

The onset of the period of ascent cannot be always defined, for the symptoms are blended with the prodromata, and in a patient seen for the first time some days after the invasion of the fever we are often much embarrassed in stating on the chart the exact onset of the disease.

The first period is characterized by an increase in the prodromal symptoms or by the appearance of fresh ones. **Headache** is severe, and may be the chief symptom for some days. It is present day and night, and sometimes assumes a neuralgic form, with painful points in the course of the suborbital and occipital nerves. Insomnia is practically constant, and is also a symptom of great value. The patient complains of pains in the neck, vertigo, and of buzzing in the ears, which increase as soon as he raises himself or sits up in bed. Epistaxis is frequent, but not profuse. The tongue is coated ; the loss of appetite is complete, and diarrhœa commences. Some patients by this time show considerable prostration. Bronchial congestion is frequent, and revealed on auscultation by scattered sibilant râles. During this period, which lasts from four to six days, the fever is continuous, the evening reading being always higher than the morning one. The temperature rises until it reaches 104° F. at night. The acceleration of the pulse is not always in proportion to the elevation of temperature. The cause of this discrepancy is discussed under the Pathological Physiology.

2. **Stationary Stage.**—This stage, so called because of the stationary character of the fever, does not deserve this name as far as the symptoms are concerned, because they generally become worse during this stage. The eruption of **lenticular rose spots** usually appears on the abdomen about the seventh day of the disease—that is, at the commencement of this stage. The spots are from 2 to 5 millimetres in circumference, papular, slightly prominent, appreciable to the touch, and fade on pressure. Each spot lasts from three to six days. It then becomes pale, and disappears without leaving any trace. The whole eruption may last two or three weeks. It is generally discrete, and is sometimes limited to a few spots ; but in other cases it is so confluent as to simulate a papular, morbilliform eruption. The rose spots are usually seen on the belly and chest. They sometimes spread over the back and the limbs. Although they are not absolutely constant, they are of considerable diagnostic value.

During this period the **nervous symptoms** become gradually more severe, with the exception of the headache, which improves or disappears. The buzzing noises in the ears are followed by dullness of hearing, which may end in **deafness.** In addition to the insomnia and disturbed dreams, quiet delirium may occur at night, and may be accompanied by restlessness and incoherent speech. During the day the patient is quite indifferent to what is going on around him, and lies in a state of somnolence, which in some cases borders on stupor (τύφος). He lies in the dorsal decubitus, with vacant look, wasted face, and mouth half open. His lips are tremulous, and his nostrils work rapidly, and at times he appears to grasp imaginary objects (carphologia, from κάρφος, flake ; λέγειν, to pluck). We shall see later how severe these symptoms become in the ataxo-adynamic forms.

The **digestive disturbances** are chiefly seen in this period. The tongue is dry, cracked, red, tremulous, and covered by dry mucus, blackened by traces of blood. Sordes are seen on the teeth, and the throat is covered with mucus or with pulpy exudate. Vomiting is rare. The **diarrhœa** is characterized by frequent, offensive, liquid stools of a yellow-ochre colour. They are sometimes passed without the patient's knowledge, and contain, among other microbes, Eberth's bacillus. In some cases diarrhœa is absent, and there may even be constipation.

As soon as diarrhœa has set in, we find in the right iliac fossa **gurgling,** which, however, is of no value in diagnosis ; but this region, and also the epigastric hollow, are usually tender on pressure. **Meteorism,** due to intestinal paresis and accumulation of gas, sometimes becomes so marked as to push up the diaphragm and embarrass respiration.

The troubles in the **respiratory system** are of moderate severity. Although the patient coughs but little, numerous sonorous and mucous râles are heard on auscultation. The **broncho-pulmonary congestion** causes fairly acute dyspnœa, and may be the origin of serious complications.

The **urine** is scanty, highly coloured, rich in extractives, and often contains albumin, while the amount of urea varies inversely to the severity of the disease. Albuminuria does not appear, as a rule, until the beginning of the second week, and disappears in the course of the third week (Gubler). **Retention of urine** is fairly common, and it is therefore necessary to watch the bladder, in order to perform catheterism if needed.

The **spleen** is enlarged, and the swelling is marked from the commencement of the case, especially in young patients. The pulse is sometimes dicrotic (*bis feriens*)—that is to say, the beat appears to be doubled—and the rate varies from 100 to 110 beats a minute. A pulse of 120 in an adult **indicates a grave condition,** especially if this frequency is maintained (Hardy). Softness and irregularity of the pulse are also unfavourable signs, and are often associated with lesions in the cardiac muscle, which, in the grave forms, favour collapse.

During this period the evening temperature may exceed 104° F., while the morning temperature shows, as a rule, only a slight remission (stationary oscillation), and the prognosis becomes graver the less marked the morning remission.

Other eruptions, including blue spots and sweat rashes, are seen, in addition to the rose spots. The blue or dusky spots which are found in many other diseases would present little interest if the question of their pathogenesis had not aroused curiosity. Mourson has shown that these blue spots are due to the presence of pediculi. This opinion has been confirmed by Duguet's experiments, in which colouring matter from the pediculi introduced under the skin gives rise to blue spots.

The sudamina met with in different stages of typhoid fever are only of moderate interest.

3. **Period of Decline.**—Between the fifteenth and the thirtieth day of the disease—rarely earlier, and sometimes later—the patient enters on the period of defervescence. The evening temperature, although it falls somewhat, remains higher than the morning temperature; but the morning remissions are well marked, and the temperature curve falls progressively. This slow defervescence by lysis (λύσις, solution) occurs in most cases. In some cases, however, the defervescence is as **sudden** as in pneumonia. Jaccoud has carefully studied this sudden defervescence, and has found it seventy-three times in 261 cases. It takes place in a space of time which varies from twelve to thirty-six hours, and the fall of temperature varies from $1\frac{1}{2}°$ to 3°; but it does not end in hypothermia. It may be seen in all the varieties of typhoid fever. We shall find later a curve showing sudden defervescence in one of my cases.

During this period the symptoms gradually diminish in severity. The insomnia is replaced by sleep; the tongue is moist; and the patient, who now takes some interest in his surroundings, has not the previous appearance of prostration and stupor. The diarrhœa and meteorism disappear; the pulse is less frequent, and tends to regain its normal characters, and the patient, although much wasted and anæmic, enters on convalescence.

4. **Convalescence.**—In this stage the wasting stops and the appetite returns, but convalescence in typhoid fever presents this peculiarity: that, without appreciable cause, the fever, which had completely disappeared, may return, last three or four days, and disappear, in order to return again. This **fever of convalescence** does not indicate a relapse, and has nothing in common with the febrile condition which sometimes follows an increase in the diet. Moreover, it is not associated with any inflammatory lesion, and presents no danger, although it may delay recovery.

If the attack has been severe, and no complication interrupts the natural course of convalescence, the patient requires months to recover. In the convalescent patient the temperature is subnormal, the pulse is often slow, the reflexes are exaggerated, and vertigo and palpitation are frequent symptoms. The first attempts at feeding are sometimes followed by vomiting. The muscular system remains weak for a long while; the patient has not the same aptitude for work, and in some cases the memory is very slow to return.

Typhoid fever often causes temporary alopecia, and sometimes leaves scars on the skin of the thighs and of the abdomen (Bouchard). In young subjects growth is quickened.

Clinical Forms of Typhoid Fever.

Mild Typhoid Fever.—Mild or defaced forms occur in typhoid fever, just as in all the eruptive fevers. In the slight forms improperly grouped under the name of "mucous fever," the symptoms are mild. This term must be abandoned, and we must remember that these cases, although usually quite benign, are not exempt from such dread complications as hæmorrhage, perforation, and peritonitis.

Abortive Typhoid Fever.—The term **abortive typhus,** coined by Lebert, corresponds to the disease named by other authors as typhus levissimus. As Griesinger has remarked, the word levissimus should not be applied to the benign nature of the symptoms, but rather to the short duration of the disease. In this form the invasion is acute and febrile, and the symptoms (epistaxis, diarrhœa, swelling of the spleen, and rose-rash) somewhat resemble those of mild enteric fever; but in the second week "the disease stops short, behaving with regard to abdominal typhus just as varioloid does with regard to variola" (Jaccoud). The fall of temperature is usually accompanied by critical sweats. It is possible, adds Jaccoud, though not proven, that in the abortive forms the intestinal changes may be limited to infiltration of the glands, and that resolution replaces necrosis and consequent sloughing.

Ambulatory Form.—The preceding or abortive form was characterized by its short duration and by its well-marked, though benign, symptoms. The **ambulatory** form, so called because patients feel such slight malaise that they continue to go about, is latent. Fever is absent or very slight. The malaise, headache, insomnia, and diarrhœa, which are usually so marked in typhoid fever, are here but little in evidence. Nevertheless, we may find swelling of the spleen, rose spots, and bronchitic râles ; but the patient, who does not consider himself ill, and has not lost his appetite, goes about and tries to attend to business. In spite of the apparently benign nature of the disease, the patient runs the risk of hæmorrhage, perforation, and peritonitis, and at the autopsy the typical lesions of typhoid fever are found.

Adynamic Form.—This term does not apply to the secondary symptoms of adynamia which supervene in severe cases. It is reserved for those cases which assume an adynamic character during the invasion. General feebleness and prostration, compressible pulse, profound and lasting stupor, quiet delirium, deafness, paralysis of the bladder, abundant diarrhœa, considerable meteorism, fœtor of the sweat and of the breath, and a tendency to hæmorrhage and gangrene, are the symptoms of the adynamic form, which corresponds to the old putrid and malignant fever. The prognosis is usually grave.

Ataxic Form.—" Prostration and enfeeblement of the animal functions are not present, as in the preceding form. It is their want of harmony that strikes us " (Trousseau). The ataxic form begins with very high temperature. Cramps and lumbar pain occur. The delirium, which appears early and is sometimes violent, may be accompanied by loquacity and hallucinations. Squint, chewing movements of the jaws, tremors of the face, of the lips, of the hands, and of the fingers, carphologia, subsultus tendinum, and convulsions are seen. This variety of enteric fever is most fatal, and carries the patients off in five or six days. In some cases symptoms of adynamia appear, and we then have the mixed Ataxo-adynamic variety. We must always feel anxious in these ataxic cases, even when the symptoms are trifling.

Sudoral Form.—The form called sudoral by Jaccoud presents special characters. Apart from the headache, which is severe, there are neither cerebral symptoms, delirium, nor stupor. Abdominal symptoms are almost absent—no diarrhœa, no meteorism ; the tongue remains moist ; the broncho-pulmonary system is less affected than in ordinary typhoid fever, and albuminuria is extremely rare. The rose spots are not present in all the cases, but their complete absence, says Jaccoud, is exceptional. Hæmorrhage from the bowels is fairly frequent. **Fever** and **sweats** are the constant and prominent symptoms in this form. The fever, though continuous, shows well-marked paroxysms, which may occur several times in the twenty-four hours, and are followed by "profuse, drenching sweats." This form is common in Italy, especially in Naples (Borelli), and is also seen in Paris.

Hæmorrhagic Form.—This form, called **hæmorrhagic putrid fever** by old writers, is marked by cutaneous hæmorrhages, purpuric ecchymoses, bleeding from the nose and gums, hæmaturia, and metrorrhagia. It is more frequent in certain epidemics. It is usually associated with changes in the liver, and with symptoms of ataxia or of ataxo-adynamia. It is always fatal.

Typhoid Fever in Children and Elderly People.—Typhoid fever in children differs anatomically and clinically from the disease as seen in the adult. The infiltration of Peyer's patches almost always takes the form of soft plaques, which rarely ulcerate. Perforation, peritonitis, and hæmorrhage are very rare in infancy. The disease is especially frequent after the fifth year, but yet cases have been seen as early as the first year, and even at the age of six months. The tongue remains moist; vomiting is frequent; diarrhœa is rare; ballooning of the belly is exceptional; convulsions, with slight delirium, may be seen; the eruption of rose spots is discrete; the wasting is rapid; and the disease often ends with critical sweats. The ataxo-adynamic symptoms which are seen in youths about the age of puberty are extremely rare in young children. Pulmonary manifestations, especially lobular pneumonia, are formidable in early life, and relapses are more frequent than in adults; and yet the prognosis of typhoid fever in the child is much less grave than at a more advanced age. In children's hospitals diphtheria, the eruptive fevers, and whooping-cough form the common complications.

Typhoid fever in elderly people presents some peculiarities. The temperature is not very high, the swelling of the spleen is slight, the rose spots are few in number; and yet, in spite of the apparently trifling nature of the symptoms, the disease rapidly ends in prostration. The course of the disease is slow, and the broncho-pulmonary troubles add much to the gravity of the prognosis.

Complications of Typhoid Fever.

Digestive System.—Numerous complications affect the digestive system. As regards the bucco-pharyngeal cavity, there is little to be said; but membranous angina, due to staphylococci or to streptococci, may be seen. Diphtheria is only present in very rare cases. We may see on the pillars of the fauces, on the tonsils, and on the pharynx **ulcers**, which at first sight resemble those of herpes and of tuberculosis. They are really due to Eberth's bacillus. Thrush is fairly frequent in the pharynx.

Violent spasmodic dyspnœa is at times seen during the course or during the decline of typhoid fever. It may be the only nervous symptom of the disease or the prelude of grave nervous troubles in convalescence (Vergely).

Gastric Troubles.—The anatomical study of the gastric lesions in typhoid fever (lymphatic infiltration, thrombosis, miliary abscesses, and ulcers) explains the symptoms present in some cases (Chauffard). I refer here to the repeated and obstinate vomiting sometimes seen in the course of the second or of the third week, or even during convalescence (Trousseau). It appears probable that this vomiting, which is accompanied by pain and a rise of temperature in the epigastric angle (Peter), is associated with infective and ulcerating lesions of the stomach. Hæmatemesis may be seen. If the reader will turn to the section on Appendicular Vomito Negro, he will see that in one of the cases the hæmatemesis (Millard's case) was due to changes in the stomach following upon paratyphoid appendicitis.

Hæmorrhage from the Bowel.—Hæmorrhage is seen in 6 per cent. of cases, and its frequency varies according to the epidemic. In some cases the blood remains in the bowel, where it is found at the autopsy. As a rule, it is passed (melæna), either in the form of pure blood (this is rare), or in the form of clots, and of brownish or blackish fœtid fluid, like soot and water, or sticky, like tar. Hæmorrhage may occur several times in the same day, or on several days following. It usually occurs at the beginning or during the course of the third week, and is due to ulceration of the intestine, to degeneration and perforation of the vessels, and to the formation of fleshy, perivascular granulations. When, however, the bleeding appears in the early part of the second week, before ulceration has taken place, we must rather admit that it is due to congestion of the gut, with or without changes in the vessel wall. The more abundant and the more frequent the hæmorrhage, the more serious the outlook. In some exceptional cases the bleeding is fulminating at the first onset. Thus, one of Trousseau's patients was carried off in an hour, and a patient whose case is reported by Leymarie was seized with such severe hæmorrhage from the bowel that he died in less than an hour, and at the autopsy the hæmorrhage was found to proceed from a small artery opening into an ulcer. Several authors regard hæmorrhage from the bowel as relatively benign. Graves called it an almost critical phenomenon, and Trousseau did not consider it to be very formidable. Griesinger says that it is fatal in only 33 per cent. of the cases.

Some authors have distorted Trousseau's statement, making him say

Diphtheritic angina appears during the second, third, or fourth week of scarlatina, when the patient is on the road to recovery or is convalescent. In some cases the disease is relatively benign, and recovery takes place ; but in other cases croup occurs (four times in ten cases in Bourges' statistics). Other cases run a malignant course, and are always fatal.

It would be well to quote as a whole Trousseau's admirable account of malignant diphtheria in scarlatina. " Individuals are taken ill with scarlatina of moderate severity. They have slight delirium at night, and perhaps some nervous symptoms. The pulse is rather quick, and the pain in the throat is of moderate severity. Recovery appears certain about the eighth or ninth day. The fever has fallen and the eruption has disappeared, so that the physician reassures the family. Suddenly considerable swelling appears at the angle of the jaw, and is not confined to this region, but extends to the neck, and sometimes to a portion of the face. Very abundant and fœtid, sanious fluid flows from the nostrils ; the tonsils are much swollen ; the breath is fœtid ; the pulse suddenly becomes very rapid and small ; the delirium reappears, and other nervous symptoms set in. Then, while the delirium is persistent, coma appears, and at the same time the skin. becomes cold, the pulse more and more feeble, and the patient dies after three or four days, or is suddenly carried off by syncope. How can we explain the course of events ? These phenomena so closely resemble the terrible forms of diphtheria, which kill patients before the membrane has had time to spread to the larynx, and are so like in character to these fulminant forms of malignant diphtheria, that we are tempted to believe that it is not scarlatina, but rather this latter and deadly affection, which has carried off the patient. Indeed, the patients succumb with every symptom of diphtheritic poisoning—coldness of the body, smallness of the pulse, fœtor of the breath, and universal pallor of the skin, which are seen in no other species of grave disease."

We know that this malignant diphtheria is most often due to the association of the diphtheria bacillus with the streptococcus. This angina supervenes as a secondary infection, the diphtheria developing on a soil already prepared by the scarlatinal angina.

I must now say a word about suppurative angina. It would appear a *priori* that it should be frequent in scarlatina, seeing that the virulent streptococcus is often present in this disease. On the contrary, however, suppurative tonsillitis and retropharyngeal abscess are very rare.

Purulent rhinitis is a very grave complication, since eighteen patients out of thirty-nine died. It may be early and characterized by profuse running from the nose, as in glanders. This is the most severe form. Sometimes it does not appear until desquamation has begun. Lastly, it may be

that he considered intestinal hæmorrhage as absolutely benign. Trousseau, after giving his opinion that these hæmorrhages " are far from having the gravity usually attributed to them," took care to add : " I would not have it said that I regard these complications, which are usually considered to be serious in every case, as being absolutely harmless." For my part, I consider hæmorrhage as formidable to a moderate degree. Most of the patients in whom I have seen hæmorrhage have recovered, and I am therefore quite ready to regard them as being benign in most cases ; and yet we must reserve our prognosis, because hæmorrhage **sometimes heralds perforation of the gut,** and, on the other hand, it is particularly formidable when it forms part of a general hæmorrhagic process (hæmorrhagic putrid fever).

When the hæmorrhage is abundant, it usually, but not always, causes a sudden fall of temperature. This fall, however, is transient, and in some cases in one or two hours the temperature may exceed the point at which it stood before the bleeding. Such a course is not seen after the fall provoked by perforation of the bowel.

Peritonitis.—Two varieties of peritonitis—one by perforation, the other by propagation—are usually described. The former is more serious, and is generally due to perforation of Peyer's patches, or of the ulcerated closed follicles. The latter, less serious and more limited, is said to be due to the propagation of the infecting process through the intestine which is ulcerated, but **not perforated.**

The perforation is usually found in the lower portion of the ileum—that is to say, in the region where the ulcerative process is most severe. A perforation of the ileum is rarely found more than 2 feet above the ileo-cæcal valve, but it is not uncommon to find perforation below the valve in the cæcum, the appendix, or the colon. In Nacke's statistics, comprising 127 autopsies, perforations were found 106 times in the end of the ileum, 15 times in the appendix, and 12 times in the colon. Care must be exercised when making an autopsy not to mistake an artificial tear made during the examination for a perforation of the gut. The perforation is usually very small, being about as large as a pin's head, a hemp-seed, or a lentil. It is rounded, forming the apex of a kind of crater, which results from the ulceration of the agminated or isolated follicles. In some cases the ulcer may be as large as a florin ; in others it takes the form of a slit. As a rule, only one perforation is found, but it is by no means rare to find two, three, or even several, which have occurred simultaneously or in succession.

Perforation of the gut takes place at different times, but most frequently during the course of the third or at the beginning of the fourth week, when the ulcerative process is at its maximum. Writers have, however, quoted very early perforations, occurring between the eighth and twelfth days of the disease ; but it may then be asked whether the date of the onset was correctly determined. They have also quoted very late perforations, supervening during convalescence or after recovery. We shall see later the meaning of these facts. Perforations are far from being rare during relapses.

The frequency of perforation varies in different epidemics and countries. As a general rule, perforation is one of the most formidable complications of typhoid fever. It is not as common in children as in adults. It appears to be more frequent among the Anglo-Saxon race. Murchison has collected some interesting statistics, which show the large proportion of eighty perforations in 412 autopsies (19 per cent.) in English hospitals. In the French and German hospitals the proportion is 116 perforations in 1,300 deaths (10 per cent.).

Perforation of the gut is the result of an ulcerative process. Drastic purgatives, large enemata, the strain of vomiting, and departure from careful treatment, have been suggested as favouring perforation. There is some truth in these statements. Perforation occurs more readily in severe ataxo-adynamic cases, but cases of perforation supervening in the course of very mild attacks have also been reported (typhus levissimus, typhus ambulatorius). In the latter case peritonitis sets in suddenly, just as pneumothorax may do in the course of an almost latent tuberculosis. The cold-bath treatment should not be blamed. I think, on the other hand, that hydrotherapy lessens the virulence of the disease, and eliminates to some extent the danger caused by the ulcerative process.

Intestinal hæmorrhage fairly often precedes peritonitis by perforation, and the fact need cause no surprise, for the same ulcerative process is at work in both these complications. Homolle gives the following conclusive statistics on this point : In the cases collected by Murchison, 11 out of 69 patients who suffered from perforative peritonitis had hæmorrhage from the bowel. Goldhamer has observed the same course of events : in 13 patients suffering from peritonitis 3 had intestinal hæmorrhage. One of Grasset's patients died from perforation after intestinal hæmorrhage, and one of Buhl's patients, who had escaped the complication of perforation, died later from bleeding. The association and the succession of these complications had arrested my attention, and of the numerous patients whom I saw die from peritonitis by perforation many had previously had hæmorrhage from the gut. The most alarming feature of hæmorrhage is, in my opinion, that it is often a forerunner of perforation.

We are too prone to think that peritonitis in the course of typhoid fever is ushered in with severe symptoms. In some instances this is true, but often such is by no means the case. In typhoid fever peritonitis is often insidious in its appearance. It is somewhat rare, I repeat, for peritonitis in typhoid fever to assume the severe type, with intense pain and porraceous vomiting, so frequent in peritonitis following **perforating ulcer** of the stomach or of the duodenum. There are several reasons for this. In the first place, typhoid peritonitis often supervenes in patients whose sensations are more or less blunted by the infection; and, further, the perforation of the bowel is usually so small and so limited that the infecting agents—intestinal fluid, microbes, and toxines—reach the peritoneum very slowly and in small doses. Thus in some cases, as I have often seen, the onset of peritonitis would pass almost unnoticed if the patient were not carefully watched. He has pain, it is true, but it is only slight. He may vomit; but do not patients with enteric fever vomit, apart from peritonitis? Tympanites may be present; but is not the belly usually tympanitic in typhoid fever? There may be pain in the right iliac fossa; but is not this often the case in the course of this disease, without any reason for suspecting peritonitis? Accordingly, nausea, vomiting, pain, and tympanites, which may be more or less marked, leave us sometimes in doubt as to the occurrence of perforation and the appearance of peritonitis.

Hiccough is a sign of considerable importance in my opinion. Peritonitis is probably present when a patient in the third week of typhoid fever suffers from abdominal pain, nausea, and vomiting, while the abdomen is more distended than usual, especially if hiccough is added to these symptoms. Hiccough may, however, exist in typhoid fever as a consecutive complication, independent of peritonitis. Graves many years ago noticed this fact, and I have seen it in two of my cases, one of whom came under my care during the second week of an attack of typhoid fever, with incessant hiccough day and night. After the first few cold baths had been given, the hiccough disappeared. We should be wrong, therefore, in considering hiccough as a certain sign of peritonitis.

In my opinion the temperature curve is the most important symptom of insidious peritonitis by perforation. Perforation of the bowel in the course of typhoid fever shows itself in a large number of cases by a **sudden fall** of temperature. This fall may be as much as 5° or 6° F. in a few hours. The fall nearly always results in **hypothermia.** It is not accompanied by rigors, and may be almost unnoticed by the patient. Most writers place this sudden fall of temperature among the signs of perforation. The following cases will illustrate this point :

The temperature fell in a few hours from 103·5° to 96° F. in one of Netter's patients suffering from severe typhoid fever, which had run a normal course until the twentieth day. The patient did not vomit or complain of abdominal pain, because his senses were much dulled. The autopsy revealed fairly circumscribed peritonitis, due to perforation of a Peyer's patch. In a case reported by Dillay sharp pain, with vomiting, appeared during the decline of a case of typhoid fever, and the temperature fell to 96° F. on the morning after the patient's admission to hospital. The man died some days later, and the autopsy revealed peritonitis, consecutive to two intestinal perforations in ulcerated Peyer's patches. These perforations were situated in the ileum, 6 and 8 inches above the ileo-cæcal valve. Peritonitis supervened on the fifteenth day in a case of adynamic fever reported by Laboulbène; the abdomen was much distended; the patient was delirious. He did not vomit, but he had diarrhœa, and the temperature **suddenly fell** from 103° to 98° F. At the autopsy peritonitis, resulting from a perforation of a Peyer's patch near the end of the ileum, was found.

Martineau has related three cases of peritonitis by perforation in the course of typhoid fever, and all three showed a **fall of temperature**, which at the time of death was only 96° F.

In a work published in 1889 by Reunert on peritonitis in typhoid fever by perforation of the bowel, I find three cases in which it is said that in the first patient the temperature fell to 96° F., in the second to 97° F., and in the third to 95° F.

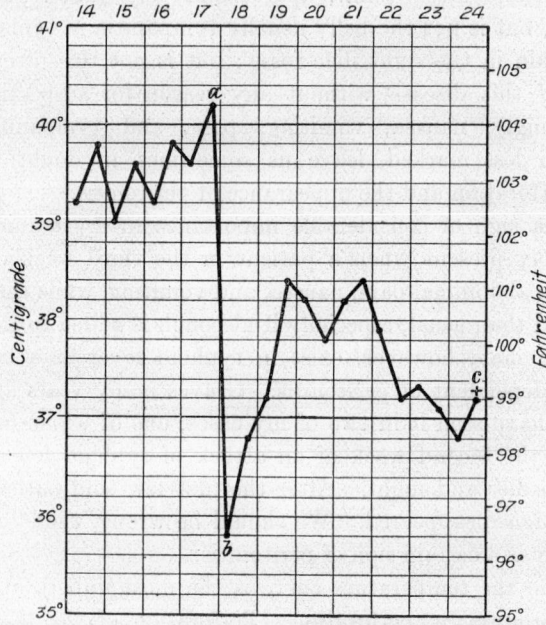

FIG. 85.—TYPHOID FEVER: FALL OF TEMPERATURE AFTER INTESTINAL PERFORATION IN A PATIENT OF MINE.

a, 104·2° F. on the evening of the seventeenth day; *b*, 96·5° F. on the morning of the eighteenth day; *c*, death on the twenty-fourth day.

I have quoted these cases because **sudden hypothermia** is a valuable sign of insidious perforation in the course of typhoid fever, and this sign is the more precious because the other symptoms of acute peritonitis—namely, pain, vomiting, and hiccough—are sometimes almost absent. In such cases, therefore, our best guide as regards surgical intervention is sudden hypothermia; but I do not say, of course, that this hypothermia always follows in intestinal perforation of typhoid origin, for there are cases in which peritonitis is accompanied by severe pain, vomiting, and a rise of temperature to 103° or 104° F.; but whether the fall of temperature be due to the hypothermic action of the coli bacillus and its toxine,* with or without the assistance of Eberth's bacillus, or whether it is due to sideration of the abdominal sympathetic, it is none the less true that this fall is a sign of undoubted value. Nevertheless, it must not be thought that sudden falls of temperature in the course of typhoid fever always indicate a perforation. In some rare cases the defervescence in typhoid fever is as sudden as in pneumonia. In the evening the temperature may be 104° F., and on the next morning only 98° F., this fall indicating recovery. I have seen an instance of this kind in one of my patients. A young woman was suffering from typhoid fever of a fairly severe type, and recovery took place by sudden defervescence, as the chart on p. 1632 shows.

There is a difference, however, between the sudden defervescence of recovery and that of perforation. The former coincides with an improvement in all the symptoms, and the temperature does not fall below normal ; the fall which announces perforation sometimes leads rapidly to hypothermia, and coincides with aggravation of the general symptoms, or with the appearance of fresh ones.

A sudden fall of temperature, with or without hypothermia, may also supervene in the course of typhoid fever as the result of profuse **hæmorrhage from the bowels,** and consequently simulate the sudden hypothermia of perforation ; in the latter case the temperature rises slowly, while as a rule a rapid rise follows in the former, so that the temperature in a few hours is as high as it was before the fall.

I have never seen a better proof of this assertion than in the case of one of my patients, whose chart is given (Fig. 57). The patient was taken ill on the twelfth day of very severe ataxo-adynamic fever, with two very copious hæmorrhages at an interval of a quarter of an hour. Just before the hæmorrhage the temperature was 105° F., but it at once fell as low as 97·5° F. This was indeed a case of sudden hypothermia, counterfeiting that of perforation, but two hours after the hæmorrhage the temperature had already gone up to 103·6° F. The patient died four days later, and it was easy to see that she had neither perforation nor the least trace of peritonitis, although several Peyer's patches were ulcerated down to the serous coat.

Peritonitis from perforation is fatal in the great majority of cases. It has a duration varying from two to eight days, sometimes interrupted by

* Sanarelli, in his experimental researches on typhoid fever, comes to the following conclusions : He injects a culture of the *Bacillus coli* and *Bacillus typhosus* into the peritoneum of the guinea-pig ; he then injects in another guinea-pig the peritoneal exudate of the first guinea-pig which has succumbed, and so on. He thus succeeds in obtaining a *Bacillus typhosus* of much increased virulence. Injection of two drops of this virus in the peritoneum of the guinea-pig kills the animal in fifteen hours, and produces in one hour a fall of temperature from 37·5° to 34° C. (*Ann. de l'Inst. Pasteur*, Avril, 1894). On the other hand, Roux and Rodet arrive at the same result with a culture of coli bacillus of increased virulence (*Arch. de Méd. Expérim.*, Mai, 1892). Boix, in a work on the pathogenesis of icterus gravis, has analyzed the hypothermic properties of the coli bacillus (*Arch. de Méd.*, Juillet et Août, 1896).

remissions or fictitious improvement, and the peritoneal symptoms are
fairly often masked by the typhoid symptoms. In a few days the face
becomes pinched, the eyes hollow, the pulse miserable and very rapid ; the
patient is cold and covered with clammy sweat, and death supervenes in
collapse or in coma.

Nevertheless, peritonitis from perforation is not always fatal, for
adhesions may be established **in time,** in which case the peritonitis becomes
circumscribed, and after two, three, or four days, during which the

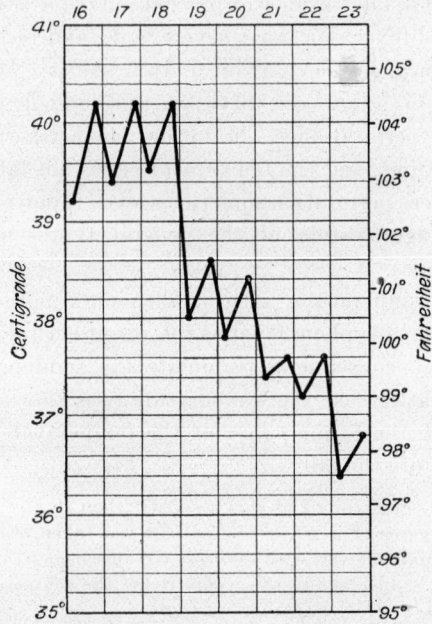

FIG. 86.—TYPHOID FEVER : RECOVERY ON NINETEENTH DAY, WITH SUDDEN
DEFERVESCENCE.

Temperature falling from 104·2° to 100·5° F.

symptoms of peritonitis from perforation have been evident, improvement
sets in, and the patient recovers.

Reunert's cases, to which I alluded above, are types of this peritonitis ending in
recovery, and in them sudden fall of temperature, vomiting, hiccough, tympanites,
dyspnœa, thready pulse, and collapse were all present. I have seen a case of this kind.
The peritonitis commenced with a sudden fall of temperature, while the distension of
the abdomen, the pain, the vomiting, and the hiccough caused me to give an exceedingly
grave prognosis; but the patient fortunately recovered.

In these cases some authors maintain that the peritonitis is caused by
propagation, and not by perforation. It appears *a priori,* that peritonitis
from perforation cannot be curable, and yet it may if adhesions limit the

perforation, and lessen or destroy its noxious effects. Positive cases of this kind have been published.

A patient of Bucquoy's with typhoid fever was doing well, but he was hardly convalescent when a relapse occurred, and proved rapidly fatal. At the autopsy Bucquoy found, among other lesions, a large ulcer at the termination of the ileum, with a **perforation** which was closed by old adhesions, and which dated from the first attack of the fever. He adds, very justly : "This is a well-marked case of perforation causing circumscribed peritonitis, which had escaped notice, and which would not have hindered recovery if a relapse of the typhoid fever had not caused the patient's death. Widal tells me that he has seen a similar case in which the perforation was situated in the cæcum ; the peritoneum had been protected by the timely formation of adhesions.

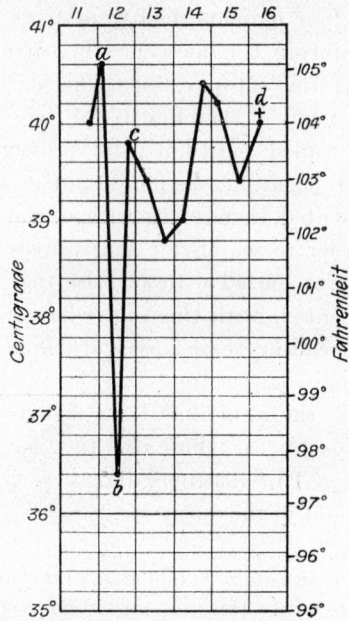

FIG. 87.—FALL OF TEMPERATURE DUE TO INTESTINAL HÆMORRHAGE.

a, Morning of twelfth day ; *b*, evening, 5 p.m., two hæmorrhages ; *c*, two hours after the second hæmorrhage ; *d*, death on sixteenth day.

We must now consider peritonitis by **propagation,** in which case the infective process is supposed to traverse the ulcerated but **non-perforated** intestine. The term "peritonitis by propagation" was coined by Trousseau.

All authorities have since admitted peritonitis by propagation, and they consider it more limited, circumscribed, and more favourable than peritonitis by perforation. It has been described by Jaccoud and by Homolle, who have called attention to Thirial's monograph.* Chantemesse reserves special mention for it in his "Treatise on Medicine," while Brouardel and Thoinot

* Thirial, *Union Méd.*, 1853, Nos. 83, 84, and 85.

give it a special place in their " Treatise on Medicine and Therapeutics." I shall try to show that this peritonitis by propagation in the form described by Thirial and others **does not exist.** The present discussion is the résumé of the lectures I have given in my " Course of Pathology " and of my communication to the Académie in 1896.

I said then that there is no longer a place for peritonitis by propagation as understood by Thirial. In the first place, if the reader will consult Thirial's monograph he will see that in the four cases which form the basis of this monograph it is not possible to find in any case a process of peritonitis by propagation. The information furnished by the autopsies is very incomplete ; we find that four patients died from acute peritonitis, and that peritonitis supervened during convalescence in three who were suffering from typhoid fever. At the autopsy, says Thirial, Peyer's patches were found to be **cicatrized.** I cannot therefore admit that the repaired intestinal lesion provoked the so-called peritonitis by propagation. Moreover, I repeat, the process of propagation was not found in any of the autopsies. The demonstrators contented themselves with opening the intestine from above downwards, in order to search for the supposed perforation, which they did not find ; they recognized with surprise that the intestinal lesions were healed, and were content with this somewhat too summary examination. My first idea on reading these observations is that the patients in question died from appendicular peritonitis. The tendency of the peritoneal lesions to predominate in the right iliac fossa and in the pelvis leads to a suspicion of typhoid appendicitis ; but attention had not been drawn to appendicular peritonitis in Thirial's time, and there is no mention made of the appendix in the account of the autopsies.

I will quote a case of Letulle in opposition to those of Thirial. A patient died from typhoid peritonitis, and the most minute examination of the intestine revealed typhoid ulcerations, but no perforation. In this case peritonitis by propagation might have been suspected, but the anatomical examination was complete, and showed a perforation of the **appendix** as the cause of the peritonitis. The lesion is thus described : " The appendix shows, 5 centimetres from its tip, a perforation extending through the anterior half of its circumference. After opening the appendix, the mucous membrane is seen to be swollen, and presents two ulcers and one large closed follicle which is not ulcerated." We have, therefore, a type of the lesion which I shall describe later as paratyphoid appendicitis. I would make the same remark regarding Millard's very interesting case, in which again typhoid peritonitis, without perforation, was found, and the intestinal lesions were completely cicatrized. Peritonitis " by propagation " might have been suspected, but Millard discovered, on careful search, appendicitis as the cause of the peritoneal infection (paratyphoid appendicitis).

We must therefore cut out " peritonitis by propagation." And, moreover, if it really existed many persons suffering from typhoid fever would die of peritonitis. Very often, indeed, the autopsy in cases of typhoid fever, in which death has been due to other causes than peritonitis, shows the intestinal wall to be so thin in the neighbourhood of the Peyer's patches, which are so ulcerated and transparent that we wonder how the tissue could have resisted the ulcerative process, and how such a fragile barrier was sufficient to prevent peritonitis. And yet it does so. This view of the question was well borne out in the autopsy on a woman who died from ataxo-adynamic typhoid, and of whom I spoke above with reference to the fall of temperature following intestinal hæmorrhage. I pointed out to my class how excessively thin the wall of the intestine was in the neighbourhood of several of the ulcerated Peyer's patches, and yet no peritonitis and no adhesions were present.

I know that two or three well-known cases (Chantemesse, Véron, and Bosquet) may be quoted in favour of peritonitis by propagation, a perforation being absent. What is there to prove to us that in these cases the peritoneal infection came from the bowel ? If the intestine had indeed been the origin of the peritoneal infection, we should have found in the peritoneum not only Eberth's bacillus, but other intestinal microbes, including the *Bacillus coli*. I find it more reasonable to admit that there may be an infection of the peritoneum by Eberth's bacillus independent of the intestinal infection, the peritoneum being invaded on its own account, like the pleura and the bones, without the necessity for invoking a process of intestinal propagation which **absolutely lacks demonstration.** I hold, therefore, to my opinion that peritonitis by propagation such as Thirial described does not exist.

The *Bacillus typhosus*, like the *Bacillus coli,* can pass through the walls of the bowel, which is **not** perforated, only under special conditions. Thus, as I have tried to show under Appendicitis, in order that migration of certain pathogenic agents may take place through the non-perforated wall of the bowel, it is necessary that these pathogenic agents be endowed with the exalted virulence which they acquire in a **closed cavity,** but which they do not possess so long as they find a free road through the intestinal track. We can find peritonitis by propagation, which I would rather call peritonitis **by migration,** or **by emigration,** whenever a portion of the intestine is transformed into a **closed cavity.** Appendicular peritonitis is the typical form, and is comparable to the peritonitis following strangulated hernia, internal strangulation, and intussusception. As this question is discussed in detail under Appendicular Peritonitis, I shall merely state the following conclusion : From the pathogenic and anatomo-pathological point of view peritonitis by propagation, such as has been understood since Thirial's time, does not exist; but this does not, of course, exclude the possibility of adhesions which localize peritonitis when the intestinal fissure is in process of formation. When a patient with enteric fever succumbs with symptoms of peritonitis from perforation, and when no intestinal lesion can be discovered, careful search must be made for the existence of an intestinal fissure, which suffices, even though small, to explain the pathogenesis of this peritonitis. Careful search must be made for peritonitis consecutive to a **glandular infection,** or to perforation of the **gall-bladder,** and it is especially necessary minutely to examine the appendix, which is the cause of peritoneal complications more often than has been previously supposed.

Paratyphoid Appendicitis.—According to the works I have examined and the cases I have seen, the appendix may be affected by the typhoid process in two different ways. In the first category I place perforation of the appendix following typhoid ulceration of its walls, the process being in every way comparable to perforation of the intestine in the Peyer's patches and in the ulcerated closed follicles. Perforation of the appendix is far from being rare, since it figures fifteen times in Nacke's statistics of 133 cases of intestinal perforation in typhoid patients, verified by post-mortem examination. Rolleston has twice found perforation of the appendix in sixty autopsies on cases of typhoid fever. The peritoneal symptoms following perforation of the appendix differ in no way from those following perforation of other parts of the intestine, either cæcum or ileum. Acute or insidious peritonitis, possible fall of temperature and hypothermia, are the same in all these cases.

In the second category of cases, which did not appear to me to have been described when I made a communication to the Académie de Médecine in 1896, it is a question—and I repeat it intentionally—not of perforation of the appendix, comparable to perforations of the intestine, but it is a question, at least in my opinion, of an appendicitis, in the true sense of the word, which may run its course with or without perforation, and with the various kinds of toxi-infection and all its consequences. I will explain what I mean. We have an individual suffering from typhoid fever, which has followed a normal course, and is entering on convalescence. Suddenly, with or without warning, sharp pain is felt in the right iliac fossa, the temperature rises, vomiting comes on, the abdomen is distended, and as the patient is convalescent from typhoid fever, a diagnosis of late intestinal perforation is made ; peritonitis by perforation is thought to be present, and the most gloomy prognosis is given.

Two or three days after this event, which has given rise to the most acute anxiety, the symptoms improve, and the patient recovers. In other less fortunate cases, in spite of the improvement in the initial symptoms, the temperature does not fall, the abdominal pains do not disappear, the belly remains sensitive in the right iliac fossa at McBurney's point, palpation is very painful, the subjacent muscles become rigid, deep matting of the tissue becomes perceptible, and in a few days a collection of pus forms in the ileo-cæcal region. Lastly, in other cases, which are much more formidable, the peritonitis is not encysted, but is diffuse, and remote complications may occur, including pleurisy, hepatitis, vomito-negro, etc.

Who will not recognize the evolution of ordinary appendicitis in its different forms in the picture which I have just sketched in broad outlines? Will he not find in it the different forms of appendicular toxi-infection, such as I have described in the section on Appendicitis? Sometimes, in typhoid appendicitis, indeed, the whole case centres in an acute appendicular attack, without infection of the peritoneum, just as in the ordinary form; in other cases the appendicular attack is followed by limited peritonitis, or by encysted abscess; lastly, the appendicular attack is the prelude of more or less general peritonitis, of remote infections and of fatal toxæmia.

How can we explain the pathogenesis of this appendicitis, which I propose to call paratyphoid? It is the result of the lesions of typhoid fever, which have converted a portion of the appendicular canal into a **closed cavity.** It may not end in perforation, and yet all the complications which arise, with or without perforation of the appendix, are comparable to those which I have described in detail under Appendicitis, and therefore I shall not labour the point here. I think that many cases, published under the title of peritonitis, supervening during convalescence from typhoid fever, and under the heading of Peritonitis by Propagation, are really cases of paratyphoid appendicitis. These cases, with the peritonitis which follows them, are often less formidable than those due to perforation of the intestine; they result more surely in adhesions with circumscribed abscess and in recovery.

Do these cases of paratyphoid appendicitis, with or without peritonitis, show signs distinguishing them from perforative peritonitis in typhoid fever? Many symptoms are indeed common to both these diseases, but I shall nevertheless try to point out the distinctions between paratyphoid appendicitis and perforation of the bowel. Appendicitis usually supervenes at a time when the convalescent is more able to describe his feelings, so that we can better analyze each symptom and localize more clearly the seat of the pain (McBurney's point), while we can also more easily estimate the defensive rigidity of the subjacent muscle and the hyperæsthesia in this region. Further, appendicitis does not set in with an abrupt fall of temperature, as is the case in most perforations; it causes, on the contrary, a **rise,** and the fever reappears, if it had previously disappeared. Accordingly, the following symptoms are in favour of appendicitis, and almost certainly eliminate the idea of perforation of the bowel, if a patient, during the decline or the convalescence of typhoid fever, is seized with pain limited to the appendicular region, and at the same time with nausea, vomiting, fever, and high temperature. Examples :

In June, 1896, I was called to see a young lady, with Bucquoy and Leval. She had fallen ill four weeks before with a fairly severe attack of typhoid fever. In the early days of convalescence she experienced sharp pain in the right iliac fossa, and symptoms simulating perforation of the bowel. A period of calm then appeared, but the improvement was only apparent; the belly remained distended, sharp pains reappeared, with violent crises in the region of the cæcum and appendix, and the pulse was much quickened. We found on examining the temperature chart that these symptoms had coincided with an attack of fever. This symptom-complex allowed us to state that the patient had had, not perforation of the belly, but paratyphoid appendicitis. Moreover, Routier, who also saw the patient, was of the same opinion. A collection of pus in the neighbourhood of the cæcum was opened by Routier, and the patient recovered.

My colleague Hue, of Rouen, has told me that he operated upon a patient who, during the decline of typhoid fever, was seized with sharp pain in the right iliac fossa, and peritoneal symptoms resembling those of intestinal perforation. This complication had been accompanied with fever, and had finally resulted in a peritoneal abscess in the cæco-appendicular region, which was operated upon and followed by recovery. The case was one of paratyphoid appendicitis. With Thomas I saw a gentleman, fifty years of age, who had just had an attack of acute appendicitis; he had not consulted his physician. He suspected appendicitis himself, and told us that he had had a similar attack some years before during the decline of typhoid fever. These cases prove therefore that typhoid appendicitis may later be the origin of fresh appendicular attacks.

The case which Millard, in 1876, brought before the Société Médicale des Hôpitaux was only one of paratyphoid appendicitis.

Zuber saw paratyphoid appendicitis in a child suffering from severe typhoid fever, which had run a normal course. After some days of apyrexia, appendicitis, followed by fatal general peritonitis, appeared four weeks after the onset of the enteric fever.

Alexandroff, of Moscow, quotes an analogous case in a child nine and a half years of age, in whom the peritonitis supervened nearly six weeks after the onset of the enteric fever.

I have said that paratyphoid appendicitis may cause a number of complications; it may also be the origin of abscess of the liver. Examples:

A young man suffering from typhoid fever was taken ill during convalescence, and after several days of apyrexia, with a severe return of the fever. The temperature rose to 104° F., the abdomen became distended, and pain was present, especially in the right hypochondriac region. From this moment general infection, with peritonitis, set in, and the patient died. At the autopsy, peritonitis, especially well marked in the neighbourhood of the cæcum, was discovered, and about a dozen abscesses, varying in size from an egg to a tangerine orange. Small abscesses of the areolar type were found in the enlarged liver. In order to explain the peritonitis we could not hold the intestinal lesions guilty, for all the ulcers were cicatrized, or in process of cicatrization, and it was one of those cases which formerly would have been labelled " peritonitis by propagation." But here **appendicitis** was present; the appendix was adherent to the cæcum, and contained a longitudinal ulcer. These appendicular lesions had been the origin, and were still evidence of the pathological process which had ended on the one hand in peritonitis, and on the other in suppurative hepatitis.

Osler relates the case of a man who, after convalescence from typhoid fever, succumbed to acute peritonitis and purulent infection of the liver. At the autopsy scars, due to typhoid ulcers, were found in the ileum. The fatal complications were due to paratyphoid appendicitis, with toxi-infection, which had caused peritonitis and phlebitis of the portal vein, with multiple abscesses in the liver.

Boulloche has reported the following case: A child convalescent from typhoid fever, and practically cured, was taken ill, with a temperature of 103° F. and pain in the right iliac fossa (this marked the appearance of paratyphoid appendicitis). Ice-bags were applied to the painful region, and the pain improved, but the general condition became worse ; the intermittent character of the fever, the profuse sweating, the earthy tint, and the rapid wasting pointed to a focus of suppuration. The little patient died in a state of collapse. At the autopsy the liver was found to be enormously enlarged, and crammed with abscesses of every size. Ulcers in process of cicatrization were visible in the ileum. Paratyphoid appendicitis, therefore, had been the cause of the trouble. The infection from the appendix had spared the peritoneum, but had been carried to the liver by the portal vein ; it was a typical case of appendicular liver. Bacteriological examination of the pus revealed the existence of anaerobic microbes.

Perrone has published three cases of paratyphoid appendicitis which were operated upon. The histological and bacteriological examinations proved that the term " paratyphoid " is absolutely applicable to this form of appendicitis ; it supervenes in connection with typhoid fever, but the appendicular infection is not due to Eberth's bacillus.

I may now state the following conclusions :

1. Peritonitis by perforation usually supervenes during the stationary stage or during relapses in typhoid fever. The perforation may affect the ileum, cæcum, appendix, or colon. These cases are seen not only in severe typhoid fever, but also in the slight forms. The symptoms which usher in peritonitis from perforation may be insidious or violent ; whatever the severity may be, the sudden fall of temperature, which goes as far as hypothermia, is often, but not always, a valuable sign. This form of peritonitis is exceedingly grave, and yet it may be checked at its commencement by adhesions which limit the perforation.

2. Paratyphoid appendicitis usually supervenes during the decline or the convalescence of typhoid fever. It is generally accompanied by an elevation of temperature ; it runs its course like a commonplace appendicitis ; the toxi-infectious process may be limited in its action to the simple appendicular attack without peritonitis, or may result in all the complications of appendicitis—peritonitis, abscess of the liver, etc.

3. The so-called peritonitis by propagation, as Thirial understood it, does not exist.

Let us next consider the treatment to be employed for peritonitis in typhoid fever. This treatment is medical and surgical. The former consists in limiting, as far as possible, the movements of the intestine in order to lessen or to prevent the passage of septic material into the peritoneum, and to favour the formation of adhesions. For this purpose all food and drink are stopped. The patient is allowed to suck small pieces of ice, and every hour a pill of $\frac{1}{3}$ grain of extract of opium is administered. Injections of morphia may be given if necessary, while ice-bags, suspended from a hook to avoid the weight upon the abdomen, are applied, or the belly may be covered with cold compresses.

Medical measures are, however, often powerless, and the important question of surgical intervention then requires consideration. Is it necessary to operate, and at what time should intervention be made? This intervention takes place under such unfavourable conditions—the operator finds the intestine so damaged, the patient himself is in a very bad condition to stand an operation and its results—that at first sight the proposed operation seems rash, to say the least. In my opinion, the question must be considered in a slightly different manner to that in which it has been previously looked upon. In future we must not include all cases of typhoid peritonitis in the same category, but distinguish as far as possible paratyphoid appendicitis from peritonitis by perforation. In the case of paratyphoid infection, the operation is indicated for the reasons set forth under Appendicitis. It is not enough to operate; the operation must be performed before the toxi-infection has had time to complete its work. The examples which I have quoted show once more that in appendicitis speedy operation may be the only means of saving the patient from fatal complications. The patient whom I saw with Bucquoy, and upon whom Routier operated, recovered, as did Hue's patient. Letulle's patient, with general peritonitis, would probably have recovered if he had been operated upon; and the patients quoted by Lannois, Osler, and Boulloche would not have succumbed to hepatic complications if the indications had suggested in time an operation for paratyphoid appendicitis. The operation for appendicular peritonitis in enteric fever is much simplified by the fact that the operator has not to suture an ulcerated and perforated bowel, and that the whole lesion is confined to the appendix.

If the problem appears to me easy of solution in the case of paratyphoid appendicitis, it is very different in that of typhoid peritonitis from intestinal perforation. First, is it quite clear that there is a perforation? The symptoms of peritonitis are sometimes so slight and so vague that the diagnosis would remain doubtful were it not for the sudden drop in the temperature. On the other hand, if we wait a day or two before coming to a decision, we deprive the patient of the few chances of safety remaining to him.

We can only form an opinion as to the value of surgical intervention by examining the cases published on this subject. Unfortunately, these observations are often incomplete. They include dissimilar cases, and the diagnosis is not always irreproachable. The first table of statistics has been published by Louis, a second one by Lejars, who has collected twenty-five cases of laparotomy, with six recoveries, of which three at least did not appear to afford material for discussion. These results, says he, are not brilliant, but yet they are not of such a nature as to discourage surgical intervention. I have reread these cases one by one, and, I repeat, most of them are too incomplete to permit of a definite opinion being formed. We shall see later the results obtained in other statistics.

The following case was under my care : .

A man suffering from typhoid fever of a somewhat adynamic character came under my care at the Necker Hospital about the twelfth day of the disease. On the fifteenth day he complained of general abdominal pain, without other symptoms, and the temperature fell suddenly. It rose again momentarily, and next day became subnormal, as may be seen from the accompanying chart. Although the abdominal pain had almost disappeared and the abdomen was but little distended, and in spite of the absence of vomiting, the hypothermia and hiccough which were also present appeared to me sufficient for a diagnosis of intestinal perforation, and I decided upon an operation, which was performed the same morning by Routier.

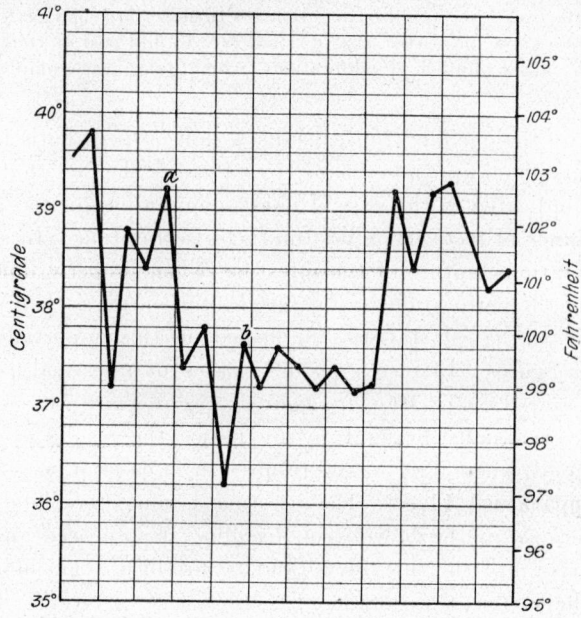

FIG. 88.—TEMPERATURE CHART OF A CASE OF INTESTINAL PERFORATION FOLLOWED BY LAPAROTOMY.

a, Intestinal perforation and subnormal fall of temperature : the perforation had, perhaps, commenced on the previous evening, and appeared to take place about the fifteenth day ; *b*, laparotomy.

We found peritonitis, with a few spoonfuls of fæcal fluid in the peritoneum. The perforation, of the size of a small lentil, was situated at the end of the ileum, 2 inches above the cæcum. The intestine was sutured in two layers, so as to form a prominent longitudinal fold projecting into the lumen. The peritoneum was dusted with iodoform. A large wick of iodoform gauze was left for drainage.

In the evening the condition had improved : the pulse was of better quality, the hiccough had not reappeared, and the temperature rose to nearly normal ; but during the next three days the pulse became quick and small, and the patient was very restless and delirious. These phenomena, in the absence of any peritoneal symptoms (pain, vomiting, and hiccough), were considered as due to iodoform-poisoning rather than to a return of peritonitis. The dressing was soiled with pus, which flowed out in fairly large amount. The restlessness soon became less, the patient looked better, the pulse improved, and the situation was markedly satisfactory, in spite of the elevation of temperature, and I thought for a time that the patient was saved. The general condition, however, became worse, and, although the abdominal wound improved daily and the peritoneal symptoms did not reappear, the patient fell into a condition of collapse, and, in spite of all our efforts, died ten days after the operation.

At the autopsy we found recent peritonitis, with pus and fæcal fluid in the right iliac fossa, and we thought at first that a tear had taken place in the sutured bowel. This was not the case, and an examination of the intestine showed that the sutured perforation had quite healed ; but, unfortunately, two fresh perforations had taken place near the first, the one as large as a pin's head and the other considerably larger. The remainder of the intestine showed the characteristic lesions of typhoid fever. I am convinced that the operation would have cured this patient if two new perforations had not occurred. We know, moreover, that it is not rare to find post mortem two, three, or even a much larger number of perforations, which take place simultaneously or successively.

What are we to conclude from this discussion on peritonitis by perforation and paratyphoid appendicitis ? It establishes the fact that an operation is clearly indicated in the case of paratyphoid appendicitis, and that it gives some chance of recovery in peritonitis by perforation. In spite of the intestinal ulcerations, suture of the intestine, when properly done, ends in cicatrization of the perforation, and surgical intervention is then justified.

I give here the latest statistics published on this important question. John Finney's figures : 13 recoveries in 47 cases of intestinal perforations which were operated upon ; Mauger's figures : 25 cures in 107 cases. Harvey Cushing has very kindly brought to my notice the results at the Johns Hopkins Hospital, where 5 recoveries resulted in 11 cases of perforation.

Biliary Apparatus—Liver.—The intestinal lesions of typhoid fever may allow the microbes in the bowel (coli bacillus, streptococci, and Eberth's bacillus) to pass into the bile-ducts, and to produce angiocholitis, cholecystitis, and hepatitis.

Cholecystitis.—The inflammation of the gall-bladder may be slight or severe, catarrhal, muco-purulent, purulent, ulcerative, or perforating. Ulcerative cholecystitis is often associated with angiocholitis of the cystic duct, which may cause obliteration of the canal. Typhoid cholecystitis is often latent in its evolution, and is found unexpectedly at the autopsy. In fourteen cases after post-mortem examination reported by Hagenmüller the cholecystitis had on eleven occasions caused no symptoms. Pain, swelling, and jaundice are sometimes noticed.

The acute process often seems to become extinct, and suppurative or non-suppurative cholecystitis only appears several months after the typhoid fever. I will quote some examples :

In Gilbert and Girode's case a patient suffered from typhoid fever and symptoms of cholecystitis, but the pain and swelling soon improved, as though the cholecystitis were cured ; they appeared, however, five months later. The operation, performed by Terrier, who thought the cholecystitis was due to a calculus, showed that the inflammation of the gall-bladder was due to Eberth's bacillus. In Tuffier's case a young woman suffered from typhoid fever and from symptoms of cholecystitis, from which she recovered. Some days later the symptoms of acute cholecystitis reappeared; an operation was performed, and calculous non-suppurative cholecystitis was found. The bacteriological examination revealed the presence of the *Bacillus typhosus* and of the *B. coli.* Dupré's case is that of a woman suffering from severe typhoid fever, with recovery. She suffered four months later from attacks of hepatic colic, which recurred on several occasions, with persistent decoloration of the fæcal matter, fever, symptoms of obstruction and of biliary infection. An operation was decided on by Letulle, and performed by Monod. The gall-bladder contained a calculus, but no pus was present. The bacteriological examination gave pure cultures of Eberth's bacillus.

Typhoid cholecystitis is fairly often accompanied by **perforation,** which causes circumscribed or general peritonitis. I have seen a case of this kind which ended fatally, and several analogous cases have been reported.

Liver.—The hepatic complications are rarely well marked, except in the case of jaundice or of pyæmia (suppurative angiocholitis).

In some cases the microbes and their toxines cause more or less complete degeneration of the liver cells. The functional affection of the liver diminishes the formation of glycogen, disturbs the formation of bile, and gives rise to the presence of urobilin in the urine, a jaundice colour of the skin, and a series of symptoms which resemble those of *icterus gravis*.

Abscess of the liver is a very rare complication in typhoid fever. Lannois gives Romberg's statistics : hepatic abscess once in 667 autopsies in typhoid fever. Dopfer, in 927 autopsies, found abscess of the liver present on ten occasions. Lannois has seen only one case in seventy-one autopsies, and expresses surprise at its rarity. " It is well calculated," says he, " to astonish us, if we think of the direct venous connections between the intestine and the liver, and of the deep lesions of the intestinal wall, resulting from the ulcerative process of typhoid fever." For my part, I am less surprised, for I am convinced that in typhoid fever in our climates the abscesses of the liver do not result from the intestinal ulcerations, but from typhoid appendicitis, which is a somewhat rare complication. Such was the case in the patients of Lannois, Osler, and Boulloche. The infective process which ends in abscess of the liver **(appendicular liver)**, with or without pylephlebitis, is elaborated in a **closed cavity,** just as in ordinary appendicitis.

In addition to abscesses of the liver, which are nearly always the result of paratyphoid appendicitis, we may also find hepatic abscesses from other sources. Some form part of a purulent infection, with parotiditis, perichondritis, and cutaneous abscesses, while others are the result of pylephlebitis of ill-known origin, as the autopsies on this subject are incomplete or silent as regards appendicitis. Let us further take note of hepatic abscesses in typhoid fever in tropical climates. We may ask whether dysentery is not associated with typhoid fever in this last variety.

Different bacilli, including that of Eberth, may remain for a long time alive in the gall-bladder, but in a latent state. Perhaps they give rise to biliary calculi—a question discussed under Biliary Lithiasis.

Respiratory System—Laryngeal Complications.—Diphtheria of the larynx is excessively rare in typhoid fever, but laryngeal erosions and ulcerations are, on the other hand, so common that Louis considered them as almost constant, and Griesinger has found them in 20 per cent. of fatal cases. This development of ulcers in the larynx need not surprise us, since Coyne has shown that the mucosa of the larynx is formed of reticular tissue and adenoid follicles, comparable in structure to that of the intestinal mucous membrane. Ulceration of the larynx appears in the course of the second or third week. It affects the epiglottis, the aryteno-epiglottic ligaments, the neighbourhood of the arytenoid cartilages, and the posterior wall of the larynx—in short, everywhere, except on the vocal cords—at least, in its initial stage—which explains why it is usually latent in its progress, without vocal troubles, and why the patient recovers from ulceration of the larynx, as from that of the gut. Sometimes, however, the vocal cords are invaded, and aphonia results. At times œdema of the larynx appears, and asphyxia becomes imminent.

The ulceration of the larynx may sometimes be subacute. It extends deeply, invading the perichondrium and the cartilage, which it destroys, and gives rise to suppuration, abscess, perforation of the larynx, œdema of the glottis, and laryngeal stenosis. In some cases perichondritis and necrosis **at once** attack the cartilages of the larynx.

Perichondritis nearly always ends in suppuration and detachment of the subjacent cartilage, which, being deprived of its nutrient membrane, finally necroses. Necrosis frequently attacks the cricoid cartilage, more rarely the arytenoid, and the thyroid cartilage only in exceptional cases. The necrosed cartilages form sequestra, which tend to be eliminated. As a result of this necrotic process, abscesses infiltrate the submucosa and the articulations, and, with their sequestra, open into the larynx, pharynx, or on the skin. This laryngo-typhus is a very formidable complication, and although patients escape œdema of the larynx, they are exposed either to emphysema following the perforation of the larynx, or to the dire results of stenosis of the cavities of the larynx.

Ulceration of the cartilages of the larynx may be compared to the ulceration and perforation of the nasal septum. In Roger's case the perforation of the septum was as large as a sixpenny-piece. The lesion persisted, and the patient had a somewhat nasal twang. I saw an analogous case in a young woman in whom the perforation of the septum was as large as a small lentil.

Broncho-Pulmonary Inflammations.—Bronchial catarrh in typhoid fever is a common and generally benign phenomenon, but it may be very formidable. We may also find pulmonary congestion, atelectasis, and splenization, which are very grave and fairly frequent lesions, since atelectasis has been noticed thirty-two times in 118 autopsies (Griesinger). Lobular and pseudo-lobar pneumonia chiefly appear in the last stage of the disease, the rise of temperature and the severe dyspnœa indicating the imminence of the danger. In these cases dry-cupping has rendered material service.

Lobar pneumonia appears at different stages. I have already spoken of the pneumonia which may mark the onset of typhoid fever, and in which the prognosis is usually good. Pneumonia supervening during the course of the disease is more frequent. It is insidious, bastard in its course and symptoms, and usually very serious.

These pulmonary complications are started, and in some cases (congestion, splenization) consummated, by the *Bacillus typhosus*. Pneumonia is the result of a parallel or associated infection due to the pneumococcus. The streptococcus and staphylococcus favour the appearance of bronchopneumonia.

Pleurisy is much less common than pneumonia. It is accompanied by fever and prostration, which are in relation to its origin. Typhoid pleurisy may remain sero-fibrinous throughout, but it is sometimes purulent, and often hæmorrhagic. The effusion may be loculated, being purulent in one pocket and sero-fibrinous in another. Cultivations taken at different intervals may be sterile or may swarm with Eberth's bacilli. This intermittence in the presence of the *Bacillus typhosus* proves that apparent sterility of an exudate in typhoid fever does not make it certain that it is not of a typhoid nature.

The frequency of pleuro-broncho-pulmonary inflammations varies in different epidemics. Gangrene of the lung has been seen in seven out of 118 autopsies (Griesinger).

Tuberculosis.—Typhoid fever and tuberculosis are not at all antagonistic, as was formerly said. It is by no means rare for a tubercular patient to be stricken with enteric fever, and the course of the latter disease is in no way influenced, but the phthisis undergoes a recrudescence (Vulpian). In some cases tuberculosis appears during convalescence in a patient who was not tubercular, or who at least showed no signs of it. The patient appears cured of typhoid fever, but the fever reappears, and a relapse is promptly suspected, when it is really a question of more or less rapidly progressive tuberculosis.

We may in such a case accuse contagiousness, but most frequently we find, on making careful inquiry as to the cause, that the patient comes of suspicious stock. Tuberculosis is sometimes clearly marked in the parents, or at other times the disease of the father or of the mother is hidden under

When the intoxication has been of long duration, irregular patches of fibrosis are seen in the myocardium. In the human heart these patches are attributed by classical writers to the presence of adult connective tissue. Regaud and Mollard, in their experiments with the diphtheritic toxine, also regard the zones of fibrosis as a neo-formation of connective tissue, and consider the lesions to be purely inflammatory. Chantemesse, who has experimented with typhoid toxine, holds a different opinion. He considers that the fibrosis is not formed of connective tissue, but results from a peculiar hyaline change in the muscular tissue, so that the lesion is not inflammatory, but degenerative. He has been able to follow step by step the process of this change in the hearts of animals who were submitted to typhoid intoxication, and survived from one day to two years.

When the intoxication is slow in its progress, we find in the heart hyaline degeneration of the muscular fibres (staining by Van Giessen's method). This degeneration first shows itself by a modification in the staining properties of the fibre, which assumes a reddish colour instead of the yellowish tint of normal muscle. The nucleus is still recognizable, although increased in size. Later, the fibrillæ which constitute the fibre swell up, and become homogeneous. They are often separated from one another, and are increased in thickness and length. They become tortuous, and very closely simulate small bundles of connective tissue. The contractile substance has undergone hyaline degeneration, while the nuclei preserve their vitality for quite a long while.

According to Chantemesse, this is the chief cause of the formation of patches of fibrosis, but he admits that connective tissue, newly formed by organization of immigrant leucocytes, is found in these hearts. The lesion of experimental fibrosis would, therefore, consist in a mixture of connective tissue of inflammatory origin and of hyaline degeneration of the contractile fibre.

The change in this variety of fibrosis is not localized to the ventricles ; the degeneration affects the wall of the auricles with as much severity. The vessels chiefly show the attack in their tunica media, which becomes thick and hyaline. The change sometimes extends to the aorta. It is then thickened, and shows zones of aortitis, projecting into the lumen of the vessel. The culminating-point of these patches in contact with the blood is also affected by hyaline degeneration.

The intracardiac nerve fibres are most probably affected, although no direct observation of this has been obtained. In return, Chantemesse has found in the hearts of guinea-pigs submitted to typhoid intoxication two years previously changes in the nerve cells of the ganglion in the articular wall behind the septum. These cells were less numerous, their volume had diminished, and some of them showed immigration of leucocytes similar to that seen in the ganglion cells of the nervous system as the result of microbic poisoning (rabies, typhoid fever, etc.).

This last discovery—namely, the change in the intracardiac nervous system—explains the pathogenesis of the sudden crises of asystole in individuals suffering from fibrosis of the myocardium. In spite of grave lesions of the cardiac muscle, the functional power of the organ may be sufficient for a long while, but the resistance of the nervous system of the heart, already materially affected, may suddenly yield under the influence of a poison upon the nerve cells (various intoxications, fatigue, moral shock, etc.).

Arteritis.—In the course or in the convalescence of typhoid fever, which may have been severe or benign, more or less acute pain appears in the foot, calf, bend of the knee, Scarpa's triangle, hand, arm, or axilla. This pain is not accompanied by œdema, as in phlebitis, and sometimes follows the course of the inflamed artery. When the artery is accessible to the touch (dorsalis pedis, popliteal, femoral, radial, or temporal), we can feel an indurated cord. The pulse disappears, the whole limb undergoes a hard swelling which is not œdema, and the skin supplied by the obliterated artery becomes cold and mottled with violet patches. The pain continues to be extremely acute, and if the permeability of the vessel is not re-established, dry gangrene, of which I quote examples, may result.

CASE 1 (Bourgeois): Following a slight attack of typhoid fever, gangrene of the right limb below the knee; loss of the leg, and recovery. CASE 2 (Patry): Dry gangrene of the leg and moist gangrene of the thigh; crural artery found obliterated at the autopsy. CASE 3 (Gigon): Œdema and gangrene of the right arm; at the autopsy a clot was found plugging the subclavian artery. CASE 4 (Hayem): Dry gangrene of the feet and of the left leg; at the autopsy, clots in both femoral arteries, extending into the aorta; endocarditis and laminated clots in the heart.

These cases of infective arteritis are due to endarteritis obliterans; fortunately, typhoid arteritis does not always end in obliteration of the vessel, but may occur as a parietal non-obliterating arteritis. Barié, in his monograph, reports ten cases, in which the signs of arteritis comprised pain, diminution in the pulse, more or less marked swelling of the limb, and coldness of the skin; but the absence of a hard cord and the persistence of the pulse indicated that the vessel was not completely obliterated. Under these conditions recovery took place without further complications.

Phlebitis.—Phlebitis in typhoid fever is, like arteritis, a common complication in convalescence from typhoid fever. Phlegmasia alba dolens affected the left leg forty-five times in seventy cases collected by Veillard.

In ten cases under my care the phlebitis affected the left leg. The phlebitis is sometimes bilateral; it may affect the iliac veins, the innominate vein, the axillary vein, the veins of the arm, the cerebral sinuses, and the sacral veins. It is usually ushered in by a rise of temperature ; pain and œdema occur, as in phlegmasia alba dolens, but the œdematous skin is always rosy.

The chief danger lies in the possibility of pulmonary embolism. The large emboli produce sudden death by syncope and by asphyxia ; the small emboli provoke infection of the lung, a curable though grave condition. The phlebitis may be followed by general infection and septicæmia. It appears that phlebitis obliterans may cause gangrene of the limbs without any concomitant arteritis. Nevertheless, gangrene of the limbs in typhoid fever is usually the result of arteritis obliterans alone, or combined with phlebitis obliterans ; the infection perhaps spreads from the artery to the vein. These combinations (gangrene, phlebitis, and arteritis) are nowhere more common than in typhoid fever, and I do not know of any disease showing a greater predilection for the vascular system. The pathogenesis of phlebitis in typhoid is still obscure ; account must be taken of the dyscrasias and of secondary or specific infections.

The phlebitis is followed by œdema and trophic troubles, consisting of permanent hypertrophy of the muscles of the calf. In Burlurcaux's case the whole of the right leg was hypertrophied ; œdema was absent, and the hypertrophy appeared to affect the muscles and the bones. In Lesage's case the hypertrophy affected the left leg, and the softness of the muscles appeared to indicate an excess of fat in the muscle. In Cerné's case the left leg was involved ; the muscular power was increased, and the examination of the muscles appeared to indicate genuine hypertrophy of the muscle. Babinski has told me of two cases of persistent hypertrophy of the left calf in patients who had previously suffered from phlebitis in the course of typhoid fever. These trophic disorders should be looked for in every case of phlebitis. I have seen them in a woman who had had puerperal phlebitis four years previously. Chantemesse has employed a diet free from salt in the treatment of typhoid phlebitis.

Dropsy.—Dropsy in typhoid fever is of mechanical or of dyscrasic origin. The former is the result of phlebitis. Dropsy of dyscrasic origin is more frequent in certain countries and epidemics. Although it is very rare in Paris, it has frequently been noted at Rouen (Leudet), and in an epidemic in Germany (Griesinger) 25 per cent. of the patients were attacked. Its cause is not known, but possibly some cases are associated with the nephritis which at times accompanies typhoid fever.

Genito-Urinary Organs.—Albuminuria is often the only symptom of typhoid nephritis, which, as a rule, is not serious. The nephritis is sometimes associated with hæmaturia ; the urine is of a rosy or brownish colour, and may contain clots. At the autopsy ulcerations are found in all parts of the urinary system, including the bladder. In some cases the nephritis is so marked, and the albuminuria is so severe, and the symptoms are so prominent, that the course of the typhoid fever is altered, uræmic symptoms being added to those of the original disease, and the renal condition becoming a very formidable complication. In some cases of typhoid nephritis miliary abscesses may be present.

The nephritis is due either to the *Bacillus typhosus* or to toxic substances.

Rendu has published the case of a young woman suffering from typhoid fever, with albuminuria, hyperpyrexia, and a raspberry-like erythema. Death from uræmia supervened on the fifteenth day of the disease. The ordinary lesions of typhoid fever were found post mortem. In addition, the kidneys were congested with numerous subcortical ecchymoses. The histological examination revealed the typical lesions of epithelial nephritis. The interest of this case lies in the fact that Eberth's bacilli were collected *en masse* in the interior of the tubules.

The morbid process in the kidney does not always become completely extinct; it may be the starting-point of Bright's disease.

Orchitis.—Orchitis may occur during convalescence in typhoid fever. I have seen eight cases, of which one ended in suppuration. The orchitis shows itself by very acute pain in the testis, or in the groin along the spermatic cord; the testis becomes heavy and large; the epididymis is also affected, and resolution does not occur for two or three weeks. If we study these symptoms in the testis, which sometimes show an ephemeral congestive character, and at other times an inflammatory character, sometimes ending in suppuration, we see that the process is analogous to that seen in the parotid glands during the decline of typhoid fever.

Several characteristics differentiate this orchitis from that of mumps. Thus, typhoid orchitis is unilateral; it may suppurate and leave limited induration of the organ, but it never ends in atrophy and impotence. Orchitis in mumps is more often double; it does not suppurate, and fairly frequently results in atrophy of the testis. Typhoid orchitis is due to Eberth's bacillus, which has been found in the testis, and the suppuration is caused either by this bacillus or by secondary infection.

Oöphoritis and salpingitis, mastitis and inflammation of the labia majora, have been seen on several occasions.

Pregnancy is not incompatible with typhoid fever. The frequency of miscarriages varies with the duration of the pregnancy and the severity of the fever. The child succumbs in most cases of premature birth, but the prognosis is less serious for the mother.

Infection of the foetus results from the fact that the *Bacillus typhosus* is transmitted from the mother to the foetus through the placenta. Eberth's bacillus has been found in the placenta (Chantemesse), and also in the spleen of the foetus (Ernst).

Nervous Complications.—We sometimes see during the course of the disease, or during convalescence, especially in patients predisposed by personal or hereditary antecedents, mental troubles, attacks of acute mania, delirium with ideas of persecution, hallucinations, and tendency to suicide, to such an extent that some patients have been considered insane. These attacks of mania last only a few days or weeks.

Sometimes the delirium assumes an ambitious character, and simulates general paralysis. In other patients stupor is the chief symptom; the expression is vacant, the eyes are half-closed, and the patient is in a condition of torpor, which simulates idiocy or imbecility. This condition may last months and years. In other cases delirium is associated with symptoms of meningitis, which proves fatal.

The symptoms of delirium in typhoid fever are sometimes associated with the cerebral lesions, characterized by a hydrangea tint of the grey matter, with capillary congestion, with punctate hæmorrhages, and with œdema of the brain and ventricles. Phagocytic reaction is seen around the nerve cells which are more or less degenerated, and the *Bacillus typhosus* is frequently found in the brain. In some autopsies suppurative meningoencephalitis, with Eberth's bacillus, has been found (Fernet).

Typhoid fever is sometimes followed by loss of memory, dullness, imbecility, and dementia, which may last for several months, or even for the remainder of the patient's life.

Aphasia in typhoid fever deserves close attention. It is more common in children than in adults, both in the severe and the slight forms of typhoid fever, and in the stationary stage, or during the onset of convalescence.

When we read the cases published on this subject, we see that they may be divided into two classes. Aphasia of the first class occurs in children, and is nearly always a pure aphasia, without hemiplegia. The loss of speech is absolute, but the aphasia is transitory, rarely lasting more than a week or a fortnight, and disappearing without leaving any traces. In a child of ten years of age with typhoid aphasia, the aphasia partially disappeared after the first cold bath, and definite recovery soon followed. Whatever be the explanation of this infantile aphasia, we can exclude, considering the benign nature and the rapid disappearance of this complication, arteritis obliterans, and any lesion of Broca's convolution. The symptoms are different in the aphasia of adults, and most of the cases show that it is associated with right hemiplegia, with or without hemianæsthesia. The aphasia disappears very slowly, and the hemiplegia is even more persistent. In these cases endarteritis obliterans of the Sylvian artery is present.

The **spinal cord** may be affected by the typhoid infection, and in some cases rachialgia, hyperæsthesia of the dorsal and nuchal muscles, contractures, convulsions, and oculo-pupillary troubles indicate invasion of the spinal meninges. These symptoms, which constitute the spinal form of some writers, are early or late. When they are associated with rachialgia and vomiting, we can hardly eliminate the idea of cerebro-spinal meningitis, and the diagnosis is the more difficult in that in some cases observers have found post mortem myelitis or cerebro-spinal meningitis, which has supervened during the course of the typhoid fever. I refer the reader for the study of this question to the section on Cerebro-Spinal Meningitis. Myelitis in typhoid fever may assume different types, including the focal, ascending, and disseminated forms.

In some cases contractures of the extremities have been noted. Tetanus has also been seen.

Paralysis.—Paralytic troubles are rare during the onset of typhoid fever, being especially seen in convalescence. They are sometimes general, and affect to an equal degree the special senses, the power of movement, and sensation ; at other times they occur in the form of paraplegia and of hemiplegia (endarteritis or embolism of the Sylvian artery). They may be limited to a single organ (bladder), to the territory of a single nerve branch, or to a single group of muscles. These different localizations show that the paralyses result from different causes. Thus, those which affect the paraplegic form are due to changes in the spinal cord, while the more limited paralyses of a cranial nerve or one arm are due, on the one hand, to peripheral neuritis, and on the other hand to muscular changes, which are sometimes marked in typhoid fever. Most of these paralyses are transitory, and end in recovery.

Eschars—Suppuration.—The tendency to sloughing is especially marked in the adynamic forms of typhoid fever. Bedsores appear on the sacrum, on the trochanters, on the occiput (Chomel), as well as on the surface of blisters or in the neighbourhood of leech-bites. Gangrene of the mouth, vulva, penis, face, ear, cheek, and pupils, has been seen.

The sacral bedsore may extend deeply, and affect the coverings of the spinal cord. The gangrenous ulcerations of the skin are at times the starting-point of erysipelas.

During convalescence a tendency to suppuration shows itself by a succession of boils, and by abscesses. Chauffard thinks that in some cases the boils and abscesses are due to the entrance of the staphylococcus, which is facilitated by the baths. The fact is possible, but boils and abscesses of convalescence were seen before typhoid fever was treated by cold baths.

Suppuration sometimes appears in the form of purulent effusion into the joints, or into the serous cavities; of abscesses in the muscles (rectus abdominis, psoas) ; and of suppuration in the thyroid and parotid glands.

Parotiditis.—Parotiditis may supervene in typhoid fever, as in the course of serious infections. It is somewhat rare, but indicates a grave prognosis. Louis quotes only two examples in fifty-nine cases of typhoid fever, and Bouillaud has seen it only five or six times in many hundreds of patients.

On the other hand, it appears that parotiditis was more frequent in former epidemics (Hildenbrand, Pinel), while in a recent epidemic in Paris (1899-1900), remarkable for the variety of complications, I saw one case at the Hôtel-Dieu.

Parotiditis may appear in the course of the fever, or during convalescence. Hippocrates divided these cases into critical and acritical, attributing a favourable influence to the former. This division has long dominated the history of parotiditis, but Trousseau was one of the first to show the error. " What the ancients," says he, " called a crisis or a metastasis I call a very gloomy complication. I regard parotiditis as a most serious complication." Bacteriology has classed parotiditis among the secondary infections of typhoid fever. It is only a complication.

The onset is more or less clearly marked, and is generally ushered in by dryness of the mouth. Such was the mode of onset in my patient.

She came under my care for severe typhoid fever, with persistent hiccough, which yielded to cold baths. The temperature had been normal for four days, when one evening the thermometer registered 104° F., but the patient made no complaint, except of dryness of the mouth. Two days later she experienced acute pain at the angle of the jaw, in front of the tragus, and in the anterior process of the parotid gland. The right side of the face was slightly swollen, but there was neither tension nor redness of the skin. Palpation was painful, and I found slight brawny swelling of the parotid gland, while the lymphatic gland in front of the tragus was slightly enlarged. The cheek was dry on the right side, and the gum red and swollen, especially opposite the second upper molar. The orifice of Stenson's duct projected, and seemed to open in a papilla which was larger than that of the opposite side. Pressure on the gland caused one or two drops of sero-purulent fluid to issue from the duct. Bacteriological examination revealed the presence of the *Staphylococcus aureus*, to the exclusion of Eberth's bacillus. During the next few days the temperature fell, the swelling diminished, the pain disappeared, and in a week there was no trace of parotiditis.

Such is the slight form of parotiditis in typhoid fever, and it would rather deserve the name of stensonitis. In the severe cases the symptoms, instead of diminishing, become worse. The pain in the temporo-maxillary articulation increases. A hard and painful nodule, which rapidly enlarges, appears at some point of the parotid region, most frequently near the angle of the jaw. The swelling may invade the whole of one side of the face and neck, corresponding to the inflamed gland. The face becomes unrecognizable, and the movements of the jaw are almost impossible. The parotid tumour soon becomes tense, painful, and tender on pressure. The skin over it is shiny, red, or sometimes of a violet colour, and presents a certain softness, which soon gives place to well-marked fluctuation. The patient complains of pain in the neck and shoulders. The opposite side is sometimes affected. The pulse is small and quick, the dyspnœa is acute, the mouth is dry, and the general condition is very grave. Deafness supervenes, and the patient dies in an adynamic condition.

At the autopsy Stenson's duct and all the excretory channels of the gland are distended with pus. Their wall is destroyed in many places, and the bands of connective tissue separating the acini oppose but a feeble obstacle to the ever-increasing invasion of the suppuration. The lesion commences in the excretory duct of the acinus, and is always due to ascending infection, caused by the micro-organisms of the mouth, and especially by the *Staphylococcus aureus* or by the streptococcus. Eberth's bacillus is said to have been found in two cases.

The microbes do not normally enter Stenson's duct, and the saliva is sterile. This asepsis is explained by the direction of the duct, and by the fact that the saliva forms a bad culture medium (Sanarelli). In typhoid fever the sordes on the teeth and on the mucous membrane of the mouth afford the organisms the favourable medium. In addition, the salivary secretion is notably diminished, as in all forms of pyrexia. The physiological equilibrium is broken, and the microbes, no longer finding obstacles, are able to pass along Stenson's duct. My patient suffered from well-marked gingivitis on the right side three days before the first signs of parotiditis. It seems probable that this gingivitis may have marked the first stage of the ascending salivary infection; it may have been the immediate cause of it.

It is, therefore, necessary in infection of the mouth to take prophylactic measures and to institute rigid antisepsis. These antiseptic measures are sufficient in slight cases, but in the severe ones early surgical intervention must be resorted to.

Hæmatoma and Muscular Abscesses.—Lesions of the muscles in typhoid fever are various.

I had in the Hôtel-Dieu a patient suffering from suppurating hæmatoma of the rectus abdominis. The man was convalescent when fever reappeared, and I found a somewhat painful swelling in the suprapubic region. The skin was of an ecchymotic colour, and pressure gave blood crepitus, due to hæmorrhage in the rectus muscle. On the next day the swelling and the ecchymosis had increased, and exploratory puncture gave exit to hæmorrhagic and purulent fluid, in which the *Bacillus typhosus* alone was found. The tumour was incised, and 6 ounces of purulent blood-stained fluid, enclosed in the sheath of the muscle, were let out. The patient recovered some days later.

As a general rule, the infection due to Eberth's bacillus and its toxine causes fatty, waxy, and vacuolar degeneration of the muscles. The degeneration attacks the fibre itself, and limits its action to the contractile substance. "This change consists in a modification of the contractile fibre, probably due to coagulation of the myosin. Complete loss of muscular elasticity results, and is followed by very marked friability of the muscle" (Chantemesse). These changes show themselves by ruptures, hæmatomata, or abscesses, chiefly found in the rectus abdominis and in the adductor muscles of the thigh.

Ruptures may be painful or painless. Rupture of the rectus abdominis has been mistaken in some cases for the onset of peritonitis.

Hæmatoma of the muscle is generally consecutive to rupture. The hæmatoma often remains in a pure state, without purulent change, so that the blood found on incision is fluid or clotted, without any trace of pus.

Letulle has given me notes of a case of this kind in which, on the sixteenth day of typhoid fever, sharp pain appeared in the region of the rectus abdominis on the left side. The painful region was prominent, ecchymosis appeared, and hæmatoma of the muscle was diagnosed. The patient died of intestinal perforation, and rupture and hæmatoma of the muscle were found at the autopsy. The histological examination by Letulle may be thus summed up: Diffuse hæmorrhage in the rectus abdominis, separation of the muscle fibres by masses of red corpuscles with interstitial œdema, and infiltration, with innumerable lymphatic cells, for the most part mononuclear.

Rémy told me of the following case:

In a young man suffering from a relapse in typhoid fever a hæmatoma appeared, occupying the whole of the thigh, from the knee to Scarpa's triangle; the skin was of a violet colour. The swelling appeared a few minutes after a strain, and cure was obtained by pressure, without incision. Boisson and Simonin published a case of hæmatoma, without suppuration, in the course of typhoid fever.

The hæmatoma often suppurates, as in my case, to which I may add other examples. Tollemer communicated the following case to me:

A patient with typhoid fever, under Brissaud's care, raised himself and separated his legs in order to sit down on the stool, when he experienced a sharp pain on the inside of the left thigh. On the next day swelling appeared, with great pain and ecchymosis of the skin. The brawny induration became fluctuating, and incision gave exit to hæmorrhagic and purulent fluid, and brought about recovery of the lesion.

In some cases the suppuration invades the muscle from the first, without previous hæmatoma. On closer inspection, however, we see that a small quantity of blood is present in addition to the pus.

Lastly, the muscle may become gangrenous (Millard).

These muscular lesions—rupture, pure hæmatoma, suppurating hæmatoma, or suppuration without hæmatoma—are sometimes more or less painful at first, and are then followed by brawny induration, ecchymoses, and fluctuation. These various forms may be due to Eberth's bacillus, without other microbes, or to streptococci and staphylococci. Surgical intervention is almost always indicated.

Osseous Lesions.—Many osseous and articular lesions may be seen during convalescence from typhoid fever—rapid growth of the bones, rheumatic pains, fixed pain in the tibia or the femur, swelling of the bones and joints, deformity of the long bones, hypertrophy of the epiphyses, exostoses, acute osteomyelitis and suppurative periostitis, chronic osteomyelitis and periostitis.

In the first place, it is certain that in mankind, as in experimental animals, the bone-marrow is, next to the spleen, the seat of election of the

Bacillus typhosus (Wyssokowitch, Chantemesse, and Widal), which causes more often than any other microbe disease of the marrow in typhoid fever. If pure cultures of Eberth's bacillus are injected into the blood of rabbits, the microbe is found most often in the bone-marrow and the spleen, although observation has long since proved that children and adolescents, when convalescent from typhoid fever, show exaggerated growth of the limbs, proving rapid increase in the length of the bones. It is certain, therefore, that the typhoid infection causes hyperactivity of growth in the bones, and especially in those which are in process of growth. This hyperactivity is shown anatomically by increased proliferation of the bone-marrow and of the subperiosteal layers. The bone-marrow and the periosteum are equally infected by the *Bacillus typhosus*, but the lesion (osteomyelitis) appears to commence in the marrow, and spreads thence to the periosteum. Accordingly, we see osteomyelitis and osteoperiostitis, but the former is sometimes the more important lesion.

The bone infections generally take place during convalescence, or some time after recovery from typhoid fever. They are especially frequent in children and youths, in whom the skeleton has not reached its full development. It assumes the following forms :

A rheumatoid form has been described by Déhu. In this form the infective process is not localized, but causes pain in the limbs and joints which are like the so-called " growing pains." Pressure on the bones and joints is painful. Walking and standing rapidly induce fatigue. The condition lasts some weeks, and is accompanied by rapid increase in stature.

In other cases the infective process may be localized to the tibia, to the femur, to the bones of the arm, to the sternum, or to the ribs, in the form of acute osteomyelitis or osteoperiostitis. The first symptoms are pain and fever, and the patient complains of a painful spot, which is at first very limited. The least pressure on the diseased bone sometimes causes most acute pain, which is increased by movement. The pain is continuous or paroxysmal, and more marked at night. This acute febrile period, however, with or without rigors, does not always end in suppuration. The skin in the painful region is somewhat œdematous, but shows no change in colour. Palpation reveals a swelling of the bone, over which the skin slides freely. The pain and swelling disappear, and recovery results after a period which is sometimes very long. Relapses may occur.

I had under my care a case of osteomyelitis of the ribs. The patient was a young man, eighteen years of age, who was convalescent from severe typhoid fever. Acute pain in the right side came on a fortnight after defervescence ; it was exactly localized to the seventh rib, 2 inches from the chondro-vertebral joint. No swelling was present at this spot. I made a diagnosis of commencing osteomyelitis, and, in fact, swelling and pain made their appearance in a few days ; there was no rise of temperature. Slight fluctuation was thought to be felt on the sixteenth day, but the process remained stationary, resolution took place, and at the end of a month the patient was discharged with a small painless exostosis. The costal localization of this osteomyelitis was interesting, for it corresponded with the centre of ossification for the tuberosity which appears at the eighteenth year.

When osteoperiostitis ends in suppuration, the pain is very severe, the œdema of the affected region increases in amount, the skin becomes red and shiny, and the pus forces its way outwards if surgical interference is not forthcoming. The pus is thick, brownish, and odourless. The fever and pain cease, or improve with the free exit of the pus, and a probe introduced into the fistula shows the condition of the bone. In the case of necrosis, however, very troublesome fistulæ occur, and do not close until the sequestrum is removed.

In some cases the osseous infection passes into a chronic condition, or assumes from the first a slow course. It lasts for months and years under the mask of syphilitic osteopathy or tubercular cold abscess (Chantemesse and Widal). Even when the lesion is chronic from the outset it is always painful at some period. The pain at times coincides with the onset of the lesion, but in other cases it supervenes months or years later. The bony tumour increases very slowly in size, and ends in resolution, in exostosis, or in suppuration. The exostosis may become as large as a nut or an orange, causing deformity of the limbs, or hampering their function.

In a case reported by Achard and Broca the fluctuating swelling of the bone lasted for eleven months ; the pus which was drawn off contained Eberth's bacillus. Péan has published a very interesting case of a patient who was attacked, during the decline of typhoid fever, with osteoperiostitis of the right femur, which was operated upon and drained. Pain had at this time also appeared in the left femur ; it gradually disappeared, and did not reappear until some years later. This fresh lesion ended in osteomyelitis, which was operated upon ; the *Bacillus typhosus* was found in the pus.

The **diagnosis** presents no difficulty when the osteomyelitis or the osteoperiostitis supervenes in a classical manner during or after convalescence. When they do not appear until long afterwards, the lesion having remained for a longer or shorter period in the latent state, we must not confuse the lesion, when accompanied by induration or by softening of the bone, with syphilitic or tubercular osteitis. The osteomyelitis of adolescents must also be differentiated from them.

The **prognosis** is very rarely serious. In most cases, says Schwartz, the superficial nature and the small extent of the damage is very striking.

Medical treatment consists in relieving the pain and limiting the lesion as far as possible. For this purpose leeches, inunction of mercury, rest, and fixation are employed. Surgical treatment is often indicated, and good results may be looked for. Bacteriological examination at the time of operation gives valuable information as to the nature of the pathogenic agents. Eberth's bacillus is sometimes associated with staphylococci or streptococci. In other cases it may no longer be present at the time of operation.

Organs of the Senses.—Ulcers of the cornea, panophthalmitis, and inflammation of the orbit have been seen. In one of Panas's cases the *Bacillus typhosus* was present in a pure state.

Deafness is a frequent symptom in the stationary stage of typhoid fever. It may depend on nerve trouble, or on catarrh of the Eustachian tube and of the middle ear, coincident with the laryngeal catarrh. These auditory troubles are not serious. In some cases they are due to purulent otitis, which may cause perforation of the membrana tympani, spread to the mastoid cells, and induce caries of the petrous bone, with all its consequences.

The **skin** may be affected by multiple eruptions resembling those of measles or of scarlatina. In some cases it is not a question of simple eruptions, but of infective erythemata, which may carry off the patients in thirty-six or in forty-eight hours.

Course—Relapse.—I have mentioned in the description of the disease the possible irregularities of the onset and the slowness of convalescence, which is sometimes excessive, but there are other peculiarities deserving of notice. Typhoid fever may at its onset simulate an intermittent fever, with tertian or quotidian attacks. The fever then, from being intermittent, becomes remittent, and assumes the type of typhoid fever. Typhoid fever chiefly assumes an intermittent character in countries where malaria is endemic, or in persons who have recently left these countries. Old writers knew these facts, but, in their opinion, the intermittent marsh fever became transformed into ataxic or malignant fever. In this they were wrong, for the disease does not change its nature, although it presents a change of type (Trousseau).

I have said that convalescence in typhoid fever may be interrupted by innumerable complications, and I have reserved the question of **relapses** in order to speak of them here. The relapse must not be confounded with the **second attack.** The latter—very rare, because typhoid fever confers immunity—only concerns cases which supervene several months or several years after the first attack. The relapse, on the contrary, is a fairly frequent complication, and affects the patient during convalescence, after some days of complete apyrexia, just as though the disease ran its course in several distinct attacks, relapses occurring in from 6 to 10 per cent. They are more common in children.

The relapse may give no warning of its onset. It often begins with vomiting, and the temperature rises and the rose spots reappear, although in very small numbers. The relapse usually lasts eight to twelve days, and generally ends in recovery. Complications, however, may occur. As many as four and even five relapses have been seen (Jaccoud).

It is not rare, especially in children's hospitals, to see a patient suffering from typhoid fever contract scarlatina, measles, or variola ; but the reciprocal condition is extremely rare, because the typhoid fever is far from being as contagious as the eruptive fevers.

Prognosis—Sudden Death.—The foregoing descriptions give an account of the various modes of termination in typhoid fever. Its gravity and its mortality vary in different epidemics, countries, and surroundings (hospital, town, country). The mean mortality varies from 18 to 20 per cent. (Murchison, Griesinger, Jaccoud). We shall see later that the mortality has been much lowered.

The **prognosis** in this disease must always be reserved, as the most terrible accidents (peritonitis, sudden death) may supervene in apparently slight cases, and also because the most serious complications may appear during convalescence, when the patient is looked upon as cured.

Sudden Death.—This pathological fact had been almost ignored until my first publications on *Sudden Death in Typhoid Fever*, and the few scattered cases in various writings had passed unnoticed. In less than a year I was able to collect fourteen cases, which served as the theme of my inaugural thesis.* Some years later, in a fresh work on the same subject,† I collected sixty-three cases, and I am now in possession of nearly eighty. These figures are, in my opinion, more than sufficient to establish the fact that sudden death is far from being exceptional in typhoid fever, and is almost as common as intestinal perforation or peritonitis. I place its frequency at 2 per cent., which gives it an important place in the history of this disease.

Two questions belong to the study of sudden death, the one purely clinical, and the other theoretical, which seeks for the cause and mechanism of this accident.

Sudden death usually occurs without warning in mild or moderate cases, when all danger appears at an end. When we compare cases with one another, we find that the circumstances accompanying sudden death usually occur under the same conditions. We see that the two first weeks are passed without mishap, the temperature begins to fall, the patient feels better and begs for food, and convalescence commences,‡ when suddenly,

---

* Dieulafoy, " De la Mort Subite dans la Fièvre Typhoïde " (*Thèse de Paris*, 1867).
† *Gaz. Hebdom.*, 1877, Nos. 20 and 21.
‡ In twenty-three cases sudden death occurred as follows :

2 cases on the 17th day.
2 „ „ 18th „
4 „ „ 19th „
6 „ „ 20th „
5 „ „ 21st „
2 „ „ 23rd „
2 „ „ 24th „

without pain or warning, the patient becomes exceedingly pale, suffers from a few convulsive movements, and dies. Death is evidently due to syncope, but what is the explanation of this syncope ? It has not been difficult for me to collect a fair number of cases in which sudden death, **apart from typhoid fever,** is due to trifling circumstances, such as drinking a glass of iced water, cauterization of the pharynx, etc. We know, on the other hand, that foreign bodies in the intestine, such as worms, fruit-stones, etc., may cause epileptiform troubles,* which are sometimes followed by syncope and death. I have, therefore, fixed my base, on the one hand, upon clinical facts, and, on the other hand, upon the experiments of Brown-Séquard and Goltz, which show the special excitability of the intestine, and the mechanism of syncope following such excitation, and I have put forward the following theory : Syncope in typhoid fever is partly due to a reflex action starting in the diseased intestine. The stimulus is transmitted by the centripetal fibres of the great sympathetic to the cells of the spinal cord and bulb, and produces a fulminant action upon the nuclei of the vagus.

Hayem has defended a theory which attributes sudden death to the changes in the cardiac muscle seen in typhoid fever, as well as in most severe fevers. This theory is seductive, for it appears based upon pathological anatomy ; but if we admit that sudden death is due to cardiac degeneration, we ought to find this degeneration in all cases of sudden death. It is, however, often absent. In the seven cases so far published histological examination has shown no change in the heart. Accordingly, if sudden death has occurred seven times without any change in the heart, we must look elsewhere for the cause. Sudden death from syncope is not, then, the end of the so-called cardiac form. As I have already said, it is quite a different thing. The study of the typhoid toxine on the nerve ganglia of the heart may perhaps elucidate the pathogenesis (Chantemesse).

Diagnosis.—Any **typhoid condition** may simulate typhoid fever—as, for instance, the condition caused by lumbricosis, to which Chauffard has just drawn attention afresh in the case of a little boy who had all the symptoms of typhoid fever. In this case recovery occurred after the passage of thirty-nine worms.

The diagnosis of typhoid fever by clinical methods alone is often very difficult, and the exceptional cases which commence with angina, gastric catarrh, lobar pneumonia, or intermittent fever are well calculated to puzzle the clinician. The same remark applies to the slight forms and to the ataxic form, with early delirium, which simulates meningitis or acute mania. According to Wunderlich, any disease in which the temperature

* I saw, with Krishaber, a child, eleven years old, who had swallowed plum-stones. He was seized with convulsions, and died. At the autopsy we found the plum-stones accumulated in the latter part of the ileum.

has not reached 104° F. by the evening of the fourth day is not typhoid fever, and every disease in which the temperature reaches 104° F. on the first day is not typhoid fever. The latter proposition cannot be accepted, and the former is subject to many exceptions.

Cerebro-spinal meningitis has many symptoms in common with typhoid fever, more especially as the typhoid infection may at the same time cause cerebro-spinal infection. I will ask the reader to turn to the section on Cerebro-spinal Meningitis, where he will find this difficult question discussed in detail.

Malignant hypertoxic syphilis may simulate typhoid fever. Fournier has described this condition under the name of **syphilitic typhosis.** I have seen a case at the Hôtel-Dieu which ended in death. Letulle has given me the following notes :

A young woman came into hospital suffering from secondary syphilis, the temperature varying between 102° and 104° F. ; the spleen was enlarged and the abdomen distended, just as in typhoid fever. Three days later the temperature fell, the general condition improved, and the syphilis ran its course.

In syphilitic typhosis (hypertoxic form) the secondary rash appears with symptoms which sometimes recall the invasion of an eruptive fever, and at other times of typhoid fever. The temperature reaches 103° or 104° F. Prostration, adynamia, headache, vertigo, epistaxis, vomiting, and dyspnœa are the symptoms usually seen in syphilitic typhosis. In my patient, to whom I alluded above, the symptoms of hypertoxia reached a maximum, and the hæmoglobin was diminished to 50 per cent. The tachycardia, dyspnœa, and adynamia ended in fatal collapse, although at the autopsy we were unable to discover the slightest lesion.

Influenza, cerebral meningitis, infective endocarditis, and acute tuberculosis may closely simulate typhoid fever. Everyone in his hospital career or in his private practice has often found himself in the awkward situation where it was impossible to say whether a patient had or had not typhoid fever. For example :

A young man, twenty years old, has been taken ill a few days before with fever, severe headache, and vomiting. He is troubled with cough, and auscultation of the chest shows some scattered, whistling râles. The evening temperature is 104° F., there is no diarrhœa, the insomnia is persistent, and we wonder whether the case is one of typhoid fever, likely to end in recovery, or whether it is commencing miliary tuberculosis, which is nearly always fatal. On what can we base the diagnosis ? On the temperature curve ? Unfortunately, it rarely, in any special case, follows the well-known classical form. Can we rely upon the appearance of spots ? Unfortunately, they have not yet appeared, and perhaps they will not do so. The râles, however, become general, dyspnœa appears, and our fears of acute tuberculosis increase, while time runs on and the diagnosis still remains indefinite.

We shall see later that it is necessary to think of paratyphoid fever. Bacteriology has been employed as an aid to diagnosis. The method consists in examination of blood withdrawn by puncture from the spleen, but this is a very complicated and often impracticable method. Elsner proposed search for the bacillus in the stools, which is an unpractical and, furthermore, an insufficient method. Widal made a most important communication at the Société Médicale des Hôpitaux.* He showed how to make in a few minutes an accurate diagnosis of typhoid fever.

I was anxious to confirm these results, and I at once made a communication to the Académie de Médecine.† This method of **sero-diagnosis** is based on the fact that the serum of persons suffering from typhoid fever, or even of convalescents, possesses the power of immobilizing and agglutinating *in vitro* Eberth's bacilli suspended in broth.

Accordingly, if we place a young broth culture of Eberth's bacillus under the microscope, we see that the bacilli are **isolated,** and endowed with extreme **mobility.**‡

* F. Widal, "Séro-diagnostic de la Fièvre Typhoïde " (*Soc. Méd. des Hôpit.*, 26 Juin, 1896 ; *Congr. de Nancy*, 1896 ; *Pr. Méd.*, 8 Avril, 1896).

† Dieulafoy.   Communication faite à l'Acad., le 7 Juillet, 1896.

‡ Widal adopts the following method : " I begin with the extemporaneous microscopical examination, after mixing serum with an active culture in the proportion of 1 to 10, or even 1 to 5.   When the preparation is disturbed by Brownian movements, we must let it remain for a quarter or for half an hour in order to see the agglutination.   We should always examine, for the sake of comparison, a preparation of the culture made before the addition of serum.   The employment of a young culture which is only one or two days old is preferable.   I may even say that if the development of a culture is sufficiently rich, **the younger it is the better.**   A broth culture which is quite neutral and several days old may give the reaction, provided that we carefully follow the indications stated later.   Practically, in a hospital laboratory we can always have cultures some days old which are sufficient for immediate examination.

" If the extemporaneous examination shows numerous confluent masses, made up of bacteria, and scattered all over the preparation like the islands of an archipelago, the diagnosis is certain.   If the masses, though characteristic, be not especially confluent, or if I find only mobile or isolated bacilli, I examine the mixture again several hours afterwards, both with the naked eye and with the microscope.   After this time the reaction is often apparent.   In case of a negative result I repeat the examination several days following, as long as suspicious symptoms last.

" If we only possess a very old culture, or, indeed, one some days old, which under the microscope shows precipitation of false masses before the addition of serum, we must not hesitate to make a fresh culture, and to delay the answer to the next day.   The serum may be mixed with broth, sown, and put in the oven.   In fifteen hours, or even less, the microbes are found in masses at the bottom of the tube, forming small whitish flakes, and leaving the broth almost clear.   On shaking, these flakes do not dissolve completely ; they always leave a precipitate floating in the liquid as a very fine dust.   I constantly employ this procedure concurrently with the extemporaneous one when I am dealing with a serum taken under conditions of absolute purity.   If I am not sure of the asepsis of my serum, I make a new culture by sowing it on simple broth. In less than twenty-four hours I have a fresh culture sufficiently turbid to give the phenomenon under the microscope immediately after the addition of the typhoid serum.   I may add that, some hours after mixing, the clots may be visible to the naked eye."

On the other hand, if we mix in a test-tube ten drops of a culture of Eberth's bacillus and one drop of serum from the patient, and then examine this mixture under the microscope, we notice very striking changes. The bacilli no longer remain isolated and mobile, as in the preceding preparation. They tend to lose their mobility, and agglutinate in masses, separated by vacant spaces. These empty spaces are still traversed by some bacilli, which are less mobile, and, as it were, siderated, and are finally attracted to one of these masses, in which they in turn are engulfed.

If a patient yields serum capable of causing agglutination in a broth culture of typhoid bacilli, he is suffering from typhoid fever.

The reaction has been found by Widal in patients who had been suffering from typhoid fever for seven, twelve, fifteen, sixteen, nineteen, and twenty-one days. On the other hand, the serum of patients suffering from other diseases, such as nephritis, tuberculosis, pneumonia, jaundice, rheumatism, etc., when mixed with a broth culture of Eberth's bacillus, leaves the micro-organisms mobile and isolated.

Sero-diagnosis has been adopted both in France and abroad. We have " a simple and rapid method, which requires no elaborate material, not even stains. All that is required is a pure broth culture of Eberth's bacilli, which can be kept for weeks, a microscope with an immersion lens, and a drop of blood or of serum from the patient " (Widal).

The experiment may also be made in another manner. If typhoid serum is added to a broth culture of active bacilli, or if virgin broth is impregnated immediately after the serum has been added, and kept for some hours in the oven, we see that the broth becomes clear, and little whitish flakes collect at the bottom of the tube.

The agglutinating property appears to belong to the albuminoid matter of the blood, or of the fluids which form a kind of chemical precipitate around the microbes (Widal and Sicard). Further, the agglutinative reaction is obtained not only with typhoid serum, but also with other secretions from typhoid patients — serous fluid of blisters or of œdema, tears, bile, and exceptionally urine (Widal and Sicard).

The agglutinative reaction has been seen in the milk of wet-nurses suffering from typhoid fever (Achard and Bensaude).

In a case published by Étienne the reaction did not take place with the blood of a fœtus, although the mother was suffering from typhoid fever, and gave the agglutinative reaction. This observation should not be set up as a precedent, for the passage of the agglutinating property from the mother to the fœtus occurs in rabbits (Widal and Sicard).

In short, as I said in 1896 at the Académie de Médecine, we can foresee the services which sero-diagnosis will render. We shall now know how to regard these fevers, called in turn synochal, gastric, autumnal, mucous, or typhoidal, febrile, and infectious diseases, which, according to the current teaching, helped to increase or diminish the balance-sheet of typhoid fever.

We can now diagnose cases of influenza resembling typhoid fever and presenting insuperable obstacles to correct diagnosis. We can understand the cases in which typhoid fever appears to localize itself in a typhoid lung, and those in which pneumonia assumes a typhoid course, although it has nothing in common with infection due to Eberth's bacillus. We can tell whether patients who come to us with obscure symptoms of typhoid fever and a cardiac murmur are suffering from typhoid fever or from endocarditis of the typhoid type.

We can promptly decide the diagnosis of typhoid fever and acute tuberculosis. We can form a correct opinion of typhus ambulatorius, typhus levissimus, and abortive typhoid fever, which will take a properly defined place in the list of diseases.

In future we shall not hesitate in deciding whether the disease is meningitis, cerebro-spinal typhus, or typhoid fever of a meningeal type.

Hæmo-Diagnosis.—In the severe form of typhoid fever Courmont and Lesieur have always found Eberth's bacillus in the blood up to the end of the third week. To carry out this examination, it is sufficient to sow 2 to 4 c.c. of blood immediately after withdrawal on 300 to 500 c.c. of broth. As a rule, the culture is positive in the first few days. The following table indicates the dates :

Positive culture on the 1st day	..	..	11 cases.
„ „ „ 2nd „	..	..	17 „
„ „ „ 3rd „	..	..	4 „
„ „ „ 4th „	..	..	8 „
„ „ „ 5th „	..	..	4 „

In 60 per cent. of the cases the culture is positive in from twenty-four to forty-eight hours. The delay seen in the development of cultures is most probably due to the hindering action of the typhoid serum, rather than to the small number of microbes present in the blood. The discovery of the bacillus in the blood may be useful in cases where the serum reaction is delayed. Thus, the bacillus existed in the blood four times in thirty-three positive cases, although agglutination was not appreciable. Nevertheless, " sero-diagnosis is more easily carried out, and remains the favourite method whenever it gives positive information." There is no relation between the agglutinative power of the blood and the rapidity of growth of the cultures. In any case, we do not find other microbes in the blood. Eberth's bacillus is present in a pure condition.

Gelo-Diagnosis.—This method, proposed by Chantemesse, is based on the discovery of the *Bacillus typhosus* in the dejecta. It depends on the properties of Eberth's bacillus.

(1) This bacillus can stand a fairly large dose of carbolic acid (Chante-messe and Widal) ; (2) it does not cause fermentation of milk-sugar, while the *Bacillus coli* gives rise to lactic acid (Chantemesse and Widal, 1892) ; (3) on plates of agar, to which milk-sugar and litmus have been added, the *B. typhosus* gives blue colonies with lactic acid, and the *B. coli* gives red ones (Würtz, 1893) ; (4) this microbe is agglutinated by a specific serum (Pfeiffer, 1894) ; (5) before looking for it in the dejecta, it is an advantage previously to cause its multiplication, and to make the search easier, the material should be sown on an extremely thin layer of agar (Chantemesse, 1901) ; (6) in order to find these bacilli in the suspected fluid, it is useful before analysis to collect them in masses by means of a specific agglutinative serum (Chantemesse, 1902).

Chantemesse and Decobert* have found by the aid of gélo-diagnosis typhoid bacilli in the stools of all those suffering from well-marked typhoid fever, and have controlled their observations by sero-diagnosis. They have also found them in some patients who have been well for a month. Finally, they have been able to prove the presence of the *B. typhosus* in the dejecta at the onset of the typhoid fever before the agglutination reaction could be obtained.

Ophthalmo-Diagnosis.—This method, employed by Chantemesse, con-sists in dropping into the eye a solution of the toxines of the *B. typhosus*. The technique is as follows : He dissolves in a drop of water the typhoid toxine precipitated by alcohol, and reduced to a dry powder. The dose is $\frac{1}{50}$ milligramme. This dose is instilled under the lower lid. The reaction reaches its maximum in six to twelve hours. It is characterized by redness and lachrymation, with sero-fibrinous exudate. The reaction lasts for one or two days. Fifty persons free from typhoid fever gave no reaction, while the test was positive in seventy persons with typhoid fever. It was also positive at a time when sero-diagnosis was negative.

Diagnosis from Paratyphoid Infection.—Some patients appear to have typhoid fever, when they are really suffering from a paratyphoid infection. Sero-diagnosis is negative in these cases. When a patient is in the typhoid state, we may suspect paratyphoid infection if sero-diagnosis and ophthalmo-diagnosis are negative. Paratyphoid infection, however, is not certain, unless the patient's serum agglutinates a culture of paratyphoid bacilli. These are the bacillus of Brion and Kayser, that of Conradi, and the *B. enteritidis* of Gärtner. The proper method of examination for para-typhoid bacilli is hæmoculture, similar to that used in the case of Eberth's bacillus. The *B. typhosus* and the paratyphoid bacilli are sometimes associated, the infection being mixed. Aside from typhoid conditions, the

* Decobert, " Du Gélo-diagnostic des Selles et de son Emploi au Diagnostic Précoce de la Fièvre Typhoïde " (*Thèse de Paris*, 1903).

paratyphoid bacilli give rise to gastro-intestinal, pyæmic, and remittent infection, to infective jaundice, and to cholecystitis.

Ætiology.—Eberth's bacillus is the specific agent in typhoid fever. The pathogenic conditions of the disease are those which govern the hatching of all infectious diseases due to micro-organisms : (1) It is necessary that the microbe introduced into the economy be present in such numbers or be endowed with such virulence that it can overcome the resistance of the body ; (2) this more or less feeble resistance in the economy constitutes the *occasio morbi*.

The bacillus of typhoid fever may be present in the stools of healthy individuals, or may exist in a **latent** condition, like the pneumococcus or the *B. coli*, becoming a pathogenic agent under the influence of certain causes (armies in the field, fatigue, overwork). In this way the old dogma of **morbid spontaneity** is in part explained, and the motto " *Multa renascentur quæ jam cecidere* " applies.

Typhoid fever has been seen in practically every country, but still it shows a marked predilection for the Temperate Zones. It is endemic in large towns.

It reaches its maximum in the autumn (Besnier). It is **epidemic,** but only to a slight degree **contagious,** and the first attack, as a rule, confers immunity. In this disease, as in all epidemic diseases, each epidemic may present special forms and characters, distinguishing it from other epidemics. Typhoid fever by choice attacks young people, and especially those who have come to a city from the country, and who are in a special state of receptivity, favoured by bad hygienic conditions, home-sickness, worry, and excess of fatigue or of work.

Bacteriology.—The pathogenic agent in typhoid fever was discovered by Eberth in 1880. Since this time numerous observers, including Friedlander and Meyer (1881), Letzerich (1885), Gaffky (1884), Artaud, Brieger (1885), etc., have verified Eberth's discovery, and have added many interesting facts.

Eberth's bacillus can be cultivated on broth, gelatine, agar-agar, and potato. Colonies of Eberth's bacillus, obtained by culture on gelatine-plates, and examined with a low power, present the form of islets with cut edges. " They appear traversed by wrinkles, which are more or less marked throughout their whole extent. Their surface is often irregular, and the whole colony resembles the twisted coils of the small intestine. The combination of these two aspects, joined to the shining colour, sometimes causes the colony to look like a mountain of ice " (Chantemesse and Widal).

In cultures the *B. typhosus* is polymorphous. It is exceedingly mobile, and shows no tendency to agglutination. As a rule, it has the shape of a small rod, with rounded ends, while its length is three times its breadth.

the guise of hæmoptysis, of pleurisy, and of chronic bronchitis, which have recovered without further complications. The disease—or, at least, the morbid predisposition—has, however, been transmitted to the child, in whom it has been present in a latent state, only waiting for a favourable opportunity, such as whooping-cough, measles, or typhoid fever, to offer to the microbes a suitable culture medium.

Cardio-Vascular System.—Endocarditis is exceptional, but myocarditis is fairly common in typhoid fever. The change in the heart muscle is often shown by no appreciable symptom, and yet, when the lesion is sufficiently marked, the precordial shock is less forcible. A murmur is sometimes discovered, but as this murmur is frequently modified by the respiratory movements and by the position of the patient, it is probable that it is more often an extracardiac bruit, which can give no information as to the state of the myocardium (Potain). The change in the heart in part explains the softness and the irregularity of the pulse, and favours the pulmonary congestion, the coldness of the extremities, as well as the state of **collapse** which appears at an advanced stage, and is generally of evil omen.

The degeneration of the heart muscle is due to the *Bacillus typhosus,* to its products of secretion, to the phagocytic reaction, and to the secondary infections. It may produce the symptom-complex known as the **cardiac form** of typhoid fever. These cardiac troubles, which contribute to the fatal ending by their progressive severity, are not the true cause of sudden death.

Experimental Typhoid Myocarditis.—Various opinions had been enunciated as to the nature and pathogenesis of fibrosis of the myocardium before the question was experimentally treated. We know to-day that it is the result of an intoxication which is, as a rule, slow and progressive in its course.

If small and repeated doses of typhoid toxine are injected under the skin of animals (guinea-pigs, rabbits, and dogs) (Chantemesse), various lesions are produced, and in particular the appearance in the myocardium of spots, patches, or zones of fibrosis, comparable to those of the hypertrophied heart in the cardiac forms of arterio-sclerosis.

The survival of the animals depends on the doses of toxine administered. They may succumb in twenty-four hours, or may live for several years with cardiac fibrosis (Chantemesse). In those which succumb rapidly we find in the heart an inflammatory reaction, characterized by slight leucocytic infiltration, congestion of the vessels, and perivascular œdema ; but the chief lesion consists in acute degeneration of the muscular fibre, which has lost its regular striation, the discs being blended together and the fibre having a " watered " appearance. The protoplasmic zone around the nuclei has undergone more or less marked vacuolar degeneration. At certain points the striation is no longer recognizable.

In addition to the usual forms, the *B. typhosus* is sometimes very short, or at other times elongated in the form of threads, which are two or three times as long as the bacillus. The stained bacillus often presents at its centre or at its extremities clear spaces, wrongly taken for spores.

After staining, we may see cilia, which may be very numerous and tuft-like, and which proceed from the ends of the rod or from its body. Eberth's bacillus is found in the fæces, the walls of the intestine, Peyer's patches, the mesenteric glands, the liver, the kidneys, the lungs, and the spleen, from which organ it may be obtained during life by puncture with a capillary trocar after the tenth day of the disease. It is not found in the blood, except in that from the rose spots. It is sometimes found in the urine, as was shown by Bouchard before its morphological characters were known.

Cultures of Eberth's bacillus yield a specific typho-toxine, which, on injection into a guinea-pig, produces marked secretion from the intestinal and salivary glands, and deprives the animal of the power of voluntary motion. The microbe of typhoid fever secretes a vaccine, which is still under study.

Water offers an excellent natural culture medium, and most epidemics of typhoid fever at the present day may be explained by this property.

The infiltration of cesspools and manure-heaps, upon which the dejecta of typhoid patients are sometimes thrown, are quite enough to pollute the water of wells, cisterns, streams, etc., with the result that a local epidemic is seen, or, on the other hand, an epidemic appears in a town far from the primary focus of contagion, but situated on the same river.

This fact is proved by the recent epidemics at Zurich, Auxerre, Plymouth, Pierrefonds, Clermont-Ferrand, and Havre. It also explains how inhabitants in a town who drink the water from one source may be attacked, while those whose reservoirs are supplied by a different water may escape contagion. This fact has several times been seen in Paris (Chantemesse and Widal), where the water of the Seine above and below the city (Thoinet) constantly contains typhoid bacilli, while the water of the Vanne and of the Ourcq, as a rule, does not contain them.

At certain seasons of the year, when the water in these two rivers is low, some quarters then receive their supply from the Seine, with the result that typhoid fever appears there almost at once in an epidemic form, and it has been proved that the water supplied for consumption contains pathogenic bacilli. Oysters may harbour the *B. typhosus*, and cause typhoid fever, just as they may transmit cholera. Flies have been held guilty as propagating agents.

The air may also carry the contagion. The fæces of patients with typhoid fever, mixed with the soil, are finally transformed into dust. The bacilli, by reason of their great vitality, preserve in a latent state their pathogenic properties for a more or less lengthy period, and then, mingling with the air, they finally enter the bronchi, and contagion takes place, although much less frequently than by ingestion of polluted water. In a similar way linen impregnated with the fæcal matter from typhoid patients has formed an important element of contagion in some families.

The *B. typhosus* can be inoculated in some animals, such as mice, guinea-pigs, and rabbits. The soluble products of various microbes, when injected into animals, favour infection by Eberth's bacillus, even though it is of slight virulence (Chantemesse and Widal, Sanarelli). The disease produced in this manner is not a copy of the disease in man, but is a kind of experimental septicæmia, which allows us to manipulate the virulence of the microbe, and to make attempts at vaccination and serotherapy in animals.

The experiments of Chantemesse and Widal have shown that the serum from animals vaccinated with the soluble products of cultures of Eberth's bacillus possesses immunizing properties against the action of the virus, and that the same serum also possesses curative properties in experimental typhoid infection which is in process of evolution. The serum from an individual who has recovered from typhoid fever weeks, months, and even years previously possesses preventative and therapeutic properties against experimental infection, while the serum of an individual who has not had typhoid fever is not, as a rule, endowed with the same power.

An attempt has been made to identify the *B. typhosus* with the *B. coli*, a micro-organism always present in the bowel (Rodet and Roux). Chantemesse and Widal have answered the various arguments brought forward, and, while confining themselves to clinical study and pathological anatomy, have shown that the *B. coli*, in passing through the human organism, does not assume the characters of Eberth's bacillus, as had been supposed, but that it preserves its own proper characters. It causes in man common-place lesions, and never those which are special to typhoid fever. We know that the *B. coli*, which is an ordinary inhabitant of our digestive tube, may, like the pneumococcus, become pathogenic, and cause acute pleurisy, suppurative peritonitis, cholera-like complications, and even suppurative infection of the urinary tract, according to Krogius, Renaut, and Achard.

From the technical point of view, Chantemesse and Widal have always maintained that the *B. typhosus* and the *B. coli*, though apparently similar, present only differences. In order to distinguish these two microbes, they give a simple and easy method of procedure, which consists in sowing the one or the other upon broth to which lactose has been added. Under these conditions, the *B. coli* causes bubbles of gas, which are always absent when the broth is inoculated with Eberth's bacillus.

The coagulating property (Widal), discussed under Sero-Diagnosis, closes the epoch of these discussions, and proves the specific nature of the *B. typhosus*.

Pathological Anatomy.—"Considering only the first steps in the pathological anatomy, we notice the invasion and the multiplication of the bacilli, and the struggle on the part of the phagocytes. Further, the fixed cells of the tissues, being incapable of destroying the microbe, submit to its attacks, and show granular, fatty, waxy, pigmentary, and other degenerations of varying nature and gravity. In addition to these lesions, we find changes depending on the physiology and structure of the vessels.

" The course of this process, when studied in any organ, may be summed up as follows : infiltration with bacilli, phagocytic reaction, circulatory changes, degeneration of the parenchyma, normal or abnormal repair (Chantemesse).

It is impossible to give a better sketch of the process. The characteristic changes in typhoid fever affect the small intestine, and are most marked in the isolated follicles and in Peyer's patches.

The mucous membrane of the small intestine is composed of reticular connective tissue, containing in its meshes a large number of lymphatic cells (His). The isolated or agminated closed follicles belong to this mucous membrane ; the former are rounded, and measure ½ to 1 millimetre in diameter, while the latter are flattened one against the other, and arranged in groups of twenty, thirty, fifty, or sixty, to form the Peyer's patches, which commence in the ileum, and become more numerous towards the termination of the small intestine. They are situated on the free border of the intestine, opposite to the insertion of the mesentery ; their prominence and their opaque nature render them conspicuous with transmitted light. They are elongated in form, and parallel to the long axis of the bowel ; their long diameter varies from a few millimetres to several centimetres, and their number from thirteen to fifty. Both the isolated follicles and the Peyer's patches are composed of reticular lymphatic tissue, which is very vascular and continuous with the adjacent tissue, without any limiting membrane.

Post mortem the intestinal lesions vary, according to the stage of the disease. They present the following peculiarities :

1. During the first, or so-called catarrhal, period, which lasts from four to five days, the mucous membrane is congested, and secretes diarrhœal fluid ; the isolated follicles stand out, as in cholera (psorenteria) ; and the Peyer's patches are swollen. During this period the bacilli, which abound in the mucus, enter the glands of Lieberkühn, and reach the deep layers of the mucous membrane either individually or in colonies. Some days later the follicles assume the appearance of hard and prominent buttons, and the Peyer's patches present two different forms—namely, hard and soft (Louis). The hard patches are resistant to the touch and very prominent, thus bearing witness to the severity of the process, which involves most of the follicles in the patch. The soft patches are less prominent and more supple to the touch, because the follicles in the patch are only in part affected. It is possible that they may represent a more advanced period

of the process. The patches called crimped, or reticular, owe their appearance to the unequal distribution of the inflammation in the follicles which make up the patch.

On section, the follicles and patches present an appearance resembling the tissue of the lymphatic glands. There is abundant proliferation of the adenoid tissue, and the lymphatic infiltration extends to the connective tissue around the glands, and to the deep layer of the mucous membrane. The tubular glands are elongated, doubtless because of the development which the septa undergo ; the vessels and the capillaries are engorged with blood, and thrombosis is frequent. During this period the bacilli have penetrated the follicles and Peyer's patches, and the phagocytes are present in abundance, but the most virulent bacilli are difficult to ingest and digest. The lymphatic vessels are blocked with leucocytes and bacilli. The bacilli enter the vessels, and are found in the submucous and even in the muscular coats.

2. **Ulceration** begins about the tenth day of the disease. The bacilli and their toxines, and the dystrophy consecutive to obliteration of the vessels, affect the fixed cells of the tissue and the leucocytes, which have accumulated there in numbers, causing granulo-fatty and vitreous degeneration, followed by necrosis and ulceration.

The ulceration takes place in successive stages, and often commences in the patches nearest to the ileo-cæcal valve. The mortification of the soft patches is slow and molecular, so that the resulting ulceration is not very deep. In the hard patches, on the other hand, the mortification seizes on the most prominent parts of the patch, and forms cores, markedly stained with bile, which is secreted in abundance at this period of the disease. Next, the dead portions become detached, and leave deep ulcerations, which sometimes reach the number of six or seven in a single patch, and which usually rest on the muscular coat of the intestine. The small ulcers are cupuliform, or oval ; the large ulcers are aligned in the long axis of the intestine, and may measure some inches.

The ulcerated surfaces are covered with fleshy buds. They are poor in typhoid bacilli, whose part is played, and rich in other organisms, which sometimes cause secondary infections.

The inflammation also attacks the connective tissue between the two muscular layers and the subserous tissue, and the intestinal peritoneum over the ulcerated hard patches is sometimes red, congested, and thickened. " It is certain that the infiltration of all the coats of the intestine by cells, as well as the softening and friability of the fibrous bundles, favour ulceration, which extends in depth towards the serous coat, and subsequent perforation (Cornil and Ranvier). The elimination of the sloughs and the embryonic structure of the vascular walls favour hæmorrhage.

In sixty out of 200 autopsies (Leudet) the large intestine presents typhoid ulcers, because it also possesses lymphoid tissue, and there are cases in which the lesion is exclusively situated in the colon (coleo-typhus).

3. Cicatrization of the intestinal ulcers takes place slowly, but complete repair occurs. It is sometimes followed by fibrous change, but stenosis of the bowel is never found. The surface of the cicatrized patches may remain pigmented for several years.

In some exceptional cases the intestinal lesions may be absent, or scarcely appreciable. In the fœtus they are wanting.

The **mesenteric glands,** which normally are no larger than a lentil, and are separated from one another, may be as large as a walnut in the first week of the disease. They form a tumour, composed of a chain of glands, in front of the vertebral column. During this period the glands are usually hard and globular. The microscope shows that the lesion consists in dilatation of the vessels, with considerable proliferation of lymphatic cells. At a later period, during the second week, the glands become soft and decrease in size. Those which correspond to the most diseased portions of the bowel are themselves the most affected. The change in the glands, however, appears to be independent up to a certain point, for very large mesenteric glands are met with, although the intestinal lesion is trifling. The retroperitoneal glands, and in some cases the bronchial and peripheral glands, are affected by the typhoid poison. The bacilli and the phagocytic reaction are seen in the glands, just as in the Peyer's patches.

The **spleen** is large, soft, friable, congested, and engorged with lymphatic cells. It is sometimes the seat of small hæmorrhages. Its normal weight is 5 ounces, but it may exceed 12 ounces in this disease. The lesions include infiltration by phagocytes, changes in the arteries, marked congestion, and swelling. They are caused by the bacilli, which swarm in the parenchyma from the very first. A drop of blood drawn from the spleen during the first ten days of typhoid fever always yields colonies of the B. typhosus.

The **liver** is slightly enlarged. Its colour resembles that due to advanced fatty degeneration. The cells show cloudy swelling or fatty degeneration. Numerous lymphoid nodules are found. The bacilli are present in large numbers in the portal vein and its capillaries. The bile-ducts and the gall-bladder show catarrhal changes, suppuration, or ulceration (B. typhosus and B. coli).

The changes in the **muscular system,** though frequent, but not constant, are vitreous (Zenker, Weber) or granulo-vitreous degeneration (Hayem), changes also found in other diseases, but rarely as marked as in typhoid fever. This muscular dystrophy, which has a predilection for certain muscles, does not always spare the heart, and two concomitant lesions are found on histological examination, the one affecting the muscular fibre and the other the small vessels. The muscular fibre loses its transparency and its striation. It becomes granular, and is infiltrated with fatty elements. The surrounding connective tissue and the perimysium are the seat of active proliferation, which fills the surface of the primary bundles. The tunica externa of the small vessels participates in this proliferation, and the tunica interna shows endarteritis (Hayem, Laveran). These changes are doubtless of importance in the production of the intramuscular hæmorrhages sometimes seen in typhoid fever. The *B. typhosus* is often found in the cardiac muscle (Chantemesse and Widal).

Pathological Physiology.—The discordance existing at the onset of the disease between the pulse-rate and the rise of temperature is an interesting peculiarity. The pulse beats less frequently than we should expect, considering the height of the fever. In some cases the rate may be diminished. Murchison saw a patient whose pulse was only sixty during the early stages of the fever. In the later stages of the disease, when the pulse becomes quickened on the verge of severe complications, this sign is so valuable that examination of the pulse has been considered as the keynote in the prognosis of typhoid fever (Liebermeister). To what are these two successive conditions in the working of the heart due ?

According to Chantemesse and Courtade, the action of the typhoid toxine is more clear in cold-blooded animals, because it is not disturbed by the severe phenomena of reaction that occur in warm-blooded creatures. A dose of typhoid toxine (fatal in a few hours) injected under the skin of a frog causes after a quarter of an hour general sluggishness, which hampers the animal's movements. They become more and more difficult, and the animal does not respond to any sensory stimulus. If the thorax is opened, the heart is seen to beat very slowly, and then to stop in diastole. While the paralysis lasts, we can show that the muscles react well to the faradic current. The poison attacks neither the terminal end-plates of the motor nerves (as can be proved by the classical experiment of Bernard) nor the nerve filaments, the excitation of which brings about the usual muscular contraction. The toxine first acts upon the spinal cord, and we know that section of the frog's head increases the reflex irritability of the cord. If this section is made on a frog poisoned with typhoid toxine, we see that the reflex irritability has disappeared, and yet the electrical excitation of the cord through the white tracts still causes strong contractions in the limbs. In the living animal, therefore, the typhoid poison at first acts upon the grey matter of the cord. We shall see that it affects later the nerve cells of the cerebral centres and of the cardiac ganglia.

Chantemesse and Lamy, employing defibrinated blood from a normal rabbit, in order to produce an artificial circulation through the heart of a tortoise, have found that the cardiac contractions remain perfectly regular for more than twenty-four hours. If the blood is taken from a rabbit which half an hour previously has received a fatal dose of typhoid toxine, it behaves, as regards the heart of the tortoise, in practically the same way as normal blood. Further, the same dose of toxine added (*in vitro*) to normal defibrinated blood no longer produces any effect. If the dose of toxine added (*in vitro*) is two or three times stronger, we witness after several hours the slow appearance in the heart of the tortoise of disturbances, characterized by slowness and feebleness of the beats, and, finally, arrest of the heart in diastole. These phenomena result from slow poisoning of the heart. When the heart is arrested in diastole, electric stimuli, massage, and the passage of fresh blood are unable to cause it to beat again. When the results have been less marked, the substitution of normal blood for the toxic blood allows the heart gradually to resume its work. The addition to the blood, *in vivo* or *in vitro*, of typhoid toxine then produces cardiac symptoms, characterized by slowing, enfeeblement, and arrest of the heart in diastole.

These effects of pure typhoid poison upon the heart explain the cardiac symptoms at the onset of typhoid fever. As regards the cardiac phenomena in the later stages of the disease, the experiments of Chantemesse and Lamy also furnish some information on this point. Indeed, if we take blood from an animal sufficiently long after the injection of typhoid toxine, while the animal is in the reaction stage—for instance, in the sheep when the fever reaches its maximum point, or in the rabbit when the temperature finally begins to fall—the effects of the artificial circulation through the heart of the tortoise are diametrically opposite to those above mentioned. This blood acts rapidly. It causes marked tachycardia and short systole, and the effects gradually disappear as if the blood, possibly through the influence of oxygen, lost the property of exciting the heart. It is sufficient to add a fresh dose of blood, taken from the animal suffering from fever, in order to reproduce the same effects of excitation in the heart of the tortoise.

Chantemesse and Lamy draw the following conclusions from their researches : (1) As the result of reaction, toxic substances are produced in the organism, but their properties are distinct from those of the toxine. These substances manifest themselves physiologically by effects which are opposite to those caused by the primary typhoid poison. (2) These new substances, once formed, are not amenable to treatment with antitoxic serum, which neutralizes only the primary typhoid poison.

Treatment.—The cold bath may be regarded almost as a specific in typhoid fever. I have studied carefully the action and the results of the cold bath for many years, both in hospital and in private practice, and I am ready to do the fullest justice to Brand's method. I am quite convinced that the cold bath is as efficacious in typhoid fever as is quinine in malaria or mercury in syphilis.

I would state, as the first principle, that every patient suffering from typhoid fever should be treated with cold baths. At the onset of typhoid fever, even though the rose spots have not yet appeared, every individual who is taken ill with fever, accompanied by headache, insomnia, epistaxis, loss of appetite, prostration, and a rising temperature, which reaches about 102° F. at night, is probably suffering from typhoid fever, and should be treated with cold baths. If we delay giving cold baths until spots have appeared and the temperature has reached 104° F., we lose valuable time.

Cold baths are most efficacious when they are given **at the very commencement** of the disease. I have often proved the truth of this statement. When we receive in hospital a patient who has had typhoid fever for twelve or for thirteen days, cold baths are not as efficacious as in a sufferer who has been treated at an earlier period. Cold baths have not only a beneficial action upon **the symptoms of the moment,** but they also have an action upon **the symptoms of the future**—that is to say, they change an attack of fever which would have been very severe into one of moderate severity. Unfortunately, we are often too slow in making our decision, especially in private cases.

The bath treatment does not only aim at removing complications which have already appeared ; it is employed to moderate the disease, to modify its course, and to lower the virulence of the bacillus. Accordingly, it is not a method of treatment reserved for special symptoms ; it practically comprises the whole treatment.

The bath is placed near the patient's bed, the temperature of the water being 75° F. The patient is placed naked in the bath, and water is added until the temperature gradually falls to 68° F. As the cold water is added, an equal quantity of water is drawn off from the bath. This procedure has the advantage of avoiding or lessening the discomfort and chill which accompany the bath given at 68° F. on commencement. The patient should remain in the bath twelve to fifteen minutes. Cold compresses are applied to the head, and the body and limbs may be rubbed.

On leaving the bath the patient, who has not been dried, is placed in a blanket, and well covered up. He is given warm tea with a teaspoonful of brandy, and then left quiet. The bath is nearly always followed by a feeling of comfort, sleep, perspiration, and marked fall of temperature.

Another bath is given three or four hours later, according to the case, the patient taking six or eight baths in the twenty-four hours. The number of baths is regulated by the condition of the patient and by the height of the temperature. If the general condition is good, if nervous symptoms are absent, and if the temperature does not exceed 104° F., or if it does not rise rapidly after the temporary fall which follows the bath, it will be sufficient to bathe the patient four times in the twenty-four hours. On the other hand, if the temperature is very high, and if it remains so in spite of the baths, or if the patient shows a tendency to ataxo-adynamia, the temperature of the bath must be lowered, and a bath given every three hours at 68° F., the temperature being gradually lowered to 60° F.

Balneotherapy must be continued during the whole period of the disease, but the number of baths is diminished and their temperature gradually raised in proportion as the fever falls and convalescence approaches.

If the patient has soiled the bath-water with fæces or with urine, it must be changed for the next bath. In the opposite case, it is unnecessary to change the water more than once in twenty-four hours. In the interval between the baths it is useful to place upon the abdomen of the patient cold compresses, changed frequently; but the patient should not be wakened if he is sleeping comfortably.

Let us next consider the contra-indications.

Are we to place the patient who is perspiring freely in the cold bath? In such a case, it is better to wait till the perspiration ceases.

Are we to put a patient suffering from bronchitis or from broncho-pulmonary congestion in the bath? Bronchitis in typhoid fever forms part of the morbid process, with or without secondary infection, and is, therefore, to be treated in the same way. In typhoid fever, as in measles of the typhoid form, I have remarked that the broncho-pulmonary symptoms are improved by cold baths.

Are we to place a patient who has intestinal hæmorrhage in the bath? I do not hesitate to do so. I have lost only three patients suffering from hæmorrhage and treated by cold baths. According to my experience, intestinal hæmorrhage is neither brought on again nor increased by the baths. Improvement follows, and success may be obtained even in cases which appear desperate. Accordingly, except for special reasons, and unless the hæmorrhage by its extreme abundance threatens to carry off the patient with syncope, I am of opinion that intestinal hæmorrhage is not a contra-indication to the cold bath.

Are feeble heart action, intermittence, and signs of myocarditis a contra-indication to the use of cold baths? They are if these signs be very marked, but we can modify them by treatment, and the cold baths are then again indicated.

Balneotherapy does not comprise the whole treatment of typhoid fever, and another indication of the highest importance must be fulfilled —namely, that of nourishing the patient. For this purpose, **nothing is better than milk diet,** which is at once food and drink, as well as being diuretic. In hospital my patients take in twenty-four hours 3 pints of milk, to which lime-water has been added. In addition to the milk, they are given 2 or 3 pints of pure fresh water, to which lactose, with citron, orange, claret, or champagne may or may not be added. If the patient cannot take milk, he is given meat, or vegetable broth and raw eggs, but nothing is so good as milk diet.

As the result of this treatment with cold baths, milk diet, and abundant fluid, the urine is clear, and the patient, who was passing only 12 or 13 ounces of thick urine, now voids 3 or 4 pints of practically normal urine. This abundant diuresis is one of the best features in prognosis. As long as the kidneys act well, even though the symptoms are severe, we may be quite satisfied, for the poison is almost eliminated, and severe complica tions are usually absent.

This method of treatment has changed the classical picture of typhoid fever. We rarely see the dry red tongue, sordes on the teeth, tympanitic abdomen, and general condition of stupor. The disease has changed its appearance, and its two great factors, **intoxication** and **infection,** are practically conquered. I may even say that, as a result of cold baths **given in good time,** severe complications have become much less common, thus lowering the death-rate. Laryngo-typhus, peritonitis, perforation of the bowel, and ataxic symptoms are seen much less frequently than formerly, and I have not seen a case of sudden death for several years, although I did so fairly often prior to this method of treatment.

Are these fortunate results due to the treatment itself, or do they result from a natural change in the cyclical evolution of the disease ? Is not typhoid fever less fatal than it was twenty years ago ? Has it become less virulent in nature ?* These hypotheses are admissible, for the history of medicine tells us that epidemic diseases appear to undergo not only changes in different years and seasons (medical constitution), but they also appear to undergo more lasting changes (Stoll's stationary fever). I am quite willing to admit this hypothesis, and I have respect for certain traditions which have been handed down to us by our forebears ; but I cannot forget that in a number of circumstances, and notably in the treatment of typhoid fever, the greatest progress has been realized. Systematic balneotherapy, when properly applied, has reduced to 5, 6, or 7 per cent. the mortality in typhoid fever, which was formerly 18 to 20 per cent., and in this respect immense progress has been realized.†

For the early headache we may give antipyrin or aspirin, cold compresses being applied to the head, and frequently changed.

Purgatives are indicated at the onset of the disease, but later, when ulceration is present, we must give only enemata or gentle laxatives, such

* I find that the epidemics of typhoid fever which we have dealt with in Paris have been more severe and fatal.

† It must, however, be remembered that in the last few years we have had in the country, as well as in Paris, very severe epidemics, with high mortality.

as manna, in doses of from 3 to 5 drachms in milk. In the case of constipation, I usually prescribe this mixture of milk and manna, and have often seen its beneficial action.

Diarrhœa is checked by lime-water, Sydenham's decoctum album, in doses of 5 ounces daily, or salicylate of bismuth in a daily dose of 30 to 160 grammes. Intestinal antisepsis (Bouchard), if rigorously employed, is very difficult to carry out, and is sometimes ill borne by patients.

In case of pulmonary congestion, dry-cupping of the thorax and of the legs may be employed. The cupping-glass is applied thirty or forty times morning and evening. Wet-cupping and leeches may also be used. Care must be taken to raise the bed, so that the patient is in the sitting posture.

The following draught, in spoonful doses, may be employed for intestinal hæmorrhage :

Water	℥cxx.
Syrup of rhatany	℥xxx.
Rabel water	℥ii.

If the heart is weak and the pulse is feeble and irregular, subcutaneous injections of caffeine should be given.

Musk (10 grains), ether, chloral, and bromide of potassium are of considerable service in the nervous forms with ataxia.

In **adynamic** cases, with a tendency to collapse, we must employ tinctures of kola, coca, or cinchona, acetate of ammonia, brandy, subcutaneous injections of ether, and rubbing with alcohol.

I would recommend, provided the kidneys are normal, injections of serum, repeated several times during the day. I usually add benzoate of caffeine. For further details, see the Appendix on Therapeutics.

Quinine should be reserved for special cases in which the fever appears to show a malarial type. As I have explained the treatment of typhoid peritonitis and of paratyphoid appendicitis in detail, I shall not refer to it again.

Bedsores should be washed with a weak solution of hot boric acid, or with a solution of sublimate (4 in 1,000), and dusted with powdered cinchona.

The details given as to the pathogenesis of typhoid fever show clearly what prophylactic measures must be employed. As soon as an epidemic appears in a house, in a camp, or in a school, the patients must be isolated, the healthy removed, and an active search made for the origin of the disease, in order to remove it.

Serotherapy.—Serotherapy in typhoid fever is based on the experimental fact that animals may gradually become accustomed to doses of typhoid poison capable of killing healthy animals, and that from this time their blood has acquired properties antagonistic to those of the typhoid virus.

The problem at issue is to know whether the serum of immunized animals may profitably be injected into persons suffering from typhoid fever, and what is the measure of its efficacy.

Several poisons are present in the bacillus of typhoid fever, just as in all pathogenic microbes. The poison upon which the peculiar symptoms of typhoid fever in man depend was isolated first by Chantemesse. It has the characteristic of being very sensitive to oxygen. It multiplies rapidly in certain culture media, and is destroyed very quickly by contact with air. The effects produced by injecting it into animals have been studied by Chantemesse and Balthazard. The soluble toxine, when injected into the blood, has little effect on the red corpuscles, but shows an energetic action on the white blood-corpuscles, and especially upon the polynuclear cells. If a rapidly fatal dose is given, it produces hypoleucocytosis, which increases till death. With a smaller dose, the initial destruction of polynuclear cells is followed by a hyperleucocytic reaction.

In the **spleen** the toxine produces a double series of changes. In the first place, it increases the number and the size of the macrophages which are present in the pulp and in the lymphatic follicles, and causes them to ingest and to destroy the white and red corpuscles poisoned by the toxine.

In the second place, it causes a new formation of the elements of the lymphogenous series in the follicles and in Billroth's cords, thus constituting an act of repair.

In the **lymphatic glands** and **Peyer's patches** the poison produces the same hypertrophy as in the spleen (Balthazard), calling into activity the macrophages, which are soon filled with red cells, and causing enlargement of the lymphocytes and rapid multiplication of the cells of the follicles.

The **bone-marrow** becomes the seat of great activity. Its usual yellow tint gives place to a reddish-violet colour when the intoxication is fatal, and blood flows out on section. The red corpuscles pass through the broken cells of the capillaries, invade the intravesicular bands, and check the cellular proliferation. In the slighter forms of poisoning, however, we find that the marrow rapidly gives birth to polynuclear corpuscles destined to replace those destroyed by the toxine.

In the **intestine,** besides abundant diarrhœa, we may note dilatation of the vessels, œdema of the connective tissue of the villi and of the sub-mucosa, as well as an increase in the epithelial cells of the mucous membrane.

In the **liver** congestion is seen, with cloudy swelling and fatty degeneration of the cells. The amount of glycogen is diminished, and the lecithin accumulates (Balthazard).

The **kidney** is especially affected by the typhoid toxine. The most frequent changes comprise degeneration of the cells of the convoluted tubules, abrasions, blocking of the tubules with amorphous débris and cylindrical casts, glomerulitis, and in chronic cases fibrous changes.

If we compare the preceding lesions with the pathological anatomy of human typhoid fever, we cannot mistake the close resemblance.

Immunization of horses by repeated injection of a similar toxine requires much time if we desire to avoid all danger, and if we are anxious to make certain that the blood of the animal furnishing the material is quite free from any toxic property.

Serum thus obtained possesses great agglutinative power, and on injection into animals immunizes them against doses of living bacilli or of soluble toxine which prove fatal to the control animals.

If we inject the same dose of typhoid bacilli under the skin of the ear in several rabbits, of which some have been given 2 or 3 c.c. of serum nine hours previously, while others **have been given the serum several hours previously,** we notice after eight to ten hours that the microbes swarm in the ear of the control rabbits just as in broth culture. In the rabbits which have been given serum the bacilli are for the most part engulfed by the leucocytes, and undergo rapid destruction. The preventive injection of serum, which renders the microbes sensitive, constitutes, therefore, an anti-infectious as well as an antitoxic treatment. Serum injected as a preventive from two to twenty-four hours before the toxine protects the rabbit against three or four times a fatal dose. The animals then behave as regards leucocytic changes just as do rabbits immunized by small and repeated injections of toxine.

When the serum is injected **at the same time** as the toxine, its action is less efficacious, since animals which have received more than twice the fatal dose succumb. The initial destruction of the leucocytes is not immediately prevented. The leucocytic reaction, however, takes place earlier and to a greater extent than in the control animals. The intense congestion which impedes the production of leucocytes in the control animals is much less marked, and the bone-marrow shows considerable activity at the end of ten hours. Consequently, the antitoxic serum renders the leucocytes less sensitive to the noxious action of the toxine, and increases the reaction of the blood-forming organs.

When the serum is injected **after** the toxine, it is less efficacious in proportion as the time elapses between the penetration of the toxine and that of the serum increases. When the intoxication of the elements of resistance is too advanced, the favourable blow produced by the serum no longer occurs with the same power, whence the indication to inject the serum into man as early as possible. This essential point has been brought out in all the experimental researches.

The **duration of the preventive action** of the serum, determined experimentally, is over six and under fifteen days. The duration of the immunity conferred by an injection of serum is not longer than ten to twelve days.

We have still to examine the action of this serum on a patient with typhoid fever. From the first, however, the physician must bear in mind two points which result from experimental facts. On the one hand, the serum shows its full power only when it acts upon an organism which has all its forces, and which is not profoundly intoxicated, whence the indication to intervene as early as possible ; on the other hand, in the case of profound intoxication, it does not appear useful to inject large doses. Again, we must be afraid of preventing the reaction, and we must give a small dose which will not disturb the leucopoietic apparatus, which is incapable of making suddenly too great an effort. The recovery of the patient will be slower, but it will result from the assistance given to the normal processes of defence. The resistance will be increased. It is evident that the employment of this serum demands accurate clinical knowledge on the part of the physician, as well as a knowledge of the proper technique and of the resources of the remedy. We must remember that it is chiefly effective against the cause of the disease. This serum is anti-infectious and antitoxic, but less so than in the case of antidiphtheritic serum ; and therefore the toxic symptoms, properly called, should be treated with cold baths in addition to the actual serum. The two modes of treatment are not exclusive, but rather interdependent.

The treatment of typhoid fever by serotherapy and by cold baths has been carried out in Chantemesse's wards for some years past. Every patient, without exception, to the number of 350, has been treated by this method. Thirteen died, giving a total mortality of less than 4 per cent. In Josias's wards eighty children were thus treated in a systematic manner. Two died—one from perforation of the intestine, on the same day as the injection, and the other from laryngo-typhus. Patients treated before the seventh day have always recovered, and the fever has been shorter and the cure more rapid the sooner the injection of serum has been made after the onset of the disease. We thus become reconciled to the experimental results of so-called preventive injection, since typhoid fever in man only causes gradual changes in the organs.

In his communication to the Congress of Hygiene at Berlin (1907), Chantemesse gave his latest figures. In six years 1,000 cases of typhoid were under treatment in his wards. The death-rate was 4·3 per cent. These figures are conclusive.

Independently of the results furnished by the diminution in mortality, the action of the serum, says Chantemesse, shows itself in the course of the various symptoms. In sixty-one cases treated on the fourth or on the fifth day, apyrexia resulted in a few days. In the severe forms the defervescence is less rapid, but it is exceptional if the patient cannot begin to **dispense with baths** three or four days after the injection. The duration of the cold-bath treatment, which is sometimes very long in patients treated by the baths alone, is thus much shortened. After the injection the blood-pressure rises and the quantity of urine increases. Accordingly, it is necessary with serum to stop all medication which increases the blood-pressure, and especially caffeine. The serum does not cause albuminuria. The general condition improves as soon as the temperature falls. Perforation does not occur in patients who receive injections before the seventh day—at least, it has never been seen in the large number of persons thus treated.

The bridle action of the serum on the course of typhoid fever is seen with great clearness in relapses. After twelve days, the benefit of immunity secured by treatment disappears, and a relapse occurs. A fresh injection of serum then prevents its development or moderates it, giving rise to defervescence by lysis. A fact worthy of notice was present nine times in 350 cases. Some patients suffering from typhoid fever were given serum at the commencement of the disease—about the fourth or the sixth day. The disease ended in less than a week, the temperature fell to normal, and the recovery was apparently perfect.

Nevertheless, after two months in two cases, three months in three cases, and six months in four cases, following a chill, overwork, or poisoning by tainted meat, the typhoid fever reappeared, and ran quite a benign course. This example, in which the microbes were checked and rendered latent by the injection of serum, deserves attention from the point of view of the pathological physiology of the disease.

Whatever may be the future of antityphoid serum, which must still be submitted to prolonged observation, we cannot forget that it forms a powerful method of treatment, attacking the very cause of the disease.

II. TYPHUS FEVER.

Ætiology.—The principal centres of typhus in Europe are Ireland and Silesia. The disease readily spreads from Ireland to England, where typhus and typhoid fever are both found. From Silesia it spreads to neighbouring countries, and the epidemics of typhus in Berlin were, in Virchow's opinion, due to this source. We have had typhus in France at different times, but it was imported from abroad. In 1856 it followed the return of our soldiers from the Crimea.

It has appeared several times in Brittany since 1870 : at Riantec (1870-1872), Rouisson (1872-1873), the Isle of Molène (1878), the Isle of Tudy (1891); lastly, in 1891-1892, it broke out in the prison of Nanterre, and from there spread to Paris. Some months previously Leloir had seen cases at Lille, and its presence was ultimately notified at Beauvais, Amiens, Havre, etc.

Typhus is both epidemic and contagious. The contagion has been proved on many occasions. In the Crimea the mortality from typhus was 12·88 per cent. among the medical staff, while it was only 0·47 per cent. among the combatant officers (Laveran). In the last epidemic in Paris the hospital attendants especially suffered. Netter believes that the contagion is effected by contact, but Chantemesse, on the other hand, puts it down chiefly to drying of the sputum and to the inhalation of the dust thus produced.

Hava (1888) traced the development of typhus to a strepto-bacillus, but Cornil and Babès think that it is only an organism of secondary infection. Calmette and Thoinot, in the epidemic of the Island of Tudy, found in the blood from the heart and from the spleen abnormal elements, including mobile granules and threads which were mobile or united with the red blood-corpuscles. These elements resemble those found in the blood of patients suffering from typhoid fever, erysipelas, anæmia, and even of healthy persons. It is possible that they are formed at the expense of red corpuscles in process of destruction.

Typhus breaks out among armies in the field, in convict stations, in prisons, and on ships, where no previous cases have occurred. Overcrowding, poverty, dirt, privation, and fatigue are generally potent factors in the hatching of typhus.

Jaccoud, in a remarkable report on an epidemic of typhus which he saw during a long voyage, arrived at a conclusion " that the accumulation of animal products in a state of fermentation or decomposition may cause an outbreak of typhus, apart from any human overcrowding."

Symptoms.—After an incubation period lasting about ten days, the disease appears suddenly in most cases, although it may be preceded by a prodromal period.

Invasion.—The onset is sudden, with a chill, immediately followed by headache, tremors in the limbs, and vertigo. Vomiting is not rare. The prostration is extreme, the conjunctivæ are injected, the pulse frequent, and the temperature may reach 104° F. on the evening of the first or of the second day. Insomnia, restlessness, delirium, and suicidal mania may be added to the above symptoms. The course of events is not always continuous. Alternating improvement and aggravation may occur. Bronchial catarrh is often added to the nervous complications which dominate the clinical picture. We sometimes see broncho-pulmonary symptoms, which may induce error as to the nature of the disease. The temperature shows but a slight morning remission.

The period of invasion is sometimes preceded by prodromal symptoms :

lumbar pain, headache, lassitude, injection of the face, and hesitation in speech.

Eruption.—The eruption of typhus appears between the third and fifth days, commencing in the abdomen, and invading all the body, except the face. It is characterized by flat or papular rose-coloured spots, which are usually isolated, being confluent only in rare cases. They fade for a moment on pressure. The exanthem changes in character after two or three days, many of the spots being transformed into small petechiæ, which do not fade on pressure (petechial typhus). In some cases slight desquamation follows the eruption. In certain epidemics, and especially in mild cases, the eruption is absent. All the symptoms increase in severity at the time of the eruption. " Violent delirium, with a tendency to suicide " (Jaccoud), is frequent in the severe forms of typhus, though very exceptional in typhoid fever.

A typhoid condition of torpor and stupor follows the period of restlessness. The patient lies on his back, hardly recognizing those around him, and mumbles in an unintelligible manner. Constipation is the rule, and the abdominal symptoms, which are almost constant in typhoid fever, are absent in typhus. The urine is scanty, and often contains albumin.

Combemale has noticed upon the skin a whitish dust, formed of dry fatty acids, in those patients who are affected with acute nephritis.

Typhus lasts from eight to ten days in mild cases, and from twelve days to a fortnight in severe ones. Defervescence is often sudden, and takes place within twenty-four hours. It is accompanied by perspiration, sleep, and a feeling of comfort—it is, in fact, a true crisis. In other cases defervescence takes three or four days. Typhus may cause various complications in the nervous system; motor troubles, such as paresis of the upper or of the lower limbs ; abolition of the patellar or of the plantar reflexes ; inco-ordination of movements ; and trophic troubles, with acute bedsores. These nervous troubles appear to be due to spinal lesions, characterized by microscopic interstitial hæmorrhages, and by a vesicular condition of some of the motor cells in the anterior cornua.

In spite of the sudden return to health, convalescence is, as a rule, long, and the patient is liable to pleuro-pulmonary inflammation, multiple abscesses, otitis media, gangrene of the extremities, parotiditis, and erysipelas, which may, moreover, supervene in the course of typhus.

Diagnosis—Prognosis.—The principal elements in the differential diagnosis between typhus and typhoid fever are the sudden onset and the stupor, which is more marked than in typhoid fever ; the absence of meteorism ; the constipation ; the abundance and the general distribution of the rash, its petechial character, and the rapid recovery which often takes place by crisis. Further, typhus attacks patients at a more advanced age than typhoid fever. It is much more contagious than the latter, and it especially affects vagrants, prisoners, and armies in the field. Certain malignant eruptive fevers (measles, scarlatina) are accompanied by adynamia as marked as in typhus, but the distribution of the eruption and the course of the disease differ sufficiently to prevent error. **Sero-diagnosis** (Widal), described in detail in the preceding section, will remove all doubts, and clinch the diagnosis.

The mortality of typhus varies according to the epidemic, and to the circumstances which have given rise to the disease, thus explaining why the mortality varies from 15 per cent. to the high rate of 50 per cent. Every degree of severity is seen between the benign cases, which recover in a few days, and the severe forms to which I have alluded in my description. Death usually occurs about the end of the second week, but in severe epidemics malignant cases are seen, causing death as early as the third day (typhus siderans).

Pathological Anatomy.—The lesion of Peyer's patches is a change special to typhoid fever. Typhus presents no characteristic anatomical lesions. The spleen, as in all cases of severe pyrexia, is enlarged, the muscular fibres are degenerated, and the same change is seen in the heart muscle, which is flabby and pale. The blood is abnormally fluid.

Treatment.—Prophylactic treatment must be rigorously employed. Patients must be isolated in well-aired apartments, and all contaminated media thoroughly disinfected.

The treatment of typhus may be summed up in tonics, alcohol, cold sponging, sedatives, and restricted diet. Warm baths at 90° F. give good results. Injections of artificial serum may be employed with advantage.

III. RELAPSING FEVER.

Relapsing fever is a specific, contagious, and epidemic malady proper to man. It is due to the presence of a micro-organism of the blood—**Obermeier's spirillum**—and is characterized clinically by the succession in a well-defined cycle of two acute febrile attacks, with a regular temperature curve.

History.—The old descriptions confounded relapsing fever with the other continuous fevers, and in particular with typhus, to which, indeed, it has some relation ; the chief centres of both diseases are found in the same regions, and their epidemics are almost always associated. They differ clinically in numerous points, and there is not the least doubt as to the specific nature of relapsing fever at the present time, because we know the infectious agent concerned.

Craigie and Henderson, of Edinburgh, definitely separated this disease from typhus during the Scotch epidemic of 1843. Since that time recurrent fever has been studied by Irish, Scotch, German, and Russian physicians, who have been able to watch it in the countries where it is especially prevalent. The discovery of the spirillum by Obermeier has been followed by numerous experimental researches, which I shall have occasion to quote in the course of this section.

Ætiology.—Recurrent fever has a special geographical distribution. Its chief endemic centre is Ireland, and it has been imported thence in epidemic form into Scotland in 1843, into England, and even into the United States. Another more extensive centre comprises the shores of the Baltic, Finland, the Western Provinces of Russia, Poland, and the North-East of Germany. From this centre certain epidemics invaded Galicia, Bohemia, Saxony, and Bavaria, spreading to the banks of the Rhine, and appearing even in the Belgian portion of Flanders. At the present time the number of cases seen in Germany is constantly diminishing, and France, Switzerland, Italy, and Spain have so far remained free from the disease. The malady is, further-more, endemic in the South of Russia, on the borders of the Black Sea, and in Roumania. It has also been seen in Egypt, Abyssinia, India, China, etc.

Numerous proofs of the great contagiousness of this disease are furnished by all these epidemics. The contagion appears to proceed either directly from the patient or by contact with clothes, linen, and other articles. During the Edinburgh epidemic of 1843 the physicians and the hospital attendants suffered to a marked degree. During epidemics it is common to see small centres, limited to a house or to a family, which show clearly the mode of contagion. Overcrowding and famine were looked upon by Murchison as the cause of this affection (**famine disease**), but they are only predisposing factors, preparing the soil for the infective germ, which must enter the organism in order to produce the disease.

Symptoms.—Recurrent fever is chiefly seen in young people, and its onset is extremely violent. A healthy individual is seized with a sharp chill, and feels sudden general malaise, which, as it were, roots him to the spot. He is sometimes quite incapable of standing upright. He suffers from violent headache, severe backache, and acute pains in the trunk and in the limbs. Nausea and vomiting appear, the skin is burning hot, the face is injected, the pulse is quickened, and the temperature rapidly rises to 104° F.

The nature of the attack is clearly marked upon the first day of the disease. The headache and the pains in the limbs are persistent and intense, producing most troublesome insomnia. The patient is anxious, and sometimes restless. The mental powers, however, are clear, and the con-dition of stupor present in typhus and typhoid fever is not seen, although in a few days transient delirium may supervene. Nausea and vomiting of bile may be only slight. Constipation is the rule. The patient's face is red and injected, and his eyes are bright. The respiration is at times slightly quickened, the tongue remains moist, and is covered with a thin fur, and some vesicles of herpes may in rare cases appear upon the lips. The skin is dry and burning; the pulse is full, bounding, and rapid, the rate being about 120.

No eruption is seen, but a few insignificant petechiæ or rose-coloured spots may appear upon the abdomen. The epigastric region is particularly tender on palpation, especially near the border of the ribs, both on the right and left sides. The **spleen** undergoes rapid and marked increase in size. It can be felt below the false ribs. The stethoscope may reveal a soft systolic murmur. The liver is but slightly increased in size. Auscultation of the lungs sometimes reveals the signs of pulmonary congestion.

The urine is of a dark colour, and the excretion of urea is much increased. In about a third of the cases albuminuria is found, and the microscope shows red corpuscles and cylindrical casts, which are said to be fairly common (Obermeier). Kannenberg has found the spirillum in the urine. Jaundice is frequent, and is usually seen in severe cases accompanied by delirium. It commences on the third, fourth, or fifth day, appearing first in the conjunctivæ, and rapidly becoming general, but it diminishes very quickly, and soon disappears. It is sometimes accompanied by a general bilious condition, with vomiting of greenish and blackish matter. It is important to remember that the jaundice is not due to retention. The bile continues to flow into the intestine, and the stools remain coloured.

During this time, whether jaundice is or is not present, the temperature remains between 104° F. and 106° F. It may even reach 107° F. The morning remission is slight, and does not exceed 1°. There is often recrudescence of fever before the appearance of the phenomena which will mark the terminal crisis of the attack. The thermometer may then show a reading of 108° F.

These symptoms usually last a week, but the attack may last only three days, or may be as long as twelve days. The final **crisis** then takes place as suddenly as the onset of the attack appeared : profuse sweating, abundant urine, and a fall of temperature to 98° F., or sometimes to 95° F. The pulse becomes normal, the pains disappear, and the patient experiences only a somewhat marked feeling of fatigue. The appetite returns, and after two or three days the patient thinks that he is cured. The spleen may have diminished in size, but it often remains much hypertrophied (Griesinger).

A fresh phase, which is quite characteristic, and which has given the disease its name, appears five, six, or seven days after the end of the crisis (sometimes earlier—viz., two or three days; sometimes later, as long as two weeks). The patient is again seized with a chill, extreme malaise, headache, pain, and nausea. The pulse is quickened, and the temperature rapidly rises to 104° F. This second attack is an exact reproduction of the first attack. As a general rule, the second attack does not last so long as the first one, and after three, four, or five days the terminal crisis appears suddenly.

The crisis of the second attack in most cases means the end of the disease. The fever has been **once recurrent,** and there has been only a single relapse. In some cases, however, after a fresh period of apyrexia, a second relapse occurs, which is shorter than the first one. Four or five successive attacks may be seen in exceptional cases (Moszutkowsky).

Recurrent fever generally ends in recovery, and death only results from complications. The immunity acquired by a first attack is not always lasting, as recurrence may be seen after some months. In this case there is sometimes only a single attack.

Forms—Bilious Typhoid Fever of Hot Countries.—Griesinger, who has studied this affection during an epidemic in Egypt, has shown its relation to relapsing fever, and has demonstrated that it is a form thereof, modified by the appearance of certain severe typhoid symptoms, with jaundice. The onset is as sudden as in the ordinary form, and the jaundice appears about the fourth or the fifth day, being accompanied by nervous symptoms. The patient soon falls into a state of prostration. The tongue and lips are dry, and covered with sordes, diarrhœa appears, the pulse becomes slow, and death usually takes place in a typhoid condition, being often due to the complications so frequent in this form.

Complications—Prognosis.—Epistaxis, cutaneous hæmorrhage, bleeding from the gastro-intestinal tract, cerebral hæmorrhage, and metrorrhagia may occur in the course of relapsing fever. Uterine hæmorrhages are especially serious in pregnant women. Detachment of the placenta and miscarriage, which is a characteristic feature of relapsing fever, may be followed by profuse and fatal hæmorrhage, and the fœtus almost always succumbs.

During convalescence we may see ocular symptoms, which are usually unilateral (Mackenzie), and comprise retinitis and **iridochoroiditis,** which are transient affections, receding slowly, but leaving no other results.

Acute **myocarditis** may cause fatal syncope. **Rupture of the spleen** is another complication special to relapsing fever, and worthy of notice because it accounts for 20 per cent. of the fatal cases. The patient dies from intra-peritoneal hæmorrhage. In other cases the ·presence of small abscesses in the tissue of the spleen produces general peritonitis.

The other complications are sacral bedsores, subcutaneous abscesses, diffuse cellulitis, parotiditis, arthritis, etc.; they are due to common secondary infection. It is necessary to dwell upon the complications which may arise in the respiratory tract. In 12 per cent. of the fatal cases œdema of the glottis results from laryngeal perichondritis, but broncho-pneumonia, and more often lobar pneumonia, are fatal in relapsing fever, and about 20 per cent. of deaths must be attributed to them (Ponfick). Pneumonia generally appears about the end of the first attack, and then runs its own course in a soil which is profoundly weakened.

It is well to remember that all these complications are exceptional in the ordinary form, and that the prognosis of recurrent fever is rarely grave except in the delirious form of tropical countries. The mortality varies much in different epidemics, of which some are remarkably benign, while others are very fatal (St. Petersburg, 1864, 10 per cent.). The mean mortality is given as from 2 to 5 per cent., and the German statistics show that these figures have a tendency to progressive diminution.

Pathological Anatomy.—Post-mortem examinations of persons who have died from relapsing fever show, in the first place, lesions which have been the direct cause of death (pneumonia, broncho-pneumonia, laryngeal lesions, etc.). At times small foci of cerebral hæmorrhage, hæmorrhagic lesions in the stomach and in the small intestine, and exceptionally in the large intestine, are also found. But the lesions special to relapsing fever affect other organs. The kidneys are large and soft, and the medullary substance is of a greyish colour. The myocardium is flabby, friable, and of a dirty grey colour, like that of dead leaves. The other striated muscles show similar changes. Small yellowish, softened nodules are found in the bone-marrow. The liver is large and altered in colour, but the most characteristic lesions are found in the spleen.

The **spleen** is commonly five or six times larger than normal. The capsule is stretched, and sometimes torn near the hilum. On section, the parenchyma is softened, of a bright red, and studded with grey or with yellowish points, which are the corpuscles of Malpighi. The appearance is, therefore, somewhat analogous to that of the typhoid spleen. These little yellowish points are sometimes true miliary abscesses. Hæmorrhagic infarcts (attributed to obliteration of the vessels by masses of degenerated cells) may also be found, and may end in suppuration, with the formation of large abscesses.

The spleen in relapsing fever shows two kinds of histological changes— hypertrophy of the corpuscles of Malpighi, and formation of leucocytic masses in the spleen pulp. The cells of the corpuscles of Malpighi multiply exceedingly. Those in the centre sometimes undergo degeneration, which results in the formation of a small miliary abscess. The leucocytic masses (inflammatory lymphomata of Roudnef), which are scattered through the pulp, and are very variable in size, are said to appear in each attack (Sondakewitch). They are considered by Ponfick as characteristic of relapsing fever. In some cases they disappear, but in others their centre necroses (in 40 per cent. of the cases, according to Griesinger), and in this manner other small abscesses are formed. The spirillum is very abundant in all these foci.

Diagnosis.—The sudden onset, with prostration, general pain, rapid rise of temperature, marked swelling of the spleen, absence of eruption, co-existence of jaundice, attacks of apyrexia, and relapse, are such characteristic symptoms that there can scarcely be doubt in the diagnosis of relapsing fever, especially during an epidemic. In the absence of any epidemic, however, the sudden onset may be set down to influenza, dengue, gastric trouble, etc. Attacks of intermittent fever also commence with a severe chill, and the spleen is large and hard, but inquiry into the patient's past history at once decides the question of malaria. The coexistence of jaundice, especially in warm climates, may closely simulate the biliary form of malaria or even of yellow fever. **Typhus** is especially liable to be confounded with relapsing fever, and this is the more likely, because both diseases are seen in the same regions, and epidemics of them are usually associated. And yet the distinction is not really a matter of difficulty. The onset of typhus is less violent, and is preceded by slight prodromata. The temperature reaches a high degree much less rapidly ; the abdominal rash is generally present on the fourth or on the fifth day ; the spleen is rarely enlarged ; lastly, the temperature curve is different, and the duration of the disease is longer.

Besides, in any doubtful case the diagnosis can be readily established by examination of the blood, in which the spirilla swarm during the attacks.

Bacteriology and Pathological Physiology.—During an epidemic of relapsing fever in Berlin in 1868 Obermeier discovered the pathogenic parasite in the blood of patients examined during the febrile attack. This was the first discovery of a pathogenic microbe in man. It was only in 1873, however, on the occasion of a fresh epidemic, that Obermeier published his discovery. He pointed out the filiform appearance, spiral shape, and great mobility of this micro-organism, and remarked that it is only met with during the febrile attack, and that it disappears in the apyretic stage.

Obermeier's discovery has been verified by numerous observers, and the parasite has been constantly found in relapsing fever, and, as it is present in no other disease, its special pathogenic action is therefore established beyond a doubt. Cohn gave it the name of *Spirochæta Obermeieri*, or *Spirillum Obermeieri*, because the morphological characters of this organism place it in the bacterial family of the spirochætæ.

To confirm the diagnosis of recurrent fever by discovery of the spirillum, it is necessary to examine the blood during the febrile attacks. After puncture with a needle, we can make two sets of preparations, which are examined in the fresh state without staining, and also after drying and staining. In the former the parasites which remain alive preserve their mobility. We see under the microscope, among the elements of the blood, long filaments of remarkable fineness, varying in length from 15 to 45 μ (from two to ten times the diameter of a red corpuscle), twisted in spirals, with eight to twenty turns, exceedingly mobile, altering their position by turning on their long axis, moving laterally, and pursuing the corpuscles which are in their way. At a temperature of 37° C. the spirilla preserve their mobility for a fairly long period. When the spirilla are scanty, preparations dried in air thould be examined. Günther's method is the best. A 5 per cent. solution of acetic acid is employed for a few seconds to dissolve the hæmoglobin of the red corpuscles, and is then neutralized by exposure to ammonia vapour. The preparation is stained with aniline gentian violet for a long time. The red corpuscles remain unstained, but the nuclei of the leucocytes and the spirilla appear of a violet colour. The latter are very numerous, clearly outlined, and are sometimes isolated, or at other times interwoven in groups.

By these methods we can follow from hour to hour the presence of the spirilla in the patient's blood. It has also been proved that, speaking generally, the spirilla are found in the blood of the peripheral veins only during the febrile phase. They are found at the onset of the attack, and sometimes, indeed, a few hours before, their number increasing up to the last day, and attaining its maximum on the day of the crisis, sixteen hours before the sweating stage. They diminish rapidly in numbers, and disappear at the moment of the precritical hyperthermia. Half an hour after the onset of the sweats they are no longer visible, although some authors have found them during the stage of apyrexia. During the relapse they reappear again in large numbers, and disappear afresh after the final crisis.

Every attempt to preserve cultures of the spirillum has so far failed, and we are therefore ignorant as to the phases of its development. Metchnikoff, however, has seen reproduction by transverse division, without any formation of spores. Its habitat is also unknown, but Klebs thinks that the parasites (fleas, bugs, etc.) so frequent in the rooms or the night-shelters occupied by the usual victims of relapsing fever play a part in the transmission of the spirillum. Tiktine has found the spirillum in the digestive tube of bugs. Klebs's opinion, however, remains hypothetical.

Apart from the usual **contagion,** the mechanism of which still evades our knowledge, the pathogenic action of Obermeier's spirillum in the blood of patients has been proved by a series of accidental and experimental discoveries. Pricks received at the autopsy of patients who have died from this disease have been sufficient to cause it. We may remember the fact that the phase of incubation—or, in other words, the interval between the prick introducing the spirillum into the blood and the clinical onset of symptoms—varies from three days and a half to eight days and a half.

Munch, in 1874, after inoculating himself with the blood of a patient in the stage of pyrexia, was attacked by relapsing fever. Moszutkuwsky, in 1876, performed inoculation upon a number of lunatics. The results were in every case positive, and the mean period of incubation was from five to eight days.

Relapsing fever is seen spontaneously only in man. The various laboratory animals are refractory to inoculation. Monkeys have been successfully inoculated (Koch, Carter, Metchnikoff, Soudakewitch, etc.), and experimental studies with this animal furnish very interesting information as to the pathological physiology of the disease. The inoculation, of course, only succeeds if made with blood taken during the febrile phase. After an inoculation period of about four days, symptoms analogous to those of relapsing fever in man appear—the same sudden onset, high temperature, etc.; but the attacks are shorter, and the second attack or relapse is very rare. During the febrile phase the blood of the inoculated animals contains spirilla in large numbers, and the animals, like human beings, acquire more or less lasting immunity after the first attack.

Metchnikoff, by killing inoculated monkeys at different phases of the disease, has proved the action of phagocytosis in recurrent fever, and the important rôle of the spleen in the defence of the organism against the infection. Ponfick was of opinion that if the spirilla, which are so numerous in the peripheral veins during the attack, disappear during the apyretic phase, a certain number of them are lodged in the abdominal viscera and especially in the enlarged spleen.

Metchnikoff has proved that the spleen contains a very large number of spirilla at the end of the attack and during the first days of apyrexia, but it is a particularly interesting point that the spirilla are then included in the leucocytes. During the attack the spirilla are extracellular, and phagocytosis does not appear to take place in the blood. When the precritical rise of temperature occurs, they disappear from the blood, and crowd into the spleen. Although alive and mobile, they are **engulfed by the microphages** (leucocytes with multilobular nuclei, etc.), which fight them, and bring about their gradual disappearance. This **intrasplenic phagocytosis,** which is exceedingly active, may bring about the end of the attack. Experimental research agrees well with the facts revealed by histological examination of the spleen in fatal cases of relapsing fever, and this examination has shown us the development of leucocytic masses in the pulp, and the proliferation of the Malpighian corpuscles, which are leucocytopoietic organs, and assist in phagocytosis. At this time the liver, kidneys, glands, and bone-marrow do not contain spirilla. The spleen, therefore, is said to be the exclusive seat of the phagocytosis.

Certain spirilla, however, preserve their virulence for some time after ingestion, as proved by the positive result of inoculation of a small portion of the spleen of an animal killed during the apyretic period (Metchnikoff); these active spirilla may determine the second attack in man.

Soudakewitch has confirmed the essential rôle of phagocytosis in the spleen by the following experiments : On the one hand, he inoculated nine monkeys with blood containing spirilla ; and, on the other hand, nine monkeys, in which splenectomy had been performed, with blood containing spirilla. The former recovered, but the latter died, and their blood contained enormous numbers of free spirilla, phagocytosis being absent.

Tiktine, on the other hand, has shown that inoculated monkeys may recover, even after previous splenectomy, and that animals immunized by a previous attack preserve their immunity even after removal of the spleen. The splenic phagocytosis, which is not doubtful, because it has been directly observed, would not, therefore, be the only means of defence of the organism against the spirillum.

Gabritchewsky of Moscow thinks that the principal rôle in this struggle may be attributed to the **bactericidal power of the serum.** He tries to prove the presence of bactericidal substances by test-tube experiments. He has found the spirilla immobile and deformed one to four hours after mixing a drop of blood taken from a patient during the crisis, and containing spirilla, with a drop of serum from a monkey during the period of apyrexia. He has studied the coefficiency of this bactericidal power with regard to the spirillum in man, and also the different phases of infection. He concludes that this coefficient increases during the disease, especially on the two days previous to the crisis, and that it reaches its maximum during the crisis by a prompt accumulation of bactericidal substances. According to Gabritchewsky, splenic phagocytosis commences only after this attenuation by fluids, although the spirilla may be already modified as regards their vitality ; certain germs, moreover, may assist in producing a relapse, favoured by the rapid enfeeblement of the bactericidal power of the serum after the crisis. This power reappears during the second attack, and persists, though more or less weakened, after recovery for months and years. In order to complete his theory and to make use of this bactericidal power, Gabritchewsky attempted serotherapy by means of a serum from a monkey which had just entered the stage of defervescence, and in which the blood might be considered to possess this immunizing power. Two other monkeys were simultaneously inoculated with blood containing spirilla : the one not treated by serum was sick for seventy-two hours, and had a relapse ; the other, to whom serum had been given, showed in forty-eight hours rapid defervescence, the spirilla were less abundant in the blood, and no relapse appeared.

Metchnikoff has criticized the experiments of Gabritchewsky, and thinks that they are not sufficiently clear to justify the conclusions of the

Russian author ; the results have been too variable to allow the deduction of general laws applicable to the process **in the living.** Metchnikoff has found that the spirilla do not lose their vitality in the blood before the crisis and the splenic phagocytosis. He considers, therefore, that it is not yet demonstrated that the refractory state (immunity) depends on the bactericidal power of the serum. Lastly, it may be remarked that, as regards serotherapy, we cannot deduce general results from the single experiment performed by Gabritchewsky.

Treatment.—It is of the highest importance to guard against contagion by every possible means ; hygiene of apartments, isolation of the sick, careful disinfection of the clothes, of the hands, of the linen, and of the articles which have been in contact with the sick. Although further researches are necessary before we are in possession of a specific treatment for the disease, we must, nevertheless, have recourse to systematic treatment, employing analgesics when indicated to diminish the pain, tonics or alcohol to sustain the general health, and cold baths to reduce the hyperpyrexia.

CHAPTER III

INFECTIOUS DISEASES PROPER TO MAN

I.—ERYSIPELAS OF THE FACE—STREPTOCOCCIA.

Bacteriology.—The infectious nature of erysipelas (ἐρυθρός, red; πέλλα, skin) and its microbic origin are well known. The agent which produces it is the streptococcus (Nepveu, Fehleisen). This microbe is both aerobic and anaerobic.

The streptococcus of erysipelas, like all streptococci, is a micrococcus, the elements of which are set end to end, so as to form small chains.

The chain may be short, containing only three or four elements, or it may be long and tortuous, containing eight or ten. In erysipelas, however, the chains are never very long; long sinuous chains, with thirty or forty elements, are seen on certain culture media. In some cases the streptococcus is reduced to two elements, coupled in the form of a diplococcus; the elements may even be isolated. All the elements of a chain are of practically the same size, especially in young cultures, but we sometimes find larger ones in the same chain. The streptococcus stains readily with aniline dyes; it is not decolorized by Gram.

On inclined tubes of gelatinized serum or of agar, placed in the oven at 37° C., cultures of streptococci appear in less than twenty-four hours in the form of a whitish, dusty seed-plot. These colonies show little tendency to increase in size. They are sometimes confluent along the course of the inoculation streak, so that they spread out in the form of tracts which have been compared to a fern-leaf.

Cultures on broth at 37° C. show the following peculiarities : The broth becomes turbid after twelve to fifteen hours, and clear after two or three days, when the whitish clots which made it turbid have fallen to the bottom of the tube. In broth cultures the streptococcus rapidly loses its virulence, and in a few days or in a few weeks its vitality is exhausted, thus forming a serious obstacle to experimental research. Marmorek, however, has found a culture medium upon which the streptococcus may preserve its virulence. This medium is **broth serum ;** its various compositions are:

(a) Broth, 1 part ; human blood-serum, 2 parts.
(b) Broth, 2 parts ; ascitic fluid or pleuritic serum, 2 parts.
(c) Broth, 1 part ; ass's serum, 1 part.

1694

The culture of the streptococcus on broth serum does not increase the virulence, but preserves it unaltered, an essential difference from other culture media, in which the virulence of the streptococcus rapidly diminishes. Broth serum is so favourable to the culture of the streptococcus that old cultures which are apparently dead, if sown upon ordinary broth or upon agar, recover their vitality if they are sown on broth serum. We shall see later, in the treatment of erysipelas by injections of serum, how these facts have been utilized.

Experimental Researches.—The rabbit is the animal chosen for this purpose. If a culture of streptococci taken from a case of erysipelas is inoculated under the skin of a rabbit's ear, typical erysipelas appears one or two days later. The ear becomes red and swollen, and feels hot. Chains of streptococci are found in the bullæ. The rabbit is sleepy and prostrate, the temperature reaches 104° F., and death may supervene before desquamation of the erysipelatous patch has taken place.

In some cases intravenous inoculation of the attenuated streptococcus produces infectious myelitis with paralysis (in about 6 per cent. of the cases), eschars, contractures, muscular atrophy, disorders of the bladder, and convulsions, in the rabbit. The spinal cord shows diffuse myelitis in the grey matter, and degenerative lesions in the white tracts. We can increase the virulence of the streptococcus by intravenous injection of this microbe in series or in large doses in rabbits (Chantemesse and Widal).

Streptococcia.—I have so far considered only the streptococcus of erysipelas, but my remarks are applicable to all streptococci, whatever be their nature and their origin. It has long been thought, and some authors are still of this opinion, that there are grounds for separating the streptococci into different species. Thus, to quote examples, it had been admitted primarily that the streptococcus of erysipelas (*Streptococcus erysipelatis*) can only produce this disease, and that the *S. pyogenes* can only produce pus ; but the former may produce pus, and the latter may give rise to erysipelas.

A classification based upon the morphological appearance of the streptococci has also been attempted : streptococci in small chains (*brevis*), streptococci in long chains (*longus*), and streptococci *en masse* (*conglomeratus*).

In reality, the various streptococci form a single species. The proof is : streptococci are present in the human body as ordinary saprophytes of the skin. They are absolutely harmless in the general conditions of existence, but the most trifling negligence in cutaneous asepsis during the course of an operation, the least scratch, may allow these harmless streptococci to enter the economy, where they find such a favourable culture medium that their exalted virulence may be shown by erysipelas, purulent infection, or by fatal streptococcia. Nevertheless, the streptococcus is the same, in spite of the diverse nature of the lesions.

Streptococci devoid of virulence are present in the nasal fossæ, in the mouth, and in the saliva as harmless inhabitants. They appear, in fact, to belong to a peculiar species. If, however, the virulence of these streptococci is increased, pathologically or experimentally, they acquire the most virulent properties. They may then cause erysipelas, suppuration, septicæmia, and infective endocarditis in animals, as Widal and Besançon have seen.

The experiments of Widal are quite conclusive. The same microbe, by an alteration of virulence, may produce at one time suppuration, at another time erysipelas. If the streptococcus taken from the pus is passed through the rabbit, the virulence is increased, the microbe loses its pyogenic properties, and becomes capable of causing erysipelas. This fact proves that the same agent may cause erysipelas and suppuration. It explains the pathogenesis of certain cases of phlegmonous erysipelas, as well as the reciprocal coincidence and contagion of erysipelas and of puerperal infection, seen in certain epidemics.

In short, all the streptococci of human origin may be referred to the same type. They may differ temporarily from this type, according to the soil and to the medium in which they are, but at a given moment they show their special aptitudes, and give rise in different cases to "erysipelas, lymphangitis, abscess, pus, phlegmasia, with its clot, cellular degenerations, hæmorrhages, and the false membrane in certain anginæ " (Widal).

By this adaptation to different kinds of life the streptococcus becomes modified in its virulence, and in some of its biological characters. New races of streptococci may thus arise in nature or in mankind without our knowledge, but the modification is never so complete as to end in a true change of form (Widal).

Description.—Facial erysipelas is usually ushered in by chills, malaise, headache, nausea, vomiting, and high temperature. As these symptoms may precede the appearance of the erysipelatous patch, erysipelas has been compared to an eruptive fever (Borsieri). In some cases erysipelas is preceded by painful enlargement of the submaxillary glands.

Erysipelas appears as a red and sensitive patch. The aperture of the nostrils, the angle of the eye, and the external ear are the usual starting-points. If the skin of the face or the scalp presents an excoriation (eczema, herpes), erysipelas usually commences at the excoriated spot. The patch soon becomes dark red, shiny, and painful. The skin is burning, tense, prominent, dry, and parchment-like. The redness does not completely disappear on pressure, as in erythema. The patch, when taken between the fingers, cannot be raised in folds, but is resistant and gives a sensation of thickening, due to the invasion of the dermis and of the subjacent tissue.

The erysipelatous patch spreads in an irregular manner, and presents at its invading edge a prominent border, clearly marked against the healthy parts. When the border disappears, we may say that the erysipelas has reached its limit. Its course is more or less rapid in different cases. When it begins at the root of the nose, it extends in a symmetrical manner to the cheeks, like a pair of spectacles. In its progress the disease dies out upon the parts first invaded. It may be limited to a part of the face, or it may affect the whole face, which then becomes unrecognizable. The red œdematous eyelids cover the eyeballs, the swollen and deformed nostrils are almost closed, the cheeks are swollen, and the ears are red, shiny, and double their normal size. The face thus deformed recalls the appearance of certain Chinese grotesques (Raynaud). The forehead, the cranium, the nape of the neck, and the neck itself are sometimes invaded. Upon the scalp the erysipelatous tint is not as dark as upon the face, but the pain is more acute.

In some cases the skin of the face is raised by a serous effusion, which collects in the form of vesicles. The fluid in the bullæ may become turbid, purulent, or hæmorrhagic. The pus collects in the form of an abscess. After rupture, the blebs become covered with thick yellowish crusts. The skin desquamates in patches, and the hair usually falls out when the disease affects the scalp. It does not end in baldness, although the scalp is sometimes much affected. The loss of the eyebrows may be permanent.

The disease usually lasts from six to ten days. The fever is high at night, with a more or less marked morning remission. In some cases it diminishes gradually, but in others it falls suddenly in one night. In some cases erysipelas, supposed to be at an end, revives. The fever reappears, and the disease lasts from a fortnight to three weeks.

A disordered condition of the digestive tract, with anorexia and constipation, succeeds the gastric troubles of the onset ; the urine is scanty and albuminous ; the headache is severe ; and the restlessness and delirium are sometimes very marked, especially when the scalp is affected.

Erysipelas of the Mucous Membranes.—The disease usually remains localized to the face, but it may affect the **mucous membranes** either **before** or **after** it has affected the face.

Angina and Stomatitis.—The mouth is rarely invaded. At most, it is but slightly affected by erysipelas, while the pharynx is one of the most frequent seats of the disease. Erysipelas of the pharynx—or, rather, of the throat (Lasègue)—is characterized by purple, shiny redness and severe angina. It is sometimes accompanied by bullæ, gangrene, and retropharyngeal abscess. It may spread to the face, either by way of the buccal mucous membrane, the nasal fossæ, or the lachrymal ducts (Peter).

Respiratory Tracts.—Erysipelas often begins in the nasal fossæ. The coryza is very painful, and is accompanied by acute fever and by adenitis of the cervical glands.   In some cases the rhinitis extends to the middle ear (deafness), reaching the mastoid cells and the meninges.

The **larynx** is invaded secondarily by erysipelas, but primary laryngitis has been seen.   The usual symptoms, when the larynx is affected, comprise great swelling of the mucosa covering the tongue, of the arytenoid region, and of the epiglottis with more or less rapid œdema, and severe dyspnœa.

Bronchopneumonia is well recognized since Straus's case was published :

A patient suffered from a mild attack of facial erysipelas, and the fever fell, but at the same time pain appeared in the right side ; erysipelatous pharyngitis and pneumonia at the right base were discovered ; the pneumonia invaded the whole lung ; albuminuria appeared, with slight jaundice and bleeding from the nose.   The patient died.   I have seen a similar case in a workman who was taken ill with pneumonia during the decline of facial erysipelas.   In Straus's case the autopsy proved that the erysipelas had invaded the trachea, the bronchi, and the lung.   Histologically the pneumonic exudate was composed solely of leucocytes without fibrin.   Rendu has reported a similar case, in which benign facial erysipelas had commenced at the angle of the eye.

In Mosny's case the pulmonary erysipelas was primary.   A servant who was attending her master suffering from erysipelas took bronchopneumonia, which proved fatal. The bacteriological examination revealed the presence of the streptococcus.

Complications—Nephritis.—Albuminuria is very frequent in the course of facial erysipelas, and the only evidence of the renal lesion is, as a rule, the presence of casts, and sometimes of streptococci, in the urine.   In other cases œdema and symptoms of acute uræmia may also be present.   Nephritis in erysipelas recovers, but the affected kidney may at some later period become the starting-point of Bright's disease.

Joint troubles are rarely associated with facial erysipelas.   In all cases it is a question of mild pseudo-rheumatic infection.   Nevertheless, synovitis of the tendon-sheaths of the wrist (Quinquaud) and suppurative arthritis have been seen (Aubrée).

Pericarditis is very rare.   In two cases with effusion streptococci in chains were found (Denucée).

Endocarditis is more common.   Although it is usually benign and transient, it may sometimes assume the character of infective endocarditis, and may lead to embolism, aphasia, and gangrene.

Streptococci have been found in the vegetations of the endocardium (Achalme).   This form of endocarditis has been reproduced experimentally. Erysipelas appeared in a rabbit which had been inoculated with the streptococcus.   The erysipelas recovered, but the animal died from endocarditis, and at the autopsy a large vegetation containing the streptococcus was found upon the mitral valve.

Pleurisy is exceptional.   It was present in two out of six cases which were inoculated by Fehleisen.

Erysipelas sometimes attacks the eye, and the following complications have been seen : Conjunctivitis, chemosis, keratitis, iritis, suppuration of the eyelids, and atrophy of the papilla, following obliteration of the central artery of the retina.

The ear may also suffer in erysipelas, which causes purulent catarrh of the tympanic cavity.

Meningitis is extremely rare. In three cases published by Roger the fibrino-purulent exudate contained the pneumococcus, with or without the streptococcus. Delirium in erysipelas is, therefore, due to the toxines or to alcoholism.

Prognosis.—In the great majority of cases erysipelas of the face is a benign disease. The nervous troubles and delirium need cause no alarm, and recovery is the rule. In fact, in about a third of the cases erysipelas is extremely slight and benign, so that the name primary attenuated erysipelas has been given to this form.

Erysipelas, however, may in some cases be extremely serious. Thus, erysipelas of the face may become **ambulant,** reaching the trunk or the limbs, and causing prostration and infection of the patient.

It must not be forgotten that erysipelas of the face may attack the pharynx, the larynx, the bronchi, or the lung, and cause severe inflammation of these organs, which justifies Cornil's assertion that erysipelas which goes in is more severe than erysipelas which comes out.

When erysipelas occurs in cachectic people, or in those suffering from Bright's disease, diabetes, abuse of alcohol, pneumonia, diphtheria, or typhoid fever, the prognosis is often grave, because of their impaired constitution, and the same remark applies to erysipelas contracted during the puerperium or in surgical operations.

The streptococcal infection may, then, be so intense that it shows its malignant nature either by a tendency to diffuse suppuration and gangrenous inflammation or by a typhoid condition, with ataxo-adynamic symptoms. In these infective cases of erysipelas the tongue is dry, the pulse is quickened, the patient is prostrated, the delirium is more or less violent, and retention or incontinence of urine is present. These cases are **very contagious.** They may become the origin of epidemic foci. Trousseau, with his marvellous sagacity, anticipating the explanation which bacteriological researches have now given, wrote a most lucid description of the pathogenesis of these malignant cases. "At the commencement of 1861, when a terrible epidemic of **puerperal fever** broke out in nearly every lying-in hospital, facial erysipelas, which is generally so slight, assumed severe proportions in a fair number of cases." This malignant character of erysipelas is also frequent when the contagion is transmitted from traumatic or surgical erysipelas. As a matter of fact, surgical erysipelas is, practically speaking, no longer seen, owing to the wonderful progress of antiseptic surgery ; but if we refer to former times, many persons have paid heavy tribute to facial erysipelas in the practice of surgery.

Erysipelas, in some exceptional cases, has appeared to be a fortunate complication, which brought about recovery in certain chronic diseases of the skin. Thus, in tubercular scrofula and ulcerative lupus an improvement, and even recovery, have been brought about by erysipelas. The injection of streptococcal toxines has caused a definite improvement in the local condition of lupus (Hallopeau and Roger).

As regards the prognosis of erysipelas, the blood-count (Chantemesse and Rey) gives important results. In severe cases we find general leucocytosis, so that the number of white corpuscles always exceeds 12,000 per cubic millimetre, and also an excessive proportion of polynuclear leucocytes, which may exceed 92 per cent. " The degree of leucocytosis, and especially the increase in the number of polynuclear cells, is in direct relation with the severity of the disease. On the other hand, the formation of numerous abscesses indicates a favourable prognosis. In 6,000 cases of erysipelas Chantemesse never saw death occur when abscesses supervened ; in 1,000 cases with spontaneous abscesses, or with abscess following the use of Marmorek's serum, recovery was the rule ; in 300 fatal cases observed by Chantemesse death did not supervene by reason of suppuration. Abscesses are, therefore, an indication of recovery, and may be compared to the abscesses of fixation, playing the part of the curative abscess which Trousseau described in erysipelas of the new-born.

Diagnosis.—The idea of erysipelas at once enters the mind if an individual presents a reddish and swollen patch upon the face. The face may show the gross appearance of erysipelas in other conditions—erythema produced by the application of carbolic acid, or only the emanation from thapsia plaster, dental inflammation, conjunctivitis, dacryocystitis, boils upon the lips and nose, urticaria, and impetigo. In all these conditions some portion of the face may simulate erysipelas by reason of its redness and swelling.

The **diagnosis,** however, rests upon the following signs : Erysipelas begins with fever, and, further, the erysipelatous patch has special characters. It is shiny, painful, and thickened, while it is also red, without intervals of healthy skin. This redness does not disappear on pressure, like that of erythema ; and, lastly, an essential point is that the limit of the erysipelatous patch is clearly marked from the healthy skin by a **prominent edge,** which is not found in erythema. Moreover, the streptococcus is the pathogenic agent.

Eczema rubrum, which is accompanied by redness and swelling of the face, at first sight resembles erysipelas ; but the disease, instead of gradually spreading, at once invades almost the whole of the face. The redness blends insensibly with the healthy parts. We can almost always discover some small vesicles, which itch acutely ; the fever is absent or very slight (Hardy).

Ætiology.—Erysipelas is contagious and epidemic. Any streptococcus possessing special virulence may cause erysipelas, the more surely if it grows on a soil favourable to its development. Consequently, it is not only erysipelas which may produce erysipelas. Erysipelas may also arise from puerperal infection, lymphangitis, and collections of pus. The pathogenic streptococcus may be conveyed by the fingers, by the linen, or by articles of any kind, and the germ enters more easily if the skin presents chafes, cracks, or abrasions. The flakes of skin in erysipelas are not virulent (Achalme).

The old name of idiopathic erysipelas should be preserved, because erysipelas, like many infectious diseases, may arise spontaneously. I must, however, explain this statement. Streptococci devoid of virulence are present in the mouth, in the nasal cavities, in the saliva, and in the skin. Under the influence of known or unknown causes, these inoffensive microbes may acquire a virulence which renders them pathogenic, as has been proved by experiments.

Further, our economy, our phagocytes, and our cells are not always in a proper state of defence against the hostile microbe. Consequently, on the one hand, exaltation of virulence in an inoffensive agent, and, on the other hand, weakness of the defence (overwork, diabetes, Bright's disease, menstruation, etc.), are the factors which explain the development of so-called spontaneous erysipelas.

A similar explanation is applicable to many infectious diseases, such as typhoid fever, pneumonia, and perhaps diphtheria. Morbid spontaneity, therefore, rises phœnix-like from its ashes, and will continue to occupy its place in the pathogenesis of diseases after a momentary eclipse.

Erysipelas does not confer immunity, and other attacks are frequent. " The persistence of the micro-organism of erysipelas in the tissues is as clear as that which is met with in old cultures, and its presence at a certain moment in the organism, where it is fixed, explains the pathogenesis of periodical erysipelas " (Leroy). Menstruation and the puerperal condition favour the return of erysipelas (*érysipèle à répétition*). Experimentally, vasomotor paralysis favours the rapid arrival of phagocytes, and opposes the development of erysipelas, while section of the sensory nerves favours infection.

Pathological Anatomy.—The coloration has almost disappeared from the skin of the cadaver, and the peripheral edge is but little prominent, although the skin is slightly œdematous, and preserves the imprint of the finger. The skin is thickened and adherent to the subcutaneous fatty tissue, over which it no longer moves. We find under the microscope that the skin is infiltrated with white corpuscles, the vessels are dilated, the flat cells of the connective tissue are swollen and granular, and their nuclei are divided. The adipose tissue takes part in the inflammation, lymphangitis is frequent, but not constant, and " the absence of abundant fibrinous exudate constitutes in ordinary cases a very important difference between erysipelas and inflammation of the skin " (Renaut).

Erysipelas is an **œdematous dermatitis.** The streptococci, after pene-trating the derma, produce, either by themselves or by their toxines, the following phenomena : dilatation of the small vessels, diapedesis of the white corpuscles, phagocytosis, proliferation of the fixed cells of the con-nective tissue, infiltration of the cutis by serous fluid containing a small amount of fibrin, and changes in the epidermis. The streptococci are found in the lymphatic spaces, in the channels at the base of the papillæ, and in the crevices of the derma, as well as in the connective spaces of the sheaths of the hair-follicles (Cornil and Babès).

Fehleisen has described three zones in the patch of erysipelas. The zone external to the edge, or the peripheral zone, has almost the appearance of normal skin, in which the streptococci are numerous. They prepare the soil, but have not as yet caused phagocytosis, accumulation of wandering cells, dermatitis, or œdema. The lesion is found in full activity at the edge of the patch. A considerable accumulation of migratory cells, with œdema, takes place there, the edge in erysipelas being produced through the separation of the connective tissue bundles by the œdema and the leucocytes. The central zone of the patch shows the process in retrogres-sion. The streptococci are no longer present in the derma, or, at least, only in very small numbers.

The **epidermis** also undergoes multiple lesions. The cells which form its various layers become separated and degenerated, and yield to the pressure of the œdema, forming a bleb. In some cases the lesion ends in abscess, in inflammation, or in gangrene.

Treatment.—Until recent times the treatment of erysipelas was absolutely empirical, and, it must be said, unsatisfactory. The topical remedies variously advised to arrest the progress of the disease, such as collodion, iodine, solutions of nitrate of silver, mercurial ointment, boric lotions, and solutions of mercury, had really no action. Compresses soaked in soothing applications, and frequently renewed, were the best topical applications, and gave the patient some relief.

An emetic or a saline purgative was employed for gastric trouble ; opium, bromides, chloral, and sedative draughts were given for restlessness and delirium ; tonics, such as extract of cinchona and champagne, were indicated if adynamic symptoms predominated.

Some of these latter methods of treatment are not to be despised, but they do not cure erysipelas. The rational treatment, if it realizes expectations, would consist in the injection of antistreptococcic serum, as advised by Marmorek.

In view of the growing importance of serotherapy, I shall describe in detail this treatment, which is similar to that of diphtheria by injections of serum.

The first difficulty was to obtain in sufficient quantity a very virulent streptococcal virus which retained its virulence. The method of increasing the virulence of the streptococcus is well known. It is sufficient to employ the classical method of passage through successive hosts (Pasteur).

For this purpose, a rabbit is infected with a dose of streptococcus which is sufficiently virulent to kill the animal. The blood from the heart of the first rabbit is injected into a second rabbit, which dies in its turn. The blood from the second rabbit serves for injection into a third rabbit, which succumbs more quickly in proportion as the virulence of the streptococcus increases by its successive passages. A microbe of extremely exalted virulence is thus obtained. But in order to preserve the activity which has just been conferred on the streptococcus, we must continue to pass it on from rabbit to rabbit. If the streptococcus is sown on broth, in the hope of preserving its acquired virulence, or with the desire of producing a large quantity of virus, we find our mistake, for on broth and in the first culture therefrom " the virulence falls in an extraordinary manner, and the results of the tedious series of passages are lost."

On the other hand, the virulence does not change when the germ is sown upon broth serum. I gave Marmorek's method of preparing broth serum at the commencement of the section.

By alternate inoculations in animals and cultures on broth serum the virus in two months becomes so active that a hundred thousandth part of a c.c. of the culture is sufficient to kill a rabbit.

A tenth of a c.c. of one of these very virulent solutions kills a rabbit in six hours, and at the autopsy hæmorrhagic effusions in the pericardium and the peritoneum are found. All the viscera, but especially the liver, contain masses of streptococci in long chains, and the blood also shows them in the form of short chains or of diplococci.

Immunization of Animals.—Several experimenters have succeeded in immunizing rabbits and mice (Roger, Behring) against the streptococcus by vaccinating them with living and with sterilized cultures, and Roger vaccinated a horse and a mule by inoculating them on repeated occasions with cultures heated in the autoclave to 120° C.

This difficulty was overcome by Marmorek, who employed the extremely virulent cultures above mentioned. He vaccinated large animals, and in particular the horse, with these cultures. Six months or a year elapse

" before a horse is able to furnish therapeutic serum." Subcutaneous injections are made of extremely virulent living cultures of streptococci, commencing with very small doses, such as a millionth part of a c.c., and gradually increasing the dose until 200 to 300 c.c. of culture are given at once. When we reach these large doses, it is preferable to perform intravenous injections of a small dose. An immunized horse received in five months thirteen injections, comprising in all 195 c.c. of culture. The first injections cause high fever and acute reaction. Tolerance is gradually established, but still the fever and the reaction are always fairly acute. Marmorek has always employed living cultures, and has been unable to manufacture a suitable toxine if the living elements are removed.

Antitoxic Serum.—When the horse has attained the desired degree of immunization, the serum must be promptly collected. The bleeding and collection of serum should be made only four or five weeks after the last inoculation. During the first few weeks after each inoculation or intravenous injection the serum of the horse is toxic—not because the blood of the animal contains streptococci, but because the serum is endowed with a toxic property, which only disappears three or four weeks after the last inoculation. The serum at this time is absolutely harmless, and possesses a prophylactic and curative power.

Experiments on Rabbits.—Experiments prove that serum taken from an immunized horse is harmless, prophylactic, and curative. It is harmless because it does not cause the slightest symptoms when injected into rabbits in various doses.

It is prophylactic, as is proved by the following experiments : Two rabbits are injected with a fifth of a c.c. of serum, and two others with a tenth of a c.c. Eighteen hours afterwards a millionth of a c.c. of culture is injected under the skin of each rabbit, and at the same time two other control rabbits which have not received any preventive serum are inoculated with an equal dose of culture—namely, a millionth of a c.c. The control rabbits die about thirty hours afterwards, but the two rabbits which have received a tenth of a c.c. of serum do not succumb until the tenth or the eleventh day, although cultures may not show the streptococcus in the blood or in the organs. The two rabbits which have received a fifth of a c.c. remain well, and do not show the least rise of temperature.

The serum is curative if the dose administered is large enough, and if the injection of serum is not made too long after the inoculation.

Injections of Serum in Man.—Streptococcal infections are very frequent in man. Whether the streptococcus is present alone (erysipelas, puerperal condition, inflammatory infections), or whether it acts in association with other germs (diphtheria, angina, scarlatina, influenza, bronchopneumonia, tuberculosis, etc.) ; whether it is itself a very virulent microbe, or whether this virulence is exalted by the other microbes with which it is associated, it is certain that the streptococcus plays a considerable part in human pathology. The future will show us in what manner the injections of anti-streptococcic serum will constitute a rational mode of treatment in most of the streptococcal infections which I have just enumerated ; but the subject requires further study.

Chantemesse advises the application of serum mixed with lanoline to the erysipelatous patch. This local serotherapy gives good results.

II. MUMPS.

In the first place, it is necessary to establish a well-marked difference between **parotiditis** and **mumps.** This difference is not exclusively based upon the anatomical position of the lesion, since in both cases the cellular tissue of the parotid gland may be as much involved as the glandular tissue. The difference lies in the nature of the disease itself.

The term parotiditis is applied to inflammations which sometimes supervene during the course or during the decline of severe fevers and infectious diseases, such as scarlatina, measles, variola, typhoid fever, dysentery, diphtheria, puerperal fever, and appendicitis. These cases of parotiditis, which often end in suppuration, in necrosis, or in gangrene of the gland, are the indication and the result of general ill-health, and their appearance is generally of gloomy augury. There are also cases of parotiditis which are associated with stomatitis (mercurial stomatitis), in which the inflammation is purely local, and spreads through Stenson's duct to the gland. These inflammations, though of different origins, are due to the ordinary microbes of suppuration, and have nothing in common with mumps.

Mumps, which has justly been compared with the eruptive fevers, may be placed among the infectious diseases. It is a specific, epidemic, and contagious disease.

Description.—Mumps is characterized by enlargement of the parotid glands, and usually of the salivary glands in general, for the submaxillary and sublingual glands are often affected. The incubation period varies from two to three weeks in general, and then the mumps commences on one side, and speedily invades the opposite one. It is usually ushered in with more or less pain in the parotid region, mastication becomes difficult, the secretion of saliva is decreased, the swelling affects the parotid region, and sometimes invades the neck and face, so as to disfigure the patient. It may even extend to the tonsils and pharynx. In some cases the angina and the swelling of the tonsils precede the affection of the parotid gland. The skin of the face preserves its colour, or may be slightly reddened.

In some instances rigors, headache, lassitude, and insomnia precede the local symptoms of mumps. In the stationary stage, especially in children, we often see fever accompanied by vomiting, and lasting twenty-four or forty-eight hours. The disease declines about the fourth day, and recovery supervenes between the sixth and eighth days.

Orchitis.—In young people and in adults, more often than in children, as soon as the swelling of the parotid disappears, whether the disease have been slight or severe, we may see orchitis, which is so frequent that it may be regarded as a symptom and not as a complication. Simple or double orchitis has been noted 156 times in 432 cases of mumps in soldiers (Laveran). The frequency of orchitis varies in different epidemics. Thus, at Digne, in 1892, it was noted four times in nine cases of mumps, and at Saintes, during the same year, six times in ninety-three cases. At Libourne, in 1889, orchitis was noticed once in forty cases of mumps, and at Épinal, during the same year, it was found eight times in twenty-six cases. In the Paris epidemic of 1892 Catrin saw orchitis forty-three times in 159 cases of mumps.

The orchitis may present every degree of severity. We see congestions of the testis which do not deserve the name of orchitis. The epididymis or the testis is slightly painful and swollen, but fever is absent or trifling, and these abortive cases are of particular interest, because they are not followed by atrophy of the organ (Catrin). More often the orchitis is associated with high fever and sharp pain in the testes, which may swell to three or four times their normal size ; the skin of the scrotum is red and tense. In four or five days the swelling diminishes, and resolution speedily occurs.

Lastly, orchitis may be ushered in with acute fever, restlessness, delirium, and a typhoid condition, forming the *febris testicularis* of Morton. I may mention here a case quoted by Trousseau :

"In 1832," says Trousseau, "I was attending a man, thirty-five years of age, who was suffering from mumps. The disease ran a regular course, the pain had diminished, and the swelling in the parotid region was beginning to decrease. I saw the patient in the morning, and he was as well as I could expect, but at the end of the day I was called in haste. I found him in the greatest distress—pale, drawn face ; small, frequent, and irregular pulse ; cold extremities. He had neither vomiting, diarrhœa, nor any appreciable lesions in the heart and lungs. I acted as the emergency suggested, and gave ether, warm drinks, and ordered mustard plasters, anxiously awaiting the issue of a disease which showed itself under such gloomy auspices. Next morning I was agreeably surprised to find the patient with marked fever, full pulse, and free perspiration ; his face was of good colour, and his appearance was lively. The scrotum, however, was swollen, and one of the testes, and especially the epididymis, was enlarged and painful, so that the symptoms were those of acute orchitis. I recalled the case reported by Borsieri, and the **febris testicularis** of Morton, and felt satisfied. I felt respect for the local manifestation which had freed the economy from the menacing symptoms, and a few days sufficed for the cure of this metastatic complication and for complete recovery."

Occasionally orchitis and mumps appear at the same time, and in rare cases the former may precede the appearance of the latter. In some instances the orchitis is the **sole** symptom of the disease, parotid troubles being absent. These cases are more or less frequent in different epidemics, and I may here quote an excellent example of defaced mumps reported by Trousseau :

" In 1853 I was called by Moynier to see a youth, seventeen years of age, whose case caused him the greatest anxiety. The young man had suddenly been taken ill with severe fever, rapid pulse, tendency to syncope, delirium, carphology, vomiting, and involuntary defæcation. The case thus resembled the dread period of the third week in putrid fever, or the onset of malignant scarlet fever, which kills patients in a few hours. You will readily understand the anxiety of the family and of the physician in the presence of such formidable symptoms. Andral had seen the young man in the early part of the attack, and, like Moynier, had observed the danger, without being able to account for it. These two gentlemen felt that it was, before all, essential to relieve the threatening symptoms, and with excellent judgment, had prescribed small doses of opium, with sulphate of quinine, in fairly large doses, and cardiac tonics.

" Next day, when I met my colleagues in consultation, there was no evident change in the patient's condition, though perhaps he was not quite so ill. We were told of a complication which had appeared during the night—namely, that the scrotum was swollen, and that one of the testes was enlarged and painful. This was the only organic lesion to be found, and it was scarcely of such a nature as to account for the alarming symptom-complex present. The history of my other patient came back to my mind, and I told it to my colleagues. I ran the risk of giving a somewhat less gloomy prognosis, on the supposition that the case might be one of metastasis in mumps. The parents and the principal of the institution, on being questioned, replied that the patient had shown no signs of mumps during the last few days. I was therefore obliged to yield in the face of such clear statements, and the same treatment was continued. Next day the swelling of the testis and of the epididymis **was much more marked ;** the delirium had ceased, as well as the vomiting and the diarrhœa. The fever was still acute, but the pulse was fuller and the skin was moist.

" After a few days the patient went home in good health. We questioned him carefully, and he told us that two or three days before the onset of the severe symptoms he had felt out of sorts, with pain in the throat and **swelling between the ear and the angle of the jaw,** and, further, that he had been for a walk in the forest of Saint-Germain, when he was seized with a chill. The swelling had diminished on the next day, and the day after the alarming complications noted above became manifest."

As regards the **localization** of the orchitis, we should be wrong in saying that it is always limited to the testis. It may be limited to the epididymis, and even in the numerous cases in which the testis appears to be alone invaded the epididymis is as a rule slightly affected. In forty-three cases reported by Catrin epididymitis was always coexistent with the orchitis.

Although the orchitis is only a transient affection, it is followed at times by **atrophy of the testis,** which occurs slowly and progressively, and may lead in some persons to impotence and to signs of feminism. When the atrophy is complete, the testis is reduced to a mere shell, being soft and of the size of a bean. It preserves its shape, and does not present either the induration or the irregular character of the syphilitic testis.

Very trifling orchitis (simple congestion of the organ) is never followed by atrophy, but such is not the case in severe orchitis. It is interesting to know what happens in these cases of atrophy months and years later, and we often see that the testes recover their consistency and their size after a prolonged period of atrophy. Catrin re-examined, seven to eleven months after orchitis, thirty-eight out of forty-three soldiers who had suffered from testicular atrophy. In thirteen the testes were absolutely normal, in sixteen marked atrophy was present, in five the change was slight, and in the remaining four, although the testes remained atrophied for several months, they finally recovered their functional integrity.

Malassez had occasion to examine an atrophied testis. The epididymis was healthy; the seminiferous tubules were reduced to half of their size; some were converted into cords, while others presented some epithelial débris at their centre; so that the lesion was a kind of parenchymatous orchitis, the vessels and connective tissue being practically spared.

Writers have quoted cases of mumps in which the breasts, the ovaries, and the labia majora showed congestion.

The preceding description applies to the classical form of mumps, with or without orchitis, but the so-called mumps fever does not always answer to the description just given. We see here, as in all epidemic diseases, slight or abortive forms, which are none the less very contagious. Some individuals during an epidemic of mumps have only slight malaise and swelling of the parotid gland, which may pass almost unnoticed. In other cases the parotid glands remain free, and the congestion is localized to the submaxillary and sublingual glands. This clinical picture is fairly common. We might well think of submaxillary adenitis when we see the submaxillary region swollen and painful, but here, as in other forms, orchitis may appear.

Complications.—Mumps is sometimes followed by complications. Albuminuria may be severe (Stoïcesco). Its frequency varies in different epidemics, and it is nearly always the sign of slight and transient nephritis, although in some cases the nephritis may be so severe as to cause death from uræmia. The infection in mumps may in some cases become the origin of Bright's disease.

I may mention among the **nervous complications** of mumps cerebral troubles of the preorchitic stage, with delirium, contractures, convulsions, and even coma, which disappear when the orchitis appears. The paralyses and the aphasia have been considered by Comby as related to hysteria. Finally, mumps may be followed by peripheral neuritis, with sensory troubles, flaccid paralysis of the limbs, complete loss of the muscular sense, total abolition of the reflexes, slight atrophy, and reaction of degeneration (Gallavardin).

Some patients suffer from slight pericarditis or from **endocarditis** during the course of the fever; others show pseudo-rheumatic joint troubles, which appear chiefly during the decline of the disease. They are subacute, causing but little pain and swelling of the joints, and they never suppurate.

In some epidemics œdema of the larynx, bronchial catarrh, and congestion of the lungs, have been seen. Suppuration in the salivary glands is exceptional. We may see infection of the lachrymal gland, with dacryocystitis, which resolves after a few days.

Fournié has carefully studied the auricular complications in mumps, and Eloy has given an excellent description of them. " The lesion is a special one," writes Fournié, " and is due to direct infection of the auditory centres." However this may be, the resulting deafness is generally incurable. It may be unilateral or bilateral ; it appears suddenly and at an early date ; it may or may not be accompanied by vertigo, buzzing in the ears, vomiting, and insomnia. The fits of giddiness may increase in severity and persist indefinitely.

Ætiology.—The numerous examples of contagion prove that mumps is essentially a contagious disease. It is hardly ever transmitted to a distance by a third person or by inanimate objects. The contagion is nearly always direct, and may take place at any period of the disease, but it is perhaps more active during the onset, before the appearance of the swelling in the glands. The disease chiefly affects infants and young people. Boarding-schools, colleges, orphanages, and barracks are generally the centres of epidemics. The epidemic does not strike down a large number of persons at once ; it extends by successive outbursts. A first attack generally confers immunity, but second attacks are fairly frequent.

The researches of Laveran and Catrin indicate progress in the bacteriology of mumps. They have collected serum from the parotid gland and from the testis, as well as the œdematous fluid and the joint secretion in cases of rheumatism. In sixty-seven out of ninety-two patients they found diplococci, and more rarely micrococci, united in fours or in zooglæa. The micrococci measure from 1 to 1·5 μ, and are mobile, but their movements are slight. They stain readily with the usual dyes, but do not take Gram's stain. A culture placed in the oven at 35° C. becomes turbid in twenty hours, and the turbidity increases during the next few days. On plates of gelatine the colonies only appear after forty-eight hours. They are punctiform, whitish, spread slowly, and only liquefy gelatine at a very late period. The colonies are white on agar, potato, carrot, and serum. Mumps has never been reproduced by inoculation. Moreover, the disease is unknown in animals.

Prognosis.—Mumps, though benign as a rule, may in some exceptional cases assume the malignant or typhoid form. The prognosis, however, is exceedingly benign if we only remember that in the French army, since 1887, only three deaths have taken place out of 33,445 cases (Catrin).

Diagnosis and Treatment.—Mumps will not be confounded with cases of parotiditis, although the diagnosis of mumps from certain cases of toxic parotiditis may sometimes be a delicate matter. Orchitis in mumps is clearly distinguished from blennorrhagic epididymitis, which is always consecutive to a urethral discharge.

During epidemics the patients must be isolated as far as possible, and, when the disease has appeared, rest, milk diet, gentle laxatives, and ointments applied to the parotid region, form the basis of treatment.

Antipyrin should be prescribed for pain. An ointment composed of ten parts of vaseline with one part of methyl salicylate should be rubbed into the painful region.

Orchitis during this painful stage should be treated by compresses soaked in poppy-head water, or inunction of the salicylate ointment may be used. In addition, we may employ leeches over the cord in the fold of the groin. Sedative draughts or hypodermic injections of morphia should be given if necessary.

We must not forget that mumps is contagious from its onset until three weeks after its disappearance. From the point of view of prophylaxis, we cannot be too energetic in our disinfection, for the germ of mumps is very tenacious of life, and is exceedingly resistant.

Atrophy of the testis must be carefully watched for, and the continuous current employed, as this method has given excellent results. Olivier has published a very interesting paper on this subject, and it is clear that in several cases atrophy of the testis has been arrested by the treatment.

III. CHOLERA.

In this section I shall describe true cholera, which has received the name of **Indian cholera**, from its place of origin.

Cholera, after being confined to India, where it is endemic, invaded several countries in Asia in 1818. Since this time both continents have frequently been visited by this terrible scourge, and the fearful ravages caused by cholera in France in the epidemics of 1832, 1849, and 1853 are well known. For some years past cholera, which has paid us several visits, has assumed an attenuated form. I may even say that between Indian cholera and cholera nostras a kind of promiscuity is established, which bacteriological studies have not been able to clear up.

Ætiology.—In India, where cholera is endemic, it is probable that the poison is engendered and nourished by special telluric conditions and by infection of water. From these endemic centres cholera sometimes appears in epidemic form, and the epidemic is provoked by large collections of persons living under defective hygienic conditions, as is often seen during the great pilgrimages of the Mohammedans.

The pilgrims leave the epidemic focus, and carry the cholera with them by land and sea, and, as it were, sow it in their journeys in the form of secondary epidemic centres, which may in their turn become the origin of severe epidemics. Cholera may be transmitted by numerous agents. Patients suffering from cholera or from specific diarrhœa, linen and articles of clothing or bed-clothes fouled by the dejecta, are the most important. When a focus of cholera is established, drinking-water and cesspools are active agents in its diffusion, while the atmosphere has only a very limited action. These peculiarities explain why alluvial soil, which is readily permeated by water and by organic matter, is more favourable to the diffusion of cholera than hard ground. These telluric conditions are of great importance when they concern the superficial layers of the soil, which are in close relation with houses and dwelling-places.

An epidemic of cholera may reappear in the same locality months and even years apart. These recrudescences are explained by the survival of the germ in the drinking-water and in the soil of the affected localities. In 1893 Blachstein and Sanarelli found the bacillus of cholera in the waters of the Seine eight months after the termination of the epidemic.

Small epidemics of autochthonous cholera, developing *in situ*, apart from any apparent contagion, have been noted. The frequent presence of vibrios in water (Metchnikoff), so often recognized of late years, even apart from any choleraic constitution, accounts for the origin of these epidemics, which at first sight appear to arise in an incomprehensible manner. The vibrios come from the intestine. They are poured into the water by man and by domestic animals, who may often, while in good health, carry them as saprophytes in their digestive canal.

We find refractory localities, where cholera may only produce isolated cases, and not epidemics. Lyons, and especially Versailles, are well known for their immunity. In 1893, however, Sanarelli often found the comma bacillus in water from the spring of Versailles, and Metchnikoff has seen typical cholera in man after ingestion of water containing this microbe. The comma bacillus does not comprise the whole ætiology of cholera. In addition to predisposing causes, such as the physiological, pathological, and social condition of the individual, as well as poverty, alcoholism, intestinal troubles, overcrowding in asylums and prisons, etc., we must also reckon with a predisposing cause which has its origin in the intestinal flora of individuals living in certain regions. Metchnikoff has shown that receptivity in cholera results from the association of microbes. The vibrio remains inactive or becomes dangerous according as it meets with an unfavourable or favourable microbic flora in the alimentary canal. Metchnikoff has also found that young rabbits, prepared by the ingestion of favourable microbes, such as the torula, sarcinæ, and the coliform bacillus, die much more readily when they are subsequently made to ingest the cholera bacillus.

Bacteriology.—The epidemic of cholera which affected Egypt and part of Europe some years ago furnished an opportunity of finding the micro-organism of this disease. Koch found in the contents of the small intestine, as well as in its walls, a slightly curved and short bacillus, known as the *comma bacillus.* This bacillus is found in large numbers in the stools of cholera patients, and stains very readily either with Ziehl's fuchsin or with gentian violet. It may be seen, though unstained, with very high mag-nification. It then shows extreme **mobility.** It has not always the curved form, the young bacilli being nearly straight. The comma bacilli, placed end to end, form the letter **S.** In old cultures several bacilli, when placed end to end, present the picture of the **choleraic spirillum.** The comma bacillus presents at its extremities waving cilia, which vary in number in different epidemics.

The bacillus of cholera can be cultivated in milk, broth, agar, potato, and gelatine. The culture on the latter medium is characteristic. Tubes kept in the oven at 22° C. show a kind of air-bubble on the surface of the gelatine, which becomes liquefied in a funnel-shaped form. Colonies with a fringe-like lower edge develop in the deep part of the gelatine. The liquefaction of the gelatine is complete at the end of six or seven days.

The cholera bacillus acquires its maximum vitality between 30° and 37° C., but it can also be cultivated in spite of cold. This fact explains the appearance of epidemics at any season of the year.

The reaction of indol nitrate, still called **cholera-roth,** is very typical. A rosy violet colour is seen on the addition of pure sulphuric or hydrochloric acid.

The bacillus is present in the rice-water fluid of the small intestine, especially in fulminant or very acute cases. When the disease is less acute, and the patient dies in the algid stage, the bacillus is associated with other micro-organisms, which render its discovery more difficult. Moreover, the longer the duration of the disease, the greater is the number of foreign microbes present. The comma bacillus may even completely disappear in the period of reaction. The bacillus, at first confined to the intestinal fluid, subsequently penetrates the mucous membranes, after the epithelium has disappeared. It may then reach the liver or the lungs, but it is very rarely present in the blood.

Koch was not only able to isolate and cultivate the cholera bacillus, but also to produce choleraic symptoms, by causing various animals to ingest the bacillus after the contents of the stomach had been rendered alkaline. Guinea-pigs are sensitive to the intraperitoneal injection of the comma bacillus, and die in less than twenty-four hours, with progressive lowering of the internal temperature. Post mortem, the intestine is found to be of a hydrangea colour, with a deposit of fibrin on the liver. The serous fluid in the peritoneum contains the bacillus.

Haffkine, by applying the method of exaltation and attenuation of the virus used in the study of anthrax and of chicken cholera to the Asiatic disease, has been able to obtain a remarkable attenuation of the bacillus by cultivating it in a constantly aerated atmosphere at a temperature of 39° C. A guinea-pig, after two inoculations of this attenuated virus, is immune to the infection of cholera, in spite of every attempt to produce the disease. The animal is, therefore, **vaccinated.** This method, formerly indicated by Ferran in Spain, is still under study as regards man.

In the laboratory the virulence of the vibrio is governed by inoculation of cultures into the cellular tissue, and especially into the peritoneum of guinea-pigs. The peritonitis thus produced rapidly brings about the death of the animal.

We have seen how Metchnikoff succeeded in causing intestinal cholera in young rabbits by mixed infection.

Bacteriologists who have lately studied the vibrios isolated during the course of epidemics in different parts of the world (India, Cochin-China, Massowa, Constantinople, Rome, Hamburg, Paris, etc.) have found morphological and biological differences between them. In addition to the small, short, curved type described by Koch in India, slightly curved as well as thin elongated types have been met with. The number of cilia varies. The vibrios at Hamburg and at Courbevoie had only one cilium ; those at Massowa and Calcutta had four cilia. The characters of cultures on gelatine may present variations. The virulence in animals is by no means constant, so that every intermediate form is found between the vibrio at Massowa, which was extremely virulent, and that at Rome or Lisbon, which was practically harmless. The cholera-roth reaction may in exceptional cases be absent. The microbe of cholera, therefore, is not always of a uniform nature, like Eberth's bacillus. It presents certain modifications, according to the epidemic soil, but this fact does not destroy the bacteriological unity of cholera. The different specimens are merely races of the same species.

The cholera bacillus is formidable by reason of the poison which it elaborates. In this respect it resembles the bacilli of diphtheria and of tetanus, which also elaborate toxines. " Cholera is an acute poisoning, due to the absorption of a special substance elaborated in the intestine by Koch's comma bacillus " (Metchnikoff, Roux, and Taurelli-Salimbeni).

Petri, Hueffe, and Gamaleia have described various toxines in cholera. Pfeiffer has recently maintained that the cholera toxine was adherent to the body of the vibrio, and that it only made its exit after the death of the vibrio. Behring and Ransom have stated, on the other hand, that the poison secreted by the microbe is soluble and diffusible during its life. In a remarkable work, full of therapeutic promise, Metchnikoff, Roux, and Taurelli-Salimbeni have clearly pointed out the difference. They succeeded in making the bacilli of cholera, enclosed in capsules of collodion, live in the peritoneum of guinea-pigs, and they have shown that the toxine alone was diffused through the organism, killing it, without any microbic action. This capsule is practically an artificial coil of bowel, in which they have produced a simplified cholera, without the presence of microbes, and apart from the action of the digestive juices. This experiment proves the existence of a soluble poison in cholera, and teaches us that, in order to obtain an efficient serum against experimental infection, we must employ an antitoxic serum, as in diphtheria, and not an antimicrobic one. These authors have obtained such a serum by progressive injections in horses of an active toxine produced by a vibrio with exalted virulence. The most minute dose of this serum not only cures choleraic peritonitis in guinea-pigs, but prevents intestinal cholera in young rabbits, although no other serum had so far accomplished this end.

Bacteriological Diagnosis of Cholera.—This diagnosis is a matter of extreme importance. In a suspected case we must first examine the stools for the bacillus, and then make cultures on broth or upon peptonized agar and glycerine (Koch). Upon broth a thin cloud containing curved bacilli in abundance forms after twelve hours, the temperature being 37° C. The culture on agar is less characteristic, but develops almost as quickly. On gelatine we obtain, after two or three days' exposure in the oven at 22° C., the special aspect already mentioned.

The variation in character of the cholera bacillus in different epidemics shows that the bacteriological diagnosis is often difficult. Is the vibrio obtained from the intestine of a patient at the onset of an epidemic, or perhaps obtained from drinking-water, a true cholera bacillus? Koch has lately recommended us to rely upon two points in order to prove the diagnosis: the reaction of cholera-roth and the reaction of immunity in vaccinated animals; but in exceptional cases the former reaction may be absent, and we have dwelt above on the variation of the virulence according to the origin of the microbe.

Pfeiffer and Issaëf have expressed their belief in a specific character in the reaction of immunity of guinea-pigs previously vaccinated. If fresh guinea-pigs are vaccinated with a true vibrio, the immunity lasts for about three months. If an animal, vaccinated three months previously by inoculation with a cholera bacillus, does not prove resistant to the intraperitoneal injection of the suspected vibrio, the latter should not be considered as cholerigenous; if, on the other hand, the animal proves resistant, the vibrio in question is that of cholera. In the peritoneum of the inoculated animal the vibrios become agglutinated and form small masses. According to

Pfeiffer and Issaëf, the serum of a guinea-pig vaccinated against an authentic cholera vibrio should confer immunity against all vibrios which are cholerigenous in nature. This reactino constitutes Pfeiffer's phenomenon, which may render the greatest service in the diagnosis of the cholera bacillus, but its certainty is not absolute. The Massowa vibrio, which has become classical by reason of its toxicity, kills guinea-pigs treated by preventive inoculation of serum from an animal immunized against the Hamburg vibrio. If we recognize Pfeiffer's law, we should exclude the active Massowa bacillus from the group of cholerigenous vibrios. By reason of the variety of races of the cholera vibrio, the reaction of immunity is not as exact as in typhoid fever, where the bacillus is always of the same nature.

Asiatic Cholera and Cholera Nostras.—Until 1892 the distinction between these two diseases appeared to be very clear. Asiatic cholera was contagious, epidemic, and fulminant; it was characterized by the presence of the comma bacillus in the stools and in the intestinal contents. Cholera nostras, on the other hand, was as a rule benign, rarely causing death, being but little contagious, and never epidemic, although endemic in our countries during very hot weather, and appeared to be due either to Finkler and Prior's bacillus, to the *B. coli communis* (Girode and Gilbert), or to Thiercelin's enterococcus.

The question has become more obscure since the epidemic of Paris in 1892, and I shall quote cases in proof of this assertion :

At the end of May, 1892, I saw four cases of cholera at the Necker Hospital. Three of the patients survived, and the fourth died. Rénon examined the stools and the intestinal contents in these four patients, and on two occasions found the *B. coli communis* alone, the comma bacillus once, and in the fourth case these two bacilli in association. I should have thought that the case due to the comma bacillus would be more severe than those due to the *B. coli communis*. Such was not the case, and the symptoms were equally grave in both cases. Clinically, no difference existed, and in the patient who died the *Bacillus coli* was found without the comma bacillus. At the same time Netter saw numerous deaths among choleraic patients in whom the *B. coli communis* was alone present. In 1893 Giraudeau and Rénon, who examined nearly all the cases of cholera in Paris and the suburbs, did not find in two months and a half a single case due to the comma bacillus. In all their patients the *B. coli communis* was found, and several died with the symptoms and lesions of Indian cholera. Giraudeau and Rénon have seen a case of contagion, which I will report briefly : A patient, who came from Nantes, where cholera was raging, was admitted to hospital, and died. A very virulent *Bacillus coli* was found in the stools and the bowel, since it killed a guinea-pig in eight hours. The attendants who nursed this patient died of cholera two days later, and here again the *Bacillus coli* was found **alone** in the dejecta and in the bowel.

Cholera due to the *Bacillus coli* may kill as surely and as rapidly as cholera due to the comma bacillus. The former is as contagious as the latter.

The study of the relations between cholera due to the *B. coli* and cholera due to the comma bacillus, and especially the assisting action of the former microbe on the latter, have enabled Rénon to throw some light on this obscure question. He formulates the following conclusions :

"This assisting action of the *B. coli communis* on the comma bacillus may occur just as readily outside as inside the organism, since it is proved that we can give asylum to the comma bacillus and the *B. typhosus* without being absolutely doomed to cholera or to typhoid fever. The assisting action of the *B. coli communis* becomes still more clear and immediate if its virulence has been reinforced by causes which we cannot as yet appreciate, causing choleriform diarrhœa or cholera nostras. If, however, we absorb with the ingesta a comma bacillus, whose virulence is exalted by successive passages through the human organism, such as occurs in large epidemics, the *B. coli* is not necessary to produce cholera. The invasion is rapid, and the course is fulminant. These considerations as to the ætiologic relations between these two varieties of cholera may be summed up in the following statement : Cholera nostras prepares the way for Indian cholera. The pathogenic data of a bacteriological nature are thus in perfect accord with the epidemiology and with the clinical facts.

"In the cases observed during the epidemic of 1892 the action of the *B. coli communis* was clear and precise, since the most severe cases were those in which both pathogenic agents were found. In the epidemic of 1893 the absence of the comma bacillus, noted by all authorities, coincided with the benign nature of this epidemic, which would have become terrible if the comma bacillus had also been present, seeing that the *Bacillus coli* alone acquired a fatal virulence. These data account for the immunity of certain towns against cholera, as Metchnikoff had remarked. They explain why cholera does not always exist where the comma bacillus is present. Sanarelli, in the benign epidemic of 1893, found the comma bacillus almost constantly present in the water of the Seine, and yet only one case of cholera due to the comma bacillus was discovered at Saint-Denis. In conclusion, these data explain the clinical importance of premonitory diarrhœa which occurs when the comma bacillus alone has not acquired sufficient virulence to produce Indian cholera."

Pathological Anatomy.—**Rigor mortis** is always very pronounced, and the **cyanotic tint** is as marked as it was during the last hours of life. All the tissues are bloodless, and this dryness becomes the more striking when we examine a vascular organ, such as the liver or the kidneys. The small quantity of blood contained in the vessels and in the heart is viscid, brownish, and fluid, or clotted in soft black coagula.

The intestinal lesions are constant, but, according to Kelsch and Vaillard, no relation exists between their severity and the duration of the disease. They chiefly occupy the small intestine, and become the more marked the nearer they are to the cæcum. The mucous membrane is pale and colourless, or, on the other hand, shows in spots a clear hydrangea tint. The ramifications of the bloodvessels are well marked in this membrane. Its free surface is studded with small transparent projections of the size of a millet-seed, collapsing on puncture. They contain colourless fluid. This psorenteria, regarded as characteristic of cholera by Serres, is common to every severe diarrhœa. In some cases the intestinal mucous membrane presents scattered ecchymoses, which may reach the submucous coat, and may occupy a fairly large extent.

The epithelium is detached, and floats in the contents of the intestine, thus producing the **rice-water** appearance. This desquamation is sometimes the prelude of small ulcerations, which destroy the mucous coat to a greater or less extent. It is sometimes appreciable to the naked eye, but at other times it is visible only with the microscope (Kelsch and Vaillard). The superficial ulcerations are necrobiotic in nature, since they always follow thrombosis of the vessels. We find the capillaries and small arterioles of the mucosa filled with corpuscles, which are more or less altered in shape, while the cells covering the walls of these ulcerations show granulo-fatty degeneration.

Lieberkühn's and Brunner's glands are healthy (Jaccoud), but the closed follicles are swollen and infiltrated with leucocytes. The integrity of the large intestine contrasts with the lesions in the small bowel. The spleen is always atrophied and bloodless (Kelsch and Vaillard). The follicles of Malpighi are increased in size, and present at their centre an irregular vitreous mass, which is cracked upon its surface, and formed at the expense of the artery and of the lymphatic tissue of the follicle.

Straus and Roux have described in the liver greyish anæmic areas, which are also found in a number of infectious states, and which have been attributed by Doyen to an arrest in the local circulation. This assertion appears true, for the bloodvessels are obliterated by leucocytes and by fibrin. According to Doyen, this coagulation is consecutive to the arrest of the cholera microbes. Hanot and Gilbert have found in many of the liver cells a change characterized by swelling of the nucleus and by difficulty in staining the protoplasm. They have given to this change the name of **transparent swelling.** Apart from these hepatic lesions, all authors have insisted on the distension of the bile-ducts, and especially of the gall-bladder, by thick, almost colourless bile. Hayem and Winter have found a toxic alkaloid in this fluid.

The kidneys are fairly often increased in size and congested. They sometimes show an early stage of parenchymatous nephritis. The cells of the tubuli contorti have undergone a kind of cloudy infiltration (Doyen), and the straight tubules are filled with hyaline casts.

Description.—The incubation period of cholera is from thirty-six to fifty-six hours, and the course of the symptoms in an ordinary case may be divided into three periods : period of premonitory diarrhœa, algid stage, and the period of reaction.

1. *Premonitory Diarrhœa.*—The diarrhœa commences suddenly, without colic or tenesmus. It is characterized by stools which are at first fæcaloid, but which later become bilious and serous, and accompanied by borborygmi. Fever is either slight or absent ; the appetite is good, except in cases of gastric catarrh ; the stools are frequent ; the patient feels ex-

ceedingly tired ; and after a period of from three to seven days the disease is well marked. Let me state that this **premonitory diarrhœa** is not constant, being absent in a third of the cases, and, on the other hand, it may be the only manifestation of very mild cholera.

2. *Algid Stage.*—The dejecta of the preceding period change in character, and become exceedingly frequent. The stools have no fæcal odour ; they are serous, and composed of a watery, colourless fluid, in which whitish flakes of epithelial débris float (rice-water stools). The stools contain the bacilli previously described.

Cramps now appear, with vomiting of watery matter, repeated every few minutes, and accompanied by precordial distress. The thirst is intense ; the belly is retracted; the pulse is small; the face is shrunken; the eyes become hollow ; the nose is cold and pinched ; the voice sinks to a whisper ; the skin of the hands grows pale, dry, and wrinkled ; the limbs become as cold as ice ; the nails are blue ; and the feet and hands are covered with a purple mottling. During the algid stage the temperature of the hands or of the mouth is 10° or 12° F. below normal, while the internal temperature rises, thus explaining the sensation of heat felt by the patient. If this period ends fatally, the respiration becomes embarrassed, and the patient falls into a state of stupor, and dies in collapse.

Most of these symptoms are due to the toxines and the **thickening of the blood,** deprived of its watery elements by the incessant loss resulting from the stools and vomiting. The circulatory organs fail, the secretions diminish, and hæmatosis is at a standstill. This stage, which in some cases lasts only two or three hours, scarcely ever exceeds thirty hours.

3. *Period of Reaction.*—If the patient does not die in the algid stage, the cyanosis disappears, the skin grows warm again, the rectal temperature falls and the secretion of urine is re-established. The first urine passed is albuminous, and poor in urea and chlorides. The different functions gradually become normal and recovery takes place in a few days. The period of reaction does not always run this favourable course. It is sometimes **incomplete,** and after various oscillations the patient may recover or may pass again into the algid stage. At other times the reaction oversteps, as it were, the normal line ; congestion of the chief organs, and especially of the brain, occurs and the fever reappears. The chances of recovery, however, are not hopeless ; and if improvement supervenes, it generally does so after a short period of from twenty-four to forty-eight hours.

The length of **convalescence** varies in proportion to the severity of the disease. It is sometimes interrupted by dyspepsia and paralyses, and the patient is not free from the risk of a second attack, because cholera does not confer immunity.

Rare Forms.—The above description of cholera applies in the majority of cases. It comprises the slight forms which have been called **cholerine,** and which are characterized by the first period—namely, that of premonitory diarrhœa. Between these slight and severe forms we see every intermediate form, and as regards severity, they practically correspond to the preceding description.

Rare forms are, however, seen : cholera fulminans and cholera sicca. True cholera fulminans is excessively rare, although it has been seen in India ; but we may often see in certain epidemics **rapid** forms, in which the patients may or may not suffer from premonitory diarrhœa and are carried off in less than twenty-four hours.

The form which is not accompanied by alvine evacuations is called cholera sicca. In this form the fluid is not expelled from the intestine, probably because of the paralysis of the gut.

Diagnosis and Prognosis.—**Cholera nostras** has nothing in common with Indian cholera. The evacuations are bilious and serous, but not like rice-water, because the epithelial flakes are absent. Vomiting and marked coldness of the body are not seen, and the disease is essentially one of seasons (summer and autumn diarrhœa), and presents no gravity. If the reader will refer to the remarks at the commencement of this section, he will see that in many cases clinically, anatomically and bacteriologically, cholera nostras and Asiatic cholera are often difficult to differentiate from one another, and here, as in pernicious choleraic fever, the clinical diagnosis depends upon bacteriology and sero-diagnosis.

Sero-Diagnosis.—The phenomenon of agglutination of the microbes by serum is most typically seen among animals in choleraic infection. It will, perhaps, furnish the elements for the sero-diagnosis of cholera in man, as, indeed, the researches of Achard and Bensaude lead us to hope.

The **prognosis** of cholera is so grave that in some epidemics the mortality exceeds 60 per cent.

Treatment.—Prophylactic measures should be rigorously observed, in order to prevent the importation and dissemination of cholera. Quarantine is not as efficacious in cholera as in yellow fever, which, by reason of its origin, can only be imported by sea. Cholera spread by land in the first two epidemics which ravaged Europe. The usefulness of sanitary cordons is undoubted, but, unfortunately, these measures are difficult to put into execution. We must prevent any great exodus of the population (pilgrimages and caravans), which is liable to spread the disease.

The usual measures employed to prevent the spread of cholera are : Patients and their attendants must be absolutely isolated ; pans in which the dejecta are received, latrines, linen, bed-clothes, and flooring must be disinfected with a solution of sulphate of iron or of sulphuric acid. The physician should change his clothes and wash his hands in carbolic lotion after visiting a patient.

People who live in an epidemic centre should drink only boiled water or table waters. They must avoid all excess or fatigue, and the slightest intestinal symptoms are to be rigorously checked.

What is the treatment for cholera ? In the first stage, our efforts must be directed to checking the diarrhœa by administration of subnitrate of bismuth, and opium and its preparations. Rice-water forms an excellent drink. Champagne and iced drinks may be given for vomiting. At the very first sign of the algid stage the patient must be rubbed with cold aromatic lotions or with tampons of wool soaked in chloroform liniment. Lactic acid in doses of 3 drachms daily has given good results (Hayem). Intravenous injection of artificial serum was recommended by Hayem in 1884, and was much used in 1892. It showed a larger measure of successes than had been previously obtained.

If the reaction is too acute, we must employ mustard plasters, cold compresses to the head and diaphoretics.

IV. INFLUENZA.

Description.—Influenza is a contagious microbic disease affecting chiefly the respiratory system, but presenting in addition a variety of local manifestations and symptoms, which vary in character and severity in different epidemics.

Influenza arises after a very short period of incubation, varying from a few hours to a day. The onset is often sudden. An individual in good health is struck down by violent headache, pains in the joints, chills, fainting-fits, hallucinations, and syncope. The onset is, however, less sudden in most cases and the disease begins as common cold.

I shall describe two forms of influenza—the one mild or of moderate intensity, the other severe, though, of course, every intermediate degree may be seen.

The mild form resembles an attack of bronchitis, in which the general symptoms assume an unwonted severity. The entire economy is invaded, as in the severe fevers. For several days muscular weakness and malaise are felt, with intense frontal or occipital headache, pains awakened by every fit of coughing and repeated cramps in the limbs and chills. Ocular, nasal, and pharyngeal catarrhs appear. In some cases these local symptoms are wanting, and the influenza begins with catarrhal laryngitis or bronchitis, accompanied by hoarseness of the voice and very painful fits of coughing. The expectoration is at first aerated, but later becomes more thick ; the chest is full of snoring and whistling rhonchi ; the fever is high at night, and falls in the morning. In some cases the fever is slight, and yet the headache, pains in the muscles of the neck, in the spine, in the sides, and in the lumbar region, as well as in the neighbourhood of the joints, may be of marked severity during the whole disease. In some patients the chief symptoms are nausea, vomiting, gastric catarrh, and biliousness. After about a week or a fortnight, recovery is ushered in by a crisis, with sweating, diarrhœa, bleeding from the nose, and herpes on the lips.

The severe form of influenza is characterized by the exaggeration of the symptoms just described, with a tendency to delirium and syncope, or by the predominance of lesions and symptoms which lend a special character to each epidemic.

Moreover, most epidemic diseases, such as typhoid fever, whooping-cough, dysentery, scarlet fever, mumps, etc., are subject to these symptomatic variations, which impress their special hall-mark on the epidemics (génie épidémique), and which are dependent upon the climatic, telluric, or atmospheric conditions (circumfusa), whereby the virulence of the pathogenic agents is modified or increased. The varied nature of the lesions and symptoms in different epidemics and individuals has led authors to describe severe forms of influenza of a nervous, thoracic, or of an abdominal type.

Nervous Influenza.—In some cases the cerebral or cerebro-spinal symptoms are so marked that they seem to comprise the whole disease. The headache may be intense, dull, stabbing, or like the blows of a hammer, with orbital pains and a feeling of constriction in the temples. The pain in the head is sometimes accompanied by vomiting, somnolence, and photophobia, so that meningitis is naturally thought of. In most cases this lesion is not present, and the condition is only a pseudo-meningitis. In some cases, however, true meningitis develops and the patient dies in a few days. This **influenzal meningitis** generally results from suppurative otitis (Weichselbaum), pneumonia, or broncho-pneumonia, the pathogenic agents primarily localized to the nose, to the ear, or to the lung, having spread to the brain.

Influenza may cause polyneuritis, ascending paralysis, meningo-myelitis, and polymyelitis. The numerous cases, some of which have been followed by post-mortem examination, permit the clear description of these nervous complications. Mossé quotes three cases which prove that patients suffering from influenza may show, either in the course of the disease or during convalescence, nervous symptoms due to peripheral neuritis, symptoms of bulbo-spinal meningo-myelitis, which specially affect the dorso-lumbar enlargement of the spinal cord, and progressive ascending paralysis of a mixed type, both polyneuritic and spinal, which ends in general spinal paralysis.

Polyneuritis due to influenza is, however, more frequent than myelitis.

The nervous complications, which appear *a priori* to be of spinal origin, most often end in recovery, even though they may be very marked. Paralysis of the bladder, rachialgia, and severe trigeminal neuralgia also belong to the nervous disorders.

We see in some persons symptoms of depression and prostration, which at first sight simulate coma ; others suffer from headache, fainting-fits, and syncope. I have also seen delirium, restlessness, hallucinations, and acute mania. Mental alienation following influenza has also been noted.

The innervation of the heart may be affected, so that patients are seized with arrhythmia, collapse and pains like those of angina pectoris.

Thoracic Influenza.—Broncho-pulmonary complications play a large part in the mortality from influenza. These complications include capillary bronchitis, inflammation of the chest, broncho-pneumonia, or pneumonia ; they are usually rare at the commencement of an epidemic. The severe broncho-pulmonary lesions appear later, when the epidemic is at its height. Capillary bronchitis may rapidly become purulent.

Inflammation of the chest in influenza is often serious. It is accompanied by blood-stained sputum, with intense dyspnœa, and the multiple localizations described under Inflammation of the Chest.

Broncho-pneumonia is one of the most terrible manifestations of influenza. It is characterized bacteriologically by the presence of the streptococcus, with which the pneumococcus, the pneumobacillus and the staphylococcus are often associated. Broncho-pneumonia arises in the course of influenzal bronchitis and its description is precisely similar to the classical form. In the terrible epidemic of 1837 many persons died from capillary bronchitis and from broncho-pneumonia (Nonat).

Lobar pneumonia is also one of the manifestations of influenza. It is due to the pneumococcus, and may be accompanied by pleurisy, endocarditis, pericarditis, and meningitis. " On the one hand, the study of previous epidemics shows us that pneumonia is not simply a complication ; it may appear in the primary form, thus forming a coincident epidemic ; and, on the other hand, in the influenzal pneumonia seen this year [1886], we have been able to demonstrate the presence of the pneumococcus in the sputum, in the hepatized lung after death, and in the blood during life. We may, therefore, conclude that influenza and pneumonia are two independent diseases, although presenting marked affinities. The one predisposes to the other, and both appear to be favoured by the same causes" (Menetrier).

At other times the respiratory tracts are almost unaffected, and yet the dyspnœa is acute, early, and sudden (Graves, epidemic in Ireland, 1830), as though the nervous system was directly affected by the poison. This nervous dyspnœa, formerly called *sine materia*, is similar to that seen in the malignant forms of certain diseases, such as scarlatina.

Pleurisy is by no means rare in influenza, being either sero-fibrinous or purulent, and due to the streptococcus or to the pneumococcus. It is sometimes interlobar, and is always associated with lesions of the lungs and bronchi.

Gangrene is certainly the gravest of the pulmonary complications. It may appear during the acute phase of influenza, or much later during convalescence. This terrible complication, whether it is circumscribed or diffuse, and whether it is or is not accompanied by pyopneumothorax, is nearly always fatal.

Gastro-Intestinal Influenza.—In some cases influenza takes the form of a severe gastric disorder, with vomiting, absolute intolerance of the stomach, pain in the epigastric region, and dry, red tongue.   Erythema of the pharynx, alveolo-dental periostitis, and aphthous or ulcerative stomatitis are sometimes added to these symptoms.   In some cases the symptoms of sore throat are predominant.   The patient complains of acute dysphagia, violet patches are seen on the velum palati and on the pharynx, and the tonsils are affected by suppurative inflammation.   The spleen is often enlarged and painful.

The intestinal troubles are characterized by bilious and fœtid diarrhœa, with colic, tenesmus, meteorism, vomiting of bile, epistaxis, and prostration—symptoms resembling those of typhoid fever.   The epidemic which broke out in Vienna in 1775 was remarkable for the predominance of biliary phenomena, with vomiting, anorexia, diarrhœa, and jaundice, affecting the conjunctivæ and skin (Stoll).   In the Paris epidemic of 1830 the cramps and intestinal troubles were so marked that they closely resembled cholera (Hardy and Béhier).

Influenzal Nephritis.—Nephritis is a frequent complication of influenza, and here, as in other infectious diseases, it may assume the most diverse characters.   The nephritis is, as a rule, slight and transient.   The change in the epithelium is shown only by more or less severe and prolonged albuminuria, without other symptoms.   Sometimes, however, œdema, puffiness of the face, and swelling of the lower limbs are seen in addition to the albuminuria.   At other times influenzal nephritis becomes of considerable importance.   The urine is scanty and blood-stained, and the patient suffers from slight symptoms of uræmia, viz., headache, dyspnœa, and diarrhœa. As these symptoms are often blended with similar troubles due to the influenza itself, their true cause may be unnoticed in the absence of careful examination.   Lastly, influenzal nephritis, especially in its severe form, may pass into the subacute and chronic stage, and give rise to Bright's disease, especially if the kidneys have been previously damaged by other infectious diseases.   I have several times seen all these forms of influenzal nephritis.   I have known 60 to 70 grains of albumin to be passed in the twenty-four hours. I have also seen symptoms of uræmia which dominated the scene, and I cannot count the cases in which Bright's disease has had influenza for its primary cause.

Other Local Manifestations.—I must call attention to certain local manifestations which are of great importance. The organs of the senses are often invaded, and the nasal form of influenza, which shows itself by rhinitis, epistaxis, and by discharge from the nose, may be complicated by inflammation of the frontal sinuses and of the meninges.

Otitis, previously almost unmentioned, was so frequent in the epidemic of 1889-90 that much was written on the subject (Loewenberg). The condition is one of acute otitis media, accompanied by pain and more or less prolonged discharge of pus. The pain ceases after perforation of the membrane. The most usual microbes found in these cases are the strepto-coccus and the pneumococcus. In some cases the mastoid cells are invaded, in which case it is necessary to trephine the bone.

Ocular paralyses which are not unlike those of diphtheria have been described.

Cystitis, urethritis, orchitis, epididymitis, and vaginalitis have also been seen in influenza. Exanthematous and pustular eruptions are frequent.

In certain epidemics a hæmorrhagic form may be seen. It is accom-panied by metrorrhagia (Law, 1779), hæmaturia (Voisin, 1837), purpura and epistaxis. This form was very common in the epidemic of 1889-90.

Ætiology.—Influenza is an epidemic disease, which usually spares children and by choice affects adults, and a first attack does not confer immunity. It is at present impossible to state the causes which favour its development, because it appears to disregard conditions of climate, season, and temperature (Graves). It swoops down upon a town or a country, lays low a half, two-thirds, or three-quarters of the inhabitants, and after a duration of some weeks it disappears, thus affecting immense areas, although its course has not always a definite direction (Gintrac).

Nevertheless, epidemics of influenza usually travel from north to south and from east to west. The original seat of the disease is said to be in Siberia by some authorities and in Persia by others. At any rate, it is certain that influenza is endemic in Moscow and St. Petersburg, where it appears every year in the autumn and spring, and is the result of conditions as yet unknown. It assumes an epidemic or pandemic character.

Our severe epidemic of 1889-90 furnished material for studying its conditions of diffusibility. Influenza does not exceed in its diffusion the quickness of human communications. It usually breaks out in a large town, and then spreads to smaller communities. There are, however, exceptions which remain inexplicable. Why, for example, did not the London epidemic in May, 1890, spread to the Continent ?

The contagious nature of influenza, which had long been doubted, must be definitely accepted, for the proofs of contagion are clear. Influenza appears to be transmissible by direct contact and by fomites.

Bacteriology.—The various organisms met with in influenza, such as the *Streptococcus pyogenes*, which is most common, the pneumococcus, the pneumobacillus, and the staphylococcus, are only secondary agents. They are not the prime cause of influenza.

Pfeiffer discovered the influenza bacillus in 1892. It is found in abundance in the sputum. Its presence is revealed by the usual bacterial stains, but care must be taken to expose the slide to the stain for at least ten minutes, because the influenza bacillus is slow to take the dye.

Pfeiffer's bacillus does not stain well with aniline dyes. It is preferable to use diluted Ziehl's stain. It does not take Gram's stain. After staining, the bacillus appears among the shreds of mucus and the leucocytes, or sometimes in the leucocytes themselves. It has the shape of an extremely thin rod; it, indeed, is thinner than any other bacillus. It is very short, and only about twice as long as it is broad, so that it sometimes has the appearance of a **cocco-bacillus.** When these rods are in pairs they simulate a diplococcus, and when three or four are joined end to end they resemble a streptococcus.

The bacillus of Pfeiffer is cultivated with difficulty on the ordinary media. It grows best on agar to which a few drops of blood have been added. A mixture of hæmoglobin and agar gives the same results. If the agar is impregnated with blood, and placed in the oven at 57° C., we find after twenty-four hours very small colonies, which are visible with the lens. They have the appearance of small transparent drops, which show no tendency to become confluent (Kitasato).

The bacillus may live from fifteen to eighteen days on blood agar, and from thirty to forty days on hæmoglobin agar.

If we sow Pfeiffer's bacillus on agar covered with blood, making stabs with the *Staphylococcus aureus* at intervals, the culture of the influenza bacillus is assisted in a remarkable manner. Around the fertilizing colonies of the staphylococcus we find the development of giant colonies, which may be twenty times as large as those of a pure control culture. This **cultural satellitism** (Meunier) must be employed in order to find Pfeiffer's bacillus in pathological exudates. Excellent satellite cultures of the influenza bacillus are obtained in twenty-four hours.

Diagnosis.—The diagnosis of influenza is not always simple. It may at first sight simulate typhoid fever, measles, rheumatism, meningitis, or acute tuberculosis, either by reason of well-marked lesions in a particular system or by reason of the general symptom-complex. The diagnosis from meningitis is the more indefinite because influenzal meningitis is also seen.

I would refer the reader for further details to the section on Cerebro-Spinal Meningitis. When influenza simulates typhoid fever, sero-diagnosis (Widal) will remove all doubts.

Treatment.—It is not possible to state any treatment for a disease which is so different in its course and appearance. We may employ antiphlogistic measures for the inflammatory complications and antispasmodics for the nervous symptoms. Emetics are of use in the bilious forms. Slight cases of influenza, which are happily the most frequent, should be treated in the same manner as acute bronchitis.

V. YELLOW FEVER—VOMITO NEGRO.

Ætiology.—Yellow fever has been classed both among telluric diseases and typhoid maladies, but it should certainly find a place among the infectious diseases of microbic origin.

We are not yet in possession of precise data as to the microbe of yellow fever. Lacerda has found in most of the viscera a microscopic fungus, which he regards as specific. Carmona and Domingo Freire have described a proto-organism from which they have prepared vaccine. Babès has found in the liver and kidneys micro-organisms which have not been verified by other authors. Sanarelli thinks that the *B. icteroides* is the pathogenic agent of yellow fever.

Reed, Caroll, and Agramante have attributed yellow fever to a microbe belonging to the class of invisible microbes which pass through the pores of filtering candles. This microbe is carried by a special mosquito, the *Culex fasciatus*, which is classed by Theobald in the genus *Stegomya (Stegomya fasciata)*. " Healthy men, living with those suffering from yellow fever, and exposed to the bites of mosquitoes, which settle alternately upon the patients and the healthy, have contracted the disease. This fact alone explains why the scourge remains limited in most cases to the seashore and to low-lying districts. The habits of the *Stegomya* control the spread of the disease, which is only met with in an epidemic condition where the insects themselves are found. The parasite in question swarms only in the low, damp, and warm shores of intertropical countries. Moreover, these diptera are not found on high ground above the 600-metre line or outside the zone in which the diminution of the barometric pressure considerably interferes with their flight " (Bogey).

Chantemesse and Borel speak as follows in their communication to the Academy of Medicine (1905) :

The mission of the Pasteur Institute, composed of Drs. Marchoux, Simond, and Salimbeni, has confirmed and extended these views. It is now settled that the existence of yellow fever and the presence of the

Stegomya are absolutely reciprocal. Although this mosquito is widely scattered, its habitat has something special in that it is clearly determined by the forty-third north and south parallels, and this is the reason why every region external to these two parallels remains free from yellow fever. The forty-third parallel just touches the South of France. It enters at the Department of the Basses-Pyrénées, passes through Argelès, Saint-Girons, and Foix, and reaches the coast a little above La Nouvelle. The only port of any note in this region is Port-Vendres. The same parallel passes through the islands of Hyères, and then through the north of Corsica. It would, therefore, be unwise to send soldiers coming from countries infected with yellow fever to the islands of Hyères, which have formerly been used as a quarantine station. On the other hand, all our colonies, except Saint-Pierre and Miquelon, are in the country of the *Stegomya*.

Yellow fever is endemic upon the shores of the Gulf of Mexico, in the Antilles, in Brazil (Visca), and on the West Coast of Africa, etc. It may be imported from these centres, and appear in epidemic form in both hemispheres, as the multiple epidemics in America and Europe (Gibraltar, 1828 ; Lisbon, 1847 ; Saint-Nazaire, 1861) prove.

Yellow fever only leaves its endemic centres for the purpose of invading other regions by reason of importation, which is always caused through ships. In some cases the vessel has shipped passengers who are already infected, and in whom the disease appears during the voyage. At other times the whole crew is quite well on starting, but the ship harbours the mosquito in the holds, and an epidemic appears some days after sailing.

Experience has shown that infection occurs chiefly after sunset and at night. Physicians, therefore, visit their patients about midday.

The disease does not spread rapidly, but remains at first limited to certain houses or to a single street. Visca has noted the interesting fact that the invasion often takes place by excentric zones, which spread from the primary centre. The epidemic, like the endemic form, shows little tendency to invade places remote from the sea-coast and elevated regions.

The **incubation** of yellow fever lasts from three to six days.

Description.—Prodromata do not, as a rule, occur in yellow fever, which commences suddenly in the middle of the night with a sharp rigor, followed by backache (*coup de barre*), headache, lassitude, and epigastric distress, with or without pulsation in the cœliac region. The temperature on the first day may exceed 105° F. (Naegele). The eyes are haggard and injected, the face is red, thirst is severe, constipation is the rule, the restlessness and insomnia are sometimes accompanied by delirium, and the skin is erythematous. On the second day the patient is seized with nausea and vomiting—first of food-stuffs, later of mucus and of bile. The urine is scanty and usually contains albumin.

This first stage, which is very severe, lasts about three days. The symptoms then improve, the temperature falls, and jaundice appears. Jaundice, which is the most constant symptom of the disease, and has gained for the disease the name of **yellow fever,** coincides with the remission which ends the initial period. In benign cases the disease does not pass beyond this inflammatory stage, and the fever does not reappear. In severe cases, however, the remission lasts only a few hours, and the fever reappears, though it may not be as high as in the first stage.

The jaundice varies in intensity from the palest to the deepest greenish-yellow. The urine contains bile, but the stools are not colourless, because the flow of bile is free. Jaccoud thinks that the pathogenesis of this symptom is not always the same ; he is of opinion that the jaundice is sometimes catarrhal and at other times associated with hypercholia. Vomiting of dark blood (*vomito negro*) is practically contemporaneous with the jaundice, though it is much less constant, being present in about 50 per cent. of cases. The hæmorrhage from the stomach is often accompanied by bleeding from the intestines, from the pharynx, or from the mouth, by metrorrhagia, and by purpura.

The general condition of the patient varies, and **adynamic, typhoid, and delirious forms are seen.** In some cases the anuria is complete, and we may well ask if the symptoms of dyspnœa and ataxo-adynamia should not be set down to uræmia.

Duration.—In the slight forms the remission, which usually occurs about the third day, is accompanied by profuse sweating, and recovery speedily follows. In the grave forms the disease lasts from six to ten days, or even longer. The fulminant form is fatal in three or four days.

Diagnosis.—We are not likely to confound yellow fever with icterus gravis, for in the latter disease the sudden onset of the fever, the backache, the epigastric distress, and the injection of the face and eyes are wanting. We can distinguish yellow fever from the bilious forms of malaria, which are accompanied by more or less marked swelling of the spleen, and characterized by the presence of the parasite and of melanotic pigment in the blood. The bilious form of typhoid fever somewhat resembles the typhoid form of yellow fever, but in the former the temperature rises slowly and the spleen is enlarged. The mortality varies in different epidemics of yellow fever from 14 to 50 per cent. (Dutroulau).

Pathological Anatomy.—The chief lesions are of a steatogenous nature. The liver resembles the fatty liver of phthisis (Louis). It is of a light yellow colour, bloodless and friable. The cells rapidly become fatty, but are only in part necrosed. The heart and the kidneys are also affected by fatty degeneration. The muscles, especially those of the abdomen and thighs, are sometimes the seat of ecchymoses. Ecchymotic patches, which are sometimes ulcerated, may be seen in the stomach, pharynx, and intestine. The blood is of **abnormal fluidity**—a condition found in most of the infectious diseases. The spleen is normal.

Treatment.—In countries where yellow fever reigns, prophylaxis, according to the latest data, consists in destroying the mosquitoes, isolating the patients, and protecting them against the *Stegomya*. For this purpose the beds are covered by mosquito curtains, the doors and the windows are covered with fine wire-netting. The mosquitoes are destroyed by fumigation with sulphurous acid or by the fumes of pyrethrum. Dr. Diaz Albertini, who has taken great interest in the sanitation of Havana, has given much interesting information. Each room in the house is subjected to the fumes of pyrethrum after every aperture has been hermetically sealed. When the rooms are opened it is surprising to see the number of dead mosquitoes on the floor and elsewhere. Excellent results follow this method of disinfection where mosquitoes are found.

In order to destroy the larvæ, petroleum is poured into the drains, closets, and puddles where the mosquito lays its eggs. The Americans have obtained marvellous results in Cuba by these measures. The fight against mosquitoes commenced at Havana on February 16, 1901, and during the half-year from April to October, in which the majority of cases occur, only eighteen deaths from yellow fever occurred, while the mean death-rate in previous years had been 483. For 150 years no one had ever seen such an excellent state of sanitation as during this season.

The usual treatment consists in giving gentle purgatives, such as castor-oil, mixed with lemon-juice (Fuzier), and in treating hyperthermia by means of cold aromatic applications. Acidulated drinks, quinine, and brandy are prescribed.

Prophylaxis on Board Vessels.—I quote from the communication of Chantemesse and Borel (1905): Let us take the case of a vessel leaving a country in which yellow fever is prevalent. After sailing, an antimosquito crusade must be carried on by fumigation of their local habitats, especially those in which the temperature is high (galley, engine-room, etc.). If a case of yellow fever breaks out on board, the cabin occupied by the patient must be evacuated if possible, fumigated, and then ventilated. Search must be made for receptacles likely to contain stagnant water, and the patient must sleep under a net. If the disease breaks out on a sailing-ship, the captain should steer a northerly course.

Prophylaxis against Yellow Fever in Ships on their Arrival in France. —Three hypotheses may present themselves on the arrival of a ship from an infected part. First hypothesis : Nothing has happened during the voyage. Free pratique should be given. Second hypothesis : One or two cases, obviously contracted in the infected country, have occurred on board, without giving rise to any further trouble. Pratique should be given without restrictions as to the crew and the cargo. Third hypothesis : A series of cases has appeared during the voyage. Precautions are then necessary. The vessel must be emptied, and the most thorough disinfection of all local habitats be carried out with sulphurous acid. If the cargo is of a nature liable to harbour mosquitoes (bananas, fruit, sugar, or damp timber), the holds must be fumigated with sulphurous acid.

Lastly, persons suffering from yellow fever, on arrival in ports where no quarantine hospital exists, should be placed in the local hospital. Yellow fever is not considered to be a contagious disease in France.

The most rigorous measures are, of course, necessary in countries inhabited by the *Stegomya*.

VI. PLAGUE.

Plague is a disease which, after ravaging the greater part of the Old World, remained for some years localized to certain provinces of Turkey in Asia, to Persia, and to the adjacent States. It was endemic there, but at intervals epidemics broke out, and spread by means of importation from their original centres, causing secondary centres on the borders of the Red Sea, of the Persian Gulf, and of the Caspian Sea.

Plague has lately resumed its widespread course, and after the epidemic at Hong-Kong has made constant progress. The disease appeared at Bombay in 1896, spread over India, passed through the Suez Canal, and invaded Alexandria. In July, 1899, it broke out at Oporto, and later showed itself at Glasgow. I need not speak of the epidemic at Vienna in 1898, which only occurred in the laboratory and was stamped out there.

Let us remember the epidemic on the s.s. *Sénégal*, chartered for a cruise by *La Revue des Sciences*, which ended in a quarantine at Frioul, so well known throughout the scientific world.

Epidemiology.—Plague is due to a microbe discovered by Yersin in 1884. The conditions necessary for the development of plague are well known, and the history of recent epidemics at Oporto and Bombay have yielded abundant data as to its epidemiology.

In the Oporto epidemic the breach remained unknown; plague was already present in Portugal in the early spring of 1899, when the first case was officially notified on June 5. Calmette and Salimbeni think that the disease was brought to Oporto by rats from some ship coming from the Island of Mauritius, the Persian Gulf, or from Alexandria. For a long while dead rats were found in the narrow streets of Fonte-Taurina and in the neighbourhood. The disease, disseminated by these rodents, quickly spread among the rats and mice which swarm in the vessels and in the docks of the port. The first cases of human plague did not appear until several weeks later, the first victims being the lumpers and poor people, who are herded together in the most insanitary houses of the town.

It appears certain that the disease was imported into Bombay by sea. The onset of the epidemic in the Mandvi quarter, which is close to the port and includes numerous warehouses, and the ease with which rats from ships moored in the docks could reach the land and overrun this quarter, are strong arguments in favour of this opinion. There seems to be no doubt that the infection came from Hong-Kong.

Plague is chiefly carried by the **rat** (Simond), and human agency is insufficient to explain the spread of the disease. The epidemic appears among rats before it does among the inhabitants in plague-infected towns. This fact also obtains in the case of ships, and Simond quotes a striking example :

" In February, 1898, the s.s. *Shannon* went from Bombay to Aden and back. Plague was raging at Bombay at this time, and the boat was submitted before its departure to the rigorous prophylactic measures laid down at the Venice Conference. Nothing special happened during the outward voyage, nor during the stop at Aden, but during the return voyage dead rats were found in the mail office, where the mail-bags were stored. Shortly after the postal official who worked in this room was attacked by plague. The man could not have brought the plague on board among his effects, nor could he have been in the incubation stage, for he had been taken on board at Aden, and did not come from a plague-infected area. There is no doubt, therefore, that he contracted the disease in the rat-infected cabin. It is also certain that an epidemic among rats had broken out on the boat long after its departure from Bombay, either because sick rats had come on board the ship at that port, or because the rats on board had contracted plague carried in the cargo."

The transmission of plague from the rat to man appears in most cases to be effected by means of parasites, and most writers have incriminated **fleas** (Simond), which live on corpses, and only leave them when they become cold. These facts explain why dead rats are at different times **very** dangerous or harmless (Simond).

Plague respects neither age, sex, nor race, but overcrowding, want, famine, and dirt are very favourable to its development. Its incubation period hardly ever exceeds ten days, and as a rule it is under five.

Description.—Plague usually runs the course of a malignant infection, with painful swelling of the lymphatic glands, high fever, and marked prostration. This is the classical or bubonic form of plague. In some cases it chiefly affects the lung or the intestine, bnt in other cases it runs the course of a true septicæmia.

1. *Classical Bubonic Plague.*—The onset is usually sudden, and accompanied by a sharp chill, fever, vomiting, headache, photophobia, and pains in the epigastrium, kidneys, and limbs. The gait becomes uncertain and reelin ʒ, and the patient is quickly compelled to lie down. At this period the chief symptoms are helplessness and prostration ; the power of speech is embarrassed or abolished ; the look is dull and resigned, and the patient is sometimes seized with vomiting and diarrhœa.

The temperature by the evening of the second day may reach 106° F. ; the morning remission is slight. A momentary fall of 2° is often noticed on the second or third day. The pulse rises to 120 or 140 ; the breathing becomes quick ; the tongue is black, dry, and cracked, and the lips are covered with sordes. Delirium may appear at this stage, being quiet or violent, with convulsions, carphologia, chilling of the extremities, and cyanosis of the lips. The vomiting and diarrhœa become more severe. The appearance of the tongue is characteristic. It is at first swollen, covered by a whitish coat, except at the edges and tip, which are clean. Later, the dorsum becomes dry and covered with a yellow or brownish coat, while the edges and the tip remain red. Cough and other signs of bronchial congestion are present, and, finally, various hæmorrhages help to complete the clinical picture of the stationary stage, which may last from one to three days.

The third period, or period of termination, presents two characteristic symptoms, which may, however, appear earlier—namely, **buboes** and **carbuncles.**

The buboes may affect any of the lymphatic glands, but they chiefly attack the glands in the groin, the axillæ, the popliteal spaces, and the neck. They do not always produce discoloration of the skin, unless suppuration occur. The deep glands (mediastinal and mesenteric) are often affected at the same time, giving rise to a train of symptoms which vary according to the situation of the enlarged glands. Their size varies from a hazel-nut to a walnut. They are sensitive to the touch. When the bubo is situated in the groin, the patient flexes the thigh upon the abdomen, in order to avoid stretching of the painful region. When the axilla is affected, the patient lies on his back, with the arm motionless and abducted from the trunk.

The situation of the initial bubo is of some importance as regards prognosis. Buboes in the neck are more serious than those in the groin. Each fresh invasion of glands is accompanied by a return of the fever. In rapidly fatal cases the glands remain hard and very painful. If the disease is prolonged, we find a brownish swelling of the gland and of the neighbouring region. This condition may end in resolution, or more often in suppuration, about the seventh or eighth day. When the bubo is opened, yellowish or sanious pus exudes. The sloughing of the skin is followed by an indolent ulcer, with prominent jagged edges and a greyish floor, in which the necrosed glands are exposed. These ulcers usually take several weeks to heal, and leave large and deep scars. Any gland which does not suppurate remains indurated for a lengthy period (Netter).

The appearance of buboes coincides in some patients with fall of temperature, moisture of the skin, and general feeling of comfort, which is of good omen. Events do not always run this course, and death may occur before the enlargement of the glands.

Let us now study the characteristic carbuncle of plague. These carbuncles are comparable to the first, second, and third degrees of burns (superficial lesions, eschars of the dermis, and deep gangrene affecting the muscles and even the bones). They vary in number from one to twelve, and may be found on any part of the body, except on the palms of the hands and soles of the feet. They are of evil omen, but less so than petechiæ, and the body is sometimes covered with black ecchymoses or pustules resembling hæmorrhagic variola. The cutaneous manifestations almost always accompany the very severe forms of plague. They are characteristic of the type called black plague by old writers (Calmette and Salimbeni).

Death usually appears with symptoms of ataxo-adynamia. Recovery, which is seen in half of the cases, may be interrupted or retarded by suppuration in the glands and by suppurative inflammations of the viscera and serous membranes.

2. *Septicæmic, Pneumonic, and Intestinal Forms.*—In the **septicæmic form** the buboes are absent. The onset is very severe, and the temperature rapidly rises to 105° or 106° F. The nervous phenomena are very marked. The prostration is extreme, even on the first day. Coma follows delirium, when it is present. Diarrhœa, tympanites, retention of urine, epistaxis, subconjunctival hæmorrhages, enterorrhagia, and hæmaturia have been noted. Death may occur in twenty-four hours.

Pneumonic plague, found in Bombay (Childe), was the only form seen in Vienna in October, 1898, in the laboratory epidemic, when Müller and Barish died. This terrible form of the disease is almost always fatal. It may be secondary, but it is usually primary. " The glandular enlargements are wanting, or only appear late, as a secondary result. The lesion in the lung replaces, as it were, the initial bubo, and forms the essential expression of the disease " (Cheinisse). The symptoms are those of pneumonia. Calmette and Salimbeni saw patients at Oporto with a temperature of 106° F., who had been taken ill with an initial rigor, as in pneumonia. The breathing was very laboured ; the rusty sputum became viscid, and in two or three days took on the appearance of prune-juice, as in a case of pneumonia which is passing into the stage of grey hepatization. Auscultation revealed the same signs as in pneumonia—fine crepitant râles and tubular breathing.

The diagnosis can be made only by bacteriological examination of the sputum. The prognosis is extremely grave, and recovery is exceptional. In the epidemic of pneumonic plague at Kolobovka there were twenty-three deaths out of twenty-four cases (Tchistowitch).

The **intestinal form** of plague is characterized by chills, fever, pain, and vomiting, with diarrhœa, distension of the abdomen, and backache. The glands become enlarged in a few days (Hogel).

Diagnosis.—The diagnosis of classical plague is very easy, especially during an epidemic. The sudden onset, the appearance of the tongue, the tenderness and swelling of the glands, attract attention. This does not obtain in the other forms, especially in the pneumonic form. Müller took the disease while nursing and examining his laboratory assistant, who was stricken with plague pneumonia, which remained undiscovered for thirty-six hours. He had not at that time the slightest suspicion as to the nature of the infection. The only means of diagnosis is by bacteriological examination of the sputum. The search for the plague bacillus is best made in the brawny area around the buboes. It will give the more valuable results the sooner it is made after the onset of the disease. When the bubo commences to suppurate, the *B. pestis* has given way to the agents of secondary infection.

Pathological Anatomy and Bacteriology.—The glands in plague are swollen, indurated, or softened, of a reddish, brownish, or yellowish colour, and filled with pus. They unite with the neighbouring glands, so as to form a large mass, enclosing nerves and vessels. The visceral lesions consist in congestion and hæmorrhages. The right heart is dilated; its walls may be softened to the point of rupture; and the venous system is distended and engorged with dark blood, both in the sinuses of the dura mater as well as in the veins of the limbs and trunk. The liver and spleen are enlarged and softened, while the lung is hard and hypertrophied. All the organs, and in particular the kidneys and the walls of the alimentary canal, show infiltration of blood.

Bacteriology.—Yersin has been able to isolate from the pulp of the buboes a short truncated bacillus, with rounded ends, staining with aniline dyes, but not with Gram.

The centre of the bacillus does not stain as deeply as its extremities. The bacillus is found in large numbers in the buboes, glands, and also in the blood. Cultures on broth somewhat resemble those of erysipelas. They show chains of short bacilli, which in places present nodular swellings. Cultures on agar yield transparent, whitish colonies, with radiating edges. Rats or guinea-pigs inoculated with cultures or with the pulp of the buboes die in a few days. Moreover, in plague epidemics rats are affected by the disease in plague-houses. Yersin found the same bacillus in the organs of rats which have died from plague as in man. He is of opinion that plague is inoculable and contagious, because he was able to cause plague by placing healthy mice in the same cage as inoculated ones.

"La peste, puisqu'il faut l'appeler par son nom,
Capable d'enrichir en un jour l'Achéron,"

has decimated a part of the globe for centuries, but is becoming more and more limited, on account of the energy of sanitary measures, though we cannot keep too close a watch, since it is at our doors.

Treatment.—Yersin has successfully treated patients with his anti-plague serum. On August 25, 1896, Brouardel announced that he had just received a despatch, saying that Yersin had treated and cured twenty-seven cases of plague with the serum. I give the result of the first case, which is destined to take its place among the marvellous methods of treatment which are the outcome of Pasteur's teaching :

" On June 26, 1896," says Yersin, " at the Catholic Mission School a young Chinaman called Tisé, eighteen years of age, complained, about ten o'clock in the morning, of pain in the right groin. At midday he felt very tired, fever appeared, and he was obliged to go to bed. I saw the patient at three o'clock in the afternoon, and his general condition was bad : extreme lassitude, vertigo, and fever. The characteristic bubo was present in the right groin, and this region was brawny, and formed a well-marked projection. The mass was exceedingly painful to the touch. About five o'clock I made preparations for a first injection of serum. The patient's condition was now worse. The weakness was extreme, the fever was higher, and delirium was setting in. In the opinion of all those accustomed to see patients with plague the patient was doomed to die within twelve hours.

" I gave the first injection of serum at five o'clock (10 c.c. under the skin of the flank), using serum prepared at Nha-Tsang, and successfully employed in the case of mice. It vaccinates mice with $\frac{1}{10}$ c.c. Immediately after the injection the patient vomited food and biliary matter (a frequent symptom in cases of pestis gravis). At six o'clock in the evening the general condition appeared a little better ; the eye was brighter, and the patient said that he felt stronger. I therefore gave a second injection of serum (10 c.c. under the skin of the flank).

" At half-past seven the fever had increased, and the patient was restless and wandering. He had colic and slight diarrhœa. At nine o'clock in the evening I gave the third and final injection of serum (10 c.c. under the skin of the flank). The fever was now very marked, and the patient continued to wander, but he slept in a restless manner from nine o'clock till midnight. The injection wounds were painful. At midnight notable improvement. The fever diminished, the patient regained consciousness, said that he felt better, and slept more quietly till three o'clock in the morning. By this time the improvement in his condition was manifest, the weakness and fever being less marked. The patient passed a motion (slight diarrhœa), and slept quietly from three o'clock till six in the morning, when he awoke quite conscious. The weakness had disappeared, the bubo was no longer painful and had decreased in size, and the fever had vanished.

" At eleven o'clock in the morning the patient said that he was cured. The skin was moist, and the temperature normal ; no trace of the lassitude and prostration of the previous evening remained. The brawny swelling in the right groin had completely disappeared. This region was now painless to the touch, and the only trace of the disease remaining was one or two glands of the size of a haricot-bean. The injection wounds were still painful.

" June 28 : The patient passed an excellent day and night. The injection wounds were no longer painful, and the resulting induration had disappeared. The patient's strength and appetite were returning. June 29 : I saw the patient for the last time to-day. His strength continues to return, and he is able to take a short walk in the garden without excessive fatigue. The glands of the groin are diminishing in size."

Yersin's serum has been employed at Bombay and Oporto. Calmette and Salimbeni who have obtained excellent results, advise as early as possible an **intravenous** injection of 20 c.c. of antiplague serum, followed by two **subcutaneous** injections of 40 c.c. each, repeated during the first twenty-four hours. The mortality at Oporto reached 63·72 per cent. before sero-therapy, but fell to 14·78 per cent. after the use of the serum. The difference between these two figures indicates the efficiency of the serum.

This method of treatment forms one of the greatest triumphs of sero-therapy.

Antiplague serum has a preventive action, conferring an immunity which lasts about a fortnight. It is necessary, therefore, during epidemics, to give an injection every two weeks. A dose of 5 c.c. is sufficient. The death of Dr. Pestana, who was vaccinated on September 18, and contracted plague on October 13, through omitting revaccination in the interval, is the best example of the necessity for revaccination every fortnight.

Injection of cultures of plague bacilli killed by heat at 70° C. (Haffkine) has also given good prophylactic results, but it is not free from danger during an epidemic, as it may hasten and aggravate the crisis of plague in patients already infected with the disease (Calmette and Salimbeni).

VII. TETANUS.

Tetanus (τιταίνω, I stretch) is characterized by paroxysmal contractures affecting a large number of muscles. This condition is due to the exaggeration of the excito-motor force of the spinal cord and bulb, and, consequently, to the abnormal excitation of their grey matter. Certain poisons, such as strychnine and brucine, cause tetaniform conditions, but true tetanus is a microbic disease.

Bacteriology.—The bacillus of tetanus was found in 1885 by Nicolaïer in the pus of wounds in mice and guinea-pigs which had been infected with tetanus by placing earth under their skin. Rosenbach found it later in the wound of a man suffering from spontaneous tetanus. Kitasato isolated it and obtained pure cultures in 1889.

The bacillus of tetanus is very thin and straight. It stains deeply with all the basic aniline dyes in hydro-alcoholic solution. In some cases it may be elongated into a thread which somewhat resembles the *Vibrio septicus*.

The bacillus may also occur in another form, which is much more characteristic. The bacillus, either in cultures or in wounds, passes into the sporula (Rosenbach) stage. It assumes the shape of a pin, a drumstick, or a racquet. This form is due to the spore which develops at one end of the bacillus, and often at both ends, in which case the bacillus assumes the form of a dumb-bell. In somewhat older cultures the spores detached from the rods resemble **cocci,** and do not stain as the bacillus does.   The methods used for the tubercle bacillus or for the *B. lepræ* must be employed to stain them.   The spores are very virulent and resistant.   They may remain alive for six months in cultures, in the tissues, or in the earth (Nicolaïer, Bonane, Sanchez Toledo and Veillon).

A stab culture on gelatine at 22° C. or on agar at 37° C. gives rise to colonies of the tetanus bacillus, developing in the form of small cloudy points, from which small rays extend perpendicularly, presenting the flaky appearance of a thistle.   The bacillus of Nicolaïer is anaerobic when cultivated in hydrogen or *in vacuo* in the oven at 37° C.   It yields abundant spores after twenty-four hours.

The tetanus bacillus exists in the superficial layers of the soil.   It is, therefore, a telluric microbe (Nicolaïer).   It has been met with in the soils of fields, in streets (Socin), in the dust from houses and gardens, in hay (Sanchez Toledo and Veillon), in manure (Sormani), and in animal excreta. It gains entrance by a wound or by a break in the continuity of the skin or of the mucous membrane.   Animals (especially the guinea-pig, the mouse, and the rat) can be infected with experimental tetanus by inoculation, and death almost always occurs after a period varying from one to five days. The bacillus is found at the point of inoculation, but is not met with elsewhere.   Like the diphtheria bacillus, it does not become general.   It is only diffused through the organs and the blood after death (Nicolaïer, Kitasato, Sanchez Toledo and Veillon).

The virulence of the tetanus bacillus is increased by successive passages through animals (Nicolaïer, Nocard, Dor), and by the association of the *B. prodigiosus* (Baillard).   It is diminished by the action of high temperatures (Dor, Vaillard), antiseptics, and lactic acid (Tizzoni and Cattani, Vaillard).

The **tetanus toxine** secreted by the bacillus is very active, but its chemical composition is not yet decided.   It would appear to be composed of several ptomaines, albuminoid substances, a diastasis, and a soluble ferment.   The poison is exceedingly active, and a hundredth part of a c.c. is sufficient to kill a guinea-pig.   In this case, too, as in diphtheria, the bacillus is confined to the wound, and secretes continuously a poison which has upon the nerve centres an action similar to that of strychnine or of brucine (Vaillard and Vincent).   Courmont and Dujon attribute this toxic power to a soluble ferment, harmless in itself, which elaborates a tetanizing substance at the expense of the organism.

A previous mild attack of tetanus does not confer immunity.   Immunity may be produced in animals by injecting tetanus toxine with trichloride of iodine (Behring and Kitasato).   The blood of animals treated in this manner is **antitoxic.**   Their serum, when inoculated in other animals, **vaccinates** them against tetanus (Behring and Kitasato, Tizzoni and Cattani), and

cures animals suffering from tetanus (Tizzoni and Cattani). This vaccination by antitoxic serum is transmitted from the mother to the fœtus (Tizzoni and Cattani), and is also carried by the milk (Ehrlich). The duration of the immunity produced by antitoxic serum is not very long (Roux and Vaillard). In one case Vaillard noticed its disappearance after a fortnight.

Recent researches on the tetanus toxine have allowed us to settle certain interesting points in its action, and to open up new vistas in therapeutics. Marie has shown that the toxine does not spread through the blood-stream. The intravenous injection of tetanus toxine must be eight to ten times as strong as the subcutaneous injection in order to produce death, because the poison acts almost exclusively on the nerves and fixes itself in the cells of the spinal cord or of the bulb.

The nerve cells show considerable affinity for the tetanus toxine. If the toxine is directly applied to the nervous substance (Roux and Borrel), it is immediately fixed and produces in rabbits and guinea-pigs a special form of tetanus, called **cerebral tetanus,** characterized by restlessness, epileptiform attacks, polyuria and motor troubles.

Roux and Borrel have formed the idea of injecting the antitoxine into the brain. " The antitoxine is injected at this spot in order to hinder the progress of the toxine, and to preserve the vital portions of the spinal cord before they are attacked." These injections have been successful in arresting tetanus in guinea-pigs twenty-four, twenty-eight, and even thirty-two hours after the appearance of the convulsions.

If the tetanus toxine is injected into the viscera of the guinea-pig—*i.e.*, testis, peritoneal cavity, liver, kidney, bladder, stomach, uterus, trachea, lung, or lymphatic glands—splanchnic tetanus results. It is never followed by permanent contractures and antitoxine inoculated by the subcutaneous or by the intracerebral method has no effect on it.

Ætiology.—Tetanus is always consecutive to a wound or to a scratch. The worst cases are seen in the wounds of the extremities (feet and hands), or in gun-shot injuries and jagged wounds. Tetanus may follow a physiological injury, as of the uterus after delivery, or of the umbilicus in the new-born infant. The disease is more frequent in men than in women, and is endemic in certain tropical countries (India, Madagascar, and Guiana). It is epidemic and contagious.

The inquiry pursued by Verneuil aims at ascertaining whether the horse has not something to do with the development of tetanus. The disease is common in warm countries where horses are numerous. It has developed following a wound from the lash of a whip, and Nicolaïer's bacillus was found on the lash itself (Poisson) ; but the horse is not an agent of immediate contagion between the soil and man and the telluric origin of tetanus is the only one at present admitted.

Pathological Anatomy.—The anatomical study of tetanus is as yet incomplete, for the lesions which have been seen, including ascending neuritis, granular degeneration of the cells of the spinal cord, and proliferation of the neuroglia, are applicable to but few cases and appear to be secondary changes. Hunter has, however, found in the spinal cord of man similar cellular lesions to those of experimental tetanus in animals—globular swelling of the cell, rarefaction of the chromatic elements, slight swelling of the protoplasmic processes, granular condition of the axis-cylinder, etc. Lastly, Joukowsky found in a fatal case of cephalic tetanus in man that the cells of the motor area of the cerebral cortex were impregnated with clear yellow pigment in great abundance. It was also present in the bulb and cord, but it does not appear to be a characteristic lesion. The accumulation of migratory rounded cells around the nerve cells, with penetration into their protoplasm, may be of more importance.

Description.—Tetanus usually commences with painful stiffness in the cervico-dorsal region, and, when it is of traumatic origin, the appearance of the wound changes, the suppuration diminishes and the cicatrization is arrested. As a rule, **trismus** (contracture of the jaw) is the first symptom. It is often associated with contracture of the nuchal and facial muscles (risus sardonicus). The cramp then reaches the muscles of the trunk and limbs. The trunk is bent backwards (opisthotonos), though in rare cases it may be bent forwards or to one side. The abdomen is retracted by the spasm of the abdominal muscles and the lower limbs are rigidly extended. The arms are less affected.

This tetanic contraction is not continuous. We find alternate relaxation and spasms, which are very painful. Trifling causes, such as touching the skin, contact of the bed-clothes, or any reflex excitation, are sufficient to bring on an attack. During the attack the trismus is more severe. The opisthotonos is so marked that the patient is bent in the form of a bow, and only touches the bed at the head and the toes; and the constriction of the pharynx and glottis, associated with a tetanic contraction of the inspiratory muscles, causes dyspnœa bordering on asphyxia. The patient is cyanosed, bathed in sweat, and tortured by the pains of the contractions. He is unable to speak or to make any sign, although he retains full consciousness. The attacks, which are at first short, with intervals between them, in favourable cases become gradually less frequent; but in unfavourable cases they occur at shorter intervals, and end in death.

The temperature in tetanus rises above 106° F. during the attack. This rise is not the result of fever and, in spite of some contradictory facts, it must be attributed to the heat given off by the muscles during the condition of tonic contraction. The pulse-rate and the breathing show the same variations as the temperature.

When tetanus is rapid in its course, the patient is carried off after a few days by asphyxia (tetanization of the respiratory muscles). It may be prolonged for several weeks as the result of remissions, but recovery is exceptional in this disease.

Cephalic Tetanus.—In some cases tetanus is limited to the head, several forms being seen : (1) The contraction is bilateral, the stiffness of the neck is sometimes associated with rigidity of the jaws, and the cervical opisthotonos mechanically causes dyspnœa and dysphagia (Verneuil) ; (2) the contracture is unilateral, and at first sight resembles facial paralysis ; (3) cephalic tetanus is accompanied by symptoms of dysphagia ; (4) it is accompanied by symptoms of hydrophobia (Rose's hydrophobic tetanus) ; (5) cephalic tetanus is accompanied by facial paralysis.

Tetanus in the Puerperal Condition and in the New-Born.—Epidemics of tetanus in lying-in women and new-born infants may be seen in maternity hospitals. The infection enters through the placental site and through the umbilical sore. The symptoms are identical with those described above. The gravity of the condition is extreme, and of twenty-one women suffering from puerperal tetanus, only one recovered (Rubeska). Among forty-four children only two recoveries were noted.

Tetanus by Injection of Gelatinized Serum.—The stir naturally caused by Chauffard's report and by my communication to the Académie de Médecine* leads me to give details of this question. The following case was under my care at the Hôtel-Dieu :

A woman in the Sainte-Jeanne ward was taken ill with symptoms of tetanus. The trismus had commenced suddenly about three o'clock in the morning. When we examined the patient at nine o'clock, she presented the characteristic picture of tetanic trismus. The teeth were shut so tightly that we could not separate the jaws ; the neck was stiff and painful ; the risus sardonicus was present and speech was almost impossible. It was evident that she was suffering from tetanus, but it remained to find the cause thereof.

The patient, who was thirty-eight years of age, had been under my care for some six weeks for advanced pulmonary tuberculosis, when hæmoptysis supervened. The treatment employed was chloride of calcium and preparations of rhatany. Some days later a fresh attack of hæmoptysis occurred, and my house physician prescribed an injection of gelatinized serum, a method of treatment much in vogue for hæmorrhage. The solution was carefully prepared in the dispensary, and the sterilization exceeded half an hour. The injection was given in the upper part of the left thigh with every aseptic precaution. The tetanus appeared eleven days after the injection of gelatine. As we were unable to find any other cause, it was reasonable to attribute the tetanus to the injection of gelatine.

I examined the spot where the injection had been made, but only an insignificant trace of the puncture was seen ; the skin was normal ; redness, pain, œdema, and swelling were absent ; there was no contraction of the thigh.

I gave a very bad prognosis. Treatment was at once commenced. Although injections of antitetanic serum after the onset of symptoms are not of much use, we

---

* Dieulafoy, *Académie de Médecine*, séance du 12 Mai, 1909.

gave, as a forlorn hope, an injection of 20 c.c. of antitetanic serum, and repeated the dose two hours later in the region where the injection of gelatine had been given. An enema containing 15 grains of chloral was given every hour and in the evening injections of carbolic acid were ordered. In spite of the treatment, the symptoms became worse. At four o'clock in the afternoon the head was stiff and retracted, opisthotonos was present, and the pains were continuous. The patient was much distressed, and could not spit out the mucus which accumulated in her throat. In the evening the symptoms became worse, although the temperature did not rise above 98° F., the dyspnœa increased in severity, and the poor woman died at half-past one in the morning, in a fit of suffocation.

Griffon made experiments in order to clear up this case ; on the one hand he examined the pus from a small abscess found at the spot where the injection of gelatine had been made, and on the other hand the gelatine furnished by the dispensary. The results of these experiments were :

Although a post-mortem was refused by the family, we were able, with every aseptic precaution, to incise the spot where the injection of gelatine had been given, and found under the skin a small abscess of the size of a hazel-nut. The pus was creamy, very thick, of a greyish-white colour, but without odour. The pus was collected in two sterile Pasteur pipettes, which were sealed by heat and taken to the laboratory. The pus, after staining, was examined under the microscope. Several slides were treated with different stains, and we found polynuclear leucocytes with clearly stained nuclei, but no sign of any organisms. After staining by Gram's method, the examination for micro-organisms was also negative ; neither Nicolaïer's bacilli nor other microbes were present.

Aerobic Cultures.—The pus from the pipettes was sown on agar and on broth, and cultivated in the presence of air. The culture taken from one of the pipettes remained sterile, but that from the other pipette showed colonies of a bulky rod, which liquefied gelatine and gave off a fœtid odour. This condition was evidently due to a bacterium of putrefaction, probably derived from the skin of the corpse ; this hypothesis was confirmed by the fact that the removal of pus had been delayed, and, further, that only one of the pipettes was found to be contaminated.

Anaerobic Cultures.—The pus from the pipette found to be sterile as regards aerobic cultures was then sown deeply in long tubes of agar, which was not set out at an angle, following the procedure of Liborius. We obtained pure cultures of Nicolaïer's bacillus after twenty-four hours' incubation in the oven at 37° C. The colonies were punctiform, spherical, and opaque, and scattered throughout the whole culture medium, except in the upper layer next to the air. After three or four days some of these colonies took on the flaky appearance of a tuft, and at length a few bubbles of gas burst through the agar in certain places. Under the microscope, after drying upon a slide in a drop of water, these colonies appeared to be formed of rods, which retained Gram's stain, and which showed a single spore (drumstick form), and, more rarely, a spore at each end (dumb-bell form).

Inoculation of Guinea-Pigs.—The pus was found to be very virulent. Several animals died in less than twenty-four hours, even after inoculation with a minute dose of pus taken from either pipette. A guinea-pig, inoculated with 4 or 6 drops of pus made into an emulsion with 1 centimetre of sterile broth, died in less than twenty hours with typical tetanic contractions.

The animal's body was bent to the left in emprosthotonos, the head was retracted to the side, and the four limbs were in a position of extension. Locally, the autopsy revealed in the thigh of these animals only a little serous fluid without microbes. The organs were congested, and the blood from the heart, upon microscopical examination and upon culture, contained no microbes.

After these results obtained by inoculation of the pus, we inoculated, for comparative purposes, a guinea-pig, a mouse and a rabbit, with culture of broth *in vacuo*, impregnated with a portion of a colony grown in a Liborius tube. All the animals died of tetanus.

Inoculation of Pure Spores.—The experiments of Vaillard and Vincent have resulted in the conclusion that **sporular** cultures, from which the living bacilli and the tetanus toxine have been removed by heating for three hours at 80° C., are harmless in the guinea-pig as long as they are not associated with a culture of the so-called assisting microbes or with a mechanical agent, such as lactic acid, producing negative chemiotaxis as regards the phagocytes.

" It is possible to inoculate guinea-pigs with doses of $\frac{1}{2}$ to $\frac{2}{3}$ c.c. of these cultures, which contain only spores, without the animal presenting any symptom of tetanus. The pure spores do not germinate in the healthy tissue, and therefore cannot produce the toxine which is indispensable to the development of tetanus " (Besson).

Since in my patient bacteriological analysis of the abscess from the thigh proved that the bacillus must have acted on its own account, it was interesting to place guinea-pigs experimentally under the same conditions as the patient—that is to say, to include the spores in a solution of gelatine.

Two guinea-pigs were, therefore, inoculated with $\frac{1}{2}$ c.c. of a sporular culture, to which a 10 per cent. solution of gelatine had been added. Only one animal showed symptoms of tetanus at the end of twelve days.

Two other control guinea-pigs were given injections of pure spores in the thigh ($\frac{1}{2}$ c.c. of a sporular culture, without the addition of gelatine). They also suffered from tetanus after an incubation of twelve days, just as did the guinea-pig inoculated with the first solution. The contractions were limited to the inoculated limb.

The experiments made in the laboratory justified the conclusions formulated in regard to my patient, and proved that the abscess was due to the development of Nicolaïer's bacillus in a pure state.

Search for the Tetanus Bacillus in Gelatine from the Laboratory.— Experiments upon guinea-pigs in order to find in the gelatine from the laboratory the bacillus or the spores yielded only negative results. Guinea-pigs, whether inoculated with a weak or with a concentrated solution (1 per cent. or 10 per cent.) of gelatine heated in a water-bath to boiling-point, remained healthy.

Cultures on anaerobic agar, however, gave positive results. A 10 per cent. solution of gelatine was kept boiling at 100° C. for several minutes, and a few drops were placed in a Liborius tube. After incubation for forty-eight hours in the oven at 37° C., numerous colonies of the tetanus bacillus were found. One of these colonies caused tetanus in an inoculated guinea-pig, which died in less than twenty-four hours. The experiment is, therefore, absolutely conclusive. Spores of a very virulent tetanus bacillus were found by culture in the pieces of gelatine taken from the hospital dispensary. These results confirmed the researches of Lévy and Brus, Anderson, etc., as regards commercial gelatine.

This case proves—(1) the presence of the tetanus microbe in commercial gelatine ; (2) the development of tetanus in men and animals by the pathogenic agent in a pure state without other microbes. This case of tetanus due to the injection of gelatine is not exceptional. On the contrary, several cases of fatal tetanus following injection of gelatinized serum have been published during the last two years. I give a summary of some of these cases :

On October 20, 1901, Méreau was called to see a patient suffering from severe hæmatemesis, due to an ulcer of the stomach. As several methods of treatment produced no effect, an injection of ½ litre of serum with 10 per cent. of gelatine, previously boiled for five minutes, was injected into the left flank, with every aseptic precaution. Eight days later the subjacent muscles became the seat of very painful contractions, although the injected region appeared free. During the day the patient was very restless, and complained of great discomfort in the muscles of the neck ; she could not open the jaw, because the masseters were contracted. On the following morning the patient had attacks of unbearable pain, opisthotonos was marked, and the lower limbs were contracted in the extended position. The constriction of the larynx and pharynx during the attacks brought on acute dyspnœa, and she passed away.

On January 6, 1902, a physician, called to see a woman suffering from severe metrorrhagia, which had resisted all treatment, gave an injection of 30 c.c. of gelatinized serum in the right gluteal region. On January 7 a fresh injection of 50 c.c. was made in the left buttock. Both these regions became painful, fever appeared, and the temperature during the next few days stood at 105° F. Brachet was called in consultation, and found that the left buttock was inflamed. On the evening of January 10 tetanus appeared, stiffness at the back of the neck, and retention of urine, requiring catheterization. On the 11th convulsions appeared, followed by trismus, which resisted every remedy. The back of the neck was contracted. On the 12th the gluteal abscess was incised. Soon afterwards a terrible attack came on, with spasm of the respiratory muscles, lividity of the face, and projection of the tongue between the teeth, which were tightly shut. After lasting a few seconds, the crisis appeared at an end, but the attacks increased in number, and death supervened at eleven o'clock the same night.

The cases of fatal tetanus following injections of gelatinized serum are so numerous that Chauffard succeeded in collecting eighteen in a report which he presented to the Académie. I can add five others to these eighteen, including those of Méreau and Krug, two cases reported by Doerfler (Berlin, 1903), and one case which I saw myself. We have, therefore, the large total of twenty-three cases in two years, without counting those which have escaped my notice, or which have not been published.

All these cases are very similar. Without entering into useless discussions, we know that tetanus may occur in patients because the gelatine employed in the preparation of the serum contains the germ of tetanus. In order to avoid such accidents, it is necessary either to abolish once for all injections of gelatinized serum or to employ serum from an absolutely reliable source. The difficulty, however, is to find such a source, and every care must be taken in the preparation of gelatinized serum, and also in the manufacture of the gelatine itself.

In Germany, at Merck's laboratory, fresh calves' feet are used, and boiled for an hour at 120° C. The gelatine is, therefore, absolutely pure. It is filtered and placed in tubes, which are sterilized on two successive days at 120° C. for a period of one hour. A large amount of the gelatine preparation is then injected into mice and guinea-pigs, and if the animals remain healthy for twenty days after the operation, the solution of 1 per cent. gelatine is placed on the market.

In order to obtain preparations absolutely free from danger, I agree with Chauffard that the preparation of gelatinized serum " should not be free, but should be restricted by the laws and rules which regulate the preparation of therapeutic serums." And even then, in spite of every precaution, we shall always feel anxious when we prescribe this treatment. For my part, I have never made use of gelatinized serum, and in the future I shall hold to the same principle.

Moreover, the hæmostatic properties of gelatinized serum are **nil,** as the observations and experiments of Labbé and Froin conclusively prove.

We may, therefore, abandon without regret this useless and harmful remedy.

Diagnosis.—The diagnosis of tetanus is easy when the characteristic symptoms are present. Tetanus can scarcely be confounded with acute or chronic strychnine-poisoning, as there are certain differences. We usually find in strychnine-poisoning that trismus appears later, delirium is frequent, blue vision may be present (Tardieu), and the pupils are dilated (Brouardel).

Treatment.—In order to avoid the contagion of tetanus, it is necessary to disinfect localities contaminated by individuals or by animals with tetanus, to isolate the clearly defined cases and to cleanse suspected wounds with the greatest care. When tetanus is present, isolation of the patient in the most quiet surroundings, chloral, morphia and Calabar bean have been advised. If the infected focus is accessible and if amputation does not entail too serious a mutilation, it should be performed without delay, in order to avoid the formation of fresh toxines (Berger). Lastly, the patient must be given injections of antitoxic serum, which is the only rational method of treatment. The failures resulting from Behring and Kitasato's method are explained by the extreme fixity of the tetanus toxine in the nerve cells, and by the impossibility of the antitoxine reaching them in time if it is given by subcutaneous or by intravenous injection. Accordingly, the experimental treatment proposed by Roux and Borrel in the case of the guinea-pig (**intracerebral injection** of antitoxine) has been used in man. In twenty-six cases collected last year Lereboullet found eighteen deaths and eight recoveries. Early intracerebral injection, as soon as trismus occurs, appears to be one of the conditions for success and there is then some chance of arresting the disease.

Sicard has related the cases of three patients suffering from tetanus who were treated and cured by subarachnoid injections of antitetanic toxine. In one of these cases several injections of antitetanic serum were also made into the large peripheral nerve trunks.

Preventive injections of antitoxine are very efficacious in any patient suffering from a suspected wound which has been soiled by earth (Vaillard and Roux). The injection of 10 c.c. of antitetanic serum, repeated a fortnight after the first injection, is an excellent safeguard against tetanus, and I cannot recommend its use too strongly.

VIII. MALARIA.

The researches of recent years have enriched the history of malaria with fresh and exact knowledge, which has cleared up many previously obscure questions. The infectious agent of paludism—the hæmatozoon—is well known (Laveran). We know that certain mosquitoes are extremely active agents of propagation and contagion, and this knowledge has furnished prophylactic measures which give excellent results. The discovery of the pathogenic agents and the use of sero-diagnosis helps to elucidate the obscure points in complex cases of typho-malarial fever. It is, indeed, evident that the views held twenty years ago are very different from those we hold to-day.

Malaria may assume many forms, including intermittent, remittent, continuous, pernicious, or larval fever, chronic lesions, and cachexia ; and certainly, of all the infectious diseases, it occupies the largest surface of the globe. Few countries escape ; it holds sway either in an endemic or in an endemo-epidemic form in the five divisions of the world, increasing in virulence in tropical climates.

When the infection has entered the economy, it remains there with such pertinacity that it may reappear for years in different forms, either febrile or afebrile, even after the patient has long since left the original centre of infection.

In tropical climates malaria is often associated with other infections, such as typhoid fever or dysentery, and these complications play a large part in the severity of epidemics.

At every moment in large undertakings and great enterprises mankind encounters malaria, which is his most terrible enemy. Many examples of this may be quoted. At Bordeaux, in 1805, the swamp of Chartreuse, which is close to the town, was drained in the summer ; 12,000 inhabitants were taken ill with malarial fever, and 3,000 died. The Saint-Martin canal was dug at Paris in 1811, and the Temple, Villette, and Pantin quarters of the city paid a heavy tribute to malarial fever. Epidemics of malarial fever broke out during the work upon the Suez Canal and the Panama Canal.

When it was found advisable to replant the vine in the Department of Hérault some years ago, the pick and plough opened up old swampy areas in the sand on the sea-shore, and malarial fever appeared in an epidemic form (Jeannel).

Our troops were decimated by the terrible scourge in Algeria, the Crimea, Italy, China, Cochin-China, Mexico, and Tonkin. In the United States, during the famous War of Secession, tens of thousands were attacked by malarial and typho-malarial infection.

Towns which were formerly flourishing have been ruined by their proximity to salt marshes.

The greatest disaster recorded in history is certainly the blotting out of the British army in Walcheren. This took place in 1809. "England," says Thiers, the historian, "sent to the Scheldt a formidable expedition, composed of 470 vessels, with 44,000 men, in order to capture Antwerp and the French fleet. Some anxiety was felt in Paris as to the issue of this expedition, but Napoleon, who was at Schoenbrunn, re-assured everyone; for he saw, by a flash of genius, that the British army would perish in the malarial regions of the Scheldt. He therefore ordered his Generals to hold the army in check in this region, and not to give battle. His prognosis was verified: malaria caused terrible ravages among the English, and 27,000 of their soldiers perished or were sent to hospital."

Parasitology.—Until recent years the pathogenesis and the nature of malaria was a matter of supposition, because micro-biology had not as yet revealed the intimate cause of the infectious diseases. The honour of dis-covering the pathogenic agent of malaria was reserved for a French physician, Laveran, who, on November 6, 1880, saw for the first time the flagella of the hæmatozoon, and his first publication, which dates from 1881, is several years prior to the works of Marchiafava and Celli, "who in 1889 simply verified the facts announced by Laveran between 1880 and 1882."

The parasite of malaria is a **hæmatozoon.** It shows two forms (*parva et magna*), so called from the size of the parasitic elements. When a patient returns to France after the small variety has been found in his blood in a malarial country, we find the large variety in the blood if he has a return of the fever. Accordingly, they are *not* two different species, but only varieties of the same species. Its forms may be classified in the following four types:

1. **Spherical Bodies.**—These represent the most common form of the parasite, and are composed of transparent hyaline substance. The largest ones may exceed the size of the red corpuscles. The spherical bodies show amœboid movements. They may be free in the serum, or may be incorporated in the red blood-corpuscles, which may show two or three in each corpuscle.

These parasites live at the expense of the red corpuscles. As the spherical body grows, it becomes filled with pigment, and the red corpuscle becomes pale, until it is as transparent as the parasite. The granules of pigment are often absent in the smallest spherical bodies, but they may form a regular crown of black granules in the large ones. After half an hour the amœboid movements cease, the pigment collects at certain points and the spherical bodies take on their cadaveric form. They differ from melaniferous leuco-cytes in the absence of a nucleus.

2. **Flagella.**—In preparations from fresh blood, where the spherical bodies are free in the serum, we may see excapsulation of the flagella. The flagella are mobile threads moving actively and varying in length from

20 to 28 μ. Two, three, or four flagella are sometimes attached to one spherical body, which then resembles a pseudopod. The free end of the flagella always presents a pyriform swelling. These filaments become detached from the spherical body at a given moment. According to Laveran, the flagella are the most characteristic elements of the parasite, as he found them 92 times in 432 cases. The flagella are the male elements, destined to fertilize the female elements (MacCallum, Koch, Marchaix).

3. **The crescent bodies** have a length equal to that of the diameter of the red blood-corpuscles. The horns of the crescent are tapered and curved. Grains of black pigment accumulate at the central part.

4. **The rosettes** closely resemble the shape of a rose. They are pigmented at the centre and segmented at the periphery. Laveran was at first of opinion that they were retrogressive forms of the spherical bodies. Golgi studied them carefully in 1886, and again in 1889. The peripheral segments break up, becoming free, and are converted into small amœboid spherical bodies. According to some authorities, the rosettes are more numerous in tertian than in quartan fever.

5. **Cadaveric Forms.**—We find in the blood of malarial patients immobile, irregular and pigmented hyaline bodies, which are the remnants of the hæmatozoon.

Phagocytosis.—The leucocytes are recognized by their regular form, and by their nuclei, which stains readily with carmine. These melaniferous leucocytes absorb the pigment from the dead parasite. They may even absorb it from the living organism.

Evolution of the Parasite.—The first act of this polymorphous parasitism is its appearance in the form of a transparent vacuole in the red corpuscle. The vacuole becomes a spherical body and is filled with pigment granules at the expense of the red corpuscles. After this, the spherical bodies push out the flagella. The hæmatozoon sometimes assumes the form of a crescent incorporated in a red corpuscle which has been digested, but at other times it breaks up and forms a rosette body. Segments or spores numbering ten to twenty become free and pass into the plasma, where the cycle starts afresh.

Frequency of the Types.—In the cases observed by Laveran the types of the hæmatozoon alone or combined were divided as follows :

Spherical body	..	..	..	..	389 times.
Crescent	..	..	..	..	107 „
Flagella..	..	..	..	..	92 „

It has recently been stated that the type of the parasite varies with that of the fever. According to Golgi, there is a special parasite for tertian fever, quartan fever, etc. This is an error. The flagella and the spherical bodies are more frequent in acute malaria, the crescent bodies are more often found in chronic cases, but the **parasite is always the same.**

Technique.—In order to find the hæmatozoon, we must look for it at the onset of an attack before the paroxysm, and **before the administration of quinine.** A drop of blood is withdrawn and spread upon a slide, and the cover-glass should be ringed in order to prevent currents. Laveran usually employs methylene blue as the staining reagent.

Discussion.—According to some authors, Laveran's hæmatozoon is not the specific agent of malaria, because it is present in the lizard, tortoise, jackdaw, etc. The hæmatozoon is no doubt found among the animal species (Danilewsky), but in man it is pathogenic. The proofs furnished by Laveran are : hæmatozoa are found in malaria wherever it occurs. They have never been met with in persons who were not suffering from malaria. The development of the hæmatozoa is intimately related to the production of melanæmia, which is characteristic of malaria. The salts of quinine cause the parasite to disappear from the blood and at the same time cure malaria. Malaria has been successfully transmitted from animal to man by injecting into the veins of a healthy individual a small quantity of blood containing the parasites from a malarial patient (Mariotti and Ciarrochi).

Ætiology.—The hypotheses put forward by Laveran and Patrick Manson concerning the propagation of malaria by some sucking insect, such as the mosquito, have received definite acknowledgment. Ronald Ross has found that the hæmatozoon of birds develops in the mosquito in the form of pigmented bodies and germ filaments which have recently developed in the venomo-salivary gland of the mosquito. These bodies pass with the secretion of the gland into the wound made by the insect upon the skin of a healthy subject, mix with the blood, and produce infection. Ronald Ross was able in this way to infect healthy birds, which succumbed. The liver and the spleen were filled with black pigment characteristic of the disease in birds. All mosquitoes are not capable of propagating malaria. The Anopheles must be held guilty. The coexistence of the Anopheles and of endemic malarial fever have been recognized in several parts of the world. On the other hand, the Culex is only found in healthy localities (Laveran).

In London, where this disease does not exist normally, Manson succeeded in causing malaria in the following manner : The larvæ of the Anopheles were collected in Rome, and were kept in close confinement. When they became adult, they were placed in mosquito-proof cylinders and were so far harmless. In order to make them poisonous, the cylinder was placed upon a patient suffering from malaria, and the mosquitoes, biting the patient through the meshes of the gauze, absorbed both the blood and the hæmatozoa. The cylinders containing the infected mosquitoes were sent from Rome to London. Manson's son, who was studying medicine at Guy's Hospital, allowed these mosquitoes to bite him and was attacked by malaria. The hæmatozoa were found in his blood.

Another experiment, the inverse of the preceding, clearly shows the part played by the mosquito in the spread of malaria. Sambon, Low, and three other persons lived near the mouth of the Tiber, in a locality where malaria attacks both the inhabitants and travellers. They were careful, however, to live in a wooden hut specially constructed in London, with windows fitted with such fine wire blinds that the Anopheles could not pass through them. The beds were protected by mosquito-curtains. The experimenters remained a month in their hut without going out between bedtime and sunrise. They were not attacked by malaria.

The Anopheles is distinguished from the Culex by the position of its head. In the former, the trunk and the palps are of the same length, instead of the palps being shorter than the trunk. The Anopheles does not rise above the ground, as it is a poor flier, and does not travel far from the pool where it is born. During the day the Anopheles hides on plants or in dark places, but at night it comes out on the pools. The female alone bites man at dusk. The larvæ of the Anopheles live in the water, like those of the Culex, but their shape is very different. In the Culex a respiratory tube which projects out of the water is found at the tail end; the Anopheles breathes by means of the whole surface of the body, which remains in a horizontal position just under the water. It is possible to deprive them of air and kill them by pouring on the water petroleum oil or some fatty material.

The development of the hæmatozoon in the Anopheles is exogenous and sexual. The female bites a malarial patient during the night, and injects into him some of the poison which is secreted by the salivary glands, and which has the property of preventing the coagulation of the blood. In this manner it absorbs human blood, which contains the hæmatozoon in the form of spherical bodies or of crescents. The spherical bodies are destroyed by the digestive juices of the mosquito, and the crescents alone survive. In the digestive tube of the Anopheles the latter form ovoid bodies of two kinds—one is the male (microgametocyte), and the other is the female (macrogametocyte). The male sends out several flagella, which become detached, and unite, like spermatozoa, with the female. Fertilization is followed by the expulsion of a fertile egg, the zygote, which lengthens and becomes encysted in the muscular wall of the stomach. It grows, forming a hernia upon the external wall of the stomach of the Anopheles and becomes filled with numerous fusiform bodies, the sporozoïtes. These become free, pass into the blood of the mosquito and are found in the salivary glands and in their excretory ducts. Ten thousand sporozoïtes have been counted in a single Anopheles. In human blood they are converted into spherical bodies and destroy the blood-corpuscles.

The sporozoïtes develop only at a temperature of 80° to 85° F., which explains the absence of malaria in northern countries and in France during the winter.

Badly drained marshes, the mixing of sweet and salt waters (Dutroulau), the great disturbance of soil in the cutting of canals and in the reclamation of ground, are favourable media for the development of the pathogenic agent. The marshy soils formed by thin sheets of water and mud, rich in vegetable matter and exposed to the rays of the sun, are most favourable to the hatching of malaria. It also appears in localities which are not marshy, but on closer inspection we see that, under the dry crust of these localities, damp earth, which is the origin of miasma, is found; and we can thus explain the appearance of malaria which broke out in Paris during the great disturbance of the soil in 1811 in order to cut the Saint-Martin Canal and in 1840 for the construction of fortifications.

The conditions which I have just enumerated are not, however, absolutely indispensable to the production of malaria, for it is endemic in countries which are composed of sandy, granitic, or volcanic soils.

Thus, in Algeria malaria appeared during the reclamation of our colony in a very " dry and sterile country, where neither damp nor decomposition in marshes is seen." The term palustral infection, paludism, or palustral fever, which comes from *palus*, a marsh, is, therefore, not exact : although we preserve it from custom, it does not apply to all cases.

Malaria may be caused by drinking marshy water, and the report by Boudin on the small epidemic which broke out on a Sardinian vessel, the *Arago*, leaves no doubt on this point. A first attack, instead of conferring immunity, is generally the origin of later troubles. In a country where malaria is endemic the inhabitants, by reason of their acclimatization, are little subject to acute attacks, though they often suffer from malarial cachexia, and their children are sometimes cachectic from birth. The black races enjoy marked immunity.

Malaria, while very rare in cold countries, is endemic in many warm and temperate climates, and among such I may mention France (Bresse and Sologne), Italy (the Pontino Marshes and the Roman Campagna), Greece, the mouths of the Danube, Lower Hungary, Algeria, Lower Egypt, Senegal, Madagascar, India, Persia, Cochin-China, the Gulf of Mexico, the Antilles, Central America, etc.

In countries where malaria is endemic, the fever is most frequent and most severe during the **summer,** and the disease is most severe in very hot climates and in tropical regions. Malaria sometimes assumes an **epidemic** form in countries where it is endemic, and may then extend to countries which apparently offer conditions unfavourable to its development. These epidemics have often preceded those of cholera.

Manifestations of Malarial Fever.—The manifestations of malarial fever are febrile and afebrile. The former have long been included under the name of intermittent fevers, and at the present day we are still too prone to employ this vicious synonym, as though the parasite could only cause intermittent fever. In our climate, it is true, intermittent fever is the most general manifestation of malaria ; but in tropical climates the intermittent form becomes more rare and the poison shows itself by remittent and continuous fevers. If we make intermittence the essential character of malaria, we return to the erroneous classification of Pinel. In 1828 Annesley made it known that the same miasmatic cause produces the intermittent, remittent, and continuous fevers of India; in 1836 Maillot, in Algeria, definitely established the remittent and continuous types of malaria, and noted their relation to the intermittent ones. "In Algeria we have been able to extricate the tertian and the quartan forms, to free ourselves from the nosological prejudice of the type, and thus to include them under a wider pathology, which for medical purposes is more correct and more practical. In Algeria we have been able to recognise defaced and mixed types, so that our classical intermittent fevers have changed into continuous ones, as well as to note the error of a pyretology exclusively founded on the consideration of the type " (Trousseau and Pidoux).

Malaria also shows afebrile forms, which we shall study later. We shall see that these manifestations are usually chronic and follow the primary febrile attacks.

The febrile and afebrile forms of malaria may appear alone or in association. They may succeed one another, or may be combined in different cases. For purposes of description, I shall divide them into the following groups :

1. Intermittent fevers of variable type.
2. Remittent and continuous fevers.
3. Pernicious fevers.
4. Malarial cachexia.
5. Larval fevers.

Intermittent Fevers.

Description.—Intermittent fever is the commonest form of malaria. It occurs in attacks. It is quite sufficient to have stayed for a short time, or even to have passed through a country, where malaria is prevalent, to suffer from intermittent fever. The period of **incubation** lasts six, eight, or ten days, and rarely more than three weeks. In some cases the attack of fever appears suddenly, but in other cases it is preceded for a few hours or for a day by malaise, chills, and gastric troubles, which simulate febrile gastritis, although they are really due to malaria. In some persons unusual lassitude, pains in the muscles or in the joints, turbid urine, and chills with headache, which cannot be mistaken, indicate that an attack is about to appear. Then the rigor occurs.

In the regular attack we find three **stages**—cold, hot, and sweating.

The **cold** stage—or, rather, the stage of the rigor—is characterized by a **rigor,** accompanied by **shaking,** which at first affects the muscles of the jaw (chattering of the teeth), and then the whole body, so as to shake the patient's bed. The skin is dry and the prominent papillæ give to it the appearance of goose-flesh. The face and extremities are cold and bluish, the restlessness is acute, the oppression is marked, the voice is weak, the pulse is small and rapid and the urine is scanty and watery. Although the patient feels extremely cold, the temperature in the axilla may exceed 104° F. during this cold stage.

The rigor is, however, only the apparent starting of the attack. Rise of temperature, changes in the urine, and increase in the quantity of urea (Jaccoud), as well as of the carbonic acid excreted by respiration—in short, an excess of organic combustion—appear several hours before the rigor. Chills alternate with hot flushes after a duration which varies from one to two hours. This forms the commencement of the hot stage.

During the **hot stage** the feeling of heat becomes gradually more severe, and may be extremely painful. Patients throw off the bed-clothes, and frequently change their position in bed to obtain a cool spot. The pulse becomes full, but remains rapid. The skin is dry and burning, and the face is injected. The respiration is quickened ; delirium is sometimes present ; the thirst is acute ; and the urine is high-coloured. This stage usually lasts one to two hours.

The **sweating stage** commences with moisture and a general feeling of well-being. The sweating is abundant; the temperature falls rapidly ; the skin becomes cool ; the pulse improves, but is still somewhat full ; the urine is thick, high-coloured, and sometimes contains albumin. This stage, which is the longest of the three, usually lasts from two to four hours. Refreshing sleep comes on as soon as the calm has reappeared. An eruption of herpes is sometimes seen on the face.

The above description represents a typical attack, but the malady does not always show the classical course above described. The series is not always complete. Some persons may not shiver, while others perspire but little. The attack almost always commences between midnight and midday, in contradistinction to the attacks of symptomatic intermittent fever, which commence in the evening. The pains in the left hypochondrium of which patients sometimes complain are due to the swelling of the spleen which accompanies the attack. This swelling is at first transient, but becomes permanent after repeated attacks. At the end of the attack the patient, except for a certain lassitude, feels well ; but if the period of apyrexia is short, and the attack is repeated, the patient feels ill, even during the periods of apyrexia, and suffers from weakness, which is often accompanied by digestive troubles.

I have just described an attack of intermittent fever, such as we see in France, but in different countries it presents certain variations deserving of notice. Thus, in Persia the fever is often accompanied by vomiting or by delirium, and sometimes simulates meningitis, although the prognosis is not of much gravity.

Types.—The **period of apyrexia** determines, according to its duration, a type of the intermittent fever.

Quotidian fever is characterized by daily attacks.

Tertian fever is characterized by attacks which return every two days, and show a period of apyrexia for twenty-four hours.

Quartan fever is characterized by attacks which return every third day.

We also see very rare types in which the fever is **quintan, sextan, septan,** or **octan.**

The tertian and quotidian fevers present varieties which have been called **doubled** and **redoubled fever.**

The former are more rare than the latter ; they are characterized by two attacks occurring in the same day. Both attacks come on daily in double quotidian fever, every two days in double tertian fever, and every three days in double quartan fever.

The latter forms, also called **double tertian** and **double quartan,** are characterized by attacks which occur in the following manner : In the **double tertian** form there is an attack every day, but the attack of the next day does not resemble that of the previous one, as in quotidian fever, the resemblance being confined to the attack of two days previously—that is to say, the attack on the third day resembles in its severity, duration, and time of appearance the attack of the first day, the attack of the fourth day resembles that of the second, and so on. In **double quartan** fever attacks occur every two days, the attack on the fourth day resembling that of the first, and the attack of the fifth day resembling that of the second.

The tertian and quotidian fevers are the most frequent of all these types. In our country we have the tertian or the quotidian type, but the fever is rarely quartan at its onset. The doubled and redoubled types are never primary. The type appears to depend upon the nature of the miasma which infects the particular locality.

In a patient who is not under treatment the attack of true intermittent fever returns on a fixed day, and practically at the same hour. If it occur later, it is said to postpone ; if it occur earlier, it is said to anticipate ; and if a fresh attack appear before the end of the preceding one, the fever is subintrant.

One type may be converted into another. Thus, quotidian fever becomes double tertian, then genuine tertian, and, inversely, tertian fever may be converted into quotidian fever. The tertian type changes into the quartan, especially in autumn (Van Swieten), and the quartan fever may assume the tertian type. The more the fever differs from the quotidian type, the more obstinate it is; the quartan fever is specially rebellious, as the Latin curse shows : *Quartana te teneat !*

Course—Diagnosis.—Intermittent fever may recover without treatment after a duration of some weeks, but the first attack, whether treated or not, is generally followed by a series of fresh attacks, which come on weeks, months, or even years apart, sometimes without appreciable cause, and at other times as the result of a chill, fatigue, or injury (Verneuil), or as the sequela of an acute disease. This return of malaria, following some external or internal disturbance, is highly important.

When the recurrences follow in close succession, they usually appear with such regularity that the paroxysm, according as the fever was tertian or quartan, returns on the day upon which it would have been due if the succession of attacks had not been interrupted. After several recurrences, the **short rhythms** become more frequent, the attacks at length lose their regularity, the stages are less clean and complete, the periodicity is less precise, and the type loses its clearness, so that the fever is said to be irregular.

In some cases the patient, who is wasted and anæmic, is liable to headache, to cold shivers followed by sweating, and to dyspepsia, and the febrile attacks appear at times. The **spleen** sometimes becomes very large. The liver is also bulky, the nutrition is faulty, and if remedial measures are not employed, the patient passes into the cachectic stage.

The diagnosis of intermittent fever is sometimes difficult, and we may be unable to give a correct opinion without having seen several attacks unless the hæmatozoon has been found. In countries where malaria is endemic, cases of pyrexia which are naturally continuous—as, for example, typhoid fever—sometimes commence with intermittent attacks before assuming their proper type. We cannot say in any case that malaria has been converted into typhoid fever, but we shall see later that typhoid fever and malaria may run a coincident course, forming a mixed type—typhomalarial fever.

We see in marshy countries continuous fevers which at first simulate typhoid fever, but the fever soon becomes interrupted, rigors mark the onset of true attacks, and genuine intermittence appears. In every case in which the diagnosis between the continuous forms of malaria and typhoid fever is difficult **sero-diagnosis** (Widal) will remove all doubts.

We shall not confound **symptomatic** intermittent fevers (tuberculosis, suppuration, cachexia) with malaria. They are associated with different morbid states. Hypertrophy of the spleen is absent and the attack comes on in the evening.

Remittent and Continuous Fevers.

Remittent fever is a continuous fever in which the paroxysms are more or less marked, while the remissions never show the complete apyrexia characteristic of intermittence. The terms remittent fever and continuous fever might, therefore, be blended. In the remittent forms, however, the paroxysms are fairly well marked, and are sometimes preceded by a cold stage, while in the continuous fever no periodicity is seen.

The remittent forms may be converted into intermittent ones. The fever is generally remittent from the first. In some cases, however, the remittence or the continuity is established after the intermittent attacks have become subintrant.

Remittent fever has little tendency to recur in its initial form. When it does so, it takes the intermittent type (Colin).

Remittent fever is endemic in some countries of Europe (South of France, Greece, Italy, countries of the Lower Danube), but it is chiefly found in hot climates (Algeria, Senegal, India, Cochin-China, the Antilles, centre of America, etc.). It often appears in an epidemic form, and may then disappear for some years. In some tropical countries the remittent form is found at the coast, while the intermittent form is present in the interior or upon the plateaux. The native or the acclimatized individual usually contracts intermittent fever, but the new-comer is stricken down with the remittent form (Griesinger). These facts have been discovered in Rome and Algeria by French physicians, and by English doctors in India, where the great epidemics of remittent and continuous fever chiefly appear in newly-arrived troops, while the acclimatized soldiers suffer for the most part from the intermittent forms.

The remittent and continuous fevers show several varieties, which are briefly as follows :

Solitary Remittent Fever.—An individual living in a marshy country is seized with violent headache ; fever, lassitude, lumbar pains like those of variola, epistaxis, prostration, vertigo, and insomnia, similar to that of typhoid fever, are present. Anorexia, nausea, vomiting, acute thirst, and dry tongue occur, as in gastric disorders. The spleen is large and painful, and slight jaundice is seen. The fever is pseudo-continuous, presenting exacerbations, which are sometimes preceded by a rigor, and reaching as high as 104° F. The disease lasts from eight to ten days. It may then terminate quickly, with abundant sweating, or it may drag on for a long

while if quinine be not exhibited.   It may also be converted into the intermittent form.   The above type is that of **simple** remittent fever, unaccompanied by complications.

Bilious Remittent Fevers.—In other cases the remittent fever is not
" solitary," but is accompanied by **gastric** or **biliary** symptoms, which are
of sufficient importance to create the gastric or the biliary types of remittent
fever.   Here, as in all infectious diseases, we find every intermediate grade
between benign and fatal cases.   These variations depend largely upon the
severity of the epidemic and upon the country in which the fever occurs.

Indeed, the nearer we come to the equatorial zones, the more frequent
are bilious fevers, such as biliary typhoid fever, yellow fever, and biliary
malarial fever.   It has even been asked if there may not be a climatic
biliary fever independent of other groups.   As regards bilious remittent
fever, the severe forms run the following course :

An individual living in a warm country where malaria is prevalent is at
first taken ill with remittent fever or with intermittent attacks, which
quickly become remittent.   The onset is characterized by headache, lassitude, chills, and fever.   A violent attack soon sets in, with gastric pain,
vomiting of food and of bile, vertigo, nausea, and a feeling of faintness.
The intolerance of the stomach may be so great that nothing can be retained.
The tongue is coated.   Diarrhœa is frequent.   In some cases **floods of bile**
are vomited or passed in the stools.   The jaundice may be of every degree.
It appears on the third or fourth day of the disease, and is bilipheic and
hæmapheic, but rarely one or the other.   The liver is enlarged, and at times
so painful as to cause suspicion of an abscess.   The spleen is hypertrophied
and very painful.   The symptom-complex of bilious remittent fever, therefore, comprises pain in the liver, in the spleen, in the lumbar region, in the
muscles, in the joints, and in the stomach.

The fever during the course of this trouble exceeds 104° F.   The usual
remission is 1° F., and may occur in the evening or in the morning, while the
patient remains conscious of the attack during the paroxysms.   Hæmorrhages are frequent (epistaxis, purpura, melæna).   Nervous troubles, restlessness, delirium, and ataxo-adynamic symptoms are common.   Coma is
somewhat rare.   The gastric, intestinal, biliary, hæmorrhagic, and nervous
phenomena are much intermingled in different cases.

When the patient does not succumb in these severe forms, convalescence
is long and painful.   It is at times ushered in by the change to a remittent
or to an intermittent type, by the complete remission of the fever or by
abundant sweating, but fresh attacks are always to be feared.

In other cases the bilious troubles are less marked, and the chief symptom
is the continuous nature of the fever, with only slight remissions, with predominance of **ataxo-adynamic** symptoms, such as weakness, prostration,

stupor, delirium, dryness of the tongue, distension of the belly and fœtid diarrhœa, which recall the clinical picture of typhoid fever.

Lastly, in some cases the typhoid symptoms and the bilious symptoms may be intermixed.

The **severe** forms of remittent fever present, therefore, the most different aspects. Sometimes the typhoid state is marked from the first, and the remissions are irregular, though appreciable, for some days. If at a later stage they are no longer seen, the prognosis is grave, and in this case adynamia sets in early. In other cases we see multiple hæmorrhages from the nose or from the kidneys, and in the skin, forming the **hæmaturic** type common in Senegal and the Antilles. In some instances the chief feature of the disease comprises symptoms of jaundice, dysentery, or of cholera. We may also see purulent collections in the serous membranes, abscesses of the liver, œdema followed by coagulation in the veins, and gangrene of the extremities. These terrible forms often result in death.

Typho-Malarial Fever.—I have said that malaria in many cases resembles typhoid fever by reason of the continuity of the apyrexia and of the nature of the symptoms, so that the diagnosis is at times very difficult. In other cases there is genuine association of typhoid and of malarial infection. This form develops in centres where malaria and typhoid fever are endemic. It is rare in France, though common in Algeria and in many other countries. Typhoid fever sometimes appears in a patient who already has malaria, and the two diseases run a parallel course without affecting one another ; but at other times the two diseases appear at the same moment in the same individual, forming the typho-malarial type. In the latter case each of the diseases runs its own course, and a special symptomatology, depending on the preponderance of one of these two maladies, is seen in the course of the disease.

Patients suffering from typho-malarial fever present during life or post mortem the changes special to the two diseases. Accordingly, in typhoid fever we find hypertrophy and ulceration of Peyer's patches, and in malaria we find melanic pigment in the blood and in the tissues, but I should like to know if these patients show at the same time Eberth's bacillus and Laveran's hæmatozoon. Sero-diagnosis will render great service in the case of so-called typho-malarial fever (Widal) by defining the extent of the typhoid infection.

Hæmoglobinuric Fever.—Malarial fevers are often accompanied by multiple hæmorrhages. Purpura, ecchymoses, and nasal, buccal, or intestinal hæmorrhage are seen both in the bilious and non-bilious forms of remittent fever. The bilious condition is not absolutely associated with hæmorrhages. Thus, in the Antilles, Carvajal saw cases where patients suffering from acute malaria, with hæmorrhages from the mucous mem-

branes of the eyes, mouth, or nose, and hæmorrhages into the skin from
the intestines or from the kidneys, showed no jaundice, just as occurs in
some cases of infectious purpura.

Side by side with these cases, however, in which multiple hæmorrhages are
or are not associated with bilious fevers, there are others in which hæmaturia
alone is seen.   This form, formerly called hæmaturic fever, should be called
hæmoglobinuric bilious fever, because we find hæmoglobin, and not blood,
in the urine.   This disease (Corre) is especially frequent in tropical countries,
but it has also been seen in the Mediterranean regions, in Greece and Algeria,
as the following example shows :

A man suffers from quotidian or tertian attacks, or from remittent fever,
which implies a gravity usually absent in the intermittent form.   In the
case of intermittent attacks the cold stage is accompanied by lumbar pains,
gastric distress, vomiting of bile, and dyspnœa, which becomes still more
marked during the hot stage.   The **hæmoglobinuria** appears before or with
the chill, increases gradually during the attack, and ends with the stage of
apyrexia.   The urine, which during the attack assumes in succession the
tint of claret, sherry, and brown beer, becomes clear after the attack.

The bilious symptoms commence with the attack, and the vomiting of
bile is often accompanied by bilious stools.   The jaundice appears so rapidly
that the skin is of a saffron colour in the hot stage.   The bilious attack,
which is very marked in the first attack of hæmoglobinuria, often becomes
less severe during the following attacks.   Hæmoglobinuria may appear
daily or every two days.   The jaundice does not disappear between the
attacks.   The spleen is enlarged, and the patient is very anæmic ; but in
spite of its apparent gravity, the form just described usually results in
recovery.

Hæmoglobinuric bilious fever is more severe if the hot stage is prolonged,
if the attacks are subintrant—in short, if the fever is remittent or continuous.
The vomiting is then more frequent, the jaundice is more severe, the urine
is black, the tongue becomes dry, the eyes sink in, hiccough appears, and
the patient dies, sometimes from weakness ; at other times from anuria
and uræmia.   Fulminant forms are also seen ; they carry the patient off in
three or four days (Leroy de Méricourt).

In these bilious forms the urine presents the following characters : Very
abundant sediment, with epithelial cells, hyaline casts, white corpuscles,
few or no red corpuscles, and abundant **hæmoglobin,** which can be recognized with the spectroscope.   The colour of the urine is due to urobilin,
to the chromogenes, to the bile-pigments, and to the hæmoglobin.   As
regards the pathogenesis of hæmoglobinuria, the reader will find it discussed
under Paroxysmal Hæmoglobinuria.

Pernicious Fevers.

The malarial fevers are called pernicious when they cause such disturbance of the economy as to endanger in a few days or in a few hours the patient's life. In some cases the pernicious forms show themselves by exaggeration of an ordinary symptom (algid or sweating fever), but at other times they are associated with complications which affect certain systems or organs. In this case the fevers are called "accompanied," or *comitatæ*.

The imminence of the danger, however, does not depend so much on the importance of the organ infected as on the nature and the virulence of the infective element, which causes a "true, primary, protopathic, malignant character, which in most cases is apparent from the first" (Trousseau).

The pernicious forms are more frequent in tropical regions. We may see them in some departments of France, but hardly ever in Paris. Their development is notably influenced by seasons. In Rome they are more frequent between July and October (Baccelli), and at Senegal they chiefly appear at the end of the rainy season, from August to November. They nearly always appear in an **epidemic** form. If an individual leaves a country in which malaria is prevalent, he does not avoid thereby the return of symptoms of malaria contracted in the country, but he does avoid pernicious attacks. Negroes are less susceptible than white men. Youth confers no immunity, and children are more liable than adults to the pernicious forms.

Cerebro-Spinal Fevers.—Coma, delirium, convulsions, and paralyses are the troubles seen in this group. The comatose form is the most frequent and the best known of these varieties.

The coma comes on during an attack of intermittent or of remittent fever, though in some cases it seems to be established at once, and comprises the whole attack. In the slight form it is said that the attack is accompanied by somnolence, so that the patient appears to be under the influence of opium. In severe cases the attack is said to be apoplectiform. The attack of coma is characterized by loss of consciousness and of sensation, with involuntary evacuations, immobility of the pupil, and relaxation of limbs. The attack lasts about a day. It sometimes disappears rapidly, without leaving traces; in other cases it is accompanied by hemiplegia, monoplegia, and amaurosis, and we find post mortem congestion and hæmorrhage in the cerebro-spinal meninges.

The convulsive form simulates at times epilepsy, and at other times tetanus.

These different cerebro-spinal forms may be combined. The diagnosis is simple when the symptoms appear in a patient who is known to be malarial,

but when a man suffering from contractions simulating tetanus, from convulsions like those of epilepsy, from delirium simulating delirium tremens,
or from coma which resembles apoplexy, insolation, or sunstroke, is admitted
to hospital, the diagnosis is sometimes difficult, the more so as the attack
may be larval, while fever is absent, or appears only later. A prompt
diagnosis can alone be made by the discovery of the parasite in the blood.

Algid Fevers.—Under this term Kelsch includes pernicious forms
characterized by cyanotic colour and icy coldness of the body, and we may
note the following forms : choleraic, cardialgic, dysenteric, diaphoretic,
algid, and syncopal.

The **algid** form, which is the gravest of all, does not consist in exaggeration of the cold stage, as might be supposed, for the chilling of the body
takes place and becomes accentuated during the hot stage, or even during
the sweating stage. The patient does not shiver, but the skin becomes
livid and ice-cold, the voice sinks to a whisper, cold clammy sweat breaks
out, the distress is terrible, the dyspnœa is extreme, the expired air is cold,
the pulse is small and frequent, and the face assumes a death-like expression—*cadaveris imaginem refert* (Borstieri). This chilling of the body
may end in death, or may be followed by healthy reaction. In this form
we also see cholera-like symptoms, which may give rise to the **choleraic form**
of the disease. The symptoms comprise vomiting and uncontrollable
diarrhœa, with cramps and suppression of urine, as in the algid stage of
cholera.

In the **diaphoretic** form, which is not so serious as the algid form, the
sweating stage brings the patient no relief, as it does in true intermittent
fever. On the contrary, the distress increases, the body and face are
bathed in cold sweat, the algid condition makes rapid progress, and the
patient falls into a state of collapse.

These various forms are not always isolated, and we may see them in
association in the same subject, with predominance of algid, sudoral, or of
choleraic phenomena.

In **dysenteriform** fever the troubles become so intense as to end in
collapse and the algid condition.

In the **syncopal** form the patient remains for a long while in a state of
apparent death.

The **cardialgic** form is characterized by acute pains in the epigastrium
(cardiac region), with a sensation of burning or of tearing, and with vomiting
of bile or of blood. This form is often an exaggeration of the gastric remittent form. In very grave cases it ends in syncope or in the algid condition.

Pernicious fever may also assume other forms. The peripneumonic
form is characterized by pulmonary symptoms, the breathing is laboured

and difficult as in suffocative catarrh, the expectoration is mucous and blood-stained, and subcrepitant râles are audible over the whole chest.

The **pleuritic** form is characterized by sharp pain in the side, with painful and jerky breathing and more or less considerable effusion, which is usually absorbed after the attack.

The pernicious fevers show some differences, according to their type.

Torti and Morton, who saw, on the one hand, a case in the North of Italy, and, on the other, a case in England, said that the pernicious attack assumes the tertian type, and their assertion remains in part true as regards temperate climates, but not as regards hot countries (Algeria), and especially as regards tropical regions (India, Senegal), where the pernicious fevers chiefly assume the **remittent** and the **continuous** type. We may even see in some European climates (Roman Campagna, Greece, Corsica, etc.) that the pernicious form changes from the periodic type to the continuous type (Colin).

As a general rule, in the Mediterranean pernicious symptoms do not appear, except after a certain number of previous intermittent or remittent attacks; but in some countries where **malaria** occurs in a severe epidemic form, such as India, Senegal, Tonkin, etc., the symptoms may be pernicious from the first. It is very rare that pernicious fever is fatal during its invasion. As the pernicious fevers are **anomalous** in nature and do not show the regularity of the intermittent fevers, as the paroxysms often anticipate or are subintrant, and as the pernicious form often changes from the periodic to the continuous type, the delirium, algidity, and coma sometimes last more than a day without any possibility of noting either a remission or a periodic type. The fever sometimes remains in abeyance. We should be quite wrong if we took the periodicity as a guide in cases which demand special attention and prompt intervention.

It is often difficult to appreciate the shades which indicate that a remittent or intermittent fever will become pernicious. During an **epidemic** we must be warned by the abnormal symptoms and the nervous troubles which appear during the period of remission.

The **diagnosis** of malarial fever is often very difficult, especially in warm climates, where malaria, by reason of its multiple aspects, so closely simulates other diseases (biliary typhoid fever, yellow fever, cholera, dysentery, and sunstroke). In cases of doubt, we always commence with the administration of quinine, but this means is often insufficient to clear up the diagnosis. The only real control measure is the examination of the blood, and the discovery of the parasite will, save in very exceptional cases, remove all doubts.

Chronic Malaria—Anæmia and Cachexia.

Patients who have had intermittent or remittent fever often suffer from organic troubles, which are more marked in proportion as the attacks have been severe or often repeated. The anæmia is early, and this is not sur prising when we remember that a single attack causes a loss of several hundreds of thousands of red blood-corpuscles per cubic millimetre (Kelsch). The skin assumes an earthy tint, and the patient wastes and complains of prostration, headache and palpitation.

The **spleen** is enlarged. When the hypertrophy is slight, the organ is not palpable, and does not extend beyond the edge of the ribs. On percussion, we find that its vertical diameter remains parallel with the edge of the false ribs. When the hypertrophy is considerable, the spleen forms an enormous tumour parallel with the middle line, invades the left hypochondrium and the neighbouring regions, and becomes movable if the phrenico-splenic ligament is elongated or torn. The hypertrophied spleen often gives rise to a feeling of weight. An old-standing tumour of the spleen is, however, by no means incompatible with satisfactory health.

The **liver** shows similar swelling to that of the spleen, but the hepatic lesions are more rare, and appear less slowly. I am speaking of what occurs in France, for the first attack in hot climates often causes acute swelling of the liver. The hypertrophy of the liver, though general, chiefly affects the surface of the organ (ague-cake). In some cases the hepatic and splenic tumours unite, and invade a part of the abdominal cavity.

Chronic malaria may cause lesions in the lungs and bronchi. The cases published on this point are conclusive (Frerichs, Lancereaux, Grasset). **Chronic bronchitis** and **pulmonary fibrosis** of malarial origin may either commence with acute attacks or may be chronic from the first.

Among the pulmonary manifestations, says De Brun, we see a form of chronic congestion, localized to one or both apices of the lung, and showing itself by dullness, increase of tactile vocal fremitus, tubular breathing, and exaggerated voice-sounds. This congestion is rarely accompanied by râles. It generally yields to prolonged treatment with sulphate of quinine. As it most often coexists with febrile cachexia, we may readily confound it with tubercular induration of the lung (De Brun).

Retinal hæmorrhages have been seen in chronic malaria, as well as after acute attacks. They lead to ocular troubles, which may recur and persist for several months.

The symptoms of malarial anæmia end in confirmed **cachexia** in persons who have been hard hit by the infection and in those who live under bad hygienic conditions. The colour is dark, the skin is dry, and the wasting contrasts with the size of the abdomen, due to the enlargement of the liver and of the spleen. Œdema, ascites, albuminuria, diarrhœa, epistaxis, ulcers on the legs, and amenorrhœa are often noticed. This cachectic stage, sometimes interrupted by irregular paroxysms, may end in recovery, but more often terminates fatally (hectic fever, tuberculosis, chronic hepatitis, chronic nephritis, pneumonia).

In some malarial countries a large number of the inhabitants bear the stamp of anæmia and cachexia due to malarial infection, although they have never had intermittent or remittent attacks. The **cachexia is established from the first,** like a chronic intoxication. We may even see new-born children with enlargement of the spleen and the liver, and with a cachectic colour of the skin. Fractures unite badly, and the formation of callus is often retarded (Verneuil) in persons who have suffered from malaria.

The **prognosis** in malarial cachexia is very grave, because the cachexia is the result of all the manifestations of malarial infection, and survives the endemo-epidemic recrudescences of malaria.

Larval Malaria.

A larval disease is one which assumes the appearance (*induit larvam*) of another disease with which it has little or no analogy. Malarial infection is larval when it assumes the form of neuralgia of a flux or of a neurosis. In these larval forms fever is completely absent, or is confined to slight symptoms. The febrile element is secondary and accessory, and the neuralgic or digestive element predominates.

These larval fevers, as a rule, affect the fifth pair of nerves. The **neuralgia** is usually apyretic. It may appear at indefinite times, and affect a pseudo-continuous type. The pains sometimes return at the fixed time, just as the symptoms which comprise the complex of facial neuralgia : injection of the conjunctivæ, abundant secretion of tears, etc. The paroxysms generally occur in the morning, and the attacks may assume the quotidian, tertian, or quartan type.

We also see neuralgia affecting the occipital, intercostal, and sciatic nerves, and certain neuralgias of the breast, stomach, intestines and heart are really larval fevers.

The larval fever is represented in some cases by congestion or by hæmorrhages. In this class we may place coryza, tonsillitis, cutaneous hyperæmia, urticaria, partial or extensive œdema, intermittent diarrhœa, arthralgic pains, epistaxis, purpura, and perhaps the reawakening of the rheumatic diathesis.

Among the **neuroses** seen in these forms of larval fevers I may quote spasmodic cough, pseudo-asthmatic dyspnœa, migraine, and hiccough.

All these larval manifestations have certain characters in common. They may present a certain periodicity. The individuals whom they attack have dwelt in a malarial country, and present more or less considerable enlargement of the spleen, and have very often suffered from attacks of malaria. These various considerations assist in the diagnosis of the larval fevers.

Many pernicious fevers might be considered as larval, but the febrile element usually acquires a severity not found in the forms just examined. They are really **pseudo-larval.**

Pathological Anatomy.—Let us first study the lesions of acute malaria, and the changes present in the blood during life. The number of red corpuscles diminishes by from 100,000 to 1,000,000 per cubic millimetre in twenty-four hours as the result of the attacks of fever. This diminution is proportionate to the severity of the attack, and explains the rapid anæmia. And yet, when speaking of the intensity of the attack, I do not allude merely to the severity of the fever, but to the morbid process as a whole, for some pernicious attacks destroy an enormous quantity of red blood-corpuscles, although the fever is not high.

The red corpuscles are deformed, and during the period of apyrexia many hæmatoblasts (Hayem) are found. The white corpuscles increase in number, and become three or four times as numerous as in the normal condition.

The quantity of pigment found in the blood (melanæmia) is in direct proportion to the severity of the disease. The melanæmia is not continuous. Kelsch has shown that it is intermittent, and intimately associated with the attacks. The melanæmia appears during the attack, especially at the time of the paroxysm. The pigment is very abundant in the case of severe or of pernicious fever. If the attacks are trifling, and occur at sufficiently long intervals, the pigment may entirely disappear between two attacks, and even when the attacks are severe and repeated the melanæmia does not persist for more than five or six days after the last attack. Melanæmia is absent when the malarial cachexia is not interrupted by acute attacks.

The **melanic pigment** is present in the form of grains or irregular masses, measuring at most 1 μ in diameter, and collected into small blackish masses, which may be free or enclosed in the white corpuscles. The pigment arises from the destruction of the red corpuscles, due to the parasite which lives upon them. The black pigment which accumulates in the hæmatozoon results from the digestion of the hæmoglobin. This melanæmia is characteristic of malaria, and is reproduced in no other disease.

Melanæmia induces melanosis. The melanic pigment blocks the capillaries and infiltrates the organs. In some cases the pigment is not solely intravascular, but penetrates the cells of the organ, giving them a slaty or a brownish colour. This phenomenon is seen in the spleen, in the bone-marrow, and later in the liver. In other organs (brain, kidneys, lungs, muscles) the pigment remains intravascular, and does not enter the cells (Kelsch).

Kelsch and Kiener have been very careful not to confound the melanic pigment with an ochre pigment, which is not found in the blood, but infiltrates the cells of the liver, the kidney, the spleen, the spinal cord, and the bones, where it may cause trophic troubles.

If the patient has died from acute malaria or from pernicious fever, the spleen is enlarged, and its weight may reach 30 to 40 ounces. It is pigmented, and softened to the point of diffluence. Rupture of the organ is extremely rare. The **liver** shows inflammatory hyperæmia. The capillary networks are blocked by melaniferous cells and pigment, and the hepatic cells are cloudy. The biliary vessels are intact, but the bile is thick and abundant. The meninges are congested, and the convolutions of the brain are of a characteristic slate colour. It might be said that the capillaries have been injected with black material. The kidneys, even in the absence of hæmoglobinuria, show constant lesions. The tubules are blocked with casts, mixed with pigmented granules. In the lungs pigmented granulations are found in the interior of the vessels and in the blood of the alveoli.

In short, the lesions of **acute** malaria are characterized by the presence of a melanic pigment in the blood, in the capillary network, where it forms emboli, in the parenchyma of the spleen and of the bones, where the altered red corpuscles are destroyed.

The lesions of chronic malaria must next occupy our attention. The presence of the parasites causes a congestive and irritative process, which shows itself by inflammatory lesions, especially well marked in the organs where the parasite dwells (Laveran).

The **spleen** is enlarged, and at times enormous, hard, and cirrhosed. On section, it is pigmented, slaty-coloured, and blackish, and presents fibrous bands of connective tissue. It is sometimes affected by amyloid degeneration.

The changes in the **liver** occur later than those in the spleen. The organ is enlarged, pigmented, and indurated. The hypertrophy chiefly affects the surface, and gives the organ a flattened form. The melanic pigment obstructs the capillaries of the portal vein, and finally enters the hepatic cells, especially at the periphery of the acinus. Amyloid degeneration is rare. On section, the parenchyma is sometimes mammillated, as the result of parenchymatous hepatitis, with hypertrophy and hyperplasia of the hepatic cells. The nodular form of parenchymatous hepatitis, with large adenomatous areas, has been carefully studied by Kelsch and Kiener. These lesions are associated with cirrhotic changes.

The **kidneys** show multiple lesions—fibrous changes in the glomeruli, fatty condition of the epithelium, colloid degeneration, and pigmentation of the organ.

The **lungs** present the lesions of chronic interstitial pneumonia, with or without dilatation of the bronchi.

Treatment.—The organism may struggle against the parasites by reason of phagocytosis, and recovery may occur in mild cases without any treatment, but they are the exception. In most cases it is necessary to prescribe quinine, which is the specific drug for malaria.

" It is possible to prove directly the action of quinine salts upon the parasites by mixing a drop of blood which contains them with a drop of a weak solution of sulphate of quinine. The movements of the pigmented granules, and also those of the mobile threads, rapidly disappear, and we see only the dead parasites " (Laveran).

Cinchona and quinine are the drugs in malaria. An individual is suffering from tertian or from quotidian fever. Upon what lines are we to proceed ? A purgative is ordered, and then sulphate of quinine is administered in a dose of 10 to 15 grains. The quinine should be divided into two doses, one being given as far as possible from the coming attack, and the other being given four or five hours before the supposed return of the attack. The quinine should be continued for a week, when it may be suspended, to be again given if the attacks of fever reappear.

The same treatment is applicable in remittent fever. Since the remittent form is nearly always accompanied by gastric or bilious symptoms, an emetic is prescribed, and quinine is then given in doses of 10 to 15 grains daily, choosing as far as possible the moment of remission.

In **severe and pernicious fever,** as there is no time to be lost, and as the attacks are often subintrant, large doses of quinine (30 to 40 grains) are given during the attack, either by the mouth or by subcutaneous injections of the following solution :

Distilled water	18 parts.
Alcohol	4 ,,
Hydrobromate of quinine	2 ,,

Care must be taken to make the injection deeply into a region rich in cellular tissue, and strict asepsis must be observed.

By this means it does not matter if the patient is comatose or delirious. We have not to consider whether he can swallow the drug or to think of the tolerance of the stomach, as the medicine quickly reaches its destination by means of cutaneous absorption. We may also administer quinine in an enema. In acute malaria of the pernicious type, however, it is well to administer quinine by every possible means at once—by the mouth, by subcutaneous injections, by enemata, and by inunction. The above comprises the treatment of acute malaria with quinine. In persons who cannot take the sulphate well we may give the lactate or the hydrobromate of quinine.

Quinine has not the same efficacy in all cases, especially when the disease is of long standing and when the patient has already suffered from several attacks. It is then necessary to substitute **cinchona,** which is, under these circumstances, **superior to quinine.** I have often been able to help soldiers who had returned from Cochin-China or from Tonkin suffering from inveterate and irregular fever to shake it off by means of cinchona when quinine had no action. We may prescribe every morning 120 grains of powdered yellow cinchona in black coffee or in lemonade, care being taken to stir the powder, so that it is well mixed with the fluid. Slight diarrhœa sometimes follows the exhibition of cinchona, and in such cases a pill of opium may be given in conjunction with it. We may also give cinchona in the form of an electuary (powdered cinchona and *conserve de rose*), or mixed with orange syrup.

The exhibition of quinine or of cinchona must be repeated for eight days in succession. After this period we may spread the doses out according to Trousseau's method by giving them at successive intervals of two, three, four, and up to eight days.

In the treatment of fever which resists cinchona or quinine I have obtained good results by the subcutaneous injection of **carbolic acid.** I employ a 2 per cent. solution, so that each Pravaz syringe contains 4 centigrammes of carbolic acid. Several injections are given daily, so as to comprise a total dose of from 10 to 20 centigrammes of carbolic acid.*

Arsenical preparations (Boudin) give good results. Cacodylate of soda and arrhenal have been advised in the form of subcutaneous injections, repeated for a more or less lengthy period, according to the obstinacy of the fever.

Hydrotherapy also renders the greatest service, but the douches should not be too cold at first, lest they should cause fresh attacks.

Prophylaxis.—Prophylaxis comprises the following measures : To render marshy lands healthy, but not to undertake drainage works during the hot season and during epidemics. Inhabitants should remove from the plains, and seek high levels, or leave the country in which malaria is prevalent. In cachexia it is absolutely necessary for the patient to change his residence, and to leave the country in which the disease is endemic.

Neveu-Lemaire has given an excellent summary of the method of general and individual prophylaxis. It is necessary to do away with pools, wells, cisterns, and water-butts in the neighbourhood of dwelling-houses, since the larvæ of the Anopheles swarm in the water, where they are promptly hatched, and invade the neighbouring house.

The direct means consist in the destruction of the larvæ in the water,

* Dieulafoy, *Gazette Hebdom.*, Octobre 17, 1884.

In large ponds rearing of fish should be encouraged, as they eat the larvæ of the mosquitoes. When the mass of stagnant water is not large (reservoir, pool, or well), rag impregnated with petroleum and tar is placed on the surface of the water ; 10 c.c. of this mixture are sufficient per square metre of surface. This operation should be performed in the springtime, and repeated every fortnight.

As regards individual protection, care should be taken to protect all the openings of the house, such as windows and chimneys, etc., with a wire network, the meshes of which are so fine that the mosquitoes cannot pass through them. Beds should always be covered with mosquito-curtains. When the individual goes out, the face and the neck should be protected with a veil, the hands covered with gloves, and the trousers securely fastened at the bottom. The Anopheles are most formidable at nightfall.

The Italian Railway Companies on the Mediterranean and Adriatic coasts have reduced the number of cases of malaria among their employees by fitting all windows of their stations, gate-keepers' houses, and switch-point cabins with wire gauze, and insisting on their employees wearing a special mask and gloves, in order to avoid mosquito-bites. These results are the more interesting, as on the parts of the railways where these pre-cautions have not been taken malaria has not diminished in severity.

Quinine and cinchona taken daily in malarial countries may act as **prophylactics.** It is necessary to avoid going out in the morning when the dew is still on the ground, or in the evening after sunset.

IX. SLEEPING SICKNESS.

The history of sleeping sickness dates from the clinical studies of Winter-bottom (1803), Moreau, Jonnès, and Guérin. The pathogenesis has been elucidated by the researches of Forde, Dutton, Castellani, and Brumpt. This peculiar affection is due to the invasion of the organism by a flagellated parasite, the next of kin to the trypanosomes, which in animals determines dourine, nagana, and surra. The parasite is called the *Trypanosoma Gambiense.* Sleeping sickness is transmitted to man by the bite of the tsetse-fly.

Geographical Distribution.—The disease is endemic in a region extend-ing from Gambia to the Portuguese Congo. French Guinea, Benin, the French Congo, and the Congo Free State are the chief seats of the disease. It has extended across Africa as far as Uganda. The basins of the Senegal, Niger, Congo, and Upper Nile have been thus infected. The disease is becoming more frequent in the European colonies of the Congo. " Sleeping sickness is as terrible in its results as the most severe epidemics of plague reported in history " (Blanchard). Men and women, old and young, may fall victims. Persons of every station are liable to the disease, and if negroes are more affected, it is simply because they work all day in places where the flies are more numerous.

Parasitology.—In 1901 Forde, an English physician residing in Gambia, found in the blood of one of his patients a parasite whose nature he could not determine. It was recognized by Dutton as belonging to the trypanosomes. Other cases were published, and the existence of a special fever caused by the *T. Gambiense* was established. Two years later Castellani found a trypanosome in the cerebro-spinal fluid of a patient with sleeping sickness. This discovery was confirmed by Castellani, Bruce, Nabarro, Wiggins, and Brumpt. Lumbar puncture in cases of sleeping sickness almost always yielded trypanosomes. The results were always negative in other persons. Was Castellani's parasite identical with Forde's trypanosome ? The answer is affirmative. It has been proved that sleeping sickness is the terminal stage of Gambia fever, that both diseases have the same field of distribution, and that their parasites are identical. Finally, sleeping sickness has been reproduced in monkeys by inoculating them with blood from persons with Gambia fever.

The trypanosome is a flagellated organism. Its length is four times that of a red blood-corpuscle, while its breadth is less than a third of the diameter of a corpuscle. Appropriate methods show that the parasite possesses a protoplasmic body, studded with granulations, and having an oval nucleus. The posterior extremity is rounded ; the anterior extremity ends in a fine flagellum. A kind of crest (*membrana undulans*) unites the flagellum to a centrosome, situated at the opposite end of the parasite. In fresh blood the parasite is mobile, and advances rapidly by turning on its long axis. The undulating membrane then assumes the shape of a spiral.

The trypanosomes multiply in the blood by longitudinal division. They may be cultivated on liquid media rich in hæmoglobin. Inoculation of the trypanosome produces a fatal disease in the dog, the rat, and the guinea-pig. If the parasites are inoculated under the skin of a monkey, they appear in the blood a fortnight later, and the animal suffers from febrile attacks, anæmia and wasting; death follows within two months, all the symptoms of sleeping sickness being present.

The Tsetse-Fly.—Since the rôle of the trypanosome in sleeping sickness has been known, it has been suggested that the contamination might result from the bites of the tsetse-fly. It was already known that another form of trypanosomiasis—" nagana "—was transmitted by this dipteran. Brumpt proved that sleeping sickness was met with in the regions where a special species of tsetse-fly—the *Glossina palpalis*—was found, and Bruce and Nabarro were able to transmit sleeping sickness to monkeys by the bites of this fly. The Glossina, which is intermediate in size between a house-fly and a bee, is readily distinguished by its wings—" folded over its back like the blades of a pair of scissors." It lives on the banks of rivers, and flies quickly, producing the noise which has given to it its name (tsetse). It bites during the day, and the bite is somewhat painful. In about twenty seconds the insect's belly is filled with blood. The trypanosomes which the insect has thus imbibed from the patient's circulation multiply in its stomach, and enter the salivary gland. They are then injected during the bite, and thus transmit the disease.

Symptoms.—The disease comprises two successive phases. During the former the infection is limited to the blood; during the latter the parasites invade the nerve centres, and sleep results.

First Period.—It is only seen in white people, and is characterized by a syndrome which Forde, Dutton, Manson, Daniels, Laveran and Mesnil, and Nattan-Larrier have studied. The fever is characterized by attacks lasting about two days. The attacks may succeed one another at brief intervals, or may be separated by months of apyrexia. "The rise of temperature is rarely preceded by chills, and when a chill occurs it is often very slight. The temperature begins to rise about midday, and reaches its maximum about 6 p.m. Defervescence takes place during the night; sweating is absent, and slight hypothermia may be noticed." The fever does not yield to quinine. In the intervals between the attacks the pulse is quick, irregular, and compressible. This tachycardia is not always in direct proportion to the rise of temperature.

The epitrochlear glands, the chain along the sterno-mastoid, and the supraclavicular glands are always affected. The glands are painless, hard, mobile, quite isolated, and rarely larger than a hazel-nut. Erythema is a very characteristic feature of the disease, but it is not seen in every case. It is usually of the circinate variety, and comes out in successive crops. The spots vary in size, and are seen on the shoulder, at the upper part of the chest, and in the hypochondriac regions. Acceleration of the respiration-rate and hypertrophy of the spleen are constant. Pruriginous erythema and pseudo-phlegmonous œdema are sometimes met with. In most cases the syndrome is incomplete, and the disease would pass unnoticed if we did not find the tachycardia and the glandular enlargements. In some instances, on the other hand, the patient during the first stage is apathetic and asthenic, severe and obstinate headache is present, the upper limbs are affected by tremors, and the eyelids and the face are swollen.

Second Period—Sleeping Sickness.—The duration of the first period varies. In some cases it does not exceed ten or twelve months; in other cases it lasts for years, although the patient's health is not deeply affected. The second period is characterized by the appearance of nervous symptoms, and in particular of lethargy. "At first it is a question of drowsiness rather than of sleep. The patient sleeps for a couple of hours after his midday meal. He then wakes up, and perhaps attends to his business. The drowsiness is not very deep, and the patient at once wakes up when spoken to. After a certain time a second spell of sleep comes on in the evening before dinner, and finally the patient sleeps nearly all day. The sleep is very profound, and it is possible to drag the bed about the room without awakening the patient. In order to awaken the sleeper it is necessary to shake him. He raises his eyelids with difficulty, and answers in monosyllables to the questions asked. If food is given the patient forgets to swallow it, and goes to sleep with it in his mouth. The sleep becomes more prolonged and more profound, and finally ends in coma " (Le Dentec).

As a matter of fact, the patient does not sleep during the onset of the second period. He suffers from extreme asthenia, with headache, pain in the back, and cutaneous hyperæsthesia. He dreads the least movement. The eyelids, too, are shut as the result of ptosis, which he may attempt to overcome by contracting the frontalis muscle. In some cases mental troubles take the place of the lethargic symptoms, and the patient commits lawless acts, and suffers from attacks of mania with homicidal impulses, followed by a stage of coma.

Tremor is never absent. It affects the tongue and the upper limbs. In the tongue it simulates the tremor of general paralysis, and causes disturbance of speech. In the upper limb it assumes the alcoholic type. It is rapid, persists during rest, and is increased by movement.

The patellar reflex may be abolished. The loss of the light reflex and the existence of Argyll-Robertson's sign at times cause the disease to resemble tabes. Confusion is, however, impossible, on account of the presence of lethargy and fever. At this stage the fever appears daily, the temperature at night being very high, but falling to normal in the morning. The tachycardia, the enlargement of the glands, and the erythema still persist; œdema of the face and of the eyelids is often present.

The terminal period generally supervenes at the end of ten or twelve months. The fever gives place to hypothermia, the tachycardia disappears, the breathing becomes slow and sighing, micturition is involuntary, alimentation becomes impossible, and the wasting is extreme. The patient is plunged in coma, interrupted at times by epileptiform crises or by contractures of the face, arms, and legs. He dies in a state of cachexia. " It is exceptional for the disease to be prolonged for a year after the onset of the nervous symptoms " (Laveran and Mesnil).

Pathological Anatomy.—The essential lesion is a chronic meningitis. " In some cases the meningitis is well marked—meninges injected, thickened, and adherent to the brain—in others we find hyperæmia, which is but little characteristic if we are content with a macroscopic examination " (Laveran and Mesnil). The histological lesions are characterized by lymphocytic

infiltration of the perivascular spaces, in which we may see stained trypanosomes. These changes are found in the brain, in the bulb, and in the spinal
cord. The cerebro-spinal fluid is always very rich in albumin, and cyto-
diagnosis reveals numerous mononuclear cells.

Diagnosis.—We may suspect trypanosomiasis if we find tachycardia,
enlargement of glands, and circinate erythema. Moreover, the nature of the
febrile attacks and their resistance to quinine will be of much value. The
clinical diagnosis should always be confirmed by the examination of the
blood. This examination is difficult if we only employ smears, because the
trypanosomes are always very few in dried films prepared by the ordinary
methods. Other methods have, therefore, been proposed. We take from
the arm 5 c.c. of blood rendered incoagulable by the addition of any equal
quantity of a 5 per cent. solution of sodium citrate. The mixture is centrifugalized, and dried preparations are made from the thin layer of leucocytes
which settles above the red corpuscles. Grieg and Gray have attempted to
procure the parasite from lymph obtained by puncture of the enlarged
glands. Nattan-Larrier has found the parasite in blood obtained by scari-
fying the erythematous areas.

In the second period, the tremor, the dysarthria, the mental troubles,
and the absence of the reflexes slightly resemble the conditions seen in
general paralysis, but the attacks of sleeping prevent any confusion. In
any case, the discovery of the trypanosomes in the cerebro-spinal fluid will
remove all doubt, but we must remember that the parasite is only found in
nine out of every ten cases. If the direct examination is negative, we must
employ inoculation of a monkey or of a rat.

Prophylaxis and Treatment.—Proper prophylaxis can only be realized
by an international agreement between the colonies concerned. Early
diagnosis of the disease is essential, and the administration of each colony
must try to prevent the migration of infected natives into healthy regions.
It is necessary, whenever possible, to isolate the sick in regions where the
tsetse-fly is not found. The bush should be destroyed on the banks of
rivers where the Glossina exists. It is, unfortunately, very difficult to
apply these measures in vast tracts of unexplored country. The covering
of doors and windows with netting is more useful in the case of the Anopheles
than in that of the tsetse-fly.

Serotherapy has so far given no results. Arsenious acid delays the
progress of the disease, but does not cure it. Improvement appears to have
been obtained with atoxyl. The adult dose is 50 centigrammes by hypodermic injection. This is gradually increased to a gramme. The injections
are given every five days, then every eight days, and continued for several
months. "It is probable," says Laveran, "that success will be obtained,
provided the disease is not in an advanced stage."

X. LEPROSY.

History and Geography.—Leprosy is by common accord regarded as a Biblical malady, but it is probable that the leprosy of the Hebrews included the most diverse affections of the skin. The disease is, in any case, of great antiquity, and was imported into Europe from India and from Egypt some centuries before our era. It became a scourge during the Crusades. At this time the number of leper-houses which had existed since the seventh century multiplied to a remarkable extent; the order of Saint Lazarus was formed, in order to take care of lepers, and these unfortunate people were subject to severe measures of isolation, which saved Europe from contagion.

It must not be thought, however, that leprosy is completely extinct in our country; it is always ready to make an invasion upon the least defect in our watchfulness. The rare cases of leprosy seen in Paris are all of exotic origin, but some discrete centres exist along the Corniche and the Riviera. It exists in Brittany, where the cases of Morvan's disease described in recent years are considered by Zambaco to be cases of leprosy. More important centres exist in Spain and in Portugal in the Baltic provinces of Russia, and in Sweden and Norway, where prophylactic measures have considerably diminished the number of cases in the last few years. The most important exotic centres are found in Persia, India, China, Tonkin, the Antilles, Brazil, Louisiana, the Sunda Islands, and the Sandwich Islands.

Ætiology.—Leprosy is an infectious disease caused by a special bacillus. Heredity and contagion are considered to be the most frequent agents in the propagation of the parasite.

Danielssen laid most stress upon heredity. As a matter of fact, about a third of the patients are descended from lepers, but it is difficult to prove that the individual has not been infected during infancy by contact with his parents. The disease may be transmitted from the mother to the fœtus in leprosy, as in tuberculosis, but this is a case of simple direct contamination.

Heredity is, therefore, possible, but contagion is certainly the usual cause of the disease. Leprosy follows changes of domicile and large migrations. It entered Europe with the Crusaders, and the Sandwich Islands with the Chinese immigration. It may be transmitted by direct contact, as by sleeping in the same bed or following on a cut with an instrument soiled by the discharge from a leprous ulcer. Although these cases are exceptional, they are nevertheless incontestable. We know that long residence among leprous patients rarely gives rise to the disease, whence comes the immunity of physicians and of hospital attendants. The arrival of lepers in localities previously free from the disease may cause an outbreak among the population. Lastly, the rapid decline of leprosy in countries where patients are rigorously isolated forms a decisive argument in favour of contagion. Kalindéro (of Bucharest) in 1897 made a series of interesting communications on the distribution and extension of leprosy in Roumania.

Symptoms.—Leprosy, although a specific disease, does not always present an identical symptomatology. We meet with three principal forms: tubercular, anæsthetic, and mixed.

The incubation period is always very long; it may be as long as thirty-two years (Hallopeau), but its mean duration is from two to six years.

The invasion is often marked by lassitude, rigors, and fever at night. The patient is a prey to a physical and moral apathy, which may last months and years.

Mariano and Wurtz have shown that the affection may commence with an isolated spot some years before other symptoms. In the stationary stage the symptoms of the tubercular form differ from those of the anæsthetic form.

1. **The Tubercular Form.**—We find two phases—the macular and the nodular.

Macular Stage.—The macular stage is essentially characterized by the appearance of vascular or pigmentary spots, which vary in colour from grey to pale rose or to bright crimson. They may in time change to yellow or even to brown. Their edges are polycyclical and slightly prominent; their centre is often shiny, as though varnished. Parts which are uncovered (face, hands), or parts which are exposed to pressure (elbows, buttocks, or knees), form their seat of election.

The spots are sometimes the seat of sensory and trophic troubles, which become more marked in the nodular stage. The sensory troubles are most varied, and characterized by hyperæsthesia and hypo-anæsthesia. The trophic troubles are shown by persistent alopecia in certain regions, such as the eyebrows, by hyperkeratinization of the nails, and by absence of sweat.

The maculæ gradually become infiltrated, and the disease passes progressively into the second stage.

Nodular Stage.—The nodule is the characteristic lesion of the second period. It attacks both the skin and the mucous membranes, and develops either in the maculæ above described or in the healthy skin. It corresponds to the tubercular *leproides* of Bazin and to the *leprides* of Besnier. The projections formed by the nodules may be isolated or confluent. They may infiltrate the hypodermic tissue (hypodermic leproma of Leloir) or the dermis (pure dermic leproma of Leloir). They are firm and elastic in consistency; they vary in colour from red to violet and bistre, and may be as small as a pin's head or as large as a small nut. Their seat of election is the face (throat, outer part of the superciliary region, nose, lips, chin, cheeks, and especially the lobule of the ear), the hands, the forearm, and the lower limbs. The whole thickness of the skin may be invaded. When the disease has reached this degree, the mucous membranes are generally affected. We may also see conjunctivitis, keratitis, and iritis, which may end in indelible opacities and even in panophthalmitis. Hansen's bacillus is found in the interstitial keratitis of leprosy (Jeanselme and Morax).

Beneath the inflamed pituitary membrane the septum is perforated, the cartilages are eroded, and foul-smelling pus flows from the nasal fossæ. The mucous membrane of the tongue is ulcerated and covered with vegetations. The changes in the mucosæ of the pharynx and larynx may end in more or less complete aphonia, with stridor, dyspnœa, and attacks of suffocation.

Among the visceral changes orchitis has been noticed (Hallopeau and Jeanselme), and lepromata have also been found in the lungs and intestines.

The leper presents a characteristic facies, due to the mutilating effect of the disease. The bloated face, the thickened and irregular forehead, the semipendent eyelids, the swollen and flattened nose, the enlarged chin, the thick lips, the ears with large infiltrated lobules, form a striking symptom-complex, which includes in the same hideous deformity all lepers, whatever their age, their sex, or their race may be.

The course of the disease is characterized by acute febrile attacks, interrupted by more or less lengthy periods of calm. After each attack the tubercles increase in size and number. The lepromata finally break down, and form deep foul-smelling ulcers. Bones, tendons, and joints may be exposed. The natural tendency of the disease is to cause destruction of the tissues by ulceration. Death occurs ten, twelve, or fifteen years after the onset of the infection, either from marasmus or from some intercurrent malady, tuberculosis being the most frequent.

2. **Anæsthetic Form.**—The principal symptoms of this form are pigmented spots, bullous eruptions, trophic, sensory and motor troubles, thickening of the nerves, and especially of the ulnar nerve, the lesions being symmetrical.

The spots at the commencement of this stage resemble those of the preceding period in their morphology, and can only be distinguished by their more symmetrical disposition, by their greater number and size, by their rapid and well-marked pigmentation, and by the more early decoloration of their centres. The achromia of the centre and the hyperchromia of the edge combine to give them the appearance of vitiligo or of black morphœa, according to the nomenclature of old writers. Bullous eruptions may develop on the surface of these spots, and form a leprous pemphigus. The bullæ may continue to appear for months. After they have burst they may form the starting-point of intractable ulcers upon the limbs.

The sensory troubles are very marked from the onset. They are usually ushered in by paroxysms of severe pain along the course of the nerves, by sensations of heat and of cold, and by cutting and gnawing pains in the flesh. The patient screams with pain on the slightest touch, but typical anæsthesia may accompany or may follow this hyperanæsthesia. The anæsthesia is often so marked that wounds and burns are unnoticed by the patient. A pin may be pushed into the tissues or the cautery point may be applied to the skin without producing the least suffering.

The trophic troubles are the most interesting. They are characterized by thickening of the nerve trunks and amyotrophy. The **ulnar nerve,** which might be called the nerve of reaction in leprosy, should be examined from its origin in the brachial plexus as far as the olecranon groove, where we can feel the regular or moniliform thickening so valuable in diagnosis.

The thenar and hypothenar eminences and the interossei are chiefly affected by the amyotrophy. The hand finally presents the claw-hand of the Aran-Duchenne syndrome. The flexors of the feet, the peronei, and the extensors of the toes are chiefly affected as regards the lower limbs. Finally, as in syringomyelia, amyotrophic lateral sclerosis, or progressive muscular atrophy, the pectoral, deltoid, and gluteal muscles may be affected simultaneously or progressively. The muscles of the face no longer remain free. The paralysis of the orbicularis palpebrarum, characterized by ptosis of the upper lid and by ectropion of the lower lid, is of great importance in diagnosis.

We may see lesions in the skeleton, and especially in the fingers, shedding of the nails and teeth, perforating ulcers, and anæsthetic lesions, which may destroy whole segments of the limbs.

The motor troubles generally depend upon the muscular atrophy, and true hemiplegia or monoplegia is rare. Some authors have, however, noticed paralysis of the extensors of the lower limbs, giving rise to the steppage gait.

The patient finally succumbs from suppuration, prostration, and stupor, or may be carried off by some secondary infection, such as pneumonia or tuberculosis.

Mixed Form.—This form, which results from the combination of the two preceding ones, is most typical. The association may exist at the onset of the affection, but in most cases anæsthetic leprosy follows the tubercular form.

Bacteriology.—The bacillus of leprosy was first discovered by Hansen in 1871, stained by Neisser in 1881, and has since been studied by numerous bacteriologists, and especially in France by Cornil and Suchard, Hillairet and Gaucher, and by Leloir.

The bacillus measures from 3 to 5 μ in length, and 1 μ in breadth. It is very mobile, straight or slightly curved, and stains, like the tubercle bacillus, with Ehrlich's reagent. After staining it shows small clear points in its substance. It is surrounded by a capsule, and appears either alone or grouped in masses.

The bacilli are enclosed in the large cells of the dermis and in the interior of the nerve cells. They closely resemble those of tuberculosis, having nearly the same form and staining reaction. The bacilli of leprosy form closely packed masses in the centre of old nodules.

Attempts at inoculation have so far remained ineffectual, and uncertain results have been given by culture experiments.

Pathological Anatomy.—The lesions of leprosy resemble those of tuberculosis and of glanders. The tissues are infiltrated with leucocytes and epithelioid cells, and with elements comparable to the giant cells, although the nuclei are not so numerous. **Virchow's cell** is histologically characteristic of leprosy. It is four or five times as broad as a leucocyte. Its single or double nucleus is large and clear, and closely resembles that of the epithelial cells. The protoplasm shows numerous small vacuoles (*protoplasma en écumoire*), which may later invade the whole cell. The bacilli nearly always form masses of five or six rods placed side by side, like " bundles of cigars," or more compact masses are seen, in which the bacilli lie in various positions.

The bacilli are more numerous in the larger and older cells. In the most advanced stage the protoplasm is replaced by the bacilli. Virchow's cell is always present in the central and oldest parts of the leproma. It is especially frequent in the lymphatic glands, the bone-marrow, and the spleen.

The dermis at the site of the lepromata is infiltrated throughout its whole extent by cells, which are often grouped in islets along the blood-vessels and lymphatics. The epidermis is generally intact, and only becomes affected when the tubercles ulcerate. Some authors have found bacilli in the sweat-glands and around the orifices of the hair-follicles.

The bacilli are situated in the **interior of the cells** which make up the leproma. They often form emboli in the central vessels of the erythematous spots, and are sometimes present in the fluid from the bullæ. They have also been found in the Pacinian corpuscles, in the epithelioid cells of the cornea, and in their interstices, in the different layers of the vessels, and in the lymphatic glands.

The changes in the nerves are constant in the anæsthetic form. They commence in the cutaneous nerves, and then spread to the nerve trunks, which become enormously enlarged. The swelling of the nerves is sometimes regular, sometimes uniform. The perineurium is inflamed, and numerous bacilli are found in the cells which occupy the interstices. These cells may, by compression, cause atrophy of the myelin sheaths and of the axis-cylinders.

Bacilli have been found in the cells of the seminiferous tubules, and also in the cells of the bone-marrow. During acute attacks Hoëbna found them in the blood.

As regards pathogenesis, the following view is generally adopted : The

II.   113

bacillus, entering by the lymphatic channels, multiplies at first in the skin, where it forms nodular new growths. It then causes changes in the nerve endings, and finally determines ascending inflammation of the nerve trunks.

Diagnosis.—The diagnosis, impossible during the period of invasion and difficult during the onset of the disease, becomes easy in the stationary stage. The chief elements in diagnosis are : present or former residence in a country where the disease is prevalent ; sensory troubles, characterized especially by well-marked anæsthesia ; the presence of nodes upon the ulnar nerve ; and especially the discovery of the bacillus in a snip, in the blood withdrawn by cupping, in the serous exudate of a blister, or in the excised fragments of nerves (Pitres and Sabrazès).

During the period of onset the leprous patches may be confounded with those of vitiligo, morphœa, and mycosis fungoides. Leprosy can be eliminated by the fact that sensation is preserved in the first case ; the discovery of the lilac edge in the second, and the coincidence of eczematous or lichenoid eruptions in the third, will prevent error. Syphilides and cutaneous tuberculosis may at first sight cause confusion. Careful inquiry into the previous history and close examination of the lesions present will speedily remove all doubt.

Between anæsthetic leprosy and Morvan's disease, or syringomyelia, the diagnosis is often a very difficult matter. Anæsthesia and loss of the phalanges are present in both diseases, and Zambaco has stated the identity of the two diseases. The question can only be decided by repeated bacteriological examination.

Sero-diagnosis of leprosy, proposed by Spronck, who attempted to cultivate Hensen's bacillus, is an interesting method, but its value is not yet confirmed.

Leprosy ends fatally after several years. Life is more prolonged in the case of the anæsthetic form. Besnier and Hallopeau admit attenuated forms, characterized by simple macules.

Treatment.—We possess no efficient treatment for leprosy. Chaulmugra oil given in capsules is the remedy most often employed. Chrysophanic and pyrogallic acids and Guyun's balsam are usually employed as local remedies. It is of some service to cover the affected parts with a protective sheath in order to avoid the exciting action of air.

Sero-Therapy of Leprosy—Cytotoxines—Hæmolytic Serum ($a\hat{\imath}\mu a$, blood ; $\lambda\acute{\upsilon}\sigma\iota\varsigma$, dissolution).—Carrasquilla, employing in man serum from a horse treated with blood from lepers, has seen diminution in the size of the tubercles, cicatrization of the ulcers, and improvement in the general condition. Laverde has obtained similar results by employing serum from goats treated by injections of finely crushed human lepromata. The serotherapy of leprosy has been taken up by Metchnikoff. His results are so important that I shall describe in detail his method, which is based on the knowledge of **cytotoxines.**

Cytotoxines, or poisons produced by the cells, have attracted much attention in the medical world. Their discovery dates from the experiments made upon the transfusion of blood from the mammiferæ to man. This form of transfusion has been followed by fatal results, attributed to the solvent action of the animal fluids upon the corpuscles of human blood. The phenomenon is really due to natural cytotoxines, which have since been described by Daremberg and Büchner.

In 1898 Bordet, at the instigation of Metchnikoff, made known the first artificial cytotoxines. He found that the serum from one animal injected into an animal of another species acquires the property of dissolving the red corpuscles in the latter. Thus, serum from the guinea-pig dissolves the red corpuscles of the rabbit. This fact led Metchnikoff to think that it might be possible to prepare artificial cytotoxines which would be specific against the corresponding cells. The following examples will explain this idea :

If spermatozoa from the bull are injected into the peritoneum of the guinea-pig, they are digested and absorbed alive by the white corpuscles, microphages, and macrophages. A substance which immobilizes the spermatozoa is formed, therefore, in the peritoneal fluid and in the blood-serum of the guinea-pig.

If an emulsion of a rabbit's kidney is injected into the guinea-pig, the serum of the latter becomes toxic as regards the kidney of the former, and it is quite sufficient to inject into the rabbit a little of this serum in order to cause marked albuminuria and death from uræmia. Post mortem necrosis and marked changes in the tubuli contorti are found. We have, therefore, a **nephrolytic** serum (νεφρός, kidney ; λύσις, dissolution).

If ducks are injected with an emulsion from the dog's liver, we obtain a serum which has a markedly toxic action upon the hepatic cells of the dog ; injection of this serum causes rapid death, with all the signs of hepatic insufficiency (diminution of urea, increase of ammonia salts, alimentary glycosuria, etc.). We find post mortem the lesions of acute yellow atrophy of the liver or of phosphorus-poisoning, so that we have here a true **hepatolytic** serum (ἧπαρ, liver ; λύσις, dissolution).

Lastly, if an emulsion of a rat's spleen is injected under the skin of a guinea-pig, we obtain a serum which dissolves the leucocytes of the rat (Metchnikoff). It was therefore reasonable to hope that the macrophages might alone be destroyed, without injury to the microphages, and there were visions of the possibility of removing the macrophages which produce fibrous tissue, and perhaps of being able to delay the appearance of senile atrophy (Metchnikoff). The antiphagocytic serum, however, destroys all the white corpuscles without making any distinction.

All these cytotoxines are **specific.** They dissolve only the cells which give rise to them. Thus, nephrolytic serum attacks the kidney, and spares the other organs ; hepatolytic serum attacks the liver, etc.

The application of hæmolytic serum in man depends on the very curious fact that **cytotoxines in weak doses are capable of producing a stimulating action upon the corresponding cells** (Metchnikoff). Small doses of hæmolytic serum prepared by inoculation of rabbit's blood into the peritoneum of the guinea-pig increase the number of corpuscles and the quantity of hæmoglobin in the rabbit (Cantacuzène). Small doses of leucocytic serum prepared by the inoculation of an emulsion from the mesenteric glands of the rabbit into the peritoneum of the guinea-pig produce in the former animal a marked hyperleucocytosis (Besredka).

Metchnikoff made the first experiments with hæmolytic serum on man, because he was convinced that the improvement seen in the treatment of lepers by injections of Carrasquilla's and Laverde's serum must be attributed, "not to some products of Hansen's bacillus, but to the cytotoxines developed in the animal organism after injections of blood or of human tissues." He chose lepers from the St. Louis Hospital, and inoculated them with very small doses of hæmolytic serum prepared by the injection of defibrinated human blood into the goat. These injections, given only in stimulating, and not in solvent, doses, in every case brought about an increase in hæmatopoiesis and in the hæmoglobin.

The results upon leprous lesions have not been as well marked as the results obtained by Carrasquilla and Laverde, but Metchnikoff hopes for improvement by employing leucocytic, and not hæmolytic, serum. In any case, these facts prove that **small doses of cytotoxines produce hyperactivity of the corresponding cells,** and open up new vistas in the treatment of the anæmias. It is not rash to state that the employment of small doses of cytotoxines in diseases of different organs may be a new departure in therapeutics.

CHAPTER IV

INFECTIOUS DISEASES COMMON TO MAN AND TO ANIMALS

I. RABIES.

Ætiology.—Rabies in man does not develop spontaneously. It is always preceded by the bite of rabid animals (dog, wolf, cat). Many people, however, are bitten by a rabid animal without rabies resulting, because they are not all in the same state of receptivity ; and, moreover, bites upon parts covered by clothing are much less dangerous than those upon the hands or upon the face.

Up to 1881 it was known that rabies was a contagious disease usually communicated from one animal to another by means of bites, and especially affecting dogs, ruminants, carnivora, rabbits, and guinea-pigs. It probably never developed spontaneously ; it appeared after a variable period of incubation, and often ended in death.

Pasteur has succeeded in changing this gloomy prognosis by his excellent work on **antirabic vaccination.** I shall rapidly sketch the various stages which have led to this marvellous result.

The nervous symptoms are so constant in individuals suffering from rabies that the attention of pathologists had long been fixed upon the nerve centres, though without much result. Duboué had put forward the theory that the poison reached the spinal cord by way of the nerves, and then involved the bulb ; Jaccoud had placed the receptacle of the poison in the mesencephalon ; but these statements were not sustained by any experimental proofs. Pasteur conceived the idea of injecting dogs with the diseased spinal cord, which had been diluted in sterile broth. When injections were made in the subcutaneous cellular tissue, the period of incubation was long and uncertain ; when, on the other hand, they were made under the dura mater, after previous trephining, the duration was shorter, and the animals took the disease within a definite time.

Seeking for a convenient and expeditious method of procedure, he conceived the idea of comparing the virulence of spinal cords taken from various animals, and was thus able to prove that the spinal cord of a monkey was less virulent than that of a dog, which, again, was less virulent than

1781

the cord from a rabbit. He showed also that the virulence increased in proportion as the poison passed from one rabbit to another, and that it diminished in proportion as it passed from one monkey to another. The virulence remained stationary in each series after reaching a certain point.

Pasteur thus obtained two poisons, the one attenuated and the other exalted, which he employed for the inoculation of dogs. He commenced by inoculating them with the most feeble virus, and progressively increased the virulence until the most active poison was inoculated.

The dogs thus prepared were brought in contact with dogs suffering from furious rabies. Though bitten on several occasions, they did not take the disease against which they had been **vaccinated.** These experiments were performed before a Commission nominated by the Ministre de l'Instruction Publique, and the results announced by Pasteur were confirmed.

Pasteur shortly afterwards discovered another method of **antirabic vaccination,** which was simpler and quite as certain. It is based upon the attenuation of the virus in the spinal cords of rabbits by the aid of **desiccation.** The activity of the virus is completely destroyed by this procedure at the end of a fortnight, but this attenuation takes place progressively, so that the virulence varies inversely as the time of desiccation. Pasteur used for inoculation cords of successively greater virulence, and succeeded in rendering a series of dogs absolutely refractory to rabies.

Such was the condition of affairs when a young man named Meister, who was terribly bitten and doomed to almost certain death, came to Paris. Pasteur, in conjunction with Vulpian and Grancher, treated him with a series of subcutaneous injections from rabid cords of progressively increasing virulence, with the result that he felt no inconvenience, and rabies did not develop.

Numerous individuals bitten by rabid animals proceeded to Paris, attracted there by the hope of a radical cure.

Some failures occurred, especially in those bitten by wolves, and it was conclusively proved that rabies in the wolf is more virulent than in the dog, and that the most active treatment must be employed against it. The **intensive method** was then created.

According to the statistics of the Institut Pasteur, the mortality from the bite of rabid dogs, which was formerly 14 per cent., fell between 1886 and 1889 to 0·67 per cent., in 1890 to 0·57 per cent., and in 1892 to 0·22 per cent. Between 1886 and 1899 23,245 bitten persons were treated at the Institut Pasteur, with a total mortality of 103, or 0·44 per cent. The mortality following bites of rabid wolves has fallen from 60 to 14 per cent. (Dumesnil).

From the present-day knowledge of rabies, of its course and propagation, and the attenuation of the poison, there is no doubt that the disease is a microbic one, although the special micro-organism is as yet unknown.

Roux, Bouchard, and Gibier have seen extremely fine points in the tissue of the spinal cord, bulb, and nerves. Hermann Foll has given a description of this microbe, but at present it has been neither isolated nor cultivated.

Description.—The incubation period of rabies is extremely variable. Its usual duration is from three to eight weeks, but authentic cases have been quoted in which the incubation period was more than eighteen months.

Some importance has been given to the presence of elliptical vesicles which develop at times on the sides of the frænum linguæ, but these vesicles, called **lyssæ** (λύσσα, rabies), do not possess the properties attributed to them.

After its incubation period, rabies is ushered in by a prodromal stage, characterized by a tendency to **melancholia.** Patients are sad and depressed, even though they are ignorant of the danger which threatens them. Those who understand the situation suffer from intense restlessness, with insomnia, nightmare, and alternate excitement and depression. These prodromata are absent in some cases, and the disease appears suddenly, with the following symptoms :

The patient suffers from extreme **hyperæsthesia,** so that light, the least noise, and smells cause much distress. Satyriasis is seen in some cases. The chief symptom is **hydrophobia,** which does not mean that the patient is afraid of water, as the term would appear to convey, but the least attempt at swallowing produces such painful spasms that the unhappy patient prefers the torments of thirst to the terrible sense of strangulation and suffocation caused by the laryngo-pharyngeal spasm. The spasms are sometimes brought on by the sight of water or of a shining object. The saliva is instantly spat out in order to avoid the least movement of swallowing.

Later, these laryngo-pharyngeal spasms appear spontaneously in the form of paroxysms. Shivering fits, horripilations, epileptiform and tetaniform contractions are also seen. The attacks, which are exceedingly painful, become longer and more numerous ; the remissions are shorter and less frequent. The patient is a prey to terror between the attacks. Attacks of **mania** or ideas of suicide are sometimes present, but the affected person has no tendency to bite those around him, contrary to the common belief. The temperature during the attack rises to 106° F., and may remain high after death (Peter).

This stage usually lasts about two days. The next stage—that of **paralysis** or of **asphyxia**—only lasts a few hours. It is characterized by a loss of strength, which leads to collapse and death, though the end may also occur during the preceding period from suffocation. In some cases the course of rabies appears to be checked for a few days, and the disease shows several successive attacks.

The **diagnosis** of rabies must be made from diseases such as hysteria or mental alienation, in which hydrophobia may be present. In delirium tremens the dysphagia and spitting are not accompanied by the characteristic laryngo-pharyngeal spasms of rabies. The diagnosis can be readily made in the suspected animal by **histological examination** of the spinal cord, of the bulb and of the peripheral cerebro-spinal and sympathetic ganglia. The spinal cord and the bulb (Babès), as well as the ganglia (van Gehuchten), show nodules, which appear to be characteristic of rabies. It is preferable, however, to perform intracerebral inoculation with the nerve tissue from the suspected animals.

Pathological anatomy shows but few changes. The congestion of organs (lung and meninges) is consecutive to the convulsions and to the respiratory distress. Some writers have noted a granular condition and diffuse myelitis of the spinal cord.

Prophylactic treatment consists in immediately destroying any rabid animal, and in keeping any animal suspected of rabies in close confinement for observation purposes.

The following measures should be employed for an individual who has been bitten by a mad dog : The wound should be cleansed with especial care, and **vigorously** cauterized with the actual cautery. These measures should be carried out as quickly as possible. The mortality in wounds which had not been cauterized was 84·84 per cent., but it was only 31·34 per cent. in those which had been burnt (Bouley). Pasteur's method of treatment by vaccination has been described at the commencement of this section.

II. ANTHRAX.

Bacteriology.—The early work of Pasteur on fermentation led Davaine to ask whether the disease, studied by Chabert from the symptomatic point of view, was not produced by the presence of a low form of organism in the blood. Davaine, in his early researches (1852), noticed the presence of small transparent rods, which he called bacteridia, in the blood of infected animals, and he established a causal relation between the existence of these bacteridia and the development of anthrax.

Some years later Pollender (1855) and Brauell (1857) confirmed this discovery, and the latter deserves the honour of first observing the bacillus of anthrax in man. Davaine showed that inoculation of infected blood, even in very small doses, gives rise to the same affection, and the idea of contagion was thus experimentally established.

The pathogenic history of anthrax, however, did not advance until Pasteur and Koch, profiting by the previously acquired knowledge as to the microbic nature of this disease, undertook the study of anthrax.   The results obtained by these two observers have been far more important than was at first supposed ; they have served as the basis for the bacteriological study of the infectious diseases.

In the blood the bacteridia form short rods, with clearly marked breaks ; in broth cultures they appear in the form of long, interwoven filaments. The bacilli are single, or are placed end to end in pairs or in triplets.   Each bacillus is rectilinear, flexible, cylindrical, and immobile, with a clearly-marked fracture.   The cement substance which joins the bacillus in pairs (diplo-bacilli) or in chains (strepto-bacilli) is loose and incomplete.

If a culture is made upon any sort of nutritive broth, the bacilli, after some hours in the oven, assume the form of very long and much interwoven filaments.   These filaments are cylindrical, wavy, and very flexible.

They never show any branches, and though they appear to be long and homogeneous, they are really composed of a series of bacilli, placed end to end, and separated from one another by clear spaces, remaining unstained and indicating the division between the elements.   The filaments are immobile, like the bacilli ; they stain well with aniline dyes, and in cultures which are twenty-four to forty-eight hours old they show spores.

The **spores** do not appear as long as the germ is in living blood.   After forty-eight hours on a culture medium ovoid granules are seen at the centre of each small segment of the filament.   The bacteridium arises from the spore, which often passes unnoticed, so that the blood of an infected animal may at first sight appear to be free from infective elements, when in reality it contains them.

Cultures on gelatine plates at a temperature of from 15° to 20° C. yield sinuous colonies, which after thirty-six hours (magnification of 60 diameters) resemble a cluster of threads, and after three to four days the lashes of a whip.

The bacteridia are found in the blood, in the lymph, in the urine, and, indeed, in all the fluids of the body.   They are essentially aerobic—that is to say, they absorb oxygen readily whenever they come in contact with it. The blood thus deoxygenated assumes a brownish colour, which gives a cyanotic tint to the tissues.

The bacteridia are very easily cultivated, providing the experimental media are kept at a temperature of about 40° C.   They no longer multiply below 12° and above 45° C.   In solutions of glycerinated peptone they produce a toxine which may prove fatal to animals (Marmier).

Pathogenesis.—The spores are very resistant and preserve their infective properties for some years, and they are usually the cause of the infection.

Animals are infected from the corpses of dead animals buried in the earth and from the fluids which may have escaped from the body before burial. In fields where the burials have taken place earthworms bring to the surface particles of earth loaded with bacteridia and spores, which are spread over the pasture lands. The persistence of anthrax in an endemic state in *les champs maudits*, as well as the possibility of apparently spontaneous epidemics, are thus explained. The germs enter in animals through small wounds of the throat caused by the leaves of dried thistles, by the beards on the ears of barley, by the dried leaves of almond trees, and also by the introduction of the elements of contagion into the digestive tube. This mode of contagion is very rare in man and has even been denied, but yet undoubted examples exist (Bouisson). Inoculation in man usually occurs through a scratch upon the skin.

It was long held, as the result of Brauell-Davaine's opinion, that the bacteridia of anthrax do not pass through the placenta, but this is not so, as Straus and Chamberland have proved.

Let me also mention that in chicken cholera Pasteur employed the bacteridia of anthrax in order to study the **attenuation of the virus** and the **preventive vaccination** of infectious diseases. This attenuation of the virus in anthrax is everywhere admitted, although it was at first rejected by Koch, and vaccination against anthrax has for several years been performed by the farming community in numerous countries.

In the study of anthrax it is important to distinguish the disease which Chabert had described under the name of symptomatic anthrax. Arloing, Cornevin, and Thomas have shown that the latter is quite a distinct disease.

Malignant pustule, malignant anthrax, and malignant œdema may be united in a single description as manifestations of the same disease.

Anthrax is particularly common in sheep (blood of the spleen), bullocks, goats, and horses, but here I shall describe only the disease in the human race. Anthrax is transmitted from animals to man in many ways. Farmers and shepherds who look after infected animals, butchers who skin them, and knackers are more liable than others to contract anthrax. The dried hides of infected animals, the skins, the wool, and the hairs may harbour the infection for years, so that tanners, workmen who handle skins, dressers and curriers, and mattress carders are especially liable to contract the disease. I may quote the following examples : A young woman who had worked for six weeks in a hair factory was pricked by a hair in the right cheek ; a malignant pustule developed, and death followed in a few days (Straus). A malignant pustule ended fatally in an individual whose work was to pull the old hair stuffing out of cushions in the railway carriages (Orth). These cases prove that the spores which reproduce the bacteridium are endowed with great resistance to changes of temperature and to desiccation (Pasteur).

The transmission of the poison also takes place indirectly, and flies may carry and deposit it.

In the cases above quoted the anthrax entered the economy by a breach of surface, and a chafe or a wound of the skin was always present. This mode of entrance, which is the rule in human beings, is exceptional in animals. The latter are especially subject to internal or **spontaneous** anthrax. They become infected after eating food (sainfoin, maize) impregnated with **spores** or after feeding in fields where infected animals have been buried. Experiments have been undertaken in order to elucidate the question of this so-called spontaneous anthrax, and it has been found that foods soaked in fluid containing bacteria are more likely to cause anthrax if the beards of barley or of thistles are added, because these plants are capable of causing wounds and abrasions of the digestive tract.

Whatever theory we may adopt, anthrax of external origin is the rule in man, while that of internal origin is the rule in animals. The latter form has so far been seen only in a few rope-makers (Wagner), in a leather-dresser (Bouisson), and in certain cases of pulmonary or of gastric anthrax. In every case the spores are absorbed together with the dust in which they are contained (Bouisson), thus allowing them to escape the noxious action of the gastric juice.

Description.—After the poison has been introduced into the economy the disease shows an incubation which varies from a few hours to six days. In nearly every case (I speak of man) the malignant pustule is the first manifestation, and precedes the general symptoms. Intense itching commences at the point of inoculation, followed by the appearance of a vesicle. This vesicle has the appearance of a small phlyctena or pustule, and bursts, leaving in its place an ulcer with a livid or with a blackish base, which is sometimes covered by a small eschar. The scab is usually only a few millimetres in diameter. The cellular tissue beneath it is indurated, and an inflammatory areola, studded with small vesicles, develops at the periphery. The neighbouring tissues are swollen and œdematous; the **œdema in anthrax** sometimes extends to a great distance. In some cases lymphangitis is seen, and the neighbouring glands are swollen. The above description pertains to the **malignant pustule**; it is not painful, and has its seat of election upon the face, the neck, or the hands—that is to say, upon the uncovered parts.

The local lesion does not always present the foregoing appearance. The *charbon* is only a malignant pustule in which the dark and bulky eschar is surrounded by a highly coloured areola.

A true pustule is not present in some cases; we may see simply an abrasion of the skin, with diffuse redness, swelling, and lymphangitis. In other cases the œdema is the chief feature (**malignant œdema**), and the pustule passes practically unnoticed, or may even be absent (malignant œdema of the eyelids).

The **general symptoms** appear within one to three days after the appearance of the pustule ; nausea and vomiting are sometimes present, the face is covered with sweat, the pulse is small and irregular, the patient complains of prostration, and in some cases the temperature is raised. The clinical picture is characterized by prostration, dyspnœa, asphyxia, cyanosis, and anæsthesia, and the patient dies in an adynamic condition. The general symptoms may precede or may accompany the appearance of the malignant pustule in exceptional cases.

Pulmonary anthrax nearly always commences suddenly with rigors, headache, vertigo, vomiting, and pains in the side or in the epigastrium. The cyanosis is very marked, and is accompanied by acute dyspnœa ; the pulse is small, rapid, and irregular. Auscultation at first reveals only moist râles, but pleuro-pulmonary signs soon appear, indicating an effusion, which is often bilateral. The temperature, which may be as high as 104° F. at the onset, falls progressively to subnormal by the third day. The sputum is bloodstained and swarms with bacilli. The disease runs a very rapid course, and death occurs between the third and sixth days (Schottmuller).

Anthrax of the tongue presents the general characters of the disease. The tongue, which is ulcerated at one point, much swollen, and of a livid colour, protrudes from the mouth, and is locked between the teeth. The tonsils, the uvula, the velum palati, the floor of the mouth, and the face are enormously swollen. The bacilli are found in the ulcerated parts. The affection, although very serious, may end in recovery (Rammstedt).

Intestinal anthrax very closely resembles cholera. The chief symptoms are cyanosis, asphyxia, vomiting, and diarrhœa. Cramps appear, the urine is suppressed, and the patient dies in an algid condition (Bouisson). **Anthrax of the stomach** presents practically the same symptoms ; it is often found as a surprise at the autopsy (Nebolioubov).

The **diagnosis** of the malignant pustule is based upon the signs already enumerated. The pustule is not painful and does not suppurate, while the bacteridia are found both in the pustule and in the serous effusion of the neighbouring tissue. These signs constitute the points of difference between anthrax and boils, carbuncles and wasp-stings. The diagnosis is more difficult when the pustule is ill-developed and the œdema is the chief lesion, and careful inquiry must therefore be made as to the patient's occupation.

The **prognosis** is very grave. Anthrax, when untreated, is nearly always fatal. Death supervenes between the second and fourth days, sometimes even within twenty-four hours.

Pathological Anatomy.—The pustule and the surrounding œdematous tissue are poor in leucocytes ; we know also that the malignant pustule has no tendency to suppurate, but that the chief lesion in the œdematous tissue is an excess of coagulable lymph.   The bacteridia are not found in uniform numbers in all the organs ; the malignant pustule, which is the initial seat of the disease, and the gelatiniform œdema which surrounds the pustule, contain but few bacilli, while the neighbouring lymphatic glands, which communicate directly with the seat of the primary infection, are swollen and hyperæmic, and their sinuses and follicles are packed with bacilli.   The infective germ finds in their tissue its first centre for multiplication, and its progress is for a moment retarded by them (Toussaint).

The mucous membrane of the stomach and of the intestine presents prominent ecchymotic patches, which are usually situated on the free edge of the valvulæ conniventes of the small intestine.   The tissue of the villi, the submucous connective tissue, the bundles of the muscular coat, and the subserous cellular layer are infiltrated by the bacilli.   A similar condition is found in the coats of the stomach.

In the spleen, liver, kidneys, pancreas, breast, and salivary glands the bacilli are distributed in and remain confined to the capillary vessels, and, accordingly, the cells of the liver and the canaliculi of the kidney, together with the tubuli recti and tubuli contorti, are unaffected, while the capillary vessels and the glomeruli are invaded.   The blood, both before and after death, presents special characters : the red corpuscles agglutinate, and have little tendency to form rouleaux, the white corpuscles are exceedingly numerous, and the bacteria, in more or less large numbers, are found in the serum.

Treatment.—The prophylactic measures consist in the destruction and the deep burial of infected animals.

The pustule in man must be promptly treated by injections around the pustule, and for this purpose a solution of 50 per cent. carbolic acid or a solution of iodine may be employed.   The pustule is cauterized, either by the thermocautery or with sublimate of mercury.

Serum, which is preventive and curative in experimental anthrax (Marchoux), may perhaps be of service in man.

III. GLANDERS—FARCY.

Glanders is an infectious disease fairly common in ungulate animals (horse, ass, mule), and transmissible from man to animals, from animals to man, and from man to man.   Farcy, formerly described as a separate disease, should be included under glanders.

Bacteriology.—Glanders is a microbic disease.   The bacillus, which was discovered at the same time by Bouchar, Capitan and Charrin, and by

Löffler and Schüly, presents the form of a small rod, with straight or slightly curved, rounded ends; it is a little thicker than the tubercle bacillus, to which it bears a close resemblance. It grows well on the ordinary culture media, but the growth on potato is characteristic. The culture, after three days in the oven at 37° C., assumes an amber colour, and during the next few days a reddish colour, with greenish-blue edges—a feature not seen in the cultures of any other microbe.

The virulence of the cultures is not great; it becomes attenuated on exposure to the air for a few days; *in vacuo* it may last for three or four months (Löffler, Sanarelli). Of animals, the donkey, the mule, the horse and the guinea-pig are the most sensitive to inoculation. In the male guinea-pig we find, after two or three days, enormous swelling of the testes, which is of use in the early diagnosis of glanders (Straus). The early diagnosis can also be made in suspected animals by the injection of mallein, which is a soluble product of the cultures of the bacillus. Mallein has as great a diagnostic importance in glanders as tuberculin has in tuberculosis (Nocard).

Ætiology.—Transmission from animals to man takes place by inoculation or by infection. The nasal discharge in animals and the secretion from the farcy buds or ulcers may impregnate the straw or the blankets, and become a powerful agent of contagion.

Inoculation requires a scratch or an abrasion of the skin or of the mucous membranes. Stablemen become inoculated with the disease from the straw, the blankets, and the bandages soiled by the nasal discharge of the glandered horses. The secretion of the farcy buds or ulcers, and the skin and hides of animals which have died from glanders, contain the bacillus. Indirect transmission probably takes place by absorption of the dried nasal discharge.

Description.—In man glanders is usually acute, and farcy is more often chronic.

Let us first study acute glanders. In some cases, after an incubation which varies from two to eight days, the disease commences with lymphangitis, adenitis, and diffuse inflammation, which correspond to the seat of inoculation, and are often found on the hands or on the feet. The disease, however, more usually begins with general symptoms, like those of acute septicæmia. The patient is seized with a rigor, fever, headache, vomiting, and pains in the muscles and joints, which at first sight resemble rheumatism. Erythematous patches soon appear on the face and in the neighbourhood of the joints; they take on a livid tint, and are converted into blebs, with a tendency to sloughing. A **pustular eruption**, which is generally discrete, appears on the face about the twelfth day (Rayer); it may spread to the trunk, the limbs, and the respiratory tract.

Before or at the same time as this eruption, ulcers, with fœtid discharge of blood and of mucus similar to that seen in horses, may develop in the nasal fossæ. The enlargement of the maxillary glands, which is almost constant in horses (glandage), is wanting in man. As the eruption affects various parts it may cause dysphagia, dyspnœa, cough, and expectoration of blood-stained sputum.

The fever is continuous, with an evening rise, the dyspnœa is progressive, and the patient dies with adynamia or with delirium from the twelfth to the twentieth day.

Acute farcy differs from glanders in the **local** troubles, which are more marked, and include suppurating angioleucitis, ulcers, the presence of farcy buds in the muscles and in the subcutaneous tissue, and in the absence of nasal discharge.

Primary chronic glanders is very rare ; it usually follows farcy (*morve chronique farcineuse* of Tardieu). This description will, therefore, deal with chronic farcy, rather than with the acute form. **Farcy** in the chronic condition is a disease which is at times purely local, so that we may see a chronic angioleucitis which ends in recovery, or a chronic ulcer which also recovers, unless the increasing cachexia carries the patient off (Tardieu). In other cases chronic farcy is characterized by abscesses, with or without ulceration, and by general symptoms of fever, diarrhœa, wasting and hectic, which render the prognosis fatal. The symptoms of chronic glanders resemble those of very mild acute glanders, and appear during the course of chronic farcy.

The **diagnosis** of these affections is generally revealed by the occupation of the patient. In acute glanders the nasal discharge is a valuable symptom, but it appears late in man, and is sometimes absent. In difficult cases inoculation of a male guinea-pig (Straus) will rapidly clear up the diagnosis.

Pathological Anatomy.—The pustules of glanders and those of variola are almost identical in structure. The inflammatory process in the former is more extensive, and affects all the layers of the dermis, as well as the subjacent cellular tissue. Ulcers are also present in the swollen nasal mucous membrane. The lesions of the laryngeal and tracheal mucosa are less marked than those of the nose. The abscesses in the lung resemble the metastatic abscess of septicæmia. In the parenchyma of the lung we find yellowish or greyish areas, which resemble the lesions of lobular pneumonia. The tubercles in glanders, which resemble true tubercle in their anatomical characters, are not found in man. Bloody or purulent fluid is found in the abscesses of the cellular tissue and of the muscles. The bacillus is found in all these lesions.

Treatment.—The prophylactic measures consist in the isolation and destruction of horses suffering from glanders or from farcy. Their corpses should be buried deeply in the soil, and the stable furniture should be burnt. In man any suspicious scratch should be immediately burnt with the actual cautery.

IV. ACTINOMYCOSIS.

Parasitology.—Actinomycosis (Harz) is an infectious disease common to man and to many domestic animals. The infective agent is a fungus, which resembles the rays of a star, whence the name "actinomyces" (ἀκτίς, star; and μύκης, fungus) given to it by Harz in 1876. In the tissues and in the fluids from the infected regions the actinomyces is present in the form of yellow grains, which may be as large as a pin's head. The elementary granule, or the actinomyces, is composed of a central part made up by an inextricable network of filaments. This network is the mycelium. The peripheral part is formed of divergent rays, set like a crown around the central network. Each of these rays is bent at its extremity into the form of a club.

These two parts, however, vary in importance. The constant element is the mycelium. The rays are a superadded element, and the result of a

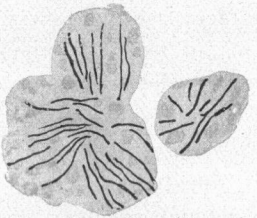

FIG. 89.—ACTINOMYCES: TUFTS WITHOUT CLUBS.

defensive reaction on the part of the actinomyces. For this reason, the clubs are practically constant in the grains taken from the tissues, while they are usually absent in cultures where the actinomyces is not in the presence of live cells, and therefore has no need of defence by a crown of clubs.

The essential part, therefore, is the mycelium, which occupies the centre of the grain. The crown of clubs is the rampart. We often find tufts of mycelium without clubs in the infected tissues or in the discharge from them.

According to certain writers, the club is said to be due " to a product of hyaline degeneration of the exoplasm condensed at the edges of the mycelium filament, and appearing to constitute a sheath, which in reality does not exist in the plain state. Each club is at first hung on to a filament, which pierces it like a pedicle; later, the extremity of the filament is destroyed and the club is set free " (Poncet and Bérard).

As the mycelium is converted into clubs, the staining reactions change. Instead of staining with blue and violet dyes, as the mycelium does, the club takes up the red colours. In specimens, therefore, the mycelium is stained blue or violet (gentian violet), and the crown of clubs is coloured red (eosin).

I have said that the mycelium is composed of entangled filaments. The filaments are larger and two or three times longer than Koch's bacillus. If these filaments are placed in a suitable broth culture, they become longer still, giving off branches, breaking up into segments, and producing numerous spores.

The parasite develops in the ordinary culture media. It assumes the form of greyish tubercles, which penetrate into the depth of the substratum, and do not form spores. The latter develop almost always in broth cultures of a month old. On this medium Sauvageau and Radais have obtained a "thin superficial pellicle, which soon showed an appearance like white velvet, and became a pale, clear yellow, following the formation of the spores."

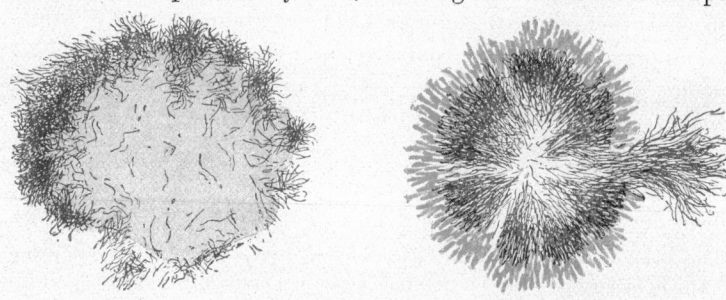

FIGS. 90 AND 91.—ACTINOMYCES.

On potato cultures the fungus forms large masses, which are very prominent, and covered by a pale yellowish dust, characteristic of the presence of spores, and clearly marked from the deep parts, which are of a rusty colour. The spores may be single or united in chains ; the latter may hang from the end of the filaments or remain quite free, so that the actinomyces can be definitely classed among the Oöspora.

Figs. 90 and 91 are taken from Cranwell's work on Actinomycosis. The former figure shows the section of a grain without clubs. The mycelium is very scanty in the central part of the section. It is almost absent at some points.

The latter shows a section with the mycelium and the radiating crown of clubs. The mycelium is somewhat rarefied at the centre, and much tufted at the periphery. At one point a tuft of mycelium is escaping through the crown of clubs.

The parasite can be inoculated in calves, rabbits, and guinea-pigs, but its transmission is somewhat difficult, as actinomycosis becomes attenuated in its passage through the human body and through animals. In some cases it is necessary to pass it through a plant before it becomes pathogenic (Liebman).

The special appearance of actinomycosis is not always confined to this affection alone; it has been met with in certain cases of tuberculosis due to favus, as well as in cultures from human tuberculosis (Metchnikoff) and in aspergillary tuberculosis, when it sometimes indicates spontaneous cure of the disease.

Ætiology.—This disease is fairly frequent in Russia, Germany, and especially in Austria. It was very rare in France, where only fourteen cases were recorded in 1894. Since this period many more cases have been seen, and the Lyons School of Medicine has succeeded in collecting several. Although it is much more common in animals (bovine) than in man, the same ætiology holds good in both cases. Contagion from animals is exceptional, in spite of the frequency of the disease in horned cattle and its existence in other domestic animals. The contagion usually results from grasses impregnated with the parasite, and actinomycosis may sometimes result from a splinter of corn or oats getting under the skin, into the pharynx or into the cavity of a hollow tooth, from scratches or abrasions received during harvest-time, from contact of a wound with a mouldy mattress, or from inhalation of hay-dust.

Poncet and Bérard record the following cases :

A child swallowed a small ear of barley, and after a while felt severe pains in the back. Abscesses formed between the spine and the scapula. On opening the abscesses, the remains of the ear of barley, covered with actinomycotic granules, were found. In three cases of actinomycosis of the tongue, Schartan and Jürinka found, on incising the affected tissue, small fragments of barley-ears, covered with the actinomyces. In five cases Bostrom has found the vegetable fragment buried in the yellow grains or in the masses of mycelium. In a case of actinomycosis of the ovary of intestinal origin sheaves of mycelium were seen bursting from an ear of barley.

The fungus may also be present on large plants and on a piece of worked-up wood, which explains the inoculation from a prick with a fragment of wood or with a splinter from a shrub (Poncet).

The time of year appears to have some influence on the evolution of the disease. It is much more frequent between August and January, during the thrashing of the harvest (Boström).

Pathological Anatomy.—The lesions of actinomycosis sometimes take the form of a sarcomatous or myxomatous tumour (Bollinger), at other times that of a sero-purulent pocket containing chocolate-brown pus. The yellow granules of the actinomyces are found in the interior of the tumour and in the pus. The bones, lungs, mouth, pharynx, intestine (Chiari), and testis may be affected, and the parasite may extend to the pleura, mediastinum, peritoneum, spinal meninges, and spinal cord (Dor, Macaigne, and

Raingeard). Abscesses have also been noted in the Fallopian tube, in the ovaries, in the bladder, in the kidneys, etc.

Description.—The disease presents such different aspects that its description is a matter of great difficulty. In some cases a neoplasm is found in the temporo-maxillary region, and presents a close analogy with a sarcoma ; in other cases we find inflammation of the cervical region, Ludwig's angina (Roser, Kapper), or a tumour of the inferior maxilla, of the parotid gland, or of the tongue (Hochenegg). The neighbouring parts are as a rule invaded. The skin becomes ulcerated, sanious material and pus making their escape. In more rare cases, actinomycosis gives rise to bronchitis, pseudo-tuberculosis, enteritis, typhlitis, appendicitis, abscess of the liver (Boari), and meningitis. I have described actinomycosis of the ileo-cæcal appendix under Hypertrophic Tuberculoma of the Cæcum. The skin may be affected from the first by the parasite, and the affection then resembles either ordinary tubercular lupus, with or without ulceration, or certain ulcers of hot climates, such as madura-foot (Roux, Brocq).

When the actinomyces, carried by infected plant-dust, enters the air-passages, it causes primary lesions in the lungs and bronchi. The bronchial and pulmonary symptoms are then the first to appear. For months the patient coughs and expectorates as if he had chronic bronchitis or tuber-cular lesions. Auscultation reveals râles of all kinds, tubular breathing, bronchophony, and even signs of a cavity. At a later date the actino-myces invades the pleura, chest-wall, and skin.

Infection through the œsophagus is fairly common. " In many cases it determines the distribution of the thoracic lesions, even more than does infection through the lung. In Soltmann's case, a small boy, after swallow-ing an ear of barley, suffered from retrosternal pain. After some weeks abscesses appeared between the spine and the scapula. Death followed at the end of fifteen months. Slight lesions were found in the lungs, and very large abscesses in the mediastinum, vertebræ, and muscles " (Poncet and Bérard).

The entrance of the actinomyces through the œsophagus, says Cranwell, is quite in agreement with the clinical facts, for we could not otherwise explain the prolonged absence of pulmonary symptoms when the neigh-bouring organs—the pleura, the pericardium, etc.—are so often invaded.

In one of my patients at the Hôtel-Dieu, the actinomyces, after entering the cellular tissue of the mediastinum, spread in two directions. On the one hand it provoked lesions in the pleura and in the thoracic wall ; on the other hand it tracked up along the spine, infecting the vertebræ, and giving rise to multiple abscesses and lumbar fistulæ.*

* *Clinique Médicale de l'Hôtel-Dieu,* " Actinomycose lombaire et thoracique," 1906, 16me leçon.

As Cranwell observes, one of the characters of actinomycotic infection is its tendency to spread to a distance. As regards thoracic actinomycosis, starting from the pharynx or œsophagus, it may track in all directions. We find fistulæ in the mediastinum, lungs, and pleura. In one of Adler's cases the anterior mediastinum was converted into a lardaceous block of a milky colour, and studded with yellow abscesses. Clear or purulent effusion may be present in the pleural cavity. Actinomycotic pleurisy may simulate pleurisy of quite a different nature, and the pathogenic diagnosis may be impossible unless the actinomyces is found.

Actinomycosis is a terrible malady. It may be limited to regions in which surgical intervention is possible (face, appendix, and skin). When the lesions are widespread, and deep or inaccessible, the patient dies from the onslaught of the little fungus.

Diagnosis.—The diagnosis is very difficult, if we remember all the diseases which actinomycosis may simulate. When the disease is limited to the mouth, neck, face, or pharynx, we may debate the possibility of dental periostitis, sarcoma, syphilis, epithelioma, and scrofulo-tuberculosis of these regions. If the tongue is affected, there is nothing to distinguish this disease from gumma, tuberculosis, or from cancer. In the thoracic forms, doubts may be present between this disease and such lesions as tuberculosis, pulmonary aspergillosis, broncho-pneumonia, purulent pleurisy, cancer of the lung and pleura, etc. The abdominal forms may simulate local peritonitis, tubercular typhlitis, appendicitis, and bone lesions of the pelvis. Actinomycosis of the spine may simulate Pott's disease. In spite of the distinctive signs, which may help in making a differential diagnosis, we are often in doubt until ulceration takes place, and the discovery of the actinomyces clears up the diagnosis. The same difficulty occurs in actinomycosis of the chest-wall, which simulates osteosarcoma or a cold abscess of a rib. Doubt may occur until the discovery of the fungus is made. Lastly, when actinomycosis runs an acute course, it may simulate typhoid fever, purulent infection, or acute miliary tuberculosis.

When we see these clinical varieties, of which the cause appears to be obscure, we must always think of actinomycosis, and undertake a bacteriological examination of the pus and of the various secretions. The presence of the characteristic yellow granules will confirm the diagnosis. In doubtful cases cultures will be indispensable. In ordinary practice there is no need to reckon the rare cases of **pseudo-actinomycosis,** due to bacilli (Coppen, Jones, Svotchenko) or to myocotic fungi (Dor).

Botryomycosis, formed by inflammatory neoplasms, and due " to the fungus of castration " in the horse, has been met with in man (Poncet and Dor, Ten Siethoff). The neoplasm resembles a fleshy bud or a vascular papilloma, deprived of its epidermic covering. It is rounded, mammillated, and assumes the appearance of a strawberry, connected with the surrounding tissues by a pedicle. In cultures, botryomycosis is present in the form of microbes resembling staphylococci; in the tissues it assumes the appearance of granules collected into a bunch.

Treatment.—Contagion must be avoided by the complete covering of wounds and ulcers. Grains, stalks, and ears of cereals must not be put into the mouth.

Incision, scraping, and curetting of the abscess are brought to a happy ending by the employment of iodide of potassium. This drug is, however, not a specific in actinomycosis. In my patient at the Hôtel-Dieu it produced no improvement. Poncet and Bérard speak as follows: "Out of twenty-five grave cases of actinomycosis in man, iodide of potassium was quite useless in eighteen."

V. PSITTACOSIS.

The term **psittacosis** (ψίττακος, parrot) is applied to an infectious disease transmitted to man by parrots. The infection is due to a special microbe—Nocard's bacillus.

Ætiology.—Psittacosis has become endemic since the Paris epidemic of 1892. The direct transmission from the parrot to man has often been recognized. A bird affected with psittacosis is listless and sleepy; the feathers stand on end, and the wings droop. This condition lasts from a week to a fortnight, during which period diarrhœa and anorexia are present. The wasting is rapid, and the disease ends fatally in nearly every case. Contamination from the bird to man takes place in various ways. Thus, in order to make the sick bird eat, the evil habit of feeding from mouth to beak is employed—a dangerous method, which explains the frequent onset of the affection, with transient œdema of the face and diphtheroid patches in the mouth or the pharynx, or else with angina. Other persons do not go so far as to gavage, but they fondle the sick creature, and warm it under their clothes—a practice that exposes them the more readily to contagion, as the feathers of the bird are soiled by the infected excreta.

Transmission may occur indirectly through objects soiled by the dejecta (cages and perches). The disease very rarely spreads from man to man (Dujardin-Beaumetz, Peter, Nicolle).

Bacteriology.—Nocard's microbe, isolated in 1892 from the bone-marrow of the wings of parrakeets which died during the voyage from America to France, is a short, truncated bacillus with rounded ends. It does not stain by Gram. It is endowed with great mobility, and possesses from ten to twelve cilia. It is readily cultivated on the usual media, and is both aerobic and anaerobic. It rapidly makes broth turbid, producing a thin pellicle on its surface. It does not liquefy gelatine, and it does not cause fermentation in lactose or coagulation in milk. Lastly, it does not give the reaction of indol. It grows slowly on Elsner's medium, and forms small colonies. It does not develop, like the *Bacillus coli*, on agar, from which colonies of the *Bacillus typhosus* have been scraped away ; and, lastly, it multiplies in broth, together with the *Bacillus coli*. These last two characteristics distinguish it from the *Bacillus typhosus*.

In short, Nocard's bacillus resembles both the *Bacillus coli* and the *Bacillus typhosus*, although it preserves its autonomy. It is agglutinated by typhoid serum, but to a much less marked degree than Eberth's bacillus (Gilbert and Fournier, Widal and Sicard). This difference in the agglutinative power is such that Widal has set it down as one of the best differential points between the bacillus of Eberth and that of Nocard.

The bacillus is extremely virulent in parrakeets, parrots, mice, pigeons, and rabbits. These animals can be infected by mixing cultures with their food, or, better still, by inoculating them.

Gilbert and Fournier have isolated a bacillus which closely resembles that of Nocard, from the intestinal contents of healthy parrakeets or parrots. This fact permits the two following hypotheses as to the nature and origin of psittacosis : Either the bacillus of healthy parrots and Nocard's bacillus are derived from a common source, in which case the former, though harmless in the normal state, may become virulent, and cause psittacosis ; or these two bacilli have nothing in common as regards their origin, and may be considered as radically distinct.

Nocard's bacillus has been found only once in man (Gilbert and Fournier)—in a cultivation from the blood of a woman who died from psittacosis.

Description.—The general character of the disease is that of a typhoid infection, rapidly complicated by pulmonary troubles. I shall divide its course into four periods : incubation, onset, stationary stage, and decline.

The incubation seems to last from seven to twelve days. In a case published by Dubief, this period was found to be exactly nine days.

The onset is insidious. The patient complains of malaise, anorexia, lassitude, and pains in the limbs, kidneys, and trunk. The morbid process commences with peribuccal œdema, prostration, and headache, which may be accompanied by epistaxis, nausea, and vomiting. Rigors are constant, and the temperature may exceed 104° F., with a slight morning remission.

After four or five days the stationary stage declares itself. The symptoms of the onset become more marked ; the patient is prostrated, and lies in a state of muttering or of violent delirium, with restlessness and incoordinate movements. The tongue is coated, the thirst is acute, and the loss of appetite is absolute and lasts until the fever falls. Vomiting of food and of bile is frequent, the stomach is slightly distended, and diarrhœa or constipation may be present. The liver is normal, but the spleen is generally enlarged.

Pulmonary troubles are early and of the highest importance. At the onset the cough is paroxysmal, and distresses the patient greatly. The dyspnœa is severe if the pulmonary lesions are extensive. According to the case, we may find on auscultation general bronchitis, lobar or lobular penumonia, or pleural effusion. The urine is scanty, dark-coloured, and often albuminous. Nervous troubles (headache and delirium) increase during the course of the disease, especially when thoracic complications appear; and we may then note hallucinations, carphologia, and subsultus tendinum.

The disease remains stationary for eight to ten days, and then in favourable cases the fever diminishes, the other symptoms improve, the patient passes out of his stupor, and enters on convalescence, although he remains feeble and anæmic for several weeks. In unfavourable cases the patient falls into a state of deep stupor, and succumbs a few days later, without having regained consciousness. In most cases death results from pulmonary complications, such as double congestion, pneumonia, or broncho-pneumonia.

Psittacosis may assume several clinical forms : the slight form, especially among young people and children ; the nervous form, exceedingly grave, and ataxic or ataxo-adynamic ; and the pulmonary form, marked by the severity of the thoracic symptoms and by the almost total absence of sputum. In old people, psittacosis is especially grave when the heart and arteries are diseased. The disease is always exceedingly dangerous in diabetic and cardiac patients.

Diagnosis.—The diagnosis of psittacosis is based on the clinical characters of the disease, and, above all, upon the information furnished by inquiry **as to the cause.** We shall not confound psittacosis with infective pneumonia, which is also seen as an epidemic in families and houses, because the pulmonary phenomena in psittacosis supervene as complications, and are not the **substratum** of the disease. The ætiological conditions must also be inquired into carefully. Typhoid fever, however, is the disease which has most often to be excluded. In its regular forms, typhoid fever is easily distinguished from psittacosis. The course of the disease, the temperature curve (the temperature chart in psittacosis resembles that of pneumonia), the abdominal symptoms, and the lenticular spots, are evidence in favour of typhoid fever. We see, however, abnormal cases and septi-cæmic forms of typhoid fever, in which the course differs much from the classical type. The agglutinative reaction (Widal) will be of great assistance in diagnosis. Influenza begins in the same way as psittacosis, and the respiratory troubles have the same importance in both diseases ; but in psittacosis we do not see the oculo-nasal catarrh, which is one of the most constant symptoms in influenza. The diagnosis becomes very difficult if influenza is complicated with severe pulmonary trouble. A decision can be reached only after the most careful ætiological inquiry, completed, if need be, by bacteriological examination of the bone-marrow from the suspected bird.

Researches as to the agglutinative property of serum in patients suffering from psittacosis at first gave negative results (Gilbert and Fournier, Achard and Bensaude, Sicard). Psittacosis runs, in most cases, such a rapid course that the blood has scarcely time to acquire any agglutinative power. The researches of Nicolle, however, show that **sero-diagnosis** is possible in psittacosis. The agglutinative power was manifest in two patients; it reached a fiftieth in one case and a tenth in the other. The method is carried out in a similar manner to Widal's reaction.

Prognosis.—The mortality amounts to 30 per cent., and the prognosis is made worse by pulmonary complications. The age of the patient must also be taken into account. The disease is relatively benign in children, but is very deadly in old people.

Treatment.—Prophylaxis depends upon general measures, such as the examination of parrakeets and parrots on arrival, and, among special measures, it is important to buy neither parrots nor parrakeets from hawkers. It is always unwise to feed a parrot from one's own mouth. When the creatures are sick, they should be left in their cage, especially if they have been recently bought. If they die, they must be disposed of at once, and the cages disinfected. If the disease declares itself in a family, it must be treated as an infectious malady. We must insist upon the danger of contagion, isolating the patient, and carefully carrying out the disinfection of all articles which in any way may come near him. Milk diet, cold baths, and injections of serum, comprise the chief methods employed.

PART VI

DISEASES OF THE SPLEEN

HYDATID CYSTS OF THE SPLEEN—DIAGNOSIS OF ENLARGE-MENTS OF THE SPLEEN

BEFORE I describe the history of hydatid cysts of the spleen, I will quote cases from two of my clinical lectures on this subject.*

Clinical Cases.—On January 7, 1899, Dr. Gillebert-Dhercourt sent me a patient with the following note : " Kindly examine the policeman who brings my card. There is a question of splenomeglia and surgical intervention. I should like to have your opinion before it is carried out." I told the man to take off his clothes, and I examined him.

The bulging of the left hypochondrium struck me at once ; the tumour was evident both in full face and in profile. The ribs were bent outwards, the hypochondrium and left flank showed deformity, and the projection affected both the thorax and the abdomen, although it was rather thoracic than abdominal.

In order to appreciate the lesions causing this projection, it was necessary to examine the patient in the upright, supine, and right lateral positions. On palpation of the abdomen, I found, in the left flank, an oval, painless tumour. Its indented edge gave the feeling of two lobes. This tumour, which could be circumscribed by the hand below and internally, measured 4 inches in a vertical direction. It extended inwards nearly to the linea alba. It was not mobile. Above, the tumour passed up behind the left ribs, which it pushed outwards ; the diaphragm and the lungs were pushed up as far as the third intercostal space, and the heart was displaced to the right of the sternum. In its vertical diameter the tumour gave a total dullness of 11 inches—that is to say, 8 inches in its thoracic portion behind the ribs, and 3 inches in its abdominal portion. The thoracic portion of the tumour was, therefore, much larger than the abdominal one.

What was the nature of this tumour, and in what organ was it situated ? It was not in the liver, which normally takes up the right hypochondrium, but it was necessary to eliminate the kidney, which did not appear to have left the lumbar region of the left side. Everything, therefore, pointed to a tumour of the spleen, which accounts for most of the tumours in the left hypochondrium. It remained to be seen what was the nature of this tumour. Speaking generally, very large spleens, due to malaria, leukæmia, tuberculosis, and primary splenomeglia, are especially abdominal tumours. They commence in the left hypochondrium, and their weight and their size drag them downwards towards the abdomen, while their upper part is situated behind the ribs in the hypochondrium, where they cause deformity. In any case, only the smaller

---

* *Clinique Médicale de l'Hôtel-Dieu*, " Les Kystes Hydatiques de la Rate," 1899, 5me et 6me leçons.

1801

portion of the tumour is situated here, the principal part being in the belly. The shape of the tumour in my patient was quite different, and in the abdomen I felt only the small part of the tumour, which measured 3 inches, while the large part of the tumour, which measured 8 inches, was hidden behind the ribs, bending them outwards, pushing up the diaphragm and the lung, and displacing the heart to the right of the sternum. The tumour was therefore abdomino-thoracic ; but it was much more thoracic than abdominal. Such is not the case in the enlargements of the spleen which I have just enumerated.

If the tumour had been on the right instead of on the left side, there would have been no hesitation in diagnosing hydatid cyst of the liver, and I should have thought of those large cysts on the convex surface of the liver which push up the thoracic organs, so as to simulate pleural effusion. In this patient, as the tumour was situated on the left side, it seemed logical to diagnose hydatid cyst of the spleen, the abdominal portion of the tumour being formed by the spleen and by the cyst, the thoracic portion being formed by the cyst alone. One more point, however, remained to be cleared up. Was it quite certain that the patient had not a large effusion in the left pleura ? He showed all the principal signs : Dullness, reaching as high as the third intercostal space ; disappearance of resonance in Traube's space ; absence of tactile fremitus ; silence on auscultation ; and displacement of the heart, which was felt to the right of the sternum.

I put aside the idea of a pleural effusion for two reasons : first, the bulging of the lower ribs was better explained by a tumour of the hypochondrium than by fluid in the pleural cavity ; and, second, the left nipple was 1 inch higher than the right one. In the case of pleural effusion, however much the heart may be displaced, the two nipples remain, practically, in the same horizontal line. In the case of hydatid cysts of the spleen, as the pressure acts from below upwards, the whole of the skin, including the nipple, is affected, and hence the marked difference of level between the two nipples in this patient.

Many other reasons were in favour of hydatid cyst of the spleen. There could be no question of malaria, because he had never shown any symptoms of this disease. We could also reject the hypothesis of leukæmia, because the blood was normal and the corpuscles numbered 5,180,000 red, and 6,800 white. Further, the general symptoms agreed with the diagnosis of hydatid cyst, which is for a long time compatible with good health. The disease in this man had commenced four years previously, with pain in the hypochondrium and the left shoulder. He could not exactly state the time when the thoracic bulging appeared, but the increase in size had become so marked in the past six months that his clothes did not fit, and movement was difficult. Subsequently the chief symptoms had been dyspnœa and pain.

The man was fairly well, apart from the pain and dyspnœa ; his appetite was good, and the wasting was slight. I therefore made a diagnosis of hydatid cyst of the spleen, which had extended upwards. It had displaced the ribs outwards, forming a marked bulging in the left hypochondrium, pushing up the diaphragm and the lung, and displacing the heart to the right of the sternum, just as a large pleural effusion would do, but the pleura was free. The absence of fever and of any infective symptoms showed that the cyst was not suppurating, and that the fluid would be as transparent as water.

I was careful not to perform an exploratory puncture, in order to confirm my diagnosis, because the so-called exploratory punctures (extraction of a few ounces of fluid) should be forbidden in hydatid cysts. Exploration of a cyst, even though made with a fine aspirating needle, may have the most terrible results. It is a control method in diagnosis which should be left alone, because the hydatid fluid, being under pressure, may pass into the peritoneum, through the breach left by the needle, and give rise to the fatal troubles described in detail under Hydatid Cysts of the Liver.

I gave a favourable prognosis and advised immediate operation. Delay would be fatal in such a case, for there was nothing to prove that the cyst, already of long standing, might not become infected, and thus make the prognosis far worse. Moreover, there was nothing to prove that the cyst, in its expansion upwards, might not perforate the diaphragm and pleura, and thus bring about formidable complications.

The operation was performed by Gérard Marchant, who agreed with me as to the diagnosis of hydatid cyst of the spleen. After opening the abdomen, we found that the spleen was free from adhesions and reached very low down in the abdominal cavity. It was large and partly surmounted by an enormous cyst, which extended up under the ribs and encroached upon the thorax, by pushing up the diaphragm. Through the wide incision we perceived the lower end of the spleen and the cyst, which bulged like a hemisphere between the spleen and the stomach. The cyst was inlaid in the spleen, and was only adherent at the hilum. The finger could be passed all round the spleen, except at the hilum, where the cyst originated. The cyst-wall was slate-coloured, and so thin as to be translucent.

A large trocar plunged into the cyst gave exit to about 4 pints of clear fluid. The patient was then turned on to the left side, and another quart of fluid evacuated, so that at least 3 quarts of fluid were contained in this unilocular cyst. After the fluid had been evacuated, Gérard Marchant at first thought of seizing the spleen and drawing it out, together with the greater portion of the cyst. Splenectomy, followed by incision of a portion of the pocket, appeared to be impracticable, because of the thinness of the wall, as well as from its deep situation and its adhesion to the deep parts. He found it better to marsupialize the pouch to the wall, although this was a difficult task, because of the friability and the depth to which the wall extended. The results of the operation were excellent, and the patient recovered.

By one of those chances which are not rare in clinical medicine, we had, in the St. Christopher ward, another patient also suffering from hydatid cyst of the spleen. There were, however, some differences between the second and the first cases. In my second patient the bulging of the hypochondrium was much less marked than in the first, but the abdominal tumour was very much larger. It could be taken in both hands, and reached below the umbilicus and to the right of the linea alba. The dullness, indicating the upper limit of the tumour, did not reach as high as in the first patient, and only extended as far as the fifth rib instead of the third. The heart was not displaced, and the two nipples were practically on the same level.

The symptoms included pain in the chest and abdomen, heaviness and dragging sensations, of three years' duration. The deformity of the hypochondrium and the swelling of the abdomen had been noticed for only about a year. From this period onward, dyspepsia, loss of appetite, pain, and constipation had been present. With the exception of these symptoms, the general health remained good, the patient had wasted but little, and had never suffered from fever. I made a diagnosis of hydatid cyst of the spleen, and was careful, for the above-mentioned reasons, not to perform exploratory puncture. I felt that it was necessary to intervene without delay, and asked Gérard Marchant to undertake the operation.

The abdominal wall was opened by an incision on the left side, extending from the false ribs to 1 inch below the level of the umbilicus. We then found an enormous spherical cyst, covered almost entirely by the spleen, which was spread over it like an envelope. Adhesions were present only at the level of the phrenico-splenic ligament. The cyst was punctured at its thinnest point. It contained 4 pints of typical fluid, in which hooklets were found. In proportion as the cyst became empty, it was pulled out of the incision, and after some manipulation the spleen was removed. The operation resulted in recovery.

Such, then, was my second case of hydatid cyst in the interior of the spleen. From its tendency to extend downwards into the abdomen, it belonged to the clinical variety which I have called cysts of the **descending type.**

I may here recall its chief characters. It differed from the preceding case in that the tumour did not reach so high into the thorax, and caused less displacement of the ribs, so that the bulging in the hypochondrium was less marked. On the other hand, in the abdomen it formed an enormous tumour which invaded the iliac fossa, and reached beyond the linea alba. The symptoms were therefore of the abdominal rather than of the thoracic type.

Anatomical Classification.—All hydatid cysts of the spleen are far from being alike, and we have just seen the proof in the history of my patients, in whom the cysts from the anatomical and clinical point of view were absolutely different. The cyst developed in the pulp of the spleen, in the second case, and the splenic tissue was pushed aside excentrically, so as to form a cap ; Marchant was therefore obliged to perform splenectomy. In the first patient, on the other hand, the cyst was only attached to the spleen, and had commenced in the hilum, leaving the rest of the organ free. The spleen was therefore left alone by the surgeon. It is evident, then, that the anatomical conditions may lead to different indications as regards treatment. Accordingly, it appears advisable to class cysts of the spleen according as they answer to the nature of the facts, rather than to unite them in one description.

From the **anatomical** point of view, I may describe three varieties. In the first variety the cyst develops in the tissue of the spleen, more or less near to the centre of the organ. In this case the spleen tissue is pushed aside excentrically, forming a cap for the cyst. A tumour results, formed at its centre by the cyst and at its periphery by the spleen tissue. Such was the case in my second patient, where the spleen was spread out over the cyst, and formed an envelope, thin at certain spots, but elsewhere much hypertrophied. The hypertrophy in this case (compensatory hypertrophy) was so great that the spleen tissue weighed 25 ounces.

I have been able to collect cases of hydatid cysts which commenced in the spleen tissue, and pushed it aside like an envelope. The following case is reported by Rambeau :

A woman was admitted to the Hôpital de la Charité, under Velpeau, for dyspnœa, fever, and pain in the left flank. On examination of the patient, it was found that the left hypochondrium and flank were bulging outwards. This bulging formed a tumour with ill-defined limits. The patient said that the tumour had increased three-fold in eight months. The pain, dyspnœa, and fever were only of a fortnight's duration. The patient died some weeks later, and the autopsy gave the following results : The spleen was converted into an enormous tumour, which filled the left half of the abdomen. It yielded, on examination, the feeling of a thin covering, formed of the spleen tissue, and spread out over a fluid tumour in the centre of the organ. The organ was punctured, and 3 pints of purulent fluid came out. The finger was introduced into the cavity, and withdrew a large spherical membrane, which was really the covering of a hydatid cyst. The spleen tissue was expanded over the surface of the cyst, and formed an adventitious tissue, more or less thickened at different points.

The following case was published by Hartmann :

A woman, twenty-nine years of age, was suffering from an abdominal tumour, with pain, dyspepsia, and dyspnœa. Examination of the abdomen showed a large tumour, resembling the shape of a bean. Its convexity corresponded to the left iliac fossa, and its hilum looked towards the umbilicus. On palpation the tumour presented a rounded outline with marked nodulations. In its left superior portion it was tense, painless, and very mobile in all directions. When it was pushed upwards, or when the patient was placed in the Trendelenburg position, the tumour was partly hidden in the left hypochondrium. The sensation of ballottement, comparable to that of the kidney, was felt, with this difference, that, instead of being caused by succussion at the costo-vertebral angle, the ballottement was produced by pushing in the costo-iliac space. The tumour, which encroached upon the hypochondrium, fell back as soon as the patient sat down, and the patient then experienced a dragging sensation. It was possible to push the tumour considerably to the right of the umbilicus, but not quite so far as the right hypochondrium. When the tumour was drawn forcibly downwards, pain to the left of the umbilicus resulted. From these various symptoms Hartmann made a diagnosis of a cyst in a movable spleen. The blood-examination was practically normal.

Hartmann performed splenectomy. The tumour was formed by a hydatid cyst of the spleen, which had pushed aside the spleen tissue in an eccentric manner, so as to form an incomplete cap. At the upper end of the cyst the spleen tissue had the appearance of a small flattened tongue, resembling in shape the end of a bullock's tongue. The spleen tissue was thin over an extent of two fingers' breath, and was spread out beyond into a large rounded and lobular mass. The whole inferior part of the spleen was spread out, and contained a large hydatid cyst with numerous small hydatids.

Snéguirew (of Moscow) has seen a case which comes under the category of intrasplenic cysts. After the abdomen had been opened in the linea alba, a splenic tumour, as large as a man's head, was withdrawn. He caused the spleen tissue to shrivel up by means of a jet of steam, and then made an incision, 3 inches long, across the spleen. By this incision he opened up the interior of a hydatid cyst, situated in the depth of the organ. After removal of the cyst, the spleen was two or three times its normal size. He decided to remove the spleen. The task was difficult, but recovery resulted without any febrile reaction.

In Jejebherg's case the spleen formed a sac around the cyst. The wall of this sac was composed of two layers : an external thickened layer of splenic tissue, and an internal thin layer of fibrous tissue. After opening the sac, numerous hydatids of various sizes escaped.

Lyons has reported the case of a young woman suffering from an abdominal tumour which extended from the epigastrium to the left iliac region. On opening the abdomen, he found an enormous spleen, which was incised and about 8 pints of hydatid fluid drawn off. This case was also one of intrasplenic cyst, as the spleen " was completely hollowed out by the cyst, and resembled the uterus after accouchement."

I have applied the name of " intrasplenic hydatid cyst " to this anatomical variety, in which the cyst develops near the centre of the spleen, and in its growth pushes aside the spleen pulp, which forms a cap of unequal thickness. In the specimen from my second patient the thin parts of the cap were partly converted into fibrous tissue ; elsewhere the splenic tissue was considerably thickened.

The hydatid cyst during its intrasplenic development preserves a spherical form. The whole tumour may be oblong, curved, and nodular at its extremities through the unequal amount of spleen tissue over the surface of the cyst, but the cyst preserves its spherical form.

Let us now consider another anatomical variety of hydatid cyst in the spleen. In this form the cyst does not develop at the centre of the organ, but at the periphery, at one end, or at the edge, and not far from the surface. In such a case the splenic tissue is not spread out over the cyst like a cap, for it is affected in only a small portion; the cyst expands outwards, and the spleen practically preserves its normal shape, with or without subsequent hypertrophy. I have been able to find a few cases which come under this category. Gras writes: "The hydatid cyst developed at the upper end and at the posterior portion of the spleen, which was hypertrophied."

In a case published by Jayle, the spleen was much hypertrophied (apart from the cyst), measuring 7 by 6 inches. It assumed a triangular form, with its apex downwards and its base upwards, supporting an enormous hydatid cyst, which was "implanted upon the upper and internal part of the organ." The splenic tissue was spread out over the cyst for a distance of 4 inches. I find, in a case published by Fink, that the hydatid cyst developed "at the lower part of the spleen," while the upper part was normal.

The tumours in this second variety are generally bilobular and of an irregular shape. The larger part of the tumour is formed by the cyst, which grows externally, and the smaller part belongs to the spleen, which is sometimes hypertrophied. I have reserved for this variety the term of **exteriorized** hydatid cyst of the spleen.

In the third variety I have placed hydatid cysts which develop, not in the tissue of the spleen, but in contact with it, either at the hilum or under the capsule, and I have given to this variety the name of **juxtasplenic** cyst, in order to distinguish it from **intrasplenic** and **exteriorized** cysts.

In the case quoted above, a juxtasplenic hydatid cyst surmounted the spleen, and appeared at first sight to be a part of that organ; but the spleen was affected only as regards its pedicle, and its tissue was free, as the cyst had originated in the hilum.

James Oliver has published a case which belongs to the category of juxtasplenic cysts:

A lady came to consult him for a tumour which filled the lower part of the abdomen. It was palpable in the left cul-de-sac on vaginal examination. Bimanual palpation gave the feeling that it was the same tumour. As the pains were very acute in the left ovarian region, the tumour was thought to be a cyst of the broad ligament, and an operation was decided upon. The abdominal incision revealed an enormous cyst, bound down to the interior wall of the abdomen by dense adhesions, which extended from the pubes to the umbilicus. On dissection it was found that the tumour was adherent to the omentum in the left hypochondrium. The cyst, which was of the shape of a leather bottle, was firmly bound down by a pedicle to the right edge and to the lower part of the spleen. The cyst was first evacuated, and contained 5 or 6 pints of fluid with several hydatid vesicles, of which some were as large as a nut. The wall of the cyst was clearly felt, passing into the pedicle adherent to the spleen. The case was therefore one of pedunculated juxtasplenic cyst. The pedicle was ligatured and cut off, as in an ovarian cyst, and the patient recovered without mishap.

This variety of juxtasplenic hydatid cyst is analogous with cysts of the kidney, as the following case proves :

A young girl consulted a physician for acute pains, and a tumour was found in the left hypochondrium. Two years later the tumour, which was very painful, caused a bulging in the flank and in the left hypochondrium. The diagnosis remained doubtful between a tumour of the left kidney and one of the spleen, but an operation was not even thought of, which is not astonishing, as the case occurred some sixty years ago. The unfortunate patient died, and at the autopsy a tumour as large as the fœtal head was found in the left flank and hypochondrium. It weighed 2 pounds, and was a hydatid cyst of the kidney which had developed, not in the renal tissue, but between the capsule and the tissue proper of the kidney, which was atrophied, so that the cyst was only separated from the calices and pelvis by a very thin layer of tissue. The case was therefore a juxtarenal cyst, analogous to the juxtasplenic cysts which I have just described.

I therefore propose to admit, from the anatomical point of view, three varieties of hydatid cysts of the spleen. The first variety, which is the most numerous, comprises the **intrasplenic** cyst of the spleen. The spleen, pushed back in an excentric fashion by the cyst, forms a cap or envelope, atrophied in some places and hypertrophied in others.

In the second variety the cyst develops, not in the deep tissue of the spleen, but at some point near the surface ; it grows outwards, and forms a bilobed tumour, of which the large lobe is formed by the cyst, and the small lobe is formed by the spleen. The cyst is **exteriorized.**

The third variety concerns the **juxtasplenic** cyst, which is sessile or pedunculated. It develops under the capsule of the spleen, at the ends, at the edges, or in the hilum, but the splenic tissue remains free. The tumour is irregular and bilobed ; the large lobe is formed by the cyst, and the small lobe is formed by the spleen.

Pathological Anatomy.—There is no need for me to describe here the formation and the structure of the hydatid cyst, with its coverings, its vesicles, its fluid, and its echinococci ; these details are given under Hydatid Cysts of the Liver. I need not dwell upon the adhesions, the suppurations, and the perforation, which may result during the evolution of the cyst, but there are some pathological peculiarities which I desire to mention. Whatever the general shape of the tumour may be, whether it be oval, elongated, or fusiform, the cyst itself remains absolutely spherical, in spite of the resistance of the tissue in which it develops.

In my case the pericystic tissue of the spleen was not of the same thickness at all points. The tissue was very thin and reduced to a cap at the centre of the spleen, while it had undergone such hypertrophy at the extremities that the spleen, after removal of the cyst, still weighed four times its normal weight.

In the thin portion forming the cap, fibrous tissue (perisplenitis) had taken the place of the normal splenic tissue, but at the extremities of the spleen the tissue had hypertrophied to a considerable extent, and the two histological preparations reproduced in my clinical lectures show the hypertrophy of the spleen pulp and the fibrosis of the capsule (perisplenitis).

What is, then, the signification of this hypertrophy which more than compensates for the partial loss of spleen tissue, due to atrophy ? This variety of hypertrophy, which has, as far as I know, not as yet been described in the spleen, is comparable to the compensatory hypertrophy of the liver described by Hanot, Chauffard, and Kahn in several diseases of the liver (large alcoholic liver and hydatid cysts) ; and in some diseases of the kidney (Albarran, Chauffard). These conditions are described in the sections on these diseases.

The spleen, when it contains a hydatid cyst, appears to me to undergo marked compensatory hypertrophy. Further, this variety of splenic hypertrophy cannot be rare, if I judge by the few remarks regarding it in cases of hydatid cysts of the spleen, as observers have not specially dwelt on it. Snéguirew's case : after removal of the cyst the spleen was double or treble the normal size ; Robert's case : the spleen was hypertrophied ; Jayle's case : the spleen was hypertrophied, and measured 17 by 14 centimetres ; Arnozan's case : the spleen was hypertrophied, and weighed 250 grammes after removal of the cyst.

Compensatory hypertrophy of the spleen in the case of cysts appears to me, therefore, to be clear, and it must take its place with the compensatory hypertrophy of the liver and of the kidney.

Hæmatology.—An interesting question is the comparative study of the blood before and after splenectomy. Wlaëff, professor at the Military Academy of St. Petersburg, has kindly communicated to me some interesting researches which he made while my first patient was under Gérard Marchant's care :

After removal of the spleen, examination of the blood yielded 4,400,000 red corpuscles and 10,560 white corpuscles. Relative proportion, 1 in 417.

Twenty-four hours after splenectomy, 3,820,000 red corpuscles and 21,200 white corpuscles. Relative proportion, 1 in 181.

Five days after operation, 3,610,000, red corpuscles and 12,600 white corpuscles. Relative proportion, 1 in 286.

Twelve days after operation, 3,520,000 red corpuscles and 13,600 white corpuscles. Relative proportion, 1 in 258.

Twenty-eight days after operation, 3,500,000 red corpuscles and 8,400 white corpuscles. Relative proportion, 1 in 410.

Thirty-five days after operation, 3,637,000 red corpuscles and 12,000 white corpuscles. Relative proportion, 1 in 303.

Forty-six days after operation, 3,800,000 red corpuscles and 11,700 white corpuscles. Relative proportion, 1 in 324.

Sixty-one days after operation, 4,000,000 red corpuscles and 12,000 white corpuscles. Relative proportion, 1 in 310.

Eighty-six days after operation, 4,250,000 red corpuscles and 14,000 white corpuscles. Relative proportion, 1 in 304.

This comparative table shows that the number of red corpuscles is considerably lowered directly after the removal of the spleen ; the number of white corpuscles is doubled. During the next few days the red corpuscles continue to diminish up to the twentieth day ; they then increase progressively until the eighty-sixth day, when they regain their normal count. The white blood-corpuscles, on the contrary, are not diminished in proportion, and their number remains decidedly higher after the operation.

For some weeks after splenectomy Wlaäff found in the patient a transient enlargement of the thyroid body, as well as transient hypertrophy of the lymphatic glands in the neck, axilla, and groin.

The examination of the blood in my patient also dealt with the condition of the red corpuscles, and the relative numbers of their different varieties.

The enumeration and the relative proportions of the elements of the blood, counted before splenectomy, gave practically normal results : Red corpuscles, 4,400,000 ; white corpuscles, 10,560. The white corpuscles were divided as follows : Small mononuclear leucocytes (lymphocytes of the Germans), and large mononuclear leucocytes, 15·4 per cent. ; intermediary leucocytes, 7·6 per cent. ; polynuclear leucocytes, 77 per cent. ; eosinophile cells, 4 per cent.

For the better understanding of the changes in the blood cells figured in the plates on p. 1811, it is necessary to remember the varieties of white blood-corpuscles in the normal condition. In order to avoid repetition, I would ask the reader to turn to the section on Leucocythæmia, where he will find a detailed description.

In Fig. 92, which shows the blood films **before** removal of the spleen, we see that the condition is normal, both as regards the number and the relative proportions of red and white corpuscles. We also see some lymphocytes (small mononuclear leucocytes), as well as the mononuclear, intermediary, polynuclear, and eosinophile forms.

In Fig. 93, which shows the blood film **a month after** removal of the spleen, we see an absolute change as regards the red and white corpuscles.

The former have diminished in number (3,820,000), and the shape of some is altered. Their outline, instead of being circular, assumes the appearance of an almond, a pear, a comma, and a heart.

Nucleated red blood cells are also present in the proportion of 1 to 20,000. The variations in the leucocytes chiefly affect the mononuclear cells

II.

and the staining reactions of their protoplasm ; while some remain well stained, the others no longer take the dye.

A white blood-corpuscle undergoing karyokinesis, which is not found in all blood, is also seen.

Fig. 94 represents an examination of the blood **three months** after splenectomy, and shows that the normal appearance has been regained.

It is evident that a substitution has taken place in the blood-forming organs.

The normal forms of the red blood cells, as well as the deformed and nucleated corpuscles, and the abnormal forms of white corpuscles showing karyokinesis, have disappeared. The relations between the different varieties are normal, as Fig. 94 shows.

I shall refrain from drawing conclusions as to the formation and changes in the red and white corpuscles. It is, however, certain that after removal of the spleen a disturbance occurred both in the quantity and quality of red corpuscles, and it is also certain that this disturbance was only transient, that substitution took place in the blood-forming organs, and that in three months the blood regained its normal morphology, the equilibrium being re-established.

Description.—Let us first consider the clinical side of the question. We find hydatid cysts in the spleen, just as in the liver, but we cannot say when they commence to develop, because in both cases there is a latent period of indefinite duration. Pain is generally the first symptom. It lasted four years in my first case, and several years in my second. Similar facts obtain in most of the cases which I have collected. It is rarely early, but more often occurs late. The pain, especially at the onset, is neither acute nor continuous ; it is rather dull and deep-seated, with paroxysms and periods of calm. Its situation is variable. In one case it may simulate left intercostal neuralgia ; in a second it is abdominal ; and in a third the left shoulder and scapular region are painful, especially if the cyst lies close to the diaphragm. The pain in some cases becomes very acute, and requires special treatment—antipyrine, morphia, blisters, or applications of iodine.

The course of events proceeds in this manner for one or two years, or longer, as in my patients, with feelings of weight and dragging in the left hypochondrium and in the abdomen, but without the appearance of clearly defined signs. During this lengthy period the appetite remains good and the strength does not diminish ; slight dyspepsia or dyspnœa may be present. The cyst, however, grows, pushes aside the neighbouring organs, hampers their function, gives rise to deformity, and excites fresh symptoms. From this time, according as the cyst develops in one direction or another, the clinical picture becomes so modified that it is desirable to classify cysts of the spleen in two categories.

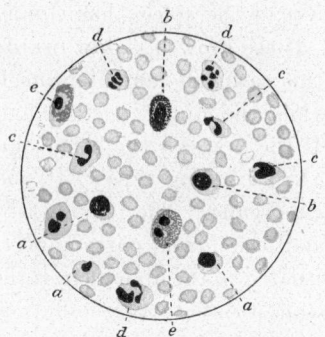

FIG. 92.—BEFORE SPLENECTOMY.

A, Small mononuclear lymphocytes; *b*, large mononuclear leucocytes; *c*, intermediary leucocytes; *d*, polynuclear leucocytes; *e*, eosinophile cells.

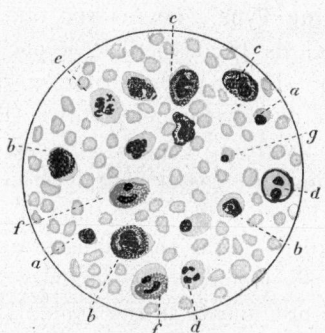

FIG. 93.—A MONTH AFTER SPLENECTOMY.

A, Small mononuclear lymphocytes; *b*, large mononuclear leucocytes; *c*, intermediary leucocytes; *d*, polynuclear leucocytes; *e*, leucocyte showing karyokinesis; *f*, eosinophile cells; *g*, nucleated red corpuscle.

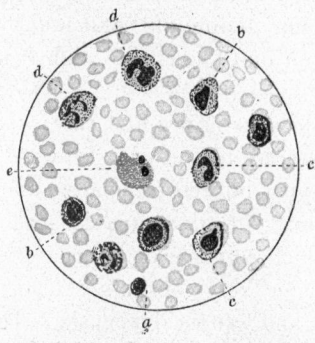

FIG. 94.—THREE MONTHS AFTER SPLENECTOMY.

A, Small mononuclear lymphocytes; *b*, large mononuclear leucocytes; *c*, intermediary leucocytes; *d*, polynuclear leucocytes; *e*, eosinophile cells.

When the hydatid cyst of the spleen has commenced to grow, it may take several directions. If the growth is downwards, we have a cyst of the descending type. In this case the tumour projects into the belly, and is especially abdominal, while the upper portion hidden behind the ribs is of minor importance. If the cyst, on the other hand, grows in an upward direction, it belongs to the ascending type. It pushes up the diaphragm, and displaces the thoracic organs. The bulging is chiefly found in the left hypochondriac region and the lower portion of the thorax. The lower portion of the tumour, situated in the abdomen, is then of minor importance.

It is therefore necessary to study the evolution and the symptoms of hydatid cysts of the spleen, according as they grow downwards, towards the abdomen (descending type), or upwards towards the thorax (ascending type). I feel the more justified in admitting these two clinical varieties, as they form a faithful reproduction of the two cases above described.

Cyst of the Ascending Type.—Let us first take the case in which the splenic cyst grows upwards from the left hypochondrium towards the thorax (ascending type). The hypochondrium, in this case, first feels the effect. The tumour, in its development, raises the diaphragm and displaces the lower ribs outwards. The patient complains of thoracic and scapular pains, simulating intercostal neuralgia and scapulalgia. At the same time the thorax becomes deformed, and its base is enlarged ; the lower ribs bulge outwards. So far the changes are evidently confined to the hypochondrium ; nevertheless, the tumour commences to become abdominal, and forms a prominence in the flank.

As the cyst continues to grow, the symptoms become more marked. The breathing is hampered, and the oppression is greater the more the diaphragm and the lungs are pushed up, and the bulging of the lower part of the thorax is the more marked in proportion as the ribs are more pushed outwards. Moreover, by this time, the tumour is no longer retrocostal and thoracic ; it has become abdominal, and may be felt in the belly. It is painless, with a regular outline, and is only slightly movable, being clamped above in the thorax.

At length the time comes, as in my first case, when the symptoms reach their maximum. The cyst, by reason of its upward growth, pushes up the left lung, as far as the upper intercostal spaces, and displaces the heart to the right of the sternum. The dyspnœa is severe, and interrupted by attacks of oppression, which coincide or alternate with crises of neuralgia. Certain movements become very painful. As regards the abdomen, the tumour increases in size, and causes dyspepsia. The bulging is no longer confined to the hypochondrium, but also affects the flank. When we place the patient in the upright position and take a full-face view, the bulging and the deformity become more apparent on making him turn to his left side.

In short, the dominant feature in a cyst of the **ascending type** is not the abdominal symptoms, but the thoracic ones. At first sight the cyst may simulate a pleural effusion, since it pushes up the diaphragm, compresses the lung, and displaces the heart. We find, on percussion, dullness as high as the fourth, or even the third, intercostal space, according to the size of the cyst. Dullness is also present in the axilla and at the back of the chest, although it does not coincide exactly with the anterior limit of dullness. The thoracic vibrations are absent over the whole of the dull area. On auscultation, we can hear neither the normal respiration nor any abnormal sounds. There is complete silence. Râles, due to pulmonary congestion, are heard both in front, behind, and above the dull region. In a word, the examination of the chest yields the signs of a large pleural effusion.

Certain slight differences, however, give the diagnosis between effusion into the left pleura and displacement of the thoracic organs by a splenic cyst. In pleural effusion the thorax may undergo an enlargement which is perceptible both on inspection and on mensuration. Some other cause than pleural effusion, such as a tumour of the hypochondrium, is, however, necessary, in order to push out the lower ribs and form a bulging limited to the lower part of the thorax. Ægophony, pectoriloquy, and tubular breathing, which are the usual signs of pleural effusion, are absent or excep-tional when the thoracic organs are displaced by a cyst of the spleen.

In both pleural effusion and in a cystic tumour the heart may be displaced beyond the right edge of the sternum ; but in pleural effusion the two nipples remain practically on the same level, whereas in the case of a cyst the left nipple, which is raised up together with the skin, is found to be higher than the right nipple.

Such are the chief symptoms in a case of hydatid cyst of the ascending type. They are somewhat more striking than the abdominal signs, of which I shall now speak. While the cyst encroaches upon the cavity of the thorax, it is also dragged down towards the abdomen by reason of its weight and its growth. We find, therefore, an oblong or a rounded tumour in the flank or in the belly. This tumour, which is not movable, because it forms part of the cyst clamped under the thorax, does not assume a large size in the abdomen. It rarely descends lower than the umbilicus or beyond the linea alba.

We find, on palpation and percussion, that the abdominal and thoracic tumours are really one, and measure 10 or 12 inches in length, the sub-costal portion being much more limited than the supracostal portion. This feature permits the elimination of splenic enlargement due to malaria, leukæmia, or to bacillary infection, etc., for the principal trait of these enlarged spleens is that they do not reach high up into the thorax, but descend low down into the abdomen, forming tumours which are abdominal rather than thoracic. When we come to the subject of the descending type of splenic cyst, we shall have to distinguish between a cyst and these various forms of splenomegaly.

I do not like to leave the description of splenic cysts of the ascending type without speaking of certain severe complications which may result. These cysts, in their upward growth towards the thorax, sometimes cause such complications as perforation of the diaphragm, invasion of the pleura and lung by the hydatids. The following cases are excellent examples :

The first of these cases deals with a young woman admitted to hospital under Arnozan's care for acute and long-standing pain on the left side of the chest.

Marked bulging of the left hypochondrium was found. This region was dull, and tactile fremitus was absent. The breathing was scarcely perceptible on auscultation ; bronchophony and ægophony were not audible. The heart was displaced to the right side of the sternum. Exploration of the abdomen revealed a large, painless tumour, which extended to within two fingers' breadth of the iliac crest, while the sharp edge reached almost to the umbilicus. Percussion showed that this abdominal tumour, diagnosed as splenic, was continuous with the dull area in the thorax. A puncture was made in the eighth left intercostal space, and a few drops of purulent fluid drawn off, the cannula being obliterated by a whitish membrane. On microscopic examination the membrane showed hydatid structure, and the purulent fluid contained hooklets of the echinococcus.

Arnozan and Demons, considering the situation and the abdomino-thoracic develop-ment of the tumour, made the diagnosis of suppurating cyst of the spleen. An operation was therefore decided upon, and Demons performed it. After resection of the ninth rib, the incision of the subjacent tissue led into a cavity from which an enormous quantity of purulent fluid, with numerous hydatids, flowed out. The finger, intro-duced into this cavity in order to explore the vault of the diaphragm, passed into a hiatus, which was, in part, obliterated by hydatid membrane. The membrane was drawn out with forceps, the orifice of communication was enlarged, and the hand then passed into an abdominal cavity. A quantity of hydatid vesicles were withdrawn, the cavity was washed out, and two drainage tubes introduced—one into the pleural cavity, and the other into the abdominal cystic cavity.

The patient died a few days later, and the autopsy revealed a suppurating cyst, which had developed in the upper three-quarters of the spleen. The tumour, in its as-cending course, had perforated the diaphragm, and opened into the left pleura. The left lung contained numerous hydatids. As regards our anatomical classification, the case was a typical one of intrasplenic cyst, and the spleen tissue covered it everywhere, except at the perforation. Furthermore, the spleen had undergone a certain amount of compensatory hypertrophy, since it weighed 8 ounces after removal of the cyst.

A woman had suffered for four years from a tumour in the left hypochondrium. A large tumour occupied the flank, the left hypochondrium, the hypogastric, and umbilical regions, and descended into the iliac fossa. The tumour was most prominent at the epigastrium and the umbilicus. It reached upwards under the false ribs, causing dullness in the fifth intercostal space. Tactile fremitus and breath sounds were absent over the whole of the dull region, which corresponded to the lower part of the thorax. The diagnosis of a splenic cyst invading the left pleura was made.

The operation was performed by Reboul. The abdominal incision revealed an enormous tumour beneath the ribs in the left hypochondrium. The tumour fluctuated, and, in the parts accessible to view, its covering was formed of spleen tissue. Puncture of the tumour gave exit to a large quantity of sero-purulent fluid, with hydatid débris. The wall of the tumour was incised with the thermo-cautery. The cavity was then explored, and the operator found that the cyst reached upwards under the diaphragm, and communicated with the thoracic cavity by a large opening. After alternate periods of improvement and relapse, the situation became definitely better, when left hemiplegia and apoplexy set in and ended fatally.

At the autopsy the spleen was found to be hypertrophied (compensatory hypertrophy). The hydatid had developed at the upper end of the organ, thus explaining its tendency to push up the diaphragm and the thoracic organs. Sections of the brain revealed, on the inner surface of the right hemisphere, two suppurating hydatid cysts, which opened into the lateral ventricle. The apoplexy and death were thus explained.

Splenic Cysts of the Descending Type.—Cysts of the descending type spread downwards, and involve the abdominal cavity. The ribs in this case are less displaced, the hypochondrium does not bulge as much as in the preceding variety, and the chief growth of the cyst takes place, not in the hypochondrium or in the thorax, but in the abdomen. The tumour, as a whole, is abdomino-thoracic, but it is more abdominal than thoracic. The tumour commences in the left hypochondrium, and spreads chiefly to the abdomen. In a few years it may acquire an enormous size, filling up the flank, and encroaching upon the epigastrium and the umbilical region, or descending into the iliac fossa. The tumour is generally somewhat irregular, resistant, and painless—at any rate in the early stages. It is usually mobile and less bound down by adhesions. On palpation and percussion we find that the tumour reaches behind the ribs, but does not cause the great displacement of the diaphragm and of the thoracic organs seen in cysts of the ascending type.

The symptoms of this variety are chiefly abdominal: dyspepsia, nausea, and vomiting, with pain in the stomach and intestines; digestion is delayed, and constipation is the rule. The patient complains of heaviness and weight in the abdomen, and notices that his stomach becomes larger, that his clothes feel too tight, and that his movements are hampered.

The chief symptoms of hydatid cysts of the abdominal type are as above. If the cysts spread upwards (ascending type) as well as downwards (descending type), we find a combination of thoracic and abdominal symptoms.

Diagnosis.—I have discussed the diagnosis of splenic cysts which grow upwards towards the thorax and simulate pleural effusion; let us now discuss the diagnosis of cysts which closely resemble other tumours of the abdomen. The diagnosis between a cyst of the spleen and one of the kidney is by no means simple. Thus Nélaton was twice wrong, and mistook a cyst of the spleen for one of the kidney, and Potain diagnosed a cyst of the spleen, when the lesion was really a left hydronephrosis. These quotations are sufficient to show the great difficulty in diagnosis.

Splenic cysts have many points in common with those of the mesentery. Braquehaye has thus presented this question : If the surgeon has to deal with an abdominal tumour which was primarily lateral, but which has rapidly become median, growing towards the umbilicus, and especially if the tumour is accompanied by Tillaux's three signs (free mobility in every direction, resonant zone between the walls and the tumour, and another resonant zone above the pubes), it is highly probable that the tumour is mesenteric. I may add that a splenic cyst arises in the left hypochondrium ; tumours of the mesentery have not this origin.

What are the diagnostic elements between hydatid cysts of the spleen and the splenic enlargements due to malaria, leukæmia, and tuberculosis ? As a general rule, every enlarged spleen, whether due to malaria, to leukæmia, or to tuberculosis, shows a natural tendency, by reason of its weight and of its size, to extend from the hypochondrium into the abdominal cavity. Every enlarged spleen forms a well-developed tumour, of which the smaller part is situated behind the ribs in the hypochondrium, and of which the larger portion projects into the abdomen. The portion of the tumour hidden behind the ribs in the left hypochondrium cannot be palpated. It reveals itself by dullness and by bulging of the hypochondrium. The abdominal portion of the tumour can be easily palpated, and we are thus enabled to estimate exactly the situation, shape, consistency, size, and degree of mobility of the tumour.

These facts are equally applicable to abdominal cysts of the spleen and to other enlargements of the organ. In both cases the smaller portion of the tumour is hidden behind the ribs, and the larger portion forms a marked projection in the abdomen. How, then, can the diagnosis between splenic cyst and splenomegaly be decided ? In order to do so let us review the different enlargements of the spleen, and see what are their distinctive characters.

Let us commence with the **malarial** spleen. The spleen may be enormously enlarged in persons suffering from malaria, especially in the chronic forms and in cachexia. The organ bulges in the left hypochondrium, and forms in the abdomen a tumour, which is sometimes exceedingly large. The malarial spleen, although it is much hypertrophied, practically preserves its form, and is not bilobed, in contradistinction to the splenic cyst. Further, while the cyst runs its course without fever and without affecting the general health for a long while, the malarial spleen is preceded by attacks of fever of different kinds, and becomes larger with the febrile attacks and with the appearance of cachexia ; and the liver is, moreover, generally hypertrophied.

Let us consider the enlarged spleen of **leucocythæmia.** I had a remarkable example under my care some years ago :

The patient was admitted to hospital in an advanced stage of cachexia. His appearance resembled that of a cancerous patient : earthy tint and colourless mucous membranes, œdema of the legs and purpura. The patient complained of extreme weakness and felt ill. On examination we found in the abdomen an enormous tumour. It was hard and painless, and caused deformity of the left flank and the hypochondrium. It reached almost as low as the umbilicus, and was wedged in above, beneath the ribs, where the dullness extended as high as the fifth intercostal space. The diagnosis of an enlarged spleen was made, but it remained to determine the nature of this tumour. If the cachectic patient with this enormous spleen had also presented glandular swellings in the neck, groin, and axilla, we should at once have thought of leucocythæmia, but he had no apparent glandular hypertrophy. And yet this fact was not a reason for abandoning the diagnosis of leucocythæmia, for examples of splenic lymphadenia exist, without apparent glandular tumours.

In order to decide the question, Apert examined the blood, and the diagnosis of a leucocythæmic spleen was confirmed. The patient had 50,000 white corpuscles to 1,900,000 red corpuscles, or a proportion of 1 to 40, instead of 1 to 500 in the normal condition. Nevertheless, in leucocythæmia it is not sufficient to find considerable excess of the white corpuscles ; we must also know to which variety they belong. This case was one of leukæmia, with small mononuclear leucocytes (the lymphocytes of German authors, and the globulins of the old French authors). The diagnosis was verified at the autopsy. The hydatid cyst of the spleen is for a long while compatible with good health, and does not modify the normal condition of the blood. The leucocythæmic spleen, on the other hand (with or without participation of the lymphatic glands), is accompanied by considerable excess of white corpuscles in the blood, with predominance of leucocytes, or of lymphocytes according to the case.

Let us now see how it is possible to arrive at a diagnosis between hydatid cysts of the spleen and **primary tubercular splenomegalia.** In addition to the secondary infection of the spleen resulting from other localizations of the tubercle bacillus (broncho-pneumonia, miliary tuberculosis, micropolyadenia, etc.), primary tuberculosis of the spleen has been described by Rendu and Widal, Moutard-Martin and Lefas, and by Guiliani. This disease does not appear, as was formerly supposed, in the course of advanced phthisis ; it develops during good health in persons whose tubercular taint has passed unnoticed. The only symptoms for some time are pain in the left hypochondrium, and a sensation of weight and dragging ; but dyspnœa may also appear in some cases.

After this indefinite phase has lasted for some months, the splenic tumour has become large ; it projects into the hypochondrium, descends into the flank, and invades the abdomen, forming an ovoid or oblong mass, which is indurated and nodular. The hypochondrium and the flank bulge. The disease, sometimes apyretic and at other times febrile, may last for several years and end fatally. The autopsy reveals an enormous spleen, weighing from 3 to 8 pounds. Its shape is practically normal, its large diameter is from 6 to 12 inches, and its surface presents nodular masses, varying in size from a cherry to an orange. The cut section of the tumour shows fibrous tissue, infiltrated with caseous masses. It is rare to find Koch's bacilli.

How are we to diagnose a tubercular spleen from a hydatid cyst ? The differential signs are : The tubercular spleen is more nodular than the cyst ; it affects the health much more quickly, and is accompanied by hypertrophy of the liver. Lastly, though this might not be expected, it sometimes excites such an increase in red corpuscles that the count shows 8,000,000 to the cubic centimetre, with or without leucocytosis. It is true, however, that in a case reported by Achard and Castaigne this increase of red corpuscles was not present.

Let us now consider the diagnosis between hydatid cyst of the spleen and so-called primary splenomegaly. In the first place, what is meant by splenomegaly ? This term, coined by Debove, is applied to an affection characterized by hypertrophy of the spleen, followed later by enlargement of the liver, by absence of glandular tumours, and by progressive diminution of the red blood cells, without notable increase in the leucocytes. Anæmia, loss of strength, and wasting coincide with the enlargement of the spleen, which may weigh from 4 to 6 pounds. Certain rare cases of this " hypertrophic cirrhosis of the spleen " have been confounded with the lesion formerly described by Gaucher under the name of primary epithelioma or idiopathic hypertrophy of the spleen without leukæmia. In any case primary splenomegaly is distinguished from hydatid cyst of the spleen by the following signs : In splenomegaly the surface and outlines of the spleen do not present the deformity of the cystic spleen ; the liver is enlarged, the anæmia is constant, and the general health, which remains good for a long time during the development of the splenic cyst, is rapidly affected in primary splenomegaly.

There are certain cases of greatly enlarged spleens which do not enter into any of the preceding categories. A lady student of medicine recounted her own case to me :

For eleven years the spleen had increased in size, until it became as large as the head of a three-year-old child, but it never caused any symptoms. She had no pain, no œdema, no signs of pressure, and no change in the composition of blood. As the tumour was becoming troublesome, it was removed by Routier, and was found to be a spleen weighing 8 pounds. The splenic tissue was semitransparent on section. Histologically the hypertrophy was due to a primary fibrous degeneration, probably dependent upon some unknown infective process. Hæmorrhages, which were most likely secondary, were found in the spleen tissue. Such a case of splenomegalia is not always easy to differentiate from a hydatid cyst.

After having reviewed the enlarged spleens, which simulate more or less closely a hydatid cyst of this organ, let me say a few words as to its evolution, which is very slow, the first phase being insidious, and the symptoms usually indefinite. The cyst takes two or three years before it acquires the size seen in my two cases. The general health remains good, except for pain, dyspnœa, and dyspepsia, and we are surprised to see such an enormous tumour compatible with apparent health. Very serious complications are, however, to be feared in the long run, especially infection and suppuration of the cyst, with perforation of the diaphragm and invasion of the pleura, as in the two cases which I have just quoted.

Danger also arises from the invasion of other organs by the hydatids. As long as the spleen alone is infected, we may, by a well-timed operation, remove the trouble, but if the hydatids affect the liver, the kidneys, the lungs, the brain, etc., the situation is far more formidable.

My second patient who recovered from the splenic hydatid had also a cyst in his left kidney. Here the pain in the left lumbar region, and the colic produced by the passage of the hydatid membrane, revealed the diagnosis.

I have collected a fairly large number of cases in which the splenic cyst was complicated by cysts in other regions : Hydatid cysts of the spleen and liver ; hydatid cysts of the spleen, liver, and lung ; hydatid cysts of the spleen, liver, and pelvis ; hydatid cysts of the spleen and right pleura ; hydatid cysts of the spleen, right pleura, and brain ; hydatid cysts of the spleen and pelvis ; hydatid cysts of the spleen, liver, gall-bladder, omentum and of the right Fallopian tube ; hydatid cysts of the spleen and the omentum.

The multiplicity of hydatid cysts, and especially the localization of some of them, cause special complications as regards prognosis. It is always necessary to think of the possibility of general hydatid infection.

Treatment.—Apart from cases in which several organs are attacked, we may say that hydatid cyst of the spleen, which was formerly a most formidable disease, is now curable, thanks to the marvellous progress of surgery. And yet it is highly necessary that surgical intervention should not be delayed too long, for here, as in all cases, it is not sufficient to operate : the operation must be performed in time. The duty of making a correct diagnosis and of deciding as to surgical intervention is incumbent upon the physician. The surgeon's duty is to perform the operation of choice. Intra-splenic cysts necessitate splenectomy, while the spleen may be preserved in the case of juxtasplenic cysts.

PART VII

PATHOLOGY OF THE BLOOD

I. CLINICAL EXAMINATION OF THE BLOOD.

THE clinical examination of the blood may afford valuable information in diagnosis and prognosis. Physicians were formerly content with the gross physical and chemical examination of the blood withdrawn from a vein. This study was rendered easier by the frequency of bleeding as a therapeutic measure. It is sufficient to-day to withdraw a few drops of blood by pricking the finger in order to obtain the necessary clinical information, which depends upon the histological condition of the blood, its chemical composition, and its bacteriological features.

The **enumeration of the blood-corpuscles** is made with Malassez's or with Hayem's instruments, but we cannot here enter into the details of the technique.

The **percentage of hæmoglobin** is estimated by the colorimetric apparatus of Malassez, Hayem, or of Hénocque. Malassez's instrument gives the weight of hæmoglobin in 100 c.c. of blood. On dividing the amount by the number of red blood-corpuscles, we easily obtain the weight of hæmoglobin contained in a single red blood-corpuscle, which is called the **colour index.** This information is of the highest importance in clinical medicine.

Normal blood contains 4,500,000 red blood-corpuscles per cubic millimetre, and 10 to 15 grammes of hæmoglobin per 100 c.c. of blood, while the colour index is from 28 to 30. Malassez's system of counting is the best, but other authors express the quantity of hæmoglobin in percentages, employing a comparative standard of so-called normal blood to which they assign a value of 100. Others, again, including Hayem, estimate the quantity of hæmoglobin (which they call the globular richness) by the number of healthy red blood-corpuscles.

Spectroscopic examination gives information as to the state of the blood in certain pathological conditions, such as carbonic oxide asphyxia.

Bacteriological examination of the blood comprises the direct examination upon the slide of fresh blood, and of fixed and stained blood, as well as the cultivation of the blood on various culture media and inoculation in animals. We have frequently had occasion to speak of this method during the course of this treatise.

The **histological examination** of the blood should be made upon fresh preparations, as well as upon fixed and stained films.

For the examination of fresh blood, it suffices to place a drop of blood upon a slide, to put a cover-glass over it, and to seal the edge with paraffin, but we may also employ Malassez's air-chambers or Hayem's hollow cell. These consist of thick glass slides, upon which a disc of glass is isolated by means of a circular trench. If the preparations are examined under the microscope, we find a large number of small, yellowish corpuscles floating in a colourless fluid—the **blood plasma.** These are the **red blood-corpuscles,** which have the shape of a biconcave disc. They often form rouleaux, and present their edge to the observer. These rouleaux are united by their extremities, and enclose spaces in which the plasma contains only the white corpuscles, or leucocytes.

The white corpuscles are present in much fewer numbers. They have the appearance of colourless, shining, mobile cells. Lastly, we see small, colourless granulations, or Hayem's hæmatoblasts, united, as a rule, in small groups. These extemporaneous preparations, which should always be examined, indicate approximately the richness of the blood in red and white cells. They may reveal the presence of dark pigment grains and of parasites. If the preparation is left alone, fibrin is precipitated, and forms a network of fine fibrillæ, so that we may estimate in an approximate manner the richness of the blood in fibrin.

It is necessary to fix and stain the blood if we wish to obtain permanent preparations. The most widely employed method consists in collecting a drop of blood on the end of a slide, spreading it out over the slide, and drying the thin layer of blood by shaking in the air.

If the process of drying lasts for some weeks, the blood is fixed, and remains unaltered by water. In the contrary case, it is necessary to complete the fixation by the action of different reagents (absolute alcohol, mixture of absolute alcohol and ether, or a 1 per cent. solution of chromic acid), or by dry heat at 120° C., according to Ehrlich's method.

In exceptional cases, as in myelogenic leukæmia, we may advantageously employ for comparison Jolly's method, which consists in employing the fixative agent (Fleming's solution) to the blood, which has been spread out, but not dried.

Hæmatoxylin and aniline dyes are the usual stains employed in staining the blood. The aniline dyes are divided by Ehrlich into acid and basic. The former comprise eosin, orange and acid fuchsin, and act upon the eosinophiles, granules, and the red corpuscles ; while the basic dyes comprise thionine, methyl violet, and methylene blue. They stain the so-called basophile granules, the nucleus of the leucocytes, and the nucleated red blood cells. Lastly, Ehrlich has distinguished in the neutral stains those which are produced by the admixture of acid and basic dyes, and also neutrophile granules. Jolly has shown that the neutrophile granules may take the acid stains, though more feebly than the eosinophile granules. The examination of fixed and stained preparations shows the nucleus of the leucocytes, marks out their various granulations, indicates the percentage of the varieties, and distinguishes the changes in form and the staining reactions of the red corpuscles, the presence of nucleated red corpuscles, and the increase or the diminution in the hæmatoblasts.

The histological lesions of the blood cannot be properly understood, unless we know the varieties of leucocytes normally present. It is, therefore, advisable to mention these points in hæmatology. Normal blood contains about 7,000 leucocytes per cubic millimetre, or one white corpuscle to 600 red corpuscles. Jolly has classified the leucocytes as follows :

The first variety comprises the small mononuclear leucocytes. I would prefer to call them microlymphocytes, in order to distinguish them from the leucocytes proper. They form the most important element in the lymphatic glands, but they are rare in normal blood, amounting to 2 per cent. of the white corpuscles. They are smaller than the red corpuscles, and the nucleus is at times so large that it appears to fill the whole cell, leaving but little room for the protoplasm. We shall see later that the accumulation of lymphocytes in the blood is the characteristic feature of one of the varieties of leucocythæmia.

The second variety comprises the large mononuclear leucocytes. The cell contains one nucleus, but the protoplasm is more abundant than in the preceding variety.

This variety includes the so-called intermediary leucocytes, in which the nucleus is, as it were, strangulated. The nucleus looks as if it were about to divide, and the leucocyte is, therefore, said to be intermediate between the mononuclear and polynuclear leucocytes. The large mononuclear and intermediary leucocytes form 36 per cent. of the white corpuscles.

The third variety comprises the polynuclear leucocytes. The nucleus is sometimes bent in the form of a rod, constricted at certain points ; at other times there are several distinct nuclei, as though the rod had broken at different points. These leucocytes amount to 60 per cent. of the total number of leucocytes in normal blood.

The fourth variety comprises the eosinophile cells. In normal blood they amount to 1 or 2 per cent. The protoplasm contains granules, which stain deeply with eosin.

Abnormal Elements.—Certain rare or abnormal elements are found in the blood. Their number does not exceed 1 or 2 per cent., but it is greater in pathological conditions. Some are about as large as a lymphocyte, and the protoplasm stains deeply with the blue dyes. They are called plasma cells. The nucleus is sometimes clear, and scarcely stained. The cell is a mononuclear basophile. Others are also mononuclear, but they also contain neutrophile or eosinophile granulations. They have been called granular myelocytes, because they originate from the bone-marrow, and appear to give rise to the normal polynuclear cells. Lastly, we have the mastzellen, in which the nucleus is multilobar or regular, and in which the protoplasm contains basophile granulations.

Some writers, by means of artificial hæmolysis, have found abnormal pigmentary and neoplastic cells in the blood. The latter are often difficult to distinguish from the large mononuclears of normal blood. In cases of cancer their presence in the blood indicates the generalization of the disease.

Variations in the Leucocytes.—The leucocytes show more or less constant variations in the course of the different morbid processes. In some cases we find an increase in the number of leucocytes or leucocytosis; in others there is a diminution or leucopenia. Leucocytosis is more common than leucopenia, and marked leucocytosis often follows recovery from transient leucopenia.

Leucocytosis is most marked in the inflammatory affections: acute rheumatism, pneumonia, erysipelas, suppurative troubles, and scarlatina.

Leucopenia occurs in typhoid fever, in certain forms of malaria, in severe and fatal infections or intoxications, etc.

Great importance is attached at the present day to the qualitative variations in the leucocytes in the course of disease. In most cases we find an increase in the number of polynuclears (polynucleosis); in some cases the increase is in the mononuclears (lymphocytosis), and in others it is in the eosinophiles (eosinophilia).

Polynucleosis is met with in inflammatory and suppurative affections: pneumonia, empyæma, acute meningitis. The percentage may be as high as 85 or 90. It is also seen in scarlatina (95 per cent.). It may help to distinguish between pneumonia and typhoid fever, between acute tubercular pleurisy or bacillary meningitis, and purulent pleurisy or meningitis, between measles and scarlet fever. In certain affections — pneumonia (Loeper), erysipelas (Chantemesse and Widal)—a polynucleosis of more than 95 per cent. indicates rapid death.

In polynucleosis the presence of glycogen in the leucocytes may be shown by the iodine test. Brown granules are seen in the protoplasm of the leucocytes. The reaction indicates acute inflammation.

Mononucleosis is seen in the stationary stage of typhoid fever, in mumps, and in malaria.

Lymphocytosis, which is always marked in the infant, is almost constant in the following conditions : whooping-cough, measles, acute tuberculosis of the organs and serous membranes, syphilis, and lead-poisoning.

Eosinophilia is common in convalescence from rheumatism, typhoid fever, scarlatina, and erysipelas. In this case it has been called critical eosinophilia. On the other hand, reactionary eosinophilia has been described in certain intoxications (mercury, iodine), in diseases of the skin (Dühring's dermatitis), and in helminthiasis.

Plasma cells are common in the critical stage of diseases. Granular and non-granular myelocytes are found in the blood in certain morbid conditions : purpura, hæmorrhagic typhoid fever, hereditary syphilis, and variola.

These leucocytic variations are not specific, because they depend chiefly on the gravity of the affection, on the anatomical process which characterizes it, and not upon the nature of the micro-organism or poison which is at work.

Moreover, polynucleosis, mononucleosis, and eosinophilia are often mere phases of a more complex reaction. On closer study, the leucocytic formulæ appear to be traced on the same type : at the onset, polynucleosis, primary reaction ; in the stationary stage, mononucleosis, more profound reaction of immunity ; in the stage of convalescence, eosinophilia, stigma of recovery. Accordingly, the early appearance, the persistence, and the abundance of the different forms of leucocytes, rather than their presence, are of use in hæmo-diagnosis and hæmo-prognosis.

II. ANÆMIA.

Any change in the respiratory function of the blood is called an anæmia (Jolly). This change may consist in the diminution of the number of red blood-corpuscles, in the diminution or the alteration of the hæmoglobin, in the lowering of the colour index, etc., and these different lesions, which are associated in various ways, affect the chief function of the blood—namely, its power of distributing oxygen.

In slight anæmia we see, as a rule, some diminution in the number of red blood-corpuscles ; in more severe cases the lowering of the colour index is also present, in addition to the diminution in the number of the red corpuscles. In chlorosis, the lowering of the colour index predominates. It may coexist with the normal number of red corpuscles. In pernicious anæmia, the number of red corpuscles is always diminished to a considerable degree, but the colour index is, on the contrary, normal or even increased.

Anæmia following hæmorrhage has served as the basis for the study of anæmia, and for researches as to the repair of the blood. It has been studied experimentally, because it can be readily produced in animals. In man, it is exceptional to meet with it under such conditions that the result may not be produced by the disease which has caused the hæmorrhage. Nevertheless, it is sometimes possible.

In one of my patients blanched by severe hæmatemesis, following **exulceratio simplex** of the stomach, and having, on his admission to hospital, only 650,000 red blood-corpuscles per cubic millimetre, Jolly was able to follow the repair of the blood under the most favourable conditions.

He showed that this repair took place in the same manner as in animals which had been bled. After an acute hæmorrhage, we find a first period, in which the number of red corpuscles and the quantity of hæmoglobin continue to fall on parallel lines. The colour-index, therefore, remains stationary. In the second period, the number of red corpuscles increases rapidly. Nucleated red corpuscles appear in the blood, but the hæmoglobin remains stationary, and rises again very slowly ; consequently, the colour-index is lowered. In the third period, the number of red corpuscles continues to rise, though slowly. The hæmoglobin count increases rapidly, and the colour-index rises. These results are interesting, because they have a general application, and because the repair of the blood takes place in the same manner in all cases of symptomatic anæmia, as well as in chlorosis.

In the experimental anæmias, just as in the traumatic anæmias in man, we may see in the blood during the period of repair nucleated red cells, which are sometimes present in large numbers (Jolly).

The various diseases of nutrition, the acute and chronic infectious disorders, and, in particular, acute rheumatism, malaria, variola, chronic tuberculosis, the intoxications such as lead-poisoning, intestinal parasites, syphilis, and cancer, most often cause anæmic conditions, which are grouped together under the term secondary or symptomatic. We look on them as the opposite of the so-called **essential** anæmias, in which the blood lesion is not a secondary symptom, or a simple consequence, but comprises practically the whole disease. Such are pernicious anæmia and chlorosis, which will form the subject of special sections.

III. PROGRESSIVE PERNICIOUS ANÆMIA.

Biermer deserves the merit of having described in 1868 and in 1872 pernicious anæmia as a morbid entity, but it must not be thought that the clinical type was unknown before his day. Andral, Piorry, Beau, and Addison had previously noticed it, and Trousseau had given a masterly description, which has hardly been added to by the researches of hæmatology.

While numerous authors have contributed to individualize pernicious anæmia by researches as to the ætiology, pathological anatomy, and hæmatology, others have asked whether the anatomy of this morbid type is real, and whether it is not always symptomatic of cancerous, tubercular, or other lesions. The truth is that, in addition to the extreme deuteropathic anæmias, there is room for a grave essential anæmia, of which the primary cause will doubtless be revealed to us some day, just as it has been in miners' anæmia.

The disease occurs chiefly in certain very poor districts of Switzerland, Prussia, and Sweden, and especially in pregnant and nursing women. It is most frequently caused by insufficient nourishment, physical or intellectual overwork, excesses, or trouble.

Pathological Anatomy.—Post mortem, the tissues are extremely pale. The skin, the mucous membranes, and the parenchyma are œdematous, or studded with small hæmorrhages. The heart shows partial fatty degeneration of its muscular fibres. The liver is pale, the cells are atrophied, and the nuclei no longer stain (Hanot and Segry).

Certain authors have recently attempted to place the initial lesion of the disease either in the stomach or in the bone-marrow.

The glands of the stomach are often affected by fatty degeneration and by extreme atrophy, and the organ itself may be so thin as to resemble a serous membrane (Gilbert). Fenwick, Quincke, and Nothnagel have insisted on the presence of this lesion, but before we can admit with Fenwick that pernicious anæmia is only a symptom of **gastric atrophy,** we have to prove that this atrophy is not the result of the anæmia.

The bone-marrow is often red, rich in nucleated corpuscles, and thus shows a return to the embryonic condition. Pepper would make this change in the marrow the *primum movens* of the disease. It is possible, says Gilbert, that pernicious anæmia is a myelogenous lymphadenia; but would it not be better to reverse the proposition, and consider the return of the marrow to the embryonic condition as the consequence of the extreme anæmia? In pernicious anæmia we find diminution, not only of the red corpuscles, but also of the hæmatoblasts. This anhæmatopoiesis, as Hayem calls it—that is to say, the sterility of the blood—would cause a resurrection of the fœtal hæmatopoietic functions of the liver, of the spleen, and especially of the bone-marrow.

The bacteriological researches of recent years have thrown no light upon the pathogenesis of the disease. Feltz and Engel have seen small rods in the blood, and Henrot has noted little granulations. The elements with a rounded body and furnished with a tail described by Pétrone and Frankenhauser are, perhaps, only poikilocytes which had become mobile by reason of the extreme anæmia.

Symptoms.—The onset is insidious. The disease commences with pallor, breathlessness, palpitation, and digestive disorder. Extreme feebleness soon appears, and compels the patient to take to his bed.

The anæmia is sometimes accompanied by a slightly jaundiced tint of the conjunctivæ, œdema of the legs, and ascites. The skin and mucous membranes are often covered with hæmorrhages. Epistaxis, stomatorrhagia, and hæmatemesis may occur. Hæmorrhage into the retina is one of the most important symptoms.

The temperature may remain normal, or may reach 104° F. in the febrile form of the disease. It has been seen to fall as low as 91° F. in the last stages of the malady. Palpitation is frequent, and the cardiac dullness is sometimes increased. The stethoscopic signs are less frequent than in chlorosis, but we may find a *bruit de diable* with a thrill over the internal jugular vein. The mind often becomes weak towards the end of the disease, which may end in coma.

As regards the stomach, we often find very marked troubles, as the anatomical lesions would lead us to suspect. They reveal themselves by anorexia, distension of the abdomen, vomiting, and diarrhœa. The disappearance of the hydrochloric acid has been recognized in one case by Cahn and von Mering.

The blood undergoes very marked changes. The red corpuscles fall to a million, and often as low as some hundreds of thousands. Their diameter is increased, and the giant cells, measuring $8 \cdot 5 \mu$ to 16μ, may represent an eighth part of the total count (Hayem). The colour-index is increased, or, in other words, in opposition to what is seen in chlorosis, the number of red cells is more reduced than the proportion of hæmoglobin.

The red blood-corpuscles are deformed, and assume a racquet or a spindle shape. These deformities, as well as the mobility of the cells, result from their abnormal contractile power. The altered cells may, indeed, present amœboid movements of rocking, oscillation, and propulsion, which have led writers to look upon them as parasites.

The hæmatoblasts and the leucocytes are diminished in number. The presence of nucleated red cells, and the increase of their colour-index, form the characteristic features in this anæmia. These nucleated cells are thrown into the blood by the spleen and by the bone-marrow in order to compensate for the insufficiency of hæmatopoiesis by the hæmatoblasts.

The course of the disease is progressive, as its name indicates, and death occurs in a year or even in a few months. The disease in some cases shows remissions, followed by relapses at more or less short intervals. Cases of definite recovery have been recorded (Quincke).

Diagnosis.—The disease is characterized by extreme anæmia, in which the patient's stoutness is preserved, and in which retinal hæmorrhages and special corpuscular changes are present; but yet this affection is so rare that the clinician should always ask whether he is not dealing with a symptomatic anæmia. The question is sometimes in doubt until the autopsy.

Extreme anæmia of the fourth degree may be met with after severe hæmorrhage, or in the course of chlorosis, tuberculosis, and cancer of the stomach and of the liver. The relations or the general evolution of the disease are generally sufficient to settle the diagnosis. Miners' anæmia, caused by the duodenal ankylostoma, or the anæmia caused by the *Bothriocephalus latus*, is not, as a rule, extreme, and does not reach the fourth degree. The eggs of the ankylostoma or of the bothriocephalus will be found in the stools, and will remove all doubt.

Treatment.—The stomach and the general health furnish us with indications for treatment, which should be based upon a diet composed of milk, eggs, grilled meat, vegetables *en purée*, stewed fruits, bread in very small quantities, light beer, white wine mixed with water, and a change of air from the town to the country. Iron may give good results, but **arsenic,** in the form of Fowler's solution, in doses of from 10 to 20 drops daily, appears to be the specific drug for the disease, and Padley's statistics attribute a large number of recoveries to it. Opotherapy with bone-marrow, radiotherapy, and injections of antidiphtheritic serum have caused improvement (Rénon and Texier).

IV. LEUCOCYTHÆMIA.

Discussion.—When Bennet and Virchow, in 1845, described the disease which forms the subject of this section, they were, without doubt, especially impressed by the colour which the blood took from the exaggerated and permanent formation of its white corpuscles, whence the name **leucocythæmia**, given by Bennet (λευκός, white; κύτος, cell; αἶμα, blood), and **leukæmia**, created by Virchow.

This change in the blood, though important, represents only one feature of the disease. The changes in the **adenoid tissue** are also of much importance. In the normal condition the adenoid tissue, scattered through the economy, is formed of a reticular connective tissue, the meshes of which are filled by lymphatic cells (His); and it is sometimes necessary to brush out the lymphatic cells, in order to show the delicate reticulum. We find, however, in leucocythæmia, such exuberant growth of this adenoid tissue that it not only multiplies in the organs where it is normally present (hypergenesis)—such as the spleen, the lymphatic glands, and the bone-marrow—but the more serious matter is, that it appears somewhat like a malignant growth in organs which are normally free from it (heterotopy), such as the liver and kidney, serous membranes, etc. These lymphoid growths have been called lymphadenomata (Virchow), whence the name of *lymphadénie*, given by Ranvier to the morbid process.

In some cases this overgrowth of adenoid tissue, or lymphadenia, invades the organs, especially the lymphatic glands and the spleen (Barfils, 1856; Cossy, 1861), without a corresponding increase of the leucocytes in the blood. Accordingly, when the question was not clearly understood, authorities attempted to separate these cases of leucocythæmia, and described them under the name of **adénie** (Trousseau), or **pseudoleukæmia.** Jaccoud rendered good service by proving the unity of lymphadenia, but the terms of "leukæmic" and "aleukæmic" lymphadenia have not the former signification, since the question of leucocythæmia has been recast.

When we see a patient with enlarged glands, with or without an enlarged spleen, the question is not solely to know to what extent the white corpuscles have increased in the blood ; we must also learn what varieties are present. In short, from a more exact knowledge of the morphology of the white corpuscles, physicians have recognized that they occur in very different forms, and we know that in leucocythæmia the morphological changes in the blood are certainly as important as the numerical ones. It is the quality of the leucocytes and not the quantity alone which matters.

At the present moment, however, we look upon leucocythæmia as only the reaction of the organism which shows itself by the changes in the blood and by the lesions in the hæmatopoietic organs, with symptoms dependent to these lesions. We know perfectly well that this reaction of the organism is not always the same, but it is as yet impossible to say whether the lesions and symptoms correspond to a single disease or belong to different maladies.

Ætiology.—The causes of leucocythæmia are unknown. It is more frequent in men than in women, and develops chiefly in the middle period of life. Splenic lymphadenia in **nurslings** has, however, been described (Jaksch, Luzet). In the patient's previous history we find malaria, typhoid fever, syphilis, and alcoholism ; but this so-called ætiology is subject to variations. Privation, grief, and repeated pregnancies appear to play some part, and in some cases the onset of the affection seems to date from an injury in the left hypochondrium, from a chill, a local lesion, an osteomyelitis following on amputation, or from chronic otorrhœa (Virchow). " Possibly we may be right in suspecting in these facts the forgotten existence of some mucous or cutaneous irritation, giving rise to primary adenopathy which precedes the outburst of the general disease " (Trousseau). There is, however, no proof on this point.

For some years past the infective origin of leucocythæmia has been suggested by many authors (Bard, Delbet), but contagion has not been proved in any case, and experimental reproduction in animals has failed (Gilbert and Cadiat). As regards the infective nature of the disease, the multiplicity of the organisms suspected shows that it is not a specific affection, but at most a commonplace process of secondary infection.

Pathological Anatomy.—Let us consider (1) the changes of the blood ; (2) the changes in the tissues and organs.

1. Changes in the Blood.—The blood in leucocythæmia presents alterations appreciable to the naked eye only when there is considerable increase in the white corpuscles. In such a case the blood is almost colourless, and its shade is sometimes like that of pus. Leukæmic blood, defibrinated and placed in a test-tube, separates into three layers : the lowest is formed of red blood-corpuscles ; the white corpuscles form the intermediary layer ; and the serum floats above. The clots produced by bleeding, and those removed from the cadaver, are separated into two layers—a lower red and an upper greyish one.

From this point of view we must consider two chief forms of leucocythæmia : the one is lymphocythæmia—in this case the lymphocytes of the blood are similar to those of the lymphoid tissue of the glands ; the other is myelocythæmia, and in this case the cells resemble those found in the bone-marrow.

Lymphocythœmia.—The number of lymphocytes may reach 600,000 per cubic millimetre ; the increase is, however, far less in most cases. To this variety belong cases in which the number of leucocytes is but little increased or practically normal (Jolly, Vaquez). The increase chiefly affects the lymphocytes, which may then reach as high as 90 per cent.

Myelocythœmia.—This variety of leucocythæmia includes most of the cases in which the number of leucocytes is considerably increased. They may exceed the total of 600,000. Instead of 1 leucocyte to 600 red corpuscles (normal condition), the relative proportion may be 1 to 20, 1 to 10, 1 to 9, and even be 1 to 1. All the varieties of white cells found in normal blood are represented in variable proportions in this variety of leucocythæmia. The special point is the appearance of large numbers of cells not present in normal blood, including rounded cells, with a large, rounded, oval, or slightly-curved nucleus. These cells in their general appearance resemble the large mononuclear cells of normal blood, but their protoplasm, instead of being clear, is filled either with fine granulations (" neutrophiles ") or with large refractile granulations (" eosinophiles "). We may also find cells in which the protoplasmic granulations stain with " basic " dyes, such as thionin and methyl violet, and answer to the " mastzellen " of Erhlich.

The nucleus of the myelocytes appears diffuse in the usual preparations ; these cells were therefore looked upon as degenerate or dead elements. Such is not the case, and Jolly has shown that the myelocytes and the lymphocytes are living and mobile cells. Relying on these facts, Ehrlich has tried to maintain that, in the different varieties of leukæmia, the various species of leucocytes come from the hæmatopoietic organs of the blood by diapedesis.

In some cases the large mononuclear cells (myelocytes) predominate in the blood, and the polynuclear cells are the exception.

These cases have sometimes been classed under the term of **splenic leukæmia,** or wrongly confounded with lymphatic leukæmia. In reality they belong to **myelocythæmia.** In myelocythæmia, as in lymphocythæmia, the red corpuscles are less numerous, and their colour-index is lowered. Lastly, this anæmia is often accompanied by the presence of nucleated red cells.

Chemical Examination.—Chemical analyses of the blood in leukæmia show the presence of glutin, hypoxanthin, leucin, and tyrosin. The peculiar crystals described by Charcot in the blood of anæmic patients are probably due to the latter substance or to some closely allied substance. These crystals, known by the name of Charcot-Leyden crystals, are only found in the blood after death.

2. **Lesions of the Connective Tissue and of the Organs.**—These lesions consist in the hypertrophy of the lymphoid tissue in the places where it exists normally, and in the formation of lymphoid tissue which is not present in health. Lymphoid or adenoid tissue is the tissue of the lymphatic glands. It is formed by a reticular connective tissue, the meshes of which are filled with lymphatic cells. "Capillaries run through this reticular tissue, being themselves surrounded by a condensed layer, from which the fibrillæ of the reticulum take their origin" (Cornil and Ranvier).

In leucocythæmia the normal adenoid tissue may be hypertrophied in every organ.

The **lymphatic glands** of the neck, axilla, groin, mesentery, and of the bronchi are often invaded, and form tumours as large as a hazel-nut, a walnut, or an egg. They may form considerable masses in such regions as the neck and the axilla.

In some cases, even apart from any scrofular or tubercular ætiology, the glands may become caseous. The predominance of the lesion in the lymphatic glands has led to the admission of a variety of lymphadenia known as the glandular form.

The spleen may weigh over four pounds, but is not altered in shape; it is hard, its capsule is thickened and often adherent to the peritoneum, and, on section, we see the corpuscles of Malpighi, which are whitish and sometimes as large as a lentil, clearly marked against the red ground. The lesions are similar to those in the lymphatic glands.

The **intestinal mucosa** is frequently affected. Three chief lesions may be present (Gilly): Folliculo-hypertrophic form, which develops at the expense of closed follicles and Peyer's patches, but, so to say, never leads to ulceration; diffuse hyperplastic and neoplastic forms, which originate in the submucous adenoid layer and ulcerate very rapidly. The neoplastic form is chiefly found in the lower part of the ileum, without narrowing of the lumen of the bowel; it is nearly always aleukæmic.

The tonsils, the closed follicles of the tongue, the thyroid body, and the bone-marrow participate in the increase of lymphoid tissue. The atrophied thymus sometimes regains its ordinary size.

When the liver is affected, the hypertrophy involves the whole of the organ, and its area of dullness blends with that of the spleen. The capillaries are dilated with blood crammed with white cells. A true apoplexy of leucocytes may be seen. New formations are not found.

In the connective tissue of the portal spaces we find a neo-formation of lymphoid tissue. Strictly speaking, this lymphoid tissue most often consists in an infiltration of the connective tissue by cells, like those of the glands, although this connective tissue may assume the appearance of true reticular tissue. It is also found in the lymphomata of the cortical substance of the kidney. The bone-marrow is sometimes converted into lymphoid tissue. Finally, we may find it in the skin and in regions where it is not present normally.

The accumulation of white blood-corpuscles in the vessels explains the hæmorrhages which may take place in the liver, kidney, brain, retina, meninges, nasal mucous membrane, gums, internal ear, or in the skin (purpura). In the intestine ulceration of the lymphoid tumours also gives rise to hæmorrhage.

I have just described in general terms the various lesions of leucocythæmia, but for some years past physicians have noticed the production of certain lymphoid growths, which differ somewhat in structure from that of the lymphatic glands. They form leukæmic tumours, which are especially frequent in the liver and spleen, and which are composed of cells larger than lymphocytes. These cells have a large round nucleus, and their protoplasm often contains granulations, like those in the cells of the bone-marrow. Under these conditions the tissue is not, properly speaking, lymphoid, but rather myeloid.

It has furthermore been noticed that these growths of myeloid tissue are allied to the hæmatological forms which we have learnt to know under the name of " myelocythæmia." These facts, joined to our knowledge of the morphology of the blood and of the structure of the bone-marrow, contribute to new ideas as regards the pathological physiology of leucocythæmia.

If myelocythæmia and lymphocythæmia do not exactly correspond to distinct clinical types, they yet form special anatomical types, in which the lesions of the blood are different. In lymphocythæmia the lymphocytes of the blood come from the glands and from the new lymphatic tissue, formed at various points, and even in the bone-marrow. In myelocythæmia the leucocytes—or, at any rate, the majority of them—come from the hyperplastic bone-marrow and from the newly-formed myeloid tissue in various organs, but especially in the spleen.

Such is the new conception of leucocythæmia. According to Ehrlich, the masses and the myeloid tumours are formed by metastasis ; the bone-marrow sends to the spleen its own cells, which are grafted there (heterotopy), in this point resembling malignant tumours. According to Dominici, the process depends, not upon metastases, but on the revival of a myeloid tissue which existed in the organ during the fœtal state.

In the cases which we have just examined the formation of the new lymphoid and myeloid tissue is accompanied by important changes in the blood. These changes, however, appear to be non-existent in some cases which answer to the names of adenia, aleukæmic lymphadenia, pseudo-leukæmia, Hodgkin's disease, etc. It is practically certain that these descriptions have been applied in error to varieties distinct from leucocy-thæmia. According to Jolly, these varieties are as follows : " (1) Chronic adenitis, with or without polynuclear leucocytosis, adenopathies of undeter-mined nature, infective and especially tubercular ; (2) glandular tumours, primary or secondary, and running their course with or without polynuclear leucocytosis ; (3) true cases of lymphocythæmia, in which the absolute number of white corpuscles is not increased, or increased only to a slight extent ; (4) cases of cutaneous lymphadenia and of mycosis fungoides which belong to the category of lymphocythæmia ; (5) lymphadenic lesions analo-gous to those of lymphocythæmia, without other change in the blood except a polynuclear leucocytosis. Certain facts tend to show, moreover, that these cases may represent only a passing stage in the evolution of lympho-cythæmia."

Often, too, we include wrongly in the category of lymphadenia various kinds of splenomegalia without blood changes.

As regards the infantile pseudo-leukæmic anæmia of Jaksch and Luzet, we do not know whether it is an infantile form of leukæmia or an anæmia due to different varieties of hypertrophy of the spleen with leucocytosis.

Symptoms.—The onset of leucocythæmia is often insidious. The patient suffers from increasing feebleness, fatigue, pallor, and breathlessness. In some cases no enlargement of the glands is as yet visible externally, the spleen is not increased in size, and yet, if the blood is examined, diminution of the red cells and considerable increase in the leucocytes or lymphocytes will be found. In some circumstances the contrary obtains. One or several lymphatic glands undergo an enlargement which appears at first immaterial, but the hypertrophy soon becomes general, although the blood does not show any excess of leucocytes.

In glandular leukæmia the hypertrophied lymphatic glands are painless and distinct from one another. In the lateral regions of the neck they form by their agglomeration enormous tumours, on which the head seems to rest. When the chain of the tracheal and bronchial glands is invaded, we may note the onset of compression symptoms, such as dyspnœa, spasm of the glottis, tubular breathing, stridor, dysphagia, and œdema of the face and arms, described under Mediastinal Tumours. The lymphatic tumours of the axilla and of the groin hamper the movements of the arms and legs. The hyper-trophy of the mesenteric glands causes compression of the veins, ascites, and œdema of the legs. The glandular tumours of lymphadenia have no ten-dency to become inflamed and to suppurate.

In splenic leukæmia the **spleen** finally attains a considerable size. It causes an enormous projection in the abdomen. It may participate alone in the process, or else the process may affect both the spleen and the glands.

The general symptoms become more marked as the disease progresses: the feebleness increases, the appetite is lost, and anæmic murmurs are heard in the heart and in the vessels. The patient complains of headache, vertigo, nausea, visual troubles (leukæmic retinitis), and dysphagia (ulcerative, leukæmic pharyngitis); he is liable to hæmorrhage, epistaxis, purpura, and bleeding from the gums.

The wasting of the face and of the limbs contrasts with the mass of the glandular tumours and with the abnormal size of the abdomen. After a duration which varies from some months to two years the period of cachexia commences, the tendency to hæmorrhage becomes far more marked, the œdema becomes general, the diarrhœa is continuous, the wasting progresses, the hands are the seat of erythematous eruptions, and fever often appears.

The patient is carried off by the incessant progress of the cachexia or by some intercurrent trouble, excessive enlargement of the bronchial glands or cerebral hæmorrhage, which may supervene long before the period of cachexia.

Acute Leucocythæmia.—The first cases were reported by Ebstein in 1889. Since that time numerous researches have been published. At the last Congress of Internal Medicine in Berlin Fraenkel and other authors brought forward cases which established the existence of super-acute leucocythæmia, and they called it **acute leukæmia or lymphocythæmia,** for the very reason that it is characterized, as regards hæmatology, by the superabundance of lymphocytes or small mononuclear cells. Their almost exclusive presence in the blood makes the prognosis grave and the rapid course of the disease foreseen.

This variety of leukæmia is perhaps not yet established with certainty. I have, however, been able to verify its extreme gravity in one of my cases.

The patient was admitted to hospital in a condition of advanced cachexia. His colour resembled that of a patient with cancer: earthy pallor, colourless mucous membranes, œdema of the legs and purpura. He experienced no suffering, but complained of great weakness. His health had always been excellent, and in his past history we found no disease worthy of note. The present condition was of a few weeks' duration.

On examination we found an enormous tumour in the belly. This swelling was hard and painless, and deformed the left flank and hypochondrium. It descended almost to the umbilicus, and was wedged above under the ribs, where the dullness reached as high as the fifth intercostal space.

The diagnosis of an enlarged spleen was evident, but the nature of the lesion remained to be proved. There could be no question of malaria, because the patient had never suffered from that disease. Hydatid cyst of the spleen was also eliminated, because it never causes such marked cachexia in a few weeks. If a patient is cachectic, with an enlarged spleen and glandular tumours in the neck, the groin, or in the axilla, we must first think of leucocythæmia; but this patient had no apparent hypertrophy of the glands.

And yet this was not a reason for abandoning the diagnosis of leucocythæmic spleen, because splenic lymphadenia may exist without obvious enlargement of the glands.

In order to decide the question, Apert examined the blood, and the diagnosis of an enlarged leucocythæmic spleen was confirmed. The patient had 50,000 white corpuscles to 1,900,000 red ones—*i.e.*, a proportion of 1 to 40, instead of 1 to 60, as in the normal condition.

In leucocythæmia, however, it is not sufficient to find a considerable excess of the white corpuscles; we must also know to which variety they belong. Preparations of the blood showed that the leukæmia was in this case due to small mononuclear leucocytes. It was therefore a case of lymphocythæmia.

Fig. 95 shows a film dried and stained with eosin and methylene blue. We see numbers of small leucocytes, stained blue and smaller than the red corpuscles, as well as two large mononuclear leucocytes and a polynuclear leucocyte.

A fortnight after the patient came under my care the number of lymphocytes increased from 50,000 to 90,000, and the proportion of the lymphocytes to the red corpuscles varied between 1 to 40 and 1 to 20. The glands of the neck, which were scarcely perceptible on the patient's admission, formed, in a fortnight, swellings similar to a bag of nuts. A little later the axillary glands hypertrophied, and we also found

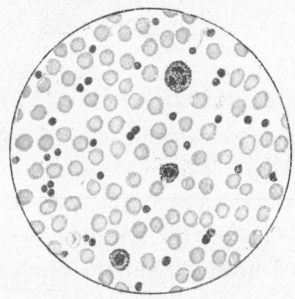

Fig. 95.

glands (where they are not found normally) in a continuous chain along the inner edge of the biceps. A hard, subcutaneous nodule appeared on the anterior surface of the right thigh. It was adherent to the skin, and was rightly considered to be a cutaneous lymphoma. At the same time the spleen became more enlarged, the strength diminished progressively, the cachexia increased, and the patient finally died five weeks after his admission. A few days before death the lymphocytes had reached 150,000, and their relation to the red corpuscles was an 1 to 10.

The autopsy showed the lesions of leucocythæmia. The spleen was enormous. It weighed nearly 5 pounds instead of 6 ounces. It had therefore increased in size tenfold. The hypertrophy affected all its diameters. The length was 10 inches instead of 5 inches, the breadth was doubled, being 6 inches instead of 3 inches, and the thickness was trebled, being $3\frac{1}{2}$ inches instead of $1\frac{1}{4}$ inches.

In spite of this marked hypertrophy, the organ had preserved its normal shape, although the upper end was curved inwards, forming a kind of hook, with its concavity internal and below. It seemed to have been hindered in its growth by the resistance of the diaphragm, and consequently it had continued to grow towards the middle line; while the rest of the organ, finding only the viscera, which were easily displaced, grew *in situ*, and without modification of its general shape. On longitudinal section of the organ the parenchyma appeared normal. It was of violet colour, with some whitish streaks; it was perhaps a little more firm than usual, but really differed from the normal appearance only to a slight extent. The only abnormal condition in the spleen, apart from its size, was the marked thickening of the capsule, which was whitish, hard, and bound down to the neighbouring organs by fibrous adhesions.

Besides this enormous spleen, we found everywhere enlarged glands : the mesenteric glands, the glands of the hilum, of the liver, and of the spleen. The prevertebral and the mediastinal glands formed large masses. Some of the glands were as large as an apple, being white and firm on section, while others showed, in their centre, violet spots, due to interstitial hæmorrhage. The viscera, liver, kidneys, lungs, and heart presented nothing worthy of note ; the follicles of the intestine and the tonsils were not hypertrophied. It was important to take count of the lesions of the bone-marrow, where changes are usual in leucocythæmia. The right humerus was sawn through at two different levels, and a tube of marrow extracted. It had lost its usual fatty appearance, and presented the same aspect as the substance of the glands, with violet spots in the middle of a dull white parenchyma.

Histological examination of the diseased organs showed a very interesting peculiarity. In the histological sections made by Apert, we found lymphocytes almost exclusively— not only in the glands, where the lymphocyte is the normal white corpuscle, but also in the pulp of the spleen and in the bone-marrow, where the lymphocytes, by reason of their abundance, masked the polymorphous cells, which are normally the most numerous. As in cancer, whatever the situation in which the secondary growths are formed, we always find the same kind of cell. So here, whatever organs are infected by the lymphoid infiltration, the lesions, both in the organs and in the blood, are characterized by the presence of lymphocythæmia. This resemblance to cancer has led writers to call leucocythæmia cancer of the blood.

Such, then, are the anatomical and clinical varieties of leucocythæmia. We cannot say whether acute leucocythæmia is only a clinical variety or a distinct disease, but it is certain that the increase in number of the white blood-corpuscles chiefly concerns the lymphocytes. The symptom-complex resembles that of chronic leukæmia, but the rapid course, sometimes accompanied by fever, gives the disease a special appearance.

Death is the constant end of acute and of chronic leukæmia ; the acute form lasts only a few weeks, the chronic form some months or years. The streptococcus appear to be fatal in leukæmic patients.

Diagnosis.—The diagnosis of leucocythæmia is often difficult, and sometimes the disease remains undiscovered. Accordingly, we must always examine the blood in patients with enlargement of the spleen, of the liver, or of the lymphatic glands, as well as in patients suffering from purpura, and in any case of abnormal leukæmia, or of cachexia of unknown origin.

Examination of the blood will remove all doubt, and will prevent confusion between leukæmia and other leucocytoses. Physicians, however, have recently discovered in the leucocytosis of variola a type which recalls in an attenuated manner the changes of the blood in myelocythæmia. This fact is a link between the leucocytoses and leucocythæmia.

The diagnosis is sometimes difficult in patients who have chains of enlarged glands, without specific changes in the blood and without myelocythæmia or lymphocythæmia. In such a case we must think of adenitis, due to tuberculosis, cancer, syphilis, etc. We must bear in mind malignant lymphadenoma if we find chronic adenopathy which runs a progressive course, especially if it commence in the cervical region.

Treatment.—No benefit has resulted from surgical measures, such as removal of the spleen and of the glandular tumours. It is therefore preferable to abstain from operations of this nature in patients suffering from leukæmia. There is no medical treatment for the disease.

Extracts of spleen tissue and of bone-marrow, preparations of arsenic, and injections of cacodylate of soda have produced some transient improvement.

V. CHLOROSIS—CHLORO-BRIGHTISM.

Chlorosis and anæmia should not be included in a single description, because the two terms are not synonymous. Anæmia is only a symptom of many and complex origins and varieties. It is caused by hæmorrhage, by various losses undergone by the organism, and by many infectious or chronic diseases. The study of anæmia, or, rather, the study of the anæmias, is, therefore, a question of semeiology, and cannot find a place here. Chlorosis, on the other hand, is a more definite morbid entity, being related, on the one hand, to the anæmias, and, on the other, to the neuroses ; not that the dyscrasic and nervous elements are forcibly subordinated one to the other, but their association and their origin give rise to a morbid type which has its own autonomy.

Ætiology.—Chlorosis owes its name to the colour of the skin. It is seen in young girls about the age of puberty (*cachexia virginum*), and its appearance seems to be intimately bound up with the evolution of the genital organs. It exists, however, before puberty—doubtless when the physical growth of the child is not in relation with its means of repair (Sée). Chlorosis may be present in young boys, just as hysteria, though a disease special to the female, is seen in men.

Heredity plays an important part in the development of chlorosis, and as occasional causes we may mention menstrual troubles, disturbances of the nervous system, emotion, grief, weakness, and dwellings which are dark and wanting in sunlight.

Pathogenesis—Pathological Anatomy. — The pathogenesis and the pathological anatomy of chlorosis have for some years been the subject of numerous researches, and it has been asked whether the blood-changes seen in chlorotic patients do not suffice to differentiate chlorosis from the anæmias.

The number of red corpuscles in chlorotic blood shows nothing characteristic, as it is normal, increased, or decreased, according to the case.

The exaggerated size of the red corpuscle has no importance, for in every anæmia the disturbance occasioned in the formation and development of the cells gives rise to abnormal forms of red corpuscles, which recall more or less clearly the fœtal condition of the elements.

Is it, then, the composition of the blood or the diminution of the hæmoglobin which produces a change special to chlorosis ? This change in the hæmoglobin is not absolutely special to chlorosis, since it exists in other anæmias, and especially in the anæmia of cancer (Hayem). The nature of the changes in the blood cannot, therefore, establish a distinction between the anæmias and chlorosis. The diminution of the hæmoglobin in chlorotic patients is, no doubt, an important element of which we must take count, but it is the symptom-complex, and especially the ætiology of the affection, which gives to chlorosis its distinctive place. The opinion, formerly expressed by Sée, that the distinguishing-point between chlorosis and the anæmias is its origin, has thus been realized.

The lesions in the blood are not the only ones seen in chlorosis. We owe our knowledge of the cardio-vascular and genital lesions to the works of Rokitansky, Bamberger, and especially of Virchow. These changes have allowed the German school to enunciate an organic theory of chlorosis.

The most frequent anomaly is a want of development in the vascular system.

The aorta is sometimes so narrowed that its lumen scarcely admits the little finger ; its calibre is only as large as the carotid or the iliac artery. The coats are thinned and the vessel allows itself to be stretched like india-rubber. The intercostal and the lumbar arteries arise in an asymmetrical fashion from the descending aorta. The internal coat is studied with reticulated blotches ; it often shows fatty degeneration which is quite superficial, in contradistinction to the lesions of atheroma.

The malformations of the heart are variable in chlorosis. The organ is sometimes remarkably small, or, at other times, larger than normal. According to Virchow, who bases his opinion on a large number of autopsies, the heart in chlorosis is originally small, and remains so in case of permanent oligæmia. If the volume of blood become too large, the heart becomes hypertrophied and dilated, because it has to struggle against the narrowing of the aorta.

Changes of the genital organs are relatively frequent in chlorosis. These organs are sometimes hypertrophied, but more often atrophied. The infantile character of the uterus and of the ovaries is frequently mentioned in Virchow's cases. This author considers the genital anomalies as secondary and the vascular hypoplasia as the primary lesion causing chlorosis.

If these lesions, though rarely seen in France, are frequently noted in the protocol of German autopsies, we must remember that in Germany, without troubling about the symptoms present during life, they apply the name *aortis chloroticæ* to any aorta which is small and pale and which shows abnormal origin of its branches.

Moreover, this theory of chlorosis is applicable only to some cases, and has been invalidated by other autopsies, so that it merely deserves to be retained as an exception.

Description.—The chlorotic woman is, as a rule, not wasted ; her face and hands have a sallow and yellowish look, like old wax, while a greenish colour is sometimes added. The lips and the conjunctivæ are bloodless and pale, the look is sad and languid, the conjunctiva is bluish, the face is puffy, and the eyelids are sometimes œdematous. This œdema, which is not solely of anæmic origin, is also seen in the legs and feet. The cheeks sometimes assume a sudden and passing redness, which in some cases may be very marked (*chlorosis fortiorum*).

The **nervous troubles** somewhat resemble those of hysteria. The chlorotic patient is melancholy, irritable, and strange ; she complains of headache, vertigo, fainting, insomnia, disturbed dreams, and facial or intercostal neuralgia. She is always tired, and often feels ready to drop ; her respiration rate is increased ; and palpitation is brought on by the least exercise or by the slighest emotion. The palpitation is sometimes violent, and comes on in the form of attacks. Epistaxis, hæmoptysis, and metrorrhagia may be present. Anæsthesia and hyperæsthesia are both seen. The muscular weakness may end in paralysis.

In the chlorotic woman the appetite is sometimes exaggerated (boulimia) or at other times suppressed (anorexia) ; it is often depraved (pica, malacia). Dyspeptic troubles, such as flatulence, gastralgia, pyrosis, vomiting, distension of the abdomen, and constipation, are sometimes associated with this perversion of the appetite.

Hypopepsia, hyperpepsia, and hyperchlorhydria have also been noted (Hayem).

Functional troubles of the **genital organs** are constant. It has been asked whether they are the cause or the effect of the chlorotic state. Amenorrhœa and dysmenorrhœa are common, but menorrhagia is more rare (Trousseau). Leucorrhœa is very frequent, and the menstrual blood is serous and colourless. Chlorosis does not necessarily cause sterility, and pregnancy sometimes has a beneficial influence.

The **urine** is pale, poor in urea and phosphates, and contains urohæmatin.

The examination of a chlorotic patient gives the following results : On auscultation we often find a systolic murmur, situated at the aortic, at the tricuspid orifice, and at the other orifices. If the finger is lightly placed over the great vessels in the neck, above the clavicle, the " **frémissement cataire** " may be felt, and auscultation of these vessels, especially on the right side, reveals an intermittent, systolic murmur of arterial origin and a continuous murmur of a venous origin, which is more or less musical in tone, and has been compared to the purring of a cat, to the sound of a spinning-wheel or of a humming-top (*diable*), whence the term *bruit de diable* given by Bouillaud.

These murmurs are not confined to chlorosis, and have not the diagnostic significance formerly attributed to them. The intermittent arterial murmur is explained, but the explanation of the continuous murmur is more difficult. Writers have suggested the vibrations of the walls of the vessel, the spasmodic condition of the walls, and the vibrations of the valves in the veins (Chauveau). The veins of the neck sometimes show pulsation. Hypertrophy of the thyroid body is also found in some cases, in addition to the cardio-vascular troubles (Hayem).

The temperature may be normal or lowered. In some cases a notable elevation of the central temperature has been observed (*febris alba virginum*).

Examination of the blood, which only requires a prick of the finger, serves to complete the clinical picture in chlorosis. The blood, though very fluid, coagulates normally, because the fibrin is present in the proper quantity. The blood-serum appears chemically normal, and yet it must exercise a deleterious globulicidal action on the red blood-corpuscles.

The number of red corpuscles is not much diminished, and it is rare to find the count below 3,000,000—indeed, the number may be almost normal. The important and characteristic lesion of the blood concerns the hæmoglobin. The size of the red corpuscles is very variable. In the normal condition the diameter is about 7 μ, but in the chlorotic patient a number of dwarf corpuscles with a diameter of from 3 to 4 μ are seen, as well as giant cells with a diameter of from 12 to 14 μ.

The normal corpuscle is discoid. In the chlorotic patient we find the most varied forms, especially among the dwarf corpuscles, which may be fusiform or piriform or racquet-shaped. These changes in shape are due to the morbid contractility of the protoplasm.

The red blood-corpuscles are much paler than normal, because they contain less hæmoglobin. We know that the red corpuscle is composed of a stroma or of a felting called globulin, and of a colouring matter rich in iron and essential to the respiratory function. This colouring matter, which impregnates the globulin and is of an albuminoid nature, is called hæmoglobin. The globulin is normal in the chlorotic patient, but the hæmoglobin is altered : the individual red corpuscle is diseased, its hæmoglobin is diminished, and the saturation of the blood with oxygen is notably lowered. The researches of Duncan and Mantegazza, as well as more recent studies (Hayem, Quinquaud, Malassez), have elucidated these changes.

The change of colour in the chlorotic woman is so great that the blood, which normally contains 12 to 15 grammes of hæmoglobin per 100 c.c., contains only 5 to 8 grammes, and as the number of red blood-corpuscles is often very slightly diminished the **colour-index**—that is to say, the quantity of hæmoglobin contained in a single corpuscle—is always very low ; it may fall to 18 or 20 grammes, as compared with 28 to 30 grammes in the normal condition. This change explains the pale colour of the skin and of the mucous membranes, and perhaps has some bearing on the greenish tint seen by reflected light in women suffering from chlorosis, if we admit that their diluted hæmoglobin allows the **green rays** to pass. The loss of respiratory power in the corpuscle is in part responsible for the poverty of the organic combustion, for the feebleness of the muscular contractions, and for the respiratory troubles.

The hæmatoblasts, which must not be confounded with the dwarf corpuscles, are often increased in chlorosis (Hayem). They are considered by Hayem as elements destined to be changed into red blood-corpuscles, and are therefore charged with the function of renewing the blood. Most authors, however, reject this view. The signification of these elements is as yet unknown.

Course—Diagnosis—Treatment. — Chlorosis may develop suddenly (acute emotion, suppression of the menses) or slowly. The nervous symptoms sometimes **precede** those of anæmia, a proof that they are not subordinate to them. The duration of the disease is indefinite, and recovery takes place after a lapse of several months or of several years. Nevertheless, " it leaves an almost indelible impression, so that a young girl who has suffered from severe chlorosis feels the effects for almost the rest of her life, even though the blood has long since become normal, furnishing a further proof that chlorosis should be considered as a nervous disease, causing a change in the blood, rather than as a cachexia producing nervous disorders " (Trousseau).

The **prognosis** in chlorosis is not grave ; the possibility of Brightism, epistaxis, and metrorrhagia, to which some patients with chlorosis are subject, should, however, be taken into serious consideration.

Phlegmasia alba dolens is not a very rare complication. The phlebitis obliterans usually affects the veins of the legs, and disappears after lasting some weeks, but it may cause embolism, followed by death. Thrombosis of the sinuses (Bollinger) and of the pulmonary artery (Rendu) have several times been noted.

Certain authors consider chlorosis as being favourable to pulmonary phthisis. Although this assertion may be true in some cases, there is still a source of error which must be avoided. Tuberculosis at its onset may simulate chlorosis, and is the **false chlorosis** on which Trousseau has dwelt at length. The diagnosis is not always easy, but the following considerations,

in the absence of Koch's bacilli, will aid in the diagnosis : " When phthisis
assumes the appearance of chloro-anæmia, we can put the matter in a nut-
shell.   There is a general dystrophy, while true chloro-anæmia principally,
and perhaps solely, affects the blood.   On comparing phthisis and chlorosis
from the only common point of view—that is to say, from the change in
the blood and from the phenomena which result—we can assure ourselves
of their predominance in primary chloro-anæmia and of their less signification
in organic anæmia : (1) The vascular murmurs, which are so marked and so
characteristic of the diminution in the number of corpuscles, are almost
always absent in organic chlorosis ; (2) the cardiac murmur at the arterial
and auriculo-ventricular orifices are never present in the anæmia of phthisis
as a true murmur : there is rather an exaggerated *bruit de claquement val-
vulaire* ; (3) the circulation is constantly quickened in tuberculosis with
anæmia, and the palpitation is permanent, whether it is or is not perceived
by the patient.   In the chlorotic patient, on the other hand, the circulation preserves its special type and rhythm ; (4) the dyspnœa in the
chlorotic patient occurs later, but is more complete because of the hypo-
globulia.

Here is the positive proof of the malnutrition, which at once strikes the
phthisical patient and spares the chlorotic one : (1) Muscular fatigue is early
and complete, hindering walking, especially up-hill.   Moreover, it is this
fatigue, due to the malnutrition, which produces dyspnœa, so that the
phthisical patient at length cannot make the least movement without
breathlessness.   (2) The skin, instead of being colourless and pale (on
account of the diminution in the hæmoglobin), presents, in the phthisical
patient, a dull greyish tint, as in cachexia.   (3) The menstruation, after
certain irregularities, is suppressed, although later than in chlorosis, but
then the menstrual troubles are totally and definitely compromised.
(4) Chlorosis is apyretic, or, rather, it never presents the same degree of fever
as does tuberculosis.   (5) Wasting appears from the first, while in chlorosis
the embonpoint is usually preserved.   In short, the condition of the muscles
and of the skin, the oxidation and the general nutrition, indicate an immediate
failing which, in the case of the chlorotic patient, affects only the blood
(Sée).

The disease, described under the name of **progressive pernicious
anæmia** (Biermer), does not appear to have, as yet, an indisputable nosological value.   It closely resembles chlorotic cachexia, and it may possibly
be an exceptionally grave chlorosis (Jaccoud).   The anæmic symptoms are
excessive : retinal hæmorrhages, epistaxis, petechiæ, and fever are seen ;
diarrhœa and œdema appear later.   The disease is not absolutely fatal, but
it is extremely grave.

Iron occupies the first place in the treatment of chlorosis.   It may be given in the form of pills or of syrup, but it should always be taken at meals. Syrup of iodide of iron and the syrup of the ammoniacal citrate are usually the best tolerated. The iron waters of Saint Moritz, Spa, etc., are useful. Preparations of iron must be continued for several weeks, and repeated at intervals. Inhalations of oxygen, hydrotherapy, and sea-baths are indicated in some cases. I cannot recommend too strongly preparations of arsenic, and especially injections of cacodylate of soda, as described in the Appendix. The chlorotic patient should live in the open air, where it is bright and sunny. Chlorosis often improves, and may be cured ; but it is, I repeat, subject to relapses.

Ovarian extract has been suggested in the treatment of chlorosis, but the number of cases is still too restricted to form any definite opinion as to this method, which, *a priori*, would appear to be useful.

Chloro-Brightism.

I shall discuss here the association and relations between chlorosis and Brightism which I pointed out in my communication to the Académie de Médecine.* I have given the name of **chloro-Brightism** to this association, to which my attention was called many years ago. In order to avoid misunderstanding, let me state the question clearly.

Under the denomination of " chloro-Brightism " I do not allude to patients in whom Brightism, especially when associated with syphilis, is accompanied by more or less marked anæmia. Chloro-Brightism, in my opinion, should be confined to patients, either women or girls, who show the symptoms, the attributes, and the mask of chlorosis, the characteristic tint of the face, the decoloration of the skin and of the mucous membranes, the varied uterine troubles, dysmenorrhœa, amenorrhœa, leucorrhœa, menorrhagia, breathlessness and palpitations, as well as dyspepsia with or without anorexia, cardiac and vascular murmurs, considerable diminution in the number of red blood-corpuscles, and more or less marked lowering of the colour-index.

I think that in this case there is no possible error as to the interpretation of the facts, and, whatever be the theoretical idea adopted as to the pathogenesis of chlorosis, we can affirm that every young woman presenting the above symptoms is either chlorotic or chloro-anæmic.

Many of these patients also suffer from Bright's disease. I shall attempt to show the truth of this opinion by applying these considerations to some forty cases, mostly taken from my clinique at the Necker Hospital and at the Hôtel-Dieu, but I shall first show by an example the nature of the association in chloro-Brightism.

* Dieulafoy, *Académie de Médecine*, Séance du 20 Juin, 1895.

A physician is called to see a girl from fifteen to twenty years of age, who has, for some time past, attracted the attention of her parents by symptoms of chloro-anæmia, and the following dialogue takes place between the mother and the physician :

"See, doctor, how pale and colourless the child is ! She looks like old wax ; and if you look at her hands, lips, and gums, you would say that she is bloodless."— "Certainly, madam, she has the appearance of chlorosis."—" She has not been regular for the past four months," continues the girl's mother, " but she suffered from a loss of blood several months ago, and since then the menses have not reappeared. However, she has leucorrhœa, which quite wears her out."—" Yes, madam, such is the case in chlorosis."—" And her appetite, doctor ! She eats nothing, and prefers only salad and acid food. Just see how she has wasted ! A trifle fatigues her. She cannot walk quickly, or go upstairs without experiencing breathlessness and palpitation of the heart."—" It is chlorosis."—" She has incessant headache, vertigo, and neuralgia." —" It is chlorosis."—" She was examined, and the doctor said that she has murmurs." —" It is chlorosis."—" The blood has been examined, and the number of the red blood-corpuscles was found to be diminished by half."—" It is chlorosis."—" Often, too, her eyes are puffy and her limbs are swollen."—" It is chlorosis."

And this dialogue, which recalls somewhat that between Toinette and Argan in the " Malade Imaginaire," ends with the following question on the part of the mother : " But, doctor, what treatment are you going to prescribe, in order to cure the chlorosis ?" —" Your daughter has need of underdone meat, strong soups, meat-juice, jellies, generous wines, extract of quinine, preparations of iron or of arsenic, and we shall succeed in overcoming the chlorosis."

Before the end of his reply the physician has, however, been interrupted. " It is no use to advise that diet, because it has been prescribed ten times already, and each time it has had to be abandoned. My daughter gets worse as soon as she commences it."

The treatment, indeed, had been of no use, and had been badly borne, because the patient in question was suffering from chloro-Brightism. If we make careful inquiry as to Brightism, we shall find that for several months she has been compelled to get up two or three times at night to pass water, has cramp in the calves and in the legs, sensation of dead fingers, and experiences electric shocks on lying down. The cryæsthesia is of long duration, and she cannot keep her legs and feet warm ; she has slight morning epistaxis ; the urine is of feeble toxicity, and sometimes shows a cloud of albumin. In short, the girl is suffering both from chlorosis and Brightism. The headache, set down to chloro-anæmia, may be due to Bright's disease ; the œdema of the eyelids, face, and legs, which has been put down to chloro-anæmia, is really due to the kidney mischief. Brightism is the chief feature in this case.

My conclusions on chloro-Brightism are confirmed by the fact that, in thirty cases mentioned by me at the Académie, as well as in those which I have since collected at the Hôtel-Dieu, I found chloro-Brightism in all its forms, often without albuminuria, but sometimes with it—chloro-Brightism against which the tonic and strengthening treatment of simple chlorosis completely fails and in which milk diet nearly always succeeds. For it is a fact worthy of remark that most of these women and girls suffering from chloro-Brightism, in which the symptoms are aggravated by a meat diet, improve rapidly, and in some cases completely, under the influence of a milk régime.

As a result of this diet the colour returns, the red blood-corpuscles increase in number, the colour-index rises, the œdema disappears, the breathlessness and the palpitation diminish in severity, the strength comes back, and menstruation is re-established. I therefore feel convinced that, of the two factors which enter in the association of chloro-Brightism, the greater part is often played by the Brightism.

At the Hôtel-Dieu I had an opportunity of giving a lecture on a case of chloro-Brightism, and I give here the résumé of it :

A woman, twenty-two years of age, came under my care for chlorosis. She was as pale as old wax, the gums and conjunctivæ were colourless, and the hands as white as ivory. She could scarcely walk up to the ward without feeling palpitation and such severe breathlessness that she was compelled to sink into an arm-chair. She complained of headache, palpitation of the heart, and continual oppression. The picture of chlorosis was completed by auscultation of the vessels of the neck, revealing *bruit de diable* and *frémissement cataire*. And yet the case was clearly one of **chloro-Brightism** and not of pure chlorosis, by reason of the puffiness of the face, the œdema of the legs, the clearly marked sensation of dead fingers, the frequent epistaxis, the itching, the buzzing in the ears, the electric shocks, and the cramps in the calves.

This history was as follows : The breathlessness and palpitation had appeared before the age of fourteen, so that the patient could not play with her friends. She menstruated at fourteen, but she soon became pale. Amenorrhœa appeared, and lasted for some months. The chlorosis was treated most successfully for six years by tonics and strengthening medicines. At this time Brightism appeared with œdema of the face and legs. A physician found a marked quantity of albumin in the urine, and prescribed milk diet. As the result of this diet the improvement was so marked that the physician, in order to make it complete, considered it advisable to order a return to underdone or to raw meat, and so-called generous wines. The new diet, however, failed, the dyspnœa and the palpitation returned, and the patient felt herself becoming weaker daily. Then everybody gave her advice, and the paler and weaker she became the more was she compelled to take kola and coca wines, quinine with iron preparations and confection of Saint Vincent de Paul. The situation became worse, and the girl was admitted to the Hôtel-Dieu in the condition above described. I therefore prescribed milk diet, because the Brightism was of more importance than the chlorosis.

In about a week the colour began to come back to the skin, the dyspnœa improved, the headache disappeared, and the patient gained 4 pounds in weight. After a fortnight of milk diet the improvement was even more manifest. The patient suffered no longer from breathlessness or palpitation, and she took 6 pints of milk with bread. In a month she had put on 12 pounds, her strength had returned, and as she was considered cured, I allowed her to leave the hospital, on the understanding that she continued the milk diet for several months.

The following table, compiled by Jolly, shows clearly the progressive increase in the red corpuscles, in the hæmoglobin, and in the colour-index. This case forms an excellent demonstration of the importance of milk diet in chloro-Brightism.

March 23, before the milk diet	red corpuscles	..	..	..	.. 3,150,000
	hæmoglobin	..	..	..	.. 4·3
	colour-index	..	..	..	.. 13·6
April 3, milk diet	red corpuscles	..	..	..	.. 4,200,000
	hæmoglobin	..	..	..	.. 8
	colour-index	..	..	..	.. 19
April 15, milk diet	red corpuscles	..	..	..	.. 4,760,000
	hæmoglobin	..	..	..	.. 9
	colour-index	..	..	..	.. 18·9
April 28, milk diet	red corpuscles	..	..	..	.. 4,400,000
	hæmoglobin	..	..	..	.. 8·5
	colour-index	..	..	..	.. 19

It may be asked what becomes of these patients in the long run, and what future is reserved for them as regards the evolution of Bright's disease. Gubler, who had considered the matter, and had noted albuminuria in chlorotic patients, asked whether this condition, composed of chlorosis and of albuminuria, might not at some time end in Bright's disease.

I think I can answer both these questions. In the great majority of cases chloro-Brightism does not end in confirmed Bright's disease. The morbid condition only shows itself by the minor symptoms of Brightism with or without albuminuria. In some cases, however, as I have myself reported, chloro-Brightism finally ends in severe uræmia, and even in death.

A young girl had been under treatment for two months for chloro-anæmia. The symptoms of this so-called chlorosis increased, her sight became affected, and Galezowski found albuminuric retinitis. I also saw the patient and found uræmia, following the troubles of chlorosis and Bright's disease, which had run a slow course. Death was the result.

In consultation I saw a patient whose case has been reported by Hays. This young girl was attacked by fatal symptoms of uræmia, with multiple hæmorrhages. The disease in this case had begun about six years before with symptoms of chloro-Brightism ; the albuminuria did not appear until four years later.

These cases prove that chloro-Brightism, although benign in general, may in some cases result in uræmia and end fatally.

In a case of chloro-Brightism published by Hanot, a young girl was seized with uræmic convulsions, which yielded to bleeding and milk diet. Labadie-Lagrave's case deals with a young girl, who in the course of chloro-Brightism, was seized with an acute uræmia during influenza. The uræmia ended in recovery. A case of chloro-Brightism, reported by Boudet, ended fatally.

Pregnancy and Chloro-Brightism.—The relations between the puerperal condition and chloro-Brightism are highly important.

I had under my care a woman, twenty years of age, suffering from chloro-Brightism without albumin. She married shortly afterwards ; the pregnancy was uneventful ; there was no albuminuria, but three days after her confinement acute attacks of eclampsia supervened, with total anuria for twenty-four hours, and some days afterwards albuminuria. The patient recovered.

With Got, I saw a young woman who had had chloro-Brightism when a young girl. During her first pregnancy she suffered from albuminuria, and a miscarriage took place at the third month. During her second pregnancy she suffered from anasarca, and was prematurely confined at the seventh month.

The question of Brightism and pregnancy has been well put by Pinard. A woman suffering from Bright's disease may become pregnant, as occurs daily. While impregnation does not appear to be influenced by the renal lesion, it is quite otherwise as regards the pregnancy. We may say that every pregnancy in a woman with Bright's disease or with chloro-Brightism will be disturbed by the appearance of complications affecting the mother or the child.

In the Mother.—The complications will depend on the severity of the renal lesion on the one hand, and on the duration of the pregnancy on the other. Although they are more frequent and more serious in the later months of pregnancy, we must still remember that formidable complications may appear from the commencement of gestation.

With Pinard I saw a young woman suffering from Bright's disease, in whom complications showed themselves as early as the second month of the pregnancy, and were so severe that it was necessary to empty the uterus at the third month. Pinard performed the operation, which was completely successful. The young woman recovered, but the albuminuria did not disappear. Pinard has informed me of several similar cases.

In the Child.—Apart from cases in which therapeutic abortion is necessary, the development of the fœtus is hindered or interrupted by the appearance of placental lesions in women suffering from Bright's disease or from chloro-Brightism. This fact has been absolutely proved by the researches of Pinard and his pupils. Moir (*Edinburgh Medical Times*) in 1864, Simpson in 1874, and Chanteuil in 1879 (*Leçons Cliniques*), suspected the relations between the renal lesion in the mother and the placental lesion of the child; they were definitely established in 1885 by Pinard and Fehling.

The lesion is characterized by the appearance of hæmorrhages, which are converted into white infarcts. The primary lesion is hæmorrhagic in nature; the white infarct is secondary. Furthermore, it is always intraplacental and most often intracotyledonous. The number of foci is extremely variable; sometimes one cotyledon, or, at other times, the whole placenta may be invaded. The recent infarct containing fluid blood, or having a gelatinous consistency, is almost of a black colour, and clearly marked from the paler tint of the surrounding tissue. It resembles a truffle let into the cotyledon; hence the name of *placenta truffé*, given by Pinard to the placenta in cases of albuminuria. When the infarct is older, it becomes pale, the colouring matter of the blood disappears gradually, and the residue of the hæmorrhage presents a tint which is at first chocolate coloured, then reddish-yellow, and finally reaches the tint of the white infarct.

If the infarct is incised, it appears formed of fibrin more or less dense and homogeneous in appearance, and sometimes disposed in a series of concentric layers. In the centre we often find a small collection of more or less coloured fluid, forming the residue of the blood-serum. Nevertheless, it is not, properly speaking, a focus, but rather an infiltration. The size of these hæmorrhagic foci or infiltrations is also extremely variable ; they may vary from the size of a millet-seed to that of a pigeon's egg. The hæmorrhage in some cases may extend beyond the limits of the placenta, and give rise to retroplacental hæmorrhage (Pinard), which may prove fatal to the mother. It seems needless to add that in the same placenta we may find recent and old foci, and thus very easily follow the different degrees in the evolution of the placental hæmatoma described above.

In spite of the works of Wiedow (1887), Cohn, and especially of Rossier (Leipzig, 1888), the pathological histology of the albuminuric placenta has been hardly more than outlined. Are the intraplacental hæmorrhages related to the lesions of the vessels of the decidua, or to lesions of the fœtal vessels ? Rossier does not venture on any conclusion. Pinard says there is no doubt that the lesion is of maternal origin, and this opinion is supported by the recent histological studies of Schaeffer.

From what has gone before, it is easy to understand how and why the development of the fœtus may be interrupted in a woman suffering from Bright's disease or from chloro-Brightism. As soon as a focus occurs the field of hæmatosis is restricted. As the child lives solely upon the maternal blood, it is evident that anything which hinders the exchange of matter in the placenta diminishes the nourishment of the fœtus, and hence we find the wasted and spider-like fœtus (according to Pinard's expression). If the lesions become general, the fœtus dies of inanition, whence the frequent expulsion of a dead and macerated fœtus.

The recognition of these facts is of extreme importance from the point of view of diagnosis and of treatment.

As regards the diagnosis of Bright's disease, examination of the placenta is of the highest interest. Pinard possesses a number of records in which the placental lesion alone pointed the way to the diagnosis, the other symptoms of Brightism being unnoticed until the expulsion of the products of conception.

Numerous cases show that rigorous treatment during the whole duration of pregnancy will, in a more or less complete fashion, prevent the production of placental lesions in women suffering from Bright's disease and chlorosis, and in the same way prolong the life of the child to full term, or, at any rate, until it is viable. **It is superfluous to say that this treatment should be an absolute milk diet.**

In short, when examining a chlorotic patient we must always think of the possibility of Brightism, and look carefully for the " minor symptoms." We also have to decide the question of prognosis, especially as regards the pregnancy and the puerperium. A woman suffering from Bright's disease and chlorosis will be more liable to albuminuria gravidarum and to attacks of eclampsia.

Hygienic measures, preparations of iron and arsenic, or injections of cacodylate of soda, which have been advised in chlorosis, are also applicable in chloro-Brightism, but **in the latter case milk diet forms the basis of the treatment.**

The pathogenesis of chloro-Brightism may be interpreted in various ways. If I have personally abstained from hypotheses, I have done so because none of them are quite satisfactory. I have been content to observe the facts without proposing an explanation. Hanot has suggested the following theory : " In chlorosis the work of internal nutrition is disturbed, and the incompletely oxidized products of disassimilation accumulate in the organism, are eliminated by the kidneys, and may finally produce an epithelial nephritis. The noxious action is often facilitated by the coincidence of arterial aplasia in the kidneys, as has been noted by Lancereaux, and in this way the kidney becomes an organ of least resistance."

Chatin has attempted to verify the question of diminished oxidation in chlorosis. We should suppose, says he (if the theory previously presented be true), that the toxicity of the urine would become increased in the chlorotic patient by reason of the elimination of insufficiently oxidized products, and that this urinary toxicity would, on the other hand, fall below normal when once nephritis has declared itself—that is to say, in the case of chloro-Brightism. Experimental facts have not confirmed this hypothesis. The toxicity is always diminished in chlorosis, and this diminution of toxicity " does not appear due to a diminution in the causes of auto-intoxication. The state of latent renal insufficiency, which manifests itself by the slight signs of Brightism, may play a large part in the matter " (Chatin).

In short, whatever be the theory invoked, it is certain that chlorosis has a tendency to cause renal insufficiency. We may say of every chlorotic woman that her urinary depuration will become insufficient at some time or other. Chloro-Brightism is made up clinically of the symptoms of chlorosis, to which are added, at some time, the minor troubles of Brightism, with or without albuminuria. The albuminuria is not constant ; it may be transitory, and does not constitute an absolute sign as regards diagnosis, considering the possible dissociation of the morbid processes in the kidney, but its importance is of the first order.

Chlorosis may precede the appearance of Brightism by several months or even by several years. Chloro-Brightism rarely ends in severe uræmia. Every patient should, however, be under careful supervision, because she is threatened with uræmia. Any infectious disease, such as influenza, tonsillitis, pneumonia, syphilis, etc., may give rise to uræmia in these patients, and in their case pregnancy, deserves special attention. The therapeutic indications are merely formal, and **milk diet sums up the treatment.**

VI. PURPURA—SCURVY—INFANTILE SCURVY.

1. Purpura.

The word **purpura** (purple), taken in its truest sense, signifies " eruption of blood spots "—that is to say, hæmorrhage into the skin. The red and purple spots are of various sizes, and are situated in various regions. They are rounded, prominent, discrete, or confluent. More or less diffuse and extensive ecchymoses are often found, in addition to the petechiæ.

The purpuric spots differ from congestive spots, in that they do not fade on digital pressure or on distension of the skin. Histological examination shows that they are formed by an extravasation of red blood-corpuscles in the dermis and hypodermis. This extravasation may be the only lesion. We sometimes find enormous dilatation of the capillaries in the papillæ and in the dermis, with an accumulation of blood-corpuscles in their interior. The extravasated red blood-corpuscles show the same changes as the traumatic ecchymoses ; the hæmoglobin is converted into hæmatoidin, which becomes gradually reabsorbed. The tint of the petechiæ indicates this conversion. It changes from a reddish-violet to dark brown, faded green, greyish-green, and chamois-yellow; it disappears completely at the end of from six to ten days. Desquamation of the epidermis is often seen.

Such is a concise description of the cutaneous hæmorrhage called pur-pura. Purpura is called *simplex* when it is limited to the skin, but another idea is attached to this term purpura. It is that the patient suffering from this disease has a more or less marked predisposition to other hæmorrhages (nasal, buccal, intestinal hæmorrhages), and this idea is clearly formulated in the term *purpura hæmorrhagica*, which indicates the tendency of the disease to multiple hæmorrhages.

There is, however, no clearly defined line between *purpura simplex* and *purpura hæmorrhagica*. No one can say whether a case which begins with the symptoms of purpura simplex will not become one of purpura hæmor-rhagica.

The pathogenic processes put forward to explain purpura comprise fragile character of the capillaries, capillary embolisms, changes in the blood, and the action of toxi-infectious agents.

Purpura is sometimes present as a symptom in the course of various diseases ; at other times it becomes a morbid entity. Classifications are not lacking as regards the different varieties of purpura (Rayer), but I cannot reproduce them here, for it is rather a question of semeiology, and I shall content myself with enumerating the chief varieties of **symptomatic purpura,** relying on their apparent ætiology. I say "apparent," for many factors are often united in this rough-and-ready ætiology.

Purpura is frequent in the **infectious** diseases. It is at times limited to the skin in the form of petechiæ and ecchymoses, with or without exanthemata, and at other times it is the prelude of multiple hæmorrhages, which are of the worst augury.

In most of the **cachectic** conditions, such as Bright's disease and lymphadenia, purpura is not always limited to petechiæ on the skin. The purpura of **tuberculosis** deserves special mention. It is more frequent in acute tuberculosis than in chronic phthisis, and it also betrays itself by general hæmorrhages.

Purpura may supervene in **nervous troubles,** which vary exceedingly both in origin and nature. In some cases it is associated with lesions of the spinal cord: tabes, myelitis, or cancer of the spine. The purpuric spots are usually symmetrical, and accompanied by anæsthesia, hyperæsthesia, or by multiple and fugitive arthralgias.

Certain **drugs,** such as mercury, copaiba, belladonna, and iodine, give rise to eruptions of purpuric spots, preceded or accompanied by exanthematous eruptions. Purpura due to iodine almost always attacks the anterior surface of the limbs in the neighbourhood of the hair-follicles.

We must now consider two other varieties of purpura with fairly well-defined characters.

Exanthematic Purpura.—This term includes a group of cases in which purpura appears as a congestive exanthema of the skin (polymorphous, infective, or seasonal erythemata). Sometimes, also, this form of purpura is in reality an erythema rendered hæmorrhagic by the severity of the cutaneous congestion or by a special predisposition of the organism to hæmorrhage. This feature is evident when both eruptions are associated in the same attack.

Exanthematic purpura is most often seen in children, and especially in those who have a fine white skin, and come of an arthritic stock. In adults, the female sex is more often attacked. The purpura reappears at the menstrual periods, and may return every month. I have seen a case of this periodic purpura in one of my patients, who for four years suffered almost every month from an attack of purpura and a hæmorrhoidal flux.

Rheumatoid Purpura.—Rheumatoid purpura, or peliosis rheumatica (πελιός, livid), is rarely associated with acute articular rheumatism. In the majority of cases it is an association of purpura with pseudo-rheumatism rather than of rheumatism with purpura (Besnier).

This form, which is more frequent in children than in adults, is especially prevalent in spring and summer, just like the polymorphous erythemata or erythema nodosum with which rheumatoid purpura has many points in common. Pain, œdema, and gastro-intestinal troubles are associated with the purpuric exanthem, as in the following example : A youth, after fatiguing exercise, or without apparent cause, is seized with pains in the joints and in the muscles, in the knees, insteps, calves, thighs, and arms. The pains are reawakened by pressure, and are sometimes accompanied by slight effusion in the joints. At the same time, gastro-intestinal troubles, with vomiting of bile and food, pains in the stomach, colic, and diarrhœa, which is sometimes streaked with blood, supervene. We may see associated with these symptoms white œdema, which is more or less limited around the joints, and more or less extensive over the rest of the body, sometimes attacking the face, and simulating the œdema of Bright's disease or of cardiac lesions.

The purpuric eruption appears during these symptoms, which are more or less marked according to the particular case. The purpuric spots are chiefly seated on the lower limbs. They are sometimes symmetrical, and are usually petechial, but rarely ecchymotic. The disease is sometimes accompanied by slight fever, which may occur in successive attacks, and last several weeks or several months. It is rarely followed by other hæmorrhages. If it is accompanied by itching it takes the name of *purpura urticans*.

We may find, in addition to the purpuric eruption, an eruption of erythema papulosum or of erythema nodosum, which shows the affinity existing between rheumatic purpura and the polymorphous and urticarial erythemata.

Infectious Purpura.—This variety of purpura sometimes supervenes in the course of well-defined infectious diseases. Variola, scarlatina, varicella, erysipelas, and typhoid fever may be complicated by purpura. Septicæmic conditions of surgical or of obstetrical origin, infective endocarditis, pyæmia, and various suppurative infections often give rise to purpuric eruptions. In some cases this purpura is limited to the skin in the form of petechiæ and of ecchymoses, with or without rashes ; at other times it is the prelude of multiple hæmorrhages, which are very serious as regards prognosis.

Apart from these cases of secondary infectious purpura, we may also see *purpura hæmorrhagica* in the course of ill-defined infectious conditions of unknown origin. These cases constitute the most perfect type of the so-called primary infectious purpura.

The following example is quoted by Hutinel :

A boy thirteen and a half years old, hitherto in good health, was seized with repeated epistaxis, which required plugging. The child was brought to the hospital. On examination the skin was pale, an eruption of petechiæ was present over the front of the tibiæ, and, furthermore, there were deep ecchymoses. The temperature and the urine were normal. Colic suddenly appeared, and was accompanied by blood in the stools, slight delirium and incoherence, but no fever. The melæna continued, and hæmaturia now declared itself. A few hours later death supervened. The absence of fever proves that we cannot judge the severity of the disease by the height of the temperature. The autopsy revealed ecchymoses and hæmorrhagic foci in the lungs, liver, spleen, kidneys, stomach, cerebellum, bulb, and testis. It was indeed a fulminant case of primary infectious purpura.

In these forms of *purpura hæmorrhagica*, whether febrile or apyretic, hæmorrhage occurs on every side (stomatorrhagia, epistaxis, hæmaturia, hæmoptysis, metrorrhagia). Ecchymoses appear on the surface of the body, and the trunk and the face are not spared, which is not the case in exanthematic purpura. Visceral hæmorrhages are common, especially into the meninges. I have seen several cases at the Necker Hospital.

One of my patients had been attacked by severe infectious purpura. All danger appeared at an end, when she was found dead in her bed. The autopsy revealed meningeal hæmorrhage. Another patient with infectious purpura was seized with vomiting. She raised herself up to get the spittoon, and fell unconscious, with her head over the bedside. She was raised up and died some hours afterwards. The autopsy revealed meningeal hæmorrhage.

Infectious purpura may be complicated by gangrene. In some cases the purpuric spots necrose (necrotic purpura); in others the gangrene is diffuse, and attacks extensive areas. Let us also note the appearance of suppuration in the purpuric spots (ecthymatous purpura) or in the form of diffuse phlegmon.

In addition to the rapid forms just described, we also find cases of primary infectious purpura in which the course is less rapid and the symptoms are less severe. They correspond to the old description of Verlhoff's disease (*morbus maculosus Verlhoffii*), and may last for months and years.

In some cases purpura assumes a typhoid character, with an insidious onset—fever, rise of temperature, prostration, and hæmorrhages into the skin and mucous membranes.

Pathogenesis.—It is probable that the different varieties of purpura— purpura simplex, purpura hæmorrhagica, rheumatoid purpura, fulminant purpura, and typhoid purpura—have not clearly defined limits. They depend for the most part on infectious causes. Attempts to discover the pathogenic agent have not been successful. Micrococci (Pétrone) and a bacillus (Letyerich) have been found, but they have not any specific character. Hanot and Luzet have published a very interesting case :

A woman suffering from meningitis and purpura gave birth at term to a dead fœtus. She died herself two days afterwards. At the autopsy on the mother streptococci were found in the meninges, in the spleen, and in a bleb which had developed in a purpuric spot. At the autopsy on the fœtus there was no trace of purpura in the skin, but ecchymoses containing streptococci were found in the pleura, peritoneum, and pericardium.

Nervous lesions influence the localization of the eruption. In Hallian's case the purpura was confined to a limb atrophied by infantile paralysis ; in Gilbert's case it had spared the healthy half of the body in a person suffering from hemiplegia.

The visceral changes favour the production of purpura, and in the grave hæmorrhagic forms we find hepatic lesions, first noted by Apert, and confirmed by later researches. Purpura is often seen in affections which accompany changes in the blood—leukocythæmia, chronic malaria, and pernicious anæmia. Lastly, in the hæmorrhagic forms of purpura we may meet with a curious lesion of the blood. The clot does not retract, and the blood-serum does not separate from the clot. This lesion, however, is neither constant in hæmorrhagic purpura nor special to this affection. It may be met with in the absence of purpura, especially in typhoid fever (Widal, Apert).

The **prognosis** of exanthematic purpura is good. It recovers, but it is prone to relapse when the convalescent begins to get up. Verlhoff's disease may recover in a few days, but infectious purpura is, on the other hand, a severe affection, both on its own account, as well as on that of possible complications.

The **treatment** is as follows : abundant nourishment, composed of meat, fruit, and fresh vegetables, and beverages containing a large amount of orange-juice. Perchloride of iron, ergot, extract of rhatany, and Rabel water may be given for the hæmorrhage.

Chloride of calcium, introduced by Wright, gives good results in the hæmorrhagic forms and in the chronic form of Verlhoff's disease. Injections of artificial serum are indicated in grave cases, but should be given with the greatest care.

In the following severe case of hæmorrhagic purpura I employed adrenaline with success :

A woman, thirty-two years of age, came into the Hôtel-Dieu on June 22, 1903. Saliva, mixed with blood, flowed incessantly from the mouth. This stomatorrhagia had appeared twenty-four hours before her admission to hospital, commencing suddenly without any prodromata. Uterine, cutaneous, and possibly also intestinal hæmorrhages were present. Although the flow of blood from these various channels had been present only since the previous evening, the hæmorrhage from the gums was so incessant and copious that the patient was very anæmic, and had already the classical facies of severe hæmorrhage. The usual medication was ordered.

Next day the lower limbs, the elbow, and the face showed very extensive ecchymoses, but there was no injury which could have given rise to them. The limbs were mottled with red blotches. The temperature was slightly above normal, and the pulse was but little accelerated. The arterial tension appeared to be lowered. A diagnosis of grave hæmorrhagic purpura was made.

I painted the gums with a solution of adrenalin, 1 to 1,000, and gave chloride of calcium and sulphate of quinine without obtaining any improvement. The anæmia became worse. Fresh hæmorrhages, including hæmaturia, appeared from the mucous membranes, and the situation became threatening.

The examination of blood showed intense anæmia (1,800,000 red corpuscles) and very slight leucocytosis with a normal formula. The coagulation of the blood took place as usual, but the clot retracted badly, and the serum was laky. I then prescribed daily 1 milligramme of *rénaline française*, which is the same as adrenalin. Next day the bleeding from the mouth was much less. A day later there were no more hæmorrhages. Some vesicles of herpes appeared on the lower lip.

From this time the situation improved rapidly, and the patient might be considered as cured, eleven days after the onset of the affection and six days after the administration of the rénaline (4½ milligrammes in five days). On July 20 the patient left the hospital. One of the most remarkable points in this case was the marked blood reaction which the adrenalin caused. The number of leucocytes rose in forty-eight hours from 18,000 to 26,000. The number of polynuclears increased, and nucleated red cells, as well as myelocytes, appeared in the blood. The red cells gradually regained their normal count. These various phenomena in hæmatology are, without doubt, the index of a reparative action on the part of the adrenalin in the blood of a patient suffering from purpura.

Experiments undertaken in my laboratory by Loeper and Crouzon have also proved the existence of variations in the red and white corpuscles in animals following injections of adrenalin in non-toxic doses.

2. Scurvy.

Scurvy is usually an epidemic disease, which for centuries has developed under absolutely identical conditions. As a matter of fact, in the ætiology of scurvy it is always a question of besieged towns, crowded populations, armies on short rations, overcrowded gaols, and passenger ships in which the hygienic conditions are bad. The prime cause of scurvy has not been discovered. Damp cold, bad water, deprivation of fruit and fresh vegetables (insufficiency of potash), and the abuse of salt meats (too much chloride of sodium) have been suggested. It is certain that in a besieged town scurvy ceases after revictualling.

Pathological Anatomy.—The changes in the blood are not well understood. The fibrine has been increased in some cases, and diminished in others. The red blood-corpuscles are less numerous, and the salts of sodium appear to be in excess, while the quantity of potash salts is lowered. The blood is dark and very fluid. Infiltrations of blood may be found in all the tissues—in the cellular tissue, in the muscles, under the periosteum, in the space between the diaphyses and the epiphyses, in the serous cavities, in the joints, etc. Bacteriological examinations (Murri, Babès) have not given exact results.

Description.—Apart from the exceptional cases in which scurvy commences with local changes in the mouth, there is a period of weakness characterized by progressive loss of strength. During this period pains are felt in the legs, in the joints, and in the base of the chest. The face becomes pale and the skin dry, but the patient has no fever. The changes in the mouth then supervene. The swollen and softened gums become ulcerated and bleed, the breath is fœtid, the buccal mucous membrane is swollen and covered with ecchymoses and blebs containing blood, and mastication becomes extremely painful.

Petechiæ appear, especially around the hair-follicles. The lower limbs are covered with purpuric spots and ecchymoses, but the upper limbs are not so much affected. The skin becomes of a dark livid or greenish-yellow tint, according to the age of the ecchymoses. The cellular tissue is sometimes invaded by hard œdema. Blood tumours develop, and form sanious ulcers (**scorbutic ulcers**). Hæmorrhages also occur in the cellular tissue, in the popliteal space, in the groin, and in the interior of the muscles. The infiltration of œdema and of blood cause extreme hardness in certain parts of the calf and thigh.

The pains are increased by the slightest movement. Muscular efforts readily cause rupture of the muscles and hæmorrhage. The patient experiences a feeling of constriction at the base of the chest, and dyspnœa, independent of any lesion, in the respiratory organs. The pulse is small, constipation is usually present, but the urine does not contain albumin.

If the disease reaches its final stage, the symptoms increase in severity, the teeth become loose, and may fall out, giving rise to alarming hæmorrhage. In young patients the epiphyses of the long bones become detached, and the ribs are separated from their cartilages. The sphincters are relaxed, constipation gives place to bloody diarrhœa, fever appears, the skin is covered with cold sweat, and the patient dies from adynamia or from syncope.

Other and more rare forms are seen, in addition to these classical ones. Scurvy may be characterized only by the changes in the gums, hæmorrhage being absent. In other conditions—as in the Crimea, for example—the swelling of the gums was often absent, and the scurvy revealed itself by muscular pains, with œdema of the lower limbs, and by the formation of tumours in the popliteal spaces (Laveran). Scurvy is often associated with typhus or with dysentery in armies in the field. Pneumonia, pleurisy, and hæmorrhagic pericarditis are frequent complications.

Scurvy lasts the longer in proportion as its causes are the more lasting, and its gravity varies in different epidemics and according to the ætiological conditions. Even after recovery the patient remains feeble for a long time, suffers from pain, and shows a notable tendency to relapse. Sporadic scurvy is much less grave.

We must not confound scurvy with purpura, which usually arises without prodromata. The usual causes of scurvy are absent, and we do not find fungous stomatitis, ulcerated hæmatomata, or the infiltrations of the muscles proper to scurvy.

The presence of lymphatic tumours and the leukæmia will distinguish the lymphogenous diathesis from scurvy, although lymphadenia may sometimes be accompanied by swelling and hæmorrhage of the gums.

Treatment.—Prophylactic measures consist in giving fruits, fresh vegetables, and lemon-juice. Persons must avoid as far as possible damp and gloomy dwellings.

The same measures should be employed when the disease is persistent—namely, fresh fruit and vegetables, watercress, lemon or orange juice, wine, and alcoholic beverages. The gums may be touched with a mixture of citron-juice and alcohol, or with diluted hydrochloric acid. The hæmorrhages should be treated by rhatany, Rabel water, perchloride of iron, and ergot.

Injections of artificial serum may give good results.

3. Infantile Scurvy.

Scurvy may occur in very young children. It differs notably from the disease in the adult, but yet the two affections are identical in nature. The divergences depend only upon the differences of the soil in which the disease arises.

The disease was first described in Germany in 1859 by Uroller under the name of acute or hæmorrhagic rickets. In 1883 Barlow showed that this so-called rickets was really scurvy occurring in children fed on tinned foods, and cured by antiscorbutic treatment with fresh food. The name of Barlow's disease has been given to infantile scurvy.

Description.—Infantile scurvy hardly ever appears before the age of five months or after the age of eighteen. It usually appears in infants apparently healthy, in the sense that they are large, fat, and well developed ; but they are pale, the flesh is soft, and there is more fat than muscle under the skin. The first symptoms consist in an increased pallor of the skin. The lips become colourless; the little patient cries out when his legs are touched, and if he is on his feet, walking and standing become difficult, and he lies in bed with his legs semiflexed. The pains are more acute in the neighbourhood of the joints than in the legs. Later, similar symptoms appear in the arms.

Bony swellings are seen on the femur, tibia, or fibula—sometimes at the upper apophysis, and at other times at the lower epiphysis. Similar swellings may also appear at the anterior extremity of the ribs. Radiography reveals in these swellings simple rarefaction of the bony tissues, an epiphyseal separation, or a fracture in the continuity of the bone (Renault).

The periosteum is stripped off by an effusion of blood, which gives the sensation of blood crepitus.

II.

118

The orbit may be the seat of a similar swelling. Ecchymosis is seen in the lower eyelid. The gums are not affected unless the patient has teeth. The root of the tongue shows little fungous growths, which bleed easily. In severe cases petechiæ may be seen on the mucous membranes and on the skin. The temperature rarely exceeds 100° F. The disease, when left to itself, is progressive and fatal. The pallor increases, the feebleness becomes more and more marked, and the child dies.

Ætiology.—Infantile scurvy is never seen in a breast-fed child. The disease is also quite exceptional in children fed on fresh cow's milk or on milk sterilized in the water-bath at 212° F. according to Budin's method. Cases have been seen in infants fed on factory milk sterilized at 120° C., and preserved for a more or less lengthy period. The great majority of these cases of infantile scurvy have been seen in children fed upon condensed milk or on farinaceous foods sterilized at high temperatures. The disease is caused by skimmed or by diluted milk, by milk containing lactose, by centrifugalized or dried milk, sold commercially as humanized milk, the concentrated milk so frequently used in England and Germany, and the special foods prepared for young infants. This fact has been clearly brought to light in the recent discussions at the Société de Pédiatrie de Paris.

Diagnosis.—We must always think of infantile scurvy if a bottle-fed infant becomes pale, gradually loses strength, and suffers from pain in the legs. Rickets never begins so suddenly. The syphilitic pseudo-paralysis of Parrot (epiphyseal separation by syphilitic changes in the bone) is not likely to be confounded with scurvy. The former is seen during the first months of life, and is almost always accompanied by stigmata of syphilis, especially purulent coryza.

Treatment.—The use of fresh and "living foods," to use Barlow's term, brings about recovery with marvellous rapidity. Raw milk in the case of very young infants, and *purée* of boiled potatoes, as well as a little raw meat, in children of more than a year, should be substituted for the farinaceous foods and tinned milks. We may also give a few teaspoonfuls of lemon-juice, or the juice of green vegetables, after each meal. It is remarkable to see how quickly the bony swellings disappear and the child regains its usual health.

PART VIII

RHEUMATIC AND DYSTROPHIC DISEASES

CHAPTER I

RHEUMATISM

WHATEVER place we assign to **rheumatism** in our list of diseases, it must be admitted that its limits are somewhat ill-determined and its nature ill-defined. And yet rheumatism lends itself to methodical description, and its importance in pathology is considerable.

As I am compelled to divide the subject for purposes of description, I shall describe:

1. Acute articular rheumatism, a disease most probably due to microbes; it is the most typical manifestation of the rheumatic affection, and is often accompanied by changes in the viscera.

2. Chronic rheumatism, which comprises several varieties, according as there is a tendency to become general (progressive polyarticular rheumatism), or to be limited to a small number of joints (partial chronic rheumatism).

3. Visceral and muscular rheumatism.

4. Pseudo-rheumatism, or infective rheumatism, which occurs in blennorrhagia, scarlatina, puerperal conditions, erysipelas, mumps, pneumonia, etc.

I hasten to say, however, that this classification is in part artificial, and that, except for infective rheumatism or pseudo-rheumatism, of which the origin and nature are known to us, the varieties of acute and chronic rheumatism which appear sometimes distinct, when present as extreme types, have such close relationship that it is necessary to place them in the same family.

I. ACUTE ARTICULAR RHEUMATISM.

The acute manifestations of rheumatism show a special liking for the joints, and although they often attack a number of organs at the same time, it is usual to describe all these manifestations under the name of acute articular rheumatism. As a rule, the morbid series commences in the joints, and only affects the organs secondarily; but there are exceptions, and we shall see in the course of this article that the so-called articular rheumatism may affect the pleura, the lung, and the heart before attacking the joints.

Ætiology.—Although acute rheumatism occurs in all countries and at all seasons, it shows a marked predilection for temperate climates and for the summer season (Besnier). Stoll has described summer epidemics of rheumatism. Kelsch, while studying rheumatism in the French army, saw recrudescences often coincide with the end of winter and the commencement of spring. The most common occasional cause is cold, and especially damp cold. Sometimes the chill acts violently upon the perspiring body, and rheumatism appears at once ; at other times the economy becomes gradually impregnated, as may happen to persons who live in damp places, in a freshly plastered room, or in a new house. Fatigue and excesses are predisposing causes, and a sprain or a dislocation has several times been the cause of an attack of rheumatism (Verneuil, Potain).

Must we admit an hereditary or an acquired predisposition in patients who suffer from rheumatism ? The answer to this question would presuppose the pathogenesis of the rheumatic diseases. The pathological affinity which rheumatism bears to gout, gravel, obesity, and diabetes make it fairly clear that nutritive troubles of similar kind play a great part in the evolution of these morbid conditions ; but while admitting that rheumatism results from the uric acid diathesis, it does not help the question much, and the intimate nature of the disease is still unknown.

Acute rheumatism has, however, all the attributes of an infective microbic disease. Its local manifestations in the endocardium and in the serous membranes bring it into close relation with the so-called infective rheumatism, in which the microbic or toxi-infectious origin is known ; but although some authors have classed rheumatism with the microbic diseases, its pathogenic agent has yet to be found, and the microbes so far discovered, though including staphylococci and streptococci, the anaerobic bacillus of Achalme and Thiroloix, or the diplococcus of Triboulet and Coyon, are not specific. They are only factors in the secondary complications. The first attack of rheumatism appears between fifteen and thirty years of age. Relapses are frequent.

Symptoms.—Acute articular rheumatism, or rheumatic fever of English authors, rarely has a sudden and violent invasion. The patient often experiences wandering pains, with or without rigors. Fever appears, and the articular troubles declare themselves. In about a third of the cases at least rheumatism begins with a sore throat, accompanied by fever, and perhaps by albuminuria. The angina, which is more or less painful, and accompanied by redness of the throat and swelling of the tonsils, may precede the appearance of pains in the joints by several days. The instep and the knees are usually first attacked ; the elbows, shoulders, and wrists are involved later. When the small joints—i.e., those of the hand, of the feet, or of the spine—are invaded, the attack of rheumatism is generally long and severe.

Pain is the chief symptom, even from the onset. It soon becomes severe. It disappears with the effusion, passes from one joint to another, reappears in a joint thought to be well, and sometimes becomes general in the small joints of the spine, of the ribs, and of the jaw, inflicting acute suffering upon the patient. The pain is brought on by the slightest movement of the diseased joint, even by the pressure of the bed-clothes or by shaking of the bed.

The joints affected by rheumatism are swollen. In the large joints—as in the knee, for example—the superficial tissues are the seat of *fluxion blanche* (Trousseau), while in the wrists and instep the skin is rosy, and shows a tracing of reddish tracks, which indicate the course of the tendon-sheaths invaded by the rheumatic effusion. As regards the hands, the dorsal surface is œdematous and rounded, the fingers are spread out, immobile, and swollen like a spindle. The **local** temperature is higher by two or three tenths of a degree in the diseased joint. The effusion is very abundant in some joints, and in the knee the amount may exceed 2 or 3 ounces. When it reaches these large proportions it causes acute pain, which disappears on aspiration of the fluid.*

If articular rheumatism is closely studied, we see in most cases that the bursæ, the tendon-sheaths, and the tendons of the muscles are invaded in the same manner as the joint itself. Accordingly, in the knee we find painful foci around the joint, which are rendered evident by the slightest pressure on the inner side of the articulation. The tendons of the sartorius, gracilis, and semitendinosus unite on the crest of the tibia, after having passed over the internal tuberosity of this bone. At this point two tendon-sheaths are present—the one beneath the sartorius, and the other below the tendon of the ham-strings. We also find on the inner surface of the knee a painful point on the head of the fibula, where the tendon of the biceps muscle is inserted with an intervening bursa. Painful points are very common in the popliteal space, and we may also find a painful centre at the insertion of the tendon of the triceps into the patella, where there are two serous bursæ—the one between the superficial and the deep fibres of the tendon, and the other between the tendon and the capsular membrane. These painful points form a kind of crown around the knee-joint, so as to give rise to the belief that the articulation itself is diseased, when it is free or only slightly invaded. Similar remarks apply to the instep. The tendons of the lateral peronei pass behind the malleolus, and the common synovial membrane bifurcates in order to accompany them. We may sometimes follow the painful track as far as the base of the fifth metatarsal bone, into which the peroneus brevis is inserted, and to the base of the first metatarsal, where the peroneus longus is inserted.

In some cases the periarticular pain affects the insertion of a muscle,

* Dieulafoy, " Traité de l'Aspiration," p. 354.

although neither a tendon nor a bursa is present—for instance, at the insertion of the deltoid into the humerus. Further, the muscles themselves are often painful above and below the diseased joint.

In short, articular rheumatism not only attacks the synovial membrane and the intra-articular ligaments, but also the tendons, bursæ, tendon-sheaths, muscular insertions, and cellular tissue.

The face of a patient suffering from rheumatism is of a dull white, which is explained by the rapid and great diminution of the red corpuscles. This rheumatic anæmia is also revealed by a cardiac murmur. The sweat is, as a rule, very profuse, and characterized by a sour smell, due to the high acidity. Œdema of the hands and feet is common. It may be general. The fever varies in intensity. The pulse is full and hard, and the rate is from 90 to 100. In severe cases the evening temperature may rise to 104° F., and the morning remission is slight. In less severe cases the evening temperature is not quite so high, and the morning remissions are more marked ; but the cycle has no regular course. The urine is scanty, of a dark colour, sometimes albuminous, and rich in urea and urates. The digestive functions are but slightly disturbed. The tongue remains moist, and the appetite is often good. One patient may suffer from constipation, and another from serous diarrhœa, resembling a " true intestinal perspiration " (Peter). The cerebral functions are normal, and the patient does not suffer from headache or from delirium, but retains the full control of his senses. Epistaxis is frequent, either at the onset or during the course of the attack.

The **duration** of the attack depends on the severity of the disease, and varies from two to several weeks. Each joint affected remains so for only a few days, but it is by no means rare for the same joint to be alternately deserted and revisited by the rheumatic inflammation. Symmetrical joints are usually invaded simultaneously or in succession. When the fever has fallen and the pain has disappeared, the patient still experiences marked discomfort in moving his joints, which depends partly upon the muscular weakness caused by the disease.

Visceral Localizations of Acute Rheumatism.—In addition to cases in which the attack of rheumatism remains limited to the joints, we see others in which the disease also affects the viscera, and gives rise to the most diverse clinical forms. As a rule, the joints are first attacked, and some days later endocarditis, pericarditis, and pleurisy appear. Rheumatism of the nervous centres, of the digestive and urinary tracts, are also seen. Some of these forms are common, others are rare.

In some cases, however, the usual course of the disease is reversed, and the patient first suffers from sore throat, pleurisy, or from endocarditis, and the joint troubles do not appear for some days.

Rheumatism of the Heart.—The heart is the organ most affected by rheumatism, and it is remarkable that rheumatism, usually so transient in its nature, tends to fix upon the heart with an obstinacy which causes most of the diseases of this organ. The history of cardiac rheumatism was only in its infancy prior to Bouillaud. In 1832 he described **rheumatic endo-carditis,** and showed that it passes into the chronic state, and becomes the origin of organic lesions in the heart. He also stated the laws of coincidence, according to which changes in the endocardium or in the pericardium are almost constant when the articular rheumatism is severe and general, and are exceptional when the disease is partial and slight. According to different statistics, endopericarditis has been stated to be present in the proportion of 30, 40, or 50 per cent. Amid these different opinions, that of Bouillaud remains true, and when articular rheumatism is severe and general, there is the greatest likelihood of endopericarditis supervening. In children cardiac lesions are to be feared, even in slight attacks.

Endocarditis is more frequent than pericarditis. The inflammation of the heart usually supervenes about the second week of the articular disease, though it is sometimes later, and in exceptional cases it may precede the joint troubles.

There is no need for me to describe endocarditis, for I have treated the question elsewhere. I only mention the fact that rheumatic endocarditis usually spares the aortic valves, and especially affects the mitral valve. Its onset is insidious, and it is revealed by a systolic murmur, most marked at the apex. We must, however, be on our guard against mistaking the anæmic murmurs so common in the course of rheumatism for the murmur of endocarditis. Endocarditis may recover after a period which does not exceed two weeks, but the disappearance of the murmur is not always a sure sign of recovery. In such a case, where recovery is apparent, the patient is liable to chronic endocarditis, which is slow and latent in its course, and the mitral lesions may not reveal themselves for years.

In rare cases the endocarditis may be infective, and may then give rise to immediate danger.

Rheumatic pericarditis is rarely accompanied by effusion. It is revealed by friction sounds, which often have a gallop rhythm. Severe pericarditis is often associated with left pleurisy, which is followed by right pleurisy, with or without effusion. Slight pericarditis is not serious, but severe pericarditis, accompanied by effusion or by pleurisy, is formidable.

Rheumatic **phlebitis** is well known. Trousseau has quoted some remarkable examples. It appears in mild as well as in severe rheumatism. It may be localized to one vein or may affect several, and may simulate *phlegmasia alba dolens*, with its train of symptoms. More frequently, says

Vaquez, rheumatism "chooses a superficial venous segment without obliterating it, and strikes the inside of it." Periphlebitis is more common than endophlebitis.

Rheumatism of the Respiratory Organs.—**Pleurisy** usually appears about the second week of the articular disease. It may precede the joint troubles. Rheumatic pleurisy is at times insidious, and at other times severe and painful. It may be single or double, and is often associated with endocarditis or with pericarditis. Effusion is the rule. The fluid increases rapidly, and often disappears just as suddenly.

Congestion of the lung of rheumatic origin may occur in the condition of simple hyperæmia or of inflammatory hyperæmia. The latter form is often described under the name of **rheumatic pueumonia,** although it is not a pneumonia in the true sense of the word. As a matter of fact, the pneumonia has but little tendency to pass into hepatization, and the congestive element always gains the day over the inflammatory one. Congestion of the lung is more or less severe and more or less general. Although it is usually transient and benign, and is often associated with pleurodynia or with pleurisy, it may develop into suffocative catarrh, invading both lungs, and proving fatal in a few days or even in a few hours.

Rheumatic pneumonia may appear and disappear several times in the course of the articular disease. It sometimes alternates with pains in the joints.

Cerebral Rheumatism.—Articular rheumatism, whatever may be the severity of the pain and of the fever, does not as a rule cause mental troubles. When cerebral troubles appear in a rheumatic patient, we must look out for some complication.

Cerebral rheumatism assumes many forms. In some rare cases (five times out of seventy-nine cases in Ball's statistics) the cerebral troubles are fulminant, and supervene without prodromata. This variety is known as **apoplectic** rheumatism, and I quote here an example from Trousseau :

A strong man who had been a heavy drinker was attacked by cerebral rheumatism on the eighteenth day of the joint disease. He complained suddenly of not being able to see clearly, shouted and cried for help, threw himself from his bed, struggled with two attendants, was put back to bed, grew weak and died. The whole affair lasted less than a quarter of an hour.

Cerebral rheumatism is more often ushered in by prodromata—headache, hallucinations, and incoherence of ideas. The prodromata may last for a few hours or for a few days, and the cerebral troubles then appear. The patient is no longer conscious of articular pains, which in some cases absolutely **disappear.** The temperature may exceed 106° F. The delirium, which is more or less violent, resembles that of confluent smallpox or of severe typhoid fever. It lasts two or three days. It is sometimes interrupted by remissions, and may be accompanied by convulsions, which indicate danger. In unfavourable cases it ends in coma.

The delirium, however, may follow a chronic course, and last several weeks. The patient becomes taciturn, melancholy, and lypemaniacal, but finally recovers, as a rule.

The way for cerebral troubles is sometimes paved by the previous condition of the patient. Brain-fag, grief, and depressing emotions, alcoholism, or hereditary predisposition, appear to be favourable to the outburst of cerebral rheumatism. In affecting the brain, rheumatism brings about its usual disorders—sometimes simple congestion, which leaves no trace at the autopsy, and at other times persistent hyperæmia, revealed by vascular injection of the meninges and of the brain substance, with effusion in the ventricles and in the subarachnoidal space.

We must not confound with cerebral rheumatism the cerebral complications (embolism, hemiplegia, aphasia) which are caused by acute or chronic rheumatic endocarditis.

Rheumatism may also affect the spinal cord and its coverings. It is revealed by lumbar pains, spreading to the lower limbs, with symptoms of paraplegia and of contracture (opisthotonos). The sphincters are intact, and we find neither anæsthesia nor trophic troubles. Spinal rheumatism presents this peculiarity—that it may **precede** the articular manifestations by several days. It is evident that the pathogenic diagnosis may be difficult in the absence of joint pains. Spinal rheumatism ends in recovery.

Chorea, disseminated sclerosis, and neuritis are also to be numbered among the nervous manifestations of rheumatism.

Rheumatism of the Digestive Tract.—Tonsillitis is a common manifestation of rheumatism, and often precedes the joint troubles (Lasègue). Rheumatic affections of the stomach and of the intestine are very rare. They occur in the form of gastric catarrh, colic, serous diarrhœa, or dysenteriform stools (Stoll). Congestion of the liver, with or without jaundice, is also very rare.

Rheumatism of the Genito-Urinary Tract.—Albuminuria in the course of acute rheumatism indicates slight nephritis. In some cases, however, severe nephritis has been noticed, but this is exceptional. Speaking generally, we may say that rheumatism, which, like the infectious diseases, is so prone to attack other viscera, as a rule spares the kidneys. Rheumatic hæmoglobinuria has been noted (Hayem and Robin), and after the following case, which I had in the Necker Hospital, I am tempted to think that **hæmaturia** may occur in rheumatism :

A man came under my care with acute articular rheumatism and hæmaturia. They had both appeared at the same time, and were of a fortnight's duration. The rheumatism was acute, general, and accompanied by fever. The hæmaturia was rather

striking, for the urine was highly coloured, and threw down a fairly copious deposit
of blood.   The patient told us that during his first attack of articular rheumatism,
ten years before, he also suffered from hæmaturia, which lasted for several weeks—
in fact, as long as the rheumatism.   Some years later he suffered from a severe attack
of subacute rheumatism, which brought him under Rigal's care, and for nine months
the hæmaturia persisted and disappeared with the rheumatic pains.   The patient had
hæmaturia in the true sense of the word, and not nephritis with hæmaturia ; for as long
as the attack of rheumatism and the hæmaturia lasted, there was no symptom of
nephritis, and as soon as the hæmaturia came to an end, we could find no traces of inflammation of the kidney or of Brightism.   The kidney bled during the attack of rheumatism, but showed no after-effects.

Rheumatism may also affect the bladder (tenesmus, dysuria) and the
testis.

Cutaneous Manifestations of Rheumatism.—Erythema, purpura, and
urticaria are the commonest dermatoses in acute articular rheumatism, but
they are especially prevalent in pseudo-rheumatism.

The erythema may be papular, nodular, or polymorphous.   It sometimes precedes the joint troubles.   The urticaria exists alone, or may
coincide with erythema.   The purpura is simple, and does not fall under
the category of hæmorrhagic and cachectic purpura.   Its seats of election
are the forearm, the legs, and the inner surface of the thighs.   The purpuric
eruption is often called **peliosis rheumatica.**

In the cutaneous cellular tissue the rheumatic congestion reveals itself
by more or less local œdema.   It forms patches or **nodules** (Jaccoud),
which disappear as rapidly as they appear.   Sometimes, however, these
rheumatic nodules are of long duration.   In some cases of rheumatism the
œdema may invade the eyelids, the cheek, the scrotum (Ferrand), and a
portion of the limbs.

In **young children** rheumatism presents some peculiarities (Roger).   The
general symptoms are less severe.   The fever is slight, the sweats are not
so profuse, cerebral troubles are extremely rare, and but few joints are
invaded ; and yet, in spite of this apparent benignity, the heart is often
affected.   Cardiac troubles may appear, even though only one joint has
been affected.

Course—Prognosis.—In the slight forms acute articular rheumatism
lasts from two to three weeks.   In certain very mild cases the disease
merely touches a few joints, and ends in a week.   It may be prolonged for
more than five weeks in the severe forms, which are characterized by high
fever and invasion of the small joints.   The disease often shows successive
attacks.   After a momentary improvement, the fever increases and other
joints are invaded.   Defervescence is slow, and during the first period of
convalescence fever sometimes reappears at night.   After the disappearance of the pain and of the fever the patient remains weak and anæmic.

In some cases we find not only muscular weakness, but **acute amyo-**

trophy (Gubler), which may last for two or three months. Creaking and grating in the joints are fairly frequent after an attack of acute rheumatism. Relapses are common, and may supervene in spite of every hygienic precaution.

The convalescent patient is not absolutely free from the risk of visceral complications, and **chorea** may appear in young subjects at a more or less distant date (Sée, Roger).

The visceral troubles considerably increase the gravity of rheumatism. In some cases they lead to immediate danger (ulcerative endocarditis, cerebral embolism, cerebral rheumatism, endopericardo-pleuritis, congestion of the lungs), but as a rule the danger is more remote, and the cardiac troubles only appear after some months of apparent immunity. The lesions of the heart, at more or less remote intervals, form a most formidable danger in an attack of rheumatism.

In some cases the rheumatic affection does not follow the classical forms which I have just described. The acuteness of the fever, the rise of the temperature, and the simultaneous appearance of endopericarditis, of pleurisy, or of congestion of the lungs, may give rise to a grave condition, but this is not an anomaly. As a matter of fact, an attack of rheumatism in which the general symptoms rapidly become **ataxic** and **adynamic,** as in severe cases of typhoid fever, is an anomaly. The attack, which scarcely affects the joints, but acts with redoubled violence upon the viscera, or which ends in **suppuration** of the joints, is an anomaly. These various anomalies, which are generally the indication of extreme gravity, must be included under infective pseudo-rheumatism, whether the infection be absent or whether the rheumatic patient have the germs of this auto-infection previously present in his economy.

Pathological Anatomy.—The changes in the blood are of great importance. The fibrin may be as high as 10 parts per 1,000 (Andral and Gavarret), as in true inflammation, and therefore the blood-clot is much retracted (Bouillaud). The solid elements of the serum may fall to 60 per 1,000 (Quinquaud). The hæmoglobin, and consequently the oxidizing power of the blood, are much diminished. The number of red corpuscles may fall to 3,000,000 per cubic millimetre.

The following lesions are found in rheumatic arthritis : Both the intra- and extra-articular parts of the joints are more or less affected. The effusion is clear, and holds in suspension flakes of mucus or of fibrin. Very few leucocytes are present. The synovial membrane is red, thickened, and sometimes velvety. The synovial fringes are injected, and their cells show abundant proliferation (Cornil and Ranvier). The **cartilages** show signs of nutritive irritation, and proliferation of the cartilage cells is found. The periosteum and the bones may, according to some authors, present changes which are at present ill understood. The lesions in the various organs affected by rheumatism do not require description in this section.

Treatment.—In a person suffering from severe acute articular rheumatism the following treatment should be employed : Salicylate of soda is of considerable service (Sée), and the patient takes from 60 to 120 grains in the twenty-four hours, the dose being continued for several days, and progressively diminished as soon as improvement becomes manifest. Another method which has given good results consists in administering antipyrin in daily doses of 30 grains, together with the salicylate.

Aspirin (acetyl-salicylic acid) has been employed with some success in acute articular rheumatism. It is a useful substitute for the salicylate, as it does not cause gastric disturbance, buzzing in the ears, etc. (Growitz, Rénon).

Methyl salicylate may be of benefit. It is used in the form of an ointment, composed of 10 parts of vaseline with 1 of the salicylate.

The patient should drink lemonade, milk, and Vichy water. The articular pains are relieved by subcutaneous injections of pure water in the neighbourhood of the diseased joints, and **very small** injections of morphia may also be given morning and evening.

The joints may be painted with a liniment of the following composition :

Oil of camomile	..	..	..	..	.. 24 parts.
Chloroform	..	..	..	..	.. 8 ,,
Laudanum	..	..	..	..	.. 2 ,,

When hyperpyrexia appears, with threatening cerebral troubles, we must employ cold baths (Raynaud). The patient is placed in a bath at a temperature of from 68° to 72° F. for ten to twenty minutes, unless the chills are so severe as to necessitate a shorter immersion. As a result of the bath, the cerebral symptoms diminish in severity, and the temperature falls. The treatment may be repeated three, four, or five times in the twenty-four hours, and for several days following if necessary. This method has certainly saved the life of patients suffering from cerebral rheumatism.

II. CHRONIC RHEUMATISM.

It is customary to describe the following affections under the heading of chronic rheumatism :

1. Simple chronic rheumatism.
2. Nodular rheumatism.
3. Partial chronic rheumatism.
4. Fibrous rheumatism.

1. Simple Chronic Rheumatism.

This variety may be chronic from the first, or may follow attacks of acute and subacute rheumatism, so that the description of chronic rheumatism in part concerns that of the subacute disease. We do not see here, as in the acute forms, severe pain and high fever, but the joints are painful on pressure, movement is difficult or painful, and often accompanied by intra-articular creaking. The patient also complains of muscular pain and of neuralgia, which alternate or coincide with the joint manifestations. The painful points are often seated in the palms of the hands or in the soles of the feet (fascia), in the heel (bursa), and in the tibial and peroneal muscles (tendon-sheaths). When subacute rheumatism fixes itself upon a joint, it is not rare to see muscular atrophy in the neighbouring regions, but the atrophy shows no invading tendency, and yields in a few weeks to the induced current.

Chronic rheumatism sometimes recovers after a duration of several months. In some cases it is interrupted by subacute attacks with fever ; the remissions are incomplete, the movements become more difficult, the muscles waste, the joints show deformity, and the patient at length becomes helpless.

The sufferer from chronic rheumatism is extremely sensitive to atmospheric changes, and the least change in temperature or barometric pressure brings on the pain. The integrity of the other functions is not incompatible with chronic rheumatism. Cardiac troubles are, however, by no means rare, even though the patient has never suffered from acute rheumatism.

2. Nodular Rheumatism.

Nodular rheumatism is also described under the name of primary chronic rheumatism, polyarthritis deformans (Jaccoud), multi-articular osseous chronic rheumatism (Besnier). The term " gouty rheumatism " (Fuller) should be abandoned, for the disease is not a hybrid between rheumatism and gout. Some authors would hold it to be independent of rheumatism, and would include it under the group of pseudo-rheumatism pending definite classification.

Nodular rheumatism is chiefly seen between forty and fifty years of age ; it is more frequent in women, especially at the menopause period, and is more common in the poorer classes. The slow and progressive action of damp cold favours its development.

Description.—Nodular rheumatism is chronic from the first, though there are exceptions, especially in young children, who may suffer from an acute form. The disease presents a progressive mode of invasion—that is to say, when once it has appeared it shows the greatest tendency to pursue its invading course. It usually commences in the small joints of the hands and feet, and then proceeds towards the trunk, affecting the larger joints of the limbs.* It is often symmetrical, and causes considerable deformities, which are due to a process to be described later.

The disease is sometimes preceded by fugitive and wandering pains, which follow the course of a nerve trunk or which attack the muscles and the joints. As a rule, the pain invades some joints, especially those of the hands, lasts for a more or less lengthy period, and is accompanied by transient' swelling of the joints. Later, fresh attacks supervene, the crises of pain become longer, the remissions are less complete, and the deformities of the joints, at first transient, become marked and persistent.

The most marked deformities are seen in the **fingers** and in the **hand.** The disease attacks the index and middle fingers ; the thumb is fairly often spared, in opposition to the course of events in the foot, where the big toe is frequently invaded.

Several causes contribute to the marked deformities seen. From its onset the disease causes in the neighbourhood of the invaded joints muscular contractures, which play a great part in the production of the deformities. These contractures, at first transient and later permanent, are usually very painful. Some authors suppose they are allied to rheumatoid arthritis, while in the opinion of others (Trousseau) they are independent of the articular lesions, run a parallel course with, and may, indeed, be antecedent to, them. In any case, the muscular contractures are soon followed by **persistent contraction,** and fix the phalanges and the hand in faulty positions, which are very varied, but which usually take the form of flexion and of extension.

In the type known as **flexion** the phalanx and the terminal phalanx are in forced flexion and the second phalanx is extended. The articular surfaces stand out in marked relief ; in some cases they may be dislocated. Accordingly the fingers represent broken lines, the metacarpo-phalangeal articulation projecting on the back of the hand, while the joint between the first and second phalanges projects towards the palmar surface ; the hand is semi-flexed and deflected towards the ulnar side. In the type known as **extension** the second phalanx is flexed, while the phalanx and the terminal phalanx are extended.

Other causes play a part in these deformities. We may note the retraction of the fibrous tissue, tendons, and aponeuroses, and in many cases,

* Statistics of forty-five patients in whom the joints were primarily invaded (Charcot, " Maladies des Vieillards ") :

Small joints of the feet and hands	.. .. ..	25 times.
Big toe	..	4 ,,
Hands and feet invaded at the same time as a large joint	..	7 ,,
Large joint invaded before the fingers	.. ..	9 ,,

especially when nodular rheumatism has run a slow course, the swelling of the articular ends of the bones, which are covered with osteophytes. The bony lesion then becomes the chief cause of the nodules.

The muscles gradually become atrophied (simple atrophy), and their prominences disappear, as in progressive muscular atrophy (Vidal). In some cases the skin becomes thin, colourless, and indurated, somewhat as in sclerodermia. The functional troubles increase with the severity of the lesions, and extreme difficulty of movement, or even complete impotence, follows the early stiffness. The other joints of the upper limb are progressively invaded in nodular rheumatism : the wrist is flexed, the forearm is pronated, the elbow is more or less bent, the shoulder is rigid, and the upper limb is, as it were, fixed to the thorax.

The lower limbs are sometimes free. The lesions are symmetrical, the big toe is displaced outwards so as to lie over the others (Charcot), the foot is displaced into the position of valgus or of equino-varus, the knee is much deformed, and the lower extremity of the femur is in front of the head of the tibia. As a rule the hip-joint is free, and this fact is the more remarkable, as this joint is the seat of election of the partial rheumatism, known under the name of *morbus coxæ senilis*. Nodular rheumatism may also affect the spinal and temporo-maxillary joints. The functional troubles depend upon the joint invaded.

Apart from a few exceptions, the disease runs a very slow course. From the clinical point of view we may distinguish an essentially chronic form which is progressive and apyretic ; it is the nodular rheumatism of elderly persons. We also see a more acute form, which runs a more rapid course (puerperal fever, suckling) ; it has not the same invading tendency, and may end in recovery. Numerous intermediary forms exist between the extreme cases.

Nodular rheumatism does not immediately threaten life if complications do not supervene. The blood does not contain an excess of uric acid, the nutrition is fairly maintained, and bedsores are extremely rare, in spite of the fact that the patient cannot move. We may note among the possible complications cardiac lesions, especially pericarditis, albuminuria, interstitial nephritis, and pulmonary phthisis.

The **diagnosis** of nodular rheumatism sometimes presents serious difficulties. Congenital atrophy of the brain and atrophy of the interosseous muscles are followed by deformities of the fingers and of the hand, which very closely resemble those of nodular rheumatism. In the latter case we find changes in the joints and symmetry of the lesions. The same statement applies to the deformities of paralysis agitans, and it must be added that the two diseases may coexist. In some cases gout determines muscular contractures and deformities like those of nodular rheumatism, but in gouty patients they are accompanied by tophi, which are not present in rheumatic patients.

Pathological Anatomy.—All the constituent parts of the joints are affected. The synovial membrane is covered with vegetations and villi; the cellular tissue which lines it is indurated and thickened; the synovial fluid is scanty or absent (arthritis sicca). The intra-articular ligaments have in part disappeared, and the joint cavity is divided up by bands of fibrous tissue. The cartilages become eroded and ulcerated, and finally disappear. The articular ends of the bone present at the centre the lesions of rarefying osteitis, and eburnation at the periphery. Bony processes, or osteophytes, often form a kind of crown around the ends of the bone. The small bones of the carpus are sometimes ankylosed together. Subluxations and luxations are frequent. The ligaments, the tendons, and their sheaths, are invaded by the inflammatory process, which has a sclerous tendency.

From the histological point of view the changes in the cartilage are those which have been described under the name of **villous condition,** the ground substance being pushed aside, and reduced to a shreddy condition by the falling out of the cartilaginous capsules. The eburnated layer at the extremities of the bone is due to the conversion of the deep embryonic cartilage cells into bone cells. Enchondroses develop by the same process.

The treatment of nodular rheumatism may be thus summed up : Internally—preparations of iodine and arsenic ; externally—painting with tincture of iodine over the diseased joints. Hydrothermal cures, sulphur, or arsenical baths may be prescribed.

3. Partial Chronic Rheumatism.

This variety of chronic rheumatism, which produces deformity of the bones, is confined to a few joints, and has but little tendency to become general. Partial chronic rheumatism and the swellings upon the fingers known as Heberden's nodules belong to this variety.

(a) **Partial chronic rheumatism,** or senile arthritis, is almost special to old age. It affects the large joints ; the knee and the hip are most often affected (*morbus coxæ senilis*). The lesions are practically the same as those described in the preceding section. The disease is almost always chronic from the first, although it may follow acute rheumatism (Adams) or acute arthritis.

The joint affection, which is often painless at its onset, is sometimes the seat of acute attacks of pain ; they are not provoked by palpation and percussion. The diseased joint is deformed, and the **deformity** is due to hydarthrosis, to foreign bodies, to bony growths, which are sometimes large, and to swelling of the epiphyses. Movement is difficult, and is often accompanied by intra-articular creaking. The lesion may result in anky-losis, from fusion of the articular surfaces, or by reason of the peripheral osteophytes.

(b) Another form of chronic partial rheumatism is described under the name of chronic rheumatism of the phalanges or Heberden's nodes. This variety has no connection with gout. It is characterized by small nodes, situated at the joints of the terminal phalanges; these nodes are due to an enlargement of the bony nodules normally present in this region. The extremity of the finger is usually displaced to the right or to the left; the joint is rigid, but does not creak. The other joints of the hand are generally but little affected. The disease is more special to old age; it is hereditary, and often coexists with migraine, asthma, or sciatica.

4. Fibrous Chronic Rheumatism.

The lesions of the fibrous tissues (tendons, ligaments, bands, and aponeuroses), which have only a secondary importance in the forms above-described, may become of the highest importance in some cases, and cause the disease to assume the character of a fibrous rheumatism. The faulty positions and the deformities of the fingers and of the hand are very marked —as, for instance, in a remarkable case published by Jaccoud. The ends of the bones are displaced and form prominences, but we find here neither swelling of the epiphyses nor osteophytes, as in nodular rheumatism. Intra-articular creaking is absent.

The treatment of chronic rheumatism, and especially of cases with a tendency to deformity, consists in the **application of superheated air** at 130°, 180°, or 200° C., and the results obtained are sometimes remarkable. In the obstinate forms of gonorrhœal talalgia this treatment produces rapid improvement.

Abarticular Rheumatism.

If it be difficult to define the limits of rheumatism, even when the joints participate in the morbid changes, this delimitation is much more difficult when we are dealing with abarticular rheumatism—that is to say, rheuma-tism which affects the organs, the muscles, or the nerves, and spares the joints.

While studying acute articular rheumatism we have already reviewed the visceral manifestations which may occur during the rheumatic attack, and we have seen that almost all the organs and systems may be attacked by acute rheumatism, but we had there the troubles in the joints as the criterion of the rheumatic nature of these visceral affections.

On the other hand, in the condition now under discussion the joint localizations are wanting, and we then ask ourselves what must be included in the category of true rheumatic affections and what must be excluded.

One individual suffers from facial neuralgia or from sciatica, and the trouble reappears as the result of chills or variations in the weather. Is this a sufficient reason for admitting the rheumatic origin of the neuralgia ? Another suffers from muscular pains, such as torticollis, pleurodynia, or lumbago. Is it right to say that he is suffering from muscular rheumatism ? Confusion has arisen in consequence of an ætiological idea which has been imperfectly interpreted. As chill is one of the causes of neuralgia, and also one of the most active causes of rheumatism, we have readily fallen into the habit of attributing to rheumatism all troubles arising from the common influence of chill.

Do we not daily speak of rheumatic facial paralysis when rheumatism often has nothing to do with the pathogenesis of this paralysis ? And the same statement applies to certain forms of tetany.

What part has not been assigned to the **rheumatic diathesis** by including under this denomination a crowd of morbid conditions and functional troubles of digestive, uterine, nervous origin, etc., while their nature and origin were by no means clearly elucidated !

In truth, I do not say that these troubles may not be of a rheumatic nature, but we must be strict in the appreciation of ætiological ideas before admitting that an abarticular morbid change is essentially rheumatic ; we must have good reasons for doing so, and inquire into the heredity, the previous medical history, and the constitution of the patient.

The previous medical history furnishes valuable information. If a patient, at some period of his life, has suffered from acute or from chronic rheumatism, we have some reason for considering the abarticular troubles which he may show later as being related to the rheumatism. If a child born of rheumatic parents suffers from eczema, sycosis, psoriasis, headache (Bazin), muscular pains, nervous spasms (tics), we may, up to a certain point, put these troubles down to rheumatic heredity. If a patient presents abarticular troubles of a rheumatic nature, although he has never had articular symptoms, we may prejudge the rheumatic nature of these troubles if the patient, by reason of his constitution, form one of the great family of arthritics (diabetes, biliary lithiasis, obesity). It must be added that the possibility of gouty troubles (gout being also a member of this morbid family) sometimes complicates the diagnosis.

We find muscular rheumatism, but it is often difficult to allow for this **muscular rheumatism,** inasmuch as the muscle is not the only tissue at fault, and we do not always know whether we are dealing with myositis, neuritis, or with neuralgia. Thus, in the affection described under the name of **atrophic deltoid rheumatism** (Duchenne), and characterized by sharp pains in the shoulder and the deltoid, with paresis and rapid atrophy of the muscle, we find lesions of myositis, neuritis, and periarthritis, so that the name **atrophic scapular rheumatism** is preferable (Sabourin). Lumbago, torticollis, and pleurodynia are often rheumatic in nature.

Neuralgia is common in rheumatic patients; **sciatica** is the most recent form.

I have already mentioned certain eruptions in acute rheumatism. " Dry circumscribed eczema, pseudo-sycosis of the upper or of the lower lip, simple sycosis of the upper lip, solitary or very discrete psoriasis, psoriasis with large patches affecting the palm of the hand or the sole of the foot, and scarlatiniform psoriasis, limited to the genital organs, acne rosacea, cicatricial acne pilaris, etc., stand in the forefront of the affections which we have recognized most frequently in rheumatic persons, and present such definite characters that we can prejudge their rheumatic nature and the arthritic condition of the patient " (E. Besnier).

Acute iritis sometimes supervenes between attacks of acute rheumatism; **chronic irido-choroiditis** accompanies the chronic disease.

Œdema is one of the most interesting of the abarticular manifestations. We have already noted the œdema which accompanies congestion of the periarticular tissues during an attack of acute or of subacute rheumatism, and the more or less coloured œdema associated with the rheumatic exanthemata. The articular manifestations may be insignificant, and yet the œdema may be of considerable extent. This **hypercrinia** of the cellular tissue belongs to the course of rheumatism. In other patients, although the rheumatic diathesis be never betrayed except by some chronic and more or less painful swellings of the joints, rheumatic œdema may, at a given moment, invade a region, a limb, or the legs, and remain there in an obstinate fashion. This œdema has nothing in common with the œdema of cardiac lesions or of nephritis; it is the result neither of cachexia nor of venous obliteration. It does not make the prognosis grave, and it represents one of the manifestations of the rheumatic diathesis in the subcutaneous cellular tissue (Potain).

Again, in rheumatic patients we see a prominence which fills up the supraclavicular hollow, where it stands out in relief to the extent of an inch or more. This swelling, which is elastic, but not painful, does not take the imprint of the finger; it is neither reducible nor fluctuating; it is accompanied by no change in the colour of the skin. It has been called **supraclavicular pseudo-lipoma** by Verneuil. It is probably due to the accumulation of adipose tissue (Verneuil), or to serous infiltration (Potain).

III. PSEUDO-RHEUMATISM DUE TO GONORRHŒA, TUBERCULOSIS, ETC.

Under the name of infective rheumatism writers have described troubles of rheumatic character which supervene in the course of general and infectious diseases, such as scarlet fever, dysentery, blennorrhagia, mumps, erysipelas, and pneumonia, or which are associated with different conditions, such as pregnancy and the puerperium. These infective forms of rheumatism are really varieties of arthritis—blennorrhagic arthritis, puerperal arthritis, etc.

Gonorrhœal Rheumatism.—This form occurs during the course or about the decline of blennorrhagia. It assumes various aspects, according as its chief manifestations are articular or abarticular. The articular manifestations sometimes reveal themselves by single or double hydrarthrosis of the knees; the hydrarthrosis is insidious in its course, generally abundant, causes but little pain, and is slow in resolving.

Gonorrhœal rheumatism often affects several joints, but even when several joints are affected from the onset the disease usually fixes itself in a single articulation (knee, instep, elbow). The fever is fairly acute, but transient; the pain is often **very severe**, and may last for several weeks; the joint is swollen and brawny, and the synovial sheaths are painful and inflamed.

It is not a question here of more or less transient articular congestion, as in true rheumatism. Gonorrhœal arthritis may last for weeks and months, and in some cases the patient suffers for a long time from creaking in the joints, and the movements are considerably hampered. In some cases, indeed, the arthritis ends in ankylosis. Termination by suppuration and by white swelling is excessively rare.

I would ask the reader to refer to the section on Gonorrhœa, where this question is treated in detail.

In the abarticular manifestations the infection affects the tendon sheaths and the bursæ (trochanteric, ischiatic bursæ). It also causes sciatica, and gives rise to eye troubles, such as iritis and conjunctivitis. These, of course, have nothing in common with the purulent ophthalmia produced by contact with the blennorrhagic pus.

These manifestations of the gonorrhœal infection differ so notably from true rheumatism that confusion is not possible. In such a case, true rheumatism and gonorrhœal pseudo-rheumatism form two absolutely distinct morbid groups.

In addition to these cases, which are the most numerous, we find others in which gonorrhœal pseudo-rheumatism has some analogy with genuine articular rheumatism. We may find general articular rheumatism, visceral manifestations, such as endocarditis, pericarditis, pleurisy, or cerebral troubles, and in this case it has been asked whether gonorrhœa is not capable of exciting or of reawakening the rheumatic diathesis (Peter).

If the reader will turn to the section on Gonorrhœa, he will find that these various visceral manifestations are caused by the gonococcal infection, and not by the rheumatism. Articular and visceral infections depend upon toxi-infection due to the gonococcus.

The morbid troubles which take place in the serous cavities and in the joints do not belong, then, exclusively to the disease called acute articular rheumatism, but are also found in a modified form in various infective conditions, such as gonorrhœa, scarlatina, dysentery, mumps, etc. From the point of view of their nature and their origin, the forms of infective pseudo-rheumatism must be clearly distinguished from true rheumatism, which is also most assuredly an infectious disease.

If, however, the distinction is clearly marked from the pathogenic point of view, it is not always so complete from the clinical one, and in some cases gonorrhœal rheumatism runs such an abnormal course that, apart from the discovery of gonorrhœa, it would be very difficult to say whether the case were one of true rheumatism or of pseudo-rheumatism.

Tubercular Rheumatism.—Since 1897 pseudo-rheumatism has formed the subject of a series of researches by Poncet, of Lyons, and his pupils, Bérard, Maillant, etc.

Tubercular rheumatism presents two chief varieties — primary or secondary. The primary form " opens the pathological scene, and is the first manifestation of the tubercular infection." The secondary form appears in a patient who " has previously been attacked by tuberculosis or is actually tubercular " (Poncet). I shall examine these two forms of tubercular rheumatism, laying stress on the first variety, which is by far the more interesting.

Primary Tubercular Rheumatism.—The joint troubles are the first indication of tuberculosis, which so far is latent, and their symptomatic value may be considerable. The joints are affected by Koch's bacillus or by its toxines, and the lesions may run the course of a tuberculization of the joint or may resolve completely, as in one of my cases, where, remarkable to relate, in spite of the presence of the bacillus in the joint, resolution took place just as completely as in the case of ordinary tubercular pleurisy.

This tubercular rheumatism sometimes begins like acute or subacute rheumatism, and generally attacks several joints. It is not, however, frank in character. " It presents great fixity in its localization, disappears slowly, and very often leaves traces of its passage. It does not return in the joint first affected, as in the case of true rheumatism. It usually affects two or three joints, rarely more, and is **oligo-articular** " (Maillant). While less mobile than rheumatism, it is also less transient, and tends to become fixed. The salicylate treatment has no action upon it.

The duration is variable. Although the fever may be moderate, the general condition is quickly affected, and the affection often terminates in one of the following ways : The joint troubles disappear, but the tuberculosis invades the viscera or the serous membranes. The joint becomes more and more involved, with fungous arthritis, white swelling, and possibly with multiple ankyloses (Poncet). Sometimes the rheumatism passes into the chronic condition, affecting the small joints of the hand and of the feet, as in chronic arthritis deformans. Lastly, recovery is possible without ulterior tuberculization, as in the case of my patient in the Hôtel-Dieu. It is probable that cases of this kind are not very rare, but they have so far passed unnoticed. We see a patient suffering from fluid in the knee-joint, and we think of arthritism, "which has a broad back," and we make a diagnosis of rheumatic arthritis. Nowadays we are not content with such a superficial diagnosis. We withdraw some of the fluid from the joint, examine for lymphocytosis, and inoculate guinea-pigs. In short, we act as in a case of pleural effusion, and we find that the so-called rheumatic hydrarthrosis is sometimes a tubercular hydrarthrosis of a curable nature.

The diagnosis of primary tubercular pseudo-rheumatism is often difficult, and we must always think of tubercular rheumatism when we cannot determine the cause of an infective rheumatism. Laboratory researches, examination of the articular fluid (cyto-diagnosis), inoculation of guinea-pigs, and Arloing and Courmont's sero-diagnosis, are indispensable procedures in forming an opinion.

The articular lesions vary in proportion to the tuberculization of the joint. They may result in miliary tuberculosis of the serous membrane or in white swelling, or they may continue to be inflammatory, and run the ordinary course of rheumatism (Poncet).

If the quantity of fluid in the joint is considerable, aspiration is performed. In other cases cryogenin, in doses of $\frac{1}{2}$ to 1 gramme daily, has a beneficial action upon the joint lesions, and also upon the pain. We may at the same time employ counter-irritation in all its forms, and prescribe general tonics—arsenic, lecithin, and glycero-phosphates. In chronic cases the thermal cures of Salies-de-Béarn, Biarritz, Bourbon-l'Archambault, and Dax give good results. Here, as in other forms of pseudo-rheumatism, salicylate treatment produces no appreciable effect.

Secondary Tubercular Rheumatism.—In this case the joint troubles occur in a patient who is already suffering from tuberculosis of the serous membranes (rare cases) or of the viscera. We must, however, be on our guard against "labelling as tubercular every case of acute arthritis in individuals suffering from a tubercular lesion, and in particular phthisical patients " (Bezançon).   Experimental verification, with the assistance of all the means at our disposal, must contribute largely to the diagnosis.

The evolution of secondary tubercular rheumatism has nothing to distinguish it from the primary form.   Simple arthralgia, acute, subacute, or chronic and deforming joint lesions comprise the principal varieties. Recovery may occur, although the primary focus continues its course, as in the cases of Bentz, in which the initial lesions, Pott's disease, and osteitis of the tibia remained active, while the joint troubles disappeared without ending in definite articular tuberculosis.

Scarlatinal Rheumatism.—The rheumatism of scarlatina may simulate true rheumatism, although it more often assumes the characters of infective pseudo-rheumatism.   It appears, as a rule, during the decline of the disease, and its seats of election are the wrist and the instep.   It is often so slight that the pain is only revealed by pressure on the parts.   Pyogenic bacteria are frequently associated with scarlatina, and scarlatinal arthritis may sometimes end in suppuration.   Pleurisy and pericarditis, which may develop simultaneously with the joint lesions, also show a tendency towards purulent change.   For further details, I would refer the reader to the section on Scarlatina.

Dysentery.—Dysentery is sometimes accompanied by arthritis.   This is Stoll's rheumatic form.   The joint manifestations supervene at an advanced period of the disease, sometimes, indeed, during convalescence. According to the particular case, one or several joints are affected simultaneously or in succession.   The arthritis is sometimes transient; at other times obstinate, as in gonorrhœal arthritis.

Mumps are sometimes accompanied by joint troubles, and even by endocarditis, as has been pointed out in the section on Mumps.

Pregnancy leads to such changes in the economy that rheumatism may be notably modified in the pregnant woman (Hanot).   The **puerperal condition** constitutes a favourable state for the development of secondary arthritis, which sometimes ends in suppuration and ankylosis.

Pneumonia may also be accompanied by simple or by suppurative arthritis, due to infection by the pneumococcus or to secondary infections.

Erysipelas may also be accompanied or followed by joint troubles of various kinds, such as hydrarthrosis and simple or suppurative arthritis.

Typhoid fever is another infectious disease, in the course of which simple or suppurative arthritis may supervene.

Certain **intoxications** (iodism, plumbism, food-poisoning) and autointoxications are capable of giving rise to rheumatic symptoms.

In many of the cases of infective arthritis just reviewed we find the pathogenic agent in the diseased joint—gonococcus, pneumococcus, *Bacillus typhosus*, streptococcus.

In other cases we find only agents of secondary infection. Sometimes, indeed, the fluid from the joint is sterile, and we then ask whether we must hold the toxines guilty, or whether it is not more correct to admit the disappearance of the microbes.

Treatment.—As a general rule, we employ the drugs used in true rheumatism. Gonorrhœal arthritis and puerperal arthritis, which so frequently assume the subacute type, must be treated from the onset by energetic local measures, such as bleeding, leeches, cupping, blisters, and the cautery. These cases may well be treated by the measures which I saw Trousseau employ, and which I have myself used with success. I have described it* under the name of Trousseau's Cataplasm. Its composition is as follows :

Take, according to the size of the diseased joint, 3 or 4 pounds of bread, 4 pounds being necessary for the knee, while 2 pounds are sufficient for the wrist. Cut the bread in pieces, taking care to remove all the crust, and soak the pieces in water for about five minutes.

When the bread is taken out of the water, it is quite soaked. It is then placed in a cloth or in a serviette, and a portion of the water which has been absorbed is expressed by twisting the cloth. The bread is then only damp.

It is next placed in a bain-marie, where it is allowed to remain for three hours. When it is taken out of the bain-marie we have a kind of dryish paste, which is gradually softened by the addition of camphorated alcohol. The cake is kneaded until it has acquired the consistency of plum-pudding or of putty. This is the most delicate part in the manufacture of the plaster, and this degree of consistency must be obtained. If the cataplasm be too soft, it softens down under the pressure exercised over the joint, and if it be too hard, it is no longer homogeneous, but forms small lumps, and the dried parts may excoriate the skin. It is, therefore, essential to exercise great care as to the consistency of the cataplasm. When we are unaccustomed to use it, we are always liable to make it too soft, either because the bread has not been sufficiently squeezed before placing it in the bain-marie, or because too large a quantity of camphorated alcohol has been added too quickly.

The paste prepared in the above manner is spread out on a linen compress in the form of an elongated rectangle of such a size that the whole joint may be covered. The cataplasm should be nearly $\frac{1}{2}$ inch thick at its edges, in order to avoid too rapid drying of the thinner parts. A solution of the following composition is then poured over the surface of the poultice :

Camphor	..	..	..	..	..	7 parts.
Extract of opium	..	..	..	..	..	5 ,,
Alcohol	..	..	..	..	..	Sufficient to make it liquid.

---

* Dieulafoy, *Gazette Hebdom.*, No. 48. 1879.

The cataplasm is now finished, and the application is more simple. It is placed directly upon the diseased joint, and covered over by oiled silk to prevent evaporation. The whole is fixed firmly by a flannel bandage several feet in length, and secured with tapes. The length of the tapes varies according to the size of the joint, and consequently to the size of the poultice.

The diseased joint, thus enveloped, is kept at rest. The compression should be fairly firm, but not so firm as to produce œdema in the subjacent parts. We may prevent œdema by taking care to surround these parts with a roller bandage. A reverse may be used in order to prevent displacement of the turns.

The cataplasm is thus applied, and allowed to remain *in situ* for from eight to ten days. It is removed after this period, and it is surprising to find the cataplasm as fresh and as moist as if it had just been applied. The strong smell of camphor is still present, and not a trace of mustiness is to be seen. The skin which has remained so long in contact with the cataplasm is absolutely healthy. It is only excoriated if the cataplasm, being too thin at its edges, has become dried or has been spread out by ill-applied compression. A second or a third application must be made if one does not suffice.

IV. GOUT.

Following the example of old writers, it is customary to describe regular and irregular gout.

Regular Gout.

Acute Gout.—The attack of gout is only an episode in the life of the gouty, especially in the **hereditary** disease, which is the most common. A patient who will some day become gouty usually experiences from an early age some of the manifestations which form part of the gouty diathesis.

At the age of fourteen or fifteen years he is subject to migraine or epistaxis. Hæmorrhoids and eczema appear somewhat later, and then, about the age of twenty-five and for a series of years, he complains of dyspepsia, with flatulence, heaviness in the stomach, distension of the abdomen, acid eructations, constipation, pruritus ani, and urine which contains thick deposits of urates or of uric acid.

Some patients have attacks of asthma, which reappear at more or less lengthy intervals ; others suffer from hepatic colic, renal colic, and attacks of boils, or show early baldness and a notable tendency to obesity. The gouty diathesis may appear in these different forms without ending in articular gout, and when the attack of gout appears it does not do so before the age of thirty or forty years.

The **attack of gout** is usually ushered in by some premonitory symptoms. The patient becomes morose and irritable without reason, his temper becomes worse, and he complains of inaptitude for work, of vertigo, and of dyspepsia. The gout is at hand, and the economy is, as it were, saturated with it—*totum corpus est podagra* (Sydenham)—and the gouty person who has had several previous attacks knows perfectly well what is pending.

The attack of gout, whether it has or has not been preceded by premonitory troubles, runs the following course : The sufferer goes to bed and falls asleep, but between midnight and three o'clock in the morning—for it is almost always in the middle of the night that the first attacks of gout appear—he is awakened by a sharp pain situated in the metatarso-phalangeal articulation of the big toe **(podagra)**. The **pain becomes intolerable** in three or four hours ; the patient is a prey to absolute torture, and cannot bear the contact of the clothes, dreads the vibration of the bed caused by persons walking about the room or by carriages passing in the street. These agonizing pains are not confined to the joint invaded. They sometimes extend to the foot and the leg, and the patient compares them to boiling oil or to molten lead flowing along the affected limb. Towards morning—" at cock-crow " (*sub galli cantu*), says Sydenham—the pains diminish, the chills which accompany them disappear, the patient falls asleep, there is slight perspiration, and the day is less painful ; but towards evening and during the night the pains reappear with all their severity, to lessen again in the morning ; they alternate in this fashion for four, five, six, or eight days.

Let us now study the appearance of the diseased parts. The veins of the invaded and of the neighbouring regions are extremely swollen ; the skin of the big toe is bright red, shiny, and recalls the appearance of onion-peel (Trousseau). The redness spreads and fades insensibly. It reaches its maximum on the second day, and then gives place to a violet tint. The tissues are swollen, and œdema, lasting some days, is seen. After the attack the skin desquamates to a slight extent, and itching is felt.

The attack of gout is accompanied by general symptoms, known as gouty fever. The congestion of the face and the headache of the onset yield after two or three days. The skin is dry, and the morning sweats have neither the abundance nor the acidity seen in articular rheumatism. The temperature increases up to the fourth or to the fifth day. It may reach 103° F. at night, and falls about a degree in the morning. The fever is accompanied by thirst, anorexia, and constipation. The urine is red, loaded with urates and uric acid, and sometimes contains albumin. If a blister is applied, the serous fluid usually contains crystals of uric acid, though less in the neighbourhood of the invaded joints than at other points. The blood, which during an attack of gout contains an excess of uric acid, only contains traces after the attack.

After the attack the patient has difficulty in walking, and the diseased joint does not regain its suppleness for some weeks ; but the general health remains excellent—**better,** indeed, than before the attack. It might be said that this acute episode has played the part of a salutary emunctory. Perhaps it is true to say that the gouty fever has played a useful part in determining more intense combustion, and in eliminating and destroying the uric acid (Bouchard).

The attack of gout does not always run the foregoing course. I have so far considered only the first or the early attacks, but in some patients, especially in those who have had several previous attacks, the course of events is somewhat different. In the first place, the gout does not remain limited to one toe, but invades both big toes in succession, and then other joints—foot, knee, hand, elbow, etc. The attacks, instead of coming on during the months of January and February, appear in the early spring-time or at the end of the autumn. These attacks appear in the form of **successive paroxysms**—that is to say, the patient experiences a series of attacks, each of which is slight, and separated by a few days of improvement.

The muscular form of gout has been carefully described by Grandmaison, and the attack may be isolated or be concurrent with articular gout. I have seen it limited to the calf, with intense congestion and painful œdema, and distension of the venous network.

An individual may have only one attack of gout in his life, but this is rare, and the subsequent attacks are sometimes separated, especially the first ones, by an interval of several years.

Chronic Gout.—Chronic gout, as a rule, attacks old people. It is rarely chronic from the first, and is preceded by more or less frequent attacks of acute gout. Chronic gout resembles the acute disease, with successive paroxysms, " with this capital difference—that its attacks are longer, and that in the intervals the patient is never completely free " (Trousseau). Further, the disease attacks several joints at once, and the joint swellings persist indefinitely. Thus, while the patient suffering from acute gout regains after the attack complete freedom of movement, the sufferer from chronic gout becomes helpless—his feet, knees, and hands are deformed ; walking is difficult or impossible. Acute attacks may supervene in chronic gout.

The history of the tophus belongs to chronic gout. The tophus is a concretion formed of urate of soda, of urate and of phosphate of lime. These concretions develop in the subcutaneous cellular tissue and in the thickness of the skin. They form small nodular tumours, which are sessile or pedunculated, and which vary in size from a small pea to a pigeon's egg. They usually develop in the hands, in the neighbourhood of the joints of the fingers, which they help to deform. They are not symmetrical. The tophi appear after the attack, during the remission stage. They are at first composed of a semifluid mass, which raises the skin, without causing changes in it. In a short time the mass becomes solid and hard, and increases in size with each fresh attack of gout. In some cases the tophus is reabsorbed; the skin sometimes ulcerates, and the contents of the tophus are discharged externally. Some gouty patients suffer for a long time from chalky fistulæ, which may become inflamed.

The tophi develop in points other than in the neighbourhood of joints. They are frequent in the external ear, at the edge of the helix, and on the inner surface of the pinna. They have also been seen on the eyelids and on the alæ nasi. Although tophi develop, as a rule, after attacks of articular gout, it must be added that they may appear in persons who, though of the gouty diathesis, have not shown articular troubles. This **gravel of the skin,** as Trousseau calls it, is a certain sign of the gouty diathesis.

I had under my care in the Avenue Gabriel a lady of gouty stock, who had never had an attack of gout. She was subject to renal colic, and had a large tophus in the forearm.

Chronic gout is very serious, because it tends to weaken the organism to such an extent that it has received the names of atonic and asthenic gout. This cachectic condition, which comes on more or less early, according to the patient, is hastened by multiple complications, such as diabetes, dyspepsia, and changes in the kidneys, heart, and great vessels.

Irregular or Visceral Gout.

Larval gout, retrocedent gout, and organic changes of gouty origin are included under this heading.

Larval Gout.—The articular changes which constitute the attack of acute or of chronic gout are the most genuine and evident expression of the gouty diathesis, but this diathesis also reveals itself by other manifestations, such as migraine, asthma, gravel, hæmorrhoids, diabetes, and eczematous eruptions.

These various forms may appear in an individual who has not suffered from an attack of articular gout, and they may, indeed, remain in the condition of larval gout, without ending in the more genuine manifestations of the articular disease. As a rule, articular gout is preceded many years previously by some of the manifestations of larval gout. In adolescence we find migraine and hæmorrhoids; in adult age asthma, dyspepsia, gravel, and eczema; later, the articular disease appears. In some cases articular gout alternates with attacks of asthma or of renal colic. These different varieties form so clear a part of the same diathesis that the parent with articular gout begets children who will present the manifestations of larval gout, and, *vice versa*, parents suffering from larval gout beget children who inherit the articular disease.

Retrocedent Gout.—The name of retrocedent or metastatic gout has been given to troubles which are more or less sudden, and which supervene in the course of an attack of articular gout.

A patient is attacked by gout, and, as a result of untimely treatment, or of some disturbing cause, or even without any appreciable reason, the articular congestion is aborted at its onset, and the gout, seizing on some organ, causes certain complications.

In the **digestive** system we may find œsophagism, dysphagia, attacks of cardialgia, characterized by terrible cramps of the stomach, and by uncontrollable vomiting, with cold sweats, algidity, and a tendency to syncope. Sometimes the gastric manifestations assume the inflammatory form, fever appears, and hæmorrhagic or phlegmonous gastritis supervenes. Let us note also intestinal colic, with or without enteritis.

In the **nervous centres** we find troubles similar to those of cerebral rheumatism—violent headache, delirium, epileptiform convulsions, stupor, apoplectiform conditions, and coma.

Aphasia forms part of these cerebral troubles. In some cases it might be said that gout strikes the mesencephalon or the bulb. The patient suddenly experiences palpitation, laryngeal spasms, respiratory distress, lipothymia, and may die suddenly in syncope.

The Visceral Lesions of Gout.—Permanent lesions occur in certain organs as a result of the gouty diathesis. We may note segmentary myocarditis (Renaut and Landouzy); fatty degeneration of the heart, favouring fatal syncope; aortitis and atheroma of the aorta, which is associated with angina pectoris; arterio-sclerosis and atheroma of the arteries, which pave the way for cerebral symptoms and gangrene of the limbs; phlebitis and emboli, chronic congestion of the liver, and the manifestations of gout in the kidney, which, on account of their importance, I discuss in detail.

Gout and the Kidney.—In the gouty person the kidney is the organ most often attacked. In the gouty, or in the individual born of gouty stock, whether he may or may not have had an attack of articular gout, the disease may show itself in the kidney under various forms, of which gravel, renal colic, nephritis, albuminuria, and hæmaturia are the principal ones.

Gravel.—As a matter of fact, gouty persons suffer from gravel to a more or less marked degree and for a more or less lengthy period. Every individual who is tainted with the gouty diathesis passes uric acid in excess, either in the shape of sand or of gravel. It is, indeed, because he passes this excess of uric acid that he is to a certain degree free from articular gout.

If the gouty person were able to pass this excess of uric acid in the form of sand all would be well, for the uric sand does not cause renal colic ; but, in addition to sand, the patient passes gravel, as a rule, at the expense of renal colic.

It is certain that three-quarters of the persons who suffer from renal colic are of the gouty diathesis, and it may be said of renal colic that it is an attack of renal gout. Out of 150 gouty persons, 48 had suffered from renal colic (Lécorché).

In most cases the trouble commences with renal colic, and the articular disease appears later. It may come on ten, twenty, or thirty years after the first attack of colic. Lécorché quotes the case of a patient who had his first attack of gout thirty-four years after his first attack of colic. During this long space of time he had had twenty-five or thirty attacks of colic. It might be said that the expulsion of sand or of gravel, with or without colic, removes the risk of articular gout up to a certain point, and the more the patient suffers from gravel, the less has he to fear an attack of gout ; but if the passage of sand or gravel cease, the gout may become articular. " It is precisely because the uric acid no longer takes the renal channel for its elimination that the joints become affected. As long as the excess is eliminated by the kidneys, the joints are free from an attack " (Lécorché). This assertion, without being absolute, contains a large degree of truth.

In other cases, which, it is true, are more rare, the attacks of articular gout are the first to occur, and the colic appears later. It may be remarked that in certain gouty patients the attacks of articular gout cease or diminish in severity when renal colic appears. One of Lécorché's patients, who had had attacks of articular gout for thirteen years, did not suffer from a single one after the appearance of the renal colic. Lastly, we find cases in which the articular attacks alternate with the renal attacks.

In spite of the close relations between articular gout and renal calculus, a patient born of gouty stock may only have lithiasis and renal colic, and may recover without suffering from articular gout.

Gouty Kidney—Nephritis.—The morbid series often commences with gravel, and goes on to nephritis. Renal lithiasis and colic occur at first, and the lesions of nephritis, which chiefly affect the interstitial tissue, supervene later. In other cases, on the contrary, gouty nephritis arises insidiously, without having been preceded by the severe symptoms of renal colic. The formation and the elimination of the uric acid occur in silence, but they pave the way, nevertheless, for fibrous lesions in the kidney. The gouty person, therefore, has his kidneys somewhat exposed, and if attacks of renal colic, thanks to the prolonged expulsion of the uric acid in the urine, may, up to a certain point, relieve the patient from the risk of an attack of articular gout, the reverse side of the question shows the possible prospect of nephritis, with all its consequences. Nephritis is the more to be dreaded, as the arterioles of the kidney are the more rapidly damaged, **arterio-sclerosis** being the appanage of the gouty.

Two chief causes dominate the evolution of gouty nephritis : On the one hand, the presence and the elimination of irritating substances, such as uric sand and gravel ; on the other hand, the arterio-sclerotic degeneration of the renal vessels.

The **lesions** of the gouty kidney are well known (Garrod, Charcot, Cornil). Their evolution is very slow. At the end of the process the gouty kidney is a type of the contracted kidney. The capsule is thickened and adherent. Cysts are frequent. We find on section that the cortical substance is almost completely atrophied. The histological examination reveals interstitial nephritis. Fibrous tissue predominates everywhere. At various spots, but especially in the glomeruli, arterio-sclerosis is very marked.

The characteristic of the gouty kidney, however, is the presence of crystals of uric acid and deposits of urate of soda. Uric acid, in the form of sand or of yellowish or brownish concretions, is deposited in the excretory apparatus of the kidney—that is to say, in the straight tubules, papillæ, calyces, and pelvis—and also, though more rarely, in the secretory apparatus of the kidney—that is, in the convoluted tubules and in the periphery of the labyrinth. The urate of soda is deposited chiefly in the region of the pyramids, either in the interior of the uriniferous tubules or externally in the connective tissue.

The **symptoms** of gouty nephritis are similar to those of chronic interstitial nephritis, with the predominance of arterio-sclerosis. The major complications of Bright's disease are slow in showing themselves, and are usually preceded by the minor symptoms of Brightism, with or without albuminuria. We see gouty persons who have not albuminuria, and in whom the renal lesion reveals itself by the minor complications of Brightism, or by some severe symptoms of Bright's disease.

Some of these patients consult us for dyspepsia, with or without vomiting ; for headache, which they term migraine ; for continuous or for paroxysmal dyspepsia, which they look upon as asthma. And, as gouty persons often suffer from dyspepsia, migraine, and asthma, we are liable to agree too readily with their diagnosis, and we sometimes wrongly attribute their troubles to the gouty diathesis. On closer inspection, however, we see that these troubles are neither asthma nor migraine ; they are symptoms of Bright's disease. The urine may for the moment be free from albumin, but it matters little : the gouty person in question is none the less a case of Bright's disease. When we make a careful inquiry, we find the minor complications of Brightism—pollakiuria, cryæsthesia, dead fingers, cramps in the calves, and electrical shocks. We find an increase of the arterial tension, or a *bruit de galop*. If we investigate the toxicity of the urine, we find it diminished.

Lastly, the symptoms of Bright's disease dominate the situation in some gouty persons. The other manifestations of gout appear to be extinguished, and these patients succumb to renal disease and uræmia.

Gouty Albuminuria.—I have said that in a gouty person albuminuria may be present as a transitory or as a permanent condition, without being absolutely associated with the progressive renal lesions of Bright's disease. It is, therefore, essential to state exactly the prognostic value of gouty albuminuria. A person who suffers from articular gout may pass albumin for years without showing symptoms of Bright's disease. I know gouty persons who have passed large quantities of albumin for three, five, and ten years, and yet they have never shown the minor troubles of Brightism.

At the Necker Hospital I have often talked with a physician who was gouty, and who had for several years passed large quantities of albumin in the urine, without having ever experienced any symptom of Bright's disease. I have seen a young man who is subject to attacks of articular gout, and who has passed albumin for three years, the urine containing, when I examined it, more than 2 grammes of albumin per litre, but its toxicity was absolutely normal. This patient has not the least sign of Brightism. There is, therefore, a gouty albuminuria, which may last for years, without resulting in Bright's disease. From the point of view of the prognosis, these facts are of great importance.

This analysis of cases proves that in the gouty diathesis, as in the infectious diseases, the **morbid acts of the kidney may be dissociated,** as I have tried to prove in my communication to the Académie de Médecine.* On the one hand, albuminuria may be absent—at least, for a time—in gouty nephritis, and, on the other hand, albuminuria, as we shall see later, may exist alone, to the exclusion of any symptom of Bright's disease, and it may acquire importance as regards prognosis only by its conjunction with signs of urinary insufficiency.

Hæmaturia.—Hæmaturia in the gouty is associated with gravel and with renal calculi. If the reader will turn to the section on Renal Calculus, he will find a description of this hæmaturia. Gouty persons may suffer from hæmaturia which has nothing to do with a calculus, and the hæmaturia appears in their case just as epistaxis or hæmorrhoids do in other persons, because the congestion affects the kidneys instead of affecting the hæmorrhoidal vessels. Lécorché has reported five cases of this gouty hæmaturia, and I have seen one case at Troyes in a patient who feared renal cancer. Gouty hæmaturia is preceded or accompanied by pain in one or in both kidneys. The pain is due to the congestion of the organ or to

* Séance des 6 et 20 Juin, 1893.

the passage of clots through the ureter, and perhaps also to the momentary obstruction of the ureter. The urine is brownish, reddish, or bloody, according to the quantity of blood passed. The hæmorrhage may be repeated several times daily for several days or weeks.

Gouty Congestion of the Kidney.—As I have said above, gouty congestion of the kidney exists. In some cases the congestion coincides with renal colic ; in other cases it is independent. It must be said, however, that it chiefly affects kidneys already damaged by lithiasis. The course of events is as follows : The patient has a feeling of swelling and of heaviness in one of the kidneys. This feeling spreads to the ureter and to the testicle. The testicle becomes tender, congested, and swollen. The onset of renal colic is then feared, but the symptoms do not increase in severity. The urine takes on a yellow colour, and a deposit of uric acid is found. The look of the water subsequently passed is cloudy, as though a few drops of ink had been added. The brownish urine in the specimen-glass has a cloudy look, and a dark deposit of uric acid and blood forms at the bottom of the glass. The renal congestion may be accompanied by painful swelling of certain joints—in the knee, in the foot, and especially in the big toe. The symptoms then cease in an abortive manner.

Ætiology—Pathogenesis.—Gout—or, rather, the gouty diathesis—may be acquired, but it is **hereditary** in two-thirds of the cases.

Gouty heredity means the heredity of the diathesis as a whole. Thus, gouty parents beget children who may have all the other manifestations of the diathesis except gout. They may be asthmatical or may suffer from urinary and biliary lithiasis, to which I have added sabulous typhlo-colitis and appendicular lithiasis, but yet they escape articular gout. On the other hand, parents who suffer from asthma, gravel, or renal troubles, but who have never suffered from the articular manifestations of gout, beget children who are affected by true articular gout. These facts have been clearly stated by Trousseau.

Gout is more frequent in men than in women. It is the appanage of the wealthy classes, and it is probable that good living, excessive use of wine, and want of exercise favour its development. Gout may appear from an early age, but this is exceptional. The first attack of gout occurs earlier when the disease is hereditary than when it is acquired, and usually shows itself between the ages of thirty and forty years. In gouty persons an injury, . a shock, a strain, a long walk, or tight boots suffice to bring on an attack.

It has been said that gout is due to an excess of uric acid in the blood, but this uric dyscrasia alone is not sufficient to explain gout, for in many cases the dyscrasia appears in an acute state (acute diseases) or as a chronic condition (cirrhosis, leucocythæmia), without the slightest manifestation of gout supervening.

According to Bouchard, the causes of the exaggerated formation of uric acid are of less importance than the causes of its retention in the blood. The latter are diminution of the alkalinity of the blood, and the predominance of oxalic and lactic acids. The predominance of acids is a condition favouring the precipitation of the uric acid, whether in the free state or in the form of urates. This dyscrasic condition, with the predominance of acid, is said to result from the fact that in gout an exaggerated formation, or too slow a destruction of the organic acids, takes place. It is, therefore, a manifestation of delayed nutrition.

Diagnosis—Prognosis.—The diagnosis between acute gout and acute rheumatism presents no difficulty, but we cannot say the same with regard to the chronic forms of these two diseases. I have discussed the explanation under Nodular Rheumatism. I must say that, in addition to the common cases, in which each of these diseases shows its normal character, we find mixed or **intermediate** cases, in which gout and rheumatism appear to occur together.

The diagnosis of irregular gout is often difficult. The patient's antecedents must be inquired into, and the question of heredity must be examined.

The gravity of gout depends upon the possibility of the complications of retrocedent gout and metastatic troubles, and upon the development of visceral changes (gouty nephritis, arterio-sclerosis, fatty degeneration, and rupture of the heart).

Pathological Anatomy.—It may be said that the gouty person is impregnated with uric acid and urates. The uric acid is in excess in the blood. It increases at the approach of the attack, and diminishes or disappears for a time after it. This uricæmia, however, is met with in other conditions (lead-poisoning, albuminuria), and is not special to gout.

Urate of soda is found in the form of crystals in the cartilages of the diseased joints, in the ligaments, tendons, and bursæ, under the periosteum, and, lastly, in the cellular tissue and in the skin, where the accumulations of urate of soda receive the name of tophi.

The excess of uric acid in the blood is easily demonstrated in the serum taken from a blister or from dry-cupping. In each case a few drops of acetic acid are added to the serum on a watch-glass; some threads of cotton are placed in the fluid. After twenty-four hours the threads are covered with crystals of uric acid. It must be stated that during an attack of gout the serous fluid in a blister from the region of the congested joint does not contain uric acid, while the serum from a blister at any other point shows the opposite condition. We find urate of soda in the secretions of the gouty person, in the serum of the pleura, or of the pericardium.

When the joint lesion is studied from the histological point of view, we find that the deposits of urate of soda which impregnate the cartilages are first laid down around the cartilage cells, without changing the structure of the cartilage.   Later, in chronic gout the cartilages change, and we sometimes find the lesions of arthritis sicca, but the articular and periarticular incrustations of urate of soda predominate.

The incrustation of the cartilages begins during the first attack of gout, and persists in the intervals between the attacks. This change is special to gout, and is not found in any variety of rheumatism. Whether the deposits of urates which occur during an attack of gout come from the blood or are formed in the tissues of the joint is a question which has not been cleared up.

Treatment.—The first care of the physician in the case of a person who is born of gouty stock, or who has presented some of the symptoms of the diathesis, is to delay or to prevent the outburst of the gouty attack. This prophylactic treatment should, if possible, commence in infancy, and measures to increase nutrition, such as exercise in the open air, cold baths, rubbing, and massage, should be ordered. The patient must be forbidden to take large meals, to eat fatty substances, to drink fermented liquors, or to indulge in excess of any kind. Alkaline preparations for dyspepsia and Vichy water should be taken in moderation.

What treatment, however, should be employed in the attack of gout ? Must we treat the attack, or must we leave it to nature ? We have all the desired measures at hand to lessen the attack or even to abort it. The preparations of colchicum are wonderful agents in this respect. Tincture of colchicum seeds, given in doses of from 8 to 10 drops, repeated two or three times a day, extract of colchicum seeds, and colchicum wine will relieve the acute pains of gout, and shorten the duration of the attack.

Similar results may be arrived at with all the more or less famous preparations, such as Lartigue's pills and Laville's solution, in which veratrine and colchicum are the chief ingredients. Salicylate of soda in large doses, antipyrin, alone or with salicylate, and aspirin may be efficacious.

Such, then, are the drugs which may be employed for the attack of gout, but it is necessary to know precisely how far intervention must be carried. Sydenham was careful not to intervene during the attacks of gout to which he was subject, and Trousseau and many others have followed the advice of Sydenham. The attack must be considered as a kind of emunctory which must be respected, especially in elderly persons. If we cut short the attack of gout, **we may expose the patient to the terrible complications of retrocedent gout.** The gouty person who moderates the severity and cuts short the duration of his attack of gout does not, as a rule, experience the same after-feeling of health as does the gouty patient in whom the attack has run its ordinary course. He is more subject to early recurrence, is more troubled by other manifestations of the diathesis, and is more exposed to the conversion of his disease into chronic or into atonic gout.

It is, therefore, necessary to respect attacks of acute gout, to avoid local measures (leeches, injections of morphia, blisters) which may suppress the articular congestion, to withhold violent purgatives at the onset of the attack, and to be content with mild anodyne treatment.

For the latter purpose, I employ antipyrin in doses of from 30 to 120 grains daily, given in cachets, alternated with cachets of salicylate of soda in a daily dose of from 30 to 120 grains.

There are, however, cases in which it is necessary to intervene more energetically, as when the gout tends to show **a chain of paroxysms,** which, by its duration, weakens the patient. We must also employ energetic treatment when the disease affects the organs, " since nothing worse than this can happen," and this is the time to have recourse to antigouty medicines. The principles formulated as to the danger of energetic treatment in an attack of acute gout are not accepted to-day by all observers. Sée, from his experience, is of opinion that the attack of gout may be treated vigorously, and he found that salicylic preparations gave excellent results, provided, of course, that the **condition of the kidneys** is watched, and that we do not expose the patient to incomplete elimination and accumulation of the drug.

The hygiene of gouty persons is similar in every way to the prophylactic measures above indicated. To avoid excesses of every kind, to take moderate exercise, to use cutaneous stimulants, such as baths, lotions, or massage, to avoid heavy meals, " high " foods, game, truffles, acid foods and drinks, sorrel, tomatoes, vinegar, and fatty foods, which, combined with proteid matter, may become a powerful excitant of uricæmia. Generous wines and alcoholic drinks should be forbidden, and pure water, with the addition of white wine, or with cider, must be the usual drink. Beer is not allowed. Alkaline waters, taken after meals or in the morning on an empty stomach, are of undoubted value. In short, the gouty person must be careful during his whole life. The cures of Vichy, Carlsbad, Contrexéville, and Vittel give excellent results.

V. DIABETES MELLITUS.

Pathogenesis.—Sugar is indispensable to life. It is fixed in the anatomical elements of the body, and undergoes changes therein. It serves for the repair of the tissues ; it is utilized for combustion, and is a source of heat and energy.

The blood normally contains sugar in proportion of about 1 per 1,000.

This physiological condition is called glycæmia. Glycæmia results from the equilibrium which exists in the economy between the supply and demand for sugar. By reason of this equilibrium the quantity of sugar remains practically the same, although the quantity of sugar taken with the food may be variable, and although there be no emunctory for the excretion of the saccharine principles.

In the pathological state, however, the equilibrium between the supply and the demand for sugar is disturbed : glycæmia gives place to hyperglycæmia, and the sugar in the blood amounts to 3, 4, or 5 parts per 1,000 ; indeed, 5·3 parts per 1,000 (Pavy) have been found—and symptoms of diabetes appear with this hyperglycæmia.

The following problem requires solution from the point of view of the pathogenesis of diabetes : By what means does normal glycæmia give place to pathological hyperglycæmia ? In attempting to answer this question, let us study the chemistry of the sugar in the organism—a study which had been absolutely ignored before the great discoveries of the illustrious physiologist, Bernard.

The sugar in the economy and that in the blood have different origins. In the first place, they come from the starchy and saccharin material of the food—starch, dextrin, cane-sugar, and the sugars from milk and fruits. These materials, converted into glucose by the saliva and by the pancreatic and intestinal juices, are carried by the portal vein to the liver. But they may neither remain in the liver nor pass through it in the condition of sugar. They are converted and fixed there (Pavy) in the form of animal starch or **glycogen,** which is converted into glucose, and is carried away in the hepatic veins (Bernard).

Starchy foods, however, are only one of the sources of glycogen. The albuminoid foods are also utilized by the liver. Thus, in animals fed exclusively on meat for several months the liver cell continues to form glycogen (Bernard).

Fats, glycerin, and gelatin also serve for the production of glycogen.

Furthermore, it is not solely from the recently ingested food that the liver obtains the elements of glycogen, for, in addition to the **direct** nutrition, which is renewed daily with the food, we find an **indirect** nutrition, which takes place at the expense of **reserve foodstuffs previously stored up** in the tissues and organs. The anatomical elements are the seat of incessant changes. The waste of living cells is not all destined to be excreted by the emunctories. The larger portion of this waste is taken up by the circulation, and the liver contains a part of the elements necessary for the elaboration of the saccharin principles of the economy. Glycogen " is thus an intermediary stage by which certain substances of disassimilation may again become assimilable " (Bouchard).

Such, then, is the origin of glycogen suggested by Bernard, and studied by Pavy and Rouget under the name of liver-starch and zoamilin.

The glycogenic function of the liver is comparable to the function of vegetables. They both form saccharin material, and the formation of starch is effected in the whole animal series by a mechanism analogous to that which is seen in the vegetable kingdom (Bernard).

There are two distinct phenomena in the formation and in the evolution of the immediate saccharin principle: (1) The creation of amylaceous matter in the hepatic cell—that is to say, secretion of glycogen; (2) the chemical phenomenon which produces successive transformations in this immediate principle. Glycogen is an assimilation product of the hepatic cell. It is fixed and stored in the liver as a reserve element of the economy. It probably undergoes there the action of a ferment produced in the liver; by the action of this ferment the glycogen, which is **converted into glucose,** passes into the veins and into the whole economy. During life these two orders of phenomena—the formation of glycogen and its conversion by the ferment—take place at the same time; but after death the formation of glycogen, which is the vital act, is arrested, while its decomposition into secondary products, which is the chemical act, continues. And therefore we may wash the liver of an animal repeatedly, and find that it still contains traces of glucose after successive washings (Bernard).

An attempt has been made to generalize the glycogenic function. Rouget, having found glycogen in other tissues—the muscles, for example, although in small proportions—thought that glycogenia was a general nutritive act, and not a special function of the liver. The presence of glycogen in a large number of tissues has not, however, the importance which some would assign to it. " These are phenomena subjected to all the eventualities of alimentation, and to all the varieties seen in the accidental phenomena of the economy, which must be distinguished from the constant functions " (Bernard). "Without doubt, sugar as well as glycogen exists in the muscle, but in the muscle, left to itself, the glycogen disappears without the sugar increasing. In the muscle, which contracts, the glycogen disappears, and lactic acid forms, but not sugar. Further, by contraction the sugar disappears at the same time as the glycogen " (Bouchard). Normal glycogenia, therefore, which is the constant, invariable, and necessary function, is **imposed upon the liver,** which, by its glycogenic function, regulates the glycæmia.

The liver-sugar, which is continually poured into the blood, is used in various ways. One part becomes fixed in the tissues, there to undergo fresh changes and to serve for their repair. It is not exactly known in what form the glucose of the blood is fixed in the tissues. In some cases—as in the muscles, for example—it is probable that it passes back again into glycogen.

Another part of the sugar serves for combustion, for the functional activity of the organs, for muscular contraction, and becomes an agent of energy and heat. Sugar is a plastic and respiratory food, and just as glycogen is converted into sugar, so sugar may pass back into glycogen. The question is one of hydration and dehydration.

Normal glycæmia results from the equilibrium which occurs in the economy between the supply and demand for saccharin principles. When this equilibrium is upset, and too much sugar is produced or too little sugar is used up, an accumulation in the blood results. We have hyperglycæmia, with all its consequences. An excess of sugar is produced if the liver, by reason of functional hyperactivity, elaborates too large a quantity of glycogen, or if the tissues of the economy, by reason of an exaggerated disassimilation, furnish an excess of materials for glycogen. Too little sugar is used up if the assimilation of the saccharin principles is turned aside from its true end, or if the consumption becomes insufficient. At this point the theories of diabetes commence.

These theories are very numerous, and no one is applicable to every case.

According to Bernard, the question is one of degree, between transient glycosuria and diabetes. This is the idea which Jaccoud has always expressed, when he says any case of glycosuria may end in diabetes. Bernard thinks that diabetes is due to an exaggerated production of glycogen, without, however, reducing the diabetes to a simple hyperactivity of the liver, as writers have been too prone to repeat by wrongly stating his theory under the name of the hepatic theory. Bernard looked at the question from a more extensive point of view, and admitted the general trouble in nutrition, with special reaction on the liver. " If, by a process of excessive disassimilation, the organ wastes the reserve depôt, of which the liver is the seat, the sugar is poured into the blood in abnormal quantity, and hence hyperglycæmia and glycosuria appear. The hepatic source, however, is not exhausted. It continues to assimilate the materials requisite for the formation of glycogen, and consequently of sugar. It redoubles its activity in order to replace the sugar eliminated, and exhausts the organism in order to provide for this exaggerated demand for saccharin material."

The present tendency is to attribute diabetes to a general perversion of the nutritive processes, without giving the liver the importance which was assigned to it by Bernard. Are we on the right track ?

This perversion of the nutritive processes has been variously interpreted. According to some authorities, there is an abnormal decomposition of tissue, by which an excess of glycogen is set free. According to other authorities, it is the normal glycogen which is not sufficiently used up by the economy, because of the diminution in the glycolytic ferment (Lépine); thence arises the residue and excess of glycogen.

The former theory admits the decomposition of the proteid substances into glycogen and urea (Jaccoud). According to the other theory, the sugar is not properly burnt up (Mialhe) in the tissues, or the ferment which effects the decomposition of sugar is wanting. According to Bouchard, the nutritive trouble which leads to diabetes is characterized "primarily and essentially by a lack or insufficiency of assimilation, and in particular by an absence of the consumption of the sugar in the anatomical elements." The excess of sugar which is not utilized accumulates in the blood, and hyperglycæmia results. Diabetes would therefore enter into the class of morbid conditions, due to a "slackening in the nutrition." This slackening of the nutritive processes affects the elaboration of sugar and constitutes diabetes, just as it favours biliary or renal lithiasis and obesity, when it depends on the defective elaboration of cholesterin or nitrogenous matter and of fat.

At the present time the hepatic theory of diabetes has somewhat returned to favour (Glénard, Triboulet). **Hyperhepatia** appears to account for diabetes in undeniable cases where the liver, whether hypertrophied or not, not does present any lesions (Gilbert and P. Lereboullet).

In Germany a renal theory of diabetes exists (Klemperer). The discovery of phloridzin-glycosuria has appeared to give it a certain basis, but we must await fresh researches.

Ætiology.—Diabetes may be divided into **essential** and **symptomatic** (Lécorché). The so-called symptomatic diabetes is rarely a true diabetes.

Symptomatic diabetes of nervous origin is sometimes caused by lesions of the bulb and of the brain, such as tumours of the fourth ventricle, traumatism of the occipital region, general concussion from carriage or railway accidents. These lesions produce glycosuria more often than diabetes. In other cases diabetes is associated, not so much with a lesion of the nervous centres, as with a neurosis (epilepsy, paralysis agitans).

One form of symptomatic diabetes is partly associated with lesions of the liver or of the pancreas. We shall see later what opinion should be held of bronzed diabetes, associated with a certain form of hepatic cirrhosis.

Changes in the pancreas are, according to Lancereaux, the origin of a wasting diabetes. This pancreatic diabetes, resulting from functional inactivity of the pancreas, has as its special characters early appearance of intestinal troubles, frequent fatty stools, and rapid wasting. I shall refer to it under the Symptoms of Diabetes.

Malarial fever appears to play some part in the development of glycosuria and of diabetes (Burdel, Verneuil).

Essential or true **diabetes** is hereditary or acquired. Heredity is manifested when the diabetes appears in children born of diabetic parents, between the ages of six months and one to two years.   In the great majority of cases diabetes is associated with the gouty diathesis, or with a nervous heredity.

To the **arthritic source** belong the various manifestations which Bazin has collected under the name of **arthritism,** and which Bouchard has described under the name of disease caused by **slackening of nutrition.** In this group we find gout, asthma, rheumatism, gravel, gall-stones, obesity, and diabetes.   Manifestations of this morbid group are frequently met with in the same individual or in the same family.   They are transmissible by heredity, and may undergo changes in their transmission.   Thus a gouty individual who has or has not had diabetes himself begets children who suffer, on the one hand, from diabetes, and, on the other hand, from asthma, gout, or calculi.   These cases are extremely frequent.

To the **nervous source** belongs the diabetes which, in the same family, is associated with dementia, epilepsy, hysteria, tabes, general paralysis, or exophthalmic goître.   I have often found this nervous heredity, with its mutations.   It is sufficient to glance at the table of statistics published on this subject to see the frequency of this nervous association, with its hereditary mutations.   To quote examples : An epileptic father had five children, of whom four were epileptics and one diabetic.   A diabetic father, who died from diabetic coma, had three children : the first diabetic, the second tabetic, and the third, for the time being, free.   A grandmother of unsound mind had a nervous daughter, who begot an epileptic son and a diabetic daughter.   I may repeat that the most usual origins of hereditary diabetes are the arthritic and the nervous sources, which are sometimes united.   In other cases diabetes is acquired, although it may be difficult to establish the pathogenesis.

The **social position** has a great influence upon the development of diabetes.   Worms has published interesting statistics on this subject. He found that the urine in 607 persons doing heavy manual work, which, as a rule, demands great muscular and respiratory activity, did not contain sugar in appreciable doses.   Of those given to more or less severe intellectual labour—such as scientists, physicians, artists, and statesmen—he found glycosuria in 10 per cent.   In these persons repeated analyses have proved that the condition is not one of simple alimentary or transitory glycosura, but rather a true diabetes.

A **conjugal** form of diabetes has been described, the husband and the wife both suffering from the disease.   Lécorché has seen conjugal diabetes six times in 114 cases.   Debove has seen it five times in fifty-nine cases. Marie has published a very interesting case.   Several theories have been proposed to explain conjugal diabetes.   Teissier is inclined to believe in contagion, but other authors invoke the similarity of the mode of life in husband and wife, who are nourished in the same manner, participate in the same occupations, in the same mode of existence, and in the same vicissitudes.

The onset is usually insidious, and many persons pass an ounce of sugar daily without knowing it—that is to say, they are diabetic for months or for years before the warning symptom appears. Sometimes this symptom is striking : the thirst is acute and the urine is abundant, or perhaps a carbuncle appears, and the patient is himself put on the track of the diagnosis by this warning symptom (Jaccoud). The warning symptom in diabetes, however, is often quite different. The patient complains of obstinate balanitis, of sexual incapacity, of visual troubles (amblyopia), of gingivitis, or of falling out of the teeth, of itching, of neuralgia, or of muscular pains. One patient wastes, another loses strength without apparent cause. Women frequently suffer from pruritus vulvæ, with or without eczema. In the presence of these various symptoms, although the thirst is not exaggerated, the urine should always be analyzed, and diabetes, the hidden cause of these troubles, is often discovered, to the great astonishment of the patient.

In order to draw attention to these symptoms, I have grouped them under the name of the **minor symptoms of diabetes.** They are comparable to the **minor symptoms of Brightism,** and, like them, they are apparently of small importance. So, too, they pass unnoticed in those who do not know of them, and yet in both cases, if they are well known, they give an immediate clue to the diagnosis.

Salivary Symptoms.—In the diabetic patient the saliva is acid, because of the presence of lactic acid, produced by the fermentation of the sugar. The *Leptothrix buccalis* finds an excellent culture medium therein. As the result of these new conditions, the mouth becomes dry (it is noticed when speaking), the tongue becomes pasty and studded with papillæ, the gums soften and bleed easily (noticed on cleaning the teeth). In some cases alveolo-dental periostitis appears (expulsive gingivitis), and causes displacement, loosening, and falling out of the teeth. These various symptoms, which may be isolated or associated, and which are sometimes incomplete, often permit the discovery of diabetes in persons who have neither polyuria nor polydipsia, and who have no idea of their condition.

Ocular Symptoms.—I do not allude here to diabetic cataract, which is a symptom of the highest importance, and cannot escape notice ; nor do I allude to ocular paralysis, or to lesions of the fundus oculi. We shall have to consider them later among the complications. I allude to those apparently insignificant troubles, which consist in weakness of the sight, following diminution in the power of accommodation (**premature presbytia**). "A healthy man tells you that his sight, previously good, has become markedly weak ; that for some time he has been obliged, when reading, to hold the book at a distance, and, later, to employ spectacles ; that he has been forced to change his glasses every month for stronger ones. This fact alone will give us cause to ask whether the patient has albuminuria or diabetes.   In default of other symptoms which may not exist, this one will show you the way, and the examination of the urine will clear up the diagnosis " (Trousseau).

Cutaneous Symptoms.—Here, again, I do not allude, of course, to the most marked symptoms, such as carbuncles or eruption of boils, which at once point to diabetes ; I speak of more trifling symptoms, which, for this reason, deserve to take a place among the minor troubles of diabetes.   We find, on the one hand, severe general pruritus, in which no cutaneous eruption is present, but which is so obstinate as to dishearten the patient. On the other hand, we find eczema, which may be limited to the genitalia, and which produces most severe itching.   An attentive observer has, from these symptoms, recognized diabetes in persons who had neither polyuria nor excessive thirst.

Nervous Symptoms.—Nervous symptoms are met with at every turn in the history of diabetes.   I shall here content myself with reviewing the milder symptoms, which are of an indefinite character.   Many persons, in the absence of a thorough examination, are said to be suffering from melancholia, neurasthenia, or other neurosis, when they are really suffering from diabetes.   One patient complains of lassitude, for which he can give no reason.   He becomes lazy, and everything tires him.

Another patient complains of muscular pains, lumbago, pleurodynia, sciatica, and hyperæsthesia ; and the condition is put down to rheumatism instead of diabetes.

A third patient has sensory troubles in the lower limbs, and a syringo-myelic dissociation of sensibility, which at first gives the idea of some disease of the spinal cord (Vergely).

A fourth patient suffers from psychical symptoms, loss of memory, tendency to sleep, inaptitude for work—symptoms put down to the onset of a cerebral lesion, when they are really due to diabetes.

Genital Symptoms.—Age or excesses are too often held to account for sexual weakness which is due to diabetes.

Urethritis, balanitis, and phimosis belong to the diabetic manifestations which are especially obvious.   The prolonged contact of a few drops of altered urine and the acetic, alcoholic, lactic, and butyric fermentation in the saccharin urine, and the possible appearance of small fungi, analogous to the aspergillus (Friedrich), explain these genital diabetides.   The urethritis, localized to the anterior part of the urethra, causes a whitish or colourless discharge, accompanied by acute pruritus, and too often mistaken for gonorrhœa.   Sometimes the glans is red and swollen, and we find balanitis, which may last for months without the patient suspecting the cause. The prepuce is often red, inflamed, and covered with ulcerated vesicles, which resemble those of herpes, and are painful on contact with the urine. A degree farther and phimosis appears. Many patients who have diabetes, urethritis, and balanitis do not speak of it, because they think that they are suffering from syphilis, and the condition goes on to phimosis. If they consult an inexperienced physician, the nature of the phimosis is misunderstood, and an operation is advised, which may lead to grave results (because the patient has diabetes), when medical treatment would have relieved the condition, even though it is of long-standing. With Terrier I saw a diabetic patient in whom phimosis of two months' duration was cured by diet and medical treatment.

Such are the **minor troubles of diabetes,** which, either grouped or isolated, may give the diagnosis in the absence of the more important revealing signs.

The initial period of diabetes, which is more or less latent, lasts as long as the diabetes is moderate. If the sugar increase, the disease shows itself by symptoms which may be more or less marked, but which are rarely wanting. These symptoms include unusual dryness of the mouth and throat, unquenchable thirst, and abundant urine, which presents special characters. These symptoms will now be described in detail.

(a) **Glycosuria,** or the presence of sugar in the urine, depends upon hyperglycæmia. In the normal condition the sugar in the blood (1 per 1,000) has no tendency to pass into the urine, but as soon as the hyperglycæmia reaches 2·50 per 1,000 glycosuria appears. The passage of sugar in the urine is favoured by the quantity of water which the sugar takes up from the blood, each gramme of sugar fixing 7 grammes of water. In extreme cases the quantity of water taken up into the blood may reach 400 grammes.

At the onset of the disease the glycosuria is transient and intermittent. In ordinary cases the quantity of sugar passed in the twenty-four hours is from 25 to 60 grammes. It may exceed 1,000 grammes in very severe forms of diabetes. " If there is hypergenesis, the quantity of sugar lost within twenty-four hours is truly without limit, and it has no other boundaries than those of the abnormal formation, which may be double, treble, or quadruple the physiological formation. This quantity may be fixed approximately at 200 grammes a day (Jaccoud). The glycosuria is increased by taking saccharin and farinaceous foods. When we suppress these foods, the glycosuria improves or disappears if the diabetes is slight; in grave cases the glycosuria persists. This caused Jaccoud to say that in the first stage the diabetic makes sugar from starchy food. At a more advanced period he elaborates sugar from his own tissues (autophagia). Sugar may disappear momentarily from the urine as a result of an inflammation or of a febrile disease. It diminishes markedly in the consumptive stage.

In diabetes the quantity of sugar passed from day to day is extremely variable, apart from variations in diet and hygiene. Worms has clearly shown this variability in the quantity of sugar passed. As a matter of fact, no fixed relation exists between these quantities.

A diabetic patient goes to his doctor and says " I pass 52 grammes of sugar " as unconcernedly as he would say I am fifty-two years old, and he shows an analysis giving this amount. The urine is examined, and is found to contain 10 or 80 grammes of sugar. On the evening before we might have found 20 or 10 grammes, and on the next day we might find perhaps 2 or 75 grammes (Worms). I have often seen diabetic patients who thought themselves ill because they had had their urine analyzed two or three days apart in different laboratories. They had come to their physician and told him, with some emphasis : " I have had my water examined by two analysts— one found 18 grammes and the other 45. One of the two is quite in the wrong." It is not the analyst who has made a mistake, but the patient, who wrongly interprets the facts. The glycosuria may be absolutely different on different days. The urine passed after meals contains the largest quantity of sugar.

The urine is colourless, acid, and of a specific gravity which increases from 1018, the normal amount, to 1032 or 1060, because of the dissolved sugar. We often find marked increase of the urea (60 grammes instead of 25 grammes), of the chlorides (36 grammes instead of 10 grammes), and of the phosphoric acid (10 grammes instead of 2 grammes).

Diabetic sugar is practically analogous to vegetable glucose. It turns polarized light to the right, but it disappears more quickly than vegetable glucose when it is injected into the blood. It is easy to discover the sugar in the urine. The reagent most used is Fehling's solution, which yields a red or orange-yellow precipitate on boiling. Quantitative analysis is made by means of the saccharometer.

Diabetic urine, in contact with linen or with clothes, often leaves dusty spots when it dries.

(b) **Polyuria** (abundance of urine) accompanies glycosuria, but does not exactly follow the variations of the latter. It is probably due to an excess of intravascular tension caused by the water in the blood. The diabetic who passes 50 grammes of sugar in the twenty-four hours may not pass more than 2 litres of urine. The polyuria rarely reaches 10 to 12 litres, and is less than in diabetes insipidus.

(c) **Polydipsia** (increase of thirst) is associated with the preceding symptoms. Hyperglycæmia, by modifying the normal conditions of osmosis, attracts water from the tissues to the blood. This dehydration produces thirst, dryness of the mouth and throat, and diminution of the pulmonary and cutaneous excretions. It probably enters largely into the production of the cutaneous, muscular, and nervous troubles. Certain diabetics who suffer from incessant thirst, drink 20 to 30 pints of fluid in the twenty-four hours. The polydipsia is, however, less in diabetes mellitus than in diabetes insipidus.

Some patients pass large quantities of sugar in the urine, and yet their thirst is practically normal.

(*d*) **Polyphagia** (increased appetite), which is less constant than poly-dipsia, depends upon the marked loss of sugar, salts, and urea by the organism. This exaggeration of the appetite compensates for a time the losses sustained by the diabetic, and some persons remain well nourished. After a time, however, dyspeptic troubles supervene, the enormous quantity of food taken is not digested, the wasting progresses, and the period of cachexia commences.

Pancreatic diabetes, which is one of the forms of wasting diabetes, appears suddenly, without prodromata. The patient can state the month, and even the day, on which the first symptoms appeared (Lapierre). This sudden onset is marked by gastro-intestinal troubles (vomiting and abundant diarrhœa), by jaundice, or, lastly, by lumbar and epigastric pains. The usual and cardinal signs of diabetes appear rapidly, and the disease is severe from the first (Lancereaux).

The polyphagia, and especially the polydipsia, are marked. The thirst is unquenchable, and the hunger is generally very great. Polyuria is excessive, and patients pass 5, 10, or 15 litres of clear urine in the twenty-four hours. The specific gravity is almost always over 1030. The glycos-uria may exceed 1,000 grammes a day, and the enormous quantity of 1,800 grammes of sugar has been noted. It is diminished neither by diet nor by treatment. This glycosuria is, in exceptional cases, accompanied by lipuria (Thirolat), rarely by albuminuria, but constantly by azoturia (Lancereaux), independent of nourishment and general treatment.

The general condition is rapidly and profoundly affected. The wasting, which always appears early, results in extreme emaciation; the incessant loss of sugar and of urea produce a true autophagism. The skin becomes dry, wrinkled, and scaly, while the hair and the nails usually fall out. The strength diminishes from day to day. Fatigue renders walking at first distressing, and later impossible. The exhausted patient often suffers from profuse diarrhœa, which is horribly fœtid and sometimes fatty. A profound state of cachexia, with some pyrexia, soon follows, and in the immense majority of cases death is caused by pulmonary tuberculosis, the natural end of this form of diabetes. Coma is rare.

The course of pancreatic diabetes differs from that of constitutional diabetes. The disease does not last for ten, twenty, or thirty years, but runs its course, on an average, in two years, though death may supervene in a few months. The gravity of the prognosis is therefore self-evident.

Complications.

The secondary or inconstant symptoms and the complications which may supervene in the course of diabetes are so numerous and varied that it is necessary to divide them into groups.

Cutaneous Symptoms.—Retraction of the **palmar fascia** is often seen. The skin is rough and dry; eczema, simple or gangrenous ecthyma (Hardy); erythema of the vulva and of the groin; intertrigo of the labial commissure (Hardy); friability of the nails; and preputial, vulvar, or cutaneous pruritus are frequently seen. Zona has been noted by Vergely.

Carbuncle, Cellulitis, Gangrene.—Boils, carbuncles, cellulitis, and diabetic gangrene may appear as early or late complications. They may be seen in patients who do not pass more than 30 to 60 grammes of sugar daily.

Moreover, diabetes induces a liability to parasitism. The lung of a diabetic patient is a favourable medium for the tubercle bacillus. The skin and cellular tissue are readily invaded by the microbes of suppuration. The multiplication of these microbes, which have most often entered through a graze or through a scratch in the skin, is singularly favoured by the presence of sugar in the tissues (Bujvid). Necrosis and gangrene result from circulatory troubles, but the saprogenic microbes frequently assist in the development of inflammatory moist gangrene.

Boils and carbuncles are very frequent in diabetes.

The **carbuncle** is almost always single, and is situated on the nape of the neck, on the back, or on the buttock. Its onset is insidious, without sharp reaction or acute pain. It may be complicated by gangrene and cellulitis, but yet it recovers fairly often after elimination of the sloughs. In 123 cases of diabetes Marchal saw carbuncles on seventeen occasions. Cellulitis, which is quite as frequent as carbuncle, is rarely primary; but a simple scratch, a prick (Verneuil), erysipelas, or some wound, may in a diabetic become the starting-point of the cellulitis.

Diabetic cellulitis does not present the acute reaction of a true inflammation. It is often diffuse, and may end in gangrene of the cellular tissue or in phagedæna, with fatal infection and adynamia. The cellulitis may appear at any period of the disease, although it usually occurs at a late stage. It develops with such rapidity that it demands the greatest attention on the part of the surgeon who is performing an operation on a diabetic patient. Intervention is, however, necessary.

Inflammations in diabetic patients show a notable tendency to end in gangrene, both in cases of visceral and cutaneous lesions (lung, tonsils, genital organs). Sometimes, indeed, the initial inflammatory stage presents such a slight reaction that only gangrene appears to be present; but, in addition to these gangrenous troubles, which appear to be secondary, and

which follow pneumonia, carbuncle, erysipelas, or other causes, we find in
the diabetic a primary gangrene which is somewhat similar to the so-called
senile gangrene.

Diabetic gangrene chiefly affects the lower limbs, and may assume
various forms. In some cases it is dry and superficial. It chiefly invades
the toes in the form of painful erythematous patches, which are sometimes
symmetrical. The patches end in dark eschars, which may heal or may
extend, causing mummification of large areas of skin. Gangrenous patches
may also appear on other parts of the body.

In some cases the gangrene invades all the tissues of the limb. The
toes are painful, the skin becomes bluish and cold, œdematous swelling
appears, blebs form, sanious fluid flows away, and the eschar invades the
deep parts, laying bare the muscles and the tendons.

The pathogenesis of this gangrene is multiple. We may incriminate
arteritis obliterans, blood conditions, the lower resistance of the diabetic
tissues, and the presence of saprogenic and pyogenic microbes.

Gangrene of the penis is a more rare complication. It sometimes runs
a fulminant course.

Œdema in the course of diabetes has various origins. It may result
from concomitant albuminuria, from venous thrombosis, or from cachexia.
In other cases it runs a rapid course, and is probably of neurovascular
origin (Sée).

Perforating Ulcer.—Among the trophic troubles of diabetes I may
specially mention perforating ulcer of the foot. As we shall see later, the
disease may limit its action to the soft parts, but in other cases it attacks the
bones and joints. A benign and a grave form may, therefore, be described.

In a diabetic patient perforating ulcer of the foot may appear under-
neath the little toe and at the heel, but its seat of election is beneath the
big toe. The onset is usually painless, and the condition resembles a corn.
This corn exfoliates, a pustule forms, and is gradually followed by an ulcer.
The ulcerated parts are painless, and a zone of anæsthesia is sometimes
found. The patient takes some precautions, but continues to walk about,
and the perforating ulcer thus lasts for months and years. The ulceration
recovers under influence of rest and of treatment, but is subject to recurrences. The above is the benign form of perforating diabetic ulcer. The
soft parts alone are affected. The skeleton is intact, and we find neither
gangrene nor secondary infection.

The disease, however, does not always run this course. In some cases
perforating ulcer spreads deeply, affecting the bones and joints. It gives
rise to necrosis, and results in sequestra—fistulæ, ankylosis, and deformity
of the affected parts. In other cases perforating ulcer is associated with
secondary infections—suppuration, gangrene, cellulitis, and erysipelas.

This fact proves that the prognosis of perforating ulcer in diabetes must be given with reserve.

The perforating ulcer in diabetes must not be confounded with that seen in tabes. In the former case it accompanies symptoms of diabetes; in the latter, those of tabes.

Digestive Troubles.—In the diabetic the mouth is dry, the salivary secretion is diminished, the tongue is thickened, red, sometimes pilous or cracked. The pilous appearance is due to an exaggerated proliferation of the epithelium which surrounds the papillæ. Dental caries is frequent, and is the result of alveolo-dental periostitis. The teeth, although healthy, are pushed out from the alveoli (Magitot). These phenomena are due to changes in the saliva, and probably to the presence of an acid derived from the fermentation of the sugar.

Dyspepsia is rare—or, at least, slow to appear—in spite of the quantity of fluid taken by the patient. The liver is fairly often hypertrophied, and in some cases shows the lesions of pigmentary cirrhosis described elsewhere.

Ocular Troubles.—We have already noted the diminution in the power of accommodation. Let us also note paresis of the sphincter (mydriasis). The cornea is sometimes affected (neuroparalytic keratitis, ulcerations of the cornea). The iris is often attacked (iritis—sometimes plastic, sometimes with hypopyon).

Cataract is one of the more frequent and more important complications of diabetes. It is usually double. While it is soft in young patients, it does not differ in the elderly from the ordinary senile cataract. Its course varies in rapidity according to the severity of the diabetes.

The fundus oculi may also be affected. Diabetic retinitis is characterized by more or less extensive hæmorrhages, and by exudation in the form of white rounded spots scattered over the retina. Contrary to retinitis in Bright's disease, the spots are not formed of large patches, and do not assume a star shape around the macula. The affection is sometimes complicated by white atrophy of the optic nerve; this atrophy marches progressively, and is not preceded by œdema of the papillæ. The atrophy may exist alone, independent of glycosuric retinitis (Lécorché). Lastly, we sometimes see transient amblyopia, which is not accompanied by ophthalmoscopic lesions. It is transient, and appears to be due to troubles of innervation.

Paralysis of the Motor Muscles of the Eye.—I have devoted to these paralyses a clinical lecture, of which the following is the summary : I have been able to collect 59 cases of paralysis of the oculo-motor nerves in diabetics—to wit, 33 cases of the sixth pair, 13 of the third pair, 5 of the fourth pair, and 6 of external ophthalmoplegia. In all the cases which I have just quoted diabetes alone was the cause. No other ætiological factors were present, and the patients were free from syphilis, tabes, and hysteria, as well as from general paralysis and cerebral tumour—in fact, they were affected only by diabetes.

The first point to note is that in diabetics paralysis of the sixth pair of nerves is three times as frequent as paralysis of the third pair. In syphilis and in tabes partial or total paralysis of the third pair is most frequently seen ; hence the precept that in paralysis of the sixth pair of nerves diabetes must first be thought of. Paralysis of the oculo-motor nerves in diabetes is most often transitory. They supervene suddenly, and then improve and disappear. Their mean duration is about three months. In the three cases which I have seen they lasted two and a half months and three months respectively. They may recover, however, more quickly ; but, on the other hand, they may persist longer. Recurrences are not rare. The diabetic person, who some months or some years previously has had paralysis of the sixth pair, but who has completely recovered, may suffer later from paralysis of the sixth, of the third, or of the fourth nerve, either in one or both eyes.

In five cases the paralysis extended progressively to all the motor muscles in the form of unilateral or bilateral external ophthalmoplegia. In Blanc's case, quoted by Sauvineau, ophthalmoplegia affected both eyes, and was followed by paresis of both hypoglossal and inferior facial nerves. In one of Sauvineau's cases the ophthalmoplegia was progressive and unilateral ; in another case the patient had paralysis of the left third nerve, and eighteen months later right progressive ophthalmoplegia which lasted for eight months.

There are cases in which the ocular palsies of diabetes may be the prelude of severe complications and of fatal polioencephalitis (Koenig).

Such, then, from the point of view of their evolution, are the various appearances which the ocular paralyses of diabetes may assume. The appearance of paralysis of an oculo-motor nerve in diabetics is not necessarily related to the severity of the glycosuria. In seventy-four cases which I have collected I find patients who have been affected by paralysis while they passed 200, 100, 50, 20, 12, and 3 grammes of sugar a day. Sometimes, indeed, the glycosuria disappeared when the paralysis supervened. There is no direct relation between the abundance of the glycosuria and the appearance of the paralysis.

I must next describe some special symptoms which I have seen in certain cases. Thus, one of my patients at the Hôtel-Dieu (550 grammes of sugar in twenty-four hours) was affected for a week previous to the development of sixth-nerve paralysis with severe and continuous temporo-orbital neuralgia. The pains were clearly localized to the temporal and periorbital region, and did not encroach upon the rest of the face. They increased on pressure, lasted day and night without respite, and ceased only when the paralysis declared itself. There was no question of ordinary headache in this case, but of a clearly localized neuralgia, which seemed to depend upon the same provoking cause as the paralysis. In short, it was my opinion that the patient was suffering from painful paralysis of the sixth nerve. I know that this coupling is scarcely classical, but my case is not isolated. Although pain accompanying paralysis of the oculo-motor nerves has not, as far as I know, attracted special attention, I find this symptom noted in several cases which have very kindly been placed at my disposal.

Thus, in one of Lapersonne's patients paralysis of the sixth pair was accompanied by neuralgia. In one of Galezowski's patients paralysis of the third pair of nerves was accompanied by such acute pain that ophthalmic zona was at first thought of. In one of Koenig's patients paralysis of the sixth pair was preceded and accompanied by a constricting pain around the right eye. In Nattan-Larrier's case the paralysis of the sixth pair was preceded by severe temporo-orbital neuralgia, which lasted during the whole period of the paralysis, and did not disappear until the paralysis was cured. In a diabetic patient of Buge paralysis of the fourth pair was accompanied by pain in both temples. In a diabetic patient of Charcot paralysis of the third pair was accompanied by facial neuralgia. In one of Sauvineau's diabetic patients paralysis of the left third nerve was accompanied by slight pains in the left side of the head.

We have, then, several diabetic patients in whom paralysis of an oculo-motor nerve has been preceded, accompanied or followed by neuralgic pains in the temporal region, with or without periorbital radiation on the side of the paralysis. This is not a simple coincidence, and the two symptoms (pain and paralysis) are associated here, as in painful paralysis of the seventh pair (facial nerve).

Pulmonary Complications.—The respiratory function is especially disturbed in some diabetics. Their breathing resembles that of the tree-frog. They absorb less oxygen, give off less carbonic acid and less water-vapour, and their lungs are in a state of receptivity favourable to the agents of suppuration, gangrene, tuberculosis, and pneumonia.

The larynx may be affected in the diabetic. The laryngitis declares itself by dryness in the throat (Leichtenstern), and loss of voice if conversation is prolonged. On laryngoscopic examination, the larynx and the vocal cords have a dry look.

Diabetics are exposed to congestion of the lungs, to broncho-pneumonia, which is sometimes so severe that the patient may succumb in one or two days (Bouchardat's fulminant pneumonia). As a rule, pneumonia in diabetics does not run a frank course or cause a high temperature. It may readily give rise to suppuration and gangrene, because the pathogenic agents of these complications have, as we have said, a marked predilection for the lung.

Nevertheless, true pneumonia may occur in diabetics, the sugar disappearing from the urine during the pneumonia, defervescence taking place classically on the ninth day, and the sugar reappearing immediately after recovery.

Diabetes Mellitus and Pulmonary Tuberculosis.—I believe pulmonary tuberculosis to be one of the most frequent and severe complications of diabetes mellitus. Every individual, whether young or old, who suffers from diabetes is liable to pulmonary tuberculosis.

According to Bradsley, nearly all diabetic patients die of phthisis. Bouchardat says that he found tuberculosis nineteen times in nineteen autopsies upon diabetic patients. Contour, in his thesis in 1844, considers tuberculosis as the inevitable consequence of diabetes. According to Lécorché, tuberculosis is the most frequent complication of diabetes, and Griensinger has said that out of 100 diabetics 43 die of phthisis.

Tuberculosis does not affect only the wasted and cachectic diabetics, whose daily loss of sugar amounts to some hundred grammes, but it also strikes down those whose health is apparently excellent, and whose daily loss of sugar may not exceed 30 to 40 grammes.

In one of Hanot's cases, relating to a diabetic with a large liver who became tubercular, the quantity of sugar was only about 15 grammes. In one of Tapret's cases a strong man, suffering from gout and such trifling diabetes that the glycosuria only amounted to a few grammes, nevertheless became tubercular.

In my lecture devoted to tuberculosis in diabetics* I have quoted examples of a similar nature.

Sometimes, indeed, the diabetes is so slight that the patient who comes to consult us for tuberculosis (or for so-called bronchitis) is ignorant of the fact that he is a diabetic. His thirst is in no way increased, and the quantity of urine passed does not exceed the normal. Indeed, we only discover the revealing signs of diabetes, such as genital eczema, gingivitis, and boils, by careful examination. An analysis of the urine then reveals a daily quantity of from 20 to 25 grammes of sugar. The patient has had diabetes without his knowledge, and tuberculosis has been grafted upon the diabetes.

The examples of this kind concern the most common form of pulmonary tuberculosis in diabetes—namely, the insidious apyretic form, which simulates ordinary bronchitis. The patient, who thinks that he is suffering from a cold, commences to cough and to spit, and feels so little anxiety that he does not seek advice. The cold, however, is obstinate, the sputum is thick and sometimes streaked with blood, the appetite fails, strength declines, and the patient then decides to seek advice. Before any examination the patient, who has been coughing for some weeks, already awakens our suspicions, and we find jerky expiration, with some moist and crackling

* Dieulafoy, *Clinique Médicale de l'Hôtel-Dieu*, 1905, 13me leçon.

sounds at one of the apices. Examination of the sputum reveals bacilli. The patient has become tubercular.

The tuberculosis has scarcely become installed when the scene changes. A diabetic who, without losing his strength and without wasting, has borne severe diabetes of some duration grows weak and wastes after the appearance of tuberculosis. As a rule, he does not know that he has become tubercular, and believes that he is suffering from an ordinary bronchitis, and yet he is astonished at the change in himself. He feels anxious, blames the diet and the treatment prescribed, when the condition is really due to tuberculosis.

We must, therefore, be on guard if a diabetic patient develops a cough. As far as I am personally concerned, I do not like the onset of coryza in diabetes, for I always dread the hatching of diabetic tuberculosis, which is far more severe than the ordinary form. I do not say that diabetic tuberculosis is absolutely incurable, since some cases respond to treatment, and may even recover, but they are the exception. Diabetic tuberculosis is difficult to dislodge, and the association of tuberculosis in diabetes creates a very threatening situation.

Let us next consider acute miliary tuberculosis, which may be grafted upon diabetes, as the following examples show :

One of Tapret's patients, with 200 grammes of sugar, was stricken down with acute febrile tuberculosis, which in **three weeks** caused cavernous lesions, and death in three months. A patient of Hutinel, with 100 to 120 grammes of sugar, was taken ill with tubercular broncho-pneumonia of both lungs, which proved fatal in a few weeks. Letulle's patient, with about 400 grammes of sugar, was stricken down with miliary tuberculosis, and died in eight days. The autopsy revealed tubercular nodules in most of the organs, but especially in the lungs, liver, and kidneys. Further, the apex of the right lung and one of the glands at the hilum of the lung showed older tubercular lesions.

Some authors have thought that tuberculosis in diabetes predisposes less to **hæmoptysis** than ordinary tuberculosis. This idea is wrong. Schmidt found hæmoptysis in twenty-six cases of diabetic tuberculosis. Lécorché has seen hæmoptysis sometimes at the onset, sometimes at an advanced period of diabetic tuberculosis, and in four cases the amount of hæmorrhage was considerable. For my part, I have fairly often seen abundant and repeated hæmoptysis in diabetic patients with tuberculosis. In my clinical lecture I have reported a case which, for want of room, I cannot reproduce here in detail.

A man, fifty-five years of age, had suffered from diabetes for several years. He had only passed from 25 to 30 grammes of sugar and a small quantity of albumin. One day he was seized with profuse hæmoptysis, as the revealing sign of tuberculosis in the apex of the right lung. The sputum, though scanty, contained bacilli. From this time on the hæmoptysis reappeared fairly frequently, and two years later he succumbed during an attack of hæmoptysis.

Diabetes of traumatic origin may favour an outburst of tuberculosis. Hutinel has communicated the following case to me :

A youth, born of healthy parents, had enjoyed excellent health, until one day, in a railway collision, he received a violent shock. Shortly after the accident he was taken ill with polyuria and polydipsia. The urine was examined, and showed the presence of 150 grammes of sugar. Rapid wasting supervened, and signs of pulmonary tuberculosis appeared. The phthisis, which defied all treatment, ran a rapid course, and the young man died in eight months from pulmonary tuberculosis grafted upon traumatic diabetes.

Such, then, are the various forms that pulmonary tuberculosis may assume in diabetes. The fact which surprises me is that the diabetic patient is so rarely attacked by tubercular **pleurisy,** whereas he is so often affected by pulmonary tuberculosis ; and the contrast is the more astonishing as pleurisy is one of the commonest manifestations of tubercular infection. It is difficult to explain why the pleura in the diabetic is spared to such an extent when his lung is spared so little. We meet with any number of cases of diabetic phthisis, whereas cases of tubercular pleurisy in diabetes are comparatively rare. To quote cases :

A man came into the Bichat Hospital for severe diabetes. The glycosuria mounted to 800 grammes daily. The disease was of four months' duration. At this time the man was suffering from polydipsia, polyuria, polyphagia, and rapid wasting. The diabetes improved to a marked extent as the result of diet and of antipyrin. Pain appeared, however, on the right side of the chest, the cough was frequent, the expectoration was abundant, and signs of phthisis were evident at the right apex. Some days later an effusion appeared in the right pleura. The patient became cachectic and died. The autopsy revealed a cavity in the lung. The pleura contained 3 litres of serous fluid.

With Ramon, I saw a lady suffering from diabetes and pleurisy, and at the Hôtel-Dieu I have had a diabetic who was taken ill with right hæmorrhagic pleurisy of a tubercular character, from which he recovered.

It follows, therefore, that pulmonary tuberculosis in all its forms may complicate diabetes mellitus, and we may see slow, rapid, miliary, or hæmoptoic tuberculosis. This terrible complication is seen in diabetics of all ages—children, adults, and elderly people. The most common form is ordinary tuberculosis, which at first simulates bronchitis, or a cold " which has no end."

The pathogenesis of the tuberculosis is difficult to explain. Writers were formerly inclined to consider phthisis in diabetics as the final expression of severe and cachectic diabetes. We know that it is often quite otherwise, because tuberculosis is grafted upon slight diabetes and also upon diabetes of traumatic origin. All this proves that the **saccharin medium** constitutes in the diabetic a soil extremely favourable to the fixation and growth of Koch's bacillus. I am content to note the fact without propounding theories. A healthy individual becomes diabetic. He is then more likely than another to become tubercular, no matter what is the cause and origin of the diabetes.

According to Bouchard, " diabetic phthisis exists almost exclusively in patients who also suffer from albuminuria. I have seen, says he, albuminuria absent only once in diabetic phthisis, and I have seen phthisis supervene in 18 per cent. of diabetic patients with albuminuria, while, in the total number of cases of diabetes phthisis only supervened in 8 per cent." My opinion differs from that of Bouchard, and I do not attach the same prognostic value to albuminuria. It is, of course, better if a diabetic has not albuminuria, but in many cases albuminuria is an epiphenomenon without grave results, and, in my opinion, without direct association with tuberculosis. Thus, out of twelve diabetics with tuberculosis mentioned in my clinical lecture, **eight did not suffer from albuminuria.** We must also take into account the frequent cases in which the diabetic patient already had tuberculosis when the albuminuria appeared.

As regards treatment, prophylaxis should occupy a very large place, Diabetes produces a soil favourable to the fixation and growth of Koch's bacillus, and the diabetic ought, therefore, as far as possible, to avoid all causes of contamination. A diabetic patient placed in a hospital ward with tubercular patients is more liable than others to take the infection. A diabetic who has a tubercular wife or child in his family should carry out strict hygiene in order to avoid contagion. Diabetics born of tubercular stock offer a soil doubly favourable to the hatching of tuberculosis, and should take precautions in consequence.

Nervous Complications.—The sensory or motor troubles of peripheral origin may be set down to **neuritis.** As regards the sensory troubles, anæsthesia and hyperæsthesia have both been seen. Neuralgia may affect the intercostal, sciatic, trigeminal, and vagus nerves (Peter). It is sometimes symmetrical (Worms). In a series of learned monographs, Vergely has called attention to attacks of angina pectoris associated with diabetes, to diabetic zona, and to the syringomyelic dissociation of sensibility in diabetics.

The **motor** troubles are very varied. Some diabetics experience painful lassitude and excessive muscular fatigue, principally in the muscles of the legs and of the loins. This muscular atony is explained by the dehydration of the muscles and by the insufficiency of oxygen destined for muscular respiration (Sée). It is probable that a diminution in nerve power is also associated with it. We find paralyses which are sometimes partial and limited to one arm or to a group of muscles, such as the muscles of the face, of the tongue, or of the larynx, or which are at other times general, and take the form of hemiplegia or of paraplegia. These paralyses may supervene at all periods of the disease. They have the characteristic of being incomplete and transitory.

In certain cases the paralyses depend upon cerebral arteritis obliterans, atheroma, softening, and cerebral or meningeal hæmorrhage. These various lesions, according to the case, provoke apoplexy, hemiplegia, or aphasia.

The cerebral troubles occupy an important place in the history of diabetes. The patient becomes apathetic, lazy, and has attacks of somnolence, lacking "the appetite for thought" (Lasègue). The symptom-complex of the cerebral troubles includes restlessness, delirium, aphasia, which is generally transitory, and coma. Coma is one of the most dread complications of diabetes (Kussmaul). In Frerichs' statistics, of 250 deaths caused by the complications of diabetes coma figures 153 times.

Diabetic coma is usually ushered in by vomiting, diarrhœa, abdominal pains which simulate peritonitis (Jaccoud), or by dyspnœa, and this fact gives it the greatest analogy with uræmia, from which it differs, however, in the absence of convulsions and of contractions, and in the condition of the respiration, which does not assume the Cheyne-Stokes type. The dyspnœic phase is usually preceded or accompanied by restlessness, which gives place to progressive depression. The temperature drops, the patient falls into collapse, and death occurs in a few days.

In a second variety (vertiginous form) headache and vertigo are the chief symptoms. In the third variety the symptoms comprise a small and irregular pulse, cyanosis, and coldness of the body, so that Jaccoud has called it the cardiac form. These two last varieties also end in coma, and carry off the patient in a few days or in a few hours. Coma appears at all periods of diabetes, but is more frequent in young patients, and especially as the result of travelling, fatigue, violent exercise, or overwork, whence the precept that the diabetic patient should abstain from every cause of fatigue. The pathogenesis of these cerebral troubles has been variously interpreted. Among the theories, of which no one is absolutely satisfactory, dehydration of the nerve centres and acetonæmia have been invoked.

Acetonæmia is said to result from the absorption of acetone formed at the expense of the glucose. The partisans of this theory depend upon the fact that acetone has been found in the breath (odour of chloroform), in the urine, and in the vomit of patients with diabetic coma. The theories which attribute the intoxication to acetone or to acetic acid are, however, insufficient.

In some cases sudden death occurs. It is probably due to cardiac syncope (cardiac form of coma).

Course—Termination.—Diabetes is generally insidious in its onset. There is, however, an acute form, which is sudden in its onset, and which runs a rapid course. In the slow and chronic form of diabetes the first

period is of indefinite duration.   I say indefinite, because for several years
we may find 10, 20, and 30 grammes of sugar in the urine, although the
severe symptoms of diabetes, such as polydipsia and polyuria, are not sufficiently marked to sound the alarm.   Often, too, the appetite is increased,
the patient grows stouter, and we hear these diabetics congratulating themselves on their excellent health.   In spite of this apparent health, and in
ignorance of their malady, they are exposed to many complications—
balanitis, phimosis, sexual weakness, expulsive gingivitis, attacks of boils,
carbuncles, muscular fatigue, cataract, erythema of the vulva and of the
groin, pruritus vulvæ, and intertrigo of the labial commissures (Hardy).
If they escape pulmonary tuberculosis, they are none the less liable to
gangrene, abscesses, cerebral troubles, and coma.   At this period appropriate treatment and suitable hygiene may keep them in a state of adequate
equilibrium.   It is often sufficient to regulate the diet in order to lessen the
glycosuria.

As the disease progresses the symptoms become marked; the polydipsia
and the glycosuria increase; treatment has less effect; the quantity of sugar
in the urine sometimes remains high, in spite of the suppression of saccharin
and starchy food, the sugar forming at the expense of the proteids (Jaccoud).
Examination of the urine often reveals albumin, and phosphates and sul-
phates in excess, pointing to a more general perversion of the metabolism.
The proteid matter amounts to as much as 50 and 60 grammes daily.
Azoturia is, therefore, present.   In spite of these losses in sugar, mineral
salts, and urea, the patient practically maintains his equilibrium if the
digestive functions allow him to compensate for the loss by taking abundant
nourishment.

We must now turn our attention to azoturia and albuminuria, which
have been variously interpreted from the point of view of pathogenesis and
of prognosis.

Albuminuria appears at a given moment in two-thirds of patients with
diabetes.   We may see it **just as much** in the slight as in the severe cases.
It is evidently a somewhat dangerous complication, but it has not quite
the gravity attributed by Rayer and others, who thought that it indicated
Bright's disease.   Bright's disease may certainly complicate diabetes, and
render the prognosis gloomy in arthritics with diabetes. We find post
mortem the lesions of the small gouty kidney, but this is an exception.
Albuminuria in diabetics has another origin, and it is probable that it arises
" in a more profound change of nutrition, the anatomical elements allowing
the expulsion of the albuminoid material without having caused it to
undergo the chemical changes which should reduce it to the condition of
crystalloid matter " (Bouchard).   Albuminuria has no direct relation
with azoturia.   I have often seen albuminuria supervene in diabetics

who were on too rigorous a diet. I shall return to this question under Treatment.

Azoturia, or excess of urea in the urine, is usually regarded as a constant and serious fact. Bouchard is not of the same opinion. In 100 diabetics, he found the urea normal in 40, lowered in 20, and increased in 40. Azoturia is present in slight as well as in severe diabetes. It must be remembered that marked azoturia (80 to 100 grammes daily) makes the prognosis very grave, unless these losses are compensated by rich and abundant nourishment. According to certain authors (Jaccoud), glycosuria and azoturia are two phenomena which have a common origin. Bouchard, on the other hand, considers them as independent, and having no relation " either in the series of cases or in the successive phases of a single case."

Azoturia intervenes on its own account gradually or suddenly, with marked oscillations. It represents, like diabetic albuminuria, a superadded trouble of nutrition.

Recovery from diabetes is fairly frequent in adults. On the other hand, we see cases of diabetes which treatment holds in check for several years, though finally they end fatally. When a diabetic patient wastes, when digestive troubles appear, and glycosuria persists in spite of all treatment, the prognosis becomes very grave. In some cases the patient succumbs from cachexia. The wasting becomes extreme, the temperature is subnormal, the albuminuria increases, and the sugar often **diminishes or disappears.** The patient, as a rule, succumbs before this period of cachexia. Cellulitis, carbuncles, gangrene, pneumonia, phthisis, and diabetic coma are among the many causes of death.

Pancreatic diabetes, as we have seen, runs an extremely rapid course.

Defaced Diabetes.—Under this term, Achard and Weil have described a constitutional diabetes without glycosuria analogous to Bright's disease without albuminuria. This diabetes is revealed by glycosuria consecutive to the subcutaneous injection of glucose. If a small quantity of glucose was already present in the urine, the glycosuria shows a very marked increase ; if glucose was not present in the urine, the appearance of glycosuria denotes defaced diabetes.

Diabetes in Children.—Diabetes, though rare in children, is extremely grave, because it assumes from the first the wasting form, with rapid course, and because it frequently terminates in tuberculosis or in coma. It is in children especially that we may recognize the importance of heredity in the ætiology of diabetes.

Diabetes and the Puerperal State.—Simple glycosuria is here an incident without special consequences. While it is rare during pregnancy, it is more frequent at the commencement of the nursing period, and shows itself by a loss of sugar which varies from 50 centigrammes to 3 grammes.

When a diabetic woman becomes pregnant, what happens to her and her child ? Diabetes causes premature births in 30 per cent. of cases. Labour usually comes on at the seventh month. Reciprocally, pregnancy makes the diabetes active, and the quantity of sugar may be doubled about the sixth month of pregnancy.

Maternal diabetes is most serious, both to the premature and to the full-term child. In the latter case the child dies in the proportion of 50 per cent., either during labour or shortly after birth. Labour in diabetic women is so serious that from 30 to 40 per cent. die, either from coma or from ulterior complications. In the face of such results, a diabetic woman should be advised not to marry—or, at least, she should be warned of the serious dangers of pregnancy.

Traumatic diabetes will be discussed in Section VII. **Bronzed diabetes** has been discussed under Pigmentary Hypertrophic Cirrhosis.

The Liver in Diabetes.—The liver is normal in a large number of cases. It is neither hypertrophied nor cirrhosed. This integrity of the liver is found both in mild and in severe diabetes. I had the following case under my care :

A man was suffering from very severe diabetes mellitus. The urine had a specific gravity of 1039. It contained no albumin. The amount of urea was 62 grammes. The glycosuria was considerable, and in one analysis 120·50 grammes per litre were found—that is to say, 1,084·50 grammes in 9 litres, or more than a kilogramme in the twenty-four hours. I was anxious to know how much alcohol this sugar represented, and I asked Corlay to undertake the necessary examination. A test was made one day when the patient had passed 9 litres of urine containing 800 grammes of sugar. The result was 350 grammes of alcohol.

In spite of the enormous quantity of food and drink taken for several months, the stomach was not dilated, and the digestive functions did their work perfectly. **The liver was normal,** measuring barely 11 centimetres in its vertical diameter, and **showed no hypertrophy.** He had not escaped one of the most grave complications—namely, tuberculosis. I could not define the exact onset of the lung trouble, because it took the insidious form of a simple bronchitis. For a year he had been subject to " bronchitis," and had several times been compelled to lie up. The cough was followed by thick and abundant expectoration, the strength was failing, and the wasting was marked, although the polyphagia had in no way diminished. The patient had no fever, and did not suffer from night-sweats. Auscultation revealed at the apex of the right lung, both in front and behind, signs of softening ; large râles, dry and moist crackling sounds. The region was dull on percussion, and the vibrations were increased. The sputum was muco-purulent, and bacilli were present in large numbers.

For seven months the patient continued to pass 600 to 700 grammes of sugar daily, and the liver **remained normal.** Finally he died, and the results of the autopsy were as follows : **The liver was absolutely normal** ; it weighed 1,450 grammes, and presented no trace of cirrhosis. The bile-ducts were healthy. The pancreas was absolutely normal, and Wirsung's duct was patent from its origin to its opening in the duodenum.

In some cases of diabetes the liver is hypertrophied or cirrhotic. I am not speaking, of course, of complex cases, in which the patient is both diabetic and alcoholic, tubercular, malarial, or syphilitic. In such cases we are frequently in doubt as to whether the hypertrophy and the cirrhosis are due to diabetes alone, or to other previous or concomitant diseases. I am not speaking here of bronzed diabetes, described in detail under Pigmentary Cirrhosis, but I allude to the hepatic complications of diabetes mellitus alone. Bernard, extending his discovery of hepatic glycogenesis to the pathogenesis of diabetes, declared that diabetes mellitus must be " localized in the liver," and yet treatises on diabetes have for the past fifteen or twenty years made only passing mention of the condition of the liver (Frerichs, Durand-Fardel, Griesinger).

Lécorché was the first to call attention to the frequency of hepatomegalia in diabetes. We might almost, says he, consider hypertrophy of the liver as one of the constant symptoms of diabetes mellitus. This hypertrophy usually affects the whole liver. It is rarely partial.

The researches of the physicians at Vichy, who have seen a very large number of diabetics, have helped to clear up the question. Glénard and Frémont have often found this hypertrophy of the liver (60 per cent.; and 44 in 105). The researches of Glénard comprise the examination of 324 cases. He found that hepatomegalia is the most frequent of the organic changes in diabetes, and thinks that it is most often partial. In 68 per cent. of the cases observed by Glénard one lobe, usually the right, was hypertrophied. The liver was indurated in the proportion of 38 in 200, and sensitive to pressure in the proportion of 23 in 100.

Chauffard says that we may find changes in the liver of diabetics varying from congestive lesions similar to those of the cardiac liver to typical cases of porto-biliary and bivenous cirrhosis, and this idea agrees well with that of hepatic phlebitis in diabetic cirrhosis.

In my clinical lecture on the liver in diabetics* I have had occasion to quote facts concerning hypertrophy and cirrhosis of the liver. To quote an example of hypertrophy :

One of my patients at the Hôtel-Dieu was suffering from severe diabetes. He drank from 8 to 9 litres of fluid, and passed about the same quantity of urine, which showed a specific gravity of 1032. It contained neither albumin nor indican. The analysis showed 85·50 grammes of sugar per litre, or 675 grammes daily. The quantity of urea was slightly increased. The appetite was in proportion to the thirst. In spite of the enormous quantity of food and drink ingested, the digestive functions were perfect, the tongue had quite a rosy colour, the teeth were not exposed, the stomach was not dilated, and there was neither constipation nor diarrhœa. **The liver in this patient was very large,** reaching three fingers' breadth below the false ribs ; but it was not painful, indurated, or deformed. As we found no other cause to explain the hypertrophy of the liver—for the patient was neither alcoholic nor suffering from malarial fever nor cardiac disease — we thought of pure diabetic hypertrophy. This hypertrophy was not complicated by cirrhosis, for not a sign of cirrhosis or of precirrhosis

---

* Dieulafoy, " Le Foie des Diabétiques " (*Clinique Médicale de l'Hôtel - Dieu,* 1903, 13me leçon).

was present. Collateral circulation and ascites were absent. In a few weeks the situation became worse, and the quantity of sugar, which was always very large, varied from 650 to 750 grammes daily. Diabetic coma then appeared, and the man died after seven months' illness.

The autopsy furnished the following results : The pancreas was absolutely normal, no gravel in the pancreatic ducts, thus proving that diabetes may be rapid and most severe, although the pancreas is healthy. The liver, on the other hand, **was very much enlarged,** and weighed 2,300 grammes. Apart from this general hypertrophy, we found no other lesion in the organ. Its consistency and its colour were normal. Induration, fatty changes, cirrhosis, and pigmentation were absent. The hypertrophy was therefore simple, and the case was one of enlarged diabetic liver without cirrhosis.

Gilbert speaks of a diabetic patient suffering from simple hypertrophy of the liver. At the autopsy the enlarged liver weighed 2,510 grammes. Fatty degeneration and appreciable cellular lesions were absent. The pancreas was normal. This case is absolutely comparable to that of my patient, who also had severe diabetes and a very large liver, without degeneration and without cirrhotic lesions.

In a diabetic patient of Tapret the autopsy revealed a large liver of 2,210 grammes. The organ was not hard on section, which appears to indicate simple hypertrophy without cirrhoses.

Some diabetics may, therefore, have a very large liver without cirrhosis, while others show hypertrophy with cirrhosis. If the patient is an alcoholic, as in Gilbert's two cases, hypertrophic cirrhosis cannot be attributed exclusively to diabetes, but there are undoubted cases of enlarged cirrhotic livers in diabetics without alcoholism, as the following examples prove :

Hanot, in a critical review on cirrhosis of the liver, reports the case of a patient admitted for diabetes. The urine contained 12 grammes of sugar per litre, and the patient also showed signs of hepatic cirrhosis. She died of coma, and the autopsy gave the following results : The liver, which was larger than normal, weighed 1,900 grammes. Its surface was nodular, but less so than in atrophic cirrhosis. On section the tissue was resistant, of a chamois-leather colour, and slightly granular. Microscopical examination showed that the intralobular vein was much dilated, being three times its normal diameter, and embedded in a fibrous coat, surrounded by a zone of embryonic cells. Hanot, in seeking to explain the pathogenesis of the cirrhosis, asks whether diabetes was not the cause. " In diabetes," says he, " the blood of the intralobular vein contains a much larger quantity of hepatic sugar than in the normal condition. It would not be impossible that this sugar in excess might, as regards the cells of the intralobular vein, play the same part as that played by alcohol or by blood-pigment with regard to the radicals of the portal vein in perilobular venous cirrhosis." Accordingly, as Triboulet remarks, this interpretation is probable, and the action of the diabetic poisoning on the internal coat of the vessels has been confirmed byLécorché and Ferraro.

Some years ago, at the Hôtel-Dieu, I saw hypertrophic cirrhosis with ascites in a diabetic patient. The diabetes appeared to me to be the sole cause of this cirrhosis. A man, fifty-two years of age, came under my care with his belly distended by a peritoneal effusion, estimated at several litres. The collateral circulation was well marked, but jaundice was absent. The ascites was three months old. It had developed slowly, without pain, and without any of the digestive troubles which almost always mark the course of Laënnec's cirrhosis. Moreover, the patient had not the appearance seen in cirrhosis : he had preserved his stoutness, his face was neither earthy nor bronzed, the conjunctivæ were scarcely tinged, and the urine was normal in quantity, and contained only a little urobilin, without any red-brown pigment. The liver, as could be felt by dipping, was hypertrophied, and reached an inch below the costal margin. The spleen was slightly enlarged. The case was therefore one of cirrhosis with an enlarged liver. The patient was not an alcoholic, and had not suffered from syphilis, malarial fever, or cardiac disease. There was nothing in his past history to explain this cirrhosis, except the diabetes mellitus, from which he had suffered for about three years, and which he had discovered himself. As he had great thirst and one day found that some drops of urine left a whitish deposit, he conceived the idea of having it examined : 140 grammes of sugar were passed in twenty-four hours. For three years the glycosuria underwent various changes, according to the diet which was taken.

When he came under my care he was passing only 12 grammes of sugar daily; polydipsia, polyphagia, and polyuria were absent. The absence of any other ætiological factor led me to conclude that it was a case of hypertrophic cirrhosis due to diabetes, but without any relation to the pigmentary cirrhosis of bronzed diabetes, in which the symptoms are very different. I considered this diabetic hepatomegalia as related to the cases of which I spoke above. The patient was put on the diet which I usually order for diabetics. He was punctured twice, and left my ward four months later, showing notable improvement.

I had under my care a patient of whom I shall have to speak presently in connection with saccharine ascites in diabetes. This patient, who was not alcoholic, had diabetes and a very large liver, with cirrhosis. Finally he died, and the histological examination made by Jolly gave the following results : The surface of the liver was granular, Glisson's capsule was somewhat thickened, and the consistency of the organ was notably increased. In sections of the liver we saw with the naked eye yellowish points of the size of a hepatic lobule, separated by parts of a clear grey colour. A fragment of liver was divided into small pieces, which were fixed by alcohol, Müller's fluid, and osmic acid. Under the microscope the normal topography of the liver was no longer recognizable. The hepatic tissue was made up of a certain number of islets, of variable sizes, and more or less rounded. These islets did not correspond to the hepatic lobules ; they were formed of hepatic cells in which the bands no longer had their usual radial disposition. In the connective tissue, between the islets, we found portal veins, bile-ducts, and also hepatic veins. In the centre of some islets, we found the cut section of a hepatic vein, surrounded by a zone of connective tissue. We also found in the connective bands masses of lymphoid cells and isolated groups of hepatic cells. A few cells were undergoing granulo-fatty degeneration. In short, the cirrhosis was hypertrophic in character, with small granules, which chiefly affected the portal system, thus closely resembling alcoholic cirrhosis, although the patient had not been a heavy drinker.

It is difficult to explain the different pathological varieties of the diabetic liver. The difficulty is quite as great when we try to estimate the respective share of the diabetes and of the hepatic hypertrophy. In a patient suffering from diabetes and a very large liver we cannot always decide whether the diabetes has produced the enlarged liver or whether the enlarged liver has produced the diabetes. Gilbert and Lereboullet, in two cases, admit that the enlarged liver, diseased through alcoholism, produced diabetes. On the other hand, Hanot admits that in his patient it was the diabetes which produced the enlarged liver.

In finding an explanation for these apparently contradictory facts, can we employ the recent researches undertaken by several authorities ? According to Gilbert and his collaborators, Weil, Carnot, and Lereboullet, there are two varieties of diabetes which depend upon a functional disturbance of the liver. The former is the result of chronic insufficiency of the liver, and is called diabetes by **anhepatia.** The latter is the result of functional hyperactivity of the liver, and is known as diabetes by **hyperhepatia.**

Diabetes by anhepatia results from the fact that the liver is chronically incapable of retaining the sugar ingested with the food or formed in the alimentary canal. In such a case the glycosuria does not come from the sugar manufactured by the liver, but from the sugar in the foodstuffs which the liver has let by. Thus, we find sugar in the urine after meals, while it disappears during periods of fasting. The glycosuria is never high, and rarely reaches more than 40 to 50 grammes. The quantity of urine passed does not exceed 1·5 to 2 litres. The amount of urea is somewhat low, and varies from 15 to 20 grammes. Indicanuria and urobilinuria are frequent. This slight diabetes does not induce severe symptoms—polydipsia, polyuria, polyphagia, and autophagia—but it may provoke numerous complications—boils, carbuncles, cataract, genital diabetides, and expulsive gingivitis—proving " that the condition is true diabetes, and not alimentary glycosuria." This anhepatic diabetes is curable. The prognosis is not grave, and it does not end in gangrene or coma. Nevertheless, it opens the door to tuberculosis. With regard to its size, the liver is normal. It may, however, be enlarged.

According to the same authorities, diabetes by hyperhepatia is different. The functional activity of the liver is increased, and the sugar passed in the urine may reach several hundred grammes. Instead of finding signs of hepatic insufficiency, with indicanuria and urobilinuria, we see a notable degree of azoturia. The urea is in excess. The liver is enlarged, with or without cirrhotic lesions. This hyperhepatic diabetes induces all the complications of the constitutional disease—namely, tuberculosis, coma, and cachexia. Opotherapy—that is to say, treatment by liver extract—is harmful in this condition, because it increases the hepatic function. It is indicated in anhepatic diabetes, in which the functions of the liver are insufficient. The diabetes called hyperhepatic may, according to Gilbert and Lereboullet, be connected with pigmentary hypertrophic cirrhosis, with certain forms of hypertrophic alcoholic cirrhosis, with some kinds of biliary cirrhosis, and with certain cases of traumatic and of pancreatic diabetes, in which the lesions of the pancreas provoke less activity in that organ, and, consequently, more activity in the liver. The latter fact is proved by opotherapy. Pancreatic extract given to a patient suffering from diabetes with hyperhepatia diminishes the production of sugar, whilst extract of pancreas given to a patient suffering from diabetes with anhepatia increases the production of sugar. " Pancreatic extract is indicated in cases of diabetes from hyperhepatia. It should not be administered in diabetes from anhepatia, which is, on the other hand, benefited by hepatic extract" (Gilbert).

These considerations are interesting, and the distinction between anhepatic and hyperhepatic diabetes is ingenious, but the liver **may be enlarged in both cases.** Further, many cases of diabetes cannot be placed in this classification, and here, as often happens in clinical medicine, the intermediary types somewhat absorb the extreme ones.

Besides, hyperhepatia or functional hyperactivity of the liver is not sufficient to explain the hypertrophy of the organ. I had under my care two patients who were not alcoholic. One of them passed an average of 700 grammes of sugar in the twenty-four hours, and died with an enlarged liver weighing 2,300 grammes. The other patient for a long time passed about 800 grammes of sugar, and his liver was absolutely normal, as the autopsy proved. How can we reconcile such divergences?

If we admit that the hypertrophy in the first patient was due to functional hyperactivity of the organ, it is difficult to explain why the liver in the second patient preserved its normal size. I know that some may answer that functional hyperactivity may exist, whether the organ is or is not hypertrophied. Furthermore, the same objection is applicable to the theory which considers hypertrophy of the liver as the result of diabetes. If diabetes in which 700 grammes of sugar are passed (as in my first patient) is capable of causing an enlarged liver, it is difficult to explain why diabetes with 800 grammes (as in the second patient) should leave the liver normal. And, however little we may wish to reconcile the two theories of diabetes capable of causing an enlarged liver, and of an enlarged liver capable of causing diabetes, we are engaged in a vicious circle which is not at all banal, and the large liver in diabetes may be at the same time the thing created and the creator. This fact proves, in short, that the pathogenesis of diabetes and of the enlarged liver in diabetes is still shrouded in obscurity.

Saccharin Ascites.—Sugar may be found in ascites of various origins. Thus, the fluid of chylous ascites sometimes contains sugar. Bahrgebuhr, in his work on chylous and chyliform ascites, states that sugar was present seven times in fifty-two cases, and as much as 8 grammes of sugar per litre has been found in the ascitic fluid. Guttmann, Strauss, and Ballmann think that the absence of sugar is a proof that the case is not one of true chylous ascites. Senator, however, observes that the absence of sugar does not allow us to deny the presence of chyle in the ascitic fluid, for the composition of the chyle may be modified by its admixture with other exudates.

The variety of saccharin ascites now under discussion is quite different.

It is consecutive to diabetes. Let me quote here a case from my clinical lecture on this subject :

A man, fifty-three years of age, came under my care with œdema of the legs and ascites, which had lasted two months. The ascites was related to hypertrophic cirrhosis of the liver, and the cirrhosis was itself associated with diabetes, from which the man was suffering. The diabetes, however, was better at the time. The quantity of sugar, which had been 150 grammes two years ago, was only 4·50 grammes when the patient came into hospital. The abdomen was tapped, and 15 litres of fluid were drawn off. The fluid reformed so quickly that in the two months preceding death eight tappings were performed, and gave a total of 122 litres of fluid. It is remarkable to note that the ascitic fluid contained sugar, and there was a fairly direct relationship between the quantity of sugar passed in the urine and the quantity of sugar in the peritoneal fluid. When the patient had only a few grammes of sugar in the urine, he had practically none in the ascitic fluid. When the sugar in the urine increased, the sugar in the ascitic fluid was proportionately augmented. Here are the comparative results furnished by several abdominal tappings :

November 14 : 16 litres of fluid drawn off. Sugar in the urine, 47 grammes ; sugar in the ascitic fluid, 45 grammes.

November 24 : 14 litres of fluid drawn off. Sugar in the urine, 50 grammes ; sugar in the ascitic fluid, 56 grammes.

December 4 : 16 litres of fluid drawn off. Sugar in the urine, 52 grammes ; sugar in the ascitic fluid, 56 grammes.

December 12 : 14 litres of fluid drawn off. Sugar in the urine, 45 grammes ; sugar in the ascitic fluid, 29 grammes.

December 21 : 15 litres of fluid drawn off. Sugar in the urine, 50 grammes ; sugar in the ascitic fluid, 50 grammes.

December 29 : 16 litres of fluid drawn off. Sugar in the urine, 160 grammes ; sugar in the ascitic fluid, 80 grammes.

January 11 : 16 litres of fluid drawn off. Sugar in the urine, 140 grammes ; sugar in the ascitic fluid, 70 grammes.

I would remind the reader that the patient had an enlarged cirrhotic liver. The histological examination has been described on p. 1918. It is clear that in this case the sugar contained in the blood (hyperglycæmia) passed through the kidneys and peritoneum, and thus gave rise to sugar in the urine and sugar in the ascites. Its passage into the peritoneum was facilitated by the slowing of the circulation in the portal veins, and by the elevation of blood-pressure in these vessels. The cirrhosis of the liver consequently favoured the transudation of the ascitic fluid and the passage of the sugar. The ascitic fluid with its sugar passed through the endothelium.

I am of opinion that the variety of cirrhosis is of little import in the production of saccharin ascites in diabetics. The important fact is the presence of cirrhosis, which facilitates ascites, and sugar is found in the ascitic fluid if the patient suffers from severe diabetes.

In short, this case proves that we may find ascitic fluid containing 40, 60, and 80 grammes of sugar in diabetics with a large cirrhotic liver. The quantity of sugar in the ascitic fluid varies with the quantity of sugar in

II. 122

the urine. It increases or diminishes in direct proportion. The sugar appears to me to favour the rapid and abundant reproduction of the ascites, just as it favours polyuria. Indeed, we may say that the sugar affects the ascites, just as it affects the urine. Saccharin ascites appears to me to be reproduced more quickly and more severely than in the non-saccharin forms, and saccharin ascites in a diabetic certainly makes the prognosis worse.

Saccharin ascites in diabetics has not been, as far as I am aware, the subject of any complete work, but yet it has been noted by certain authors. Lépine, who has made most important researches on diabetes, has given me the results of his great experience regarding saccharin ascites in diabetics. He has not had the opportunity of studying in a conclusive manner the quantity of sugar contained in the ascites of diabetics, but he has found in some cases high percentages which almost express the quantity of urinary sugar at the same time. He saw a diabetic woman who passed 70 grammes of sugar in the urine, and who had ascites. She became phthisical, and the sugar disappeared from the urine. The ascites was tapped, and sugar was not found. According to Lépine, sugar is frequent at some period in the ascites of diabetics, and it disappears when it is absent from the urine.

When pleurisy occurs in a diabetic patient it may be saccharin. I have seen two remarkable examples of this. The first case was that of a lady whom I saw in consultation with Ramon. The second case was that of a diabetic woman I had in the Hôtel-Dieu. She recovered from the pleurisy, which was at the same time tubercular, hæmorrhagic, and saccharic.

Diagnosis.—I have dwelt on the usually insidious onset of diabetes, so that we may be on our guard against an error in diagnosis. If glucose is found in the urine, we must ascertain whether the patient is suffering from simple glycosuria or from diabetes. This delimitation of the symptom and of the disease is not always possible. The question is often only one of degree, and what is thought to be a simple glycosuria is the forerunner of diabetes.

We must avoid confusion between tabes and diabetes. The abolition of the patellar reflexes, the pains in the limbs, the expulsive gingivitis, the amblyopia, and the partial paralysis of the muscles of the eye, are all symptoms common to diabetes and to tabes. In diabetics they may give rise to a **pseudo-tabes.** In other cases diabetes and tabes run a parallel course. Not that they depend upon one another, but they both belong to the same nervous source, of which I spoke under the Ætiology of Diabetes.

Prognosis.—The prognosis in diabetes should not be considered as absolutely bad. The disease is very serious in children, and it is also very formidable when it runs a rapid course and induces cachexia (pancreatic diabetes of some authors). Certain complications may give rise to serious alarm (gangrene, tuberculosis, coma), but they are exceptional.   Many patients, with care and good hygiene, survive for an indefinite period.   I have treated many diabetics, and serious troubles have appeared to me to be exceptional in those who are willing to treat the disease with respect. We must not base the prognosis on hospital results, because most hospital cases are far advanced or are suffering from severe complications.

When we examine the cases of diabetes seen in private practice, we find that the serious ones do not exceed 6 or 8 per cent.   In the benign cases, which form the very great majority, we find persons who pass 15, 20, or 30 grammes of sugar daily, and who improve as long as they take care of themselves.   " Nothing is more common than to see persons in a state of alarm because they have learnt in some way or other that their urine contains sugar.   It is very advantageous for the future of persons with mild diabetes, who constitute the great majority of cases, and take care of themselves, to know that the severe cases are rare " (Worms).   On the other hand, the gravity of the prognosis is considerable in **pancreatic diabetes,** death being the usual ending.

Pathological Anatomy.—The lesions found post mortem are not constant.   Nevertheless, the liver and the kidney frequently show changes.

The liver may show congestion, hypertrophy, or cirrhosis.

The lesions of the kidneys are important.   They have thus been summed up by Straus :

" As regards the renal lesions in diabetes, we find that, in addition to the common lesions, such as interstitial, parenchymatous, or diffuse nephritis, etc., there exists a special alteration, both as regards its nature and also as regards its topography.   As regards topography, this change clearly and exclusively affects the zona limitans, where it involves the straight tubules of Henle (large and small), and also, in my opinion, some of the collecting tubules.   This lesion does not occupy the whole of the zona limitans, but is confined to more or less numerous and extensive foci, especially in the neighbourhood of the capillaries.   As regards the nature of the lesion, it presents histologically two forms, according to the stains employed.   With ordinary stains, we find a hyaline or vitreous change in the cells lining the tubules.   This lesion was discovered by Armanni.   If we employ, with proper precautions, iodized gum, the same cells are seen to be infiltrated with glycogen.   This change was discovered by Ehrlich."

Treatment.—The treatment of diabetes has given rise to numerous works, and Robin has made important communications on the subject. My personal view of the matter is as follows :

Food.—The patient should abstain completely from sugar.   We may, nevertheless, permit him to sweeten his tea or his coffee with saccharin. He must not eat pastry, entremets with sugar, sweet fruits, and, above all, raisins. He must choose wines which are not sweet. Beer and milk are allowed. Milk is, indeed, an excellent food for the diabetic (Frémont), for lactose has nothing to do with glucose. I have often prescribed a milk cure in diabetics who also suffered from albuminuria, and they did well.

If I am extremely severe on drinks or foods which contain sugar, I am less so as regards starchy foods. I do not say, of course, that the diabetic should be allowed to eat bread, potatoes, and farinaceous foods *ad libitum*, but I do say that it is a mistake to suppress them completely. According to the particular case, we may replace bread by gluten bread, or bread made with almond meal (Pavy's bread); but this is not a reason for prohibiting wheaten bread completely, and the crust may especially be allowed. I also allow some potatoes, and I do not absolutely prohibit sauces, which assist the alimentation.

It is harmful, in my opinion, to attempt the total suppression of glycosuria by a Draconian régime. The diabetic, who has been robust and healthy, with 60, 80, and 100 grammes of sugar daily, wastes and becomes feeble if put on an absolutely rigid diet with the object of suppressing the glycosuria totally and rapidly. Under the influence of an extreme diet the sugar may indeed disappear very quickly from the urine—at least, for a time—but the patient is liable to complications, such as albuminuria, wasting, and tuberculosis, which are sometimes formidable.

I often see diabetics who have been treated, or who treat themselves, with the greatest severity by the absolute deprivation of starchy food until there is no longer any trace of sugar in the urine. Many of them waste, while the physician applauds the result of the analysis and the disappearance of the sugar. A diabetic submitted to this extreme régime recently said to me : " I was passing $2\frac{1}{2}$ ounces of sugar, and was prescribed such a severe diet that, except for meat without sauce, fish without sauce, eggs, some vegetables and gluten bread, no food was given me. The sugar certainly disappeared in four weeks, but I have lost 13 pounds in weight, my appetite has disappeared, and I feel terribly weak. Give me back my sugar. I really prefer it." And this patient was not wrong.

I have often noticed the appearance of albuminuria following upon too severe antidiabetic treatment. The sugar diminishes or disappears, and albuminuria makes its appearance.

Lastly, if we only remember that tuberculosis threatens the diabetic, we shall understand that we must beware of opening the door to it by inducing, through too severe diet, wasting, which the diabetic should always avoid.

I cannot too strongly insist upon these considerations, and for many years I have done my best to spread them in my writings and my teaching. In diabetics in whom glycosuria is obstinate I do not attempt to bring about the disappearance of all the sugar, and I prefer that the diabetic should have some sugar rather than see him lose in weight.

In short, the régime should not be too severe, especially at first. **It is necessary to know how to handle these patients.** Starchy foods, potatoes, and bread should not be absolutely forbidden. The whole question depends on the severity of the disease and the general condition of the patient.

The patient should never repress his thirst. He should drink water in sufficient quantity, because he thus prevents dehydration of the tissues and favours elimination of the sugar.

Drugs.—The drug treatment of diabetes is based on antipyrin, arsenical preparations, and alkaline remedies. Antipyrin is, in such a case, a wonderful remedy. It must not be given in large doses or for long periods. My method is as follows :

For the first week in the month the patient takes twice daily with meals a cachet composed of 5 grains of antipyrin and 3 grains of bicarbonate of soda. If the diabetes is severe, we may double or treble the number of cachets.

During the second week of the month the antipyrin is stopped, and arsenic prescribed. The patient takes with each meal a teaspoonful of a solution containing 2 ounces of distilled water and $\frac{1}{2}$ gramme of arseniate of soda. It is better, however, to give a daily injection of $\frac{1}{2}$ grain of caco-dylate of soda (*vide* Appendix on Therapeutics).

These two drugs are continued alternately for several months, together with alkaline solutions, such as Vichy water (Célestins) (8 ounces at each meal). The cures at Vichy and at Carlsbad are very efficacious.

Hygiene.—Baths, douches, and massage should be prescribed. Walking or riding, fencing and swimming, are excellent in order to increase the destruction of the muscle sugar. Profuse sweating should be avoided, and we must not forget that symptoms of diabetic coma appear after fatigue, excess, or long journeys.

Opotherapy, with **hepatic extract,** appears to have some action on the glycosuria in some patients (Gilbert and Chassevant), notably in those who have functional insufficiency of the liver, with diminution of urea, uro-bilinuria, etc. When the glycosuria appears to depend on hepatic hyper-activity, opotherapy aggravates the disease. I have attempted to ascertain the possible efficacy of subcutaneous injections of pancreatic juice in diabetics. I have not obtained any satisfactory result.

Surgical intervention is often necessary in diabetics (carbuncles, phleg-mon, gangrene). Surgeons formerly did not dare to operate on patients with diabetes for fear of the after-results. Since aseptic and antiseptic methods have been employed, we have found that these fears are greatly exaggerated. The surgeon may intervene with excellent results in diabetes, but yet we must not hide the fact that operations performed under such circumstances are not absolutely free from mishaps.

Intoxication is the more to be feared in the diabetic if the liver and the kidneys are affected. When the disease runs a rapid course, with cachexia and ascites, the patient will not be able to stand an operation as well as one in whom the disease runs a slow course, and scarcely affects the nutrition.

In any case, we have to consider the administration of chloroform, and to take account of the **erythemata** which develop spontaneously or as the result of antiseptics. We must remember that some antiseptics may cause severe toxic troubles through imperfect elimination by reason of the lesions in the liver and the kidney. Lastly, it is necessary to remember that the lowered vitality of the tissues is sometimes opposed to the firm holding of sutures and to the rapid healing of wounds.

VI. DIABETES INSIPIDUS.

1. Azoturic Diabetes — Azoturia.

The excess of nitrogenous matter in the urine is not sufficient to constitute azoturic diabetes. Azoturia is a symptom common to several morbid conditions, while azoturic diabetes (Demange), like diabetes mellitus, is a general disease characterized by an exaggerated and constant loss of nitrogenous matter and by general symptoms—polyuria, polydipsia, and polyphagia—which somewhat recall the clinical picture of diabetes mellitus.

Description.—The disease may commence suddenly. It is ushered in by ravenous hunger (Bouchard), profuse sweats (Rendu), or by unquenchable thirst. Most frequently it installs itself insidiously. The thirst and the appetite increase progressively, and the urine becomes very copious.

The **urine,** which is acid and transparent directly it is passed, soon becomes alkaline and turbid, and contains mucus and sediments (uric acid and urates), but no sugar or albumin. Its density varies from 1002 to 1015, according to the amount passed. It is azoturic—that is to say, it contains an excess of urea, of uric acid, and of nitrogenous extractives. In twenty-four hours the urea may amount to 100 grammes (Bouchardat), instead of the normal 25 grammes. The uric acid may be as much as 9 grammes (Bouchardat), and the nitrogenous extractives (creatinin, uroxanthin) may exceed 70 grammes (Bouchard). A similar excess is noticed as regards the chlorides and phosphates.

In cases of moderate severity the disease may last indefinitely without becoming dangerous, but in grave cases the muscular power decreases, the patient experiences excessive fatigue, and is exposed to the nervous troubles described under Diabetes Mellitus. He may suffer from hæmorrhages into the retina and the vitreous, which are far from being rare in azoturia, just as in phosphaturia (Trousseau). At a more advanced period the appetite is lost, the wasting becomes extreme, and cachectic œdema appears. Death supervenes by reason of this excessive denutrition or of some complications (hæmorrhage, gangrene, phthisis). In spite of the gravity of the **prognosis,** definite recovery has several times been recorded.

The **diagnosis** depends entirely on the examination of the urine. The examination is the more important as in some cases the azoturia is excessive, while the polyuria is absent (Bouchard). Azoturic diabetes is sometimes associated with phosphaturia, and, indeed, phosphaturia may assume such importance that Teissier has described a separate form of phosphatic diabetes.

Ætiology—Pathogenesis.—Azoturic diabetes is most frequent during the middle period of life. It appears to arise chiefly from nervous causes, violent emotions, grief, cerebral lesions, traumatism, and syphilis.

As regards the intimate nature of the disease, it is probable that it depends upon an exaggerated disassimilation of the tissues. In this process are we to incriminate chiefly the liver, which, according to recent theories, is the true source of urea? If, however, the liver makes urea, it is at the expense of the albuminoid material, which is split up into glycogen and urea. As Demange observes, in azoturic diabetes there is no glycosuria, and therefore the theory is at fault. Azoturia is a general disturbance of nutrition, which probably results from the nervous system. At the moment our knowledge does not extend farther.

As regards treatment, the patient must be kept at rest, and well nourished, especially with proteid food; drugs which appear to limit the denutrition should be prescribed—arsenic, valerian, and opium in large doses.

2. Essential Polyuria.

Essential polyuria is often called diabetes insipidus. I have not to describe the secondary polyuria which is associated with various morbid conditions (Bright's disease, hysteria), but I have only essential polyuria in view.

Description.—Polyuria and polydipsia, which naturally results, form the whole disease. Certain individuals drink and pass 10, 20, or 30 litres of water in the twenty-four hours, and, indeed, these figures have been exceeded. The necessity to pass water is frequent and imperative, and may cause insomnia through disturbing the night's rest. The thirst is excessive, and we see patients who swallow 1 or 2 litres of fluid at a gulp. Deprivation of fluid is so intolerable to them that they will drink anything

TEXT-BOOK OF MEDICINE

which comes to hand. They never go to bed without having made provision for the night. They do not go on a journey without taking special precautions.

This disease sometimes commences suddenly. It may last for a long while without compromising health, since the economy suffers no loss, and the clear, limpid urine, of low specific gravity, does not contain more solids in the twenty-four hours than normal urine. Nevertheless, says Trousseau, we must not rely too much on the so-called benignity of the essential polyuria.

We do not see here the nervous troubles and the disorders of nutrition which are so characteristic of diabetes mellitus. The intellectual faculties are intact and the genital functions are normal. Pulmonary phthisis, which is very frequent in diabetes, has only been found twice in seventy cases (Lancereaux).

Essential polyuria may last for years without compromising life. The digestive functions are, however, often sluggish, and constipation is very obstinate. Children do not stand this disease so well.

We know but little of the causes and of the pathogenesis of essential polyuria. In some cases the disease is hereditary. Many observations prove the influence of nervous causes, acute emotions, head injuries, falls on various parts of the body, lesions of the brain, of the bulb, and of the fourth ventricle.

As regards **treatment,** diuretic drinks must, of course, be avoided. Saccharin and starchy foods should be taken in small quantities.

Opium, valerian, and bromides have given good results. Antipyrin appears to me to have some advantages. Electricity may be employed in the form of continuous currents (Le Fort).

If the polyuria appears to be associated with syphilis, mercury and iodide of potassium may be tried.

VII. RELATIONS BETWEEN INJURY AND DIABETES.

Diabetes, diabetes mellitus, and diabetes insipidus show intimate relations with injury. A shock, a blow, a fall, a railway accident, may cause diabetes in persons who were previously in perfect health. The injury has alone been the cause of the disease, and I have quoted many examples of this in my clinical lecture on this subject.* I reproduce some of these cases here :

Traumatic Diabetes Insipidus.—A man, forty-four years of age, came under my care at the Hôtel-Dieu for wasting and severe thirst. He drank from 10 to 12 litres of fluid

---

* " Rapports du Traumatisme avec le Diabète " (*Clinique Médicale de l'Hôtel-Dieu,* 1899. 7me leçon).

daily, and had he not restrained himself, he would have drunk more. He swallowed at a gulp a litre of water more easily than I could drink a glassful. He was therefore suffering from polydipsia—that is to say, from constant and unquenchable thirst. As a corollary he had polyuria—that is to say, he passed from 10 to 12 litres of water in the twenty-four hours. The urine was always colourless, transparent, and without the slightest deposit.

With these two symptoms, polydipsia and polyuria, it might at first have been supposed that the man was suffering from diabetes mellitus. It is easy to decide this point, without employing the customary tests for sugar. The hydrometer in the test-glass showed that density was only 1003. This fact showed that the patient was not suffering from diabetes mellitus, because the sugar increases the specific gravity of the urine to a considerable degree. It rises from 1018, the normal figure, to 1025, 1030, 1050, and even more, in diabetes. A man who was suffering from diabetes, and who passed daily 10 to 12 litres of urine, ought to pass 200 grammes of sugar ; and therefore the specific gravity of his urine would be very high. On the other hand, the lowering of the specific gravity to 1003 indicated the absence of sugar, and, as a matter of fact, the analysis showed not the slightest trace of glucose.

Was this case, then, one of azoturic or of phosphaturic diabetes ? No ; for in such a case we should find a sediment in the bottom of the glass, and the specific gravity of the urine would not be so low as 1003. I ought to say, however, that the man passed more urea and more phosphates than normal. In the twenty-four hours the urine contained 44 grammes of urea and 3 grammes of phosphates. This loss of urea and phosphates was not excessive, but it was far from being sufficient to call the diabetes azoturic or phosphaturic, and it was in direct proportion to the enormous amount of urine secreted.

If the diabetes in this patient was neither glycosuric, azoturic, nor phosphaturic, what was it ? It was a simple diabetes insipidus, also called polyuria, or simple poly-dipsia. Having made this point in diagnosis, let us consider the history of the patient.

The diabetes came on suddenly in a few hours. At one fell swoop the man was taken ill with intense thirst. This seizure occurred under the following circumstances : On January 28, fifteen months before, he was working in a factory, when the lathe wheel, which weighed 40 kilogrammes, broke and struck him a severe blow on the right shoulder near the thorax. At this spot he had only a severe bruise, but the shock was so terrible that the poor man was thrown back several yards, and in his fall the nape of his neck and his head struck against the block of a vice. He remained un-conscious for five hours, and was taken in a comatose condition to the Beaujon Hospital, into Lucas-Championnière's ward. The wounds were sewn up ; the scars were still visible. It was not clear that he had fractured the petrous bone, and yet a serous and blood-stained discharge flowed from the right ear, and from this time the sense of hearing was lost. This terrible accident was accompanied by fever and delirium.

Next day the patient regained consciousness, and at once experienced the urgent thirst which has since never left him. As it was not known at the moment that he was suffering from polydipsia, his fluid allowance was quite insufficient, so that, in spite of his headache and vertigo, he dragged himself to the pantry and anywhere where he knew he would find water, in order to satisfy his thirst. " I would have drunk anything, even my urine." From this time he was given daily 15 litres of different drinks—hops, cocoa, wine and water—and he took special care to provide for the night. He remained about eight days in hospital, suffering from violent headache, and then, as he felt better, he went out, in order to resume his employment as a mechanic. He had not a trace of glycosuria.

A fresh symptom now appeared. The patient, who had formerly had a moderate appetite, was suddenly seized with boulimia. He took four or five meals a day, and got up at night in order to eat and to drink. He swallowed, without mastication, enormous quantities of meat and bread. The money which he earned scarcely served to feed him, and he spent eight francs a day on food.

He was soon obliged to give up his trade: the headache reappeared, he felt very weak and tired, and his food did not restore his strength. He then came to the Beaujon Hospital, under Fernet, where he was treated with valerian. At the end of some weeks, as he felt better, he attempted to resume his work, but his strength failed afresh. He suffered from giddiness, vertigo, and insomnia, and he went to the Charité Hospital, nuder Oulmont. Some weeks of rest and treatment appeared to produce improvement, and he made a fresh attempt to work. It was fruitless, and six weeks later he came to the Tenon Hospital, under Beclère. Finally, after going to many different hospitals, he came under my care.

Apart from the polydipsia and polyphagia, his condition was somewhat as follows: We found none of the usual symptoms of diabetes mellitus; the teeth and the gums were healthy; there were no eruptions of boils; the patellar reflexes were normal. and the sight was not affected; but the general condition left much to be desired, The patient had lost 9 kilogrammes in a year, and was quite prostrated. He also suffered from profuse sweating, especially at night. In spite of the boulimia and polydipsia, he did not suffer from dyspepsia or from vomiting, the stomach was not dilated, and the stools were normal and regular.

I gave the man as much food and drink as he wished, prescribed valerian and opium, and placed a seton in the nape of the neck. Such was the history of this patient who suddenly suffered from polydipsia following a violent injury. His case will serve as a basis for discussion, but before treating on parallel lines traumatic and non-traumatic diabetes insipidus, I think it well to quote some other cases. Several of them are given in Jodry's thesis. They are as follows:

1. A girl, fourteen years of age, fell on her feet after sliding down an escarpment 4 or 5 metres in height. When she was picked up she was apparently dead. The condition of coma lasted for four hours, with grinding of the teeth, injection of the face, vomiting, dilated pupils, squint, and hæmorrhage from the left ear, which lasted for the greater part of the day (July 11). There was some improvement during the next few days. On the 19th intelligence was fairly clear, less squint, peaceful sleep, and good appetite. On the 20th unquenchable thirst suddenly came on. The patient drank 6 litres of fluid in the twenty-four hours, and passed an equivalent quantity of urine, as clear as water, and containing no sugar or albumin. The polyuria, with the accompanying phenomena, lasted until July 29. On August 4 the thirst ceased, and the appetite was great. There remained only slight amblyopia and swimming in the head, which disappeared at the end of the month. The patient, who had lost her memory for certain proper names, recovered it, but she could not remember anything that had happened shortly before the accident.

2. A youth, eighteen years of age, came into the Charité Hospital in January, 1855. He was suffering from mild varioloid, which rapidly recovered. Soon after, to the great astonishment of his friends, he commenced to drink from 8 to 10 pots of barley-water daily. During the night he got up several times in order to drink. His appetite was voracious. The polydipsia and boulimia were of traumatic origin, for the boy had been kicked on the forehead by a horse six years previously. The loss of consciousness had lasted for only a few minutes, but the shock had been violent, as a large and well-marked cicatrix proved. On the same day as the accident the thirst became greatly increased, and had since this period never ceased troubling the patient day and night. For the past six years this condition constituted an infirmity which was bearable, and did not appear to affect the patient's health. He drank, on an average, 10 litres in the twenty-four hours. The quantity of urine was practically equal to the quantity of fluid ingested. The urine was clear, colourless, without smell, like pure

water. The absence of sugar and albuminuria was proved on several occasions. The polyuria and the polydipsia completely ceased during the acute affection which necessitated his admission to hospital.

3. A man, twenty-seven years of age, of fairly good constitution, fell from a height on June 18, 1859. He sustained a fracture, complicated by a wound, with such cerebral disturbance that he remained eleven days unconscious, and was obliged to remain in hospital for forty days. He went out too soon, his strength failed, and he was obliged to return. Condition on August 5 : Severe and almost continuous headache, not well defined, and sometimes more intense in the neighbourhood of the scar (right frontal region); dull and melancholy ; gait slow and uncertain ; frequent vertigo, giddiness, especially when walking or on making sudden movement ; slight facial paralysis on the right side ; vision completely absent on the right side, diminished on the left ; right arm a little weaker than the left. When the patient stands up he always experiences a backward movement, just before he commences to walk. Digestion good ; no vomiting ; insomnia almost constant ; **great and continuous thirst since the accident.** During his first day in the hospital he drank nearly 25 litres : urine pale, limpid, like water, without any traces of sugar. From the 11th to the 12th the patient drank 8 litres. Two grammes of extract of valerian were prescribed, and next day 2 litres less urine passed. From the 18th to the 20th urine fairly abundant and thirst somewhat acute. Extract of gentian root prescribed, and a seton placed in the nape of the neck. The headache diminished gradually, and disappeared completely during the early part of September. The paralysis, the inco-ordination of movement, and the backward motion also disappeared. The polyuria and polydipsia persisted, on the other hand, until September 5. From the 7th the quantity of urine diminished daily, and by the 17th it had regained its normal limit. On October 15 it was found that the recovery was maintained.

4. A mason fell from a scaffolding on August 30, 1859. After the fall a small contused wound was found on the upper part of the forehead, but the frontal bone was not laid bare. The right upper eyelid showed ecchymosis, and blood flowed from the left ear. No fracture was found at any part of the cranium. Both radii and the left clavicle were fractured. Loss of consciousness, which lasted five days, during which time the patient passed from a condition of stupor to one of restlessness. On September 5 he began to drink and to eat to excess. The polyuria and the polydipsia increased progressively from 5 to 14 litres. The urine was almost colourless, with a slight greenish reflection, but without any marked odour. Analysis on two occasions showed neither sugar nor albumin. On September 23 the polydipsia diminished, presenting during this decrease the same proportion as during its increase. On November 10 the patient left the hospital, completely recovered from all the effects of the fall, with the exception of a slight diminution in the hearing power on the left side.

5. A youth, eighteen years of age, who had always been in good health, received a blow from a wooden sword on the right side of the head, followed immediately by loss of consciousness, violent pain in the head, severe fever with rigors, and **acute thirst.** These troubles soon disappeared, and two days later he was able to resume his work, but the thirst persisted. Three weeks later he begged for treatment to relieve the thirst. He did not feel any weaker since the accident, but was sure he had grown thinner. His digestion was good, and his appetite had not increased. Pulse, 70. No pain in the head since the day after the accident. The quantity of water drunk was estimated at more than 30 litres in the twenty-four hours. He would have drunk continually if he had not felt his stomach swell and become painful when he drank too much. The urine was proportionate to the quantity of water taken, and was limpid, very slightly coloured, and odourless. There was not the least trace of sugar. The specific gravity was scarcely higher than that of water. After a futile exhibition of opium, valerian, in large doses, was prescribed. Progressive diminution in the thirst after three weeks' treatment.

Description.—The foregoing cases furnish material for tracing the history of traumatic diabetes insipidus. Although the disease may follow traumatism affecting any region, it is more common in head injuries. Diabetes insipidus, or simple polydipsia, may appear some hours or directly after the injury. In my patient the shock was followed by loss of consciousness, and on the next day the polydipsia was so great that 10 to 12 litres of fluid did not satisfy the thirst. In the youth kicked on the forehead by a horse (Charcot) exaggerated thirst appeared on the same day as the accident, and from that time never ceased. In the young man who fell from a height (Moutard-Martin) the thirst appeared at the time of the accident, and in the young man who received a blow on the head with a sword the polydipsia appeared directly after the accident, and the quantity of fluid was estimated at more than 30 litres in the twenty-four hours.

These examples show that traumatic diabetes insipidus may appear directly after an injury. The polydipsia supervenes at once, and the surprising feature is the sudden onset, in a healthy individual, of diabetes, which may last for the remainder of life. This sudden onset is not special to traumatic polydipsia, but is also seen in cases of diabetes insipidus which are not traumatic.

In some cases the polydipsia does not supervene until some days after the accident. Thus, in the young girl who fell upon her feet (Martin) the polydipsia appeared nine days after the accident, and in the mason who fell from the scaffolding (Debron) it appeared five days after the accident, as soon as the patient recovered consciousness.

The symptoms of diabetes insipidus are identical in traumatic and in non-traumatic cases. In those quoted the patients drank 15, 20, and 30 litres of fluid daily, and even more. Some have a thirst which is truly unquenchable. They are afraid to lie down or to go to bed without providing themselves with an abundant supply of water. My patient used a siphon-tube, so that he could satisfy his thirst during the night almost without breaking his rest. This unbridled thirst is not special to traumatic polydipsia. It is also seen in non-traumatic cases of polydipsia. Thus, Trousseau speaks of a patient who drank 40 litres daily. Aussit gives the history of a small patient, four years old, who had such urgent need for fluid that on several occasions he drank the contents of his chamber-pot. On another occasion he went down into a neighbour's cellar and drank the beer from the cask. His allowance of water during the night was 4 litres. Accordingly, whether the polydipsia is traumatic or not, the need for drink is just as urgent. Perhaps, indeed, it is more severe in simple polydipsia than in diabetes mellitus.

The polyuria is proportionate to the polydipsia, and, according to the case, the patient passes 15, 20, or 30 litres of water.

There is a symptom to which I wish to call attention—namely, boulimia or polyphagia—that is to say, excessive appetite. We are too prone to believe that polyphagia is a symptom reserved for diabetes mellitus, but this is a mistake. We see patients who have no glycosuria, and who are not suffering from diabetes mellitus, but simply from polydipsia, and yet the need for food is extreme, and we may say that their hunger is as great as their thirst—in fact, they suffer from boulimia just as much as from polydipsia. In order to ascertain the quantity of food taken daily by my patient in the Saint-Christophe Ward, his daily rations of bread, meat, vegetables, and fluid, were placed on a table, and there was sufficient to supply a whole family with food and drink. It may be said that these patients are never satisfied, and scarcely is one meal finished when they wish to start a second.

Boulimia has been noted in several cases of traumatic polydipsia. Trousseau was one of the first to call attention to it in persons suffering from polydipsia without glycosuria, and he writes as follows : " Contrary to what you will find stated by most authors, who in this respect have only repeated previous statements, the appetite as well as the thirst is, as a rule, not only increased, but very much exaggerated. You will recall my patient in the Sainte-Agnès Ward, and the enormous quantity of food which he ate in the twenty-four hours. You have heard him say that he was the terror of proprietors of those restaurants where bread was allowed free. As soon as he had taken a meal or two in one of these establishments he was offered money, so he said, not to come back again."

Whether diabetes insipidus is or is not traumatic, it may be said that, in spite of the enormous quantities of fluid and solids, the digestive faculties do not appear to be disturbed, and the digestion goes on as regularly as in the normal condition. The absence of dilatation is remarkable in the case of a stomach which for months and years receives such a quantity of liquids and solids.

An important question remains to be cleared up : Is traumatic diabetes insipidus more or less serious than the non-traumatic variety ? Let us first consider the prognosis of non-traumatic diabetes. " Althongh it may for a long while be compatible with apparent integrity of health, be on your guard," says Trousseau, " against thinking that matters will remain for long in such a favourable condition. The boulimia is soon replaced by insurmountable anorexia, the wasting becomes more and more alarming, the skin withers and takes on an earthy tint, the breath is fœtid, and, just as in diabetes mellitus, we see the symptoms of tubercular phthisis appear. I have long believed on the testimony of my predecessors that polydipsia was not as grave as glycosuria, but to-day experience has singularly modified my ideas in this respect. While in my own private practice and in my hospital wards I can record a large number of patients with glycosuria whose health was excellent for a long time, although I did not employ active treatment, I have, on the other hand, had the misfortune to see nearly all those whom I treated for polyuria waste rapidly, and come to the end of their lives much more quickly than diabetics.''

On examining the cases of traumatic polydipsia, I find that recovery has sometimes followed after a few weeks or a few months of treatment. I think, therefore, that traumatic polydipsia is less obstinate, less grave, and somewhat less rebellious to treatment than the non-traumatic form. What is the treatment ? The same indications are applicable to both varieties. Extract of valerian in large doses, extract of belladonna in daily doses of $\frac{1}{6}$ grain, and antipyrin in daily doses of 15 to 30 grains in the twenty-four hours, may be employed. Hydrotherapy is also of service, and counter-irritation with the cautery or with setons is especially applicable in traumatic polydipsia. I applied the cautery and setons in my patient. As a result, he showed great improvement : the nights were less disturbed, the thirst was less acute, the urine passed only amounted to 6 or 7 litres instead of from 8 to 10 litres. Although the therapeutic success was not complete, we may yet admit the benefit of the treatment.

Traumatic Diabetes Mellitus.—A shock or a blow upon the head or some other part of the body may bring on diabetes mellitus quite suddenly in persons who were previously in perfect health, as the following examples show :

One of my friends, who was assisting in the preparations for the fête on July 14 in Algiers, received such a violent blow on the back of the neck that he lost consciousness. When he came to, some hours later, he immediately asked for something to drink, and from this time on the polydipsia became so great that 6 to 8 litres of fluid a day scarcely sufficed to quench his thirst. The examination of the urine revealed 40 grammes of sugar in the twenty-four hours ; the urea and phosphates were also increased. In twenty years the diabetes has never completely disappeared. When the patient relaxes his diet, the sugar reaches 50 and 60 grammes. Under the influence of diet and alkaline waters, with arsenic or antipyrin, the sugar falls to 8 or 10 grammes, but the glycosuria never disappears completely, and is always ready to show an increase. Apart from polydipsia and glycosuria, this traumatic diabetes has never given rise to complications, and is not even accompanied by polyphagia. It comprises the slight yet obstinate forms of traumatic diabetes. Such is not always the case, for all the varieties of diabetes mellitus may follow trauma. The following are cases taken from the thesis of Bernstein-Kohan, Jodry, and from the work of Brouardel and Richardière :

1. A railway gatekeeper, forty-six years of age, previously in good health, received a violent blow on the head. He remained unconscious for an hour. After the accident he experienced acute thirst and ravenous hunger and passed an enormous quantity of urine. The urine was loaded with sugar, and its specific gravity was 1052. Rest in bed, blisters to the nape of the neck, and purgatives caused marked improvement in his condition : the urine became less abundant, the specific gravity fell to 1012, and the sugar disappeared completely. The man resumed his work, and the cure was permanent.

2. A farm-labourer, fourteen years of age, whose health was usually excellent, received a blow on the right occipital region from a falling tree : scalp wound, fracture of the cranium, signs of commotio cerebri, loss of consciousness, vomiting, a feeling of heaviness of the whole body, without localized paralysis. On the day following the accident the urine was abundant, and contained 5 grammes of sugar per litre. In the evening he was attacked by irresistible hunger, and ate turnip soup prepared with milk. Death followed in a few weeks. The autopsy showed a fracture of the occipital bone. The brain appeared to be healthy.

3. In the following case (Frerichs) a young man, twenty-six years of age, fell about 10 feet, striking his forehead against the ground. He was not troubled with thirst until six months afterwards. The diabetes became so severe that he passed more than 500 grammes of sugar daily. He died of pulmonary tuberculosis. The autopsy revealed several extravasations of blood in the floor of the fourth ventricle. On the right side, in the region of the nucleus acusticus, there was a brownish spot of the size of a lentil, and two others as large as poppy seeds, about 3 millimetres from the median line. After hardening the specimens, Frerichs found on the right side, at the level of the nucleus acusticus, and immediately outside the abductor nucleus, three small hæmorrhages, which could be followed in the sections. Another group was present a little higher up, 6 or 7 millimetres from the middle line of the angle of the floor of the fourth ventricle. The larger of these hæmorrhages were recent, and showed normal red blood-corpuscles. Frerichs found, on the other hand, centres composed of red blood-corpuscles, which were completely colourless, and lastly some scattered masses of brown pigmentary granules.

4. A boy, sixteen years of age, who received a blow on the occiput with a stick, was taken ill six days later with polydipsia, polyuria, boulimia, and amblyopia. The urine showed a specific gravity of 1043, and contained a large quantity of sugar. Recovery took place in a fortnight, under the influence of meat diet and alkaline medicines, and yet for two months afterwards simple polyuria was still present.

These cases deal with the appearance of diabetes mellitus after head injuries, and I shall now quote cases in which diabetes mellitus appeared after injuries to some other region of the body :

A man, fifty years of age, whose previous health was excellent, was thrown from his horse and fell on his back. He soon found that he was losing strength, his thirst became considerable, and he passed 8 litres of urine daily. On analysis, 72 grammes of sugar per litre, or 576 grammes in the twenty-four hours, were found. Treatment reduced the sugar in six months' time to 44 grammes per litre.

A man, twenty-one years of age, who was playing with one of his friends, fell on a chair and received a blow over the first two lumbar vertebræ. He did not sustain a fracture, but yet, some days later, he complained of very severe thirst and extreme weakness. The urine contained 10 grammes of sugar per litre. He died some while afterwards from coma.

Griesinger relates the case of a young man, eighteen years of age, who fell from a first story on to his feet. The accident was not followed by loss of consciousness, but during the night severe diabetes with excessive thirst appeared. The urine contained 50 grammes of sugar per litre, or an amount of 250 grammes daily. The patient was admitted to hospital in a condition of cachexia and died, covered with boils and abscesses.

Children, as well as adults, may be affected. Bouvier quotes the case of a boy, eleven years of age, who was taken ill with diabetes following a blow over the kidney. Niedergass reports the case of a young girl who became diabetic after a fall. Rossbach quotes the case of a child, eight months old, who fell from his nurse's arms, and died, four months later, in a condition of cachexia, with polyuria, glycosuria, eczema, and furunculosis (Brouardel and Richardière).

The foregoing cases prove that diabetes mellitus may follow the most varied injuries, such as blows on the head, on the nape of the neck, violent bruising of the body, falls upon the feet, etc. Head injuries, however, play the largest part. Diabetes may appear early or late after the injury. Brouardel and Richardière give the following statistics : " In twenty-five cases which state the precise date of appearance of the first symptoms, in four diabetes appeared within two days of the injury, in four it appeared during the next week, and in four others its onset was less rapid."

The symptoms of traumatic diabetes mellitus do not differ from those of the ordinary form, and in both the complications, such as carbuncles, boils, cataract, etc., may be seen. They may both result in pulmonary phthisis ; they may both terminate in coma.

As regards the question of prognosis in both cases, Brouardel and Richardière regard the question in the following manner : " Early traumatic diabetes, which follows closely upon an accident, and late traumatic diabetes, which appears a long time after the accident, have a somewhat different prognosis. The differences are important from the point of view of the gravity of the disease, because in legal medicine two distinct forms are described—the one which has a rapid and early onset is benign ; the other, which appears later and runs a slower course, is as a rule serious. Acute early diabetes always ends in recovery. Two or three weeks, or perhaps two or three months, after the appearance of the first symptoms the patient feels a return of strength, the thirst and boulimia disappear, the sugar is no longer appreciable in the urine, and plumpness returns. One symptom—polyuria—still persists, and becomes even more severe than in the stationary stage of the disease. This polyuria may amount to 5 litres daily, and may last for some weeks after the disappearance of the glycosuria. It yields at last, and as a rule recovery is complete two or three months after the injury. The late form runs a very slow course, lasting for months and years, and usually ending fatally. Death is caused by wasting or by complications, such as tuberculosis, or by coma."

These considerations regarding the early and late forms of traumatic diabetes are not absolute, and appear to me to include numerous exceptions.

Medico-Legal Study.—The question of traumatic diabetes in some respects enters the domain of legal medicine. An individual becomes diabetic after a blow or after a railway accident, and sues for damages and costs. How are we to decide that his claim is genuine, and to affirm that the plaintiff was not diabetic before the accident ? Here are two cases of this kind :

A man, forty-five years of age, who had never been ill, was in the railway accident of July 18, 1884, on the line from Puy to Saint-Étienne.   Ch—— did not lose consciousness, but was only stunned.   He did not remember how he got out of the compartment, but he remembered perfectly the condition in which he found the engine-driver and the stoker.   He noticed that he had a wound on the left leg, and he tried to follow his travelling companions.   He walked about two kilometres to reach the nearest station.   During the journey Ch—— remarked that he followed with difficulty some women who got out of the carriages at the same time as he did.

Ch—— was examined on three different occasions by Dr. Vinay, Fellow of the University of Lyons.   This physician gave him three certificates, dated July 30, 1884, December 24, 1884, and November 30, 1885, and stated : (1) That the contused wound on the leg had recovered in about twenty days ; (2) that the lumbar pains which were marked on the first day persisted and were very acute ; and (3) that the urine, increased in quantity from July 30, contained at the end of November, 1885, a notable quantity of sugar.   On February 13, at the time of my examination, Ch—— looked well.   The wound in the leg was healed, and was represented by a scar 3·5 centimetres in diameter.   The renal pain persisted.   It was absent during rest, but came on when Ch—— tried to rise, or to stand upright, or when he coughed.   It was not accompanied by any appreciable sign of fracture of the spine.   It was increased by pressure over the lumbar vertebræ, especially on the left side.   Ch——'s vision was good.   He had no cutaneous eruptions.   The specific gravity of his urine was 1032, and it contained 47 grammes of sugar per litre, but no albumin.

The second case refers to a man forty-five years of age who had never been ill, but who was hurt in a railway accident on August 14, 1883.   He lost consciousness after the accident, and felt sharp pains all over his body—notably, above the right knee and in the left lumbar region.   Since the accident he had lost 18 kilos in two years, and had become weak, being compelled to give up his duties as a commercial traveller.   He had also had hæmoptysis.   At Brouardel's first examination (two years after the accident) the patient complained of pain along the spine : the pain was increased by pressure.   The urine, a detail ignored by the patient, contained 49 grammes of sugar per litre.   The patient therefore presented a series of diabetic symptoms.

Speaking generally, the question of traumatic diabetes is often difficult to decide in legal medicine, because, in order to blame the injury, we must be certain that the plaintiff was free from diabetes before the accident. The question is the more difficult to decide because certain symptoms of diabetes are so slight as to pass unnoticed for some time.   Six months or more may elapse after the accident before some revealing sign attracts our attention, and we find sugar in the urine.

The medico-legal question may, therefore, be presented under various aspects.   If an individual who has always enjoyed good health is suddenly taken ill with polydipsia following a blow or a railway accident, and if the individual shortly after the injury presents clear signs of diabetes, including glycosuria, it is evident that the injury must be held guilty, and that the plaintiff has a right to damages.

The diagnosis is, however, not always so simple.   Traumatic diabetes, like the ordinary form, may be present for months and years without declaring itself by the cardinal symptoms of excessive polydipsia or of exaggerated polyuria, which promptly give a clue to the diagnosis. The patient often suffers from diabetes without knowing it. His appetite and his thirst are normal, but yet he experiences a certain weakness, put down to fatigue, complains of pains called rheumatism, or suffers from a nervous condition looked upon as neurasthenia, and we only find months afterwards that all these troubles should have been put down to diabetes.

This discussion is applicable to traumatic diabetes, which may remain unnoticed for a long while, and which may, for various reasons, be recognized only at a late stage. Under such conditions, how are we to affirm that the injury has been the origin of diabetes which has passed unnoticed for a year or two? I think that in such a case the plaintiff will lose his case.

Pathogenesis.—I should now like to say a few words on the pathogenesis of traumatic diabetes. It is at present a question of theory. If we refer to the memorable experiments of Bernard, we find that puncture of the fourth ventricle between the roots of the vagus and auditory nerves determines polyuria; if the puncture is slightly higher, glycosuria; and higher still, albuminuria. These phenomena of an experimental kind are, however, transient, and are in no way comparable to the pathological cases, which show us the lasting and sometimes indefinite existence of diabetes mellitus and of diabetes insipidus.

Furthermore, no lesion of the fourth ventricle is, as a rule, present in traumatic diabetes. A fall on the feet, a blow on the kidneys, or a violent shock are the injuries which may cause diabetes mellitus or diabetes insipidus. We might say that the thirst or the hunger may be caused by a dynamic disturbance of the functional powers of certain nerve cells, but what is this disturbance, and which are the cells at fault? I do not know.

The sudden and indefinite dissociation of the morbid act is still inexplicable. Why after a blow, a fall, or a bruise, should one individual suffer from simple polydipsia without showing for months any trace of sugar in the urine? Why, on the other hand, should an identical injury in another person cause not only glycosuria, but diabetes mellitus, with all its train of symptoms? The matter, some will say, is one of localization, but I should prefer to acknowledge our ignorance on the point, and to consider the question unanswered at present.

The **treatment** of traumatic diabetes mellitus is practically the same as that of the non-traumatic form. With the general treatment of the disease by diet, suppression of food and drink which contain sugar, and diminution, but not suppression, of farinaceous foods, arsenical and alkaline preparations, and antipyrin, we must also employ local treatment by blisters, setons, or the cautery to the nape of the neck, especially if the disease follows a head injury.

VIII. OBESITY.

Description.—Obesity is the pathological condition caused by the general hypertrophy of the adipose tissue. In a less pronounced degree it blends with embonpoint, and at its extreme limit it takes the name of polysarcia or adiposis. Local deposits of fat, such as lipoma, lipomatous hypertrophy of the muscles, and paralytic subcutaneous adiposis, must be distinguished from obesity.

The distribution of fatty tissue in the obese does not take place in an uniform and identical fashion. The subcutaneous and intermuscular cellular tissue, the fringes of the omentum, the mesentery, the perirenal tissue, the surface of the heart, and the cellular tissue of the orbit, may be invaded by fat. In gross feeders obesity chiefly affects the abdominal walls, and forms cutaneous pads, with stretching of the skin and lineæ comparable to those of pregnancy. In some persons fat accumulates in the neck (triple chin) or in the breasts. Adiposis does not, properly speaking, exist in the penis and the scrotum. The viscera, the liver, the kidneys, and particularly the heart, may be invaded by fat.

An important distinction should be made between **fatty infiltration,** which is compatible with the life of the tissue, and **fatty degeneration,** which, on the other hand, affects the elements which are practically dead or already necrobiotic. The former belongs to obesity, and is curable, while the latter is the result of infections and intoxications, and is incurable. When, however, the polysarcia is extreme and inveterate, it wears out the functional activity of the organs, and fatty or fibro-fatty degeneration is often added to the fatty infiltration. Troubles then commence, and finally carry off the patient.

Obesity, when less marked, recent, and unaccompanied by a visceral lesion properly speaking—as, for instance, in young persons—only causes slight breathlessness upon movement and effort. The respiration is some-what noisy, fatigue comes on rapidly, and therefore fat persons are some-what apathetic, and show but little inclination for physical exercise.

Digestion is generally sluggish after meals, sleepiness is felt, but the troubles are usually confined within the limits of health, so that obesity may be considered rather as an infirmity than as a disease.

On the contrary, when the adiposis is excessive, and the patient is no longer young, the face is usually deeply coloured and even cyanosed. The gait is slow and halting, and the breathlessness increases on the least movement. The act of walking upstairs becomes especially difficult, speech is short and broken, and the patient, when saying a long phrase, is obliged to stop and take breath. The appetite may be increased or diminished ; the thirst is always increased. Digestion is troublesome ; after meals the desire to sleep is urgent; the aptitude for mental work is not always diminished. This is, indeed, an interesting peculiarity. Examination of the liver frequently shows enlargement and tenderness of the organ.

The stools are often of a pale colour. The heart-beats are distant, feeble, and sometimes irregular. The size of the heart is increased, and the apex-beat is difficult to find.

The skin is covered with sweat on the least exertion, and gives off a fœtid odour, due to the increase of the sebaceous secretion and to the chemical changes which this secretion undergoes. The skin is readily irritated, and therefore erythema, intertrigo, and eczema are common in fat persons.

The urine presents important changes, which often serve as a guide to the pathogenesis and therapeutics of obesity.

Without speaking of polyuria, glycosuria, and albuminuria, which are often met with in obese patients, who are arthritic and neurotic, the amount of urea, and in a general way the amount of the nitrogenous products, have led to a division of obese patients into two groups, according as the nitrogenous substances in the urine are or are not increased. In some obese patients the proportion of urea is diminished.

Many patients succumb to troubles dependent upon visceral degenerations, which are almost always present at some time or other. Progressive asystolia is a very frequent mode of termination. Death also supervenes as the result of some intercurrent disease—pneumonia, general bronchitis, erysipelas, etc.—which are exceedingly grave in all fat persons. Other persons succumb to some diathetic affection of which obesity is only a manifestation. Here, again, polysarcia, by diminishing the vital resistance of the tissues, has an unfavourable action.

Ætiology and Pathogenesis.—Obesity is a disease of all ages, though more frequent in adults and rare in old people, because of the general decrepitude. Women are more often sufferers than men. The disease appears at puberty, after marriage, as the result of pregnancy, and especially of the first pregnancy, and lastly at the menopause. The genital life has, therefore, a capital importance in the appearance of obesity.

The disease is often hereditary, supervening in certain persons after an acute affection (typhoid fever and pneumonia). It is then the result of profound changes in nutrition.

Obesity, migraine, cholelithiasis, uric acid, gravel, asthma, articular rheumatism, gout, and diabetes are all manifestations of imperfect nutrition, such as are met with in arthritic subjects.

It is also to the slackening of nutrition that the fatty overgrowth in some diseases of the nervous system, and in particular hysteria and progressive pernicious anæmia, must be set down.

In the normal state the fat fixed in the tissues has a double origin—namely, **alimentation** and **disassimilation.** The pathological fat has the same origin. Increase of fatty food does not, however, increase obesity more surely than foods containing starch and sugar and alcoholic drinks (wine, brandy, beer), as is proved in the case of the Eskimos, who live almost entirely upon fat, and who are not stouter than the inhabitants of southern countries. In order that these nutritional causes may produce their full effect, they must act in persons in whom oxidation is slow and the combustion of these substances is incomplete. Want of exercise and the absorption of large quantities of proteid-sparing foods, by diminishing the quantity of oxygen used up, favour the deposit of fat droplets in the tissues. Increase of disassimilation leads to the same result, but here the source of the fat is due to quaternary substances. In the intoxications and infections the production of fat takes place at the expense of the proteid material. Such is also the case in progressive pernicious anæmia. In these patients we find in the urine an excess of urea and an albuminoid substance, which is also formed at the expense of the incompletely oxidized proteids.

The study of the variations in the saponifying ferment of the blood may perhaps clear up the pathogenesis of obesity. In one case Achard and Clerc have found exaggerated activity of this ferment.

Treatment.—The alimentary régime in obesity comprises the following indications : No sugar, no starchy foods, fluids taken in moderation at meals, avoidance of alcohol and beer. Coffee and tea are permitted. Massage, dry-rubbing, and physical exercise should be prescribed. We must avoid fatigue, especially in elderly persons.

By means of these hygienic measures we can often reduce a patient's weight by some pounds. If this treatment do not suffice, we may also employ such drugs as iodine and iodides (iodide of potassium in small doses). Tincture of iodide (3 to 5 drops in a teaspoonful of wine) may be given before meals. Purgatives and alkaline preparations have their indications. The waters of Marienbad, Kissingen, Montmirail, and of Brides, etc., act both as alkalines and laxatives.

The internal administration of thyroid gland has been recommended in obesity, because the thyroid body increases denutrition. This treatment has given good results. Ten grains of fresh or of dried thyroid gland are prescribed daily. Chaix and Rémy's tabloids, which contain 25 centigrammes of thyroid gland, may be employed, 1 or 2 grammes being taken after each meal.

IX. DIFFUSE SYMMETRICAL LIPOMATOSIS.

In this section I shall deal with the disease described by some authorities under the name of diffuse symmetrical lipomatosis, chiefly affecting the neck, and by Launois and Bensaude under the name of symmetrical adeno-lipomatosis, which chiefly affects the neck, a term which takes the glandular element into account. I shall adopt the former of these terms, and I shall give my reason later.

Here, as in all lipomata, the disease consists in tumours composed of more or less dense fatty tissue. When we speak of diffuse lipomatosis, we mean that the lipomatous masses spread without any tendency to be en capsuled, like true lipomata.

With few exceptions, this diffuse lipomatosis is a disease of adult age, and is quite exceptional in women. It is far from being rare, as more than a hundred cases are known. It is not directly associated with obesity. We see fat people without lipomata, and also lipomata in thin persons. The real cause of the affection is unknown. Heredity has not been proved, but arthritism and alcoholism have often been suggested.

The onset is insidious, the lipomatous tumours causing neither discomfort, embarrassment, nor pain. Symmetry is the rule, but it is sometimes apparent only at more or less long intervals. The lipomata, which are very small at first, do not always undergo progressive increase in size. They may remain stationary for years, and may even recede, although I do not think that they disappear. In the long run they often reach the size of a nut, an egg, or of an orange. They sometimes spread in various directions, and finally acquire a colossal size.

The first lipomata usually appear in the cervical region; sometimes in the anterior and lateral aspects of the neck; at other times in the nape of the neck, which is often the first part to be invaded. The neck swells, and the shirt-collar has to be enlarged. The lipomatous tumours are soft, painless, sometimes fused together, and having ill-defined edges. They can be moved as a whole, and are not adherent to the skin or painful. According to their disposition and extent, they form a collar or a collarette. The lipomatous collar often forms a complete circle, and rounded or oval nodules in the adipose tissues can be felt in the submental, submaxillary, parotid, preauricular, and retromastoid regions.

Above the nape of the neck two tumours develop, filling up in a symmetrical manner the retromastoid fossæ, and partly hidden beneath the hair. Lower, over the vertebra prominens, we find a lipomatous tumour, which is single or divided into two symmetrical lobes. In the lateral regions of the neck the lipomatous masses occupy the preauricular and the parotid regions, and enlarge the transverse diameter of the face.

In the front of the neck the lipomatous mass may assume the form of a double or of a treble chin ,similar to that seen in fat people (Launois and Bensaude). " As the size of the neck and of the head decreases progressively from below upwards, it follows that the cephalic extremity from the shoulders to the summit of the vertex takes the form of a truncated pyramid, with its base below and its apex above " (Hayem). The head is then said to be pear-shaped.

The symmetrical lipomata may occupy only the cervical region. More often they develop in the axillæ and in the groins, and show the same symmetry. In the axillæ they form soft, painless, mobile tumours, which run into one another, and have ill-defined edges. In the groin the symmetrical lipomata are often superposed in two stages, and form almost transverse masses, which are parallel to the fold of the groin, and which extend inwards as far as the scrotum. From a distance they might be looked on as enormous herniæ. Here, as elsewhere, cutaneous adhesions are absent, and the skin preserves its normal appearance.

The lipomata have not everywhere the same consistency, being softer and more diffuse in certain parts, especially in the region of the chin. They are firmer and more defined at the back of the neck. Sometimes the lipomatous mass is not soft through its whole extent, and we find indurated nodules, which might well be taken for lymphatic glands. I shall discuss this question later. Dystrophy has never been found. Motor and sensory troubles are not seen.

The preceding description refers to the symmetrical type, and is applicable to the majority of cases. It installs itself insidiously, and for ten, twelve, or fifteen years, or even longer, it runs its course without complications. The vessels and the air-passages are not compressed, the movements of the head are not affected, and, as the condition does not threaten life, it is simply a deformity. We find cases, however, which differ somewhat from the classical description, as is shown by the following examples :

In Madelung's case the lipomatosis assumed such proportions that the masses of fat, which were twenty-three years old, fell over the chest and the back. They had also invaded the mediastinum, affecting deglutition and respiration. Launois and Bensaude quote the following cases : In Schmidt's patient the shoulders were much enlarged by two enormous fatty masses, which covered the deltoids on each side, and descended as far as the middle of the arm. A circular lipomatous mass surrounded the umbilicus. In Virchow and Schottmüller's patient the upper part of the thighs and the scrotum as far as the perinæum, were invaded by a general fatty infiltration. In Jeanselme and Bufnoir's patient the lipomata formed mammæ on the anterior abdominal wall. In Langer's patient the belly and the back were padded with lipomata. In some cases dyspnœa, fatigue, asthenia, acceleration of the pulse, and hypertrophy of the spleen have been noted. A fatal case, probably caused by compression of the organs in the mediastinum, has been quoted.

Analysis of the blood shows nothing special. In one of my patients, of whom I shall speak later, the blood examination was normal. In Pitres' patient 6,262,000 red corpuscles and 10,800 white corpuscles were found. In Demons' patient Sabrazès found absence of eosinophiles and increase of the polynuclear neutrophiles. In Quéry's patient the number of red corpuscles was normal, and the number of white ones was slightly increased. In Hayem's patient the number of red corpuscles was slightly increased, and the number of white corpuscles was slightly above the normal. In one of Launois and Bensaude's patients the count showed: red corpuscles, 3,472,000; and white corpuscles, 6,200.

We have now to discuss the nature and the pathogenesis of symmetrical lipomatosis.

Madelung suggested that symmetrical lipomatosis might be dependent upon disease or disappearance of the thyroid body. This hypothesis does not stand the test of analysis. Several authors have thought that symmetrical lipomatosis was a tropho-neurosis of myelopathic origin. None of the partisans of this nervous theory, however, " have succeeded in establishing any exact relation between the nervous system and the adipose hypertrophy. We cannot, therefore, accept this theory, unless we are willing to place all the morbid phenomena of which we know not the nature to the account of the nervous system."

Baker and Bowlby thought that the tumours were of a lymphadeno-matous rather than of a fatty nature. Histological examinations have, however, shown their fatty character.

According to Launois and Bensaude, symmetrical lipomatosis " is a primary disease of the lymphatic glands and vessels, and has many points of resemblance with adeno-lymphocele. Such a term," they say, " does not apply to every periglandular fatty infiltration, but only to a morbid entity with constant characters, and accompanied by the production of diffuse lipomata, which are probably related to the lymphatic glands and vessels."

The lymphatic gland, which is already affected, may be surrounded by a fatty layer, and simulate a true lipoma, as in Tuffier's case. This secondary periglandular lipomatosis is comparable to lipomatous perityphlitis and perinephritis, but it does not come under the heading of the diffuse and infiltrating symmetrical lipomatosis, which we are considering in this section.

Has this diffuse lipomatosis its origin in the lymphatic system, and how can it be proved? In support of their opinions, Launois and Bensaude point out that the seat of election of the diffuse lipomatous symmetrical tumours is precisely in the region where lymphatic glands exist normally. This is true, but the lipomatous tumours are also found in regions where lymphatic glands are not present. In the absence of glands, say Launois and Bensaude, there must be a residue of lymphoid tissue, which is the orgiin of the lipomatosis. No proof exists that this hypothesis is not true, but in order to establish it, it is necessary that the histological examination of the symmetrical lipomata should show in the same specimen the presence of the lipoma and the presence of the lymphatic gland—or, at any rate, traces of it.

On reading cases we see that the palpation of the soft lipomatous masses gives a sensation of indurated nodules, which are considered to be lymphatic glands embedded in the fatty tissue, and this argument is invoked in favour of the adeno-lipomatous theory, the gland and the lipoma being side by side in the same tumour.

In Pitres' case palpation of the lipomatous tumour gave a soft and compressible consistency ; but small lobulated masses, which were firmer and rolled under the finger, were also felt. These little masses somewhat resembled hard, glandular nodules, set in a lipomatous mass. In Launois and Bensaude's case it is said that, on careful palpation of the lipomata in the inguinal region, " hypertrophic glandular masses were found in the midst of the adipose tissue."

When the value of the sensation given by examination is controlled by anatomical research, we find that the indurated nodules, which on palpation are taken for lymphatic glands included in the lipoma, are in reality condensed masses of fat, associated in some instances with fibrous tissue.

Hayem has published a case in which examination of a lipomatous mass by Delbet showed small blackish glands ; but, as a matter of fact, in all the other cases the absence of glands is carefully noted.

Thus, in Marçais' case and in two of Nélaton's cases, published by Pfestel-Mazoglu, the histological examination did not reveal any trace of lymphatic glands in the fatty mass. A case in Quéry's thesis was one of symmetrical lipomata of the cervical type. The lipomata were removed by Reclus, and histological examination was made in Cornil's laboratory by Réné Marie. " On macroscopic section of the tumours, it was found that they were composed of a mass of soft adipose tissue, which enclosed other hard masses of a fibrous appearance, and very vascular at their periphery. Microscopic examination showed that these tumours were composed of adipose tissue, without any traces of glands. The hard masses found on palpation and on macroscopic examination were therefore composed, not of glands, but of normal adipose tissue much condensed, and enclosing a large quantity of fibrous tissue."

Desmons, referring to a case of lipomatosis on which he operated, says : " The fragments of the tumour were examined macroscopically and histologically, and were found to be composed of fat alone. I have never seen or touched, much less removed, glands or fragments of tissue of a glandular appearance." Such statements make it impossible to admit a glandular origin of symmetrical diffuse lipomatosis. I know that we may call in question the part of the lymphatic glands, and more generally of the lymphoid tissue in the evolution of the fat, and if we are willing to admit that diffuse lipomatosis most often arises in a region where glandular tissue abounds, we might perhaps suppose that the glandular tissue is the *primum movens* in this affection. Only supposing that this theory were probable, the genesis of the fact would remain just as unexplicable. Why should glandular tissue thus lend itself to the production of fatty masses ?

I have, moreover, seen a case which has led me to abandon the hypothesis of the association of fatty and glandular lesions, and the reader might presume this from the title of this section. The case is as follows :

I had under my care in the Hôtel-Dieu a man suffering from classical diffuse lipomatosis, which gave me an opportunity for delivering a clinical lecture on this affection.*

---

* Dieulafoy, *Clinique Médicale de l'Hôtel-Dieu*, 1903, 18me leçon.

In this patient, as in other similar cases, the cervical region was chiefly invaded. The lipomatous tumours occupied the anterior, lateral, and posterior regions of the neck. The head rested on a lipomatous muff. The fatty masses formed tumours of various sizes. They were not genuinely lobulated, but were rather spread out and fused without any clear line of demarcation. It was possible to move them *en masse*. They were not painful or adherent to the skin, which preserved its normal appearance. In the mental region and in the lateral parts of the neck they were softer than behind. At the nape of the neck the lipomatous tumours were symmetrical, and partly hidden by the roots of the hairs. Lower there was a large lipoma at the level of the vertebra prominens.

The patient also had symmetrical lipomata in the inguinal regions. They were superposed in two stages—in the form of prominent pads, which were parallel to the folds of the groin, and extended inward as far as the scrotum. Here, too, the tumours were mobile, painless, and somewhat ill-defined. They were soft, and yet on kneading they gave the feeling of hard nodules, such as lymphatic glands embedded in the fatty mass. Nevertheless, guided by experience, I stated that these indurated nodules were not glands, and to make certain, I obtained the patient's permission to remove one. The histological examination by Jolly confirmed the absence of any lymphatic tissues in the fatty mass.

The patient had two symmetrical lipomata in the clavicular regions, and four others in the lumbo-sacral region.

The affection had begun about twelve years before in the cervical region. It made slow progress, causing no discomfort or pain, and gradually invaded the groins and other parts of the body. The general health had not undergone the least affection.

Jolly examined the blood, which was normal.*

The man left the hospital, but returned a year later, wasted, cachectic, and suffering from hypertrophic alcoholic cirrhosis of the liver and tubercular peritonitis. The diffuse lipomatosis was still present in the same regions, although the cachectic condition of the patient had caused marked diminution in its size. Death followed in a few weeks. The autopsy was especially interesting, because it is, I think, the first time that we have been able to study carefully and in several regions the lipomatous masses, and to see their true relation to the lymphatic system. Loeper found the following results :

Characteristic tubercular peritonitis without adhesions and without fibro-caseous masses was present. The liver showed alcoholic hepatitis, with hypertrophy and fatty infiltration of the cells. The spleen weighed 12 ounces. It was hard and fibrous. The pancreas was large, hard, and furrowed by fibrous bands, which pushed aside the various lobules and penetrated into the acini. The intestine showed no tubercular ulceration. Congestion was extremely well marked in the kidneys, which were filled with hæmorrhagic points in the glomeruli and tubules ; in the suprarenal capsules, the vascular network of which was very dilated ; in the thyroid body, which weighed 2 ounces ; and in the lungs, which showed splenization at the bases. The heart was dilated, and the auricles were very distended. The brain was covered with large vessels, and the Sylvian and Rolandic areas were studded with typical tubercular granules. These commonplace lesions were due to passive congestion and to the dissemination of Koch's bacillus. They had no relation to the lipomatosis.

* Red corpuscles per cubic millimetre	..	..	..	4,000,000
White corpuscles per cubic millimetre	.	..	..	4,000
Weight of hæmoglobin per 100 cubic centimetres of blood			..	13 grammes.
Colour-index	..	..	..	30·2
Varieties of white corpuscles per 100 leucocytes { lymphocytes	..	..	..	25
large mononuclears		..	..	6
polynuclears	..	..	..	65
eosinophiles ..	..	..	..	4

We carefully examined the lipomatous tumours in the regions where fat and lymphatic glands are usually present, and also in the organs which seem to play a part in the organic exchanges. These lipomatous masses were present below the parotid, along the vessels of the neck, in the supraclavicular and axillary hollows, in the pectoralis major, in the anterior surface of the latissimus dorsi, and in the inguinal and crural hollows.

We also found masses (which were not perceptible during life) in front of the iliacus muscle, along the intercostal spaces, under the pleura, and in the spaces themselves; and lastly, we found them in front of the vertebral column and in the mesentery, which was, as it were, distended with fat.

All these masses had the macroscopic appearance of the ordinary lipoma, and sections made at several parts of each of them showed **not the least trace of lymphatic glands.**

Microscopic examination of the axillary, subaxillary, inguinal, mesenteric, and intercostal tumours revealed the presence of typical adipose lobules, traversed by blood-vessels and capillaries, without any lymphatic glands and **without any cellular masses which might be looked upon as vestiges or glands.** Some bands of connective tissue, containing scattered plasma cells and connective cells, were situated in an irregular fashion in the fat. Some mastzellen were visible here and there.

The organs of internal secretion—*i.e.*, suprarenal capsules and pituitary and thyroid glands—showed, in addition to the congestion noted above, lesions which explain the blood-stasis and the infection. We must note especially the adenomatous hypertrophy of the thyroid body and the large size (80 centigrammes) of the pituitary body. The nervous system was intact. The cells of the anterior cornua were normal.

X. ADIPOSIS DOLOROSA.

Adiposis dolorosa was described by Dercum, of Philadelphia, in 1888. It is a syndrome characterized by a deposit of fat in the subcutaneous cellular tissue, with pain in the fatty neoplasms.

Symptoms.—The disease generally commences in a slow and insidious manner, with slight pains, which may be felt in any part of the body. The pains are sometimes continuous, but in most cases they are intermittent and of variable severity. Patients compare them to a feeling of " hot water running along the arm," or to " worms creeping under the skin," to " a loosening of the skin," or to " a constant sensation of cold in the knees, soon followed by dull pain." We find at first slight redness of the skin, without appreciable swelling; later, with a little care, we may discover small mobile nodules, painful on pressure, rolling under the skin, and varying in size from a hazel-nut to a walnut. The pains may precede or may be contemporaneous with the tumours.

The stationary stage comprises the cardinal and secondary symptoms. To the former belong the pains, the asthenia, and the psychical troubles. The tumours are usually nodular in form, and more rarely diffuse. Asthenia is always marked. It may be so severe as to render patients incapable of the least effort. Among the psychical troubles let me mention changes in character, cerebral instability, nightmares, hallucinations, loss of memory, and tendency to melancholy (Ballet).

To the secondary symptoms belong various hæmorrhages, vasomotor, motor, and sensory troubles, with zones of anæsthesia or of hyperæsthesia, disturbance of the special senses, and trophic troubles (arthropathies, muscular atrophy).

The disease lasts for years, and the patient succumbs to cachexia or to some intercurrent disease. Recovery is exceptional.

The **diagnosis** must be made from nervous œdema, diffuse lipomatosis, neuro-fibromatosis, and symmetrical lipomata.

Pathological Anatomy.—The neuro-fibromatous lesions and the symmetrical lipomata affect the connective tissue and the viscera. The connective tissue undergoes an œdematous swelling, which is characterized by the presence of large fusiform cells, without fatty cells, and by embryonic connective tissue. The adiposis then appears, and gives place to a final fibrosis. In a biopsy by Rénon it was easy to see the fatty change in the connective cells. The visceral lesions are but little known. Observers have found changes in the thyroid body and in the pituitary gland, atrophy of Goll's column, and the presence of myeline fibres in the pia mater, covering the posterior columns of the spinal cord.

Ætiology.—We do not exactly know the ætiology and the pathogenesis of adiposis dolorosa. It is, however, chiefly seen in women during the mature age and after injuries. Sellerin thinks that the disease may be due "in some cases to a simple dynamogenous trouble in the nervous system," since "the psychical condition of certain patients, as well as their rapid recovery, can only be set down to the possibility of troubles which are purely functional and of nervous origin, not to say hysterical."

As regards treatment, extirpation of the fatty masses, hydrotherapy, salicylate of soda, arsenic, strychnine, and thyroid extract have so far been employed with varying results.

XI. MYXŒDEMA.

General and Historical Considerations.—Myxœdema, which was practically unknown until thirty years ago, now forms one of the most complete diseases which it is possible to study in pathology. Its pathogenesis has been rapidly elucidated, and the surgeon, while operating upon the thyroid gland, has often reproduced in man the characteristic syndrome with all the exactness of an experiment. Lastly, we possess for myxœdema the most rational and specific treatment at present known. It is, then, a disease which, though rare, should be reported in detail.

Myxœdema was first described in an adult woman by Gull in 1873. It was afterwards studied by Ord, who named it, and by Charcot, who called it pachydermic cachexia.

In 1880 Bourneville showed that the syndrome of myxœdema may also appear in idiots, and described the clinical type of myxœdematous idiocy.

In 1882 Reverdin observed, after total extirpation of the thyroid body, mucous œdema similar to that described by Gull and Ord. He therefore described an operative myxœdema which Kocher called cachexia strumipriva or thyroipriva.

Experimental researches soon showed that myxœdema could be produced in animals by extirpation of the thyroid body, and the identity of spontaneous myxœdema in the adult, of cachexia strumipriva, and of myxœdematous idiocy, was speedily established. Clinical observation has shown that we may go farther, and that, in addition to these types of myxœdema, other myxœdematous conditions may supervene, as an accessory syndrome, in cretins and in certain imbeciles. The discovery of the specific treatment by injection of thyroid extract was the corollary of these researches.

Ætiology.—Myxœdema is only a syndrome consecutive to the surgical extirpation or to various changes of the thyroid gland. We are ignorant of the reason for the congenital absence of the gland which causes myxœdematous idiocy, and we have scarcely more information as to the causes of myxœdema in the adult. Writers have incriminated, though without certainty, various acute or chronic infectious diseases which are said to cause thyroiditis, ending silently in sclerosis and atrophy of the organ.

Pathological Anatomy.—If myxœdema is the result of the functional suppression of the thyroid gland, which are the changes that may give rise to it ?

Operative myxœdema necessitates the total removal of the gland. The appearance of the syndrome is exceptional after partial thyroidectomy. Cachexia does not appear if a third of the gland be left.

Congenital myxœdema almost always results from the absence of the thyroid body.

Acquired myxœdema depends on an inflammation of the thyroid body, ending in atrophy and fibrosis. The fibrosis of the organ may be complete, but more often we find, especially at the onset, masses of round cells in the walls of the vesicles—that is to say, proliferation of the epithelium. The inflammation of the gland must, therefore, be both interstitial and parenchymatous.

Any lesion of the thyroid body ending in suppression of its function may be a cause of myxœdema.

The infiltration of the subcutaneous cellular tissue by a mucinoid substance is the most constant and best-known secondary lesion. Cases of true lipomatosis have also been cited. Compensatory hypertrophy of the pituitary gland has been found.

Operative Myxœdema.—The first symptoms of operative myxœdema generally appear three or four months after removal of the gland. Sensations of weakness and of coldness in the limbs, mucous infiltration, and decoloration of the skin, suppression of the sweat, and cerebral torpor are the symptoms which gradually appear, and which we shall find complete in spontaneous myxœdema.

Operative myxœdema may be slight and curable. In these cases the extirpation of the gland has doubtless been only partial. If the myxœdema results from the removal of the thyroid body, or in a child with goitre, we see arrest of development and grave intellectual troubles, which are comparable to those of the congenital disease.

Spontaneous Myxœdema in Adults.—The onset is generally insidious, and the disease shows three periods. The first period is marked by the mucoid infiltration of the skin. The derma and the subcutaneous tissue are infiltrated with colloid substance. The skin is swollen, elastic, and loses its suppleness. It is of a yellowish-white colour. The pressure of the finger does not cause pitting. The lips are thickened, the nose is enlarged, and the face has a full-moon appearance. The hands and feet are swollen, and become pachydermic. The epidermis is dry; the sweat is diminished; the hair, eyebrows, eyelashes, and the beard become thin. The tongue and the mucous membrane of the mouth and pharynx are thickened.

At the end of a few months the stationary stage is characterized by profound muscular weakness and psychical troubles, which are ushered in by dulness, very marked intellectual torpor, and absolute indifference. The pulse becomes slow; the temperature falls to 95° or 96° F. The patient is very sensitive to cold; the urine diminishes, and the voice is rough and monotonous. In fact, as Brissaud says, in the patient with myxœdema the entire body appears to be asleep. At this period atrophy of the thyroid body is the rule, and hypertrophy is the exception. If specific treatment be not employed, the patient passes into a state of pachydermic cachexia, and death is the ending of the third phase. Specific treatment will prevent the onset of this last period.

Congenital Myxœdema—Myxœdematous Idiocy.—Congenital myxœdema may appear before the age of two years. Absence of the thyroid body and infiltration of the skin are seen in children, just as in adults. Arrest of mental and physical development characterizes myxœdematous idiocy. "It does not run a course characterized by successive periods, and does not end in cachexia. It remains the same from the first to the last day, and life is not compromised. The general nutrition, which is at a very low ebb, when it should be at its maximum, is in keeping with a dull, indolent, and passive state of existence, without initiative, without needs, and almost without instinct. The heart beats, the lungs breathe, but the brain remains plunged in its fœtal torpor, and nothing awakens it." Such is the striking picture of myxœdematous idiocy painted by Brissaud. The Pacha of Bicêtre, whose height was only 3 feet at twenty years old, is a striking example. The physical and intellectual condition remains practically in the same state as when the individual was affected, and "he is condemned to perpetual infancy" (Brissaud).

Myxœdematous idiocy, as we have already said, is reproduced experimentally in young children in whom the thyroid body is extirpated.   The myxœdema is really a trophic trouble following extirpation of the thyroid body, and its effects vary according to the age of the patient.

Cretins with goitre are most often myxœdematous, and their history closely resembles that of myxœdematous idiots.   In the cretin the thyroid body is almost always hypertrophied, but cystic degeneration, just as much as the atrophy, deprives the thyroid gland of its functions.

Brissaud distinguishes **thyroid** from **parathyroid** myxœdema.   The latter disease is said to be in man the analogue of the experimental myxœdema which follows the extirpation of the parathyroid glands in animals (Gley).   Myxœdema, properly speaking, is not complicated by intellectual apathy.   Parathyroid myxœdema, which results from a complete and total change in all the parts of the gland, is characterized by " cretinoid idiocy and the brutishness of cachexia strumipriva," in addition to the infiltration of the skin (Brissaud).

Diagnosis.—We shall not dwell on the diagnosis of myxœdema, as it is always easy to differentiate it from various forms of soft œdema in cardiac and renal diseases, from lipomatosis, or from acromegaly.   Let us only remember the relations which exophthalmic goitre and myxœdema may present in exceptional cases.   Hyperthyroidation may gradually give place to hypothyroidation.

Cretinism is special to certain regions, and the goitre from which the patient suffers is nearly always hereditary.

Pathogenesis.—Physiologists have shown that extirpation of the thyroid body in animals causes trophic troubles similar to those of human myxœdema. Horsley experimented upon the monkey.   One question remains to be elucidated : How does functional insufficiency of the thyroid body lead to myxœdema ?

Schiff, in order to answer the question, has stated the following propositions : Either the thyroid body elaborates by internal secretion a substance which is indispensable to the proper action of the nerve centres, or else in the normal condition it has an inhibitory action on certain toxic substances which are produced in the economy, and which can freely exercise their harmful powers after the annihilation of the gland.   In spite of experiments reported by physiologists in favour of the second proposition, clinical facts appear to be in favour of the first one.   Do not the marvellous therapeutic results obtained by the injection of thyroid extract appear to indicate that the gland secretes a substance useful to the proper function of the organs ?   Besides, we are commencing to recognize the intimate nature of the active principles of the thyroid juice.   Baumann has discovered thyroidin, an organic substance consisting of proteid matter and iodine in intimate combination.   This substance, which is a very active extract of the thyroid body, cures myxœdema, as very clear cases have proved.

From the practical point of view, we must always assure ourselves of its existence in the extracts used therapeutically, and the iodine which it contains renders its discovery easy. Fränkel of Vienna, has recently isolated a crystallizable substance called thyro-antitoxin, which does not contain iodine. In animals it lessens the symptoms caused by extirpation of the thyroid body. Chemistry has, without doubt, not said its last word as to the nature of the substances in the thyroid juice.

Treatment.—The specific treatment of myxœdema consists in supplying the economy with thyroid substances, the absence of which causes the disease.

Grafting the thyroid body of animals and hypodermic injections of thyroid extract were the first methods employed, but they have been abandoned.

Howitz was the first to institute the treatment of myxœdema with thyroid tabloids. This method is the only one employed to-day. We can procure ready-made tabloids of the thyroid extract, but the best preparation is the home-made one prepared from the thyroid body of the sheep; it must be administered by lobes with the greatest care in order to avoid the troubles of hyperthyroidation, which may even simulate the symtoms of Basedow's disease, and which are most frequently ushered in by headache, syncope, albuminuria, etc.

Under the influence of the thyroid juice the central temperature is raised, rapid *demyxœdemization* occurs, the cerebral torpor disappears, and the patients rapidly regain their health. Recovery is only maintained by continuous treatment, and one or two lobes weekly must be given for the rest of the patient's life.

Such are the principles of this treatment, which is, it must be said, one of the greatest conquests of contemporary medicine.

The employment of Bayer's thyro-iodine has also been advised in doses of from 50 centigrammes to 1 gramme. The results produced by this drug are most favourable.

Pierre Marie and Crouzon treated a man suffering from operative myxœdema, and found that the patient's weight fell from 99 to 88 kilos in three months. Further, the urine, which contained 1·10 grammes of albumin per litre before treatment, did not contain a trace at the end of six weeks. These authors have not obtained the same results with capsules of fresh thyroid. The weight remains high, and the patient does not experience the same benefit as with iodothyrin.

XII. SCROFULA—LYMPHATISM.

If we refer to the descriptions which have been rendered classical by the authority of our predecessors, we shall see that **scrofula** "is a constitutional dystrophy of which the manifestations are, for the most part, of an inflammatory nature, and infect the lymphatic glands, the skin, mucous membranes, cellular tissue, the osteo-fibrous tissues, and the viscera " (Jaccoud).

There is, said Bazin, in the appearance of these multiple manifestations a kind of regularity which, although not absolute, yet has some value. Thus, the skin and the lymphatic glands are the first affected even in youth ; later the mucous membranes and the connective tissues suffer ; in the third place we find the lesions of the bones and of the joints ; and, lastly, changes in the viscera.

According to the old description, scrofula commences in the first year of life. Children at the breast, or when approaching dentition, present impetiginous eruptions on the head or on the face (milk crusts). Later, we find chronic blepharitis, impetigo, crusts, discharges from the nose and ears, and chilblains, which become ulcerated.

The glandular enlargements often appear about the second dentition (lymphatic temperament). Scrofulous adenitis takes place in successive attacks. It is often limited to the glands of the neck, but it sometimes attacks the bronchial and mesenteric glands (tabes mesenterica). Cervical adenitis may be isolated or multiple ; it may end in resolution or in suppuration, which is sometimes interminable, and leaves indelible scars.

The look of the patient is characteristic. The upper lip is enlarged and projecting, the nose is swollen, the chin is flattened, the tonsils are large, and the child is subject to sore-throats and colds.

At a more advanced age we find scrofulides or dermatoses, which have their seat of election on the head and face. These lesions are chiefly erythematous, vesicular, and pustular. They often have a violet tint, and do not cause pain or itching.

The later manifestations of scrofula are chronic and ulcerative coryza, with or without ozæna, ulcerative scrofulides of the throat and lupus, ulcerative or tubercular dermatitis, which especially attacks the nose and cheeks.

At the same time cold abscesses, articular and bony lesions, such as periostitis, caries, fungous arthritis, and white swelling appear ; and, finally, the last period, according to Bazin, comprises scrofula affecting the testis, the genito-urinary organs, the breast, or the brain, and bronchial or pulmonary phthisis.

Scrofula, which is a diathetic or acquired disease, may be arrested at any point in its evolution. It rarely commences after the age of puberty, but often presents long remissions, and an adult may suffer from scrofulous lesions, although he has had no trace since infancy.

This general survey of scrofula answers to the classical picture which has been handed down to us.

But what remains of this picture to-day ? Practically nothing. The dismemberment of scrofula has profited tuberculosis and, to a slight extent, syphilis. Scrofula has therefore lost its autonomy. In many cases scrofulo-tuberculosis has replaced the old scrofula.

Some part of the old scrofula must, however, be preserved. Thus the impetiginous eruptions on the face and on the head which supervene during lactation and the approach of dentition ; the milk crusts and the scabs, as they are vulgarly called, which persist and recur with obstinacy ; the erythemata and the discharges from the nose and the ears, form a clinical picture which corresponds to the views held, if not of scrofula, at least of lymphatism. It may be said that children subject to such manifestations are more liable than others to become scrofulo-tubercular. We shall discuss later this question, which proves, in any case, the affinity of these various conditions, but not their identity.

It is certain that in the so-called lymphatic persons resolution is imperfect in congested or inflamed parts, and it appears as though the lymphatic circulation were interrupted. Catarrhs of the nasal, ocular, and pharyngeal mucous membranes persist indefinitely ; the alæ nasi and the upper lip remain indurated and thickened ; the blepharitis seems everlasting; coryza and angina occur on the least opportunity; the lymphatic glands readily suffer from the shock; the tonsils are hypertrophied and remain large. These various lesions give a characteristic appearance to the lymphatic patient.

It is also undeniable that these "lymphatic" subjects are less armed for defence; the "soil" is in their case of inferior quality; the skin and the mucous membranes are readily invaded by the pyogenic and saprophytic microbes which usually live on these surfaces, and hence the frequency of impetigo, of boils, and of cutaneous suppurations, with or without consecutive adenitis. This attenuated scrofula, or "lymphatic temperament," if we prefer to preserve an ancient term, deserves a place in our pathological descriptions, but all the remainder of the old scrofula should be transported elsewhere.

Thus tuberculosis and syphilis must claim the ulcero-crustaceous scrofulides, the so-called scrofulous adenitis, the scrofulides of the mucous membranes, and the king's evil. Most cases of adenitis which were regarded as scrofulous are really tubercular. Their tubercular nature is proved by pathological anatomy and by experimental research, for their substance produces tuberculosis on inoculation. These cases of adenitis often supervene in persons who have not had any scrofulous trouble. They may persist for a long while in the condition of **local tuberculosis**. They improve, become worse, and are followed by tuberculosis of the bronchial glands, by suspicious bronchitis, and by pulmonary phthisis. Their course is sometimes very slow. It may last for a great number of years, and yet in some cases the march of events is much more rapid. An individual (the case is common in soldiers) who has never had any past history of scrofula is taken ill with bronchitis, or with pleurisy, or perchance has a cold abscess, caries of a bone, without any trace of pulmonary phthisis; and yet his health declines, adenitis appears, and is really tubercular, though apparently scrofulous. Acute pulmonary tuberculosis, which proves fatal, soon follows.

Syphilis in the tertiary period gives rise to glandular gummata (Fournier). These gummata are seated chiefly in the inguinal, submaxillary, and cervical regions. At first they are hard and painless, but later they soften, ulcerate in the form of a crater, and give exit to thick, viscid, and purulent matter. The analogy is sometimes so great between these syphilitic adenopathies and those which were formerly called scrofulous that treatment alone can decide the diagnosis. We can therefore eliminate the group of so-called scrofulous adenopathies.

The group of **malignant scrofulous anginæ** must also be struck out; and these anginæ are due to acquired or to hereditary syphilis, or are of tubercular origin.

Lupus of the skin and mucous membrane is also a lesion of scrofulo-tubercular origin. The description of lupus has already been given.

Cold abscesses, which we are too ready to call scrofulous, must be referred to tuberculosis. Tubercles and bacilli have been found in their walls.

Scrofula, according to old descriptions, affected the joints and the bones, causing white tumours, caries with suppuration, and fistulous tracts, from which splinters of bone came out. On closer inspection, however, it has been found that these so-called scrofulous lesions (chronic arthritis, fungous arthritis, and white swelling) are anatomically and clinically tubercular in nature.

Fungous tubercular arthritis rarely commences in the synovial membrane; it almost always has its origin in tuberculosis of the bone. A tubercular focus develops in the epiphysis, softens, causes osteitis, caries, necrosis, and the joint is then invaded.

In some cases these lesions represent a local tuberculosis, which may recover with or without ankylosis—coxalgia, white swelling of the knee (Lannelongue's treatment)—but sometimes tuberculization of the joint is followed at a more or less lengthy interval by pulmonary phthisis, and reports prove that apumtation may cause an outburst of acute pulmonary tuberculosis (Verneuil). In other cases the tubercular lesions in the joints and bones develop at the same time as a more or less latent phthisis.

Other bony lesions which have the appearance of scrofula are **syphilitic** in nature. Lastly, others arise in an old osteomyelitis, which has probably fallen short of complete recovery (Lannelongue). All these changes must be abstracted from the list of scrofula.

Visceral Lesions.—Many visceral lesions which were formerly regarded as scrofula must be put under the head of tuberculosis. We are not sufficiently familiar with the course of these local forms of tuberculosis ; we are not yet sufficiently free from the famous law of Louis, which states that pulmonary tuberculosis must accompany tuberculosis of other regions or of other organs. Local or localized tuberculosis may appear primarily in a region or in an organ, where it remains localized and ends in recovery. It has not the same gravity in all organs, its evolution does not run the same course, and its tendency to become general is different.

Certain changes in the **testis,** characterized by chronic orchitis, with induration of the epididymis, softening, suppuration, and fistulæ, have long been called scrofulous. These changes are really tubercular. Not only does the lesion recover like a local tuberculosis, but in ten cases out of thirty tuberculosis of the testis has no tendency to become general (Reclus). I would say the same of tuberculosis of the uterine mucosa, of the ovary, of the bladder, of the **kidney,** and of the breast—lesions formerly considered by Bazin as scrofulous in nature.

As regards the changes in the **lung,** we know that the tubercle and the caseous products are of the same nature (Laënnec's work) ; the so-called scrofulous phthisis and tubercular phthisis belong to one single morbid process, and clinically the differences in their symptomatology are most often reduced to a question of degree.

The foregoing comparative and analytical study proves that scrofula no longer exists as a morbid entity ; some of its changes belong to syphilis, and a still larger share belongs to tuberculosis. One thing remains : I mean " the lymphatic temperament," on which I have dwelt above, and which constitutes a weakness on the part of the individual. This weakness, which we call lymphatic or scrofulo-lymphatic, may be acquired or hereditary.

It may be caused at the most tender age by defective or insufficient nourishment, and it may depend, at a somewhat more advanced age, on faulty hygienic conditions, such as damp, dark, and airless dwellings, or bad nourishment. It may, lastly and chiefly, be hereditary when the child is born of arthritic, syphilitic, alcoholic, or of tubercular parents, or when the fœtus has been conceived under adverse conditions (advanced age of the father, ill-health of the mother).

Are we to consider lymphatism as the first stage of tuberculosis ? I do not think so.

It is indisputable that lymphatic persons are specially predisposed to scrofulo-tubercular changes and to pulmonary phthisis, but this does not prove the identity of the two processes ; it proves, rather, at most, that the scrofulo-lymphatic person offers a soil favourable to the development of tuberculosis.

The **treatment** of scrofulo-lymphatism is as follows : Residence, as far as possible, in the open air, in the country, or at the seaside ; physical exercises, riding, and gymnastics. The food should be carefully chosen, and should consist of meats, fresh vegetables, fat and oily foods, such as caviare, sardines in oil, tunny-fish, and *pâté de foie gras.* Cod-liver oil in large doses, preparations of iodine, phosphates, and arsenic are the chief drugs. Hydrotherapy, sea-baths, saline, sulphur, and bromine waters should be advised (Kreuznach).

PART IX

PARASITIC INFECTIONS

I. TRICHINOSIS.

TRICHINOSIS is the disease produced by the entrance of a large number of trichinæ into the organism, and especially into the striated muscles.

Ætiology — Pathogenesis.—The trichina—*Trichina spiralis* (Owen), *Trichinella spiralis* (Raillet)—is a helminth of the order of the Nematodes and of the tribe of the Trichotrachelides (Blanchard).

The male, which is 1·5 millimetres in length, of a cylindro-conical form, and pointed in front, presents at its posterior part two appendages—" a kind of copulatory pouch" (Blanchard). The female, which is from 3 to 4 millimetres long, only attains these dimensions after pairing, when it is filled with eggs. The hatching of the latter takes place in the oviduct at the end of six or of seven days, the trichina being " ovoviviparous." The embryos are set free alive, and each female may give rise to many thousands of small trichinæ.

In man the trichinæ contained in measly pork make their way out of the muscular cysts into the intestine, where they pair, and beget an immense number of embryos. The greater part passes into the striated muscles—" their normal habitat" (Brouardel). The paths of this migration are still under discussion. According to some authorities, the fecundated females perforate the wall of the intestine, and give off the embryos during their passage. The latter penetrate into the lymphatic network of the lacteals, pass into the venous circulation, and then into the general circulation, in order to make their way through the capillaries, and to be arrested in the muscles (Cerfontaine). According to other authors, the young trichinæ, having come from the villi of the mucosa, invade the lymphatic tracts, and reach the blood-current after passing through the thoracic duct (Askanazy). In the striated muscles the embryo increases in size, becomes encysted, and commences a latent life.

Man contracts trichinosis by eating contaminated pork which has not been cooked. Severe epidemics of trichinosis have been noted, especially in the North of Germany and in America. Among the great epidemics in Germany, I may quote those of Emersleben, Deensdorf, Groeningen, and Nienhagen in 1883, studied on the spot by Brouardel and Grancher. The ingestion of raw pork which contains trichinæ is the chief cause of the disease. Cooking, however slight, removes all danger. Salting has also a beneficial influence, and salted meats appear to be less harmful than others.

Pathological Anatomy.—If the patient dies during the first few weeks we find catarrhal inflammation of the gastro-intestinal mucous membrane ; if death occurs later, the lesions in the digestive system are no longer present, but we find congestion, inflammation, and œdema of the lung, and sometimes a general œdema, without other special changes.

The specific lesions affect the striated muscles. All the muscles may be affected. The diaphragm, the intercostal muscles, the muscles of the pharynx, and those of the neck and eye, are, however, the most liable. The changes are also more frequent in the neighbourhood of the tendons. The muscles are riddled with cysts containing the larvæ. The cyst contains the trichina in its centre, and is enveloped by an external layer of myolemma, which is softened and converted into a cellular sheath (Grancher). Progressive atrophy of the muscle fibre is often present. The cysts finally undergo calcareous infiltration. The trichinæ become impregnated with chalk, and the cystic coverings with phosphate of calcium. The adult cysts, which vary from 0·3 to 0·8 millimetre in length, generally contain a single larva. In exceptional cases we may find as many as six or seven larvæ in the same cyst (Owen, Chatin). According to Soudakewitch, the larva causes phagocytic phenomena, which tend to prevent the invasion of the parasite.

Symptoms.—Following Brouardel, we may describe three periods in the clinical study of trichinosis :

1. *Intestinal or Choleriform Phase.*—This period commences three or four days after the ingestion of the infected food with signs of indigestion. The patient suffers from nausea, which is soon followed by abundant and repeated vomiting. The diarrhœa is profuse and choleriform. It is accompanied by rigors and fever, which may reach as high as 104° F. At the end of a few days these alarming symptoms become less severe, and about the end of the first week we notice the appearance of considerable but transient œdema of the face, whence the name of epidemics of big heads given to the German epidemics. We sometimes find pains in the limbs, but they are less acute than those of the second period.

2. *Rheumatic and Typhoid Phase.*—About the eighth or ninth day pains appear in the muscles. The movements are painful and difficult, and cause the patient to cry out. Sometimes the muscles are rigid and contracted. If the diaphragm is affected, respiration is rendered difficult.

The involvement of the muscles of the eye gives the patient a fixed look, as in total ophthalmoplegia. The adynamia is profound, and is sometimes followed by violent delirium. Auscultation often yields signs of œdema and of pulmonary congestion.

3. *Cachectic Phase.*—It is characterized by enormous œdema of the legs, of the abdomen, and sometimes of the upper limbs. The face is wasted, the eye is dull, and the voice is broken (Grancher).

Slight cases of trichinosis recover after a few weeks. Severe cases may last two and three months, and generally end in death. The fatal termination, which is rare before the third or the fourth week, is due to the progressive course of the disease, but especially to pulmonary œdema, to secondary pneumonia, and to ulcerative infections with cachexia.

The **prognosis** varies directly with the duration of the affection, and in prolonged cases is often fatal.

The **diagnosis** is very simple during an epidemic. The first few and isolated cases are much more difficult to recognize. They may simulate cholera, typhoid fever, and renal or cardiac cachexia. Bacteriological examination of the stools will decide the question of cholera, and serodiagnosis will eliminate typhoid fever. If we find no reason for the condition of cachexia in any organ, we may perhaps by a biopsy of the painful muscle bundles discover the trichinæ, and also trace them in the suspected foods.

Treatment.—Rigorous prophylaxis will tend to prevent contamination by food. Cooking of doubtful meat is one of the best measures. Therapeutics have but little effect when the disease is present. We may attempt by anthelmintics (calomel or santonin) and purgatives to sweep the trichinæ out of the intestine. This treatment is absolutely powerless when the parasites have already passed into the lymphatic tracts of the muscles. General treatment must be employed for the cachexia.

II. FILARIASIS.

The name **filariasis** is applied to an affection which follows the invasion of the human organism by the *Filaria sanguinis hominis* of Lewis, and by the *F. nocturna* of Patrick Manson. The troubles caused by the *F. medinensis* (subcutaneous collections of pus, destruction of the skin, centres of gangrene, etc.) should be separated from this description, and described under the heading of **dracunculosis.**

Ætiology—Pathogenesis.—Filariasis is a disease of hot countries. While it is endemic in practically all intertropical regions, it is found chiefly in Lower India, China, Japan, Australia, Lower Egypt, Mauritius, Réunion, Madagascar, on the West Coast of Africa, in Brazil, Cuba, Guadeloupe, and in the South of the United States. It is exceptional in Europe, and is found only in persons who have lived in hot countries.

The *F. nocturna* is a helminth of the order of Nematodes and of the genus Filaria. Demarquay was the first to find the embryos of the filaria in the fluid from a chylous hydrocele, in 1863.

The adult worm is found in the lymphatic vessels of man. The male is colourless, and measures 83 millimetres in length ; the female, of a darker colour, is larger and longer, and measures from 88 to 155 millimetres. The embryos, which are present in great numbers in the lymphatic vessels, pass through the thoracic duct or through the large lymphatic vein, and reach the blood-stream. The embryos of the filaria are found in the peripheral circulation only during the evening and the night, appearing about five or six o'clock in the evening, and disappearing about eight or nine o'clock in the morning. If during this time we prick the finger, we find in the drop of blood a considerable number of filaria embryos. Their length is from 125 to 300 μ, and their breadth from 7 to 11 μ. They make very rapid movements, and push the red and white corpuscles in their passage. They are surrounded by a transparent sheath, which they perforate in order to become free. They do not possess a digestive tube or a reproductive system.

In human blood the filaria embryos cannot pass into the larval state. This transformation is effected by an intermediate host, the mosquito (Manson). The female mosquito sucks the human blood, and swallows the filaria embryos, which lose their sheath, perforate the digestive tube of the mosquito, and lodge in its thoracic muscles. When the mosquito lays its eggs, falling into water and dying, the larvæ are set free from the dead insect. Until recently it was admitted that the larvæ were ingested by man in drinking water. The recent researches of Manson show that the mechanism is quite different. The embryos, taken into the stomach of the female mosquito, together with the human blood, lose their enveloping membrane, pass through the wall of the stomach, and reach the muscles of the thorax, where they grow and develop. About the fifth day the larvæ proceed towards the prothorax, collect in the head, and accumulate below the mouth and enter the proboscis. If the female mosquito bites a man at this time she inoculates him with the filaria larvæ, which will become adult. The pathogenic mosquito is the *Culex ciliaris*. The Anopheles which transmits malaria does not transmit filariasis.

Symptoms.—Filariasis may show no symptom. As a rule, this is not the case, and the troubles provoked by the parasite are very varied.

As regards the **skin,** the complications depend upon the more or less complete mechanical obstruction of the lymphatic vessels by the filariæ. We find lymphatic varices, especially in Scarpa's triangle, the scrotal region, the inguinal region, and the lower limbs. The lymphatic vessels stand out under the skin, and form large varicose networks, and the glands are much enlarged. All these parts are of a soft and fatty consistency. Lymphatic thrombosis follows the development of the varices, and œdema appears. The swelling is considerable. The skin is white, wrinkled, and covered by small warty or gelatinous projections, and preserves the imprint of the finger. The lymphatic œdema, though most often transient, is very subject to relapses, and is at length accompanied by a thickening of all the layers of the skin and of the subcutaneous tissue, which produces **elephantiasis** of the legs. The scrotum is often affected by elephantiasis, and the swelling may reach the size of an adult head. The penis disappears completely, and the meatus is represented by a small depressed slit on the surface of the tumour (Marie). Ulcerations and injuries of the skin affect the distended lymphatic tracts, and give rise to a flow of viscid greyish-white lymph, which forms crusts.

As regards the **viscera,** filariasis produces lymphatic effusions in the various serous cavities and in the urinary system.

Chylous hydrocele is characterized by a milky effusion into the tunica vaginalis. Puncture gives exit to a milky fluid composed of fine fatty granules and abundant white corpuscles. The filaria embryos are present in great numbers, and it was here that Demarquay discovered them. Chylous hydrocele may supervene during the onset of filariasis or at a later period. It is sometimes preceded by sharp testicular pains, which may resemble renal colic (Audain). These crises were very marked in one of Rénon's cases, and supervened on an average twice a year, without any prodromata. The patient was awakened in the morning with pain in the right testis, sometimes accompanied by fever, and radiating into the right iliac fossa as far as the lumbar region. The attack resembled the symptom-complex of renal colic, with sharp pain and vomiting. The only differences were the onset with testicular congestion and the complete absence of changes in the urine. The crisis yielded at the end of twenty-four or thirty-six hours, and it was only after eight years of these attacks that the hydrocele appeared. The patient was not troubled by œdema of the scrotum or of the legs, or by chyluria. The filariasis was practically confined during this time to these crises. It is necessary to remember these facts, for I cannot too strongly insist upon the difficulty of diagnosis.

Chylous ascites is rare. It cannot be distinguished from ascites of other origin except by puncture.

Chylothorax is exceptional. As a rule, only one of the pleural cavities is affected.

The chyluria may be pure. Generally we see an admixture of blood. The urine is of an opaque and yellowish-white colour. When it contains blood, the colour becomes like that of *café-au-lait*, chocolate, or of dark beer, etc. The urine contains serin, globulin, peptones, red corpuscles, white corpuscles, fine fatty granulations, and filaria embryos. The passage of chylous urine takes place suddenly, without great pain, following excessive fatigue. It ceases at the end of a few days, to reappear after fatigue, injury, or excess.

The general health is but little affected, and the course of the disease is very slow. Filariasis is characterized by acute attacks, which are followed by periods of calm. It may last fifteen, twenty, thirty, and even fifty years. Recovery is sometimes spontaneous. It follows the death of the adult filaria. The obstruction of the lymphatic channels ceases, and causes progressive disappearance of the signs of the disease. Death results from severe visceral complications and from secondary infection.

Diagnosis.—The presence of the embryo in the blood and in the pathological fluids (ascites, effusions, and œdema) will at once make the diagnosis certain. The search for the embryos in the blood should be made at night. The exudate is centrifugalized, and the deposit is examined. We can thus see the living embryos or stain them after having fixed the preparation. The method is as follows : Gibbs's borated carmine is employed, followed by washing with hydrochloric alcohol, and then staining with methylene blue. The embryo is stained a blue colour, and its cuticle is a rose-red (De Nabias and Sabrazès). The symptoms of filariasis may be confused with many affections, and I cannot enumerate them all. Hæmatochyluria is readily distinguished from hæmaturia and from hæmoglobinuria. The hæmaturia caused by the *Bilharzia hæmatobia* is accompanied by the presence of the oval eggs of the parasite in the urine. We should always think of filariasis in any abnormal case of renal colic which is complicated by early and pronounced congestion of the testis.

Treatment.—The employment of boiled and filtered water and protection against the mosquitoes of the genus *Culex ciliaris* are the only prophylactic measures which are efficacious against the disease. Parasiticide treatment of filariasis by mercury and iodine has not given good results. On the other hand, we may remove the local troubles by puncture of the chylous effusions or by dissection of the lymphatic varices of the invaded regions, but we cannot expect a radical cure unless there is a chance of removing the adult filaria.

PART X

DISEASES AFFECTING THE LOCOMOTOR SYSTEM

I. RICKETS.

Ætiology.—Rickets is a disease of infancy, characterized by faulty nutrition and growth of the tissues which are concerned in ossification. It is probable that the absence of calcification in the rachitic bones or the delay in this calcification arises from the fact that the organism does not receive or does not assimilate in sufficient quantity the materials which form phosphate of lime. In other cases, however, the absence of calcification concerns only one side of the question, and cannot explain the extreme overgrowth of the tissues. We may, therefore, say that the pathogenesis of rickets is as yet obscure.

This disease has been for some years the object of much research. Beneke and Bouchard hold it to be a disease caused by faulty nutrition, and consecutive to the non-absorption of the phosphate of lime which is necessary for the formation of the bones. In the normal condition the phosphate of lime is not absorbed ; it is split up. The chalk combines with hydrochloric acid to form chloride of calcium, while the nascent phosphoric acid combines with the glycerine produced by the action of the pancreatic juice on the fats in order to produce glycero-phosphoric acid. If the contents of the intestine become alkaline, or if the acidity of the contents is due to lactic acid, as occurs in rickets, the splitting up does not take place, and the absorption of the phosphate of lime becomes insufficient. On the other hand, the excess of lactic acid passes into the blood, impregnates the tissues, and dissolves the phosphate of lime which is already fixed. Such, then, is the primary cause of rickets, according to the two authorities just quoted.

Rickets often coexists with dyspeptic troubles, which are accompanied by dilatation of the stomach. Comby looks upon this dilatation as the real cause of rickets, in consequence of the imperfect elaboration of the food.

According to certain authors (Parrot), rickets is one of the manifestations of hereditary syphilis, but this view has not been generally adopted.

Since the publication of Parrot's monograph the bony lesions of hereditary syphilis have been more carefully studied (Fournier, Lannelongue), and it has been shown that radical differences exist between the changes in the bones caused by syphilis and those which are attributable to rickets (Berne). On the other hand, Galliard has published the case of a rachitic child born of parents who were not syphilitic, although they contracted syphilis several years after the birth of the child ; and Giraudeau has reported four cases of rachitic persons who contracted syphilis. These facts do not agree, if we admit that rickets is syphilitic in origin.

Gley and Charrin have been able to reproduce experimentally in animals by the injection of toxines into the parents lesions which resemble those of human rickets, and Mircoli has been the defender of an infectious theory of rickets. I merely state these researches, without being able as yet to draw conclusions from them.

Pathological Anatomy.—In the first period the affected bones are not deformed ; in the second period the deformities are considerable ; the third period corresponds to the consolidation of the affected bones. The parts concerned in the growth of the bone—that is to say, the epiphyseal cartilage and the periosteum of the diaphyses—are the initial seat of the lesion.

In the normal condition, when we study the epiphyseal end of a bone in process of growth, we find in the deep parts of the epiphyseal cartilage a translucent and bluish layer, in which the phenomena of proliferation go on and converge towards the points of ossification. Below this cartilaginous layer we find another layer, " formed by areolar tissue, in which the rows are composed of a ground substance of cartilage infiltrated with calcareous salts " (Cornil and Ranvier). It is below this ossiform layer that the true bone is formed.

In rickets the lesions affect the deep layer of the cartilage and the ossiform layer. The bluish cartilaginous layer, which is normally 1 millimetre or $1\frac{1}{2}$ millimetres in thickness, becomes several centimetres thick. This tissue has been named **chondroid**—a faulty term, because we are dealing with a true cartilage.

At the level of the ossiform tissue we find the spongy tissue so called, which is very vascular, and which may encroach upon the diaphysis of the bone. The overgrowth and the persistence of these tissues is the cause of the swelling of the epiphyses. The rachitic tissues do not end in the formation of bone, the osteoblasts do not ossify, the soft and little resistant epiphysis allows itself to be deformed by muscular contraction, and a node is formed.

We also find a spongy layer in the periosteum. In the interior of the bone the marrow is much congested, its peripheral layers are organized as in young connective tissue, and the medullary cavity is narrowed or filled up by the curves and deformities of the bone.

As the result of these lesions, the skeleton offers but little resistance, the epiphyses become swollen, and the nodes may even affect the extremity of bones which have not an epiphysis. The shaft of the long bones is curved, deformed, and sometimes fractured. The weight of the body, the tonic action of the muscles, the laxity of the ligaments, and other external causes, contribute to cause the deformities of rickets.

We can thus explain the curves of the vertebral column, the deformity and narrowing of the pelvis, the persistence of the fontanelles and the size of the head, the lateral flattening of the chest and its projection forwards (chicken breast), the curves of the legs outwards or inwards, and the deformities of the arms. The deformities of the legs occur in an order which differs according to the age of the patients. They commence in the legs of children who are walking, but in those who have not begun to walk the arms are the first to show deformity, because they play a more active part.

Rickets may recover without any great deformity when it is slight, but, as a rule, after the period of consolidation of the bones the patient preserves the deformities, which are in part due to the too rapid ossification of the epiphyseal cartilages. The growth of the bone is arrested, the rachitic person remains small and more or less deformed, and as the ossification of the bones of the cranium occurs late, the head is usually large.

Description.—Rickets usually commences about the end of the first year or in the first half of the second year. The bony deformities are sometimes preceded by precursory signs—the child becomes sad and peevish, and dreads every movement because of the pain which results.

The child who has been walking or trying to stand upright is now content to lie down ; the child who loved to sit in the arms of his nurse no longer does so, and weeps when he is taken up from his cot, because of the acute pain on movement. In some patients the disease commences with an intestinal catarrh ; in others the fontanelles remain open beyond the normal term, and dentition is delayed or is arrested if it has commenced (Trousseau). A little later nodes or deformities appear at various points. The nodular prominences appear at the junction of the ribs and the costal cartilages (rachitic rosary) ; the chest is flattened laterally, bulges in the sternal region, and is enlarged in the region of the lower ribs. In consequence of these deformities the costal respiration is embarrassed, the diaphragmatic respiration is exaggerated, the abdominal organs are pushed down, and the belly becomes prominent. The joint swellings are marked, the deformities of the legs and of the arms become exaggerated, and the disease is then complete. The articular deformities are the more striking if the child is emaciated.

The general symptoms increase in severity, the appetite is lost, the skin is covered with abundant sweat, diarrhœa is frequent, and the urine contains a fairly large quantity of earthy phosphates.

Rickets usually runs its course in six or in eight months, and then remains stationary for one or two years. Consolidation of the bones next occurs, and the patient recovers at the expense of the deformities previously mentioned. In several instances, however, the disease terminates in death, due either to the severity of the disease itself or to intercurrent complications, such as bronchitis or pneumonia.

Acute rickets with paralysis of the limbs, subperiosteal swelling of the diaphyses of the bones, fever, marasma, and hæmorrhages from the gums or from the nose, etc., should be distinguished from true rickets (Barlow). It is really infantile scurvy (Comby), which recovers when the child is fed on fresh milk, meat-juice, and orange or citron juice.

Cod-liver oil, butter, with iodide of potassium and chloride of sodium, preparations of the phosphates, and milk of good quality, form the basis of treatment. Salt baths or sea baths render great service.

II. OSTEOMALACIA.

Ætiology.—Between rickets and osteomalacia there is this essential difference—that in the former the bone does not reach its complete state of development, because, as the result of vicious nutrition, the elements of calcification are wanting, and the normal evolution of the bone is interrupted. In osteomalacia, on the other hand, the bone is perfectly formed, and the fault in nutrition consists in a disassimilation of the elements of calcification. The bone becomes decalcified. Rickets is a disease of growth, osteomalacia is a disease of the adult, in which the destruction of the calcareous salts induces softening of the skeleton.

The primary cause of this destruction of the calcareous salts is scarcely understood, and the theories formulated do not aptly give the reason. Osteomalacia is extremely rare in man. It is a disease of women between the ages of thirty and fifty years, and pregnancy forms its starting-point in about half the cases. Osteomalacia is more frequent in certain countries—for example, in Bavaria.

Pathological Anatomy.—During the first period the bones are not as yet rarefied, although they can be more easily cut with the knife. We find under the microscope that the edges of the bony arches no longer contain calcareous salts, which are still found in the centre. The vessels of the marrow are turgid, and hæmorrhages occur both into the marrow and under the periosteum. During the second period the bones become rarefied and softened. They change their shape, diminishing in size, and readily breaking. The bony arches are in part decalcified and in part absorbed. Ossein, which is the fundamental substance of the bony lamellæ, becomes fibrillary. It loses its properties, and can no longer be converted into gelatin.

Fractures rarely unite firmly, and if callus forms, it has in its turn a tendency to undergo the changes of osteomalacia (Bouley).

The bones become flexible and deformed. The vertebræ become weak and flattened, and the bones of the pelvis undergo changes which are of the greatest importance in pregnancy and labour. The deformities of the thorax resemble those of rickets. The bones of the limbs are often fractured.

Description.—Osteomalacia commences with pains in the vertebral column, pelvis, and limbs. These pains sometimes come on in the form of attacks, and are increased by movement, pressure, walking, and sitting. We find, in addition to the pains, feebleness and a sensation of fatigue, which prevent the patient from moving.

The softening of the bones shows itself by the deformities which I have previously enumerated—the patient is bent and shrunken, and the thorax is deformed. We often see painful contractions. Attacks of fever sometimes appear. The general functions, which were normal during the first part of the disease, commence to fail, the appetite diminishes, and the patient complains of palpitation, dyspnœa, giddiness, and formication of the lower limbs. Fractures are frequent.

Osteomalacia does not always run a continuous course. Remissions and paroxysms occur in some cases. The urine may contain an excess of phosphates and carbonates of lime, and always of albuminose. After several years the disease passes into a cachectic condition. Diarrhœa is the rule, wasting is extreme, and the patient dies from marasmus, unless carried off by some intercurrent disease. Cases of recovery are quite exceptional.

The **diagnosis** of osteomalacia is, therefore, difficult at the onset, before the period of deformities. In syphilitics fractures may easily occur by reason of the fragility of the bones. In such cases the deformities of osteomalacia are absent.

Treatment with phosphorus is naturally indicated. Castration gives encouraging results (Fehling), and total extirpation of the uterus and of the ovaries has been advised at the commencement of pregnancy (Chroback). Utero-ovarian amputation (Neumann) or Cæsarian section has been advised at the termination of pregnancy. The beneficial influence of extirpation of the internal genital organs upon the evolution of osteomalacia is undoubted, although its action is still obscure (Polgar).

III. ACROMEGALY.

Description.—Acromegaly (ἄκρος, extremity; μέγας, large), described for the first time by Marie in 1885, presents as its cardinal symptoms: (1) Considerable hypertrophy of the hands, of the feet, and of certain parts of the face, and especially of the lower jaw ; (2) cervico-dorsal kyphosis ; (3) visual troubles, which are very frequent ; (4) in women, almost constant amenorrhœa.

The disease generally commences in the hands, which become hypertrophied as a whole. Their breadth and thickness are considerably increased, whence the names of " mutton fist " or " padded hand." Their length is practically normal. The increase in size affects all the tissues. The folds of the skin are deeper than normal ; the thenar and hypothenar eminences are remarkable for the thickness of their fleshy mass ; the metacarpus is enlarged and massive ; the fingers, which are short and thick, are swollen at the level of the phalanges. The nails, encased by fleshy tabs, are narrow, flattened, often atrophied, and striated in a longitudinal direction.

The functions of the hands are preserved. The fingers remain apt in performing delicate tasks, and are not the seat of any abnormal sensation.

The other segments of the upper limb, except the wrist in some cases, are normal in size.

The feet are enormous, being increased in breadth and in thickness, though as a rule they preserve their normal length. The hypertrophy assumes the same appearance as in the upper limbs. " We find here the same deep furrows, and especially the digito-palmar folds, which separate the same fleshy pads " (Souza-Leite). The heel is hypertrophied (Verstraeten) ; the instep is often large ; the big toes and the nails show changes similar to those of the fingers. The upper parts of the lower limb are normal.

The deformity of the face is characteristic, and the **acromegalic facies** sometimes carries the diagnosis with it. The deformity chiefly affects the lower jaw. The chin is prominent and enlarged, and instead of representing the axis of an oval with its normal extremity above, as it does in the normal condition, it becomes the axis of an ellipse. The upper jaw takes but little part in the hypertrophy, and as a result the dental arches do not correspond, the lower arch standing out in front of the upper one. This prognathism is accompanied by thickening of the lower lip, which is prominent and everted. The tongue is enormous, so enlarged and thickened as to hinder swallowing and the pronunciation of the linguals.

The vault and the velum palati are usually enlarged ; the tonsils and the uvula are hypertrophied. The nose is splayed out and hypertrophied.

The cheeks and the internal apophyses of the orbit are prominent. These prominences depend on the dilatation of the maxillary and frontal sinuses. The ears are hypertrophied, thickened, and elongated. The skin as well as the cartilages participates in this hypertrophy. The forehead appears low, and is not in proportion with the exaggerated dimensions of the face. The cranium preserves its normal size. The eyes, which are as a rule small and deep-set, are sometimes more prominent. The penis, the labia majora, and the clitoris are often increased in size.

Cervico-dorsal kyphosis is found in nearly all cases. It is sometimes accompanied by lumbar lordosis or scoliosis, with a variable degree of inclination. In the antero-inferior part of the thorax a compensatory bulging is often found. The clavicle, the ribs, and the sternum are generally thickened, and the hypertrophy of the costal cartilages frequently hampers the breathing, which then assumes the inferior thoracic and abdominal type.

The early and almost constant amenorrhœa helps in certain cases to support the diagnosis at the onset of the disease.

The following phenomena have been noticed fairly often : Bistre colour of the skin, profuse sweating, elevation of the peripheral temperature, enlargement of glands, diminution in the size of the thyroid body (Bury), hypertrophy of the thymus characterized by a zone of retrosternal dullness (Erb), asymmetry of the two halves of the body, amyotrophy, creaking in the joints, erratic pains, increased sensibility to cold, and a sensation of dead fingers.

A separate place must be reserved for the visual troubles, which may vary from slight amblyopia to complete blindness. The narrowing of the visual field, the hemianopsia, the prominence of the eyeballs, which is accompanied by a certain degree of paresis in the extrinsic muscles of the eye, and the congestion of the disc, may be explained by the hypertrophy of the pituitary body, which is so frequent in this disease.

The larynx sometimes participates in the hypertrophy of the extremities, and the voice then assumes a deep tone, which is especially striking in women. The dilatation of the sinuses of the face also contributes to the echoing of the voice (Marie).

Polyuria (Balzer), slight albuminuria, peptonuria, slight glycosuria, and phosphaturia have been noted in some patients. Palpitation and hypertrophy of the heart are also seen, the latter almost always associated with arterio-sclerosis.

The intelligence is usually intact, but changes in character are frequent (sadness, irascibility, and uncertain temper). This, indeed, is not surprising, considering the profound impression which the disease produces on the sufferers.

Acromegaly commences between the ages of twenty and twenty-six years. Its course is progressive, as can readily be proved by making a comparative examination of photographs of patients taken at long intervals. Periods of arrest, followed by active progress, are frequent. The duration of the disease is generally from twenty to thirty years. Death comes from slow cachexia, or from some intercurrent disease. The patient sometimes dies suddenly, and the autopsy reveals no lesions to explain this result.

Ætiology.—The ætiology of acromegaly is quite unknown. All we can say is that it is neither hereditary nor congenital, and that it differs in these two respects from most dystrophic diseases. Cold, syphilis, grief, injury, alcoholism, rheumatism, etc., have all been found in the antecedents of patients, but they are absent in such a large number of cases that there really exists no definite relation between these pretended causes and acromegaly.

Pathological Anatomy.—Hypertrophy of the pituitary body has been found by Marie, and since then by a very large number of authors, who would seek to make this lesion the anatomical substratum of acromegaly. The tumour varies in size from a pigeon's egg to a hen's egg. It dilates the sella turcica, separates the clinoid processes, and lodges itself at the base of the cranium in a cavity which depends on its size. Compression of the optic chiasma and of the ocular vessels accounts for the visual troubles. Histologically, the lesion is rather a simple hypertrophy than a new growth.

Persistence and reviviscence of the thymus; increase in the size of the heart and of the vessels (Klebs); hypertrophy of the ganglia and cords of the great sympathetic have been mentioned.

The lesions of the skeleton are constant. In the limbs " the hypertrophy chiefly affects the bones of the extremities and the extremities of the bones " (Marie). It consists in an increase of the spongy tissue, in dilatation of the vascular orifices of the bones, and in enlargement of the canals for the passage of the arteries. Histologically, the alveoli are enlarged, and represent very dilated Haversian canals with thin walls. The marrow contains neither osteoblasts nor myeloplaxes (Renaut).

The bones of the other parts of the body, and particularly those of the face, present similar changes. The lower jaw, compared with that of a man of the same stature, appears enormous, and the various sinuses are markedly enlarged. The osteopathies of acromegaly have been studied on the living patient with the Röntgen rays.

Diagnosis.—The diagnosis of acromegaly is generally easy, especially at an advanced stage of the disease. It has, however, been confounded with myxœdema in a certain number of cases. The error is easily avoided, since the " full-moon " face seen in cases of myxœdema does not resemble the prognathism seen in acromegaly. In myxœdema the hypertrophy affects the soft parts alone. The skin is stretched and cannot be displaced, the thyroid body is atrophied, mental troubles are frequent, and kyphosis is always absent.

Paget's osteitis deformans is characterized by " considerable overgrowth of the long bones of the legs, and also of the trunk and of the head. The femur and the tibiæ present a marked anterior curve, the legs are separated, the trunk and the neck are bent forwards by the curve of the spine, the breathing is laboured, and assumes the diaphragmatic type, because of the hypertrophy and welding of the ribs. Fairly often at the onset, or in the course of the disease, severe pains, somewhat analogous to lightning pains, may be present " (Marie).

Giants have enormous hands and feet, but in gigantism the different parts of the body are in proportion to their abnormal development. The increase in growth occurs in a regular fashion both in length and in breadth, and is, therefore, unlike the growth which takes place in acromegaly. Gigantism and acromegaly are, therefore, two different conditions, and yet writers have published cases in which these two conditions were found together. The most remarkable of these cases is that of the giant of Montastruc.

This giant was at the same time acromegalic. He had the stature of a giant, but the hands, face, feet, and torso of the acromegalic. He was an example of "these two kinds of exuberant dystrophy in the human body." But how are we to interpret the association of these two dystrophies? Is their association independent, or is it dependent on the same cause? Brissaud and Meige come to the following conclusions : "Gigantism and acromegaly are one and the same disease. If the period during which the increase in the skeleton takes place belongs to adolescence or to youth, the result is gigantism and not acromegaly. If this period belongs to adult age—that is to say, to a time of life when the stature is already fixed—the result is acromegaly. Acromegaly is gigantism of the adult, and gigantism is acromegaly of the adolescent. If the process of increase in the skeleton commences during youth, at an age when the stature is still increasing and encroaches upon the age of manhood, the result is the combination of acromegaly and gigantism."

Hypertrophic pulmonary osteo-arthropathy is met with in persons suffering from old pulmonary lesions, and also in some cardiac cases. The hands are enormous, but the hypertrophy chiefly affects the fingers, which, instead of being short and cylindrical, as in acromegaly, are long, flattened, and clubbed at their tips. The thumb has been compared by most writers to the "clapper of a bell" (Rauzier).

The metacarpus, on the other hand, is scarcely altered. It does not present either the prominences or the fleshy pads of acromegaly. The size of the wrist is, on the contrary, slightly increased. The hypertrophy chiefly affects the skeleton, and spares the soft parts. The nails are enlarged, and curved both in length and breadth. In the feet the same deformities are seen, but the big toes, and especially their free extremity, attract attention, while the metatarsus is much less affected. The face is always spared, and in the vertebral column the cervico-dorsal kyphosis of acromegaly is replaced by a dorso-lumbar kyphosis, which is often accompanied by scoliosis, depending on the coexisting pleuro-pulmonary lesions.

The **treatment** of acromegaly is purely symptomatic. Some attempts have, however, been made at attacking the cause of the disease. Three patients suffering from acromegaly were treated by Marinesco with tabloids of pituitary body. Notable improvement appeared in the general symptoms.

IV. PAGET'S DISEASE—PROGRESSIVE OSTEITIS DEFORMANS.

In this section I shall describe the affection to which the name of **Paget's osteitis deformans** has been given. Sir James Paget's first memoir was published in 1877 in the *Medico-Chirurgical Transactions*. Its title is "Chronic Inflammation of the Bones," and its subtitle "Osteitis Deformans." In a later work, published in 1882, Paget calls the affection by the name of osteitis deformans. The five cases in the first monograph are not all of equal value, but some of them are so characteristic, especially the first one, that they have led to the acceptance of the morbid entity described by the author.

I have devoted a clinical lecture to this disease,* and shall give here the notes of the case :

A man, fifty-two years of age, came into one of my wards with somewhat marked intellectual decay ; his memory was often at fault, and we had therefore to send for his wife, in order to obtain the desired information.

The onset of the disease dated back some twelve years. The patient's health had previously been excellent. At this time he remarked that walking became difficult and painful ; his legs could scarcely support the weight of his body, and appeared to be growing soft, while, at the same time, they became deformed and bowed. This inward bowing of the legs gradually became well marked ; the knees were thrown outwards, and, as the legs curved inwards, they became so much the shorter. It was therefore necessary to cut down his trousers, which had become too long. About the same time the head began to increase in size, and his hat became too small.

At length the neck subsided, the head seemed to sink between the shoulders and was bent forwards, the chest was hunched up, the back became bent, the height diminished, the arms appeared too long, the hands reached as far down as the knees, walking became more and more difficult, and could only be carried out with the aid of a stick. The cerebral activity left much to be desired.

Later the respiration became embarrassed, breathlessness was frequent and accompanied by palpitation, the appetite diminished, and the patient grew thin.

The thighs and the legs, showed an anterior curve. This curve was especially well marked in the leg, where the tibia, with its thickened crest, somewhat recalled the "scabbard deformity" seen in syphilis. On palpation, we found enormous thickening of the bone, but did not discover any osteo-periosteal tumour, apart from some slight roughness ; the hypertrophy of the bone appeared to be uniform. A radiograph taken by Lacaille showed that the femur and the fibula were much less affected than the tibia. The bones of the feet appeared to be normal, with the exception of the calcaneum, which was markedly hypertrophied.

The patient's skull was enormous, and measured 22 inches in circumference just above the ears. It was neither deformed nor nodular. The thickening of the cranial bones was general, uniform, and considerable, as shown in the radiograph. The bones of the face were not hypertrophied to the same extent, and yet, as the radiograph showed, the upper and lower jaws were relatively large. The clavicles were enormous, and their curves were exaggerated. The spine of the scapula participated in the bony hypertrophy. The radiograph showed that the pelvis was narrowed below and spread out above.

---

* Dieulafoy, "Maladie Osseuse de Paget" (*Clinique Médicale de l'Hôtel-Dieu*, 1903, 17me leçon).

The patient's attitude was remarkable : The shoulders were prominent and carried forwards ; the head appeared to lie between the shoulders and to bend towards the sternum, and this was due to the pressing together of the vertebræ. The thorax had undergone similar compression, the ribs were enlarged and close together, and the result was that the height of the thoracic cavity was notably diminished. The shortening of the trunk made the arms appear much too long—they were deformed, slightly curved inwards, and the size of the bones was increased. The hands were not larger than normal, contrary to what is seen in acromegaly. Some bones of the carpus, as our radiograph showed, were, however, affected by hypertrophic osteitis. In short, in about twelve years the greater part of the skeleton had been progressively affected by bony lesions of a deforming and hypertrophic character.

The skeleton was not alone affected. The patient gradually became cachectic. Moreover, he was breathless. The dyspnœa was in part due to the bony lesions, which had narrowed the chest, and also depended on a cardiac lesion. Auscultation of the heart gave a systolic murmur, with reduplication of the second sound. The lesion was mitral.

From this time the intellectual troubles became more marked. The patient lost his memory, did not finish sentences or words, he stammered while speaking, and at times his pronunciation recalled that of general paralysis. It might be asked if these cerebral troubles were due to compression of the brain by the hypertrophied cranium, but this was not the reason, since the bony hypertrophy was not concentric and did not encroach upon the cranial cavity. Accordingly, the cause of these cerebral troubles had to be looked for in a meningeal or in a cerebral lesion.

The patient died from progressive cachexia. Jolly made the autopsy and the histological examination, and furnished the following notes as to the condition of the skeleton and of the organs : In the lungs, emphysema, and congestion of both bases with hepatization ; pleuræ normal ; larynx, trachea, alimentary canal, and peritoneum normal. The liver was engorged with blood, and was of the nutmeg variety, without cirrhosis. It weighed 40 ounces. The spleen was small and sclerous ; it weighed 3 ounces. Kidneys, suprarenal capsules, pancreas, genital organs, and thyroid gland normal.

The heart was soft and flabby. The mitral orifice was somewhat incompetent. We found at the mitral and at the tricuspid valve fibrous thickening of the walls, with nodules which were as large as a pea. The pulmonary valves were not affected, but the aortic valves were indurated, though calcification was absent. Some points of atheroma were present in the aorta. The heart, without clots, weighed 9 ounces.

In the cranial cavity there were no adhesions between the dura mater and the soft meninges, but the adherence between the dura mater and the cranium was complete. On the surface of the brain, especially the convex parts and the base, thickenings of the pia mater were found. Nothing of importance was to be noticed in the sections of the cerebrum, cerebellum and bulb.

Histological examination of the cortex of the brain, at the points where the meninges were thickened, showed the following lesions : The cerebral substance was covered by a relatively thick layer (1 millimetre to 1½ millimetres) of loose connective tissue, which contained a large number of congested vessels. This tissue was infiltrated with numerous round lymphoid cells with a rounded nucleus, scattered in an irregular manner. The lesion was therefore chronic meningitis. There was nothing in the spinal cord.

Let us pass on to the lesions of the skeleton. At the autopsy we were able to verify the bony changes which were so clear in the radiographs. Speaking generally, these changes consisted in hypertrophy with deformity of the bone, and in modification of structure. The hypertrophy was considerable and somewhat regular.

The two tibiæ were enormously hypertrophied and curved. Some slight roughnesses were present on the surface of the bone. One tibia was incised, in order to show the thickness of the bony wall, which in front was nearly an inch.

Most of the ribs took part in the hypertrophy.   In the upper limbs the hypertrophy and deformity of the bones were less marked than in the lower limbs.   The humerus and the radius were, however, large and curved.   The two clavicles were enormously hypertrophied and very much curved.

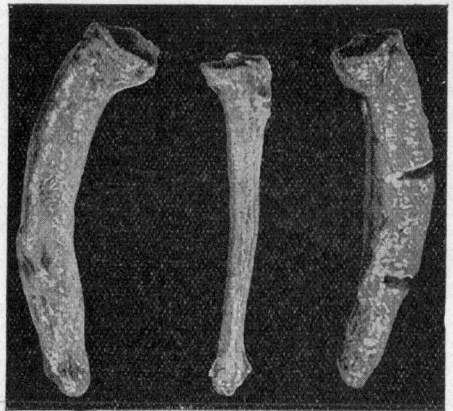

FIG. 96.—NORMAL AND DISEASED TIBIÆ.

At some points the bones of the skull were treble their normal thickness, but the cranial cavity was not encroached upon.

The structure of the hypertrophied bones was modified.   We know that in the

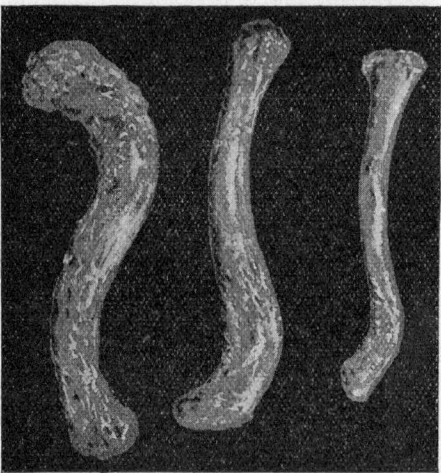

FIG. 97.—NORMAL AND DISEASED CLAVICLES.

normal condition at the diaphyses the wall of the medullary canal is formed of compact tissue, with peripheral lamellæ and Haversian systems, which are parallel to the axis of the diaphysis.   In this patient, a transverse section of the diaphysis of the tibia showed that the tissue of the bony wall was much less dense ; the Haversian canals were large and irregular, running in all directions, and giving the bony tissue a structure resembling that of the diploë.

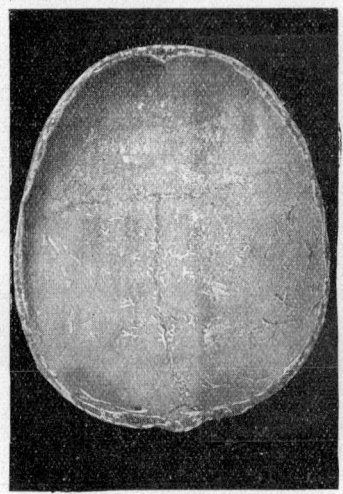

FIG. 98.—NORMAL SKULL.

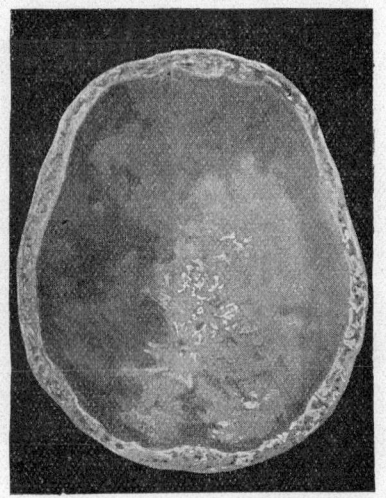

FIG. 99.—DISEASED SKULL.

Description.—Osteitis deformans is a disease of both sexes and of adult age. It is a trophic trouble which diminishes the resistance of the bones, while it provokes overgrowth of tissue. The bones, which become less

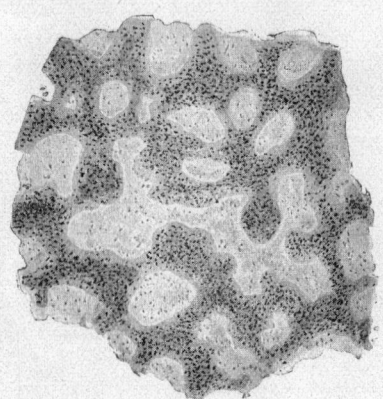

FIG. 100.—TRANSVERSE SECTION OF DIAPHYSIS OF TIBIA.

resistant, bend and are deformed. The bony deformities, which are usually symmetrical, are generally an accentuation of the normal curves, and seem to indicate softening of the bone with hypertrophying osteitis. This softening is, however, very slight, for the bones are not brittle, and fractures are exceptional.

The bones of the lower limbs are often the first to be attacked. The deformities are most marked in this situation, doubtless because these bones have to support the weight of the body. The legs form two arcs, with a double concavity inwards and backwards. In this new situation the heels may come in contact, but the knees project outwards, and cannot be brought together, being separated from one another by an interval of 6 or 7 inches. The legs sometimes show a tendency to become crossed during walking. The bending of the legs causes a diminution in the stature of the patient, and, therefore, dresses and trousers become too long; one child said to its grandmother : " Grandmother, you are shrinking." The crest of the tibia, which is broad and hypertrophied, forms a wide curved edge like a scabbard.

In Hudelo and Heitz's cases the bones of the right leg, which were hypertrophied and curved, were completely joined in their lower two-thirds. The bones of the feet, in contradistinction to what is seen in acromegaly, do not participate, or only to a small extent, in the process of the hypertrophying osteitis. In my patient the calcaneum was large.

The disease sometimes sets in without pain ; at other times the pains are sharp, continuous or paroxysmal, and simulate rheumatism or tabes.

Hypertrophy of the cranial bones is practically constant in osteitis deformans. It is rarely the earliest to appear, and it follows closely the bony lesions of the lower limbs. The head becomes enormous, and, consequently, the hats become too small. The story of larger hats is found in most cases, and is comparable to the story of the trousers or of the dresses, which have to be shortened. The circumference of the head, taken above the ears, measured 22 inches in my patient, and 24 inches in Gilles de la Tourette and Magdelaine's patient. In its general shape the hypertrophied head is often asymmetrical, the parietal eminences stand out, the parietal fossæ are filled up, and the forehead assumes, as in my patient, the appearance of the Olympian brow. On anatomical examination of the cranium, we find disappearance of the sutures, prominences and elevations on the external surface, and levelling of the inner surface. The bones of the base of the skull (petrous and sphenoid) sometimes participate in the hypertrophy.

Although the hypertrophy of the cranial bones is very frequent, they have sometimes been found unaffected post mortem, as in the cases of Hudelo and Heitz, Thibierge, Martel, and Moizard and Bourges.

The enormous size of the cranium contrasts with the condition of the face, which remains normal. Hypertrophy of the inferior maxilla and of the malar bones has been noted. In my patient the lower and upper jaws were enlarged. In a case reported by Joncheray the inferior maxilla was much elongated, and the lower incisors projected in front of the upper ones. In the superior maxilla the alveolar border was much thickened. In Gilles de la Tourette and Magdelaine's patient the inferior maxilla was hypertrophied. It would, therefore, be an error to think that the bones of the face are free in Paget's disease. The condition is, however, not comparable to that seen in acromegaly.

The neck is short and bent forward, so that the head has the appearance of emerging between the two shoulders, while the chin approaches the sternum. The spine is curved forwards, and the patient is bent. The ribs are hypertrophied, and sometimes ankylosed. As a whole, the thorax is short, and, as it were, cramped together. It has the appearance of being " pushed into the abdomen, like an opera-glass," so that the play of the diaphragm and the free activity of the intrathoracic organs are often hampered (Cadet). This is one of the causes of the respiratory distress noted in several cases. The clavicles and the scapulæ are often enormous, as in my patient. The double incurvation of the former is characteristic.

The shoulders project forwards. In consequence of the cramping and bending of the trunk, which has diminished in height, the upper limbs appear elongated, and the hands reach below the knees. The arms are less deformed than the legs. The ulna and the radius, however, are hypertrophied and curved inwards, contrary to what is seen in acromegaly. They do not, however, escape the hypertrophying osteitis completely. Thus, in my patient some of the bones of the carpus were affected; in Gilles de la Tourette and Magdelaine's patient the second and third metacarpal bones of the right hand were very large. Sometimes, as in Marie's patient, the iliac crests are much hypertrophied, and form large projections into the flank, " so that the hip-bones as a whole assume the form of a vase, which receives into its opening the thorax, which is too small for its aperture." In short, when Paget's disease is complete and confirmed, the attitude of the patient is characteristic. Large cranium ; head deeply set between the shoulders and flexed on the chest ; back bent ; thorax compressed and shortened ; deformities of the bones as regards their normal curves ; arms deformed and apparently too long ; legs bent and curved in the form of bows ; difficulty in walking, which requires the aid of one or of two sticks ; bony hypertrophy, affecting chiefly the tibiæ, the cranium, and the clavicle, make up the clinical picture known as Paget's osteitis deformans.

I have described above the lesions found on histological examination of the bones. In Hudelo and Heitz's case there was a mixture of rarefying and condensing osteitis. The most characteristic feature was " the complete derangement of the whole organization of the lamellar systems, the loss of the circular disposition of the bony arches around the Haversian canals, and the architectural structure of the whole bone."

Gombault has noted rarefaction of the bony tissue, without formation of new bone. Thibierge has found in four cases zones of rarefying osteitis alongside those of osteitis neoformans.

The chemical composition of the bone is modified, but these modifications have not much pathological value, since they are variable in different cases.   Thus, in Hudelo and Heitz's case there was an increase in the organic materials and a diminution in the mineral salts, while in Gilles de la Tourette and Magdelaine's case there was a diminution in the amount of organic matter and an increase in the salts.

Although the attention is chiefly directed to the bony system, other lesions and systems must also be considered. Thus, lesions of the heart and of the aorta are so frequent that we cannot consider them as a remarkable coincidence, and I look upon them as forming part of the morbid process.

On auscultating my patient, we found signs of a mitral lesion, which was confirmed post mortem. Paget found in his first patient signs of a mitral insufficiency, and at the autopsy the mitral valve was narrowed and atheromatous, with calcareous deposits. The aortic valves and the first portion of the aorta showed some patches of atheroma. In Lévy's patient mitral insufficiency and hard arteries were found. The autopsy showed that the heart was enlarged, the pericardium adherent, the mitral valve thickened, retracted, and wrinkled, the aortic valves calcified in places, and the aorta atheromatous. Gilles de la Tourette and Magdelaine's patient had had several attacks of asystole, and the autopsy showed that the heart was hypertrophied and dilated with atheromatous patches on the inner surface of the aorta. Moizard and Bourges' patient had atheromatous patches on the mitral and aortic valves. Marie's patient had all the symptoms of a mitral lesion—viz., breathlessness, palpitation, intermittent pulse, systolic murmur, and œdema of the lower limbs. Bonnier's patient had a mitral and aortic murmur, and died suddenly. Gaillard's patient had signs of mitral stenosis. In Sée's case there was hypertrophy of the left ventricle and atheromatous lesions. In short, in nearly every case the heart, the aorta, and the arteries are affected by atheroma or by sclerosis.

I do not know if the lesions of chronic meningitis in my patient form a direct part of Paget's disease. It is certain that meningeal lesions have been found in several cases. In one of the cases in Richard's thesis it is said that the patient became deaf in the right ear, and that his memory failed, so that he often forgot the names of the most common objects. He also suffered from vertigo. At the post-mortem examination patches of softening were found.

In short, Paget's osteitis deformans is a morbid entity which must be clearly distinguished from other affections of the bony system. From the ill-classified group in which multiple hyperostoses were formerly included Paget's osteitis and Marie's acromegaly stand out as well-defined morbid types.

Paget's osteitis deformans has certain characters which permit of a diagnosis, even though the affection is not far advanced. They are as follows : The osteitis chiefly affects the tibiæ, the cranium, and the clavicles, while the bones of the hands, the feet, and the face are practically free. The bony lesion is uniform, and affects the diaphyses of the long bones. The deformities of osteitis deformans are only an exaggeration of the normal curves of the bones. The evolution of osteitis deformans is slow, sometimes painful, and usually symmetrical. It must not be confounded with osteomalacia and with rickets, which in the time of their appearance and in the lesions produced differ so clearly from Paget's disease that further mention is needless. In acromegaly the tibiæ, the clavicles, the cranium, etc., are not affected. The feet and the hands become enormous, and the " hypertrophy shows itself chiefly in the bones of the extremities and in the extremities of the bones " (Marie). Without counting the other characteristic signs, this distinction alone would suffice to differentiate acromegaly from Paget's disease.

When we consider the course of Paget's disease, we find a progressive trophic change in the bony system. The trophic trouble causes diminished resistance in the bone and overgrowth of its tissue. The bone, which has grown less resistant, becomes bent, curved, and deformed. Although certain bones, and notably those of the hands, feet, and face, are less affected, or are even spared, and other bones, such as the tibiæ, the cranium, and the clavicle, form the seat of election in osteitis deformans, it is none the less true that the skeleton as a whole participates more or less in the lesions, which run a slow but progressive course, extending over many years. The patient at length grows cachectic, but this cachexia, which terminates in death, does not depend upon the bony lesion, properly speaking. It depends upon a complex of troubles and lesions which are directly or indirectly associated with the bony dystrophy—cardiac, aortic, cerebral, pulmonary lesions, etc.

It is certain that Paget's disease is a systematic and progressive dystrophy. By its course it approaches the group of affections which Vulpian called " systematic," and which Duchenne of Boulogne named " progressive "— progressive muscular atrophy, progressive locomotor ataxia, and progressive general paralysis. Paget's disease is systematic, for it invades almost the whole skeleton systematically, showing itself by lesions which are identical ; it is progressive, because, like the so-called progressive diseases, it pursues unchecked its fatal course. Accordingly, in the subheading of this section I have added a word to the term osteitis deformans, and have called the disease **progressive osteitis deformans.**

As regards the primary cause of the lesions, we can only conjecture. The hypothesis of an initial medullary lesion had been advanced by Gilles de la Tourette and Marinesco, who in two cases found changes in the posterior column of the spinal cord. Lévi, however, who studied these lesions in

another case, considers them to be senile lesions of vascular origin.   Hudelo
and Heitz agree with the conclusions of Lévi, and think also that these
medullary lesions, when they are found, cannot explain the bony lesions.
My patient had no medullary lesion.

The other hypotheses, such as a lesion of the vascular system, atheroma
of the nutrient arteries of the bones (Beclère), interstitial neuritis of the
nutrient nerve of the bone, do not appear to be sufficient, and I conclude
with Hudelo and Heitz that we do not know the causative lesion of the
bony malformations in Paget's disease.

According to Lannelongue (who has made a profound study of syphilis
of the bones), Paget's disease is syphilitic in nature.   Fournier shares this
opinion.

V. THOMSEN'S DISEASE.

Description.—The description of Thomsen's disease is of recent date.
It was in 1876 that a physician named Kappeln (Schleswig) published the
history of the affection from which he suffered, and which had also attacked
several members of his family.   He spoke of it in the following terms :
"Tonic spasms in the voluntary muscles, in consequence of an hereditary
psychical disposition."   This term has not been preserved, any more than
that of muscular spasms at the onset of voluntary movement proposed by
Ballet and Marie.   This latter term has, however, the merit of showing the
essential character of the affection.

When the patient begins to execute any movement, he experiences
suddenly in the muscles of the region put into action a peculiar rigidity,
which for some moments opposes this movement.   Thus, if he wishes to
walk, or to catch hold of some object, or to strike a blow, the muscles of the
leg, hand, and arm suddenly enter into contraction, and remain fixed.   If
he wishes to shake hands, he cannot for some moments loosen the hand
which he has just seized.   The same troubles may affect the muscles of the
neck, of the jaw, of the eyes, and of the tongue.   In the latter case speech
and pronunciation are much affected.   It is on the occasion of sudden
movements at a word of command, as in military service, that the spasms
reach their maximum.   At the end of a few seconds the rigidity ceases,
and the movements gradually regain their freedom ; but on the occasion of
a fresh cause, which may be insignificant, similar troubles appear, and
disappear a few moments afterwards.

On examining the muscles when they are contracted, we find that they
are hard and very prominent.   The size of the limbs is larger than in the
normal condition, but in spite of this apparent hypertrophy, the muscular
power is sometimes diminished.   Patients are easily fatigued, and although

the affection is not in an advanced stage, they are incapable of work requiring even a moderate degree of force.

All the striated muscles may be affected, but the smooth muscles are usually free.

The mechanical excitability of the muscles is much increased (Erb). The least pressure or the least blow with a percussor or with the end of the finger causes spasm in the muscle fibres. The faradic and galvanic excitability is also increased. At the commencement of the excitation the muscle contracts energetically, and then, as the current continues to pass, the muscle relaxes gradually, and behaves towards the electrical stimulus like an ordinary muscle.

The electrical and mechanical excitability of the nerves is practically normal. Isolated stimuli cause short and transient contractions; accumulated stimuli cause tonic contractions, which are persistent. This symptom-complex, furnished by the examination of the nerves and muscles, constitutes Erb's myotonic reaction.

In addition to the severe and moderate cases, we also find slight and defaced forms.

Thomsen's disease usually begins in infancy or in youth. Sometimes it has a very slow progressive course, but it usually remains stationary, and it may even recede. It is often accompanied by changes in character, such as melancholia and hypochondria, which led Thomsen to look upon the trouble as a psychosis. It is frequently hereditary, and coincides with mental, arthritic, and hysteriform manifestations in other members of the family.

The **diagnosis** is usually easy, given the mode of the appearance and the disappearance of the spasms which characterize it. In spasmodic tabes dorsalis the spasms are continuous; they are completely absent in pseudo-hypertrophic paralysis; they are painful in tetany; they may appear in hysteria, but in the latter case the question is rather one of a true " diathesis of contracture," and the hysterical stigmata are hardly ever wanting.

All the treatment employed in Thomsen's disease has been inefficient. Massage and gymnastics are the most useful measures.

The **pathological anatomy** is very incomplete, for no histological examination of the nerves and of the nerve centres has as yet been made.

Erb's researches upon fragments of the muscles removed from living subjects have shown hypertrophy of the muscular bundles, rounding off of their angles, and multiplication of their nuclei, with a watered appearance and a vacuolated condition of certain muscle fibres. The primary bundles which form the secondary bundle, instead of being straight and parallel, as in the normal condition, are wavy. Lastly, the interstitial connective tissue is usually more abundant than in the normal condition, though much less than in pseudo-hypertrophic paralysis. These characters, which were found by chance in the muscles of a cadaver, led Erb to make a retrospective diagnosis.

VI. PROGRESSIVE MUSCULAR DYSTROPHIES.

Discussion.—In describing the diseases of the spinal cord, I have already said, when referring to progressive muscular atrophy, that the troubles and the changes which affect the muscular system must be divided into two great classes. We have studied the first class in connection with the diseases of the nervous system, and we have seen that the muscular atrophies associated with lesions of the anterior cornua of the spinal cord (myelopathic amyotrophies) have sometimes only the value of an epiphenomenon; in other cases they form a morbid entity.

At the present moment we shall deal with the **primary** diseases of the muscular system—that is to say, diseases which appear to affect the muscle alone, and not the nervous system. Among these diseases we find pseudo-hypertrophic muscular paralysis (Duchenne's type) and progressive atrophic myopathy (Landouzy and Déjerine type). I say that these diseases appear to be independent of lesions of the nervous centres, and yet, when we note the symmetry, the progressive course, and the almost systematic evolution of the muscular lesion, we cannot but formulate hypotheses regarding the existence of lesions in the nervous system. With Vulpian, we may ask if these so-called primary myopathies are not comparable with the reflex muscular atrophies of articular origin, with apparent integrity of the nervous system, and whether " the weakening and disappearance of the trophic power of the motor cells of the spinal cord do not exist in all these cases as the instigating cause of the morbid process situated in the muscles" (Vulpian). We must not strain, says Raymond, at drawing conclusions from negative facts, and say that the nervous system is healthy because we find no trace of myelitis or of cellular atrophy. It seems more reasonable to suppose that some trouble has perhaps existed at the time when the central nervous system is complete and perfect, and has caused an obstacle in its regular evolution, producing a deviation of structure in proportion as the patient's age increases.

The expectations of Raymond have been completely realized, and, as I have indicated in **Diseases of the Spinal Cord,** " no insurmountable line of demarcation exists between the familiar progressive amyotrophies and the progressive muscular atrophies of the Aran-Duchenne type. The various types of progressive muscular atrophy are only variants of the same morbid entity " (Raymond).

However this may be, let us still consider as primary the myopathies which we are now about to describe.

By the side of progressive muscular atrophy (Aran-Duchenne type) Leyden was the first to describe a form of muscular atrophy which commences in the lower limbs, reaches the arms, and is often accompanied by pseudo-hypertrophy—amyotrophy of family origin, very probably due to a lesion of the muscles themselves. Since this time other analogous cases have multiplied. Moebius insists on the cases observed by Leyden, and Eichorst describes a case of muscular atrophy of myopathic origin commencing in the femoro-tibial region, but without pseudo-hypertrophy. Zimmerlin describes a case of family muscular atrophy of myopathic origin, which commenced in the shoulder and reached the lower limbs. In 1884 Erb collected all these varieties in a single group, regarding the pseudo-hypertrophy as a contingent phenomenon which may be present or absent, and he added that the onset of the disease in different parts of the body is not sufficient to stamp these amyotrophies as so many distinct diseases. Lastly, Erb insists on the early appearance of muscular atrophies, to which he gives the term of juvenile form. In the following year Landouzy and Déjerine published a memoir on progressive atrophic myopathy commencing in the face (facio-scapulo-humeral type), but they refused to consider it as a variety of Erb's juvenile form. In their opinion, the disease is distinct, and may sometimes appear in adult life.

Lastly, there are transitional forms, which present a family origin, as in the preceding muscular atrophies, but which commence in the feet, spread to the legs, and then to the hands, and are accompanied by fibrillary tremors and reaction of degeneration. This is the Charcot-Marie type. These authors believe that the disease is not a primary myopathy, but a medullary affection or a neuritis. The same may be said of the hereditary femoral form, with "claw-foot," described by Brossard. It must not, however, be held that in these latter cases the muscular atrophy may never be accompanied by pseudo-hypertrophy, for Bidard and Rémond in 1892 published a case in which certain muscles were manifestly enlarged.

In 1891 Erb reopened this question, and united all the cases under the name of **progressive muscular dystrophy.** He has shown that in this respect the histological process is the same, whether hypertrophy is present or absent. Moreover, in the same muscle we may find hypertrophic and atrophic lesions, so that the volume of the muscle may be normal, although the whole structure is really diseased. Whatever be the variety of the progressive muscular dystrophy in question, the lesions, says Erb, always run the same course. In the first degree we find hypertrophy of the muscular fibres with proliferation of the nuclei; the fibres then divide and break up, while the interstitial connective tissue presents some signs of irritation. The second degree is characterized by atrophy of the muscle fibres, which gradually disappear. At this moment the connective tissue proliferates freely, and the walls of the vessels become thickened. Lastly, in the third period the connective tissue is infiltrated with fat, so that at a given moment the muscle is replaced by fibrous tissue more or less loaded with fat. Then apparent atrophy or hypertrophy of the muscle appears.

These lesions, as we see, are absolutely distinct from the progressive muscular atrophy of myelopathic origin, and should keep the distinction which has been established between these two groups of muscular atrophy. On the other hand, the different varieties of muscular atrophy of myopathic origin which I have just reviewed are related by such close ties that, from the nosographic point of view, there is reason to unite them under the term proposed by Erb—**progressive muscular dystrophy.**

Cases published in 1891 and in 1893 by Werndig and J. Hoffmann, however, appear to show a clear relation between the two great classes of progressive muscular atrophies, and to admit the existence of a progressive muscular atrophy which at the same time is of a **myelopathic** and **family** form. This variety commences in early infancy, most often during the first year of life, in an insidious manner, without convulsions and without fever. The power and the extent of the movements of the lower limbs diminish, and the muscles of the back are affected by motor paresis. The upper limbs, the muscles of the nape of the neck and of the neck are invaded secondarily months and years afterwards. Death takes place after four or five years, and is caused by some intercurrent respiratory affection. The autopsy reveals "the existence of atrophy of the ganglion cells in the anterior cornua, along the whole extent of the neuron, with its maximum in the cervical and lumbar enlargements, and with very pronounced atrophy of the anterior roots; similar degeneration, but much less severe, of the fibres of the mixed motor sensory nerves; lastly, correlative atrophy of the muscles, and an interstitial deposit of fat, without hypertrophy, and without pseudo-hypertrophy of the muscular fibres " (Raymond).

Clinically, however, two varieties stand out prominently : (1) pseudo-hypertrophic paralysis ; and (2) progressive atrophic myopathy (Landouzy and Déjerine type).

VII. PSEUDO-HYPERTROPHIC MUSCULAR PARALYSIS.

Ætiology.—Pseudo-hypertrophic muscular paralysis is a disease of infancy, which may commence before the child has begun to walk or during the early years of life. It may be asked whether this is not an apparent onset, and whether the real onset does not date from the intra-uterine existence. In some cases the disease appears at a more advanced age, as from six to eight, and even from fourteen to fifteen years, though rarely later. It is more common in boys than in girls, and it is not rare to see several children in the same family suffering from this disease.

Pathological Anatomy.—The hypertrophy of the muscular system is only apparent, as the muscular fibres disappear, and are replaced by connective and fatty tissue. Histological examination of the muscles has been made on the living patient with small pieces of muscles removed by means of a harpoon. This examination shows that the muscle fibre has almost completely disappeared, and is replaced by cellulo-fatty tissue. As we have said above, the muscular lesion runs the following course : hyperplasia of the interstitial connective tissue, accumulation of interstitial adipose cells, and simple atrophy of the muscle fibres. Adipose tissue is substituted for muscle fibre, and the muscular tissue undergoes granulo-fatty degeneration only in exceptional cases. In its first stage the lesion is rather fibrous ; in its second stage it is chiefly fatty.

The medullary lesions which have been noted up to the present appear to be secondary or independent. They do not affect the autonomy of the muscular lesions.

The apparent hypertrophy of the muscle contrasts in a singular way with the small size of the tendons. While some muscles stand out in relief, others are atrophied.

Description.—The characteristic features of this disease are : (1) An exaggerated growth in the size of certain muscles, which appear hypertrophied, when really they are not so ; (2) a gradual diminution of the power of voluntary contraction, which ends in complete abolition of movement. It must, however, not be thought that these two symptoms are absolutely associated, and that the muscular weakness increases with the size of the muscle—in fact, the diminution of movement is proportional to the number of fibres which have disappeared ; but, while the muscular fibres disappear, the size of the muscle may undergo every possible variation. It is often increased by the addition of foreign elements, but it is sometimes wasted.

The disease nearly always commences in the muscles of the calf, which stand out in marked relief ; then in its ascending and symmetrical course the lesion attacks in succession the sacro-lumbar muscles, the deltoid, the glutei, the quadratus lumborum, the tensor vaginæ femoris, the serratus magnus, the muscles of the abdomen and of the scapula, the adductors and the flexors of the thigh, etc. The child appears to have the musculature of an athlete.

The muscles which are increased in size are sometimes firm and sometimes soft, depending upon the predominance of fibrous or of adipose tissue.

The increased size of the muscles affected by sclerolipomatosis is in singular contrast with the atrophied muscles. The atrophy may supervene at an advanced period in muscles which were formerly very large ; it may also attack **from the first** certain muscles, especially the latissimus dorsi, the pectoralis major, and the muscles of the arm.

Lastly, the disease may exist in a functional form, in which it is impossible to recognize either hypertrophy or atrophy of the muscles. Pseudo-hypertrophy is not, then, the characteristic and pathognomonic symptom of this disease. " In pseudo-hypertrophic paralysis the size of the muscle is nothing, the weakness is everything " (Marie).

The loss of movement shows a somewhat special course, which gives rise to characteristic attitudes. At the onset, when but few fibres are affected, simple weakness is present ; the child runs about less, and falls easily. Later, in the upright position, the patient assumes a special attitude, and waddles like a duck. He appears hipped, separates his legs and curves his back in a posterior direction, in order to restore equilibrium—in fact, the extensor muscles of the trunk, which, though enlarged in size, are weakened, can no longer oppose the tendency of the body to fall forward, and the patient therefore pulls his shoulders as far backwards as possible. When the muscles of the lower limbs and of the sacro-lumbar mass are very much weakened, the patient experiences the greatest difficulty in raising himself from the prone position. He is compelled to execute this movement by a series of manœuvres in which the arms are used, because he can no longer employ the muscles of the legs and of the trunk for this purpose.

In order to get up, he first turns on his stomach, which in itself is difficult. He then raises his body with his hands, and throws the trunk backwards, in order to assume the stooping position. He now proceeds to raise himself. The legs are extended, while the arms are applied to the ground to support the trunk. The hands are then brought close to the feet, pulled upwards towards the knee, and take higher points of support, the patient, as it were, climbing up himself.

The feet often show deformities, such as bilateral equinus and forced extension of the first phalanges.

In some cases the face has participated in the muscular weakness (gaping mouth and incomplete opening of the eyelids).

Course—Diagnosis.—Pseudo-hypertrophic paralysis commences without fever and without pain, but dullness of the intellect is frequently noted. The symptoms run a very slow course. The tendon reflexes are preserved, the muscles are not affected by fibrillary tremors, the muscular swellings only reach their maximum after one or two years, and the period of paralysis supervenes in a progressive manner. A period of arrest in the disease, or

II.

a remission which may last for several years, is sometimes seen when the apparent hypertrophy is confirmed. The **progressive** course of the disease is, however, practically fatal. The destruction of the muscle and the loss of power become general, and the patient, who can no longer leave his bed, lies absolutely paralyzed.

All the other functions are well carried out, and yet the patient finally becomes marasmic, or dies from some intercurrent disease (bronchitis, pneumonia).

Pseudo-hypertrophic muscular paralysis has a mean duration of from ten to eighteen years. A longer duration is exceptional.

Progressive muscular atrophy, infantile paralysis, and paraplegia will not be confounded with pseudo-hypertrophic muscular paralysis, as the signs of the latter disease are characteristic. Until matters change, we must separate from pseudo-hypertrophic paralysis cases of true muscular hypertrophy which supervene in adults, and which show only very remote resemblance to the disease just described.

Thomsen's disease is accompanied, it is true, by muscular hypertrophy, but never by atrophy. The stiffness of the muscles which characterizes it appears only after voluntary movement. It soon ceases, and the patient can then use his limbs, as in the normal condition. We never find club-foot or deformities of the limbs.

Faradization appears to be the most efficient treatment in pseudo-hypertrophic paralysis. The ingestion of thymus or of extract of thymus is indicated (Pitres).

VIII. PROGRESSIVE ATROPHIC MYOPATHY.

After his remarkable researches on progressive muscular atrophy in adults, Duchenne turned his attention to a similar condition in infancy. He clearly saw that this amyotrophy of infancy presents special characters, that it almost always commences in the face, and gives the little patient a peculiar appearance; but, in spite of these distinctive signs, and, indeed, of many others, he was of opinion that this progressive atrophy in infancy was a variety of the progressive type of muscular atrophy, which has in both cases primary and characteristic lesions in the anterior cornua of the grey substance of the cord.

After important researches, however, Landouzy and Déjerine showed that this amyotrophy in infancy is not a variety of progressive muscular atrophy, as was formerly thought. They grouped the symptoms together, adding new signs, studying the lesions ; they showed that it is a disease of the muscles, and not of the spinal cord ; and, finally, they made of it a distinct morbid entity, which they named progressive atrophic myopathy.

The condition here, then, until proof be furnished to the contrary, is one of myopathy, and not of myelopathy.

Description.—Progressive atrophic myopathy may appear at any age, but is most frequent in early childhood.   In the infant it is always ushered in by more or less marked atrophy of the muscles of the face.   The atrophy of the orbicularis palpebrarum and of the labial muscles gives a peculiar expression to the face.   During repose the child has a gaping, dull, indifferent air ; the lips project; the forehead is smooth.   In the various movements which the face makes we find that the occlusion of the eyelids is incomplete.   During the act of smiling the mouth opens very widely, and the patient grins from ear to ear.

The muscles supplied by the facial nerve are the only muscles of the head affected by this atrophy (muscles of expression), and they are attacked almost simultaneously.   The movements diminish in proportion as the atrophy progresses, but it is a question of atrophy, and not of paralysis.

The course of the facial atrophy is very slow.   It takes years to develop, and it is only after a long period that the atrophy affects the other muscles of the body.

After the face, the muscles of the shoulder and of the arm are the first to atrophy, and here, as in the face, the onset is insidious, the course very slow and symmetrical, without either sensory or paralytic troubles.   The special topography of the atrophies at this period of the disease realizes the facio-scapulo-humeral type.   The muscles of the forearm and of the hand atrophy very late ; wasting of the muscles of the lower limbs then follows.

In this disease the muscles never show hypertrophy or pseudo-hypertrophy.   The retraction of the muscular tissue sometimes produces a prominent cord under the skin.   Fibrillary contractions of the muscles are not seen, and the electrical reactions, which are normal in quality, are diminished in quantity, parallel with the progress of the atrophy.   The tendon reflexes persist for a long while ; trophic troubles are not seen.

Such is the usual picture of the disease in the child.   When the disease commences in the adult (which is far more rare), the symptoms are the same, but the localization of the atrophy presents some difference.   According to the muscles invaded, we find a facio-scapulo-humeral, a scapulo-humeral, and a femoro-tibial type.

As regards the **anatomical lesions,** the nervous system presents no change.   The muscles are affected with simple atrophy, without appreciable change in the sarcolemma.   Sometimes, however, we find interfascicular cirrhosis, but the condition is then one of atrophic cirrhosis.   In the same way as in pseudo-hypertrophic paralysis, it is the hypertrophic cirrhosis which predominates.

The tendons sometimes encroach upon the body of the muscle, and this fact explains the cord sometimes felt near the insertion of the tendons.

In order to explain the mode of invasion of the muscles, Babinski has put forward the theory that the muscles which are first developed are the first to be attacked by the disease.

As accessory or consecutive lesions to the atrophy of the muscles, Déjerine has noted antero-posterior flattening of the thorax, Hallion frequency of spontaneous fractures, and Marie considerable diminution in the antero-posterior diameter of the cranium, which contrasts with the increase in the transverse diameter.

From the description of the disease we see that it cannot be confounded either with progressive muscular atrophy (Duchenne's type, Vulpian's type) or with infantile paralysis. The face is spared in both these diseases.

The prognosis is grave, but the course is extremely slow. Collateral or direct heredity is the only factor in pathogenesis with which we are acquainted.

PART XI

VENEREAL DISEASES

I. GONORRHŒA.

Bacteriology.—The gonococcus appears under the microscope as a diplococcus, staining readily with the aniline dyes, and decolorizing with Gram's method.

The two portions of the diplococcus look like two coffee-beans, having their plane surfaces opposite to one another, and separated by a clear line.

The grouping in pairs is the special feature. The diplococci may form small masses of four or of eight elements, but they are always present in even numbers. They never form chains. Live gonococci are mobile, exclusive of Brownian movements.

The discharge in the stationary stage of the malady shows pus cells crowded with gonococci. Extracellular masses are also found. At the onset we see especially cast-off epithelial cells, with gonococci against their surface, but not in their interior.

The cultivation of the gonococcus demands the employment of special media, containing albumin. The gonococcus does not grow on the usual media (broth, agar, and gelatine). It is strictly aerobic, and so delicate that the culture-tubes must be at once placed in an oven at 37° C. Bumm has succeeded in cultivating on tubes of coagulated human serum. This method is not suitable in practice. Wertheim has improved the technique by adding agar to the serum, and the medium usually employed at the present time is known as Wertheim's medium. It is composed of a mixture of agar with ascitic or pleuritic serous fluid. This medium is solid. De Christmas has recently advised rabbit's serum, coagulated by heat. Bezançon and Griffon recognized the advantages of this medium, but they prefer blood-agar as the best medium for the practical culture of the gonococcus. The early appearance of the colonies on the surface of the blood-agar, and the morphological clearness of the gonococcus developed upon this medium, render it excellent for diagnostic purposes. As the cultures remain alive for more than six months, the medium is excellent for preserving the gonococcus.

The gonococcus is only inoculable in the human species. Attempts made to inoculate animals have always failed. Animals have been inoculated with pure cultures. Although these inoculations have been made into the urethra, the joints, and the conjunctivæ of new-born rabbits, the only result has been slight and transient inflammation due to the trauma. Hallé, using a gonococcus of exceptional virulence, has caused death in the mouse by large intraperitoneal injections of a pure culture of the gonococcus from a case of periarthritis of the elbow-joint. This case is so far unique. For practical purposes, we may consider the gonococcus as non-pathogenic in animals.

The gonococcus must not be confounded with the pseudo-gonococcus. Many diplococci show certain analogies with the gonococcus—a fact of great importance in legal medicine. When we find in the interior of the pus cells masses of diplococci like coffee-beans, and decolorizing rapidly with Gram, we can be sure that they are gonococci. Nevertheless, in a legal case, if we have only dried pus to work with, we must reserve our judgment.

Although the gonococcus is the cause of gonorrhœal urethritis, every urethritis is by no means gonorrhœal. The urethra is rich in organisms ; we find in it free cocci, cocci in the cells, cocci in pairs or in chains, bacilli, sarcinæ, etc. A urethral discharge may be due to these organisms, to gout, to rheumatism, and to the use of certain drugs, such as iodine and cantharides, but the gonococcus is not present. Septic urethritis may follow the use of an infected catheter. Urethritis may occur in syphilis, and as the result of ascending or descending tubercular infection. In each case, however, the gonococcus is absent.

In gonorrhœal pus we also find other organisms which are normal inhabitants of the urethra or of the vagina, and which play an important part in the sequelæ of gonorrhœa, especially in the chronic stage. Eraud has stated that the gonococcus may be present in the urethra of a healthy man, just as the pneumococcus may exist in normal saliva. It is said to be devoid of virulence. Straus has reported a case of gonococcic arthritis which developed apart from any contagion. The prevalent opinion is, however, that the true gonococcus is non-saprophytic. Every case of gonorrhœa results from contagion.

The inoculation of the gonococcus usually takes place during sexual intercourse. This condition, however, is not absolutely indispensable, since Bumm has experimentally produced gonorrhœa by inoculation of a man with virulent cultures of the gonococcus.

Ætiology.—The chances of inoculation vary in different persons, and in each person according to the state of receptivity. In this respect fatigue, drinking, and repeated coitus have an undoubted influences. Moreover, a first attack, instead of conferring immunity, renders a second attack more likely. In these cases revivification of germs existing in a latent state in the urethra has been suggested. The statement may be true, but it has been exaggerated. In any case, it is not applicable to attacks occurring several years apart. In women leucorrhœa appears to facilitate contagion, and to increase the virulence of the gonococcus. The menstrual period has the same effect. A woman who in the intervals of her periods is but little apt to transmit gonorrhœa becomes an active centre of contagion during menstruation. The menstrual period is also favourable to gonorrhœal rheumatism.

Description.—Let us first consider gonorrhœa in men. The appearance of symptoms is usually preceded by an incubation period of three to five days. During this time the genital organs do not present any abnormality.

On the third or fourth day a burning sensation is felt at the end of the penis. The meatus is slightly red, and the lips are swollen and moist. The glans gradually swells, and the urethral discharge appears. This discharge, which is clear and thready at first, rapidly becomes yellowish or greenish. It is sometimes tinged with blood. On the linen it leaves a stain, which is green at the centre and yellow at the periphery. On pressure, we can always squeeze out a few drops of pus, even though none is apparent at the meatus. After a few days the inflammation becomes severe, the penis is swollen, the discharge is thick and profuse, and the constant presence of the pus between the glans and the prepuce may provoke balanoposthitis. The urethra can be felt as a tender cord on the lower surface of the penis. The chordee is sometimes so painful during erection that the patient, in order to gain relief, attempts to straighten the penis by breaking the cord. The effort succeeds, but the infiltration of pus and urine into the inflamed tissues leads to serious mischief.

During micturition the burning sensation along the urethra reaches its maximum (*chaude-pisse*). In acute cases the pain is unbearable, and the patient, when passing water, goes through various contortions without succeeding in relieving the pain. He holds his water as long as possible—as a result, retention of urine is often seen. Gonorrhœa, however, is not always so painful. The patient complains of a strain. The discharge may then be the chief symptom, and the term " running " is applied ; but the nature of the disease is identical.

Acute gonorrhœa may be accompanied by fever and gastric disturbance. At night the patient suffers tortures from the incessant and painful erections. When the inflammatory process is of moderate severity it is limited to the anterior urethra ; when it is more acute it may involve the posterior urethra and neck of the bladder.

As examination of the perineum does not always reveal the exact extent of the mischief, the method of using two glasses must be employed. For this purpose the urine is collected in two portions. The portion collected in the first glass contains flocculi of muco-pus from the urethra ; the second glass is to receive the urine still contained in the bladder. If the second portion contains shreds of muco-pus, the posterior urethra is inflamed. In the latter event, between the acts of micturition a small quantity of muco-pus takes a backward course, passing through the sphincter into the bladder, where it mixes with the urine. Each specimen of urine examined will, therefore, contain muco-pus. This distinction between anterior and posterior urethritis is considered to be of importance as regards treatment.

Fatigue, walking, prolonged standing, and alcohol increase the pain and the discharge.

Gonorrhœa, when untreated, lasts from four to six weeks. The discharge gradually becomes yellow, greyish, less thick, and less profuse. The pain, whether spontaneous or provoked by micturition, is less severe. The night's rest is no longer disturbed by erections, but every morning a drop of yellowish discharge can be squeezed out from the meatus. In some cases the morning drop indicates the passage of the disease into the chronic stage of gleet. As long as this slight discharge persists, the patient is liable to a relapse as the result of walking, alcoholic excess, or of sexual intercourse. These relapses may occur more than once, and on each occasion the gonococcus is found, although it may have disappeared in the intervals between the attacks. In the latter variety the gonorrhœa is localized in the cul-de-sac of the membranous portion of the urethra, whence it is very hard to dislodge.

In women acute gonorrhœa is characterized by vulvitis, by yellowish or greenish vaginal discharge, and by burning and smarting in the vagina, which renders examination very difficult. The acute stage is usually of short duration, and the gonorrhœa rapidly becomes painless, which in part explains why contagion is spread. In acute gonorrhœa the vaginal pus contains gonococci, but after the acute stage they are not found in the vagina, although they are present in the urethra. Gonorrhœal urethritis in women provokes violent pain on micturition. A drop of pus can be squeezed out from the meatus when pressure is made on the urethra from behind forwards. Cystitis of the neck of the bladder is common.

Complications.

Complications in Man.—During the acute stage the infection may extend either deeply, causing periurethral lesions (folliculitis, cavernitis, and cowperitis), or along the surface, attacking the mucous membranes continuous with that of the urethra (balano-posthitis, prostatitis, epididymitis, cystitis, and pyelonephritis). The latter troubles are the result of ascending infection. The lacunæ, crypts, and glandular canals, which communicate with the urethra, are often infected. The result is abscesses or reservoirs containing gonococci, ready to reinfect the urethra after apparent recovery from the gonorrhœa. The prostatitis may be acute or chronic. It is usually a direct consequence of posterior urethritis. In most cases there is merely congestion of the organ ; in some suppuration occurs.

Orchitis, or rather epididymitis, appears during the third or fourth week. It is accompanied by vaginalitis, and is ushered in by acute pain in the testicle and along the cord. The scrotum is red and swollen. The pain is increased by walking and by the friction against the thighs (patients, accordingly, walk with their legs apart). It radiates into the loins. Orchitis, though usually single, may be double, the testicles being attacked simultaneously or in succession. It recovers without suppuration, save in exceptional cases. The gonococcus has been found in pus of suppurating orchitis.

The usual treatment consists in rest in bed, leeches in acute cases, and in the application of belladonna and mercury ointment, with the use of a suspensory bandage in less severe cases. The chief danger in double orchitis is sterility, due to azoöspermia. Resolution is slow in every case. Induration in the tail of the epididymis lasts for many months.

Peritonitis, though extremely rare, has been seen. It is strictly localized. The pathogenesis admits of various explanations. The ascending infection is said to take place by the lymphatics and bloodvessels of the spermatic cord ; or by the upper extremity of the vas, which, like the vesiculæ seminales, is covered with peritoneum ; or, lastly, by a special lymphatic of the vas.

The name gleet is given to the slight chronic discharge that may follow gonorrhœa. Gleet is usually painless, except for the drop of pus which can be squeezed from the meatus on rising. The patient has no trouble. The discharge may be increased as the result of fatigue, of excesses, or of the abuse of beer. Between the attacks the muco-pus may contain the microorganisms usually found in the urethra, or the microbes of suppuration. The gonococcus usually reappears only during the attacks. Stricture of the urethra, with its many complications, is a remote result of gonorrhœa.

Complications in Women.—Ascending gonorrhœa is far more serious in women than in men. It commences in the cervix. It then invades the body of the uterus, setting up acute metritis, due to the gonococcus, which may or may not be associated with other organisms. Chronic metritis may follow the acute trouble, or may occur from the first in the course of chronic gonorrhœa.

Acute bartholinitis is nearly always gonorrhœal ; the chronic is always so. Bacteriological examination reveals either the gonococcus alone or the association of the gonococcus with anaerobic organisms. The pus from the glandular abscess in the latter case is often fœtid.

In its ascending course the gonococcus, which may or may not be associated with other organisms, may lead to salpingitis, ovaritis, perimetritis, and peritonitis. Bosc has collected twenty cases in which the gonococcus was the cause. In three of these cases the gonococcus was found not only in the pus, but also in the walls of the tubes. Wertheim has thus shown that the microbes traverse the wall of the tube in order to reach the ovaries and the peritoneum. Hartmann and Morax have found the gonococcus thirteen times in pus from the tubes, and in thirteen other cases the pus was sterile. It contained the streptococcus four times, the *Bacillus coli* once, and the pneumococcus once. Raymond has shown that the infection spreads from the uterus to the tube by ascending along the mucous membrane.

It is, therefore, proved that the gonococcus is most often in evidence in many diseases of the uterus, adnexa, and pelvic peritoneum. The lesions produced by the gonococcus predispose to the development of streptococcal infection after delivery or miscarriage. We know that gonococcal infection and puerperal infection, either alone or in combination, are the two great causes of salpingitis, ovaritis, perimetritis, periovaritis, and peritonitis.

Clinically, pelvic gonorrhœa in women differs, according as it is acute or chronic. The acute form is characterized by the appearance of marked pelvic reaction a few days after contamination. The symptoms of pelvic infection are liable to supervene at the first menstruation after the contagion. The menses may be advanced or delayed. In any case, they are nearly always affected. The symptoms are acute pain in the lower part of the abdomen, extreme sensitiveness of the abdominal wall, vomiting, and constipation. Fever may or may not be present. If the lesions are marked on the right side, they may simulate appendicitis. Vaginal examination is difficult. We sometimes find in the culs-de-sac a firm mass fixing the uterus.

The acute form remains stationary during the menstrual period, and the symptoms then improve so much that recovery is expected. As the next period becomes due, the peritoneal symptoms reappear. This form is called remittent by Noggerath. It may end, when untreated, in suppuration, although at first it may be a question of serous perimetro-salpingitis rather than one of true pelvic suppuration. These forms anatomically resemble gonorrhœal orchitis in man.

The chronic form may follow acute attacks, or may be chronic from the first. It is characterized by mild peritoneal reaction and by menstrual troubles, with amenorrhœa preceding the periodic metrorrhagia. Gonorrhœa must be thought of, if a young woman, after the first few indulgences in intercourse, complains of pain and of menstrual disturbances which cannot be explained by her general condition. The peritoneal syndrome seen in the acute form is replaced by a uterine syndrome, comprising pain in the lower part of the abdomen, especially on walking, neuralgia in the pelvis, and leucorrhœa.

These forms of pelvic infection in women never endanger life, but they induce sterility and nervous troubles, rendering the woman an invalid. They demand, therefore, early and thorough treatment.

The diagnosis of these pelvic troubles is a gynæcological question. When we find inflammatory masses around the uterus and its adnexa, we must always think of gonorrhœa as the cause. In order to make sure, a minute examination of the patient is necessary, and in the absence of delivery, miscarriage, or uterine trauma, we must at once suspect the gonococcus. Young girls may, after gonorrhœal vulvitis, suffer from the foregoing peritoneal troubles, since gonorrhœa is far from rare in children. In them it may assume three chief forms—acute general peritonitis, which is sometimes grave, sometimes benign; localized peritonitis; and subacute peritonitis.

The treatment of pelvic gonorrhœa in women comprises two distinct parts—prophylactic treatment, in which the object is to prevent suppuration in the lesions present; and curative treatment, in which the object is to relieve the troubles of suppurative pelvic peritonitis, the ovaries, the tubes, and the pelvic peritoneum forming an inflammatory area around the uterus.

As regards prophylactic treatment, we must distinguish cases in which the gonorrhœal infection is limited to the uterus, with or without slight salpingitis, and cases in which the gonorrhœal infection has become general in the adnexa. In the case of gonorrhœal metritis, the uterus must be dilated and copious intra-uterine douches given daily. Bozemann's cannula is most useful. For irrigations, solutions of sublimate or of permanganate of potassium may be employed. If the irrigations do not cure the metritis, or if they do not prevent the extension of the gonococcus to the tubes and peritoneum, an injection of tincture of iodine is given with Braun's syringe twice a week. The injection should be followed by a douche of boiled water, in order to remove the excess of iodine. Absolute rest in bed is essential during the treatment. It is necessary to commence the treatment, even though the period has not completely stopped, and to suspend it only during the active stage of the flow. We know how menstruation favours the growth of the gonococcus and increases its virulence.

If the patient is already suffering from salpingo-ovaritis, the intra-uterine douches are given, and, in addition, copious vaginal douches at a temperature of 115° to 120° F. Hot compresses should be applied to the abdomen.

In more advanced cases, where the tubes, ovaries, uterus, and pelvic peritoneum are matted together, surgical intervention becomes necessary; but we must remember that gonococcal suppuration has a marked tendency to recover, and we must give the patient the full benefit of this fact. The simplest procedure, such as incision of the posterior cul-de-sac, is at times sufficient. We can by such an incision evacuate large collections, which are often aseptic, because we find in pelvic gonorrhœa serous perimetro-salpingitis, which clinically resembles the streptococcal collections of pus in the organs and in the pelvic peritoneum.

Curettage should never be advised. While this operation gives excellent results when the uterus contains fragments of placenta and pieces of membrane, yet in gonorrhœal endometritis we must not perform it. In the latter case, the infection is deeply seated in the culs-de-sac of the glands, so that the curette may favour the penetration of the gonococci.

Complications Common to Both Sexes.

Gonorrhœal Rheumatism.—This complication may appear during the acute stage, or during the decline, even after the discharge has ceased, but more often in persons with a gleet. In exceptional cases, according to Griffon, it may precede the symptoms of urethritis—that is to say, between the moment of contagion and the commencement of the discharge. Leyden has reported a case of gonococcal arthritis without any sign of gonorrhœa.

The rheumatism generally supervenes in the course of gonorrhœal urethritis, but it has also been seen in persons with gonorrhœal ophthalmia. It appears to be more common in men than in women. It is sometimes seen in children, following purulent ophthalmia or vulvo-vaginitis. It may occur in various forms. The general rheumatic form, which is very rare, at first sight simulates an attack of rheumatic fever, with these differences, however—that the profuse sweats are usually absent, that the general symptoms are less severe, and that salicylate of soda has no effect. In this acute poly-articular form several joints are affected together or in succession, but in a few days the trouble becomes limited to one or two joints, showing a marked preference for the knee, the elbow, and the wrist. In another form the arthritis is mono-articular from the first. Its seat of election is the knee and the elbow. It may, however, develop in the instep, in the wrist, in the costo-sternal joints, or in the sterno-clavicular articulation.

These pseudo-rheumatic manifestations, which are at times very painful, may affect the periarticular tissue even more than the joint itself. They are accompanied by swelling, induration, and redness of the tissues to the extent of simulating cellulitis. The effusion may be sero-fibrinous, sero-purulent, or purulent. In exceptional cases the pus may make its way through the capsule of the joint, and spread under the skin and between the neighbouring muscles. The acute arthritis may be present only in outline (arthralgia), or may change into hydrarthrosis of long duration. Gonorrhœal rheumatism may also assume the type of hydrarthrosis from the first.

Gonorrhœa may give rise to *spondylose rhizomélique* (Marie). We may find ankylosis of the vertebral column, and sometimes also of the shoulders and hips. It is strange that the other joints are spared. I have seen the following case at the Hôtel-Dieu :

The patient, on admission, walked into the ward with his back arched and his head bent forwards. When he was spoken to he raised his head a little, but his back remained bent, and he could not straighten it. When he was told to pick up anything, he flexed the trunk on the pelvis ; but this flexion being insufficient, he was compelled to bend his knees, and to lower himself stiffly, in order to touch the floor. When he was in bed, he placed one pillow under his neck and another under his knees. In this way he avoided the pain caused by straightening his spine. Percussion of the spine was painful, but the pain was not fixed, as in Pott's disease. No deformity of the vertebræ was present.

The disease was of three years' duration. It had commenced with pain in the vertebral column. The whole spine was the seat of incomplete and painful ankylosis. The shoulders and the hips were not affected. The case was therefore an imperfect example of Marie's syndrome. This case is interesting as regards its ætiology, the gonorrhœa having been surprised *flagrante delicto*. Gonorrhœa has figured in the ætiology of several cases (Léri, Bouchard), but in this case it had been present in a chronic state for four years, and the vertebral pain had come on six months after the appearance of the discharge.

Gonorrhœal arthritis often runs a subacute course. It has a tendency to pass into the chronic state, and to be followed by adhesions which limit movement or which favour dislocations. These dislocations impede the free play of the articular surfaces. Widal has shown the previous rôle of hydrarthrosis in the pathogenesis of spontaneous dislocation of the elbow due to gonorrhœal mischief. True ankylosis, which is rare, follows the so-called plastic form. Cornil has made a microscopic examination in a case of gonorrhœal rheumatism with ankylosis and deformity. The lesions were especially characterized by invasion of the cartilage by the synovial membrane, and by the tendency to fibrous and bony ankylosis.

Another feature of gonorrhœal arthritis is the early and rapid muscular atrophy, which, even in the absence of ankylosis, hampers for a long while the functions of the affected limb. Deformities of the joints are often present, especially in certain chronic forms. Chronic gonorrhœal rheumatism may assume two different types—the chronic fibrous type and the nodular pseudo-gouty type. The nodular type has a predilection for the small joints. The X rays have shown the nature and extent of the bony lesions, and Achard has demonstrated that in gonorrhœal, as in ordinary arthritis deformans, we find lesions of the bones and of the periosteum and osteophytes. When the joints of the fingers are affected, the fingers may have a peculiar fusiform shape (*doigt en radis*, Fournier). Lastly, gonorrhœal rheumatism may cause the affected joint to become a *locus minoris resistentiæ.* The tubercle bacillus may then invade the joint.

The tendon sheaths, especially those on the dorsal aspect of the wrist, and the bursæ, especially the subcalcaneal, are often affected, either alone or at the same time as the joints. Talalgia of gonorrhœal origin is now well recognized. It is very persistent, often lasting for months. It commences either as a lesion of calcaneal bursa, or in an ossification of the insertion of the plantar fascia and of the tendo Achillis into the os calcis. It is said that suppuration never occurs in the bursa (Fournier, Verneuil).

I have, however, seen an interesting case of suppuration in the bursa between the great trochanter and tensor vaginæ femoris. The bacteriological examination was most carefully made in my laboratory. The gonococcus was found in a pure state in the contents of the pocket. A woman who had suffered from very mild symptoms of gonorrhœa showed a series of joint troubles, which ran the clinical course of gonorrhœal rheumatism. The knees and the malleoli had been in turn attacked, when the patient felt acute pain in the left thigh. The upper part of the thigh was swollen, but streaked with dilated veins, and painful on the slightest touch. We succeeded, however, in making out a very tense mass beneath the glutei and the tensor vaginæ femoris. Next day the situation of the lesion was more evident : the hip-joint was free, the trouble was in the bursa, between the trochanter and the tensor vaginæ femoris. Fluctuation was evident. A puncture was made, and the pus was at once examined. Stained films and cultures on appropriate media showed that the gonococcus was alone present. This case was the first in which blood-agar, as advised by Bezançon and Griffon, was employed in order to demonstrate the gonococcus. The patient recovered after three punctures. No other troubles were observed in the synovial membranes or in the tendons heaths.

The various theories put forward at the celebrated discussion at the Société Médicale des Hôpitaux in 1867 regarding the nature of gonorrhœal rheumatism may be summed up as follows : (1) Gonorrhœal rheumatism is an ordinary rheumatism, developed on account of gonorrhœa ; (2) gonorrhœal rheumatism is the result of a special intoxication, which differs from the rheumatic diathesis.

The latter theory, put forward by Féréol, at a time when the theories of micro-organisms were in their infancy, has daily gained ground. In an individual with gonorrhœa the gonococcus may enter the circulation, and give rise to a series of complications, including gonorrhœal rheumatism. This entrance of the gonococcus into the blood-stream takes place by a kind of "microbic discharge." Thayer and Blumer have caught the process in the act by obtaining cultures of the gonococcus on media inoculated with blood withdrawn during life from the brachial vein in a case of gonorrhœal endocarditis. There is, however, no septicæmia. The gonococcus does not flourish in the blood of the general circulation. It speedily confines itself to the serous tissues, and especially to the synovial membranes of the joints and tendons. Why this affinity for the serous tissues ? Bezançon and Griffon think that, while the parenchymata can destroy *in situ* organisms brought by the blood, the serous membranes (organs of feeble vitality and of cells not highly differentiated) defend themselves feebly against this invasion, and that the struggle, which is in favour of the organism in all the other regions, is in favour of the microbes in the serous membranes.

However this may be, there is a long list of cases—twenty-nine—regarding the presence of the gonococcus in gonorrhœal arthritis. I may mention the observations of Deutschmann (1890), Lindemann (1892), Stern (1892), Rendu, Höck (1893), Neisser (1894), Bordoni-Uffreduzzi (1894), and that of Finger (1894), concerning arthritis of the left knee, following gonorrhœal ophthalmia in a new-born infant. Haushalter mentions an example of gonorrhœal rheumatism which supervened during the course of gonorrhœal ophthalmia in a child twenty-five days old. Griffon has published a very interesting case of a similar nature: A new-born infant suffered from purulent ophthalmia and multiple arthritis, in which the gonococcus existed alone or in association with other organisms. I may also quote Seiffert's case of a girl, four years of age, with gonorrhœal vulvitis and multiple arthritis. One wrist became swollen, and the gonococcus was found in the fluid removed by puncture. Cultures of this organism were also obtained by sowing the pus in the fluid from an ovarian cyst. Finally, Mercier and Metenier have seen a case of arthritis of the knee due to the gonococcus, in the course of an attack of gonorrhœa. The identity of the gonococcus was established by microscopical examination and by cultures.

The cases of tenosynovitis in which the gonococcus has been found are quite as conclusive, although they are not so numerous. I may quote that of Tollemer and Macaigne (1893), that of Jacobi and Goldmann (1894), and lastly one of my own, already mentioned.

The question is, therefore, decided. The articular manifestations of gonorrhœal rheumatism are of an infective nature, and are due to the presence of the gonococcus in the joints, synovial membranes, bursæ, and tendon sheaths. If the search for the gonococcus has often been negative in the past, it is because we did not know how to cultivate this microbe, which requires special media, and which is so delicate that it must be sown and placed in the oven as soon as it is withdrawn from the synovial fluid. On the other hand, it seems to disappear rapidly from exudates; whence the precept of making the analysis as soon as possible after the onset of the lesion. The case of peritrochanteric synovitis already mentioned is most instructive from this point of view. Three punctures were made, some days apart. In the first (made on the day after the symptoms appeared) numerous gonococci were found; in the second the result was positive, but the colonies were fewer in number; in the third the result was negative.

Burci and Bespighi have published a very suggestive case. The fluid removed from the knee was sterile. A buttonhole incision was therefore made in the synovial membrane, and the vegetations covering it were curetted. In the débris thus removed the gonococcus was found.

Positive results in gonorrhœal arthritis will become more numerous in the future. In order to explain the so-called sterile effusions, it is unnecessary to invoke the influence of the nervous system or the action of a toxine of which we have but an imperfect knowledge.

The treatment of gonorrhœal rheumatism is chiefly local. In the acute stage the joint must be fixed in good position after an ointment of methyl salicylate or Trousseau's plaster has been applied. Later, blisters, counter-irritants, and massage will hasten resolution and prevent stiffness. In the suppurative form surgical intervention is indicated.

Gonorrhœal periostitis is not uncommon. It is found in the neighbourhood of the epiphyses, either alone or in conjunction with periarthritis. Finger has found the gonococcus.

Gonorrhœal pleurisy was first described clinically (Cornil and Klippel, Baisle, Ducrey, MacDonnell), and was later called in question. Its existence has now been demonstrated by bacteriological examination. Mazza, Bordoni-Uffreduzzi, and more recently Cardile, have found the gonococcus in the pleuritic fluid.

Cardio-Vascular System.—Gonorrhœal endopericarditis may be independent of the rheumatic attack, since the articular manifestation and the cardio-vascular manifestation are both dependent on the gonococcal infection. As a matter of fact, gonorrhœal endopericarditis has occurred in some instances apart from any joint trouble. Several of these cases are mentioned in Cart's paper.

Prévost. Endocarditis appearing on the fifth day of an attack of gonorrhœa, and unaccompanied by arthritis. In a fatal case of ulcerative endocarditis, consecutive to gonorrhœa, His found diplococci resembling the gonococcus and decolorizing, with Gram. Councilman, in 1893, saw a case of gonorrhœa, with arthritis, pericarditis, and abscesses in the cardiac muscle. The gonococcus was found in the urethra, joints, pericardium, and abscesses. Winterberg, in 1894, found the gonococcus in the mitral valve in a case of ulcerative endocarditis, consecutive to gonorrhœa with arthritis. Leyden, in 1893, proved the presence of the gonococcus in the valvular thrombus of the left ventricle in a case of endocarditis following on gonorrhœa, with arthritis and epididymitis.

Thayer has reported the case of a woman who died from general gonococcal infection, with ulcerative endocarditis. The bacteriological examination revealed the presence of the gonococcus in the vegetations on the mitral valve. In one of Rendu and Hallé's cases the symptoms of the gonococcal infection were obscure. It began with metritis, and involved the elbow and the endocardium. The autopsy revealed the gonococcus in the pericardium and in the vegetations of the endocardium ; cultures showed that the gonococcus was not associated with other microbes.

Widal and Faure Beaulieu have found the gonococcus in the blood during life, while the autopsy showed endocarditis, with gonococci in the mitral vegetations.

It is, therefore, proved that the gonococcal infection may become general, and determine pericarditis, endocarditis, and abscesses in the breast, with or without concomitant gonorrhœal arthritis. The endocarditis may be simple, relatively benign, and analogous in every respect to rheumatic endocarditis, or it may be malignant and of the septicæmic or typhoid variety.

In addition to the cardiac complications, let me note gonorrhœal phlebitis, of which undoubted cases have been reported.

Other Complications.

Nervous System.—The nervous system may be attacked by the gonorrhœal infection. Peripheral neuritis is the most important lesion, and is usually found in the lower limbs. Many years ago Fournier noted the frequency of sciatica. It is usually benign, of short duration, and is not followed by atrophy. Cros has collected cases of crural and lumbo-abdominal neuralgia. I have seen two cases of intercostal neuralgia. Gonorrhœal myelitis has been described by several writers. It usually assumes the diffuse dorso-lumbar type. In the only case in which a bacteriological examination has been made staphylococci were found in the effusion around the pia mater. The gonococcus was absent (Barrié).

The cranial meninges and the brain itself may be attacked by gonorrhœa. Cerebral complications are, however, very rare. They may be of four distinct types—delirious, maniacal, meningitic, and apoplectic. In the two latter the prognosis is very grave.

Kidney.—Albuminuria is frequent. We may justly admit a gonorrhœal nephritis, dependent on the ascending migration of the gonococcus or on secondary infections. It is more often consecutive to changes in the epithelium produced by elimination of the toxines.

Sense Organs.—The gonococcus may develop on the conjunctiva, and give rise to most serious purulent ophthalmia. Two cases may be met with : (1) An individual suffering from gonorrhœa has, in addition, gonorrhœal conjunctivitis due to auto-contagion ; (2) conjunctivitis in a person who is free from urethral or vaginal gonorrhœa. In this event the conjunctivitis is due to hetero-contagion. This form is seen in the new-born from infection during delivery. The existence of a benign so-called spontaneous conjunctivitis has been admitted. It is due to infection by the blood-stream.

Auditory troubles of labyrinthine origin have been noted. The gonorrhœal erythemata may be simple, nodular, urticarial, polymorphous, or purpuric. They may occur apart from any absorption of balsams. Cutaneous horns have at times been met with.

Ano-Rectal Gonorrhœa.—This localization of gonorrhœa is extremely rare. It is more common in women than in men. The close relation between the vulvar and anal orifices make inoculations of the anus more easy in women. Ano-rectal gonorrhœa may be acute or chronic.

In the acute form, the margin of the anus is erythematous or shows geographical ulcers. The rectal mucous membrane is red, swollen, thickened, and ulcerated. It bleeds readily, and in some cases vegetations are seen. There is a constant discharge of muco-pus. The symptoms are those of more or less severe proctitis—itching, burning, pain radiating along the sacrum to the bladder, uterus, loins, and thighs. The pain on defæcation is sometimes most acute, on account of the spasm of the sphincter and of the fistulæ which are usually present. With the tenesmus and incessant desire to stool we often find a more or less extensive prolapse of the mucous membrane of the rectum. Dysuria is the rule. The anal discharge is slight at first, but soon becomes abundant, purulent, and yellow, as in gonorrhœal vaginitis. It causes excoriation of the skin at the margin of the anus. The local condition, which is exceedingly painful, may cause fever and anorexia. Gonorrhœal proctitis is similar in its course and duration to gonorrhœal urethritis. It only becomes chronic in the absence of treatment. The chronic form is exceptional, and when it is present it persists indefinitely. Gonorrhœal proctitis is not exempt from complications. Some are early—condylomata, ano-rectal abscess, and fistula ; others are late—stricture of the rectum.

The diagnosis is important. Simple rectitis from pederastia, ano-rectal chancre, fistula, piles, and polypi must be distinguished from ano-rectal gonorrhœa.

The treatment consists in lavage with solutions of corrosive sublimate (1 in 2,000) or of permanganate (1 in 3,000). Tuttle's cannula may be employed for rectal irrigation. Sitz-baths are to be recommended. In the intervals of lavage the diseased parts should be dusted with iodoform, oxide of zinc, or aristol.

Diagnosis.—In man gonorrhœal urethritis is usually easy to recognize. Urethritis, due to the passage of septic instruments or consecutive to coitus with a woman suffering from leucorrhœa, is distinguished by its short duration and by the benign nature of the local troubles. Chancre of the anterior urethra is sometimes accompanied by purulent discharge, but palpation reveals the presence of a hard nodule. As regards acute gouty urethritis, it is far from being accepted. In all these cases, moreover, bacteriology will decide the point. Microscopical examination of the pus after staining with methylene blue will give prompt information, and it will be unnecessary to make cultures with the pus. The morphological features of the gonococcus are : diplococcus, grouped *en masse*, intracellular, and decolorized after Gram's reaction. The aspect of the pus cells, crammed with diplococci, leaves no room for doubt.

It is a different matter when the discharge is scanty and matutinal, or when it is reduced to a few shreds suspended in the urine passed. We must then collect the morning drop or squeeze the shreds between two slides, repeat the examinations as long as they are negative, and especially have recourse to cultures on appropriate media. The culture is difficult to make, but the information given, if it is positive, is so important that it must be made whenever possible. The drop or the shred is at once placed on the culture medium (blood-agar)—in other words, the drop should not be kept for some hours in a pipette, as is often done in the case of pus or of exudates. The gonococcus rapidly loses its vitality. It is better to bring the patient to the laboratory, and as soon as the pus has been sown the culture-tube must be placed in the oven.

In chronic gonorrhœa, as the urethral discharge is often scanty, we may confound it with the discharge which accompanies tuberculosis of the testicle and of the prostate. All doubt will be removed, however, by examination of the testicle and prostate apart from bacteriological examination. In women gonorrhœa is far more difficult to diagnose. The discovery of the gonococcus is of great importance; the existence of urethritis is a diagnostic point of value. In the opposite event it is at times necessary to examine and even to cultivate the contents of the cervix uteri.

In a number of cases of cystitis, orchitis, and especially of arthritis, we are called upon to examine for gonorrhœa. · Without mentioning the principal differences between true and gonorrhœal rheumatism, it is well known that rest in bed may cause so great a diminution in the urethral discharge that we must squeeze the penis in order to obtain a few drops of pus. In women the diagnosis may be even more embarrassing, but the evolution of gonorrhœal arthritis permits us to make a diagnosis even in cases where gonorrhœa cannot be suspected.

Treatment.—Gonorrhœa, when untreated, shows a natural tendency to recover in a few weeks. There are, however, certain hygienic rules which the patient should follow if he does not wish the discharge to increase, and desires to escape the complications already described : rest, abstention from exercise—cycling, dancing, riding, and long walks—suppression of all alcohol, and especially of beer, of acid or spiced foods. Alkaline drinks and hot baths are all-important.

In men the bromides should be given for the nocturnal erections. When the acute stage is subsiding, we may employ astringent injections of sulphate of zinc, tannin, quinine, nitrate of silver, or resorcin. We may also give cubebs, copaiba, or sandal-wood oil. Considerable improvement may result from irrigation of the urethra with a solution of permanganate of potash (1 in 4,000). In anterior urethritis the irrigation is made with the canal open. Two litres of the warmed solution are allowed to flow over the surface of the mucosa. In posterior urethritis the pressure of the fluid must be increased, and the injection made to enter the bladder. The urethra is thus washed out from behind forwards. Microscopic examination is required in order to determine the therapeutic indications. If the gonococcus is absent, permanganate of potash should not be used. If another organism is present, we should employ injections of corrosive sublimate or of silver nitrate. We may content ourselves with ordering balsams if we do not find organisms in the exudate. The chronic nature of the urethritis may demand instillation of nitrate of silver by Guyon's method.

In women the urethral injections should be supplemented by vaginal injections of a very hot solution of permanganate of potash twice daily.

The treatment of chronic gonorrhœal rheumatism by Trousseau's plaster is given under Rheumatism (p. 1880).

II. SOFT CHANCRE.

The word "chancre," formerly synonymous with rodent ulcer, is now used exclusively to designate two varieties of contagious ulcerations, which are in most cases of venereal origin. These two varieties, clearly separated in 1850 by Hunter, Ricord, and Bassereau, are the soft chancre and the hard or syphilitic chancre. Both chancres result from infection, but in the former case the infection remains local, in the latter it becomes general.

Ætiology.—The simple chancre is rare when strict cleanliness is observed. It is, therefore, more common in hospital patients. The contagion is effected by inoculation. The pus of the chancre, even in a dilute condition, reproduces the lesion. A scratch, an erosion, or a vesicle of herpes, serves as the point of entrance, but in most cases the entrance-gate is not found. In 99 cases out of 100 the soft chancre is of venereal origin. Contamination is possible during the entire duration of the disease, not only from one subject to another, but also indefinitely in the same subject by auto-inoculation.

The soft chancre is inoculable in the monkey. In 1882 Fournier and Krishaber made 142 inoculations, with success in 60 per cent., in the macaque, baboon, and other small apes. Tomasczewski has made subcutaneous inoculations of cultures on blood-agar of the bacillus of soft chancre in two different species of monkeys. The ulcerations which developed some days later contained a bacillus which gave on culture the characters of Ducrey's bacillus. Inoculation in man produced the soft chancre.

The micro-organism of the soft chancre is a bacillus described by Ducrey. It is found in abundance in the pus oozing from the chancre. It has the following characters : Rape-seed bacillus, with rounded ends, taking the stain only at its extremities, while its central part remains colourless. It does not remain stained by Gram's method. In sections at the edges of the chancre it occurs in the form of small chains of strepto-bacilli.

Ducrey's bacilli cannot be cultivated on the ordinary media. Bezançon and Griffon, while making researches on pus taken from patients under my care, have succeeded in cultivating the bacillus on blood-agar. We have, therefore, a definite culture medium which is of practical use. In order to obtain cultures of Ducrey's bacillus for purposes of diagnosis, it is sufficient to sow on a tube of blood-agar the pus which has been allowed to collect on the surface of the ulceration after previous disinfection. The colonies are rounded, greyish, and separated from one another. The microbe shows certain peculiarities when it develops in the fluid portion of the culture medium. If we examine a drop of the liquid which bathes the sloping portion of the blood-agar tube, we find very thin chains, which are excessively long, and composed of bacilli individually smaller than those found in the colonies on the solid portion of the medium. One of these colonies, when inoculated in man, produces a typical soft chancre.

Symptoms.—The soft chancre is nearly always genital or perigenital. In men it appears on the prepuce, in the preputial fold, on the glans, within the meatus, or on the scrotum, where it is nearly always secondary. In women it is usually found on the fourchette, in the fossa navicularis, on the labia majora and minora, in the lower part of the vagina, and upon the cervix uteri. It develops secondarily on the neighbouring parts, especially on oozing or excoriated surfaces, such as hæmorrhoids. The extragenital soft chancre may be found in any part of the body, principally upon the fingers, and exceptionally on the face.

As the soft chancre is inoculable and auto-inoculable, we can readily follow its evolution by covering the inoculated area with a watch-glass. This method is an excellent diagnostic measure, but it is not superior to the discovery of the bacillus in the pus. After inoculation with pus from the surface of the chancre or from the suspected ulcer, the inoculation chancre appears in about twelve hours as a red areola. This areola gradually increases in size, and a small phlyctenule, filled with muco-pus, appears on the second or third day. Below the phlyctenule we find a superficial ulcer.

The soft chancre is an ulcer with rounded or oval reddish edges, which are clean-cut, often undermined, and rolled on themselves. The floor of the ulcer, which may be more or less deep, is dirty, greyish, pulpy, and irregular. It is important to note that the underlying tissues are supple and soft. The pain is usually trifling, and the patient continues to attend to his business.

After one or more weeks the floor of the chancre cleans up, granulations appear, the ulcer fills up, and healing follows. In some cases the soft chancre, even though carefully treated, is very persistent and rebellious. In other cases healing takes place on one side, while the ulceration extends on the opposite side. The chancre is then said to be serpiginous. The healing process leaves traces, though they may be much less pronounced than the extent and the depth of the ulceration would lead us to suppose. A white cicatrix results. It feels like a traumatic scar, and does not rest upon an indurated base.

In addition to the typical chancre, several other varieties have been described. The simple chancre may be phagedænic, acneiform, pimply, ecthymatous, or fissured.

The number of soft chancres may be considerable, on account of the liability to reinoculation. They often cause complications, which are mostly dependent on secondary infections. The soft chancre, like every ulceration, serves as a breeding-ground for micro-organisms, which cause either *in situ* or at a distance (by lymphatic infection) various troubles. Among them we may note phimosis, paraphimosis, and buboes in the glands receiving the lymphatics from the infected areas. Glandular enlargement is the rule in soft chancre. In some cases much pain and swelling are present, and suppuration follows. The ulceration thus produced has in most cases the clinical characters of a large soft chancre. Nevertheless, it appears from the researches of Straus that it is then a question of a reinoculation with Ducrey's bacillus or an ulceration at first due to the ordinary micro-organisms of suppuration. And, indeed, if the ulcerated bubo is kept well covered with antiseptic dressings, the chancre-like character is absent, and healing takes place as in an ordinary wound.

Phagedæna is not special to the soft chancre ; it is also found on the surface of many forms of ulceration. Molecular gangrene, which has been compared to hospital or to wound gangrene, is characterized by continuous extension of the primary ulceration, which gains both in depth and in extent, and exposes the patient to the risk of local and general complications in the absence of speedy and effective treatment. The proof that the phagedænic chancre is due to secondary infection is that antiseptic dressings carefully applied from the onset of the trouble limit the number and the gravity of these complications.

Treatment.—The first indication is the necessity of rigorous antisepsis. Frequent washing with antiseptic lotions should be prescribed. Carbolic acid solution, sublimate lotion (1 in 2,000) locally, baths, and dressing with iodoform, iodol, salol, etc., are indicated.

If these measures do not hasten the healing of the chancre, weak caustics should be employed—nitrate of silver in a 3 per cent. solution, carbolic acid (1 in 10), chloride of zinc paste. If these measures fail, we must use Vienna paste or the thermo-cautery.

The diagnosis of soft chancre from the syphilitic chancre and from herpes is given in the next section.

III. HARD OR SYPHILITIC CHANCRE (*TREPONEMA PALLIDUM*).

Ætiology.—Syphilis, except in the hereditary and conceptional* forms, begins with a chancre, and the virus may be furnished either by the chancre or by the mucous patches. The chancre always develops at the point of contamination. Two kinds of chancre occur—genital and extragenital. The former are nearly always of venereal origin, the latter much less often so.

The contagion in the case of extragenital chancres may take place in various ways. Let me mention suckling, whether the infant suffering from mucous patches in the mouth transmits the disease to the wet-nurse or the nurse suffering from mucous patches on the nipple infects the nursling. Articles used by a syphilitic person—feeding-bottles, pipes, spoons, or drinking-glasses—may be the origin of the chancre. Let me note buccal chancres in glass-blowers and in musicians playing wind instruments, and chancres contracted by physicians, midwives, and laundresses. These professional chancres almost always occur on the fingers. Infected instruments may give rise to a chancre (catheterization of the Eustachian tube, dental operations). Vaccination, when the vaccinator is suffering from recent syphilis, may transmit the disease, and the subject thus infected may in turn transmit syphilis ; hence arise the epidemics of vaccinal syphilis.

The hard chancre may develop on any region, and on the most accessible mucous membranes. In men it usually occurs on the inner surface of the prepuce, on the frenum, on the glans, upon the cutaneous surface of the penis, within the urethra, upon the scrotum, and at the root of the thighs. In women the hard chancre often passes unnoticed. The mucous membrane of the vagina, the cervix uteri, the vulva, the meatus urinarius, and the fourchette are the usual situations for it. Among the venereal chancres we must include those of the anal and buccal mucous membranes from abnormal coitus. Nevertheless, many buccal chancres are not of venereal origin. They are found especially on the lips, tongue, and tonsils. In 591 cases of extragenital chancres under Fournier, Nivet found 338 bucco-pharyngeal chancres, and 75 chancres of the head. The body was attacked 107 times, the limbs 54 times, and the neck 7 times.

Roux and Metchnikoff have inoculated a female chimpanzee with syphilis. The chancre appeared twenty-six days after inoculation. It then became indurated, and a typical mass of enlarged glands appeared, one large gland being surrounded by small glands. In 1882 Martineau and Hamonic produced syphilis in a large macaque monkey, " which presented a typical hard chancre, followed by secondary troubles."

* Conceptional syphilis is syphilis transmitted to the mother by a fœtus born of a syphilitic father.

TEXT-BOOK OF MEDICINE

Description.—The incubation period is from three to four weeks. Every chancre is composed of a mass of embryonic cells, forming a tumour at the expense of the derma and hypoderma. The appearance of the chancre differs on the skin and on the mucous membranes. On the skin it is covered with a crust, due in part to the presence of the stratum corneum. As this stratum does not exist in the mucous membranes, the changes in the mucous epithelium soaked in purulent fluid end in the formation of a flabby, greyish, and diphtheroid membrane.

Let us first consider the chancre of the mucous membranes, taking a chancre on the corona of the glans. At first we find a papule, which desquamates. This papule, which is not painful, and does not itch, has a dark colour like that of muscle. After a few days a very superficial ulcer appears. The ulcer is, however, more apparent than real, since it is formed at the expense of tissue which is often prominent. The ulcerated chancre may be very small ; it is usually about as large as a lentil. Its edges are adherent, thick, and regular. They never present the segments which make up the polycyclical border of herpes. The edges are not clean-cut, and there is not ulceration in the true sense of the word. The floor of the chancre is smooth, varnished, and at times greyish and diphtheroid. When the thin covering membrane is removed, the floor of the chancre has a reddish appearance, with papillæ. The secretion from the chancre is scanty and serous. The chancre rests upon an indurated base. Cicatrization takes place in four or five weeks, and the chancre is replaced by a reddish induration, which may last for several months.

The cutaneous chancre (nipple, face, scrotum, thighs) has a somewhat different evolution. At first it is a reddish erosive pimple. It then enlarges, becoming prominent, and is covered with a crust. It is always painless. This encrusted chancre resembles ordinary ecthyma, but on removal of the previously softened crust the chancre shows its special characteristics—flat or slightly convex surface, which is erosive, but not much ulcerated, smooth, reddishlike muscle, often bleeding, and studded with papillæ. A little pus-like secretion is sometimes found. The edges of the chancre are flat, and not clean-cut. Strictly, there is no edge, because there is no ulceration. The base of the chancre is indurated and parchment-like. On the nose, on the thigh, and on certain other regions, the chancre may be of large size.

Every hard chancre is accompanied by adenitis involving several glands. This adenitis does not appear before the seventh day, and its localization depends upon the situation of the chancre (groin, axilla, and neck). One gland is usually larger than the others, because it is in more direct communication with the lymphatics from the infected area. The glands are small, hard, and usually painless. They roll under the finger, and do not cause periadenitis. They show no tendency to suppurate, and as they persist for months and years after the chancre, they are of considerable value in making a retrospective diagnosis.

After a short time enlarged glands are also found in other regions, especially in the neck. Enlargement of the spleen has been noted in some cases.

The appearance of the chancre is usually accompanied by general troubles —lassitude, fever, headache, osteoscopic pains, insomnia, arthralgia, etc. The secondary troubles may appear before the cicatrization of the chancre or some weeks after it. The chancre itself may be the starting-point of a mucous patch.

The hard chancre is generally single ; nevertheless, we may find two or three, but they are nearly always contemporaneous—or, at least, when there is reinoculation, it occurs soon after the appearance of the first chancre, and not at a later date, as happens in the case of the simple chancre.

Under the microscope the chancre shows an infiltration of the dermis by leucocytes. Endarteritis is practically constant. These vascular lesions bear witness to the special predilection of syphilis for the arteries in the early as well as in the later stages.

Diagnosis.—The discovery of the *Treponema pallidum* has rendered the diagnosis of syphilis easy in doubtful cases ; but for the present let us confine ourselves to the resources of clinical medicine, taking a chancre of the genital organs or of some other region in a man or a woman, and considering the distinction from soft chancre and from herpes.

The distinctive signs of the ordinary syphilitic chancre are :

1. The hard chancre has an incubation period of three or four weeks ; the soft chancre appears one or two days after contagion ; herpes appears spontaneously, and relapses at more or less lengthy intervals.

2. The hard chancre is a projection of the dermis, erosive rather than ulcerative. It is excavated like a cup, with a crown-like contour, sometimes thickened and raised, so that the depth of the ulceration is apparently increased. It has not clean-cut edges. In the soft chancre no projection of the dermis, no hypertrophic tendency. On the contrary, a true ulceration, with clean-cut edges, and more or less deep, from the rapid and complete destruction of the epidermis and of the suppurative melting of the papillary and dermic layers. In herpes erosion of small extent, and more superficial than that of chancre.

3. In the syphilitic chancre regular outlines, never presenting the festooned segment which the polycyclical outlines of the herpetic ulcers often form.

4. The syphilitic chancre is nearly always single, never confluent, and not reinoculable ; the soft chancre is often multiple, sometimes confluent, and reinoculable to infinity.

5. The floor of the hard chancre is at times diphtheroidal and greyish, as long as it is covered by a membrane formed of the soaked and altered epithelium ; but after the removal of this membrane the floor is seen to be red, smooth, shiny, studded with papillæ, and covered with scanty serous secretion. The floor of the soft chancre is uneven, worm-eaten, anfractuous, and covered with abundant purulent secretion.

6. When we press the hard chancre between the fingers, we have great difficulty in squeezing out a little liquid ; when we knead the base of the chancreform herpes (in this form the herpes is solitary and simulates the dwarf chancre), we can squeeze out a deep amber-coloured serum, and after wiping the surface we can repeat the operation, obtaining the same serous oozing.

7. The base of the hard chancre is indurated. This parchment-like induration is one of the most striking features, and is not found in the soft chancre.

8. In the case of the syphilitic chancre the glands are hard, practically painless, and distinct from one another. They show no tendency to suppurate. In the case of the soft chancre the glands are enlarged, painful, and accompanied by periadenitis. They sometimes form masses, and have a marked tendency to suppurate.

Such are the distinctive signs between the hard chancre, the soft chancre, and herpes. Nevertheless, we may meet with very difficult cases. I allude to the mixed chancre. This variety at first presents the characters of the soft chancre. In its subsequent course the distinctive characters are not well defined, the buboes may suppurate, and later the secondary symptoms appear.

We must also make a diagnosis in the case of encrusted chancres of the skin, which are often large and hypertrophic, but in which (the crust having been removed) we find the characteristics mentioned under Chancre of the Mucous Membranes.

The chancre of scabies has nothing in common with the syphilitic chancre, except its situation on the penis. It is often multiple, papular, covered by a crust, and accompanied by the characteristic burrow of the acarus.

The pustules of ecthyma are readily recognized by their mode of development, their colour, and the absence of induration. As regards the ulcerated syphilides of the secondary and tertiary periods, the nature of the lesion, the course of events, and the absence of glandular enlargement will prevent confusion with the chancre.

Multiple Forms of the Syphilitic Chancre.—I have so far described the usual form of the syphilitic chancre. The chancre may, however, be giant, ulcerous, phagedænic, and hypertrophic.

The giant chancre may be as large as a crown-piece. In my lectures at the Hôtel-Dieu I showed a giant chancre of the thigh larger than a florin. In Gastou's case a giant chancre of the abdomen measured over 2 inches in diameter. In Fournier's case a giant chancre of the elbow was as large as a crown-piece. The giant chancre is very rare on the genital organs. It is usually found on the limbs, trunk, or face, and runs the same course as the ordinary chancre.

The ulcerous chancre is generally of large size. I said above that one of the characteristics of the ordinary chancre is that it is exulcerated without ending in true ulceration. This is true, but yet some chancres show deep and extensive ulceration. These chancres are usually extragenital. When the thickened and stratified crusts are removed, we find a somewhat excavated ulceration, with prominent edges. Sometimes, indeed, on the lips excavations occur, and at first sight we are tempted to think that the lesion will be followed by deep and deformed scars. And yet " things nearly always turn out well, and after recovery the lips become practically normal " (Fournier). This paradox arises from the fact that the ulcerative action limits itself to the specific neoplasm, and does not encroach upon the neighbouring tissues. The chancre is autophagous, and produces the ulceration at its own expense, thus differing from the phagedænic chancre.

The diagnosis of this chancre is generally easy ; nevertheless, in two cases which appeared to be ulcerous chancres the histological examination by Darier revealed a lymphosarcoma of a special species, which is not uncommon in the skin and in the glands. At the present day we can examine for the treponema.

The phagedænic chancre is fortunately very rare. The phagedæna may extend in area and in depth, destroying the tissues, and leaving behind it deformities and deep scars. In one of Fournier's cases the chancre ran a rapid but painless course, and destroyed the entire lower lip. In another case a phagedænic chancre destroyed the ear. In a case of Mencault a phagedænic chancre destroyed the inguinal region.

The syphilitic chancre may hypertrophy, reaching the size of a cherry or even of an apricot. These hypertrophic chancres form bleeding, ulcerated, and more or less encrusted tumours. We must be careful not to confound them with epitheliomata—an error that has led to an operation when the chancre would have been cured in a few weeks. Hypertrophic chancres are very rarely found on the genital organs. They have a marked predilection for the face. In one of Trélat's cases two ulcerative chancres as large as nuts were present on the chin. In a case of Mauriac the hypertrophic chancre on the lower lip formed a tumour as large as a lady-apple. I have seen a hypertrophic chancre of the size and shape of a large almond.

All the above forms of chancre are simply morphological varieties of the ordinary syphilitic chancre. The form, the dimensions, and the appearances of the syphilitic chancre may vary, but the fundamental characters of the chancre do not vary. Diagnosis is, therefore, possible. The induration of the bed of the chancre, the characters of the adenopathy, the evolution of the chancre (including the period of incubation), and the appearance of the secondary troubles, will reveal the nature of the chancre, even in the most abnormal forms. In cases of dispute the discovery of the treponema will confirm the diagnosis.

Bacteriology—Treponema Pallidum.—In May, 1905, Schaudinn discovered the pathogenic agent of syphilis. He called it first *Spirochæta pallida*, and later *Treponema pallidum*. We shall keep the term *Treponema pallidum*, which appears to be more correct.

Technique.—We can study the treponema in the blood, in the exudates, and in the parenchyma of the organs. The technique is somewhat difficult, and varies with the product to be examined.

1. In the case of papules, non-ulcerated chancres, and condylomata, a drop of serous fluid is removed from the centre of the lesion. It may be examined as a hanging-drop or may be stained by the following method :

Fix with absolute alcohol for fifteen minutes. Stain with Giemsa's mixture, 2 c.c. of the stain being mixed with 20 c.c. of distilled water. Leave in the stain from a quarter of an hour to one hour. Wash in water and mount in balsam.

2. In the blood it is often difficult to find the parasites after spreading the drop out, so that some authorities have proposed centrifugalization after the addition of oxalate. Hydro-hæmolysis has also been advised (Nattan-Larrier and Bergeron).

3. In the case of effusions into the serous cavities centrifugalization is always necessary, and it is well to stain the microbes in the centrifugalized clot spread out on a slide.

4. In the organs the technique advised is somewhat more delicate (Bertarelli, Levaditi, and Petresco) :

(*a*) Fix very small fragments in a solution of formalin, 10 per cent., from twenty-four to forty-eight hours.

(*b*) Wash in 90 per cent. alcohol for sixteen hours.

(*c*) Impregnate in a 10 per cent. solution of nitrate of silver, to which 10 per cent. of pyridin has been added, for two hours at the temperature of the room, and for five hours in the oven at 50° C.

(*d*) Wash in 40 per cent. pyridin.

(*e*) Reduce in a bath of pyrogallic acid 4 per cent. to which 10 per cent. of purified acetone and 15 per cent. of pyridin have been added. Reduction is effected in a few hours.

(*f*) Alcohol, xylol, paraffin, and sections.

(*g*) Staining of the section with Unna's blue or with toluidin blue.

The parasites are stained black, the cells blue, and the connective tissue greenish-yellow.

Differential Characters.—The *Treponema pallidum* is recognized by the following characters : It is a small filiform element from 6 μ to 14 μ in length by 0·25 μ in breadth, twisted into a spiral with from six to twenty-six extremely close and fine turns. The body is said to be cylindrical, and a flagellum has been described at each extremity. A membrana undulans is not found. We may meet with treponemata that are straight in a part of their length, while others are very short, and show only three or four undulations. It is rare to find an operculum in the length or at one extremity of the parasite. The treponema performs movements of flexion and torsion, affecting the entire organism. The disposition of the turns of the spiral is not modified during the different manifestations of activity, but is the same as it is during rest.

On examination with staining reagents, the treponema is, as a rule, somewhat pale, whence the name which has been given to it, and which serves to distinguish it from other similar parasites. Thus the *Spirochæta refringens*, which is not pathogenic, is, as its name indicates, strongly refracting, and very readily stainable. Further, the turns of the spiral are less numerous, and the thickness is greater. Its colour with Giemsa's stain is blue, and not pale rose. The spirochæte of the mouth and teeth—the *Spirochæta pyogenes*—the *Spirochæta pallidula* of Castellani, the spirochæte of Vincent (angina), Obermeier's spirochæte (recurrent fever), and the spirochæte of ulcerated carcinomata resemble the *Spirochæta refringens* in that they stain readily, and are thicker and less undulated than the treponema of syphilis.

Localization of the Parasite.—The treponema is frequently found in the chancre and in the satellite gland. It has not been discovered in the spots of the roseola, but it has been found in 90 per cent. of the mucous patches and secondary papules. The results of the blood examination are not constant. Examination by lumbar puncture is nearly always negative. Examination of the serum from a blister has been positive (Levaditi). The parasite is absent in the tertiary lesions—a fact of immense importance from the point of view of prophylaxis (Jacquet and Sevin). Sections of syphilitic tissues have sometimes yielded positive results. The treponema has been found in the suprarenal capsules (Jacquet and Sézary); in the liver in cases of hereditary syphilis (Salmon); and in the placenta (Nattan-Larrier and Brindeau).

Inoculation in Animals.—Attempts at making cultures of the treponema have so far been fruitless, but certain facts demonstrate its pathogenic action. In fact, inoculation of secondary syphilitic products has not only produced in the chimpanzee, the macaque, the gibbon, and the orang-outang such specific lesions as chancre, mucous patches, and secondary eruptions, but the parasite found in man has also been discovered in the different exudates and in the blood of these animals (Hoffmann, Metchnikoff). The parasite appears to possess but slight resistance. At 48° C. it loses its virulence, and is no longer inoculable. It preserves its virulence when mixed with glycerin. These findings deserve mention by reason of their bacteriological importance, and also by reason of the great light which they throw upon the study of syphilis in man.

Prognosis.—Is it possible, given a chancre, to say whether the resulting troubles will be benign or grave ? It is certain that extragenital chancres are usually more serious than venereal chancres, and that certain cases of syphilis derived from the same source are malignant, while others are trifling. Other facts are, however, quite opposed to this point of view. Much depends upon the question of the soil, although it may not be possible to state exactly the conditions modifying the virulence of the infective agent.

Treatment.—At all times the idea of excising the chancre has been present in the mind of physicians, but though we may thus get rid of the ulceration, we do not suppress the period of incubation. Accordingly, this method has been practically abandoned.

Leloir has reported the case of a student who, after a suspected coitus, watched most carefully for the possible appearance of a chancre. It appeared, and although excision was at once performed, the disease ran its course, the economy being already infected. Augagneur performed circumcision immediately after coitus with a syphilitic woman— that is to say, before the period of incubation ; nevertheless the chancre developed in the scar on the prepuce.

In most cases of indurated chancre we are content to prescribe cleanliness and antiseptics, such as iodoform, salol, or aristol.

In a series of experimental studies on inoculated syphilis in the anthropoid apes, Metchnikoff, after having discovered the attenuation of the syphilitic virus by passing it through certain lower species of monkeys, has employed antisyphilitic vaccination. This method has not yet been put into practice in man. Accordingly, Metchnikoff and Roux, while waiting to obtain a serum, which they believe will only be found when we can cultivate the microbe of syphilis, have sought to find a method of prophylaxis against the pox.

This method depends upon the employment of an ointment, of which the primary formula was : Calomel, 10 parts ; lanolin, 30 parts. It is rubbed in at the site of inoculation of the syphilitic virus. In monkeys it gave excellent results, and a student of medicine who submitted to the experiment has demonstrated its efficacy. The results obtained in monkeys have been disputed by Neisser, whose results were positive in only 50 per cent. of the cases. It is right to add that this authority employed an ointment of 10 per cent. instead of 33 per cent.—a fact which prevents comparison of the results. The clinical results in man have been contested by Lévy-Bing and Gaucher, because in certain isolated cases syphilis has appeared in spite of the use of calomel ointment.

At the Berlin Congress (1907) Metchnikoff did not dispute these facts, recognizing that his ointment may fail in certain cases, because, in order to gain the full effect, it must be employed within a few hours of the infectious contact. He has substituted for the primary formula one having the following strengths : Calomel, 33 parts ; lanolin, 67 parts ; vaselin, 10 parts.

Is there any other means of hindering the production of syphilis ? Metchnikoff believes in the possibility of doing so by the use of anilarseniate of soda—a drug possessing both curative and prophylactic properties. The fact that this product (atoxyl) destroys the trypanosoma, and the analogies between this parasite and the *Treponema pallidum,* have led pathologists to employ it in the treatment of syphilis. At present the matter is in the experimental stage.

The proper treatment still rests upon the use of mercury, either by inunction or by pills of protoiodide—a pill containing 1 grain of the proto-iodide and $\frac{1}{6}$ grain of extract of opium. We can double the dose if need be. The first series should be given for three weeks. An interval of one week is allowed, and the treatment is again given. At this period we may replace the pills by aqueous injections of biniodide of mercury, as described in the Appendix on Therapeutics.

IV. FULMINANT GANGRENE OF THE PENIS.*

Clinical Cases.—A young man was admitted under my care for gangrene of the penis. The odour was very offensive. The œdematous penis looked like a black-pudding ; the anterior two-thirds were as black as coal, and the rest was of a violet colour. On the dorsal surface there were vesicles, from which fœtid liquid escaped ; the prepuce resembled a bell-clapper. The glans was, so to say, set in the gangrenous prepuce. Crepitation was not present ; gaseous gangrene was therefore absent—an important point. No hæmorrhage, no purulent discharge. The urine flowed freely, but infiltrated the dead tissues. The scrotum was red and œdematous, but not gangrenous. The inguinal glands were enlarged and movable ; they were not painful. The patient was prostrated ; the temperature was 101° F.

In addition to the gangrene of the penis, rounded ulcers were present in the perianal region. A painless ulcer was present on the dorsum of the tongue. On the middle finger of the right hand we found a peri-ungual ulceration, which had given rise to lymphangitis of the forearm. The patient complained of dysphagia, and examination of the throat showed a greyish ulcer on the right pillar of the fauces. How had the gangrene of the penis commenced ? The lesion appeared to have occurred in two stages. The onset had been characterized by painless swelling of the penis, and rapid gangrene had followed.

What was the cause of this rapid gangrene ? In order to answer this question, it was necessary to review the causes of gangene of the genital organs.

Diabetes is one of the causes. Fournier and Vaquez have quoted cases.

---

* Dieulafoy, *Clinique Médicale de l'Hôtel-Dieu,* 1906, vol. v., p. 40.

Gangrene may be caused by paraphimosis, phimosis, and balano-posthitis, consecu tive to vegetations, and hard and soft chancres of the groove and of the glans. Balano-posthitis is infection of the glans and prepuce. Several pathogenic microbes have been incriminated—an inoculable and very mobile spirillum (Berdal and Bataille); anaerobic microbes (Rist); a small, thin anaerobic bacillus, giving off a fœtid odour from its cultures (Vincent). These pathogenic agents multiply the better in that they are protected from the oxygen of the air by the anatomical conformation of the prepuce. The vegetations developed in the groove and around the glans, as well as the balano-posthitis and phimosis, produce conditions favourable to gangrene of the prepuce and glans.

Simple chancres, says Fournier, by reason of their special virulence, are liable to produce gangrenous balano-posthitis. These chancres are often hidden under the prepuce, which become œdematous ; phimosis follows, foul-smelling fluid exudes from the preputial orifice, and in a few days gangrene is evident. The sloughing prepuce some-time perforates laterally, and, as Diday says, the glans shows its nose at the window. At other times the gangrene destroys a part of the prepuce, and may encroach upon the glans. Besides these partial forms, there are some, says Balzer, in which the gangrene invades the skin of the penis, the scrotum, and even the corpora cavernosa.

In my patient there was no reason to suppose gangrene consecutive to these different causes ; but might there not be a hard chancre, complicated by gangrene ? Griffon has published a case in which a hard chancre of the prepuce gave rise to gangrene, which destroyed the penis and the suprapubic region. In this case, says Fournier, it was a question of early tertiarism. Nothing similar was present in my case. In the absence of any other cause, I finally diagnosed spontaneous fulminant gangrene of the penis—spontaneous in that we knew not the cause ; fulminant in that the sloughing strikes the tissue " like a stage-trick."

The prognosis was most grave, because of the general infection, as shown by the ulceration of the nails, tongue, and throat. In such a case of septicæmia, treatment had little chance of success. Le Dentu made vigorous use of the thermo-cautery, and applied dressings of formalin to the scarifications. The symptoms grew worse, and the patient died in coma.

I saw a similar case in the Saint-Antoine Hospital. A patient came under my care with fulminant gangrene of the penis and secondary pneumonia. He died rapidly, the whole penis having been destroyed before death. The histological examination by Giraudeau revealed neither arteritis nor phlebitis. The process was one of fulminant gangrene.

Fournier's case : A healthy young man felt slight pain in the penis. He vomited, fever appeared, the penis swelled up and became red, and the pain increased. Next day patches of gangrene were visible. In three days the sloughing involved the prepuce and the scrotum, while a tract of lymphangitis started from the gangrenous region, and ended in the groin, where it gave rise to an abscess. An eruption of purpura appeared at several spots. Nevertheless, the symptoms improved, and recovery finally followed.

Troisfontaine's case : A youth felt pain behind the glans. Next day the prepuce was œdematous. During the following days the penis swelled up ; the pain was severe ; foul, bloodstained liquid flowed out from the preputial orifice ; the inguinal glands enlarged ; the temperature was 104° F. ; the general condition was bad ; and the raphe became gangrenous. A wide incision showed that the slough had invaded the sub-cutaneous tissue and fascia, and had hollowed a funnel-shaped hole in the corpus cavernosum. The sloughs were cut away with scissors. Recovery followed.

Brocq's case : On June 1 a soldier was taken ill with fever, and found that his prepuce was swollen. Next day his general condition was bad, and delirium set in on June 3. The penis was swollen right up to the pubes, the skin was blackish, and gangrene was obvious. Free incision. Although some relief followed, vomiting came on, and the temperature rose to 104° F. At night two more incisions were made. The glans was found to be intact. On June 4 the stench was fearful. On June 5 penis was black and sloughing, scrotum involved, temperature over 104° F. On June 7 improvement set in, and the fever diminished. The sloughs commenced to separate, repair took place slowly, and about the middle of July the patient left the hospital.

Description.—This variety of gangrene is not uncommon. In 1883 Fournier, who first described it, had seen five cases. In 1896 Emery, in his thesis, published twenty-three cases. Next come the cases of Fournier, Danlos, Druelle and Nicolau, Darses, Grisel, and my two cases—a total of thirty-one cases.

The disease is practically confined to the male sex. One case in a woman has been quoted by Brissaud and Sicard :

A vesicle appeared on the right labium majus of a healthy woman. On the third day of the disease pains radiating to the vulva, no glands in the groin, bloody discharge from the vulva. On the fourth day blackish slough on each side, fulminant gangrene, temperature 102° F. On the fifth day gangrene spreading, odour offensive. The patient died on the seventh day, her temperature being 106° F. The urine did not contain sugar or albumin. The blood taken on the sixth day gave pure cultures of streptococci. Anaerobes were not looked for.

This variety of gangrene has been called "spontaneous," for the reason that we do not know its cause. It is evidently an infective process, but it is hard to say whence the infectious agent comes, and why it has such virulence. In some cases it has appeared in persons who had an abrasion or an excoriation, caused by scratching in the case of eczema ; but this entrance gateway is rarely present, and, again, these small lesions are seen in many people who never show any sign of gangrene.

The disease is nearly always seen in young subjects. In thirty-one cases I find an old man and three infants. My patient at the Hôtel-Dieu was twenty-five years of age. By some writers this genital gangrene is said to form part of the specific venereal infections—gonorrhœa and soft and hard chancres—or it is said to result from excessive coitus. Fournier has rightly refuted these opinions. The disease commences in a healthy person, with itching or pain in the prepuce or in the penis. The prepuce takes on a reddish tinge and swells up. The patient and the physician are not alarmed. The swelling of the prepuce determines phimosis, and it is not rare to find slight discharge due to balano-posthitis. The appearance of these symptoms leads to a question of gonorrhœa or of soft chancres in the groove around the glans. The patient feels some alarm, but does not suspect the storm that is brewing. "The contrast is, indeed, remarkable between the apparently benign onset and the malignant character of the resulting lesion. In a few hours the scene changes. The penis, which has become painful, swells as a whole, and becomes œdematous, being converted into a pudding —at first rosy, then red, and finally livid. Bullæ often appear. Matters

II.

128

remain in this state for some twenty-four to thirty hours, and then a new symptom indicative of gangrene reveals itself " (Fournier).

Greyish or yellowish insensitive patches appear on the prepuce, penis, and scrotum. They are patches of gangrene. At this moment we cannot say whether the slough will stop or spread. Sometimes the mortification is limited ; at other times it spreads to the penis, scrotum, glans, and corpora cavernosa with astonishing rapidity. In the thirty-one cases which I have collected the regions invaded by gangrene were as follows :

In eight cases the sloughing was limited to the prepuce, which was partially or totally destroyed. These are the most benign cases. In twelve cases the slough invaded the prepuce and the raphe, with or without participation of the scrotum. Such was the case in my patient at the Hôtel-Dieu. In three cases the gangrene was limited to the glans. In five cases the corpora cavernosa and the glans participated in the gangrenous infection, and the distribution of the sloughing was as follows : Gangrene of the prepuce and glans (Cellier) ; gangrene of the raphe and of the corpus cavernosum (Trois-fontaines) ; gangrene of the raphe, glans, and corpus cavernosum, the glans being represented only by a small bud (Fournier) ; gangrene of raphe, scrotum, and glans, the latter being quite destroyed (Fournier) ; gangrene of the raphe, part of the glans, and part of the corpora cavernosa (Darses) ; gangrene of the entire penis (my case at the Saint-Antoine Hospital).

To resume the description of the disease. The dead tissues give off a most offensive odour, and become as black as coal. Greenish streaks and islets of healthy skin sometimes stand out against the black tint of the eschar. The presence of gas has not been noted, and writers upon this disease make no mention of it. This fact is noteworthy, considering the importance of fulminant gangrene in which gas is present. The general symptoms increase in severity, the temperature rises to 104° F., and the patient is plunged in a state of prostration bordering upon adynamia. The prognosis appears to be very grave—the patient seems certain to die, and if life is saved there is great likelihood that he will lose a part of the genital organs. The latter supposition is usually erroneous, since in reality this fulminant gangrene is rarely fatal, and, on the other hand, the repair of the dead tissues is so good that deformity is quite an unusual result.

The gravity of the prognosis depends upon the complications of lymphangitis, erysipelas, and cellulitis rather than upon the gangrene. As a rule, in the midst of the gangrenous stage, often about the eighth day, improvement suddenly sets in. At the same time the local condition changes. The eschar is detached, leaving in its place a healthy granulating wound, and healing takes place. In the case of the glans and corpora cavernosa the lesions may not recover sufficiently to prevent serious deformity.

The condition of the inguinal glands in hard and soft chancres is well known : in the former a pleiad of glands ; in the latter a suppurating bubo. Nothing of the kind is seen in fulminant gangrene. The glands react so little that in most cases the adenopathy is trifling. Hæmorrhages have been noted in five cases. Purpura has been seen three times. Lymphangitis has been present in several cases. The presence of lymphangitis, erythema, abscesses, and erysipelas in which streptococci have been found, had led writers to place fulminant gangrene of the penis among the streptococcal infections.

Diagnosis.—The diagnosis of declared gangrene is easy. The black colour of the integument, the œdematous swelling of the tissues, and the stench from the gangrenous region are the indications. It is, however, necessary to know the variety of gangrene present. Is it fulminant gangrene, or is it gangrene secondary to trauma, or to balano-posthitis, soft chancres, warts, phimosis, etc. ? In order to differentiate these secondary gangrenes, careful inquiry must be made as to the cause. Analysis of the urine will settle the question of diabetic gangrene. There is a variety of urinary gangrene which at first sight simulates spontaneous gangrene. It may appear as the result of infiltration of urine due to a stricture of the anterior urethra. In such a case the gangrene appears first in the penis, and closely resembles spontaneous gangrene. The passage of a catheter is the best way to decide the point.

In another variety of urinary gangrene the stricture of the urethra may not be complete. The flow of urine is fairly free, and though no stricture is present, gangrene closely resembling spontaneous fulminant gangrene supervenes. It commences in the prepuce, spreads rapidly to the raphe and scrotum, and ends in death.

How can we arrive at the diagnosis when the disease is in its early stage ? The prepuce is red or œdematous, the raphe often participates in the œdema, and the patient experiences a sensation of pain or of burning. We think of balano-posthitis, of lymphangitis following an excoriation, or of soft chancres accompanied by phimosis, but a scrupulous examination leads us to abandon these views. Bullæ form, and gangrene appears.

Treatment.—The patient should be given baths if he can bear them ; moist dressings should be applied to the gangrenous parts. The strength is kept up with stimulants, and surgical intervention is employed as soon as possible. Free incisions as well as scarification with the thermo-cautery give good results. In one of Fournier's patients the penis was gangrenous, and the scrotum appeared likely to share the same fate. Le Dentu at once made free incisions into the scrotum, and immediate improvement set in.

Pathogenesis and Pathological Anatomy.—According to some writers, fulminant gangrene of the penis is simply a gangrenous lymphangitis or erysipelas. They base their opinion upon the coexistence of lymphangitis, erysipelas, and gangrene, and on the presence of streptococci. I would refer the reader to my clinical lectures on this subject.

In several cases it appears that the streptococcus is at fault. In many other cases, however, the streptococcus is absent, and in my patient we shall see the result of the bacteriological examination.

I give first the lesions found at the autopsy. Except for a patch of meningitis, the examination of the viscera was negative. The blackish gangrenous colour extended to the root of the penis without any clear line of demarcation. The prepuce was infiltrated and gangrenous. The groove between the glans and the prepuce was of a deep red, and streaked with hæmorrhagic lines. We could not find ulcers, chancres, cicatrices, or pus at the bottom of the furrow. There was no balano-posthitis. Sections of the penis showed that the urethra and the corpora cavernosa were normal. They were sorrounded by hard connective tissue. The histological examination gave the following results : In the prepuce the necrosed tissue stained a uniform red colour with eosin. The nuclei did not stain with hæmatoxylin, and very high magnification was required to show a slight embryonic infiltration. The epidermis and the internal covering of the mucous membrane had completely disappeared. The dermis was ragged. The connective tissues were dissociated by patches of œdema and fibrin. Similar lesions were found in the balano-preputial groove. On the dorsum of the penis similar lesions were present. They did not penetrate the corpora cavernosa. At the root of the penis we found some arteritis and phlebitis, but in no part was complete or partial

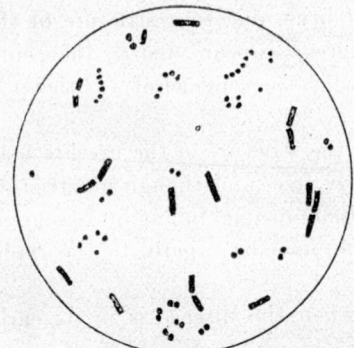

Fig. 101.—Penis : Bacillus Septicus and Enterococcus.

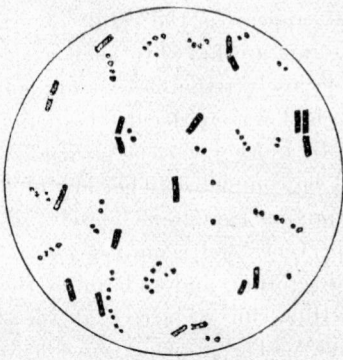

Fig. 102.—Blood : Bacillus Septicus and Enterococcus.

thrombosis present. The vascular lesions appeared to be secondary, and not primary. No line of demarcation with leucocytic infiltration was present. The transition between the healthy and the diseased tissue was insensible. The gangrenous focus in the tongue being limited, the histological picture was even more clear.

Bacteriological Examination.—I shall give a résumé of the bacteriological examination (smears, cultures, and inoculations) as regards the penis, the meninges, the anal region, and the blood. Everywhere, except in the perianal ulcerations, we found two associated microbes, which swarmed from the penis into the blood and the brain.

These two microbes showed the following characters :

1. A thick aerobic bacillus, having rounded ends, and staining with Gram. Its centre was often but little stained ; its length varied with the age of the cultures ; it was often isolated ; it occurred at times in the form of a diplobacillus or of small masses ; it grew readily on both, and gave off a fœtid odour ; it was pathogenic for guinea-pigs, in which it produced gangrene. These characters identified it as the *Bacillus septicus* of Legros and Leòène. Legros confirmed my view.

2. A facultative aerobic and anaerobic diplococcus. It stained with Gram and was

characterized by an astonishing polymorphism (small cocci, large cocci, short chains of diplococci on agar, short bacilli in old cultures). It grew readily on broth and agar, it did not liquefy gelatine, and it was very long-lived. These characters identified it as the enterococcus of Thiercelin, and, as a matter of fact, Thiercelin identified it.

In this case of fulminant gangrene the *Bacillus septicus* was the pathogenic microorganism. The other organism appeared to play quite a second part. There was no sign of the streptococcus.

What is the *Bacillus septicus?* The answer is given by the following case, taken from Legros's thesis :

A man was admitted under Pegrot for a fracture of the right leg, the tibio-tarsal joint being widely opened. The fracture was set, and an injection of antitetanic serum was given. Next morning the temperature was 104° F. On removing the dressings, the wound was blackish, and gave off an offensive odour. Reddish fluid mixed with bubbles of gas flowed out. Amputation through the middle third of the thigh was performed. In the lower part of the amputated limb the skin had a bronzed colour, and gas crepitation was noticeable. Two days after the operation the flaps were sloughing, the upper part of the thigh was crepitant, the gangrene was extending, the stench was unbearable, and death supervened six days after the accident.

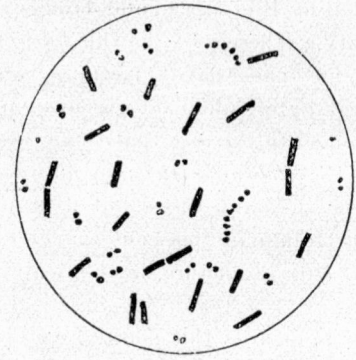

FIG. 103. — MENINGES: BACILLUS SEPTICUS AND ENTEROCOCCUS.

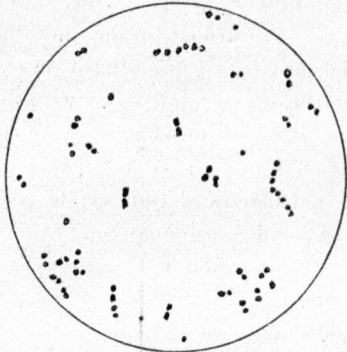

FIG. 104.—PERIANAL ULCERATION : ENTEROCOCCUS.

Some foul-smelling serous fluid had been taken from the dead muscles two days after the operation. Three species of microbes were isolated : they were aerobic by preference. They comprised a bacillus with the characters of the *Bacillus coli*, a diplostaphylococcus liquefying gelatine, and a special bacillus, corresponding in its morphological characteristics to the species predominating in direct preparations of the foul-smelling serous fluid. Of these three species the last one alone, when injected into a guinea-pig, gave rise to rapid gaseous gangrene. The animal died in forty-eight hours, the affection being characterized by its invading nature and by the enormous lesions in the muscles.

This bacillus has been described by Legros and Lecène under the name of the *Bacillus septicus aerobicus*. I shall not describe the characters of this bacillus, since they are comparable to those of the bacillus found in my case of genital gangrene, with this exception—that in one case gas was present, while in the other it was absent.

The *Bacillus septicus*, says Legros, has essential characters, which on the one hand show its relation to, and on the other hand its difference from, the *Vibrio septicus* of Pasteur. Legros has reported another case of gaseous gangrene due to the *Bacillus septicus*. Jacobelli of Naples has also published a case of acute gaseous gangrene, in which the bacillus isolated had all the characteristics of the *Bacillus septicus* of Legros.

These cases prove that the *Bacillus septicus* causes fulminant gangrene, with production of gas. In my patient, however, no gas was present. The same bacillus, therefore, may cause gangrene with the presence of gas and gangrene in which gas is not present. What is the explanation?

It is opportune at this point to discuss the question of specific microbes. Do they exist? The answer is affirmative. They cause specific diseases, and it was a stroke of genius on the part of Trousseau to have stated that some day we should discover specific germs in the case of certain maladies * Trousseau's prediction has been verified, and in the case of diphtheria and typhoid fever the specificity clinically created by Bretonneau and Trousseau has been confirmed by the microbic specificity. These views on this subject, which have shed much light on the pathogenic chaos, have sometimes overshot the mark; and since we are now speaking of fulminant gaseous gangrene, it is certain that we were too accustomed to the idea that these cases depended on a specific infection due to the *Vibrio septicus* of Pasteur. The pathogenic action of the vibrio is true in many cases, but it is not the specific organism in every case of fulminant gaseous gangrene. Other organisms may produce the same clinical picture, with identical lesions.

The writings of Legros will convince us as regards this point. We find a series of organisms capable of causing fulminant gaseous gangrene. Such are the *Bacillus emphysematis maligni*, the *B. phlegmonis emphysematosæ*, the *B. perfringens*, and the *B. septicus aerobicus*.

It is evident, says Legros, that, in addition to the cases of acute gaseous gangrene described by surgeons, we may also find more benign infections. They are due to the same pathogenic agents, and are characterized by gaseous œdema, with localized putrid decomposition. Roger ("Les Maladies Infectieuses"), forsaking the idea of specificity in the question now under discussion, has headed his chapter "Divers Agents des Gangrènes Gazeuses," and side by side with the *Vibrio septicus* he places "a series of microbes which more or less resemble it by reason of their biological or pathogenic properties."

These statements are true, and we see that the *Bacillus septicus* is capable, like the organisms just mentioned, of producing fulminant gaseous gan-

* *Vide, Lecon d'Ouverture de la Clinique de l'Hôtel-Dieu*, 1898, t. i., 1ère leçon.

grenes. Nevertheless, the gangrene in my patient was not gaseous. This fact proves that the *Bacillus septicus* under certain ill-defined conditions may engender gaseous or non-gaseous gangrene. Furthermore, the production of gas was not noted in any of the thirty-one cases of fulminant gangrene of the genitalia mentioned in this section.

There is another organ in which the gangrene is never gaseous—the appendix. I have pointed this fact out in one of my clinical lectures.* As the question is of importance, I am desirous of briefly discussing it. Appendicular pleurisy is often putrid and gaseous. It would, therefore, appear logical that the microbe which can cause putrefaction in the pleura should also cause putrefaction in the appendix. Such is not the case. I have seen 200 operations for appendicitis, but I have never seen gaseous gangrene of the appendicular focus or gaseous phlegmon in its walls. We do see fulminant gangrene in the appendix, but we do not find gas. And yet the anaerobic and aerobic flora of appendicitis is very rich. The *Bacillus septicus aerobicus* has even been found. These apparent contradictions prove that we have much to learn.

This discussion proves that fulminant gangrene of the penis cannot be included under gaseous gangrene. It is not a specific disease with a specific microbe. We must, therefore, exclude the formula which gives the streptococcus as the specific agent. It is inexact to say that this gangrene is merely a streptococcal infection. In certain cases, especially when the gangrene is associated with erysipelas, the pathogenic agent appears to be a streptococcus, but in many cases the streptococcus is absent, and we find other microbes. In my patient the *Bacillus septicus aerobicus* produced first gangrene and then fatal septicæmia.

This study in bacteriology, interesting though it be, only serves to put off the pathogenic problem, without solving it. While admitting that the streptococcus, the *Bacillus septicus*, or other organisms, may produce fulminant gangrene of the genitalia, whence come these organisms, and what is the cause of their virulence ? Why, on the one hand, fulminant destruction of the tissues, and on the other hand the relatively benign nature of the disease ? We do not know. It will be said that we must consider the receptivity of the soil. What, however, does this statement mean ? We do not know. Most of the patients were healthy and free from any previous taint, and yet fulminant gangrene set in, without appreciable cause and without proved contagion.

This form of gangrene has well-defined characters. The presence of gas has never been noted. The *Bacillus septicus*, which in surgical traumatisms produces gaseous gangrene, caused non-gaseous gangrene in my patient. Fulminant gangrene of the genitals has, then, a place beside the

* Dieulafoy, *Clinique Médicale de l'Hôtel-Dieu*, t. iv., p. 111.

various forms of gaseous gangrene. It is, moreover, far less formidable. I would add that it never extends beyond the genital organs. It is not invading, like the gaseous forms of gangrene.

It has nothing in common with gangrene due to vascular lesions, my case being an irrefutable proof thereof. In this case there was no phlebitis, no arteritis obliterans. The toxic agent appeared to have a directly necrosing action on the tissues. The pathogenesis of this variety of gangrene is not yet cleared up. For the present the term "spontaneous" must be preserved.

PART XII

THE INTOXICATIONS

THE study of poisoning belongs specially to toxicology and forensic medicine. Nevertheless, certain intoxications are intimately connected with pathological studies properly speaking. In this respect I may mention alcoholism, lead-poisoning, and hydrargyrism.

I. ALCOHOLISM.

Alcoholic drinks, in the form of wine, liqueurs, absinthe, beer, etc., are the more formidable in proportion as they are of inferior quality.

The essences (balm, mint, angelica, peppermint, etc.) which often enter the composition of liqueurs increase their toxic power, although it is not always possible to state the exact part these essences take in the morbid results. Alcoholic drinks are more harmful when taken in the morning on an empty stomach than they are at meal-times.

Acute Alcoholism.—Acute alcoholism is known as drunkenness. Drunkenness declares itself after more or less copious libations of alcoholic beverages. It commences with a period of excitation. The drunkard has a bright eye and a congested face. He becomes loquacious and noisy ; he is no longer master of his feelings, joy, anger, and sadness being pushed to their extreme limits. Vertigo soon appears ; the gait becomes unsteady ; the gastric malaise is considerable ; the face is pale ; the sweating is profuse ; and some of the fluid taken is vomited. After vomiting the malaise disappears, and sleep terminates this period of drunkenness, which leaves behind it only slight gastric distress. Vomiting, however, does not always occur, and the fluids ingested are not always rejected. The period of excitation then gives place to a phase of depression ; the drunken man falls down unconscious ; the respiration is embarrassed and stertorous, as in coma ; and the anæsthesia and the muscular relaxation are complete.

If the drunkenness results from the ingestion of liqueurs containing extracts of aromatic plants, such as absinthe, bitters, or vermuth, and especially if the patient is addicted to their use, we may witness epileptiform convulsions (Parcy's convulsive drunkenness). This condition lasts for some hours, and the patient gradually regains his faculties. In some cases, however, if the patient has absorbed a large quantity of alcohol, and has been exposed to cold for a long while, the central temperature falls progressively, and death may result.

Chronic Alcoholism.—Chronic alcoholism is slowly established, and the troubles which it causes concern chiefly the digestive tract and the nervous system.

Their predominance in one or other of these two systems depends upon hereditary predisposition. An individual born of neurotic parents, or neurotic himself, may from the first show severe nervous symptoms, while in another alcoholic such troubles will be indefinitely delayed.

Digestive Troubles.—The alcoholic person loses his appetite, experiences a burning sensation along the œsophagus (pyrosis), and in the morning vomits whitish shreddy matter (mucus). The chronic gastritis of drunkards is at times complicated by ulceration. Hæmatemesis may occur. Some authors admit that the gastric ulceration of alcoholic origin may assume the character of the round ulcer.

As the portal vein carries a portion of the ingested alcohol direct to the liver, congestion, steatosis, and fatty cirrhosis and especially atrophic cirrhosis, are frequent in alcoholics. The acute icterus of drunkards (Leudet) is of exceptional gravity.

Nervous Troubles.—The alcoholic tremor is an early symptom. It is especially marked in the upper limbs and hands, and is most severe in the early morning, when the stomach is empty. It improves during the day under the influence of fresh libations.

Sensory troubles are frequent. Alcoholics complain of headache, giddiness, formication, cramps in the calves, or anæsthesia, which sometimes invades half the body (Magnan). Hearing and sight are perverted, and some patients experience hallucinations, epileptiform convulsions, and attacks of acute mania or of lypemania ; others suffer from cerebral troubles which resemble those of general paralysis, and have been described under the name of Alcoholic General Pseudo-Paralysis. At the present day the tendency is to split these cases into two classes—in the one alcoholism (in predisposed individuals) leads to general paralysis ; in the other it ends in dementia.

The sleep is disturbed by nightmares and dreams. The patient thinks that he sees animals, such as rats, running over his bed.

Delirium Tremens is an acute episode of chronic alcoholism. Sometimes it is provoked by excess of alcoholic drinks, and at other times it complicates an intercurrent disease (pneumonia, rheumatism, injury). The patient is seized with violent, noisy, or furious delirium, requiring the employment of the strait-jacket. The insomnia is complete, and the movements are disordered. The attack lasts on an average from three to five days, and ends in deep sleep. Recovery usually occurs when the patient's temperature remains low. If delirium tremens appears apart from any febrile disease, and is accompanied by a temperature rising to 102° F., the situation becomes very grave, and the patient frequently dies (Magnan).

We may see in alcoholics, and especially in women, paralyses which commence in the lower limbs. They are localized chiefly to the antero-external group of the muscles of the legs, whence they spread to the other muscles. In severe cases the upper limbs are affected, and here, too, the paralysis commences in the extensors. The muscles of the face, of the neck, and of the eyes are more rarely affected. The paralysis is painful, and rapidly becomes complete. It is always flaccid, and is accompanied by pains in the muscles, by early muscular atrophy, by abolition of the reflexes, and by loss of the electrical contractility. It is curable as a rule, but recovery is always slow. In other cases, whether paralysis is present or absent, we find troubles of locomotion similar to those of locomotor ataxia (alcoholic pseudo-tabes).

Whether the case be one of paralysis or of pseudo-tabes, if the atrophy is very marked it leaves in its train muscular retractions which cause deformities of the limbs, and particularly of the feet. When the paralysis becomes general it may invade the muscles of respiration, attack the heart itself (Déjerine), and provoke syncope and death. It has an acute or a subacute course, and the muscular lesions are very slowly repaired. Relapses are frequent.

The peripheral nerves (peripheral neuritis) are the starting-point of these motor troubles, the nerves of the limbs being first affected (Lancereaux, Oettinger, Buzzard, etc.). No form of toxic neuritis is better established than the alcoholic form. It may also attack the cranial nerves, vagus, optic, etc.

Many authors, however, admit that these nervous changes are themselves consecutive to dynamic lesions of the cord (Erb).

Ocular troubles consecutive to chronic intoxication by alcohol are very frequent. They consist in amblyopia (toxic amblyopia), which may develop somewhat rapidly, and affect both eyes. This amblyopia is characterized by a more or less marked diminution of the central visual acuity (central scotoma), while the periphery of the visual field remains unaffected. The scotoma, before being absolute, exists only for colours—that is to say, the examination of the visual field with a white object causes no interruption, while the colour cannot be seen over the whole extent of the scotoma if a green or a red index be used for the examination. Patients see better at sundown (nyctalopia), because the sensation of dazzling disappears.

The ophthalmoscope reveals, as a rule, no lesion in the fundus oculi.

In some cases Uhthoff found decoloration of the external half of the optic papilla. If the amblyopia is treated from the onset, it disappears without leaving any traces. In older cases complete re-establishment of vision is almost always impossible.

Alcoholic poisoning may cause paralysis of the motor muscles of the eye. Acute polio-encephalitis, as I have said in a previous chapter, may sometimes be related to alcoholic poisoning.

Chronic alcoholism exercises its action on other systems. The voice is often hoarse and rough from chronic congestion of the pharyngeal mucous membrane (granular angina), of the epiglottis, of the arytenoids, and of the laryngeal mucosa. Genital weakness and impotence are not uncommon. The circulatory troubles depend upon the atheromatous condition of the vessels.

Diagnosis—Prognosis.—The characteristic odour of the patient's breath serves to distinguish the coma of drunkenness from coma or apoplexy associated with other morbid conditions.

The various troubles which depend upon chronic alcoholism will be recognized by the symptoms previously enumerated, and by the information furnished by the patient. And yet, in the face of such troubles as morning vomiting, tremor, tendency to delirium, and lypemania, the information given by alcoholic patients should be mistrusted, as some stoutly deny their alcoholic habits.

The alcoholic paralyses are distinguished from myelitis by their dissemination, by the spontaneous, and especially by the provoked, pain, by the rapid abolition of the reflexes, and by the early muscular atrophy. In pseudo-tabes the leg is never thrown to the left or to the right, as in ataxia, and the patient has the steppage gait (Charcot). The course of the disease is rapid, and not slowly progressive. Recovery is frequent, but relapses are to be feared.

The prognosis of acute alcoholism is rarely grave. Chronic alcoholism is serious, because it progressively and surely induces obstinate gastritis, cirrhosis of the liver, arterial atheroma, delirium tremens, mania, dementia, and suicide. The influences of chronic alcoholism extend to the descendants, for the children of alcoholic parentage are sometimes degenerates (idiocy, scrofula, epilepsy, etc.).

Pathological Anatomy.—Congestion of the lungs, of the meninges, and of the brain, with or without hæmorrhage, is found in those who have died from acute alcoholism (Tardieu). The blood, the liver, and the brain—in fact, all the organs—are impregnated with alcohol.

Chronic alcoholism produces two classes of lesions—chronic interstitial inflammations of the cirrhotic type and fatty degenerations of the parenchyma. The stomach is sometimes contracted, sometimes dilated. The mucous membrane is thickened, injected, and ulcerated. The liver shows **cirrhosis** or **steatosis,** either separately or in combination. The heart is fatty and the vessels are affected by endarteritis and atheroma. The kidneys present the changes of sclerosis and of fatty degeneration. The laryngeal mucous membrane is hyperæmic and thickened. The meninges are congested and inflamed. They sometimes present the lesions of pachymeningitis. The brain is affected, and its surface shows numerous foci of softening, which explain the mental troubles.

Treatment.—In a drunken man it is necessary to provoke the rejection of the ingested drink by vomiting. Acetate of ammonia (20 drops in a little water) and coffee are useful aids for stimulating the organism. In some alcoholic patients delirium tremens appears to be favoured by too sudden or too complete a suppression of alcohol. In this case beverages containing wine may be prescribed, while extract of opium, chloral, and bromide of potassium should also be administered. It is evident that we must employ all possible means to suppress or progressively to diminish the quantity of alcohol, as this is the cause of the disease. From recent experiments, the serum of a horse accustomed to alcohol is said to contain an anti-ethylin, which lessens the desire for alcoholic drinks after injection into man (Broca, Sapelier, and Thiébault).

II. MERCURIAL POISONING—HYDRARGYRISM.

Hydrargyrism comprises the pathological manifestations caused by the accumulation of mercury in the economy. This intoxication may be of therapeutic or of professional origin.

Ætiology.—The therapeutic form is sometimes consecutive to cutaneous absorption from mercurial inunction or cauterization with acid of nitrate of mercury; at other times consecutive to intestinal absorption of calomel, or proto-iodide of mercury. More rarely it follows baths of mercurial vapour.

The administration of the drug must, as a rule, be prolonged for a certain time in order to cause poisoning. In some patients, however, a single cauterization has given rise to toxic phenomena. There exists, therefore, in the case of mercury, as of many medicinal substances, a susceptibility which varies with different individuals, and which cannot be foreseen. This mode of mercurial poisoning is much less frequent than it was formerly, because saturation of the economy with mercury is no longer considered indispensable to the proper action of the drug.

Professional hydrargyrism is seen in miners (Almaden, Istria) and in workmen who handle mercury in its natural state (gilders, makers of looking-glasses and barometers), or the salts of mercury (hatters, etc.). The absorption usually takes place by the skin and the respiratory tract, but in miners the drug may also enter by the digestive tract, as the metal has been found in the stools. Idiosyncrasy plays an important part in these cases, just as in the preceding form. One miner will suffer from poisoning at the end of seven or eight hours of work, while another will resist for several weeks. The same holds good among workmen in cities.

Symptoms—Acute Hydrargyrism.—The therapeutic form usually commences with slight stomatitis, which tends to increase if the drug is continued (*vide* Mercurial Stomatitis). Such accidents are, as a rule, no longer seen, since the administration of mercury is usually stopped as soon as it produces symptoms, except in very urgent cases.

In professional hydrargyrism the first symptoms are palpitation, breathlessness, loss of appetite, insomnia, and pallor—in a word, a collection of troubles affecting the general health, and known by the name of mercurial erethism (Kussmaul). Stomatitis then appears, and runs its usual course.

In severe cases fever occurs, but the temperature does not exceed 100° F. (Hallopeau). The appetite completely disappears, and diarrhœa comes on. The urine is scanty, dark in colour, with a slight trace of albumin. The prostration is very pronounced. The number of red corpuscles is diminished (Gubler) in exceptionally grave cases, and hæmorrhages may occur from the various tracts. Hæmaturia is the most common (Kussmaul).

In this form eruptions may appear, constituting the so-called *hydrargyria.* Bazin has described three forms. The slight form is characterized by a simple erythema, localized to the inner surface of the thighs, to the scrotum, groins, and abdomen, with very small vesicles. The whole surface of the skin covered by the eruption smarts and itches most severely. The febrile form commences like the preceding one, and then extends to the whole body, reaching the face last of all. The eruption, which is of a vivid red, sometimes morbilliform, sometimes scarlatiniform, is often accompanied by sore throat. About the fourth day vesicles appear. They are larger than in the preceding form. They become filled with fluid, and then break, leaving moist and yellowish crusts. For about a week the temperature stands at 102° F. The severe form is only seen when mercurial preparations are used after the appearance of the first patches. The skin is tense and painful, the face is swollen, and the fever is severe. Grave symptoms, such as insomnia, delirium, or semi-coma appear, and in some cases death has supervened during the coma. Recovery is common, even in this form ; but during convalescence—that is to say, about the middle of the second week— abscesses, adenitis, phlegmons, and patches of gangrene often appear.

In the more severe cases of acute mercurialism the stomatitis is accompanied by swelling of the neck and suppuration of the parotid and cervical glands (Gubler), or by parenchymatous glossitis, and sometimes by gangrenous ulcers, which leave unsightly scars.

We shall study later the nervous troubles and the peripheral neuritis which result from chronic hydrargyrism. In both cases they may be due to acute hydrargyrism, and acute polyneuritis is sometimes seen during the course of active mercurial treatment, but differs from the chronic forms in that it is more generalized. The muscular atrophy is very pronounced, and the tendon reflexes are diminished.

Chronic Hydrargyrism.—This form is scarcely ever seen to-day, except in professional hydrargyrism. Mercurial erethism is here found in a complete manner, and is more marked than in the acute form. The face is pale, the breath is fœtid, the teeth are loose, and have a greenish-brown colour, being rough and rugose, with transverse striæ, which, as it were, fit into one another (Letulle's mercurial teeth). Diminution of the blood-corpuscles is constant.

At this period a tremor commences in the upper extremities, and then reaches the lower limbs, the head, and the tongue. It is sometimes more pronounced on one side than on the other, usually ceases during rest, appears on the occasion of movement, and is increased by fatigue, emotion, or by the abuse of alcohol. At first it is only slight, but it finally renders all work impossible. It lasts for weeks or for months, even after the patient ceases from work. In some cases it lasts for years after every cause of intoxication has been removed.

We sometimes see in the miners of Almaden and Istria contractures which are limited to the extremities, although they may become general. They are usually intermittent, and appear in the form of attacks. In Spain they are called by the name of *calambres,* and the workers who suffer from them are called *calambristes.*

In the moderate cases the muscular power of the patient is preserved. Letulle, however, says that he has noticed in many patients paresis of the muscles which are affected by the tremor. In exceptional cases we may see true **mercurial paralysis,** localized to the upper limbs, striking the extensors by preference, and then extending to the lower limbs. These paralyses, which are always flaccid, are not, as a rule, accompanied by muscular atrophy or by changes in the reflexes. They are incomplete and transient, and have a peripheral origin due to degenerative lesions of the nerves.

Just as cases of saturnine hysteria have been noticed, so mercury in some individuals may also give rise to nervous troubles which resemble those of ordinary hysteria in every particular. This mercurial hysteria (Letulle) can only be diagnosed by the aid of commemoratives.

The troubles of professional hydrargyrism are usually limited to the above-named affections, and after appropriate treatment nearly all are prone to disappear, or at least to improve, if they are not too inveterate and if the workman gives up his trade. Sometimes they grow worse: the maxillæ necrose, the intellectual faculties are blunted, and a general weakness supervenes, which renders the sufferer impotent. Tardieu has thus described the condition of these patients : " They stop indoors by the side of the fire, huddled up on a chair like children of tender age. Many of them cannot dress themselves or eat without assistance. Their look becomes dull, and at the same time they can only articulate a few vague and confused sounds."

Lastly, digestive troubles supervene, and are characterized by persistent loss of appetite, by constipation, or by uncontrollable diarrhœa. The gums swell and bleed at the least touch, the face is swollen, the extremities become œdematous, ecchymotic patches appear on different parts of the body, and hæmorrhages occur from the various canals. **Mercurial cachexia** thus arises. In many points it resembles the cachexia of scurvy. It often ends in collapse and death.

Diagnosis.—No one symptom of hydrargyrism is pathognomonic. The presence of several symptoms, the course of events, and the history alone allow a diagnosis to be made. Each of these troubles, if taken alone, may be confounded with similar ones due to many causes. We have already seen the varieties of stomatitis with which the mercurial form may be confounded. The mercurial tremor very closely resembles that of disseminated sclerosis, in that it is not present during repose, but only appears with movement, and increases in proportion as the patient reaches his desired object. In disseminated sclerosis we find also disturbance of sight and of speech, with permanent contractures, and sometimes also mental disorders which are not found in hydrargyrism.

Hydrargyrism, which commences on the abdomen, groin, and anterior surface of the thighs, and is sometimes accompanied by sore throat and fever, may be confounded with scarlatina. The existence of vesicles on the surface of the erythema is not always a sufficient element in diagnosis, as there exists a variety of scarlatina which is also accompanied by a vesicular eruption. The slight elevation of temperature, the absence of generalization, and especially the history, will give the diagnosis.

For a long while many syphilitic troubles, and especially changes in the bones, were attributed to mercurial treatment. Apart from necrosis of the maxillæ, mercury has no action on the osseous system. The nervous troubles, such as myelitis and encephalopathy, were formerly attributed to the influence of mercury. At the present time these discussions have only a historical interest, and the excellent effects produced by mercurial inunction in these conditions give the lie to all controversy. The therapeutic administration of mercury has, however, its limits, and in some cases examination for the presence and the quantity of mercury in the urine may be most useful.

Treatment.—This must be : (1) Hygienic or preventive—that is to say, we must attempt to ventilate as well as possible workshops and mines (Proust), to diminish the number of working-hours, and by cleanliness to check the causes of poisoning. The workmen should be made to bathe frequently, and also to brush their teeth daily, stomatitis being much less frequent in individuals who take this precaution. (2) Persons must be removed from the morbid cause, the secretion of urine must be assisted, and, in order to favour the elimination of the mercury, iodide of potassium must be administered. Hydrotherapy and electricity produce good effects.

III. LEAD-POISONING.

Ætiology.—The causes of lead-poisoning are most varied. All workers who handle lead or its compounds are more or less exposed. Those who are employed in mines, in white-lead and in red-lead works, house-painters, workmen engaged in scraping moulds for artificial ice (Rénon and Géraudel), in the setting of false pearls (Apert), in the making of frosted glass, type-setters, and glaziers, etc. The symptoms of lead-poisoning are also caused by the use of cosmetics and face-paints. The preparations of lead enter the economy by the digestive tract, by the respiratory tubes, by the mucous membranes, and by the skin.

Accidental poisoning, if we do not pay attention to it, may be the un-known cause of many morbid symptoms. Bread or meats cooked with wood painted with red lead, preserved foods, pastry covered with tinfoil, water conveyed by lead pipes, rain-water which has remained for a long while in leaden cisterns, seltzer-water, doctored wines, rooms which have been freshly painted with white lead, are all causes to be carefully looked for.

Description.—In many persons lead impresses a general deterioration upon the economy before showing itself by local manifestations. This dyscrasia chiefly depends upon changes in the blood. In **saturnine anæmia** the number of red corpuscles is diminished by 50 per cent. We may find only 2,300,000 per cubic millimetre (Malassez). The corpuscles are also altered in quality. The skin is of a pale yellow colour ; the patient is wasted ; the pulse is small, slow, and polycrotic. On examination of the mouth, we find at the edge of the gums a bluish line (**lead line**), which results either from deposit of metallic dust in the capillaries of the gum or from the elimination of the lead by the salivary glands. The breath is usually fœtid. We may note also the patches described by Gubler as a kind of tattooing of the cheeks, and situated at the level of the small and large molars. Let us mention also inflammation of the parotid glands.

Lead-colic is one of the most frequent manifestations of acute and

II. 129

chronic lead-poisoning. It is sometimes preceded by dyspeptic troubles, loss of appetite, and constipation; at other times it appears suddenly. The pain may occupy every part of the abdomen, and may radiate to the loins and to the testes. The pain is continuous, and is increased from time to time by attacks which cause the patient great suffering. His face is pale and pinched; he tries every possible position to quiet the pain, and he sometimes succeeds in doing so by squeezing the painful region. The belly is hard and retracted, the constipation is absolute, vomiting is frequent, and the urinary secretion is diminished. The apyrexia is complete, and the pulse is hard and slow. On percussing the liver we find a diminution in size (Potain), which probably depends upon the contraction of the hepatic vessels. A subicteric tint of the skin is often present. On auscultation, a systolic murmur is frequently heard at the base of the heart. Lead-colic has a duration of some weeks. It is due, according to some writers, to painful spasms of the muscular layers of the intestine; according to others, to neuralgia of the lumbar plexus.

Troubles of the Nervous System.—The general sensibility is frequently altered. Anæsthesia, analgesia, and hyperæsthesia are frequent. Sometimes there is a notable delay in the perception of sensations (Brouardel). The anæsthesia may occur in patches; it may be disseminated over the whole body, or, on the other hand, it may be localized to one side (saturnine hemianæsthesia). Lead-colic is frequently accompanied by cutaneous hyperæsthesia, arthralgia, and myalgia.

The special senses are sometimes affected, but the amblyopia and amaurosis are generally transient.

The visual troubles are not frequent. They are generally late, and of various kinds. In some cases the amblyopia is due to the appearance of a central scotoma, similar to that of alcoholic amblyopia, and without lesions of the fundus oculi. More commonly we find optic neuritis or neuro-retinitis, which, after a certain period, ends in atrophy of the optic nerve (amaurosis). In other cases albuminuric retinitis (Hirschberg, Leber) or uræmic amaurosis (Gunsburg) develops, and is consecutive to nephritis. Sometimes the oculo-motor muscles are affected by paralysis, especially the external rectus (Schroeder).

The **motor troubles** are very important (paralyses, tremors, pseudo-tabes). Lead-palsy has its seat of election in the extensor muscles of the hands and fingers. According to Duchenne (of Boulogne), it attacks in succession the extensor communis digitorum, the extensor indicis, the extensor minimi digiti, and the two radial extensors. The supinator longus is almost always spared, which is not the case in musculo-spiral paralysis. Gaucher has, however, published cases in which the supinators were affected.

Lead-palsy of the extensors is almost always bilateral. The fingers are flexed upon the hand, the hand is flexed upon the wrist, and the movements of extension are abolished. The paralysis of the extensors is complicated by the dorsal tumour of the wrist (Gubler). The tumour is indolent, and is probably due to inflammation of the synovial sheaths. It disappears upon the cure of the paralysis.

Lead-palsies have been carefully studied in the remarkable treatise of Déjerine-Klumpke. They usually are localized, and may assume the following types : (1) Remak's antibrachial type. This is the most common form, and affects the extensor muscles of the fingers and of the wrist. (2) Superior or brachial type. The paralysis affects the muscles of the Duchenne-Erb group—namely, the deltoid, the biceps, the brachialis anticus, and the supinator longus. (3) Aran-Duchenne type. The paralysis affects the muscles of the hand, the thenar and the hypothenar eminences, and the interossei, and simulates progressive muscular atrophy the more closely in that the palsy of these groups of muscles is always accompanied by atrophy in lead-poisoning. (4) Inferior or peroneal type. This is a rare form, in which the paralysis chiefly affects the peronei muscles and the extensors of the toes, while the tibialis posticus is usually, but not always, affected.

In some cases the palsies are not localized to groups of muscles. They tend to become general, and the generalization is slow or rapid. Although it may in the slow forms invade all the muscles of the trunk, it is, nevertheless, more marked in the muscles of the limbs, especially in the extensors of the fingers and of the wrist. In the rare cases in which lead-palsy rapidly becomes general it shows an ascending or a descending course, and may invade *en bloc* in a few days the muscles of the legs, of the abdomen, and of the thorax, as well as the intercostal muscles and the diaphragm, so that the paralysis only spares the muscles of the head and of the neck. In spite of the apparent gravity of these rapid paralytic forms, improvement supervenes rapidly, and termination by death is the exception.

In lead-palsy the **electrical contractility** is rapidly lost, before the voluntary power ; in musculo-spiral paralysis *a frigore* the electrical contractility is usually preserved. The muscles affected by lead-palsy have a tendency to atrophy.

The tremor, so well described by Lafont, chiefly affects the hands. It has little tendency to become general. It is usually preceded by muscular weakness, and differs from the alcoholic tremor in that it increases with fatigue, and becomes more marked towards the end of the day. This tremor is often only a hysterical one produced by saturnism.

The muscular atrophy is, as a rule, limited to the paralyzed muscles. In some cases, however, muscular atrophy of saturnine origin may exist, and become general, without being complicated by paralysis. I have seen such a case with Geoffroy. The muscular atrophy sometimes assumes in the hands the Aran-Duchenne type, so that the diagnosis can only be made from the ætiology and from the trade of the patient.

Recent writers have noted (Debove, Achard, Letulle) the existence of hysteriform attacks, which appear both in men and women, but chiefly in long-standing cases. This saturnine hysteria is identical as regards its symptoms with ordinary hysteria, and most of the cases of saturnine hemi-anæsthesia must be explained in this way. Saturnism, as a provoking agent, like syphilis and hydrargyrism, would thus prepare the organic soil for the development of the neurosis in predisposed persons (Charcot). Saturnine apoplexy is most often a manifestation of this symptomatic hysteria. It often commences in a sudden fashion, and simulates an attack of apoplexy of organic origin. It leaves behind, as a rule, motor hemiplegia and sensory hemianæsthesia, which is, as it were, the sign of hysteria.

Let us note also, among the exceptional motor troubles, hemichorea (Raymond) and pseudo-tabes (Leval, Piquechef).

The **cerebral troubles** in lead-poisoning are more serious than those just described, and are designated by the name of **saturnine encephalopathy** or **cerebro-spinal saturnism** (Jaccoud). According to the predominance of special symptoms, writers have described delirious, convulsive and comatose forms. The cerebral troubles are frequently ushered in by pro-dromata, such as headache, vertigo, squint, insomnia, hallucinations, and tendency to excitement or to depression. The condition is, as a rule, a late trouble of chronic lead-poisoning, and is, I believe, frequently associated with uræmia.

The delirious form presents no special characteristics. The delirium is sometimes quiet, sometimes noisy, and accompanied by hallucinations. The delirium is always mobile, and its duration is variable. In the con-vulsive form the convulsions may be partial and local or general, and like those of an attack of epilepsy. This saturnine epilepsy sometimes simulates the ordinary form to perfection. The precursory aura and the attacks of vertigo are, as a rule, wanting, but the attack may end in apoplexy. The comatose form is rarely primary; it usually follows one of the preceding forms. Saturnine encephalopathy is sometimes fatal after a few days. In the mixed form delirium and convulsions often precede coma.

The condition called general paralysis in these cases is considered by certain alienists as identical with Baillarger's disease. Other authors think that it is a general pseudo-paralysis, which differs from the true form by its sudden onset and its recovery under the influence of treatment favouring the elimination of the lead. Its history is connected with that of saturnine encephalopathy.

Writers have tried to explain this encephalopathy by the presence of special lesions in the brain (Renaut). The cerebrum is anæmic, yellowish, and firm to the touch, giving the sensation of marsh-mallow paste. Chemical analysis reveals the presence of lead. These lesions may, however, exist during life without saturnine encephalopathy. As a matter of fact, the tendency is to consider the encephalopathy as symptomatic either of atheroma of the cerebral vessels, or of hysteria, or particularly, let me repeat, as a uræmic manifestation.

Gout.—The attack of gout very closely resembles the ordinary form. It commences in the same manner with fever. It usually appears during the night, and the pain is localized to the big toe or to both toes, more rarely to the tibio-tarsal joint, to the knee, or to the fingers. The attack, which is very painful, improves towards the morning. Slight perspiration appears, and the patient falls asleep. The gouty region is swollen, tender, shining, and streaked with dilated veins. The pains become quite as severe again during the night, so that we find slight improvement, followed by paroxysms, as long as the attack of gout has not ended. During the attack of saturnine gout, as in the ordinary disease, the uric acid contained in the urine may be in excess. The serous fluid from a blister applied during an attack over the diseased joint contains uric acid in both cases. In saturnine gout, as in the genuine disease, we find tophi in the neighbourhood of the joints, tendons, tendon sheaths, and subcutaneous cellular tissue. These concretions develop in the cartilages of the ear. They are numerous in the neighbourhood of the small joints, which they help to deform, and are found in the serous bursæ of the knee and of the elbow, where they may acquire the size of a nut. These uratic deposits may become inflamed, forming abscesses, and giving exit to whitish chalky matter. The tophi in saturnine gout appear early, so that in gout due to lead, as in the ordinary disease, the organism seems to be impregnated with uric acid and urate of soda.

From this description it is evident that saturnine gout and diathetic gout have very great analogies, and yet they present differences which I must mention, and upon which Gallard has rightly insisted. In ordinary gout the attack is really the first episode of the gouty diathesis, and is often preceded years previously by other manifestations of this diathesis, such as gravel, renal colic, asthma, hæmorrhoids, eczema, or migraine. Nothing of the kind is seen in gout due to lead-poisoning. The articular disease and the concretions are gouty manifestations which do not depend upon a general diathetic condition. Saturnine gout appears to be of a more invading character than the common form, and although it may remain localized to the big toe after a first attack, it is rare if it does not show a tendency in the following attacks to invade the other joints, such as the knees, elbows, shoulders, and vertebræ. The duration of the attacks is longer in saturnine gout, the anæmia is more rapid, and the cachexia is earlier.

The pathogenesis of saturnine gout is still a matter of theory. Saturnine uricæmia is, perhaps, due to hyperactivity of the function of the cells of the organism under the influence of the lead (Lécorché).

Nephritis.—Renal lesions, which may end in chronic nephritis of an interstitial nature, are sometimes associated with lead-poisoning. For purposes of description I shall class the symptoms of saturnine nephritis in several groups.

In the first group I place those patients who only have albuminuria, without other symptoms of nephritis. The albuminuria is not severe. It may be transient or intermittent, but it is usually accompanied, sooner or later, by symptoms of Brightism, although it may comprise the whole lesion of the kidney. In such a case it is not very formidable.

In the second group I shall place the more numerous patients who suffer from Brightism, with or without albuminuria, the symptoms being pollakiuria, cryæsthesia, dead fingers, itching, buzzing in the ears, epistaxis, electrical shocks, and cramps in the calves. These "minor symptoms of Brightism," which are so frequent when looked for, may not be accompanied by albuminuria—at least, for a time. I have had under my care in hospital patients who came back months or years apart, and who sometimes presented symptoms of albuminuria, with or without the minor symptoms of Brightism, and at other times these symptoms with or without albuminuria. The evolution of chronic saturnine nephritis is very slow. If it is properly treated, it may not end in uræmia.

In a third group I shall place those patients who are threatened with severe symptoms of uræmia, such as violent headache, intense dyspnœa of every kind (dyspnœic uræmia), vomiting, and gastric intolerance (gastric uræmia), and every kind of nervous uræmia, etc.

Saturnine nephritis is rarely accompanied by œdema, or, if it be, the œdema is late. On the other hand, the arterial tension is always raised, the temporal artery is tortuous and distended, the heart is hypertrophied, and the gallop rhythm is present (Potain).

These patients sometimes succumb through the kidney, and we then find the lesions of the small contracted kidney. Much histological and experimental research has been undertaken in order to explain the pathogenesis of saturnine nephritis. As early as 1863 Ollivier, in an important work, studied this disease. He caused it experimentally, and found traces of lead in the urine and in the kidney. He explained the albuminuria and the nephritis by the presence and by the elimination of the lead.

In 1881 Charcot and Gombault made anatomical and experimental researches with the object of showing that saturnine nephritis is an epithelial cirrhosis, the glandular element being the first affected, and giving rise to the lesions of the connective tissue, which are secondary. This point of view has since been severely attacked, and in a recent thesis Paviot, reviewing the question from the anatomical and experimental point of view, arrives at opposite conclusions. In the fourth case of saturnine nephritis, which forms the basis of his work, " we find," he says, " the same irregularity of distribution. The saturnine intoxication does not spread, either along the epithelial system or along the vascular system, but affects the interstitial tissue at many different points in the labyrinthine spaces, preserving, however, with a somewhat regular constancy its predominance in the neighbourhood of the hilum and often of the pyramids of Ferrein." The experimental and also the histological researches of Paviot differ absolutely from those of Charcot and Gombault, for " in any case," he says, " the renal epithelia have not been found to be primarily and solely diseased. The sclerosis has often been met with, apart from any alteration of the tubules, and, on the other hand, it is never isolated."

Prévost and Binet, in 1889, in a most comprehensive monograph, state the result of their experimental researches upon lead-poisoning. They slowly produced chronic poisoning in rats and guinea-pigs. Post mortem they found that the lesions of the kidney were the more marked in proportion to the length and to the slowness of the poisoning. The kidneys were fibrous, cystic, and diminished in size, interstitial nephritis being the chief lesion. The kidneys contained much lead. The comparative examination for lead in the different viscera proved that the lead introduced into the organism accumulates **in the kidneys.** In spite of the accumulation of the metal in the kidney, the urine of the animals under experiment eliminates generally but little lead, and this fact coincides with the condition in man when suffering from lead-poisoning. The presence of lead in the urine is, indeed, difficult to recognize even when the patient is put upon iodide of potassium, with the object of converting the lead fixed in the economy into the slightly soluble iodide of lead.

We have, therefore, abundant data as to the pathogenesis and the nature of saturnine nephritis, but I must insist again upon certain considerations of importance. The patient, as we have said, is often gouty, or, at any rate, he often suffers from **uricæmia.** He may, therefore, have gouty nephritis, just like a gouty patient has. The examination of the kidney in both cases reveals traces of urate of soda. It must, therefore, be admitted that the patient has many reasons for having diseased kidneys. He is threatened by an intoxication (saturnism), and also by an auto-intoxication (uricæmia). These two processes may be in his case distinct or combined, but finally they often end in the lesions of the kidneys which cause the nephritis just described.

In the midst of this morbid complex one fact is, nevertheless, somewhat astonishing—namely, that the uricæmic process, which in the patient with lead-poisoning is an important element in nephritis, does not cause renal lithiasis and its complications (renal colic, hæmaturia, pyelo-nephritis, etc.), which are so frequent in persons of the gouty diathesis.

Parotiditis.—Hypertrophy of the parotid glands is frequent in lead-poisoning (Crontes, Achard, Claisse and Dupré). The parotid region is swollen on both sides, but it is painless both spontaneously and on palpation. Parotiditis, though essentially a chronic disease, may become acute as the result of angina, of stomatitis, or of treatment with iodides. The swelling is sometimes limited to the submaxillary glands, and the parotids are free.

The lesions of saturnine parotiditis have been carefully studied by Apert. The condition is one of simple hypertrophy, with catarrh of the excretory ducts and periglandular fibrosis. Apert has not found lead in the gland upon chemical examination. In his experiments Rénon found lead in the salivary glands of guinea-pigs poisoned with white lead.

Course—Diagnosis.—The saturnine dyscrasia decreases or increases according as the sufferer is free from or exposed to the toxic cause. Lead colic is often one of the initial symptoms. The palsies, tremors, and encephalopathy are, on the other hand, later symptoms. Nevertheless, we see some sufferers with tremor, and others with paralysis of the extensors, who have never had acute symptoms of colic.

At length the patient becomes cachectic ; the anæmia, the weakness, and the wasting progress, and the complications become more formidable.

The **diagnosis** is easy in the case of colic and in paralysis of the extensors. The diagnosis of the other troubles will be rendered easy by the trade of the patient, the attacks which he has previously suffered, and the presence of the lead-line on the gums.

Under the name of **saturnine asthma** writers appear to have confounded cardiac dyspnœa following arterio-sclerosis of the heart, uræmic dyspnœa resulting from interstitial nephritis, and attacks of dyspnœa caused by bronchitis from inhalation of lead-dust. Lastly, essential asthma may perhaps be caused by lead-poisoning in a predisposed individual.

Pathological Anatomy.—Lead is found in the blood and in the organs, especially in the liver and the kidney. The vessels are rigid, constricted, and affected with arterio-sclerosis. They are sometimes atheromatous. The heart is often hypertrophied. The muscles are diminished in size, and the microscope reveals simple atrophy, or atrophy with or without connective proliferation and fatty infiltration (Gombault). But the starting-point of lead-palsy is a periaxial segmentary neuritis, which has been recognized and reproduced experimentally by Gombault. This peripheral neuritis has been carefully worked out. The poison attacks the peripheral nerves. The spinal cord was diseased in only five cases, and these lesions were diffuse.

Treatment.—The treatment of lead-colic aims at removing the pain and the constipation. The former may be lessened by injections of morphia or by cataplasms containing laudanum, while the latter should be treated by repeated purgatives (senna, sulphate of soda, etc.).

With the object of eliminating the poison, sulphur and vapour baths may be prescribed, and iodide of potassium given, since Gubler states that it favours the disassimilation of the albuminates of lead. The continuous current is employed for the palsies. Tonics should be used for the anæmia.

Prophylactic treatment consists in preventing by every possible means the causes which favour the absorption of lead.

IV. PHOSPHORUS-POISONING.

Acute and chronic forms of phosphorus-poisoning must be distinguished.

1. Acute Poisoning.—This form is seen as the result of criminal poisoning, of attempts at suicide, or of an accident. Phosphorus from matches is the usual agent. A dose of 3 to 5 grains is almost always sufficient to cause death. Each match-head contains about $\frac{1}{10}$ grain of phosphorus, and fifty heads, therefore, represent a fatal dose. Rat-paste may be swallowed by animals eaten for food, thus rendering their flesh poisonous to man.

In children the symptoms run their course in a day, or even in a few hours ; in the adult the progress is slower. In the first phase, which lasts some hours, the patient feels a soapy taste in the mouth, and the breath is sometimes phosphorescent in the dark. The characteristic phenomena consist of pains in the throat and gullet, vomiting of food and bile, and, in rare cases, of blood ; while the vomit is luminous in the dark, and gives off a strong odour of phosphorus. The belly is distended and painful, and the patient suffers from diarrhœa, which may be luminous or hæmorrhagic.

This first period of digestive disturbance generally lasts from one to two days, and is succeeded by a deceptive remission, which may last for a few days.

The second period is more characteristic, and declares itself by the syndrome of icterus gravis, so that phosphorus-poisoning has been looked upon as an experimental reproduction of acute yellow atrophy Jaundice, the cardinal symptom, appears about the third or the fourth day The urine is scanty and rich in bile-pigment. It contains leucin and tyrosin. and is almost always albuminous.

As in icterus gravis, nervous phenomena and hæmorrhages may be the chief features. In the first case, we find more or less general pain, fibrillary contractions, hyperæsthesia, photophobia, delirium, and hallucinations. In this nervous form the phase of excitement gives place to a period of depres-

sion, which ends in coma or in collapse. The hæmorrhagic form is characterized by epistaxis, hæmatemesis, melæna, hæmaturia, large and multiple
petechiæ, and in most cases ends in collapse.

Pathological Anatomy.—When death supervenes rapidly, practically
no lesions are found. At the end of two or three days the autopsy reveals
acute fatty degeneration of the organs. It is especially marked in the liver,
which is yellow, soft, pasty, and almost diffluent.

The cells are loaded with fat, and, according to Cornil, this steatosis
commences from six to eight hours after the intoxication. The cells of the
liver refuse to act, whence the icterus gravis.

The kidneys, the heart, the vessels, and the stomach are affected with
steatosis. The cells of the tubuli contorti are loaded with fat, the fibres of
the heart lose their striation, and the epithelium of the pepsin glands is
charged with fat-drops. The gastric mucous membrane sometimes shows
small ulcerations, said by Cornil and Ranvier to be due to the phosphoric
acid formed *in situ*.

More or less general hæmorrhages may be found in the various organs.

In toxicology, in order to cause the production of phosphorescent
glimmers, the organs must be previously acidified, as alkaline matters do
not shine in the dark. Some days after poisoning this examination becomes
very delicate.

Treatment.—If the physician is called at once to a case of poisoning, he
should employ emetics and lavage of the stomach. Turpentine, administered continuously in doses of from 90 to 120 minims daily, is an excellent
antidote.

2. Chronic Poisoning.—This form is frequently seen in match-makers,
especially in those who steep the wood in the phosphorus paste or who
perform the sorting. Alcoholism, long hours in badly ventilated workshops,
neglect of personal hygiene, and dirty hands favour intoxication.

Phosphorus necrosis of the jaws and certain general troubles mark
chronic poisoning. They are seen after months or even after years of work,
according to the individual. The necrosis may affect both jaws, but shows
a predilection for the inferior maxilla.

The researches of Roussel and Magitot have shown that there was
previous dental caries, followed by penetration of the poison to the bone.
Pain in the teeth is followed by symptoms of alveolo-dental periostitis ; the
cheeks become swollen, abscesses form, and the resulting necrosis of the
bone may be very extensive. The necrosis may extend to the bones of the
face, and even to the base of the skull. It can be arrested by early surgical
treatment.

Necrosis proves fatal in one case out of every two. When it is of long
duration, it is complicated by cachexia, albuminuria, and œdema.

Grave anæmia, with vomiting and diarrhœa, may also result from chronic phosphorism.

Courtois-Suffit, who for several years has had charge of the match-makers at the Pantin-Aubervilliers, has published a profound and critical study of the troubles of phosphorism in workmen, and finds them less grave and less numerous than has been hitherto supposed. " If we except necrosis of the maxillæ, which is most certainly due to the direct influence of the vapours of white phosphorus, which gain an entrance by reason of ordinary dental caries, **we find that phosphorus has no specific action upon the general health.** It is difficult—or, rather, impossible—to distinguish in the pathological condition of the workmen what depends upon the toxine itself from what depends upon bad hygiene, anæmia, starvation, and the most ordinary pathological and toxic causes."

The replacement of white phosphorus by the sesquisulphate, which is harmless, will cause the disappearance of all troubles (Courtois-Suffit).

V. ARSENICAL POISONING.

Many years ago arsenic was the chief poison employed by criminals. Since the researches of Orfila showed how to determine the presence of arsenic in the organs, the number of cases of poisoning has markedly diminished, and at the present time criminal poisoning by phosphorus is much more frequent.

It is necessary to distinguish acute and subacute from chronic poisoning.

1. **Acute and Subacute Poisoning.**—Arsenious acid is the compound nearly always employed. In the pure state it is almost without taste, and as it is almost insoluble it is most often ingested in the form of a powder. A fatal dose varies much in individuals, and according as vomiting is or is not present. The mean fatal dose is from 1 to 2 grains.

Tolerance of the poison is readily established, so that the mountaineers of Styria and the Tyrol, in order to fit themselves for their climbs, are accustomed to take as much as 2 or 3 grains of arsenious acid daily. This habit creates a craving for the drug, and arsenic-eaters cannot give up the drug without experiencing signs of poisoning.

Clinically, we must distinguish acute from subacute poisoning.

Symptoms of Acute Poisoning.—Arsenic, if swallowed in large doses, causes symptoms within an hour. An acrid feeling in the mouth and epigastric pains open the scene. They are followed by symptoms of gastro-enteritis, with nausea, vomiting of food and bile, diarrhœa containing epithelial masses, and rice-water stools, so that the syndrome may resemble an attack of Asiatic cholera.

The heart beats quickly, the respiration becomes laboured, the skin is covered with sweat, the face is cyanosed, the urine is scanty, the patient suffers from muscular cramps, and often dies from syncope.

The nervous form differs from the gastro-intestinal one. Delirium, convulsions, and paralysis follow the headache, vertigo, and hyperæsthesia of the onset, and death often comes on with syncope.

Latent cases, in which death supervened in a few hours without agony, after some vomiting, have been noted, as well as incomplete poisoning, when the dose of the poison was insufficient. Sore throat and coryza may be the only symptoms, or, after some slight disturbances, eruptions, desquamation, and swelling of the skin of the scrotum supervene (Brouardel). Convalescence is always slow. In case of recovery the poison may be found in the urine for six weeks.

Subacute Poisoning.—This form is seen when the poison is absorbed in insufficient and intermittent doses. It causes digestive and nervous troubles.

The digestive troubles consist in vomiting, which becomes worse after each dose of the poison, in salivation, and in a bitter taste in the mouth.

The nervous troubles consist in paralyses, which appear as a rule at the end of a few weeks, and have all the characters of peripheral paralyses (Brissaud, Brouardel and Pouchet). They are chiefly motor, and affect the extensors. They are accompanied by atrophy, abolition of the reflexes, and pains in the limbs. They may present the picture of pseudo-tabes. With rare exception they recover very rapidly.

The lesions are chiefly found in the digestive tract. The stomach shows ecchymotic patches, and is covered with a thick mucus, and sometimes contains grains of arsenic in the form of a powder. The mucous membrane of the intestine is swollen, and studded with a psorenteric eruption. Steatosis is found in most of the organs, such as the liver, kidneys, heart, and muscles. Toxicological examination with Marsh's apparatus shows after sublimation traces of the poison in the viscera, in the nails, and in the hairs.

2. **Chronic Poisoning.**—This form is usually due to the patient's occupation. It is seen in labourers who extract the arseniferous mineral, and in the employés in certain aniline dye-works, or in manufacturers of green arsenic (Scheele's green and Schweinfurth's green). The making of paper coloured with green arsenic, or even living in rooms covered with this paper, may cause symptoms. The intoxication may be of alimentary origin, and it is sometimes difficult to find the cause, so complex may the ætiology be.

The changes chiefly affect the skin, the respiratory passages, and the nervous system.

The cutaneous lesions are multiple. In addition to erythemata, accompanied or not by papules and urticaria, we find vesicular and bullous eruptions, which may reach the size of a hen's egg, and become general over the whole body. I must also note the appearance of pustules and ulcerations, and especially of melanosis and keratosis. The melanosis may be general. The skin takes on a speckled appearance and the pigmentation is most marked on the trunk (Mathieu). It may also occur in isolated spots and patches. The keratosis affects the palms of the hands, the soles of the feet, and the orifices of the sweat-glands. It results from the hyper-idrosis consecutive to the employment of arsenic, which brings the poison into prolonged contact with the integument (Brouardel).

Chronic coryza, with muco-purulent secretion, chronic angina, attacks of asthma, and chronic bronchitis, comprise the changes in the respiratory passages. The coryza may end in ulceration of the mucous membrane and in the destruction of the septum and of the turbinate bones (Cartaz).

The nervous troubles are sometimes revealed by paralysis, which com-mences with pains or with changes in the general sensibility. The patient notices that he walks with greater difficulty and cannot clearly feel the ground. The paresis and the paralysis are marked in the muscles of the feet and in the extensor communis digitorum. The upper arms are often affected. The forearms are flexed, and the fingers are kept in palmar flexion.

The paralyzed muscles are more or less atrophied, but the reaction of degeneration is exceptional (Brouardel). The duration of these paralyses is very long. Improvement may not commence for some years, and recovery is rarely followed by *restitutio ad integrum*. Brouardel has been able to produce arsenical paralysis in the guinea-pig and rabbit.

Treatment.—In the case of acute and rapid poisoning the stomach must be emptied by emetics or by lavage. In less rapid cases of poisoning peroxide of iron should be taken, because it forms insoluble and harmless arsenite of iron. Magnesium hydrate, which forms arsenite of magnesia, may be given. Stimulants are indicated in case of threatening collapse.

VI. POISONING BY OPIUM, MORPHIA, AND COCAINE.

Opium.—Acute poisoning by opium is very frequent. Laudanum is often employed in suicide, and the therapeutical use of opium is liable to cause numerous accidents. Young children—especially the new-born—are peculiarly sensitive to opium, and a single drop of laudanum is sometimes sufficient to cause death. In the adult the fatal dose is about 15 grains (Hoffmann).

The poisoning may be lightning-like when it follows the absorption of huge doses of opium, and the patient becomes comatose from the first. Death supervenes rapidly in a few hours—sometimes in half an hour. Convulsions and delirium are not seen. The pupils are dilated (Tardieu).

As a rule, the course is less rapid, and the patients, who are at first excited, complain of headache and pulsation in the temples. The heart beats violently ; the pulse is rapid. The skin is often covered with patches of erythema and purpura. The tongue and throat are red and dry. Nausea and vomiting appear. The urine is suppressed, and the constipation is absolute. Delirium and restlessness are present, and we notice a symptom which is practically pathognomonic of this disease—contraction of the pupils or absolute myosis. After some hours the restlessness ceases, and gives place to complete depression. The coma lasts for a more or less lengthy period, though it may be interrupted by convulsions, and death speedily takes place. It is announced by dilatation of the pupils and by relaxation of the sphincters.

Chronic poisoning by opium is extremely rare in France and in Europe, but very frequent, on the other hand, in China, Japan, Annam, Tokin, where opium is smoked, and in Asia Minor, Persia, and Turkey, where opium is eaten. The symptoms in this intoxication reveal themselves by organic decay and complete decrepitude.

The treatment in acute poisoning consists in removing the poison from the stomach (emetics, lavage). The patient should be stimulated by coffee, given by the mouth or by the rectum.

Morphine.—Morphinism is seen under the following conditions : An individual who is suffering from an incurable and painful affection gets into the habit of relieving his sufferings with morphia. The means of relief become later a necessity, so that the patient who cannot do without injections of morphia gradually increases the doses, and becomes a morphinomaniac. Some persons seek in morphia oblivion from their troubles and griefs, or, finding the drug to be a mental stimulant, proceed to the abuse of the poison and to morphinism. Many morphinomaniacs are neuropathics, and it is very often because the patient is a neuropathic that he becomes a morphinomaniac. The quantity of morphia taken daily is very variable. It may amount to several grains.

The symptoms of morphinism take a certain time to appear, and it is only after six or eight months that the morphinomaniac shows a peculiar look. The face is pale, covered with early wrinkles, and sometimes of an earthy colour. The pupils are contracted ; the will is enfeebled. Insomnia is the rule. The mouth is dry and the thirst is acute. The appetite may be lost or exaggerated. Digestion is slow, but nausea and vomiting are absent, though pyrosis is sometimes present. Injection of morphia often causes a sensation of epigastric constriction well known to the sufferers. The constipation is obstinate and the belly is distended. Palpitation is frequent. The pulse is irregular and intermittent. The genital faculties are weakened. In women menstruation may be disturbed, and there is a tendency to abortion. The urine sometimes contains sugar or albumin.

The skin is at length covered with indurated nodules, crusts, abscesses, and ulcers—lesions due to the use of dirty syringes and septic solutions.

Psychical and mental troubles are common. Morphinism aggravates injuries and retards recovery. The morphinomaniac may be seized, either during an intercurrent disease or through the poison itself, with delirium tremens and maniacal excitement similar to that seen in alcoholism.

The only **treatment** is to leave off the drug ; but how can this be properly carried out ? The injection of morphia becomes such an imperative need that the patient would rather give up all the world than the drug. A morphinomaniac who is sad, dull, prostrate, and restless, if he have not had his injection of morphia for some time, becomes gay, talkative, and animated as soon as the injection is given. The morphinomaniac craves for the injection, and will give up drink, food, and, in fact, everything else. Whether he be at the theatre or spending an evening with his friends, he always finds means to give himself an injection. For fear of being without morphia, he lays in a sometimes enormous stock, and takes the greatest precautions to keep some of it in his wardrobe, in the drawers of his desk, and in his pockets. He keeps several syringes and spare needles. The morphinomaniac who is under treatment and is prevented from taking his morphia demands the most careful watching, as he always succeeds, by bribes or otherwise, in procuring the drug. He hides it in his bed or in his boots, and when he cannot inject it under the skin he takes it in some other way. I have seen a patient in an attack of maniacal excitement eat morphia, of which he had an enormous stock.

We can understand how difficult treatment must be in persons who would willingly submit to it, but who cannot. The morphia must not be suppressed suddenly, for this course exposes the patient to violent delirium, obstinate diarrhœa, and collapse. For two, three, or six months, if necessary, the dose should be diminished **very gradually** every week.

Cocaine.—Cocaine, even in small doses, may cause death when the patient is not accustomed to the drug. When the doses are progressive, a fatal termination is never seen ; but we find certain troubles, described under the name of " chronic cocainism."

In acute poisoning following injections given to produce analgesia (opening of abscesses, removal of teeth), the patient experiences almost at once very distressing præcordial angina. The heart beats violently ; the pulse becomes small and thready. At the same time nausea and vomiting come on, and the patient, who is pale, anxious, and weak, feels as though his life were slipping from him and death were at hand. Sometimes the muscles of the face and of the neck are affected by convulsions, which in grave cases simulate an attack of epilepsy, and may terminate fatally. In general these troubles do not last long, and recovery is rapid.

The troubles of chronic poisoning are chiefly intellectual, and give rise to *folie cocaïnique*. The delirium is of the hallucinatory type (Saury). The patients think that they have under their skin small bodies, insects, or little animals, which prick them ceaselessly, and which they are always trying to extract. Hallucinations of sight, hearing, smell, and taste are common. Sometimes delirium of persecution is also present. Loss of memory and of will-power is very frequent. Acceleration and irregularity of the pulse, profound sweats, and diarrhœa are also seen. The wasting is rapid and constant. Genital impotency is usual.

Intoxication by morphia may be associated with cocainism, especially in hereditary neuropathics, who become toxicomaniacs.

Subcutaneous injections of ether and infusion of coffee should be given for acute poisoning. The treatment of chronic cocainism demands the gradual suppression of the drug.

VII. POISONING BY TOBACCO.

Tobacco owes its toxicity to an alkaloid, nicotine, and to other dangerous compounds, such as prussic acid and pyridine bases, which are given off in the smoke.

Poisoning by pure nicotine is extremely rare. A few drops suffice to cause sudden death. When death is less sudden, it is preceded by burning in the throat, violent pains in the stomach, diarrhœa, convulsions, and coma. The autopsy reveals no lesions, and chemical analysis alone leads to the discovery of the poison in the organs.

Tobacco may cause acute poisoning. The mixture of tobacco with the food, enemata of tobacco formerly employed in intestinal occlusion, the direct application of tobacco-leaves to the skin for the cure of obstinate ulcers, are causes of intoxication. The toxic dose is uncertain; it appears to be about an ounce. The following symptoms occur : A short time after the absorption of the poison the patient suffers from burning in the throat and œsophagus, the stomach becomes painful, and vomiting, with or without diarrhœa, appears. Vertigo, intense headache, great restlessness, and cold sweats occur. The patients fall into a state of coma, and die from syncope or from asphyxia, after suffering from convulsions.

Chronic poisoning by tobacco is seen in smokers, in those who chew tobacco, and in workmen who manipulate it. Nearly all the systems are affected. Loss of memory, especially for words, tremor, and vertigo are common symptoms. As regards neuralgia, let me mention brachial and scapular neuralgias and cardio-aortic neuralgia (tobacco angina). Hysteria has also been noted (Gilbert). As regards the digestive system let me mention dental caries, stomatitis (smoker's patches), chronic pharyngitis and disturbed digestion, accompanied by acid eructations. Tobacco acts on the nerves of the heart by producing painful palpitation and inter-mittence. Genital troubles are by no means rare in the workpeople employed in tobacco factories (slight or absolute impotence, abortion).

Let me note, lastly, changes in the senses of taste and smell, catarrh of the Eustachian tube, and a form of amblyopia special to smokers (Gale-zowski and Martin).

VIII. CARBONIC OXIDE POISONING.

Carbonic oxide gas is an active poison, which rapidly causes death by its direct action on the blood. It becomes fixed with the hæmoglobin, and drives out the oxygen of the blood, in order to form a more stable com-pound than oxyhæmoglobin. The oxygen, brought to the blood by respiration, cannot act upon the red corpuscles, which become incapable of hæmatosis.

Ætiology.—Poisoning by oxide of carbon is very rarely criminal. It is nearly always the result of suicide or of accident. The charcoal stove (a very frequent means of suicide); the use of fixed stoves, in which the flue of the stove is shut, in order to keep the heat longer; the use of movable stoves, in which the draught is defective, are the commonest causes of this poisoning. Let us also mention the danger of blast furnaces, coke furnaces, plaster and tile furnaces, and foundries, in which the metallic oxides are reduced by charcoal. Carbonic oxide is also formed in explosions due to fire-damp, in conflagrations (as at the Opéra Comique), and in public carriages heated with "briquettes." It enters into the composition of gas, which largely owes its toxicity to this fact.

Symptoms.—During sleep poisoning may take place without causing any symptoms. Coma and death rapidly result.

If the patient is awake, the onset of the poisoning is marked by headache, vertigo, and visceral troubles. The patient suffers from pulsation in the head and temples, and sometimes from vomiting. The limbs become weak and walking is impossible. Dyspnœa appears, and is accompanied by acceleration of the heart and by peripheral cyanosis. Coma comes on in a very short while, and death rapidly ends the scene. It is sometimes pre-ceded by a period of violent convulsions.

Recovery is possible in cases of slight poisoning. It results at the end of a few days, after obstinate headache, which disappears gradually. In severe cases, cerebral softening, dementia (Laborde), and paralysis (Rendu, Brissaud) are often seen. The paralysis may be total, or be limited to one-half of the body (Laroche, Rendu). It is very rarely general, and death is exceptional. The extensor muscles are the most affected. The tendon reflexes are usually exaggerated. Anæsthesia is the rule. Trophic troubles, bedsores (Verneuil), and eruptions of herpes (Leudet, Rendu) may also be seen.

Poisoning by carbonic oxide may be chronic. The chief symptoms consist of anæmia, lassitude, anæsthesia or paralysis, tracheal cough (Lancereaux and Aubert), and glycosuria (Ollivier).

Pathological Anatomy.—The body in carbonic oxide poisoning remains well preserved, putrefaction developing with extreme slowness. On opening the body, the blood is fluid and of a peculiar clear red colour. On section, all the organs show this colouring, which in the lungs may be scarlet. No other lesions are apparent. The reaction of the blood with the spectroscope is characteristic. In the normal condition, when blood is treated by a reducing agent, such as sulphide of ammonia, the two absorption bands of the spectrum unite into a single band, which is the absorption band of reduced hæmoglobin. When the blood contains carbonic oxide, the addition of ammonium sulphide has no action on the two normal absorption bands, and their fusion is never seen.

Treatment.—Pure air, artificial respiration, inhalations of oxygen, and rubbing with stimulants, form the basis of treatment. Transfusion of blood may give good results.

IX. INTOXICATION BY CARBON BISULPHIDE.

Poisoning by carbon bisulphide was first noted in France by Delpech (1856).

Ætiology.—The ingestion of common sulphide of carbon in large doses is exceptional. It is usually the result of accident or of suicide. The pure drug has been used in therapeutics for diseases of the skin (itching, chronic ulcers, and sluggish wounds) and for gastro-intestinal infections (dilatation of the stomach, typhoid fever, and cholera). It has been prescribed in affections of the respiratory tract in the form of vapours and of injections. These methods of treatment are rarely accompanied by serious troubles, because pure sulphide of carbon, free from hydrosulphides and sulphuretted hydrogen, is much less toxic than the commercial product.

The poisoning is nearly always of professional origin, arising from the handling of the tube during its manufacture, and especially in the vulcanization of objects with indiarubber. It is also seen in perfumeries, where the sulphide is used to isolate the essences of flowers; in the factories where camphor and various aromatic products are made; and, lastly, in vine-growing countries, where it is used for the treatment of phylloxera.

The symptoms chiefly appear in neuropathic persons, especially women

(Delpech). The question of age is of no importance. Want, alcoholism, and excesses of all kinds have an undoubted influence.

Symptoms.—The acute accidental intoxication must be distinguished from the chronic professional form.

1. **Acute Intoxication.**—The patient shows muscular relaxation, the face is pale and moist, the lips bluish and covered with froth, the eyelids closed, the pupils dilated and insensitive to light, while the conjunctivæ show no reflex. The breathing is stertorous, and the breath has a characteristic odour (Douglas). As soon as the poison is taken, the sufferer experiences a sharp burning in the mouth, œsophagus, and stomach, with eructations, nausea, and vomiting, fœtid and black diarrhœa. The urine, which is rather scanty, is brownish or sometimes bloody. The pulse is irregular, intermittent, and quick. The respiration is rapid and laboured, and the face is covered with sweat. The nervous phenomena are never absent—headache, tremor, general restlessness, followed by somnolence and tendency to syncope. The liver may be congested and hypertrophied. The general health is profoundly affected.

2. **Chronic Intoxication.**—The symptoms appear suddenly, or after prodromata, such as violent and persistent frontal headache.

Digestive troubles, stomatitis (Rendu), a constant taste of sulphide of carbon in the mouth, a blackish line upon the gums, salivation, nausea, vomiting, and diarrhœa are seen. Persistent cough, attacks of dyspnœa and epistaxis have been noted. The hands which are " soaked " in the sulphide of carbon are swollen, painful, and covered with eczema. The skin of the limbs and of the thorax sometimes shows blackish spots and irregular maculæ, probably produced by an iron pigment (Kiéner and Engel). The urinary system is rarely affected. Such is not the case with the genital functions, which pass through phases of excitation and depression. In women menorrhagia and abortion are frequent.

The nervous system is always affected in chronic poisoning, and three chief varieties of nervous disorder have been described—psychical troubles, symptoms which resemble hysteria, and peripheral neuritis.

Among the psychical troubles I may quote a form of drunkenness in fresh workers, and especially in women. Perversion of character, neurasthenia, dementia (Ball), mania, and lypemania (Bonnet) are seen. These different varieties may be lasting or transitory (Raymond).

The hysteria produced by sulphide of carbon is shown either by hemianæsthesia, anæsthesia of the cornea and pharynx, or by hemiplegia, paraplegia, monoplegia, glosso-labial hemispasm, headache, insomnia, and tremors. These troubles commence suddenly, and are often preceded by an aura, which in man takes the form of troublesome itching in the region of the scrotum.

130—2

TEXT-BOOK OF MEDICINE

The neuritis has not any specific characters (Raymond). The localization of the paralysis to the upper extremities depends upon the contact with the poison. The flexors of the fingers are chiefly affected, and the sensibility is blunted in the zone of the musculo-spiral and median nerves. In the lower limbs the paralysis takes the paraplegic form, but it is limited to the muscles of the feet, and chiefly to the extensors.

The paralysis is flaccid, with reaction of degeneration. The atrophy is slight, and the tendon reflexes are weakened. Walking is still possible. Sensibility is affected. At first the limbs are painful ; later, hypoæsthesia, anæsthesia, or hyperæsthesia is seen. We find in exceptional cases signs of pseudo-tabes (Babès, Stadelmann), with motor inco-ordination, lightning pains, plantar anæsthesia, and abolition of the patellar reflexes. In one case Rendu found contractures of the jaw, the neck, the vertebral column, the legs, and the arms. These contractures were independent of hysteria. The nervous troubles usually recover in this form of poisoning.

The diagnosis of the acute and chronic troubles produced by sulphide of carbon is easy, as the trade of the patient at once attracts attention. The exact distinction from hysterical and toxic manifestations is sometimes more difficult.

Treatment.—The removal of the poison is the essential condition in treatment. Prophylaxis will be assured by thorough ventilation of workshops, hygienic measures, and the mechanical prehension of objects soaked in sulphide of carbon. In chronic poisoning, electricity, tonics, stimulants, and inhalations of oxygen should be employed.

X. PELLAGRA.

Pellagra is a general disease, characterized by cutaneous erythema of the parts which are uncovered, and by nervous and digestive troubles.

Ætiology.—Pellagra exists in an endemic or in a sporadic condition. The endemic condition is met with in different countries : in France, where it is very rare at the present time, after having been fairly common in Les Landes and on the frontier of the Pyrenees ; in Spain, where it is chiefly found in Asturia and Galicia ; in Italy, which furnishes a considerable number of cases in the plains of Lombardy and Venetia. In the sporadic condition pellagra is met with everywhere : in Vienna, Westphalia, and Greece. In France it has been found in Paris, in the districts of the Allier, Sologne, Normandy, the Rhone (Bouchard), and the Marne (Landouzy).

Sex has no predisposing influence, but pellagra is more common in adults and in children than in elderly persons. It is neither contagious nor hereditary (Bouchard). Some authors admit a parasitic origin in pellagra. The pathogenic agent (bacillary schizomycetes) is said to occur on decayed maize, and to have been found in the viscera and in the brain substance of patients (Majocchi); but "this opinion must be confirmed by further researches" (Gaucher and Barbe).

Pellagra is probably caused by defective nourishment. Writers have assigned a very great part to the employment of damaged maize (Balardini, Roussel). A fungus is said to develop in the interior of the grain, and to cause a disease in maize known as *le verdet*, and the granules of this affection are said to produce profound cachexia in animals (Balardini, Lombroso). Pellagra, however, may be met with in persons who do not use maize (Hameau, Bouchard, Gintrac). It develops, on the other hand, in those who are poor and live upon inferior food. Accordingly, want, insufficient nourishment, digestive troubles among lunatics and alcoholics, are most often the cause of pellagra (Hardy, Gaucher). The cutaneous erythema in a patient with pellagra is in part produced by the sun's rays, and especially by the chemical or violet rays (Bouchard).

Symptoms.—The disease commences with lassitude and prostration, accompanied by headache, diarrhœa, and sometimes by nausea and vomiting; then, towards the month of March following, the dorsal surface of the hands becomes of a bluish-red tint, which is more or less dark, and accompanied by violent itching. The dorsal surface of the two last phalanges is almost always spared (Raymond). The redness usually stops on the dorsal surface of the wrist, though it sometimes invades the forearm as far as the elbow. The erythema may be also situated on the dorsal surface of the feet, on the neck, on the upper part of the chest, and in women and children on the face. After from ten to twenty days, desquamation, which takes place in greyish layers, and more rarely in furfuraceous scales, supervenes. At the same time the erythema fades, the skin becomes brown and pigmented with small patches, which grow larger as the result of fresh attacks of erythema, so that the seats of election of the eruption finally assume a dark brown tint (Brocq). After some time the skin atrophies, and resembles closely the dry, wrinkled skin of certain elderly and cachectic persons.

In addition to the cachectic lesions very marked digestive troubles are found; the lips and the mucous membrane of the mouth are red, inflamed, and swollen. The gums are sometimes fungous and bleeding. The tongue is red, smooth, and sometimes covered by aphthous ulcerations. Gastralgia, nausea, and pyrosis are present, and may be accompanied by loss of appetite, or more usually by boulimia. Diarrhœa is practically constant, with or without intestinal hæmorrhages.

The nervous troubles consist in frontal headache, neuralgia, rachialgia, formication, buzzing in the ears, and gradual weakness of hearing and of sight. The lower limbs are often paretic (Hameau). The paralysis becomes marked and reaches the upper limbs. Cramps, tetaniform contractures, and epileptiform convulsions are present in some cases. The mental troubles may simulate those of general paralysis (Baillarger), and we often find lypemania, which sometimes leads to suicide, especially by drowning (Strambio).

The duration of pellagra varies from some months up to twenty years. Recovery is possible when the disease develops in young persons, and when it is treated in time. A fatal ending is very common, and is due to suicide, pulmonary complications (hypostatic pneumonia, tuberculosis), or to cachexia. The prognosis of pellagra is, therefore, very grave.

Diagnosis.—The erythema of pellagra is distinguished from other pellagroid erythemata by the fact that intestinal troubles and mental changes are absent in the latter. Pellagroid erythema is a benign affection, which often improves, while pellagra is subject to periodical recrudescences at different seasons (Janselme). Nevertheless, certain pellagroid erythemata may be only one of the forms of pellagra (Gaucher). Pellagrous erythema is readily distinguished from eczema on the back of the hands, which is more general and moist, and it will not be confounded with the solar erythema, which is not accompanied by general troubles.

Pathological Anatomy.—The lesions are excessively varied and but little characteristic. We find general atrophy of all the viscera, especially appreciable in the spleen; steatosis of the liver; brownish pigmentation of the pancreas and of the kidneys; frequent general hyperæmia of the mucosa of the digestive tube; interstitial gastritis; and ulcerative enteritis. The spinal cord is often affected (Bouchard), and the posterior columns of Goll show slight sclerosis. Degeneration and atrophy of the posterior group of the cells in Clarke's column have been found (Tuczek, Marie). The meninges are sometimes slightly injected and adherent. Let me quote diminution in thickness of the epidermis and disappearance of the papillæ as the chief lesions of the skin (Raymond).

Treatment.—Abundant nourishment, tonics, protection of uncovered parts from the rays of the sun, and the exhibition of arsenic (Lombroso), are the means usually employed in pellagra.

APPENDIX ON THERAPEUTICS

I. MERCURIAL TREATMENT—TREATMENT OF SYPHILIS.

EXPERIENCE has taught us that syphilis plays a considerable part in pathology. Fournier can claim a large share of this idea. The more we study syphilis, the more often do we find it—either apparent or hidden, acquired or hereditary. We must therefore be able to recognize it.

While in many morbid conditions we are in doubt when it is a question of determining the cause of the pathogenesis of the affection, with syphilis, on the other hand, even in doubtful cases, it is possible for us to find the true cause, thanks to the efficacy of treatment, and, indeed, this treatment is often a true therapeutic triumph.

A patient is suffering from severe headache, with symptoms of meningitis, from epileptiform convulsions, from Jacksonian epilepsy, or from stertor and coma. It is evident that the motor convolutions are affected, and the situation is serious. A correct pathogenic diagnosis, however, allows us to affirm or to suspect the syphilitic nature of the lesion, and we at once institute specific treatment. In a few days the symptoms improve, and in a few weeks the patient is cured.

A patient has been suffering for some months from symptoms of pulmonary phthisis : fever, night-sweats, hæmoptysis, wasting, and cavities in the lung. The situation is very grave, and the prognosis is bad. In this case, however, a correct diagnosis proves or causes suspicion that the lesion of the lung is syphilitic. Specific treatment is prescribed. In a few weeks the symptoms improve, and in a few months the patient is well.

A patient has suffered for a year or for eighteen months from Cruveilhier's **ulcus simplex** : acute pain at the xiphoid and spinal points, gastric intolerance, vomiting of food, hæmatemesis, wasting, and cachexia. The customary remedies have been employed without success, and we fear perforation of the stomach, or other complications. As a last resort we think of surgical intervention. A correct diagnosis, however, leads us to hope that the condition is due to syphilitic ulceration of the stomach. We employ specific treatment. In a fortnight the symptoms improve, and in a few weeks the patient recovers.

A patient has been suffering for fourteen years from severe trigeminal neuralgia. Treatment has failed ; large doses of morphia merely lessen the pain for a time ; the situation becomes intolerable, and beginning at the end of our resources, we discuss the question of surgical intervention. Accurate diagnosis of the pathogenesis, however again leads us to think that the neuralgia is possibly syphilitic. We employ specific treatment. In three weeks the pains improve, and in two months the patient is cured.

In the treatment of syphilis mercury and iodide of potassium are the two specific drugs. Speaking generally, it is customary to employ mercury in the early stages of the disease, and to give the preference to iodide for the tertiary troubles. I consider that iodide is often useless, and the chief point in the treatment of syphilis (secondary and tertiary troubles) is to employ mercury. It is with mercury alone that I have obtained a cure in grave, inveterate tertiary syphilis.

In what form and in what doses must we administer mercury ? As a matter of fact, we have only to take our choice from amongst the many preparations—such as pills of protoiodide of mercury, mercurial pills, Van Swieten's solution, mercurial inunctions, or injections of mercury.

The pills of protoiodide are given by Fournier at the onset of syphilis, in doses of one or two pills daily. Each pill contains a grain of the protoiodide, and $\frac{1}{6}$ grain of opium. This medicine sometimes gives rise to colic or to diarrhœa, but it is none the less an excellent remedy.

I prefer to use injections of biniodide of mercury. Like many other methods used in therapeutics, the hypodermic method of treating syphilis at first found partisans and opponents. The latter are becoming less numerous. Physicians at first proposed either solutions of bichloride of mercury, with the addition of sodium chloride, or of ammonium chloride, or combinations of the sublimate, with peptones. As the first attempts were not satisfactory, because the injections were very painful, and because peptonate of mercury did not keep, the cyanide and the sozoiodolate of mercury were employed. Attention was then turned to special preparations, such as grey oil and suspension of calomel in vaselin. These drugs have advantages and disadvantages which need mention.

The grey oil, for which several formulæ have been proposed, like the suspension of calomel in vaselin, requires a somewhat delicate manipulation. In fact, with these preparations we do not know the exact quantity of the active substance injected under the skin, and even while admitting that the mixture is as homogeneous as possible (this is always a difficult matter to obtain), the dose must be changed, for the weight of the drops is equally variable. Further, this method is not free from the following complications : Intense pain ; redness and induration around the seat of the injection ; nodes which remain so painful for a long time that absolute rest is necessary ; abscesses which supervene in spite of every antiseptic precaution ; fever, malaise, lassitude, and gastric disturbances ; stomatitis and slight salivation for the first two or three days after the injection.

For the pain, which is almost constant after the injection of grey oil, injections of cocaine have been advised ; but the improvement produced does not last—the patients soon complain, and some refuse a fresh injection.

Although the grey oil and the suspension of calomel in vaselin have drawbacks, they are none the less endowed with great activity, two or three small injections being sufficient to make up a complete treatment. The benefits of this method are no longer recognized. Writers on syphilis have extolled the effects of this method in very severe cases where other methods of administering mercury have failed. They are useful when patients cannot take pills, and they may replace with advantage the inunction of mercury, but they are by no means free from inconvenience.

Accordingly, physicians have tried to perfect this mode of treatment by using a preparation constant in its effects and free from the foregoing accidents. With this end in view, Panas has employed a solution of biniodide of mercury in sterilized olive oil. In my opinion the aqueous solution is preferable.

Aqueous Solution of Biniodide of Mercury.—The injection of oil is not always well borne locally. It is sometimes very painful, and some patients refuse to submit to it. It also has the inconvenience of leaving painful nodules. Lastly, if we desire to inject a large dose of the biniodide of mercury ($\frac{1}{2}$ grain), the oily solution is unsuitable, since it only contains $\frac{1}{2}$ grain in 110 minims. For these reasons I employ the aqueous solution, which is much less painful, leaves practically no nodules, and permits the injection of large doses of the active substance.

The watery solution of biniodide of mercury contains distilled water, the mercurial salt, and a small quantity of dried iodide of sodium. In order to prepare the solution, the two salts should be put in a small quantity of water, so that the biniodide is added to a concentrated alkaline solution of the iodide. The percentage of the solution is arbitrary. We may take it up to ½ centigramme per cubic centimetre, which is the minimum, and we may employ solutions of 1, 2, 3, or 4 centigrammes of biniodide of mercury per cubic centimetre of water. It is evident that the solutions are the more painful the more concentrated they are. With ½ centigramme per cubic centimetre pain is absent, and with 1 centigramme per cubic centimetre it is trifling.

In giving an injection, every aseptic precaution must be taken. The syringe is boiled, and the skin is cleansed with alcohol or with ether, followed by perchloride of mercury. The injection should always be given by pushing the needle deeply into the cellular tissue of the loins or of the buttocks. The liquid is slowly injected. The needle is withdrawn, and a small dressing of sterilized wool is placed over the puncture. After each injection the syringe should be cleaned with ether and alcohol, and placed in cold water, which is brought to the boil.

When the symptoms are moderate, it suffices to inject daily from 4 milligrammes to 1 centigramme of the biniodide. Twelve to fifteen consecutive injections are given, and, as a rule, improvement takes place after six or seven injections. The injections are then stopped for about from twelve to fifteen days. Several successive series may be given, if it be deemed necessary.

In severe cases, where the treatment must be thorough and quick, the dose of biniodide is increased. This can be easily accomplished with a watery solution. A solution containing 2 or 3 centigrammes of biniodide per cubic centimetre is prepared, and 3 or 4 centigrammes are injected, either in a single dose or in two doses.

This intensive treatment should be employed in cerebral syphilis, as action is necessary before the lesions become irremediable. I have also had occasion to prescribe it in rebellious cases of ulcerative syphilis of the throat, in syphilis of the aorta, etc. Consecutive series of ten injections are employed, and we must not be discouraged if we have to continue the series for several months. Tabes and general paralysis demand intensive treatment.

I have given more than 15,000 injections of biniodide of mercury, but I have never seen the least trouble; in my opinion, no preparation of mercury can be compared with it. The administration is doubtless more complicated than that of other mercurial preparations; it is more simple for the patient to take pills or Gibert's syrup than to give mercurial injections, but we are recompensed by the results obtained. In the first place, we know exactly what dose is absorbed, which we never do with inunction of mercury; in the second place, this preparation is rarely ineffectual. I may say that in most cases injections of mercury are sufficient, without the addition of iodide of potassium.

I was formerly in the habit of giving the iodide, even in very large doses, thinking that it was superior to mercury in tertiary syphilis. With further experience, I have given up this opinion. The longer I live, the less do I prescribe iodide of potash. The remarkable recoveries from tertiary syphilis reported in my clinical lectures at the Hôtel-Dieu and in the present work have been obtained in most cases by mercury alone.

The treatment of syphilis is therefore simplified in the great majority of cases; instead of prescribing iodide of potassium, which is liable to produce iodism; instead of prescribing Gibert's syrup, Van Swieten's solution, or mercury in pills, which may upset the digestive organs; instead of ordering mercurial inunctions, in which the dose is difficult to regulate, I am content to give injections of biniodide of mercury, which, with proper precautions, do not cause local troubles or symptoms of poisoning, and which give excellent results.

Nevertheless, I do not say that iodide of potassium should never be used in the treatment of syphilis. It may be useful in some cases. In syphilitic lesions of the aorta, in syphilitic arteritis of the brain and of the limbs, iodide of potassium may be of service. In such a case mercury and potassium iodide should be given alternately; twelve to fifteen injections of the biniodide are given, and iodide of potassium is then taken for a fortnight.

Let me add a few words as to possible mishaps. In some cases we think that the disease is conquered, the symptoms having disappeared, and yet they return. We must never forget that syphilis is naturally obstinate, and does not always yield easily. Let us not mistake for a definite cure what is only a transient improvement. In this case the treatment must be recommenced.

II. ARSENICAL TREATMENT—CACODYLATE OF SODA.

Three preparations of arsenic have been chiefly in vogue : Fowler's solution, pills of arsenious acid, and solution of arseniate of soda.

Fowler's solution is composed of arsenious acid, carbonate of potash, and distilled water. The dose for an adult is from 2 to 8 drops daily. We may commence with 2 drops in a little water after breakfast and after dinner, carefully increasing the dose by 1 drop daily, until the maximum is reached, when we go back again gradually to the initial dose. Fowler's solution has the drawback that it is not always well borne, and often provokes cramps in the stomach.

The pills or granules of arsenious acid are composed as follows (Trousseau) :

Arsenious acid	25 centigrammes.
Starch	5 grammes.
Syrup	q.s.

These ingredients are carefully mixed into a pill mass, which is divided into 100 pills, so that each pill contains $2\frac{1}{2}$ milligrammes of arsenious acid. Trousseau gave to this preparation the name of " pilules de Dioscorides." One pill is given to an adult before the two chief meals. Their exhibition is continued for a fortnight, and then suspended for a week, this order being maintained as long as their use is considered necessary, and according to the tolerance of the digestive organs.

An excellent preparation is the solution of arseniate of soda. The following is Trousseau's formula :

Distilled water	100 grammes.
Arseniate of soda	5 centigrammes.
Tincture of cochineal	q.s. to colour the solution.

We prescribe daily at the commencement of the two chief meals a teaspoonful of this solution, which represents $2\frac{1}{2}$ milligrammes of arseniate of soda. This preparation is excellent. I have often noticed that arseniate of soda is better tolerated than arsenious acid.

A fresh preparation—namely, cacodylate of soda—has recently been introduced.

The name **cacodyl** (κακός, bad) is given to an " organic mineral compound, in which arsenic enters into molecular combination with an organic radical." The intervention of Gautier in his communications to the Académie de Médecine has caused the speedy inclusion of cacodylate of soda among our therapeutic measures. Its good effects have been witnessed on all sides, and the frequent use which I have made of it permits me to give my personal opinion upon this subject.

Cacodylate of soda may be given in three ways : in a mixture, in enemata, and in subcutaneous injections.

Cacodylate of soda may be given in a mixture in daily doses of 5 centigrammes, but the administration of cacodylate of soda by the mouth is not free from inconveniences. In the digestive canal, says Gautier, the cacodylate of soda may be converted into oxide of cacodyl, which gives off a characteristic alliaceous odour. It may cause epigastric pain and renal congestion, with albuminuria. " On the other hand," says Gautier, " when the drug is given hypodermically, I have not noticed albuminuria, alliaceous odour of the breath, or intestinal troubles."

For my part, when I wish to give a preparation of arsenic by the mouth, I prescribe the solution of arseniate of soda, according to the formula already given. I reserve the cacodylate for injections.

Manufacturers now make sterilized glass capsules, each containing 5 centigrammes of cacodylate of soda, dissolved in 1 c.c. of water. We can keep capsules indefinitely, without any change in the solution. When we desire to use the drug, the point of the capsule is broken, and the fluid is drawn into the syringe, which has been previously sterilized.

A daily injection of from 3 to 5 centigrammes of cacodylate is given for eight, ten, or twelve days in succession. The treatment is stopped for a week, and it is then repeated as before for as long as may be necessary.

It is certain that this tonic method of treatment is to be preferred. It is applicable to all patients who, for various causes, are suffering from anæmia, neurasthenia, weakness, or wasting. Persons suffering from tuberculosis, diabetes, or cachexia derive benefit. Sometimes the result is surprising. After from twelve to fifteen injections the patient becomes fat, and his strength and colour return. Arrhenal has been extolled by Gautier in malaria.

III. INJECTIONS OF ARTIFICIAL SERUM.

In the first place, what is meant by artificial serum ? Artificial sera are saline solutions, which contain one or more of the normal salts of the blood in various proportions. Some sera are concentrated, and others are weak. Among the former we may quote that of Chéron, which has the following composition :

Crystalline carbolic acid	1 gramme.
Chloride of sodium	2 grammes.
Sulphate of soda	8 „
Phosphate of soda	4 „
Distilled water	100 „

It is injected hypodermically in small quantities of from 5 to 10 grammes. At the present day we employ dilute sera. Hayem's serum has the following composition :

Chloride of sodium	5 grammes.
Sulphate of soda	10 „
Sterilized water	1 litre.

The addition of sulphate of soda is now considered superfluous, and solutions of chloride of sodium are alone employed. The percentage composition of these solutions is of much importance. Physicians have for a long time employed a solution of 7·5 parts per 1,000, which was the " indifferent " or " physiological " solution of histologists. Malassez has shown that this solution causes marked changes in the red corpuscles, and has proposed a solution of 10 parts per 1,000. This conclusion has been confirmed by researches upon human blood-serum, and authorities are agreed in considering that the serum of human blood corresponds, from the point of view of its " molecular concentration," to a solution of chloride of sodium, with a percentage of 9 to 10 parts per 1,000.

This artificial serum is prepared as follows : 9½ grammes of pure salt are dissolved in 1 litre of distilled water. This solution is filtered through wool into a flat-bottomed flask. The neck of the flask is plugged with a tampon of cotton-wool. The flask is then placed in the autoclave at a temperature of 115° C. for ten minutes. The slight concentration caused by sterilization reduces the percentage of the solution to 9·5 per 1,000. Flasks thus prepared are easily kept. It is necessary to cover the neck with a cap of indiarubber, in order to avoid the concentration which would take place in time.

An injection may be given with various apparatus. One apparatus consists of a two-way flask, into which the serum is introduced. One of these two glass tubes is connected with an indiarubber tube, armed with a needle, which is introduced into the tissues, while the other glass tube is connected with a pump. This apparatus has several drawbacks. In the first place, it is difficult to graduate the force of the injection; in the second place, it may happen that, for want of attention, the air, instead of fluid, is injected into the tissues. Extensive emphysema may thus arise. I have twice witnessed this accident.

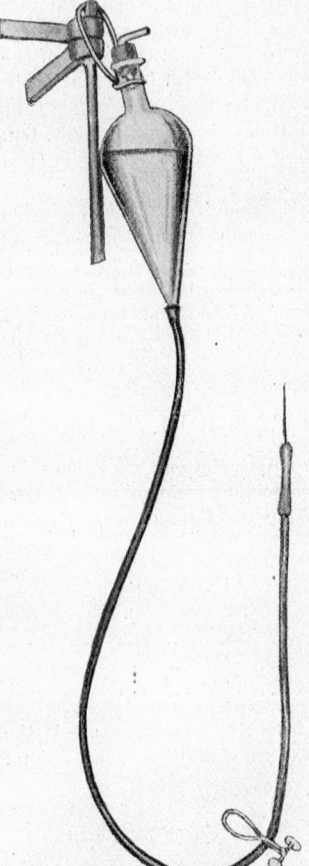

Carrion-Haillon's apparatus appears to me to fulfil the principal indications. Its management is simple. With this apparatus the injection of serum takes place, so to say, automatically and slowly, under conditions of rigorous asepsis.

This apparatus is composed of a large receiver, which will hold from 250 to 500 grammes of serum. This receiver is closed up by a stopper, and is connected to an indiarubber tube, furnished with a needle.

The injection of serum is given as follows : Before introducing the needle into the chosen region (cellular tissue of the abdomen or of the buttocks), we exhaust the air contained in the tube and in the needle. For this purpose we turn the glass tube, which is passed through the stopper, so that the position F is changed to the position O. These two letters, which are engraved upon the stopper, indicate that the tap is closed at F and open at O. The open tap allows the air, which is purified by a plug of wool, to exercise pressure on the fluid. The clip which closes the indiarubber tube is then removed, and the liquid flows out from the needle. The flow is stopped by means of the clip, and the apparatus is suspended either from the wall or from the head of the bed. The atmospheric pressure on the serum depends upon the height at which the apparatus is suspended. The needle is introduced into the cellular tissue of the region which has previously been rendered aseptic, the clip is let go, and the injection of serum takes place very slowly. An injection of 250 grammes takes about twenty minutes. We may thus give further injections in the same day, either by using a series of receivers or by recharging the same receiver with serum kept in a sterilized flask.

FIG. 105.—APPARATUS FOR INJECTION OF SERUM.

The enormous pad of œdema produced by the injection of the serum into the cellular tissue is fairly rapidly absorbed.

The injection of serum is given in the above manner. If, however, the serum is not at hand, as may happen to physicians in the country and in small towns, it is easy to make an injection on the spot, in the following manner : 9½ grammes of pure salt are put into 1 litre of water—filtered, if possible. The solution is boiled for half an hour, and the loss of fluid due to evaporation is made up by the addition of boiled water. In this way we obtain an aseptic solution, which contains 9·5 grammes of salt per 1,000.

The therapeutic indications for large injections of serum are very numerous, and are repeatedly mentioned throughout the pages of this work.

Profuse hæmorrhages (epistaxis, metrorrhagia, hæmatemeses of exulceratio simplex and of ulcus simplex, etc.) may be effectively treated by large injections of serum. Surgeons also give prophylactic injections before operating upon anæmic or debilitated persons.

At first sight large injections of serum do not appear to be logical in cases of hæmorrhage. Thus, in a patient suffering from severe hæmatemesis due to exulceratio simplex we might, a priori, fear that the rise of blood-pressure due to the injection of serum would interefere with the formation of the clot. Such is not the case. This question has been discussed under Exulceratio Simplex.

Large injections of serum may be beneficial in toxic and infectious diseases (typhoid fever, adynamic pneumonia, poisoning, etc.), since they favour diuresis and elimination of toxines. They have given good results in malignant jaundice. On account of the chloride of soda which they contain, injections of serum should be prohibited in Bright's disease, and in all diseases accompanied by œdema.

We see, therefore, from this rapid survey the importance of injections of serum, and the many indications for their use. The quantity of serum injected varies in different cases. Injections of 100, 200, 300, 400, or 500 grammes may be given. In fact, cases occur in which 2 litres may be injected, divided into four or five injections, in the twenty-four hours.

For a long while I have been accustomed to add a little benzoate of caffein to the injection of artificial serum—5 to 10 centigrammes per litre of serum. Although this dose of caffein is very small, it has a beneficial effect upon the heart and the kidneys. The mixture is readily made at the time of the injection by pouring a few drops of a solution of benzoate of caffein of known strength into the receiver.

INDEX

A.

ABASIA, 1474

Abdominal typhus, 1619

Abortion in relapsing fever, 1687 ; in small-pox, 1567

Abscess : from angiocholitis, 998 ; appendicular, 958 ; of brain, 1338 ; of cerebellum, 1301; of fixation, 139 ; in glanders, 1791 ; of liver, 951 ; of lung, 122 ; of pancreas, 1031 ; in paracholecystitis, 999 ; of parotid, 1653 ; perigastric, 757 ; perinephritic, 1180; peritoneal, 842 ; retropharyngeal, 566 ; subphrenic, 686 ; in typhoid fever, 1643

Acephalocystic cyst, 936

Acetonæmia, 1912

Acetone, 1912

Acholia, 891

Achondroplasia, 1554

Acromegaly, 1966

Actinomycosis, 1792 ; of appendix, 803

Acute bulb paralysis, 1291 ; yellow atrophy, 1012

Addison's disease, 1199

Adenia (Trousseau's), 1828

Adenitis, in scarlet fever, 1581 ; tubercular, 1955

Adenoid growths, 568

Adenoma of kidney, 1071 ; of liver, 879, 924 ; of stomach, 648, 705

Adenopathy : mediastinal, 378 ; of right iliac fossa, 241 ; scrofulous, 1954 ; supra-clavicular, 712 ; in tracheo-laryngeal syphilis, 35

Adenophlegmon of neck, 1592

Adherent pericardium, 391

Adiposis dolorosa, 1947

Adrenalin in epistaxis, 21 ; in purpura, 1854

Adrenals in Addison's disease, 1204

Adynamic typhoid fever, 1624

Ægophony, 251

Æstivo-autumnal fever, 1759

Agglutination of Eberth's bacillus, 1662 ; of Koch's bacillus, 274 ; of the pneumococcus, 124

Agoraphobia, 1472

Agraphia, 1332

Albuminous expectoration in pleurisy, 265

Albuminuria : of adolescence, 1119 ; in appendicitis, 752 ; in Bright's disease, 1085 ; not due to Bright's disease, 1118 ; in

acute Bright's disease, 1056 ; in chronic Bright's disease, 1069, 1085 ; cyclical, 1119 ; in diabetes, 1913 ; in diphtheria, 580 ; in erysipelas, 1698 ; in gout, 1885 ; in influenza, 1722 ; in malaria, 1763 ; orthostatic, 1119 ; in scarlet fever, 1587 ; in typhoid fever, 1650

Albuminuric retinitis, 2034

Alcoholic neuritis, 1431

Alcoholism, acute, 2025 ; chronic, 2026

Algid stage in cholera, 1718 ; in malaria, 1760

Alienation, mental, in epilepsy, 1437

Alopecia in typhoid, 1623

Amaurosis, hysterical, 1461 ; toxic, in lead-poisoning, 2034 ; uræmic, 1095

Amblyopia, alcoholic, 2027 ; hysterical, 1461 ; tobacco, 2049

Ambulatory typhoid, 1624

Ammoniæmia, 1092

Amnesia in general paralysis, 1368

Amœba in dysentery, 821

Amphoric breathing, 182, 375

Ampulla, cancer of Vater's, 819

Amyloid disease, of kidney, 1120 ; of liver, 949

Amyotrophic lateral sclerosis, 1251

Anæmia, 1824 ; in ankylostomiasis, 1828 ; bothriocephalic, 829 ; cerebral, 1311 ; in chlorosis, 1840 ; from hæmorrhage, 1824 ; infantile pseudo-leukæmic, 1833 ; in lead-poisoning, 2033 ; in malaria, 1762 ; pernicious, 1825 ; primary or essential, 1825 ; in rheumatism, 1867 ; secondary, 1825

Anæmic murmurs, 1839

Anæsthesia in hæmatomyelia, 1281 ; in hemiplegia, 1319 ; in hysteria, 1454 ; in in leprosy, 1775 ; locomotor, 1227 ; in Morvan's disease, 1241 ; in syringo-my-elia, 1239

Anarthria, 1337

Anasarca in cardiac disease, 413 ; in acute nephritis, 1056 ; in scarlatina, 1591

Aneurysm of abdominal aorta, 518 ; of thoracic aorta, 491 ; of aorta due to syphilis, 508 ; arterio-venous, 493 ; of brain, 1316 ; syphilitic brain, 1352 ; of heart, 438 ; of limbs, 486 ; of Rasmussen, 185

Angina : acute catarrhal, 559 ; chronic, 567 ; diphtheritic, 574 ; normal, 575 ; toxic, 578 ; symptoms, 578 ; varieties, 583 ; clinical diagnosis, 588 ; bacteriological diagnosis, 592 ; prognosis, 594 ; treatment, 597

Hypo-azoturia, orthostatic, 1119
Hypophysis, enlargement of, 1969
Hypostatic congestion of lungs in typhoid fever, 1621
Hypotension, 532
Hypothermia in typhoid fever, 1630
Hypotonia, 1219
Hysteria, 1400 ; ætiology, 1466 ; blindness, 1462 ; clavus hystericus, 1455 ; convulsive form, 1450 ; non-convulsive form, 1452 ; diagnosis, 1465 ; hemiplegia, 1453 ; organs of the senses, 1460 ; tremors, 1454
Hysterical angina pectoris, 529 ; chorea, 1484
Hystero-epilepsy, 1451
Hysterogenic zones, 1455

I

Ichthyosis, 1218
Icterus, 1004 ; benign, simple infectious, 1021 ; catarrhal, 1021 ; prolonged catarrhal, 1024 ; cholæmia, 1010 ; chronic, 820, 897, 1026 ; description, 1004 ; diagnosis, 1025 ; effects, 1005 ; gastro-intestinal troubles, 1005 ; Gmelin's reaction, 1005 ; pathogenesis, 1007, 1021 ; symptoms, 1023 ; treatment, 1027
    gravis, 1011 ; ætiology, 1018 ; course, 1017 ; diagnosis, 1018 ; pathogenesis, 1011 ; pathological anatomy, 1014 ; puerperal state, 1019 ; symptoms, 1015
Idiocy, 1344 ; myxœdematous, 1950
Idiopathic anæmia, 1825
Ileo-cæcal region : in appendicitis, 745 ; in typhoid fever, 1621
Ileus, 814
Immunization, 1703
Impotence, in diabetes, 1899 ; in locomotor ataxy, 1213
Impulses in epilepsy, 1438
Index colour, 1820
Indigestion, 761
Indol reaction, 1712
Inequality of the pupils : in aneurysm, 495 ; in general paralysis, 1369
Infantile paralysis, 1260 ; scurvy, 1857
Infarcts : of brain, 1327 ; hæmoptoic, 145, 156 ; hæmorrhagic, 412 ; of kidney, 1159 ; of myocardium, 439 ; of placenta, 1847
Infiltration, tubercular, of larynx, 37 ; of lung, 177
Inflammation of the chest, 119
Influenza, 1720 ; bacteriology, 1725 ; cerebral, 1722 ; complications, 1723 ; gastrointestinal, 1723 ; thoracic, 1722
Injections of mercury, 2056 ; of tetanus antitoxine, 1744
Inoculation preventive, against smallpox, 1571 ; in hydrophobia, 1781 ; in plague, 1736 ; in typhoid fever, 1679
Insane, general paralysis of, 1366
Insomnia in typhoid fever, 1620

Insufficiency, aortic, 425 ; mitral, 410 ; renal, 1101 ; suprarenal, 1207 ; tricuspid, 427
Insular sclerosis, 1253
Intention tremor, 1255
Intercostal neuralgia, 1505
Intermittent fever, 1751
Internal capsule, 1312
Intestinal coils, tumour formed by, 817 ; occlusion, 814 ; sand, 777 ; worms, 828
Intestines :
    diseases of, 726 ; occlusion, 814 ; strangulation, 815 ; tuberculosis of, 788
    hæmorrhage from, in dysentery, 825 ; in invagination, 817 ; in tuberculosis, 791 ; in typhoid fever, 1626
Intoxications, 2025
Intubation of larynx, 55
Intussusception, 815
Invagination of the gut, 815
Ipecacuanha : in exophthalmic goitre, 465 ; in hæmoptysis, 158
Irido-choroiditis in relapsing fever, 1687
Iritis, rheumatic, 1875
Ischæmia, 526
Ischuria, paradoxical, 1278
Island of Reil, 1312
Itching in Bright's disease, 1081 ; in diabetes, 1899 ; in jaundice, 1006 ; in uræmia, 1081

J

Jacksonian epilepsy, 1441
Jaundice, 987, 1004, 1011
Joints in locomotor ataxy, 1218 ; in syringomyelia, 1240

K

Kerato-conjunctivitis in measles, 1606
Kernig's sign, 1415
Kidney : acute nephritis, 1050 ; amyloid, 1120 ; anatomy, 1046 ; appendicular, 1058 ; in Bright's disease, 1066 ; cancer, 1154 ; cardiac, 1049 ; in diabetes, 1913 ; gouty, 1885 ; hydatid cyst of, 1152 ; large white, 1068 ; movable, 1194 ; pneumonic, 129 ; polycystic, 1148 ; small red, 1070 ; syphilis, 1133 ; tuberculosis, 1121
Klebs-Löffler bacillus, 570
Knee-jerks, loss of, in ataxia, 1210 ; in diphtheritic paralysis, 608
Koch's bacillus, 170 ; tuberculin, 193
Koplik's sign, 1608
Korsakoff's syndrome, 1433
Krishaber's disease, 1476

L

Labyrinthine syndrome, 1307
Laced liver, 930
Lacunæ of brain, 1331
Laryngeal crises, 1213
Laryngitis : acute catarrhal, 27 ; chronic catarrhal, 29 ; erysipelatous, 1698 ; glandu-

Neuralgia: of the trifacial nerve, 1496; ætiology, 1499; tic douloureux, 1498; treatment, 1500; syphilitic, 1501
Neurasthenia, 1471; diagnosis, 1473; symptoms, 1472; treatment, 1473; varieties,
1473
Neuritis: in cerebral tumours, 1348; in
diphtheria, 611; of the femoro-cutaneous
nerve, 1516; infective, 1430; œdematous
in tubercular meningitis, 1402; optic in
tabes, 1212; peripheral, 1429; toxic, 1430;
in tuberculosis, 186
Neuro-fibromatosis, 1554
Neuropathy, cerebro-cardiac, 1476
Neuroses: of the heart,. 447; occupation,
1493
Neutrophiles, 1822
Nicotine, 2048
Night-blindness, 2027
Ninth nerve paralysis, of, 1520
Nodes: Bouchard's, 721; Heberden's, 1873
Nodules in leprosy, 1774
Noma, 544
Normoblasts, 830
Nose, bleeding from, 18
Nuclei of the cranial nerves, 1288
Nucleus: caudate, 1312; Deiters', 1299;
lenticular, 1312
Nutmeg liver, 877
Nyctolopia, 2027
Nystagmus in Friedreich's disease, 1233; in
insular sclerosis, 1255; in syringomyelia,
1240

O

Obesity, 1939
Obliteration of common bile duct, 987;
diagnosis, 995; symptoms, 994; treatment, 996
Obstruction by gall-stones: of the intestine,
975; of the pylorus, 976
Occlusion: intestinal, 814; ætiology, 815;
diagnosis, 817; prognosis, 817; symptoms,
816; treatment, 819
Oculomotor nerve, paralysis of, 1532
Œdema: in Bright's disease, 1083; in cardiac
disease, 413; of the larynx, 60; of the
lung, 161; of the lung after thoracentesis,
265; malignant, 1786; in acute nephritis,
1056
Œsophageal varices, 889
Œsophagism, 637
Œsophagitis, 636
Œsophagus: cancer, 638; spasm, 637;
stenosis, 637; syphilis, 636; ulcer, 641
Oidium albicans, 539
Oliguria, orthostatic, 1119
Omentum, cysts of, in cancer of peritoneum,
860; fixation of, in cirrhosis, 896; tumour
of, in tubercular peritonitis, 840
Ophthalmia, gonorrhœal, 2001
Ophthalmoplegia, external, 1540; internal,
1540; progressive nuclear, 1293
Opium poisoning, 2045
Opotherapy: in diabetes, 1925; suprarenal,
1206; thyroid, 1952

Optic nerve, atrophy of, primary, 1349;
secondary, 1349; in tabes, 1212
neuritis: in brain tumour, 1349; in
tubercular meningitis, 1402
Orchitis: gonorrhœal, 1993; in mumps,
1706; scrofulous, 1955; in tonsillitis, 563;
in typhoid fever, 1650
Osteitis deformans, 1971
Osteo-arthropathy, hypertrophic pulmonary,
1970
Osteomalacia, 1965
Osteomyelitis, 1655
Osteophytes, 1872
Osteoporosis in tabes, 1218
Otitis:
complications: abscess of cerebellum,
1305; and of cerebrum, 1339
influenzal, 1724; in measles, 1606; in
meningitis, 1404, 1410; pneumococcal,
130; scarlatinal, 1593; tubercular,
187
Oxalate calculi, 1161
Oxide of carbon, poisoning by, 2049
Oxyuris vermicularis, 828
Oysters and typhoid fever, 1667
Ozæna: in chronic coryza, 3; in syphilitic
rhinitis, 11; tracheal, 18; true, 17

P

Pachymeningitis, cervical, 1286
Paget's disease, 1971
Pain: in appendicitis, 743; in cancer of
stomach, 707; in pleurisy, 250; in pneu-
monia, 125; in ulcer of stomach, 683
Pains, lightning, 1209
Palate, paralysis of, in diphtheria, 607;
perforation of, 10, 551
Palpitation of heart, 447
Paludism (Malaria), 1724
Pancreas: calculi of, 1031; cancer of, 1029;
cancer of head of, 989; cysts of, 1029;
diseases of, 1028; in diabetes, 1902;
hæmorrhage into, 1030
Pancreatitis and its relations to gall-stones,
1032; cytosteatonecrosis, 1039; hæmorrhage, 1041
Paracentesis: abdominis, 895; pericardii,
390
Paracholecystitis, 998
Paralyses (localization), 1391; alcoholic,
2027; alternate, 1298; diabetic, 1903;
diphtheritic, 607; hysterical, 1452; in
Jacksonian epilepsy, 1398; leprous, 1776;
of the nerves, 1517; radicular, 1546; saturnine, 2034; typhoid, 1652; uræmic, 1096
Paralysis, acute ascending, 1264; acute
spinal, in adults, 1264; agitans, 1477;
asthenic bulbar, 1292; of cranial
nerves, 1348
facial, 1516; syphilitic early, 1525; late,
1530
general, 1366; juvenile general, 1370;
anterior spinal general, 1265; pseudo-
alcoholic, 2026; saturnine, 2036;
syphilitic, 1365; in tabetics, 1217

Toxicity : of serum, in Bright's disease, 1104 ; of urine in Bright's disease, 1101 ; in chlorosis, 1849

Toxine : in diphtheria, 572 ; in tetanus, 1737 ; in typhoid fever, 1672

Trachea, compression of, 381

Tracheitis, 102

Tracheostenosis, 103

Transfusion of blood, 1109

Traube's space, 253

Trauma and diabetes, 1928

Tremors : in Basedow's disease, 454 ; in hysteria, 1454 ; in insular sclerosis, 1255 ; in lead-poisoning, 2035 ; mercurial, 2031 ; in paralysis agitans, 1477 ; in sleeping sickness, 1771

Treponema pallidum, 2012

Trichinosis, 1956

Trichocephalus, 829

Tricuspid insufficiency and stenosis, 427

Trifacial neuralgia, 1496

Trismus, 1739

Trophic disorders, 1552

Trophœdema, hereditary chronic, 1553

Trophoneurosis, facial, 1555

Trypanosomes, 1769

Trypanosomiasis, 1769

Tsetse-fly, 1769

Tubercle bacillus, 170

Tubercles of choroid, 1400

Tuberculin, 193

Tuberculocidin, 195

Tuberculoma, hypertrophic, of cæcum, 792

Tuberculosis, 169 ; ætiology, 188 ; bacillus, Koch's, 170 ; pathological anatomy, 172

    acute, of lung, 198 ; acute miliary, 203 ; ano-rectal, 806 ; of bladder, 1128 ; and cerebral abscess, 1339 ; and cirrhosis, 887 ; of choroid plexuses, 1400 ; of cranial vault, 1386 ; of intestine, 788 ; of kidney, 1121 ; of larynx, 40 ; of liver, 917 ; of lung (fibroid phthisis), 915 ; of meninges, 1399 ; of mouth, 556 ; of nasal fossæ, 14 ; of peritoneum, 837 ; of pharynx, 625 ; of pleura, 248, 268, 273 ; of tonsils (masked form), 626

    chronic pulmonary, 176 ; bacteriology, 180 ; description, 180 ; diagnosis, 190 ; hæmoptysis, 184 ; lesions in other organs, 186 ; pathological anatomy, 176 ; prognosis, 187 ; treatment, 191

Tumour : cerebral, 1346 ; dorsal, of wrist, 2035 ; of heart, 442 ; of right iliac fossa, 792 ; lachrymal, 10 ; mediastinal, 377

Twists and kinks in bowel, 815

Typhlitis, 733

Typhoid fever, 1619 ; abscess of liver, 1643 ; ætiology, 1666 ; aphasia, 1651 ; appendicitis paratyphoid, 1636 ; bacteriology, 1667 ; cholecystitis, 1642 ; clinical forms, 1623 ; complications, 1625 ; delirium, 1651 ; diagnosis, 1660 ; hæmatoma, 1654 ; hæmor-

rhage, intestinal, 1626 ; orchitis, 1650 ; osteomyelitis, 1655 ; pathological anatomy, 1669 ; perforation and peritonitis, 1627 ; phlebitis, 1648 ; pulmonary congestion, 1645 ; symptoms, 1619 ; treatment. 1673

Typho-lumbricosis, 1660

Typho-malaria, 1757

Typhosis, syphilitic, 1661

Typho-toxine, 1667

Typhus, 1681

Tyrosin, 1017

U

Ulcer :
    of the duodenum, 808 ; perforating, of stomach and duodenum in appendicitis, 695
    of the stomach, 681 ; latent form, 687 ; perforation, 691 ; perforating, in diabetes, 1904 ; in tabes, 1218

Ulceration, intestinal : dysenteric, 823 ; tubercular, 789 ; in anorectal tuberculosis. 806 ; in typhoid fever, 1670
    of the larynx, 33, 41 ; in typhoid fever, 1644
    of the stomach : general considerations, 656
    of vault of palate, tubercular, 558

Ulcers : in follicular enteritis, 727 ; in glanders, 1791 ; of nasal septum, 9

Ulnar nerve, affections of, 1548

Uræmia, 1092 ; acute, 1056 ; Brightism, minor symptoms of, 1079, 1093 ; calculous, 1169 ; in chlorosis, 1849 ; in polycystic kidney, 1150 ; prognosis, 1105 ; in scarlet fever, 1590 ; treatment, 1107

Urate of soda in gout, 1890

Urea in the sweat, 1091

Ureter, blocking by calculi, 1168 ; compression of, 1185

Ureteritis, tubercular, 1123

Urethritis : diabetic, 1899 ; gonorrhœal, 1990 ; non-gonococcal, 1990 ; gouty, 2002

Uricæmia in gout, 1890

Uric acid calculi, 1160 ; in gout, 1890 ; (gouty) diathesis, 1889 ; theory of gout, 1889

Urine :
    in acute nephritis, 1056 ; in acute yellow atrophy, 1017 ; in chlorosis, 1839 ; in chronic nephritis, 1085 ; in diabetes insipidus, 1926 ; in diabetes mellitus, 1901 ; in gout, 1885 et seq. ; in jaundice, 1008 ; in malaria, 1758 ; in typhoid fever, 1622
    cryoscopy of, 1104 ; normal composition of, 1048 ; passage of methylene blue, 1102 ; leucin, 1017 ; pus in, 1126

Urobilin, 1008

Urticaria : after aspiration, 946 ; in asthma, 112 ; in hydatid cyst of liver, 938 ; in hydatid cyst of the lung, 226 ; in jaundice, 1006

Uvula, swelling of, in diphtheria, 575 ; membrane in, 575

THE END

Baillière, Tindall & Cox, 8, Henrietta Street, Covent Garden.